BERKOWITZ'S
Pediatrics
A PRIMARY CARE APPROACH

3rd Edition

Carol D. Berkowitz, MD, FAAP

Professor of Clinical Pediatrics
David Geffen School of Medicine at
University of California Los Angeles
Executive Vice Chair
Department of Pediatrics
Harbor-UCLA Medical Center
Torrance, CA

American Academy of Pediatrics
DEDICATED TO THE HEALTH OF ALL CHILDREN™

Editor: Diane Beausoleil

Marketing Manager: Linda Smessaert

Production Manager: Theresa Wiener

Copy Editor: Kate Larson

Design and Production: Peg Mulcahy

Library of Congress Control Number: 2008925893

ISBN-13: 978-1-58110-283-3

MA0427

Preface

The role of the primary care clinician has continued to expand as the health problems facing children have evolved and become increasingly complex. Some conditions that were labeled the "new morbidities" by Dr Robert Haggerty have been replaced by "newer morbidities," some have receded in incidence, and others, such as school-related violence and disasters, have exploded. The critical role of the primary care clinician and the value of the medical home are now acknowledged not only in pediatrics but also across the disciplines of family medicine, internal medicine, and obstetrics-gynecology. Our health care system continues to challenge patients, parents, and clinicians to meet the goals of continuity and coordination of care. In response to such challenges, the clinician must remain knowledgeable about the changing demands of pediatric care. It is the goal this third edition of *Pediatrics: A Primary Care Approach* to help clinicians caring for children to meet this challenge.

My thanks to all of the contributors and to the staff of the American Academy of Pediatrics, especially Diane Beausoleil, Kate Larson, and Maureen DeRosa; the staff of Graphic World Publishing Services, particularly Leah Bross; and my assistant Mary Magee for their assistance.

Carol D. Berkowitz

Contributors

Sudhir K. Anand, MD
Professor of Clinical Pediatrics, David Geffen School of Medicine
at University of California Los Angeles; Chief, Division of Pediatric
Nephrology, Harbor-UCLA Medical Center, Torrance, CA

David Atkinson, MD
Harbor-UCLA Medical Center, Torrance, CA

Martin Baren, MD†
Attending Physician, Developmental and Behavioral Pediatrics, Children's
Hospital of Orange County, Orange County, CA

Carol D. Berkowitz, MD
Professor of Clinical Pediatrics, David Geffen School of Medicine at
University of California Los Angeles; Executive Vice Chair, Department
of Pediatrics, Harbor-UCLA Medical Center, Torrance, CA

Iris Wagman Borowsky, MD, PhD
Associate Professor of Pediatrics, Division of General Pediatrics,
Department of Pediatrics, University of Minnesota, Minneapolis, MN

Paul Bryan, MD
Pediatric Emergency Medicine Faculty, Assistant Professor of Clinical
Medicine, David Geffen School of Medicine at University of California
Los Angeles

David B. Burbulys, MD
Director, Emergency Medicine Residency Program, Harbor-UCLA
Medical Center; Associate Professor of Medicine, David Geffen School
of Medicine at University of California Los Angeles, Torrance, CA

Noah Craft, MD, PhD
Los Angeles Biomedical Research Institute, Torrance, CA

Rachel S. Darling, MD
Medicine-Pediatrics Resident, University of Minnesota, Minneapolis, MN

Robin Winkler Doroshow, MD
Associate Professor of Pediatrics, The George Washington University
School of Medicine and Health Sciences; Pediatric Cardiologist, Children's
National Medical Center, Washington, DC; Associate Professor of
Pediatrics, Georgetown University School of Medicine; Director, Division
of Pediatric Cardiology, Georgetown University Hospital

Elizabeth A. Edgerton, MD, MPH
Department of Pediatrics, Children's National Medical Center,
Washington, DC

Melissa Egge, MD
Chief Resident, Department of Pediatrics, Harbor-UCLA Medical Center,
Torrance, CA

George Gershman, MD
Associate Professor of Pediatrics, University of California Los Angeles
School of Medicine; Chief, Division of Pediatric Gastroenterology and
Nutrition, Department of Pediatrics, Harbor-UCLA Medical Center,
Torrance, CA

Rick Goldstein, MD
Assistant Professor of Pediatrics, Boston Medical Center, Boston
University School of Medicine; Instructor of Pediatrics, Harvard Medical
School; Associate Program Director, Boston Combined Residency
Program in Pediatrics, Boston, MA

Allison Golnik, MD, MPH
Assistant Professor of Pediatrics, Division of General Pediatrics,
Department of Pediatrics, University of Minnesota, Minneapolis, MN

Geeta Grover, MD
Medical Director of Developmental and Behavioral Pediatrics,
Children's Hospital of Orange County, Orange County, CA; Associate
Clinical Professor of Pediatrics, University of California, Irvine College
of Medicine, Irvine, CA

Kenneth R. Huff, MD
Professor of Pediatrics and Neurology, University of California Los
Angeles; Chief, Division of Neurology, Department of Pediatrics,
Harbor-UCLA Medical Center, Torrance, CA

Wendy T. Hui, MD
Department of Pediatrics, Harbor-UCLA Medical Center, Torrance, CA

Lynn Hunt, MD
Clinical Professor of Pediatrics, University of California, Irvine, Santa
Ana, CA

Stanley H. Inkelis, MD
Professor of Pediatrics, University of California Los Angeles School
of Medicine; Director, Pediatric Emergency Medicine, Harbor-UCLA
Medical Center, Torrance, CA

Walter Jiminez, MD
Research Fellow, Division of Pediatric Nephrology, David Geffen School
of Medicine at University of California Los Angeles

†Deceased.

Doran D. Kahana, MD
Pediatrician, Minneapolis, MN

Elaine S. Kamil, MD
Clinical Professor of Pediatrics, University of California Los Angeles School of Medicine; Associate Director, Pediatric Nephrology and Transplant Immunology, Cedars-Sinai Medical Center, Los Angeles

Kathy K. Langevin, MD, MPH
Resident, Division of Dermatology, University of California Los Angeles

Charlotte W. Lewis, MD, MPH
Associate Professor, Department of Pediatrics, General Pediatrics and Craniofacial Medicine, Adjunct Associate Professor, Pediatric Dentistry, University of Washington School of Medicine, Seattle, WA

Catherine S. Mao, MD
Pediatric Endocrinology, Harbor-UCLA Medical Center, Los Angeles Biomedical Research Institute, Torrance, CA

ChrisAnna M. Mink, MD
University of California Los Angeles School of Medicine; Department of Pediatrics, Harbor-UCLA Medical Center, Torrance, CA

Julie E. Noble, MD
Clinical Professor of Pediatrics, University of California Los Angeles School of Medicine; Director, Pediatric Managed Care, Director, Low Risk Nursery, Harbor-UCLA Medical Center, Torrance, CA

Hamid Redjal, MD
Orthopaedic Surgery Resident, Department of Orthopaedic Surgery, Harbor-UCLA Medical Center, Torrance, CA

Nasser Redjal, MD
Associate Professor of Clinical Pediatrics and Allergy/Immunology, University of California, Los Angeles School of Medicine; Director, Allergy/Immunology Managed Care, Harbor-UCLA Medical Center, Torrance, CA

Teresa Rosales, MD
Clinical Professor of Ophthalmology, University of California Los Angeles School of Medicine, Jules Stein Eye Institute; Pediatric Ophthalmologist, Private Practice, Long Beach, CA

Isidro B. Salusky, MD
Professor of Pediatrics, University of California Los Angeles School of Medicine; Director, Pediatric Dialysis Program, Program Director, General Clinical Research Center, University of California Los Angeles

Jeremy Screws, MD
Assistant Professor of Pediatrics, University of Tennessee College of Medicine, Chattanooga Unit, Chattanooga, TN

Hali Sherman, MD
Pediatrician, La Clinica de La Raza, Oakland, CA

Monica Sifuentes, MD
Professor of Clinical Pediatrics, David Geffen School of Medicine at University of California Los Angeles; Associate Program Director, Vice Chair of Education, Department of Pediatrics, Harbor-UCLA Medical Center, Torrance, CA

Lynne M. Smith, MD
Associate Professor of Clinical Pediatrics, University of California Los Angeles School of Medicine; Department of Pediatrics, Division of Neonatology, Harbor-UCLA Medical Center, Torrance, CA

Robin Steinberg-Epstein, MD
Developmental Behavioral Pediatrician, Associate Clinical Professor of Pediatrics, University of California, Irvine, CA, and the For OC Kids Neurodevelopmental Center, Orange, CA

Kenneth W. Steinhoff, MD
Associate Clinical Professor, Department of Pediatrics, University of California, Irvine, CA; Child Psychiatrist, Child Development Center, Department of Pediatrics, University of California, Irvine, CA

Sara T. Stewart, MD
Harbor-UCLA Medical Center, Torrance, CA

Wendy Y. Tcheng, MD
Assistant Professor of Pediatrics, University of California Los Angeles School of Medicine; Division of Pediatric Hematology/Oncology, Department of Pediatrics, Harbor-UCLA Medical Center, Torrance, CA

Alan Tomines, MD
Assistant Clinical Professor of Pediatrics, David Geffen School of Medicine at University of California Los Angeles; Harbor-UCLA Medical Center, Torrance, CA

Cecily L. Wait, MD
Medicine-Pediatrics Resident, University of Minnesota, Minneapolis, MN

Derek Wong, MD
Assistant Professor of Clinical Pediatrics, University of California Los Angeles School of Medicine; Program Director, Pediatric Residency Program, Harbor-UCLA Medical Center, Torrance, CA

Jennifer K. Yee, MD
Clinical Instructor of Pediatrics, David Geffen School of Medicine at University of California Los Angeles; Division of Pediatric Endocrinology, Harbor-UCLA Medical Center, Torrance, CA

Kelly D. Young, MD
Associate Clinical Professor of Pediatrics, David Geffen School of Medicine at University of California Los Angeles, Harbor-UCLA Medical Center, Torrance, CA

David P. Zamorano, MD
Assistant Professor, Department of Orthopaedic Surgery, California School of Medicine, Irvine, CA

Contents

SECTION I

Primary Care: Skills and Concepts

1. Primary Care: Introduction 3
   Julie E. Noble, MD

2. Child Advocacy 7
   Julie E. Noble, MD

3. Talking With Children 11
   Geeta Grover, MD

4. Talking With Parents 15
   Geeta Grover, MD

5. Talking With Adolescents 19
   Monica Sifuentes, MD

6. Telephone Management 23
   Iris Wagman Borowsky, MD, PhD, and Cecily L. Wait, MD

7. Informatics 27
   Alan Tomines, MD

8. Counseling Families About Internet Use 31
   Alan Tomines, MD

9. Principles of Pediatric Therapeutics 35
   Elizabeth A. Edgerton, MD, MPH

SECTION II

Health Maintenance and Anticipatory Guidance

10. Neonatal Examination and Nursery Visit 41
    Julie E. Noble, MD, and Monica Sifuentes, MD

11. Newborn Screening 47
    Derek Wong, MD

12. Caring for Twins and Higher-Order Multiples 51
    Lynne M. Smith, MD

13. Circumcision 57
    Lynne M. Smith, MD

14. Nutritional Needs 63
    Wendy T. Hui, MD, and Geeta Grover, MD

15. Breastfeeding 71
    Julie E. Noble, MD

16. Sleep: Normal Patterns and Common Disorders 75
    Geeta Grover, MD

17. Oral Health and Dental Disorders 81
    Charlotte W. Lewis, MD, MPH

18. Normal Development and Developmental Surveillance, Screening, and Evaluation 87
    Geeta Grover, MD

19. Language Development: Speech and Hearing Assessment 95
    Geeta Grover, MD

20. Literacy Promotion in Pediatric Practice 101
    Lynn Hunt, MD

21. Gifted Children 105
    Iris Wagman Borowsky, MD, PhD, and Rachel S. Darling, MD

22. Children and School: A Primer for the Practitioner 109
    Martin Baren, MD, and Geeta Grover, MD

23. Immunizations 115
    ChrisAnna M. Mink, MD

24. Health Maintenance in Older Children and Adolescents 121
    Hali Sherman, MD, and Monica Sifuentes, MD

25. Health Care for International Adoptees 129
    ChrisAnna M. Mink, MD

26. Health Care Needs of Children in Foster Care 137
    Sara T. Stewart, MD, and ChrisAnna M. Mink, MD

27. Well-Child Care for Children With Trisomy 21 143
    Derek Wong, MD

28. Well-Child Care for Preterm Infants 149
    Lynne M. Smith, MD

29. Care of Children With Special Health Care Needs 155
    Julie E. Noble, MD, and Monica Sifuentes, MD

30. Reproductive Health 161
    Monica Sifuentes, MD

31. Injury Prevention 169
    Allison Golnik, MD, MPH, and Iris Wagman Borowsky, MD, PhD

32. Fostering Self-Esteem 175
    Rick Goldstein, MD

33. Sibling Rivalry 179
    Carol D. Berkowitz, MD

34. Toilet Training 183
    Lynne M. Smith, MD

35. Crying and Colic 189
     Geeta Grover, MD

36. Discipline 193
     Carol D. Berkowitz, MD

37. Temper Tantrums 199
     Geeta Grover, MD

38. Breath-Holding Spells 203
     Geeta Grover, MD

39. Fears, Phobias, and Anxiety 207
     Carol D. Berkowitz, MD

40. Thumb Sucking and Other Habits 213
     Carol D. Berkowitz, MD

41. Enuresis 219
     Carol D. Berkowitz, MD

42. Encopresis 223
     Carol D. Berkowitz, MD

SECTION III

Acute and Emergent Problems

43. Fever and Bacteremia 229
     Paul Bryan, MD

44. Febrile Seizures 237
     Kenneth R. Huff, MD

45. Respiratory Distress 241
     David B. Burbulys, MD

46. Stridor and Croup 247
     David B. Burbulys, MD

47. Sudden Infant Death Syndrome and Apparent Life-Threatening Events 253
     Lynne M. Smith, MD

48. Syncope 259
     David Atkinson, MD, and Elizabeth A. Edgerton, MD, MPH

49. Shock 265
     Kelly D. Young, MD

50. Approach to the Traumatized Child 271
     David B. Burbulys, MD

51. Abdominal Trauma 277
     David B. Burbulys, MD

52. Head Trauma 281
     Paul Bryan, MD

53. Increased Intracranial Pressure 287
     Kenneth R. Huff, MD

54. Fluid and Electrolyte Disturbances 293
     Charlotte W. Lewis, MD, MPH, and Sudhir K. Anand, MD

55. Acute Renal Failure/Acute Kidney Injury 303
    Hali Sherman, MD, and Sudhir K. Anand, MD

56. Ingestions: Diagnosis and Management 309
    Kelly D. Young, MD

SECTION IV

Head, Neck, and Respiratory System

57. Approach to the Dysmorphic Child 317
    Julie E. Noble, MD

58. Craniofacial Anomalies 323
    Carol D. Berkowitz, MD

59. Common Oral Lesions 331
    Charlotte W. Lewis, MD, MPH

60. Otitis Media 335
    Nasser Redjal, MD

61. Hearing Impairments 341
    Julie E. Noble, MD, and Monica Sifuentes, MD

62. Sore Throat 347
    Stanley H. Inkelis, MD

63. Nosebleeds 355
    Stanley H. Inkelis, MD

64. Strabismus 361
    Teresa Rosales, MD

65. Infections of the Eye 367
    Teresa Rosales, MD

66. Excessive Tearing 373
    Teresa Rosales, MD

67. Neck Masses 377
    Stanley H. Inkelis, MD

68. Allergic Disease 387
    Nasser Redjal, MD

69. Wheezing and Asthma 393
    Nasser Redjal, MD

70. Cough 403
    Nasser Redjal, MD

SECTION V

Hematologic Disorders

71. Anemia 411
    Wendy Y. Tcheng, MD

72. Bleeding Disorders 419
    Wendy Y. Tcheng, MD

73. Lymphadenopathy 427
    Wendy Y. Tcheng, MD

SECTION VI

Cardiovascular System

74. Heart Murmurs 433
Robin Winkler Doroshow, MD

75. Cyanosis in the Newborn 437
Robin Winkler Doroshow, MD

76. Congestive Heart Failure 443
Robin Winkler Doroshow, MD

77. Chest Pain 449
Robin Winkler Doroshow, MD

78. Hypertension 455
Sudhir K. Anand, MD, and Hali Sherman, MD

SECTION VII

Genitourinary Disorders

79. Ambiguous Genitalia 467
Jennifer K. Yee, MD, and Catherine S. Mao, MD

80. Inguinal Lumps and Bumps 473
Julie E. Noble, MD

81. Hematuria 477
Elaine S. Kamil, MD

82. Proteinuria 485
Elaine S. Kamil, MD

83. Urinary Tract Infections 491
Hali Sherman, MD, and Sudhir K. Anand, MD

84. Vaginitis 497
Monica Sifuentes, MD

85. Sexually Transmitted Infections 503
Monica Sifuentes, MD

86. Menstrual Disorders 513
Monica Sifuentes, MD

87. Disorders of the Breast 521
Monica Sifuentes, MD

SECTION VIII

Orthopedic Disorders

88. Developmental Hip Dysplasia 531
Hamid R. Redjal, MD, and David P. Zamorano, MD

89. Rotational Problems of the Lower Extremity: In-toeing and Out-toeing 537
Hamid R. Redjal, MD, and David P. Zamorano, MD

90. Angular Deformities of the Lower Extremity: Bowlegs and Knock-Knees 543
Carol D. Berkowitz, MD

91. Orthopedic Injuries and Growing Pains 547
    Sara T. Stewart, MD

92. Sports-Related Acute Injuries 555
    Monica Sifuentes, MD

93. Evaluation of Limp 561
    Paul Bryan, MD

94. Musculoskeletal Disorders of the Neck and Back 567
    Carol D. Berkowitz, MD

SECTION IX

Gastrointestinal Disorders

95. Vomiting 575
    George Gershman, MD

96. Gastroesophageal Reflux 581
    Jeremy Screws, MD

97. Gastrointestinal Bleeding 587
    George Gershman, MD

98. Diarrhea 595
    George Gershman, MD

99. Constipation 601
    Doron D. Kahana, MD, and George Gershman, MD

100. Abdominal Pain 607
    George Gershman, MD

101. Jaundice 613
    Melissa Egge, MD

102. Infectious Hepatitis 621
    Monica Sifuentes, MD, and ChrisAnna M. Mink, MD

SECTION X

Neurologic Disorders

103. Hypotonia 631
    Kenneth R. Huff, MD

104. Headaches 637
    Kenneth R. Huff, MD

105. Tics 643
    Kenneth R. Huff, MD

SECTION XI

Dermatologic Disorders

106. Acne 651
    Monica Sifuentes, MD

107. Disorders of the Hair and Scalp 657
    Kathy K. Langevin, MD, MPH, and Noah Craft, MD, PhD

108. Diaper Dermatitis 663
    Kathy K. Langevin, MD, MPH, and Noah Craft MD, PhD

109. Papulosquamous Eruptions 667
    Kathy K. Langevin, MD, MPH, and Noah Craft, MD, PhD

110. Morbilliform Rashes 673
    Kathy K. Langevin, MD, MPH, and Noah Craft, MD, PhD

111. Vesicular Exanthems 679
    Kathy K. Langevin, MD, MPH, and Noah Craft, MD, PhD

SECTION XII

The New Morbidity

112. Autism Spectrum Disorders 687
    Robin Steinberg-Epstein, MD

113. Attention-Deficit/Hyperactivity Disorder 695
    Allison Golnik, MD, MPH, and Iris Wagman Borowsky, MD, PhD

114. Psychopharmacology in Children 701
    Robin Steinberg-Epstein, MD, and Kenneth W. Steinhoff, MD

115. Physical Abuse 707
    Sara T. Stewart, MD

116. Sexual Abuse 711
    Sara T. Stewart, MD

117. Failure to Thrive 717
    Carol D. Berkowitz, MD

118. Infants of Substance-Abusing Mothers 723
    Sara T. Stewart, MD

119. Substance Abuse 729
    Monica Sifuentes, MD

120. Eating Disorders 737
    Monica Sifuentes, MD

121. Body Modification: Tattooing and Body Piercing 745
    Monica Sifuentes, MD

122. Childhood Obesity 753
    Charlotte W. Lewis, MD, MPH

123. Divorce 759
    Carol D. Berkowitz, MD

124. School-Related Violence 763
    Elizabeth A. Edgerton, MD, MPH

125. Disaster Preparedness 767
    Elizabeth A. Edgerton, MD, MPH

126. Adolescent Depression and Suicide 771
    Monica Sifuentes, MD

Chronic Diseases of Childhood and Adolescence

127. Cancer in Children.. 779
Wendy Y. Tcheng, MD

128. Chronic Kidney Disease/Chronic Renal Failure 787
Walter Jimenez, MD, and Isidro B. Salusky, MD

129. Diabetes Mellitus 795
Jennifer K. Yee, MD, and Catherine S. Mao, MD

130. Juvenile Idiopathic Arthritis/Collagen Vascular Disease 801
Elizabeth A. Edgerton, MD, MPH

131. Nephrotic Syndrome... 809
Elaine S. Kamil, MD

132. Seizures and Epilepsy 817
Kenneth R. Huff, MD

Index.. 825

Primary Care: Skills and Concepts

1. Primary Care: Introduction 3
2. Child Advocacy 7
3. Talking With Children.. 11
4. Talking With Parents 15
5. Talking With Adolescents 19
6. Telephone Management 23
7. Informatics 27
8. Counseling Families About Internet Use 31
9. Principles of Pediatric Therapeutics 35

Primary Care: Introduction

Julie E. Noble, MD

Primary care is defined as the comprehensive health care that patients receive from the same health care provider over a longitudinal period. The term was first used in the 1960s to designate the role of the primary care physician in response to the abundance of subspecialists and lack of generalists among practicing physicians. It is generally accepted that primary care physicians include pediatricians, family physicians, and internists. In 1966 the Millis Committee Report to the American Medical Association on graduate medical education recognized the importance of primary care and recommended a national commitment to educating primary care physicians. Primary care was further defined in 1974 by Charney and Alpert, who separated it into component parts: first contact, longitudinal care, family orientation, and integration of comprehensive care. To understand the depth of primary care, the component parts should be explored.

First contact occurs when a patient arrives for medical care at the office of a primary care physician. The visit includes an intake history, complete physical examination, and an assessment of problems with treatment (if indicated). Of great importance is the establishment of the physician-patient relationship. Physicians become the primary medical resource and counselors to these patients and their families and the first contacts when successive medical problems arise.

Longitudinal care, the second component of primary care, implies continuity of care over a period. Physicians assume responsibility for issues concerning both health and illness. In pediatrics, such care involves monitoring growth and development, following school progress, screening for commonly found disorders, making psychosocial assessments, promoting health, and preventing illness with immunization and safety counseling programs.

Family orientation is the third component of primary care. Patients must be viewed in the context of their environment and family. Otherwise, practitioners cannot adequately care for patients. In pediatrics, a child's problems become the family's, and the family's problems become the child's. This has become increasingly apparent with the recognition that problems of poverty, drug use, human immunodeficiency virus (HIV) exposure, teenage pregnancy, and gang involvement directly affect a child's health and quality of life. The psychosocial forces in a particular child's life are intricately interwoven into their health care, and their assessment is an essential component of the primary care of that child.

As pediatric medical problems become more complex, many health and educational resources may be used to supplement care. Primary care physicians integrate and coordinate these services in the best interest of patients, thus providing **integration of comprehensive care,** the fourth component of primary care. Working with social service agencies, home care providers, educational agencies, and government agencies, physicians can use multiple resources for the benefit of patients. Understanding the resources of the community is an important part of a primary care physician's education.

Medical Home

When patients select a primary care provider, they have identified a medical home. That home incorporates the physical, psychological, and social aspects of individual patients into comprehensive health care services, thus meeting the needs of the whole person. The American Academy of Pediatrics (AAP) has defined the characteristics of a medical home to be "accessible, continuous, comprehensive, family-centered, coordinated, compassionate, and culturally effective." To make that homework for patients, geographic and financial accessibility are key elements. The most important aspect of a home is that it is a place where patients feel "cared for."

Role of the Primary Care Pediatrician

As a primary care physician, the role of the pediatrician has not only included the care of acute illnesses and injuries, but also the preventive issues of well-child care with its focus on immunizations, tracking growth and development, and anticipatory guidance. Now there is a renewed emphasis on the importance of the role of the pediatric primary care provider in assessing the psychosocial aspects of pediatric patients. Termed the *new morbidity* by Robert Haggerty, MD, in the 1970s, recognizing these social issues including family dysfunction; developmental problems, including learning disabilities; and behavioral problems, including emotional disorders, have become a significant part of the role of the provider. In 1993 the AAP stated that pediatricians are obliged to have knowledge of physical and environmental factors and behaviors affecting health, normal variations of behavior and emotional development, risk factors and behaviors affecting physical health, and behavior problems. The focus of the pediatrician should be detection, evaluation, and management, with referrals if needed. Newer morbidities secondary to the increasing complexity of our society were outlined in 2001 by the AAP. These include school problems, mood and anxiety disorders, adolescent suicide and homicide, firearms, school violence, drug and alcohol abuse, HIV, obesity, and the effects of the media on children. Other psychosocial factors such as poverty, homelessness, single-parent families, divorce, working parents, and child care necessitate the pediatrician working with social service agencies to deliver appropriate care to their patients. The role of the primary care physician is continually expanding in an effort to deliver comprehensive care to each patient.

Subspecialist Care

Medical knowledge and technology have made amazing advancements in the past several decades. Total knowledge of all fields is impossible for individual physicians. As a result, the role of the subspecialist physician has developed as an adjunct to that of the primary care physician. New fields of subspecialties, such as adolescent medicine, have arisen as a response to the increased knowledge. Primary care physicians should seek subspecialist consultation when the suspected or known disease process is unusual or complicated, when it demands specialized technology, or when they have little experience with the disease. Generally, subspecialists evaluate patients and concentrate on the organ system or disease process in their area of expertise.

Primary care physicians can use a subspecialist for either a consultation or referral. When initiating a consultation, primary care physicians send patients for advice. Consulting physicians assess the patients with a history and physical examination, focusing on their specialty. They then recommend possible additional laboratory tests, offer a diagnosis and treatment plan, and send the patients back to their primary care physicians for coordination of further care.

Use of the subspecialist is termed **secondary care.** For example, an 8-year-old girl with weight loss and persistent abdominal pain has an upper gastrointestinal x-ray series that reveals a duodenal ulcer. She is sent by her primary care physician to a pediatric gastroenterologist for **consultation,** with a request for an endoscopy to allow definitive diagnosis and up-to-date management guidelines. The girl then returns to the primary care physician with recommendations for treatment and further care.

Primary care physicians can also generate a referral to a subspecialist, which differs from a consultation. A **referral** requests that the subspecialist assume complete care of the patient. This transfer of a patient to a tertiary care site establishes a subspecialist as the coordinator of further health care for the patient. For example, a 4-year-old boy with recurrent fevers, hepatosplenomegaly, and blasts on peripheral blood smear is referred to a pediatric oncologist for diagnosis, the latest treatment, and ongoing medical care.

When requesting advice from subspecialists, whether on a consultative or referral basis, primary care physicians should outline specific questions with a probable diagnosis to be addressed by the subspecialist. For example, a consultation requesting evaluation of a child with hematuria is inappropriate. The primary care physician should perform a basic diagnostic evaluation and should make the most likely diagnosis. The child can then be referred appropriately. A child diagnosed with nephritis should be sent to a pediatric nephrologist, whereas a child diagnosed with Wilms tumor should be sent to a pediatric oncologist.

When primary care physicians and subspecialists function cooperatively and offer the 3 levels of care (primary, referral, and consultative), patients receive the highest-quality medical care. In general, care provided by subspecialists is characterized as being more expensive and procedure-driven. Laboratory studies are ordered with increased frequency by subspecialists, further inflating the cost of medical care. If patients have no longitudinal health care and see multiple providers, repeat laboratory studies are often ordered. Primary care is believed to deliver more cost-effective, improved medical care. With the spiraling cost of medical care, there continues to be a nationwide movement to produce more primary care physicians. However, it should be remembered that the role of the subspecialist is an essential supplement to the primary care physician when managing complicated disease. A balance between generalists and subspecialists needs to be maintained in the education process.

Laboratory Tests

For most conditions, the diagnosis is revealed by the history and physical examination in more than 95% of cases. Thus good communication skills are a basic tenet of primary care. Patients' complaints often concern unnecessary laboratory tests, which increase the cost of medical care and the prescription of unnecessary medications. To lessen these problems, the primary care physician should use laboratory tests and medications discriminatingly, recognizing their value as well as their potential iatrogenic effects.

In primary care, laboratory tests should be used to help confirm a condition suspected on the basis of the history or physical examination or diagnose a condition that may not be apparent after a thorough history and physical assessment. In pediatrics especially, the value of each test result should be weighed against the inconvenience, discomfort, and possible side effects in children. Tests can also be used as screening tools to prevent disease or to identify a disease early so that treatment can begin and symptoms can be minimized. Laboratory studies can provide a variety of other information, including data to establish a diagnosis, knowledge necessary to select therapy or to monitor a disease, and information about the risk of future disease. Organ function, metabolic activity, and nutritional status can also be assessed, and evidence of neoplastic or infectious disease can be provided. In addition, laboratory studies can be used to identify infectious and therapeutic agents or poisons.

Screening laboratory tests are used when the incidence of an unsuspected condition is high enough in a general population to justify the expense of the test (see Chapter 11). Subclinical conditions such as anemia, lead poisoning, and hypercholesterolemia are part of some health maintenance assessments.

Physicians must remember that there is variability in test results and that laboratory error can occur. Laboratory results should always be viewed in the context of the patient. The sensitivity of a test, the ability of the test to detect low levels, and the specificity of a test for the substance being measured must also be considered by the physician when evaluating a test result.

Challenges for the Future

The many changes in health care delivery and funding have created challenges for primary care physicians. Two of the basic tenets of primary care, accessibility and an ongoing relationship with the provider (both of which are reported by patients to be very important), are frequently interrupted secondary to changes in health care funding. When patients change health care plans, they may lose financial access to their primary care provider, negating the possibility of longitudinal care.

Because access to same-day care can be difficult in the busy schedule of primary care providers, walk-in immediate medical care clinics and retail-based clinics have arisen. Patients like the convenience, but episodic visits in a variety of settings do not deliver comprehensive care for the patient, and these short visits may not take into account the entirety of the patient's medical history. This creates a challenge for the primary care provider in being able to manage and follow up the acute care problems in the context of the family.

With the advent of hospitalists providing inpatient care, primary care physicians may not be included in in-patient management. They then face a challenge in retrieving important information regarding the care of their patients.

With a push toward managed care funding in an attempt to control health care costs, the bureaucracy of medical care has increased exponentially. This business of medicine with redundant oversight of medical care has put a tremendous burden of administrative activities in the lap of the primary care physician. There is a significant challenge to providers to provide care while answering to administrative structures.

The biggest challenge to primary care providers is the future of health care funding to ensure access and availability of health care to all children. This is a priority for child health policy reform at the national level, and universal health care for children is being advocated. The US Department of Health and Human Services includes comprehensive health care for all children with special health care needs in its Healthy People 2010 goals.

Selected References

American Academy of Pediatrics Committee on Psychosocial Aspects of Child and Family Health. The new morbidity revisited: a renewed commitment to the psychosocial aspects of pediatric care. *Pediatrics.* 2001;108:1227–1230

American Academy of Pediatrics Medical Home Initiatives for Children With Special Needs Project Advisory Committee. The medical home. *Pediatrics.* 2002;110:184–186

American Academy of Pediatrics Retail-Based Clinic Policy Work Group. American Academy of Pediatrics principles concerning retail-based clinics. *Pediatrics.* 2006;118:2561–2569

American Association of Medical Colleges. Policy on the generalist physician. *Acad Med.* 1993;68:1–6

Alpert JJ. Primary care: the future for pediatric education. *Pediatrics.* 1990;86:653–659

Cheng TL. Primary care pediatrics: 2004 and beyond. *Pediatrics.* 2004;113:1802–1809

Iglehart JK. The American health care system: managed care. *N Engl J Med.* 1992;327:742–747

Noe DA, Rock RC. *Laboratory Medicine: The Selection and Interpretation of Clinical Laboratory Studies.* Baltimore, MD: Williams & Wilkins; 1994

Showstack J, Sox H, eds. The future of primary care. *Ann Intern Med.* 2003;138(suppl):242–272

Sia CCJ. The medical home: pediatric practice and child advocacy in the 1990s. *Pediatrics.* 1992;90:419–423

Starfield B. *Primary Care. Concept, Evaluation, and Policy.* New York, NY: Oxford University Press; 1992

CHAPTER 2

Child Advocacy

Julie E. Noble, MD

CASE STUDY

A 15-year-old male is brought to the emergency department with a gunshot wound to his left leg. He says he was "hanging" outside with his friends when a random car drove by and shots were fired. He denies being in a gang, although he is wearing a large white T-shirt and oversized black pants. His physical examination reveals a shaved head, tattoos, and a gunshot wound to his left lower leg. An x-ray shows a fractured left tibia, and he is admitted for orthopedic surgical treatment.

Questions

1. What does it mean to be a child advocate?
2. Aside from caring for individual patients, what is expected of pediatricians in the community?
3. What is the role of pediatricians in child advocacy?
4. What are the levels of advocacy?
5. How do pediatricians implement advocacy?

An advocate is one who pleads the cause of others or defends or maintains a cause or proposal. It is derived from the Latin "to give voice." Children in our society have no voice, and from the beginnings of pediatrics as an independent branch of medicine, pediatricians have been the voice advocating for the health and well-being of children. The father of American pediatrics, Abraham Jacobi, MD, spent his career in the late 1800s and early 1900s advocating for children through legislation in New York and Washington, DC. He was a great teacher of pediatrics, introducing the discipline into academic medicine, but truly believed that physicians needed to be involved in public policy. Another founder of American pediatrics, Job Lewis Smith, MD, recognized the need for a clean water supply and decent housing to decrease the high infant mortality rate at that time. He worked through public advocacy to improve conditions not only for his patients but children in general. The American Academy of Pediatrics (AAP) was founded on federal advocacy principles. In June 1921 the Sheppard-Towner Act on maternal and child health legislation was introduced into Congress. It was the first involvement of the federal government on behalf of children and provided federal matching funds to states for services for pregnant women and new mothers. The American Medical Association (AMA), worried that the legislation would lead to socialized medicine, condemned the Act while the AMA Section on Diseases of Children supported the legislation. When the act was up for reauthorization in 1930 and the AMA still opposed it, the pediatric group left the AMA and founded the AAP. This organization has been advocating for children ever since.

The New Morbidity

Advocacy has become increasingly important because the new morbidities in pediatric medicine are related to community forces. As our society has become more complicated, the major health concerns are even more intertwined with the environments in which children are involved. Child health outcomes improved dramatically in the 1900s with the development of vaccines, antibiotics, and new and improved surgical care to treat the classic morbidities of infectious disease, infant mortality, poor nutrition, epidemics, overcrowding, and chronic disease. But there have emerged new morbidities that are negatively impacting child health outcomes. These morbidities of the 1960s to 1980s, as described by Robert Haggerty, MD, include family dysfunction, learning disabilities, emotional disorders, and educational problems. In the 1980s to 2000s we have developed a whole new set of morbidities. Judith Palfrey, MD, documented social disarray; political ennui; new epidemics of violence, acquired immunodeficiency syndrome, cocaine, and homelessness; and the sequelae of high-tech care as the new challenges for pediatricians. We have now expanded morbidities in the 2000s to include major health concerns with the prevalence of overweight children, increased mental health issues, significant health disparities in cultural groups, and major socioeconomic influences affecting child health. It is clear that these significant issues impacting child health cannot be adequately dealt with on an individual basis but require advocacy on a community or national scale to improve child health outcomes and life for children.

Community Pediatrics

Community pediatrics has developed as the vehicle to implement advocacy. Robert Haggerty, MD, first originated the concept in 1968 in an article published in the *New England Journal of Medicine.* His work as department chair of pediatrics at the University of Rochester, NY, developed an extensive advocacy agenda for the children of the community of Rochester. Subsequently the AAP has published a policy statement from its Committee on Community Health Services, titled, "The Pediatrician's Role in Community Pediatrics." The policy delineates 5 components of community pediatrics: a *perspective* from the individual patient to all the children in the community; a *recognition* that family, education, society, culture, spirituality, economy, environment, and politics all affect the health of children; a *synthesis* of clinical practice and public health principles directed to providing health care to a child and promoting the health of all children; a *commitment* to collaborate with the community to optimize health care for all children, especially disadvantaged children; and an *integral part* of the role of the pediatrician. All of these components are recommended as a part of pediatric practice, and training in advocacy has been instituted in pediatric training programs. Examples of potential involvement in the community include serving as a board member, developing health agendas, working with an existing organization to design and fund a community service project, and being a source of information for the community on child health issues.

Levels of Advocacy

Every pediatrician is a child advocate on a daily basis. With every patient encounter the pediatrician advocates for care in the best interest of the patient. This first level of advocacy includes treating the *individual's* immediate medical needs, performing screening tests, giving anticipatory guidance, and coordinating referrals as needed. The second level of advocacy is *community* advocacy. Pediatricians are an integral part of the community, and the community directly affects the health of their patients. Thus pediatricians have a responsibility to improve conditions in their community to benefit children. To do this, they must be familiar with the services that are available for children. They can develop relationships with child care centers, schools, community coalitions, city governments, and local organizations to advocate for the best interest of children. On a *state* level, pediatricians can work to improve health care resources or develop policies to help and protect children. Opportunities for involvement include working on legislation, budgets, regulations, and initiatives or working with the executive branch of local and state government. The next level of advocacy would be the *federal* level, where pediatricians can be involved with their senators and congressmen lobbying for child health issues. Pediatricians may also be involved in testifying before a subcommittee. The final level of advocacy is *international* level. For example, pediatricians may decide to work with the World Health Organization to improve immunizations for all children.

Becoming a Child Advocate

In becoming an effective child advocate, pediatricians first need to identify an issue that they want to change or a goal to improve the lives of children. The more specific the issue or goal, the easier it is to develop a solution. Obtaining all the information regarding the problem is necessary, and collecting the data to support the need for the change or improvement is essential. After the possible solutions are considered, pediatricians need to work with community collaborators to develop and implement the solution that is the most practical. Having credibility in the community makes the task of collaboration much easier. Everyone is more effective working with others, but collaboration necessitates the ability to compromise and be flexible in implementation plans. Decide if the issue needs to be taken to an executive, legislative, or judicial branch of government to be adequately addressed. Tools to use to advertise the cause include letter writing, public speaking, use of the media, and hiring a lobbyist to put forth the agenda. The more public support the issue has, the more likely that change will be effected. Be persistent because change doesn't happen easily or quickly.

National organizations that are available for involvement by pediatricians include the AAP with its Federal Advocacy Action Network, Docs For Tots, Children's Defense Fund, and the Child Welfare League of America among others. Toolkits for advocacy are available through these organizations.

Improving the health of all children through advocacy is considered to be the responsibility of pediatricians and can be a tremendously rewarding part of pediatric practice.

CASE RESOLUTION

In the case scenario, treating this teen for his orthopedic injury is only the first part of thorough pediatric care. His social history and the environment in which he lives are essential information for the pediatrician to obtain to be an advocate for this patient and prevent a second admission for a subsequent and potentially worse injury. A social work evaluation is performed and reveals that he lives in poverty in the inner city and does indeed belong to a gang. The patient and his family are counseled regarding his high-risk behavior, and he is referred to the police department for their Gang Alternative Program. His pediatrician becomes concerned about the high prevalence of gang activity in the community putting many teens at risk of injury. He explores coalitions in the area that recognize similar concerns. To have an effect on decreasing youth gang activity, a solution is identified to establish high-quality after-school programs to involve teens in productive activities. The Boy's and Girl's Club organization is contacted, and they have an interest in establishing a center in this community. The pediatrician volunteers to be on the board and help develop the after-school programs.

Selected References

American Academy of Pediatrics Committee on Community Health Services. The pediatrician's role in community pediatrics. *Pediatrics*. 2005;115:1092–1094

Bar-on M. The use of public education in practice. *Pediatr Rev*. 2001;22:75–80

Berman S. Training pediatricians to become child advocates. *Pediatrics*. 1998;102:632–636

Kaczorowski J, ed. Community pediatrics: making child health at the community level an integral part of pediatric training and practice. *Pediatrics*. 2005;115(suppl):1119–1212

Palfrey JS, Hametz P, Grason H, McCaskill QE, Scott G, Chi GW. Educating the next generation of pediatricians in urban health care: the Anne E. Dyson Community Pediatrics Training Initiative. *Acad Med*. 2004;79:1184–1191

Paulson J. Pediatric advocacy. *Pediatr Clin North Am*. 2001;48:1307–1318

Rudolf MC, Bundle A, Damman A, et al. Exploring the scope for advocacy by paediatricians. *Arch Dis Child*. 1999;81:515–518

Sheehan K, ed. *Pediatr Ann*. 2007;36:(entire issue)

Sia CC. Abraham Jacobi Award address, April 14, 1992. The medical home: pediatric practice and child advocacy in the 1990s. *Pediatrics*. 1992;90:419–423

Taylor D, Raman R. Look how far we've come as advocates for children—but consider where we still need to go! *Contemp Pediatr*. 2005;22:54–64

Talking With Children

Geeta Grover, MD

CASE STUDY

The moment you walk into the examination room, the 2-year-old girl begins to cry and scream uncontrollably. She clings to her mother and turns her face away. The mother appears embarrassed and states that her daughter reacts to all physicians this way. After reassuring the mother that you have received such welcomes before, you sit down at a comfortable distance from the girl and her mother. You smile at the girl and compliment her on her dress, but she does not seem to be interested in interacting with you at this point. You begin your interview with the mother and try not to look at the girl. Out of the corner of your eye, you see that her crying is easing a bit and that she is looking at you very carefully. Without moving from your chair, you hand her your stethoscope with a clip-on toy teddy bear attached to it. She accepts it hesitantly and begins to examine it as you and the mother continue talking.

Questions

1. How does children's age influence their understanding of health and illness?
2. Should physicians speak directly with children about their illnesses?
3. At what age can children begin to communicate with physicians about their illnesses?
4. How can positioning and placement of children in the examination room affect the overall tone and quality of the visit?

Effective doctor-patient communication, which is difficult enough when patients are adults, becomes even more challenging when patients are children. In pediatrics, interviewing involves balancing the needs of both parents and children. Whereas parents may be more focused on issues pertaining to disease, treatment, or aspects of parenting, children look to physicians with different needs and concerns, depending on their age. To have a meaningful and satisfying exchange with children, pediatricians must take into account children's age, intelligence, and developmental maturity because all of these factors affect their concepts of health and illness. As children grow and develop, their understanding of health and illness increases.

Table 3-1. Piaget's Stages of Cognitive Development		
Age[a]	*Stage*	*Characteristics*
Birth–2 y	Sensorimotor	Experiences world through sensations and motor acts
2–6 y	Preoperational	Egocentric thinking; imitation and fantasy play
6–11 y	Concrete operational	Mental processes only as they relate to real objects
>11 y	Formal operations	Capacity for abstract thought

[a]Approximate ages.

Developmental Approach to Communicating With Children

An appreciation of the cognitive stages of development helps pediatricians develop a healthy relationship with their patients by allowing them to communicate with the children in an age-appropriate manner. Piaget defined 4 stages of cognitive development, which occur in the same sequence but not at the same rate in all children (Table 3-1). Children in the sensorimotor stage (birth–2 years of age) experience the world and act through sensations and motor acts. They are developing the concepts of object permanence, causality, and spatial relationships. Children in the preoperational stage (2–6 years) understand reality only from their own viewpoint. As egocentric thinkers, they are unable to separate internal from external reality, and fantasy play is important. School-aged children (6–11 years) are capable of concrete operational thinking. These children can reason through problems that relate to real objects. Older children (>11 years) have the capacity for abstract thought, which defines the stage of formal operations.

An appreciation of how children's cognitive development affects their understanding of illness and pain aids physicians in developing therapeutic relationships. Bibace and colleagues have outlined a developmental approach to children's understanding of illness: Children's explanations of illness are classified into 6 categories consistent with Piaget's cognitive developmental stages. Children 2 to 6 years of age view illness as caused by external factors near the body (phenomenism and contagion). Young children engage in so-called magical thinking; proximity alone provides the link between cause and illness. Children 7–10 years of age should be able to differentiate between self and nonself. At this stage they begin to understand that although illness may be caused by some factor outside the body, illness itself is located inside the body (contamination and internalization). Children older than 11 years understand physiological and psychophysiological explanations for illness (Table 3-2).

Table 3-2. Children's Concepts of Illness[a]		
Age	Concept of Illness	Example
	Preoperational	How do people get colds?
2–6 y	Phenomenism	"From the sun."
	Contagion	"When someone else gets near them."
	Concrete Operational	How do people get colds?
7–10 y	Contamination	"You're outside without a hat and you start sneezing. Your head would get cold—the cold would touch it—and then it would go all over your body."
	Internalization	"In winter, people breathe in too much air into their nose and it blocks up the nose."
	Formal Operations	How do people get colds?
>11 y	Physiological/ Psychophysiological	"They come from viruses, I guess."
		How do people get a heart attack?
		"It can come from being all nerve-racked. You worry too much, and the tension can affect your heart."

[a]Modified and reproduced with permission from Bibace R, Walsh ME. Development of children's concepts of illness. *Pediatrics.* 1980;66:912–917.

A similar developmental sequence applies to children's understanding of pain. Gaffney and Dunne have outlined a developmental approach to this understanding. Younger children may attribute pain to punishment for some transgression or wrongdoing on their part. They may not understand the relationship between pain and illness (eg, "Pain is something in my tummy."). Children with concrete operational thought can appreciate that pain and illness are related, but they may have no clear understanding of the causation of pain (eg, "Pain is a feeling you get when you are sick."). Older children and adolescents begin to understand the complex physical and psychological components of pain. For example, they realize that although the bone in the arm is broken, pain is ultimately felt in the head (eg, "Pain goes up some nerves from the broken bone in my arm to my head.").

Guidelines for Doctor-Child Communication

Successful communication with children depends not only on spoken words but also nonverbal cues and the environment itself. A pleasant, child-friendly environment with bright colors, wall decorations, and toys helps make children feel more comfortable. Health care practitioners should be sincere, because children are extremely sensitive

to nonverbal cues. Pediatricians should take a few minutes to enjoy children; this not only gives children a chance to evaluate their physicians, but also allows clinicians to begin assessing areas of development. A general principle of the pediatric examination is to begin with the least invasive portions of the examination (eg, heart, lungs, abdomen) and save the most invasive for last (eg, oropharynx, ears). Pediatricians should maintain their self-control in difficult situations. If they approach their limit, they should step outside for a few minutes or ask someone for assistance. Overall guidelines for communicating with children are provided in Box 3-1. Age-specific guidelines follow.

Box 3-1. Physician-Child Communication	
Dos	**Don'ts**
Provide a pleasant environment.	Limit the child's participation.
Pay attention to nonverbal cues.	Threaten the child.
Be sincere and honest.	Compare the child to others.
Enjoy the child.	Get into power struggles.
Speak age appropriately.	
Get down to the child's eye level.	
Examine from least to most invasive.	
Respect the child's privacy.	
Maintain self-control.	
Have a sense of humor.	

Birth to 6 Months

Examination of children of this age is usually pleasant. Although verbal interaction is limited, it is important to play with children, hold them, and talk to them. By watching physicians interact with their children, new parents have an opportunity to learn how to behave with their infants. Infants have not yet developed a fear of strangers and can usually be easily examined either in parents' arms or on the examination table.

7 Months to 3 Years

This is perhaps the most challenging age group with regard to developing rapport and performing examinations. After entering the examination room, pediatricians should take a few moments to converse or play with children. Such actions help put children at ease and allow them to get to know their doctors. Children who are 1 to 2 years of age will probably busy themselves, exploring the room during the history taking. By acknowledging them periodically, physicians build rapport that will help later during the examination. Two- to 3-year-old children are usually very apprehensive of the examination. Physicians should get down to children's eye level when speaking to them. Reassurances such as, "You're not going to get any shots today," can help alleviate their fears. Because stranger anxiety has developed, physicians should try to do as much of the examination as possible with children in parents' laps. Distractions such as stethoscope toys, flashing penlights, or keys may be helpful.

3 to 6 Years

Children's expressive capabilities are growing at tremendous rates during this period. Children can usually be engaged in conversation. They should be given repeated opportunities for participation, but they should not feel pressured to take part. Children may doubt physicians' true intentions and will probably only speak once their comfort level has been achieved. Children should be involved; they can be asked simple questions regarding their illness (eg, "Where does it hurt?"). In addition, children should be given some control during the examination (eg, "Should I look in your mouth next or your ears?"), and they should be allowed to handle physicians' equipment. Knowing what to expect next and having some control over the examination can help to decrease fear and increase cooperation.

7 to 11 Years

Examination of children in this age group can be rewarding. Physicians should make a point to speak directly with children and not just to parents concerning the chief complaint and history. Children can usually provide a good history regarding their illness, although their concept of time may be misleading. For example, a "long, long time" may mean hours, days, or months, and parents need to clarify this. Children should be asked about school, friends, and favorite activities. Answers to such questions give physicians an idea of children's social and emotional well-being, which may be affecting their physical health. Physicians sometimes overlook children's need for privacy at this age. Drapes should be used appropriately during the examination, and physicians should be sensitive to the presence of other children or adults in the room.

Physicians should begin to involve older children in the management of their illness. Children's understanding of their illness and its management should be assessed (eg, children with asthma could be asked, "What is this inhaler for? When are you going to use it? Show me how."). Children should be given an opportunity to express their fears and anxieties, and these concerns should be discussed (eg, "Asthma can be scary, especially when you can't catch your breath. Have you ever felt like that? Tell me about it."). Children should be involved in the management of their illness, which allows them to develop a sense of responsibility for their own health and medical care.

Older Than 12 Years

Communication with adolescents is discussed in detail in Chapter 5.

Barriers to Effective Communication With Children

The manner in which adults speak to children is influenced by what they think children can understand. Clinicians tend to overestimate the understanding capabilities of younger children and underestimate those of older children. Lack of appreciation for the cognitive sophistication of children may lead to frustration for all involved. Younger children are presented with information they may not be able to comprehend, and older children may feel frustrated because they are being spoken to in a childlike manner.

Overestimating children's receptivity to medical information can be particularly problematic in the case of children with chronic illness. It is easy to assume that children with chronic medical conditions or those with more hospitalizations would have more sophisticated understanding regarding illness causation. Although these children may seem more savvy and knowledgeable regarding medical procedures, there is little research to support the assumption that they have more sophisticated understanding of illness causation than would be expected based on their age or developmental level, nor that they are better able to understand and retain medical information than their peers without chronic medical concerns.

Another potential barrier in communicating with children is limiting their participation. Physicians tend to elicit information from children but exclude them from diagnostic and management information. Older children want to know about their illness and are capable of learning about management.

All physicians have been frustrated or pushed to the limit at one time or another when working with children. In such situations, practitioners should remember that children are probably not trying to irritate physicians on purpose. Crying or lack of cooperation generally stems from fear or a sense of lack of control over the situation. Pediatricians should avoid taking part in a battle over power or control with children. Threatening remarks (eg, "If you're not good, I'll have to give you a shot.") or comparisons between children (eg, "Your brother is younger than you, and he didn't cry.") not only are ineffective but may make the situation worse. A clear perspective, empathy, and a sense of humor are much more useful.

CASE RESOLUTION

In the case presented in the opening scenario, you learn from the mother that her daughter has been in good health. The mother has brought in the child for a routine health maintenance visit. You assess that her development is normal and that her immunizations are up to date. As you and the mother talk, the child appears more relaxed and less frightened. She begins to respond to your questions and cooperate with the examination, but she chooses to remain on her mother's lap. Praising a child who is cooperative helps reinforce preferred behavior.

Selected References

Bibace R, Walsh ME. Development of children's concepts of illness. *Pediatrics.* 1980;66:912–917

Charman T, Chandrami S. Childrens' understanding of physical illness and psychological states. *Psychol Health.* 1995;10:145–153

Gaffney A, Dunne EA. Developmental aspects of children's definitions of pain. *Pain.* 1986;26:105–117

Ginsburg H, Opper S. *Piaget's Theory of Intellectual Development.* 3rd ed. Englewood Cliffs, NJ: Prentice-Hall; 1988

Krishnan B, Glazebrook C, Smyth A. Does illness experience influence the recall of medical information? *Arch Dis Child.* 1998;79:514–515

Kury SP, Rodrigue JR. Concepts of illness causality in a pediatric sample: relationship to illness duration, frequency of hospitalization and degree of life threat. *Clin Pediatr.* 1995;34:178–182

Myant KA, Williams JM. Children's concepts of health and illness: understanding of contagious illnesses, non-contagious illnesses and injuries. *J Health Psychol.* 2005;10:805–819

Perrin EC, Perrin JM. Clinicians' assessments of children's understanding of illness. *Am J Dis Child.* 1983;137:874–878

Van Dulmen AM. Children's contributions to pediatric outpatient encounters. *Pediatrics.* 1998;102:563–568

Talking With Parents

Geeta Grover, MD

CASE STUDY

An 8-month-old boy with a 1-week history of cough and runny nose and a 2-day history of vomiting, diarrhea, and fever, with a temperature of 101°F (38.3°C) is evaluated in the emergency department (ED). The mother is very concerned because her son's appetite has decreased and he has been waking up several times at night for the last 2 days.

A nurse interrupts and says that paramedics are bringing a 5-year-old trauma victim to the ED. The appearance of the 8-month-old child is quickly assessed; he seems active and alert. Bilateral otitis media is diagnosed. Before leaving the examination room the physician says to the mother, "Your son has a viral syndrome and infection in his ears. I am going to prescribe an antibiotic that you can begin giving him today. Give him Tylenol as needed for the fever. Don't worry about his vomiting and diarrhea; just make sure that he drinks plenty of liquids and don't give

him milk or milk products for a few days. Bring him back here or to his regular doctor if his fever persists, he doesn't eat, he has too much vomiting or diarrhea, he looks lethargic, or if he isn't better in 2 days."

Questions

1. How much information can most parents handle? Did this mother receive more information than she can be reasonably expected to remember?
2. How do you assess parental concerns? Did the physician address the mother's worries sufficiently?
3. How do you know whether a parent has understood all the information? Was this mother given a chance to clarify any questions she had?
4. What are some barriers to effective doctor-patient communication?
5. How does the setting itself influence communication?

Effective communication in the pediatric setting involves the exchange of information between physicians, parents, and children. In addition, observing the interaction between parents and children gives physicians an opportunity to assess parenting skills and the dynamics of the parent-child relationship. The communication needs of both parents and children are quite different; this makes the exchange of information challenging. Parental concerns should be addressed in a sensitive, empathetic, and nonjudgmental manner. A nonthreatening, pleasant demeanor and age-appropriate language help facilitate communication with children (see Chapter 3, Talking With Children).

Pediatrics encompasses not only the traditional medical model of diagnosis and treatment of disease but also maintenance of the health and well-being of children through longitudinal care and the establishment of ongoing relationships between physicians and families. Personal relationships between physicians and families create an atmosphere in which information can be exchanged openly. The pediatrician's role in such relationships is to not only diagnose and treat, but also to listen, advise, guide, and teach.

The doctor-patient relationship is truly a privilege. Patients entrust physicians with their innermost thoughts and feelings, allow them to touch private parts of their bodies, and then trust them to perform invasive procedures or administer medications. Mutual respect is essential for the development of a healthy relationship between physicians, parents, and children. Through practice and continued

awareness of interpersonal abilities, physicians can develop good communication skills. All physicians eventually develop their own personal interviewing and examination style. What seems awkward and difficult at first soon becomes routine and even enjoyable as physicians become more comfortable with patients.

Parental Concerns

Parents' preconceived ideas and concerns regarding their children's illnesses can greatly influence the exchange of information between physicians and patients. At health maintenance or well-child visits, it is important for pediatricians to address the nonmedical and psychosocial concerns of parents, such as their children's development, nutrition, and growth. Often these questions stem from discussions with other parents or information received through the media. Although such concerns may seem trivial to pediatricians, they may be extremely important to parents. In addition to addressing the needs of the child, the health maintenance visit also gives the pediatrician an opportunity to assess and address parental needs. Parental depression, substance abuse, family violence, or marital discord can all have profound effects on children's health and development. When evaluating children brought in for illness, it is important to ask parents what concerns them the most. Parental fears may be much different than medical concerns. Failure to give parents the opportunity to ask questions or to address these concerns in a sensitive manner may lead to dissatisfaction and poor communication.

The Pediatric Interview

Pediatric interviews are conducted in a variety of settings for many different reasons. The first interaction between the physician and parents may be during the prenatal interview before the birth of the child, in the hospital following the delivery, or in the doctor's office during the well-baby visit. Later, the physician may see children in the office for regular health maintenance visits or in the office, emergency department (ED), or hospital for an acute illness.

The specific clinical situation dictates the information that needs to be gathered and the appropriate interviewing techniques. During the prenatal visit, physicians should discuss common concerns and anxieties about the new baby with prospective parents. In addition, parents have an opportunity to interview physicians and evaluate their offices and staffs.

In the emergency setting, physicians must elicit pertinent information needed to make decisions regarding management within a short period. Absence of long-term relationships can make communication in the ED particularly challenging. Focused, closed-ended questions should be used primarily. The periodic health maintenance visit is at the opposite end of this spectrum. Here the use of broad, open-ended questions is more appropriate; closed-ended questions should be used as needed for clarification.

Communication Guidelines

Overall principles, applicable regardless of the setting, include interacting with the child and family in a professional yet sensitive and nonjudgmental manner. Common courtesies, such as knocking before entering the room, dressing and behaving in a professional manner, introducing oneself, and addressing parents and children by their preferred names, are always appreciated and welcomed. Taking a few moments to socialize with families develops a more personal relationship that may allow more open conversation about sensitive and emotional issues.

Family-centered care is an approach to health care in which the practitioner realizes the vital role that families play in ensuring the health and well-being of children. Family-centered care practitioners convey respect for parents' insight into and understanding of their children's behavior and needs and actively seek out their observations and incorporate their family preferences into the care plan as much as possible. Benefits of family-centered care include a stronger alliance between the practitioner and the family; increased patient, family, and professional satisfaction; and decreased health care costs.

The medical visit may be divided into 3 parts: the interview, the physical examination, and the concluding remarks. Examples of doctor-parent and doctor-child communications for each of these components are given in Table 4-1.

The Interview

The goal of the interview is to ascertain the chief complaint and determine the appropriate medical history. The interview usually begins with open-ended questions to give parents and children an

Table 4-1. Communication Guidelines and Techniques	
Techniques	**Examples**
The Interview	
Open-ended questions	"How is Susie?"
Closed-ended questions	"Does she have a cough?"
Repetition of important phrases	"She has had a high fever for four days now?"
Clarification	"What do you mean by 'Susie was acting funny'?"
Pauses and silent periods	
Limit medical jargon	"Susie has an ear infection." vs "Susie has otitis media."
Guide the interview	"Right now I am most interested in hearing about the symptoms of this illness."
Be aware of nonverbal communication	Use eye contact and phrases such as "I see."
Acknowledge parental concerns	"Worrying about hearing loss is understandable."
Empathize	"A fever of 104°F can be very frightening."
Remember common courtesies	Knock before entering.
Recognize personal limitations	"I am not an expert in this area. I would like to consult with a colleague."
Summarize	"So she has had fever for four days but the rash and cough began one week ago?"
The Physical Examination	
Show consideration for the child	"It's OK to be afraid."
Inform	"That took me some time, but her heart sounds normal."
Explain procedures	"You may feel a little uncomfortable during the rectal examination."
Avoid exclamations	"Wow! I have never seen anything like this."
Concluding Remarks	
Provide closure	"Our time is over today. May we discuss this at the next visit?"
Minimize discharge instructions	
Be specific	"I am going to treat her with amoxicillin." vs "I'll prescribe an antibiotic."
Praise	"You're doing a great job."
Confirm parental understanding	"Please repeat for me Susie's diagnosis and treatment instructions so I'm sure I've been clear in explaining them to you."

opportunity to discuss their concerns and outline their agenda for the visit. Not uncommonly, the real reason for the visit may not be disclosed until the family believes the physician is trustworthy and honest. Once the issues have been laid out, closed-ended questions can be used to clarify and further define the information presented. It often becomes necessary to guide the interview, especially when parents have several broad issues on their agenda for that visit and time does not permit their discussion.

Physicians should gently acknowledge parental concerns and define time limitations. These actions allow physicians to focus on the most salient issues of that visit. Physicians should limit their use of medical jargon (scientific terms) and be aware of nonverbal communication. Practitioners should empathize with parents; this makes them feel that their situation is truly understood even if physicians can do very little to help them. Pauses and silent periods should be used, especially when discussing emotionally difficult issues, to convey to parents and children that their physician cares enough to listen. Physicians should not underrate their own knowledge, but at the same time they should recognize their limitations and use consultants appropriately. Finally, physicians' understanding of the chief complaint and history should be summarized so parents have an opportunity to clarify points of disagreement.

Today there are increasing demands for primary care practitioners to address not only the physical but also the psychosocial health needs of their patients. Motivational interviewing (MI) offers an effective means of addressing these developmental, behavioral, and social concerns within the context of a primary care setting. Motivational interviewing is a patient-centered, collaborative, and directive interaction style that addresses the ambivalence and discrepancies between a person's current values and behaviors and their future goals. In contrast to more traditional medical approaches that rely primarily on authority and education, MI is a collaborative approach that relies on elicitation of the patient's ideas regarding change. Motivational interviewing practitioners understand that trying to move beyond a patient's readiness to change is likely to increase their resistance to treatment (eg, lecturing to an adolescent who is not yet ready to quit smoking about the dangers of smoking is unlikely to be effective and may even produce more resistance). Motivational interviewing requires that the practitioner follow 4 principles (Table 4-2). Operationally, open-ended questions (eg, "How do you feel about smoking?"), affirmations (eg, "You are tired of having to monitor your blood sugar every day and stick to your diet."), and reflective listening (eg, "You are worried about your daughter's behavior and are concerned that if it persists, she may be expelled from school.") are important tools of MI. In addition, MI practitioners ask permission before giving advice (eg. "Would it be OK if I shared some information with you?"), or the practitioner may state the facts but let the parent interpret the information (eg, "What does this mean to you?"). Motivational interviewing is not only effective with adults, but research with adolescents has shown MI to be an effective tool to increase self-efficacy to enact change (eg, adolescent smoking cessation).

Table 4-2. Principles of Motivational Interviewing[a]

Principle	Example
Express empathy.	Use reflective listening.
Develop discrepancy between patient's current behavior and his treatment goal.	Patient, not practitioner, presents arguments for change.
Roll with the patient's resistance.	Avoid arguing for change.
Support the patient's self-efficacy.	Patient's own belief in the possibility of change is an important motivator.

[a]Adapted from Miller WR, Rollnick S. *Motivational Interviewing: Preparing People for Change.* 2nd ed. New York, NY: Guilford Press; 2002.

The Physical Examination

Parents keenly observe physicians' interactions with their children during the examination. It is an important time for physicians to build a therapeutic relationship with children (see Chapter 3, Talking With Children). The transition between the history and physical examination can be made by briefly telling children and parents what to expect during the examination. Practitioners should show consideration for children's fears. Clinicians often find it helpful to speak to families at periodic intervals during the examination regarding their observations. Prolonged periods of silence as the doctor listens or palpates may be anxiety provoking for families. Physicians should be sure to explain any procedures that either they or their staff are going to perform at a level that is appropriate for both parents and children. In addition, physicians should try to avoid exclamations or comments to themselves during the examination (eg, "Wow, that's some murmur!"), which may be alarming to families.

Concluding Remarks

This portion of the visit, which is all too easy to rush through, is extremely important. Closure can be provided by either summarizing the diagnosis or outlining plans for the following visit. Parents should be asked to participate by acknowledging closure and helping to develop a management plan. It is important to assess parental readiness for knowledge (especially in emotionally difficult situations) and keep family resources and limitations in mind. Discharge instructions should be minimized; physicians should be specific and the number of diagnoses, medications, and "as needed" instructions (indications for seeking medical advice such as "return as needed for high fever") should be limited. When complicated discharge instructions are given, additional physician time may be required to ensure parental understanding. Praising parents on their care of their children can boost their self-esteem and confidence and may minimize calls and questions. Parental understanding should be confirmed; parents should be asked to repeat the diagnosis and treatment plan. Simply asking parents if they have understood is not enough, because parents often say "yes" out of respect for the physician's time or embarrassment that they have not understood what has been said. For example, the physician could say, "I want to be sure that I've spoken clearly enough. Please repeat for me [child's name] diagnosis and treatment instructions."

Barriers to Effective Communication

Barriers to effective communication may be divided into systems barriers and interpersonal barriers (Table 4-3). The primary systems barriers are the setting itself and lack of continuity of care. Because of access problems within the health care system (ie, lack of health insurance coverage), many children receive only episodic care from different physicians in acute care clinics or EDs. Without the benefit of long-term relationships, doctor-patient communication may suffer.

Interpersonal barriers include physician time constraints, frequent interruptions, and cultural insensitivity. Frequent interruptions or apparent impatience on the part of physicians conveys to parents and children that either they do not care or they are too busy for them. Language differences may pose a significant barrier depending on the region in which physicians practice. Ideally, physicians themselves should be able to speak to parents and children. If translators must be used, children should not play this role, if possible, because this places them in an awkward situation. Parents of other patients should not be used because this violates patients' privacy. Physicians should be sensitive to cultural differences (eg, gender issues, views on illness, folk remedies, and beliefs). Suggesting treatments that are not culturally acceptable or are contrary to folk wisdom simply decreases compliance with prescribed treatment plans. For example, many Eastern cultures believe in the concept of "hot" and "cold" foods and illnesses. Suggesting to a mother that she feed primarily "hot" foods to a child she believes to have an illness that is also "hot" may not be acceptable to her. Such information is rarely volunteered and must be elicited through sensitive patient interviewing.

Table 4-3. Barriers to Effective Communication	
Barriers	*Examples*
Systems	
Lack of continuity of care	Episodic care that is primarily illness driven
The setting itself	Emergency departments and acute care clinics
Interpersonal	
Physician time constraints	Appearing impatient or preoccupied
Frequent interruptions	Beeper goes off or asked to come to the phone
Cultural insensitivity	Suggesting treatments that are not acceptable within the family's belief systems

---

CASE RESOLUTION

The doctor-patient interaction presented in the case history lacks several of the points discussed here. The physician did not acknowledge parental concerns or make sure that the mother had understood the diagnosis and treatment plan. The mother was presented with more information than she could have reasonably been asked to remember. This interaction could have been improved (1) if the physician conveyed to the mother that her concerns were appreciated and (2) then reassured her that her child was going to be all right. Furthermore, the physician could have told the mother the name and dosage schedule of the antibiotic to be prescribed and limited the number of "as needed" instructions.

Selected References

American Academy of Pediatrics. *Bright Futures: Guidelines for Health Supervision of Infants, Children, and Adolescents.* Elk Grove Village, IL: American Academy of Pediatrics; 2008

American Academy of Pediatrics Committee on Hospital Care. Family-centered care and the pediatrician's role. *Pediatrics.* 2003;112:691–696

American Academy of Pediatrics Committee on Psychosocial Aspects of Child and Family Health. The new morbidity revisited: a renewed commitment to the psychosocial aspects of pediatric care. *Pediatrics.* 2001;108:1227–1230

Dixon SD, Stein MT. *Encounters with Children: Pediatric Behavior and Development.* 4th ed. Chicago, IL: Mosby-Year Book; 2006

Erickson S, Gerstle M, Feldstein S. Brief interventions and motivational interviewing with children, adolescents and their parents in pediatric health care settings. *Arch Pediatr Adolesc Med.* 2005;159:1173–1180

Grover G, Berkowitz CD, Lewis RJ. Parental recall after a visit to the emergency department. *Clin Pediatr.* 1994;33:194–201

Korsch BM, Freemon BF, Negrete VF. Practical implications of doctor-patient interaction analysis for pediatric practice. *Am J Dis Child.* 1971;12:110–114

Miller WR, Rollnick S. *Motivational Interviewing: Preparing People for Change.* 2nd ed. New York, NY: Guilford Press; 2002

Regalado MG, Halfon N. Parenting: issues for the pediatrician. *Pediatr Ann.* 1998;27:31–37

Young KT, Davis K, Schoen C, Parker S. Listening to parents: a national survey of parents with young children. *Arch Pediatr Adolesc Med.* 1998;152:255–262

Talking With Adolescents

Monica Sifuentes, MD

CASE STUDY

This is a first-time visit for a 15-year-old girl who is accompanied by her mother. The mother is concerned because her daughter's grades have been dropping since beginning high school, and she appears fatigued and irritable. The mother reports no new activities or recent changes in the home situation and no new stressors in the family. Both parents are employed, the girl has the same friends she has always had, and her siblings currently are doing well academically. The girl is healthy and has never been hospitalized. After the mother leaves the room, the girl is interviewed alone.

Questions

1. When interviewing adolescents, what is the significance of identifying their stage of development?
2. What are important areas to cover in the adolescent interview?
3. What issues of confidentiality and competence need to be discussed with adolescents before conducting the interview?
4. When should information be disclosed to others, despite issues of confidentiality?

Adolescence is a time of unique change. Unlike other periods in life when individuals have at least some knowledge or experience to guide them, adolescence can be characterized by feelings of physical awkwardness, emotional turmoil, and social isolation. In addition, the teenage years are dreaded by most parents, who often feel ill equipped to handle the wide range of children's responses. So instead of "taking the bull by the horns," parents choose the route of quiet observation. They fully intend to "be there" for their children but wait to be approached. Hence, many adolescents do not have the guidance or advice of parents during the teenage years and prefer to spend their time alone or in the company of friends or acquaintances. Fortunately, most adolescents pass through this period uneventfully. In fact, many individuals go through this period gladly, finally being permitted to drive a car or go out on a date.

Physicians must use a different approach when interviewing adolescents because information comes directly from the teenager, rather than the parents. Unlike an interview with a younger pediatric patient, the adolescent interview should focus on several psychosocial issues that may be uncomfortable to discuss with the parent present. Each teenager should therefore be interviewed alone. The goal of the interview is to discover any problems that might interfere with a relatively smooth passage through adolescence.

Stages of Adolescence

Adolescents are stereotypically labeled as difficult, complex, time-consuming patients with complicated problems or complaints that lead to uninteresting diagnoses. In addition, they are often accompanied by overbearing, demanding parents, or sometimes no parents at all.

The quality and quantity of information obtained during the medical and psychosocial interview can be greatly enhanced by taking developmental milestones into consideration. Adolescence can be divided into 3 developmental stages: early, middle, and late (Table 5-1). For example, interest in discussing long-term educational goals varies depending on the age of the adolescent. Most 18-year-olds are prepared to discuss college plans, specific vocational interests, and employment opportunities. In contrast, 12-year-olds are still anchored in the concreteness of early adolescence and often are ill prepared to discuss plans for higher education. Current school experiences are much more important to this age group and should therefore be the focus of discussion. Peer pressure is most prominent during middle adolescence; therefore, 14-year-olds with friends who smoke cigarettes and drink beer probably use the same illicit substances.

Knowledge of these developmental differences allows the interviewer to more effectively explain instructions and diagnoses to teenagers. For example, 19-year-olds can better understand the effects of untreated or recurrent chlamydia cervicitis on long-term fertility than 13-year-olds. This is not to say that physicians should not discuss these possible consequences with a sexually active 13-year-old with chlamydia, but they should use more concrete wording and

	Table 5-1. Developmental Milestones During Adolescence[a]		
	Early Adolescence (11–13 y)	*Middle Adolescence (14–16 y)*	*Late Adolescence (17–21 y)*
Thought processes	Concrete	± Abstract	Abstract
Parental supervision	+	±	−
Risk-taking behavior	+	±	−
Peer pressure	±	++	+

[a]Modified from March CA, Jay MS. Adolescents in the emergency department: an overview. *Adolesc Med State Art Rev.* 1993;4:1.

repeat the information at future visits. Age guidelines are not rigid, however, and each interview should be individually tailored to the particular adolescent and the circumstances surrounding the visit.

Issues of Confidentiality and Competence

A discussion regarding **confidentiality is essential** and can be approached in 2 ways. Each method has distinct advantages as well as disadvantages. Interviewers should use the approach that they find most comfortable; this allows conversation to flow more naturally.

The first approach involves informing adolescents at the beginning of the interview that most issues discussed are held in strict confidence and will not be repeated to anyone. Exceptions are suicidal or homicidal behavior and a history of or ongoing sexual or physical abuse. In any of these instances, other professionals are told of the disclosed information, and parents ultimately are informed of the disclosure. The advantages to this approach are that discussion of these "logistics" at the beginning of the interview is less awkward, making the ground rules clear from the start. This contributes to an atmosphere of trust and honesty. The disadvantage is possible inhibition by adolescents who are unsure about disclosing particular incidents (eg, those concerning sexual abuse); some teenagers are now almost certain not to share this information for fear of involving other professionals or family members. Interviewers should be nonjudgmental, reassuring, and empathetic to reduce the possibility of such an occurrence.

The second, less popular approach to the discussion of confidentiality involves informing adolescents at the end of the interview or when and if one of the exceptions to maintaining confidentiality arises. Proponents of this approach argue that adolescents tend to respond more honestly to questions when they do not believe physicians will inform others, including their parents or legal guardians. Physicians have a legal responsibility, however, to report sexual and physical abuse; in cases of suicidal or homicidal behavior, it is in the patient's best interest to inform other professionals of this disclosure. The disadvantage to this method is that these issues often arise at very emotional times during the interview, and it is difficult to interrupt the patient to discuss mandated reporting. If physicians wait until the end of the interview to inform adolescents about mandated reporting, however, patients may leave the office feeling deceived and probably will not return for future visits. For this reason, most health care providers prefer to inform adolescents at the onset of the interview about confidentiality with the hope that it contributes to the development of a trusting relationship.

An assessment of the adolescent's ability to make health-related decisions is another important aspect of the interview. **Competence** is the ability to understand the significance of information and assess the alternatives and consequences sufficiently to then identify a preference. Various factors besides age must be considered such as level of maturity, intelligence, degree of independence, and presence of any chronic illness. This last factor is included because adolescents with chronic conditions may have already participated in decisions regarding their health care. Regardless, it can be difficult to assess competence from just one visit. It may not even be necessary to

make an assessment emergently, except in certain cases such as with unplanned pregnancy.

Although it is imperative to interview adolescents alone, every attempt should be made to involve parents in all health-related decisions. Although specific state laws allow physicians to treat minors in emergent situations and in cases of suspected sexually transmitted infections (STIs) without parents' consent, physicians should urge adolescents to inform their parents of any problems disclosed during the interview. The ultimate decision, however, rests with the adolescent. Physicians can assist adolescents to discuss delicate issues with their parents by role-playing with the teenager or by sitting in on the conversation between the adolescent and the parent.

Psychosocial Review of Systems

A major part of the adolescent interview involves taking an adequate psychosocial history, which can be completed in 20 to 30 minutes in most cases. The approach known by the acronym **HEADDSSS** (home environment, employment and education, activities, diet, drugs, sexual activity/sexuality, suicide and depression, safety) allows interviewers to evaluate the critical areas in adolescents' lives that may contribute to a less than optimal environment for normal growth and development (Questions Box). Questions about sexuality must be asked in a nondirected, nonjudgmental fashion, giving adolescents time to respond. This information is useful to assess risks for conditions such as STIs, including human immunodeficiency virus. In addition, an inquiry about both sexual and physical abuse is indicated during this part of the interview.

Issues That Need Immediate Attention

Many issues discussed during the psychosocial interview can be a source of anxiety for adolescents. Certain problems must be taken more seriously than others, and may demand immediate attention. Suicidal ideation, with or without a previous attempt, definitely requires a more in-depth analysis of the gravity of the problem. Physicians should make sure that adolescents feel they can make verbal contact and call someone if they feel like hurting themselves. Mental health professionals should be involved in the clinical assessment of these situations. Other issues that require immediate attention include possible danger to others, possible or confirmed unplanned pregnancy, and sexual or physical abuse.

Concluding the Interview

The adolescent interview should be conducted at a time when the adolescent is relatively healthy and the interviewer has set aside ample time for a thorough, uninterrupted discussion. However, all topics need not be addressed during the initial interview if time does not permit. Issues that are not covered at this visit can be addressed at the next one. The number of appointments needed to work through or solve a particular problem is unlimited.

At the end of each visit, the interview should be summarized; any difficult topics should be mentioned, and the issue of confidentiality should be reviewed. Adolescents should then be asked to

Questions

Talking With Adolescents: HEADDSSS

H: Home environment

- With whom does the adolescent live?
- Have there been any recent changes in the living situation?
- How are things between parents?
- Are the parents employed?
- How does the adolescent get along with the parent and siblings?

E: Employment and education

- Is the adolescent currently in school?
- What are his or her favorite subjects?
- How is the adolescent performing academically?
- Has the adolescent ever been truant or expelled from school?
- Are the adolescent's friends attending school?
- Is the adolescent currently employed? How many hours does he or she work each week?
- What are the adolescent's future education/employment goals?

A: Activities

- What does the adolescent do in his or her spare time?
- What does the adolescent do for fun? Is the adolescent ever bored?
- With whom does the adolescent spend most of his or her time?

D: Diet

- What is a typical meal for the adolescent?
- Does the adolescent have any food restrictions?
- What does the adolescent think about his or her current weight and shape?
- Is there a recent history of weight loss?

D: Drugs

- Is the adolescent currently using, or has he or she ever used, tobacco?
- Is the adolescent currently using, or has he or she ever used, any illicit drugs? What about steroids? Alcohol?
- Does the adolescent ever feel pressured by friends to use drugs or alcohol?

S: Sexual activity/sexuality

- What is the adolescent's sexual orientation?
- Is the adolescent sexually active?
- If so, what was the age of the adolescent's sexual debut?
- How many sexual partners has the adolescent had in his or her lifetime?
- Does the adolescent have a history of sexually transmitted infections?
- Does the adolescent (or the partner) use condoms?
- Does the adolescent (or the partner) use other methods of contraception?
- Does the adolescent have a history of sexual or physical abuse?

S: Suicide/depression

- Is the adolescent bored all the time? Ever sad or tearful? Tired and unmotivated?
- Has the adolescent ever felt that life is not worth living or ever thought of or tried to hurt himself or herself? More importantly, does the adolescent have a suicide plan or access to a firearm?

S: Safety

- Does the adolescent use a seat belt and bicycle helmet?
- Does the adolescent participate in high-risk situations such as riding in the car with someone who has been drinking?
- Does the adolescent feel safe at home? At school? In his or her neighborhood?
- Is there a firearm in the adolescent's home? If so, what does the adolescent know about firearm safety?

For more detailed information, see the Goldenring and Cohen entry under Selected References.

---

identify a person whom they can trust or confide in should any problems arise before the next visit. In some instances, this issue may already have been discussed during the interview. Adolescents also should be given the opportunity to express any other concerns not covered in the interview and ask additional questions.

Physicians should clearly point out to the adolescent any significant risk factors or risk-taking behaviors that have been identified during the interview and assess the teenager's readiness to change this behavior. For those adolescents who are not engaging in high-risk behaviors, physicians should acknowledge that things seem to be going well, praise them with positive feedback, and review their individual strengths and accomplishments that have been discussed. Available resources such as teen hotlines and popular Web sites should be given to the adolescent prior to inviting the parent or guardian back into the examination room. General concerns should then be reviewed with the parent while maintaining the adolescent's confidentiality. The follow-up visit should be arranged at that time.

CASE RESOLUTION

The adolescent in the case history initially should be informed about confidentiality and the specific exceptions to maintaining it. Nonthreatening topics such as home life, school, and outside activities first should be explored, followed by questions regarding sexuality, sexual activity, and illicit drug use. Suicidal behavior or depression and safety issues should also be reviewed with the teenager alone. High-risk behaviors and their consequences should be discussed with the adolescent at the end of the interview, and a plan for future visits should be arranged.

Selected References

Akinbami LJ, Gandhi H, Cheng TL. Availability of adolescent health services and confidentiality in primary care practices. *Pediatrics.* 2003;111:394–401

Bravender T, Price CN, English A. Primary care providers' willingness to see unaccompanied adolescents. *J Adolesc Health.* 2004;34:30–36

Coupey SM. Interviewing adolescents. *Pediatr Clin North Am.* 1997; 44:1349–1364

Ford C, English A, Sigman G. Confidential health care for adolescents: position paper for the Society for Adolescent Medicine. *J Adolesc Health.* 2004;35:160–167

Ford CA, English A. Limiting confidentiality of adolescent health services: what are the risks? *JAMA.* 2002;288:752–753

Ginsburg KR. Viewing our adolescent patients through a positive lens. *Contemp Pediatr.* 2007;24:65–76

Goldenring JM, Cohen E. Getting into adolescent heads. *Contemp Pediatr.* 1988;5:75–90

Goldenring JM, Rosen DS. Getting into adolescent heads: an essential update. *Contemp Pediatr.* 2004;21:64–90

Green M, Sullivan P, Eichberg C. Avoid a "swiss cheese" history when psychosocial complaints are on the menu. *Contemp Pediatr.* 2002;19:115–125

Gutgesell ME. Issues of adolescent psychological development in the 21st century. *Pediatr Rev.* 2004;25:79–84

Knight JR, Sherritt L, Shrier LA, Harris SK, Chang G. Validity of the CRAFFT substance abuse screening test among adolescent clinic patients. *Arch Pediatr Adolesc Med.* 2002;156:607–614

Ott MA, Labbett RL, Gold MA. Counseling adolescents about abstinence in the office setting. *J Pediatr Adolesc Gynecol.* 2007;20:39–44

Reddy DM, Fleming R, Swain C. Effect of mandatory parental notification on adolescent girls' use of sexual health services. *JAMA.* 2002;288:710–714

Resnick MD. Protective factors, resiliency and healthy youth development. *Adolesc Med.* 2000;11:157–165

Ryan SA. Helping parents communicate with their teens Part 1: assessment and general strategies. *Adolesc Health Update.* 1999;11(2):1–8

Ryan SA, Rickert VI. Helping parents communicate with their teens Part 2: challenging clinical situations. *Adolesc Health Update.* 1999;11(3):1–8

Thrall JS, McCloskey L, Ettner SL, Rothman E, Tighe JE, Emans SJ. Confidentiality and adolescents' use of providers for health information and for pelvic examinations. *Arch Pediatr Adolesc Med.* 2000;154:885–892

Van Hook S, Harris SK, Brooks T, et al. The "Six T's": barriers to screening teens for substance abuse in primary care. *J Adolesc Health.* 2007;40:456–461

Telephone Management

Iris Wagman Borowsky, MD, PhD, and Cecily L. Wait, MD

CASE STUDY

The mother of an otherwise healthy 10-month-old girl calls and tells you that her daughter has a fever. The girl's rectal temperature has been 103°F to 104°F (39.4°C–40.0°C) for the past 2 days. Although she is cranky with the fever, she plays normally after receiving acetaminophen. The girl is eating well and has no runny nose, cough, vomiting, diarrhea, or rash.

Questions

1. How do telephone and face-to-face encounters between physicians and patients differ?
2. What are some general guidelines for effective doctor-patient communication over the telephone?
3. What historical information is necessary for appropriate telephone management?
4. What points are important to cover in home treatment advice?

Parents frequently call their pediatricians seeking medical advice about their children. It is estimated that pediatricians spend more than 25% of their total practice time engaged in telephone medicine. Telephone medicine serves 2 purposes: (1) it provides a service and (2) it controls costs and overcrowding by reducing unnecessary visits to the office and emergency department (ED). Most calls concern upper respiratory symptoms, fever, rash, trauma, or gastrointestinal complaints—the same problems most commonly seen in the office. In addition to acute illness care, triage, and advice, telephone care services provided by pediatricians include chronic disease management, care coordination, patient education, counseling, test result interpretation, illness follow-up, adherence checks, and medication adjustments.

Telephone management of illnesses differs in that it requires pediatricians to give advice based on history alone and precludes the opportunity to see the child, much less do a careful physical examination. For example, a practitioner in the ED who does not know the patient or family may choose to see the child if questions about the child's general health or the feasibility of continued contact with the family arise. On the other hand, a primary care physician who knows the patient and family and can follow the child's progress by telephone may advise home management for a child with a similar history. Pediatric practice settings, whether in an ED or primary care office, should have an organized approach to telephone care. In addition to physicians, nurse practitioners, and physician assistants, telephone care systems may include trained and supervised nurses and nonmedical office staff using protocols.

Telephone Communication Skills

Parents commonly call their pediatricians because they are worried about their child. The friendly voice of a health care worker who is ready to lend an ear goes a long way toward reassuring an anxious parent. Calls should begin with a "verbal handshake." Staff should identify themselves and the place where the call is received and offer to help. They should learn the caller's name, his or her relationship to the child, and the child's name and gender; these names, as well as the child's gender, should be used in the conversation, thereby creating a more personal atmosphere.

Telephone calls for medical advice are often received in busy environments such as EDs or clinics where patients are waiting to be seen. It is easy to be abrupt under these circumstances and not give complete attention to callers. If calls are not emergencies, practitioners can take the caller's telephone number and return the call as soon as possible. If callers do not feel that their concerns have been fully acknowledged, they are likely to feel dissatisfied, even if they are given sound advice. Furthermore, research on doctor-patient relationships suggests that lack of friendliness or warmth in the doctor-patient relationship and patient dissatisfaction are associated with noncompliance with medical advice. Studies show that the length of a patient visit does not correlate with patient satisfaction. Telephone encounters do not necessarily have to be lengthy; the average length of a call is reported to be 3 to 5 minutes, depending on the setting. Calls must be pleasant, however, and they must address callers' concerns. Open-ended questions such as "Tell me about your child's illness" or "Are there any other symptoms?" are useful at the beginning of a call because they give callers an opportunity to explain the situation without interruptions.

Establishing rapport over the telephone is more difficult than in person because the practitioner is limited to verbal communication. In face-to-face encounters, physicians can use words as well as means of nonverbal communication such as facial expressions, eye contact, gesturing, and touch to convey warmth and empathy. Practitioners should use various aspects of **verbal communication** to convey sincere interest in callers' concerns, and they should pay attention to these verbal cues in callers. Many components of verbal communication (in addition to words themselves), including vocal expression, pace, articulation, tone, volume, and pauses, affect telephone interactions. Health care professionals should speak clearly and use vocabulary that callers understand; **medical jargon should be avoided.** A friendly yet respectful tone and a calm, professional manner should be maintained.

Careful listening is crucial to obtaining the information necessary to make medical decisions over the telephone. One of the major goals of health care professionals is to recognize and respond to callers' main concerns and expectations. This can be difficult because most callers do not specifically tell their major concerns to their physicians. Researchers have found the following questions useful in the identification of parents' chief concerns: "What worries you the most about [use child's name] illness?" and "Why does that worry you?"

For callers who ramble, health care professionals may need to focus the conversation. Asking the question "What can I do to help?" should clarify the reason for the call. If information needs to be verified, practitioners can summarize what they have heard and ask if they have understood correctly.

Angry callers may elicit defensive or confrontational behavior from health care professionals. Responding to anger with arguments, however, is time-consuming, stressful, and pointless. Practitioners should be warm and understanding so that callers who want to discuss their feelings are comfortable. Acknowledging anger may encourage open discussion and problem-solving (eg, "You sound upset. Is there anything I can do to help?"). Empathizing with callers (eg, "I don't blame you for being upset." "That must have been very frustrating.") may also help.

Practitioners can build confidence in callers by complimenting them on the way they have handled things so far (eg, "You did the right thing by giving [child's name] Tylenol and a lukewarm sponge bath for the fever. That is exactly what I would have done." or "I'm glad that you called about this."). They may even be able to offer reassurance to parents who are not managing their child's illness correctly by commenting that many parents try the same treatment. A different treatment approach can then be suggested.

Before the end of the conversation, callers can be given an opportunity to ask questions and encouraged to call again if additional problems occur.

Telephone History Taking

How much history should be obtained over the telephone? Enough information should be gathered to make an appropriate decision. Questions should be directed at **determining whether an emergency exists** and **making a diagnosis.** For example, if the mother of a 20-day-old girl reports that her daughter has a temperature of 102°F (38.9°C), the infant must be seen immediately. If diarrhea is the chief complaint, some additional information would be helpful before giving advice (eg, "How many bowel movements did the girl have in the last 24 hours? Is there any blood in the diarrhea? Does she have a fever? Is she drinking less than usual? Is there any decrease in urine output?"). An older child with the same chief complaint of fever may be safely managed at home, depending on the answers to other questions about additional symptoms.

Pediatricians typically follow an organized approach to history taking for acute care visits that includes the chief complaint, history of present illness, pertinent review of systems, medical history, and family and social history. A similarly **organized framework** should be used to obtain a history over the telephone (Questions Box). Specific questions should then be asked to clarify the child's condition and obtain all the information necessary to make a good decision. A child's medical history may affect a practitioner's management of the current problem. For example, knowing that a child who has been exposed to chickenpox has asthma and is receiving steroids or has leukemia is crucial in providing the appropriate telephone advice. Practitioners can refer to several texts on pediatric telephone decision-making (see Selected References). These books outline protocols for common chief complaints to serve as guides for history taking and management over the telephone. The most efficient way to provide such medical advice is to obtain critical information that affects decisions about diagnosis and management instead of asking all possible questions. For example, with a child who is vomiting or has diarrhea, the state of hydration is critical; with a cough, the occurrence of breathing difficulty; and with head trauma, loss of consciousness. Methods of teaching telephone management skills include role-playing, listening to mock calls by "simulated" parents, and reviewing tapes of actual calls.

Because most childhood illnesses are mild and self-limited, evaluation of the safety of medical advice obtained over the telephone requires large samples to detect poor outcomes associated with mismanagement. Research has described a "wellness bias" in which practitioners, who primarily see patients with mild, self-limited illnesses, may downplay the severity of reported symptoms and choose the most benign diagnostic possibility. This bias may be more pronounced in a telephone encounter, where the physician cannot see the child. One study reported telephone encounters in which physicians seemed to make a decision early in the conversation and then "shut out" additional information that should have led to the consideration of more serious diagnoses. The safest approach is to always have a high index of suspicion for a serious condition. Questions can then be asked to confirm or dispel those suspicions.

Questions

Telephone Management

- How old is the child?
- What is the child's chief problem? What are the child's symptoms?
- How long has the child had these symptoms?
- How is the child acting?
- Does the child have any chronic illnesses?
- Is the child taking any medications?
- What is the caller most worried about?

Telephone Advice

Pediatricians should formulate an **assessment and management plan** based on the child's history. If the situation is an emergency, this should be explained to the caller, and appropriate follow-up plans should be made (ie, sending an ambulance for life-threatening conditions such as respiratory depression or uncontrollable bleeding, advising the caller to bring the child by car to the ED or physician's office within a specified amount of time for potentially dangerous complaints, such as right lower quadrant pain or possible fracture). If the call is not an emergency, then health care professionals must decide if and when the child should be seen by a physician and the appropriate home treatment.

Research shows that parents need and expect to receive an explanation of their child's illness. Practitioners should clearly state what the child's illness seems to be, what probably caused it, and what the parents can expect (eg, length of time that the child is likely to be sick, additional symptoms that may appear).

Before giving any treatment advice, health care professionals should ask callers the following questions: "What have you done so far?" "Have you given the child any medications?" and "How is this treatment working?" If the therapy seems appropriate, callers should be complimented and encouraged to continue the treatment. The regimen should be modified as indicated. Instructions for home treatment should be clear and as easy to implement as possible. If the instructions are complicated or lengthy, callers may want to write them down. When prescribing medication, ask if the child has any known drug allergies, and give the dose, frequency of administration, and information about possible side effects. Practitioners should verify that the caller can follow the telephone advice (eg, a parent has a thermometer and knows how to use it). If pediatricians plan to check up on children by telephone, they should confirm that callers (or relatives or neighbors) have a telephone and record the number.

Practitioners should confirm that callers understand the information and instructions and agree with the plan. Asking questions such as "What questions do you have?" encourages callers to raise uncertainties and ask for needed clarification. Most importantly, if the decision is to manage at home, callers should always receive specific instructions about when to call back. Caregivers should call if the child's symptoms change, persist, worsen, or cause anxiety. Also, symptoms specific to the child's condition should be followed (eg, child has fever for more than 2 days, irritability, decreased urination). Parents who seem unduly anxious or uncomfortable with home treatment should be given the opportunity to have their child seen by a physician.

Documentation

All calls for medical advice should be documented in a telephone log book or the child's medical record, for both medical reasons (eg, better follow-up, improved continuity of care) and legal purposes. The form used for documentation should include the date and time of the call; the name, identity, and telephone number of the caller; the name and age of the child; the chief complaint; other symptoms; possible diagnoses; advice given; and the name of the person who took the call.

CASE RESOLUTION

In the case history at the beginning of this chapter, the pediatrician learns several facts that lead to the recommendation that the child be seen that day (the next day if the call is made at night). These facts include the child's age, the height and duration of the fever, and lack of any symptoms of localized infection.

Selected References

American Academy of Pediatrics Section on Telephone Care and Committee on Child Health Financing. Payment for telephone care. *Pediatrics.* 2006;118:1768–1773

Brown JL. Managing legal risks of pediatric telephone care. *AAP News.* 2006;27:17

Brown JL. *Pediatric Telephone Medicine: Principles, Triage and Advice.* 2nd ed. Philadelphia, PA: J. B. Lippincott; 1994

Katz HP. *Telephone Medicine: Triage and Training for Primary Health Care.* Philadelphia, PA: F. A. Davis; 2001

Kempe A, Bunik M, Ellis J, et al. How safe is triage by an after-hours telephone call center? *Pediatrics.* 2006;118:457–463

Kempe A, Luberti A, Belman S, et al. Outcomes associated with pediatric after-hours care by call centers: a multicenter study. *Ambul Pediatr.* 2003;3:211–217

Lee TJ, Guzy J, Johnson D, Woo H, Baraff LJ. Caller satisfaction with after-hours telephone advice: nurse advice service versus on-call pediatricians. *Pediatrics.* 2002;110:865–872

Schmitt BD. *Pediatric Telephone Advice.* 3rd ed. Philadelphia, PA: Lippincott-Raven; 2004

Schmitt BD. *Pediatric Telephone Protocols: Office Version.* 11th ed. Elk Grove Village, IL: American Academy of Pediatrics; 2006

Informatics

Alan Tomines, MD

To make the best possible clinical decisions, physicians must have information about their patients' health that is current, accurate, complete, and reliable. This information should be available wherever and whenever it is needed. Where possible, the physician should be presented with information that will encourage an evidence-based approach to decision-making, and the decisions made should be communicated to other health care providers in a manner that is clear and error-free. The physician should also be able to receive feedback on the quality of care provided. Health care information technology (HIT) holds the promise of increasing access to patient health information, improving patient safety, reporting and measuring desired health outcomes, and making health care more efficient; at the same time, it holds the promise of decreasing health care expenditures. However, the implementation of HIT is not without challenges.

What Is Informatics?

Medical informatics is the science that deals with the appropriate application of information technology to the acquisition, storage, and use of health data, information, and knowledge. To apply information technology appropriately, specialists in informatics (referred to as *informaticians* or *informaticists*) focus first on improving the quality of data and the efficiency of workflow in the patient care setting; it is in this optimized environment that technology can then be applied. Medical informatics places great emphasis on non-technological considerations that can influence the successful implementation of health information systems, including information

science, cognitive psychology, project management, organizational and change management, health care policy, and ethics.

As a field, medical informatics can itself be subdivided into specific clinical domains, such as nursing, pharmacy, veterinary medicine, dentistry, and imaging. *Biomedical informatics* is a term of broader scope that encompasses medical informatics, bioinformatics (having the primary domain of genomics and bioengineering), and public health informatics. Outside of the United States, *health informatics* is the term more frequently used to convey the same breadth.

Basic Concepts

Although the terms *data, information,* and *knowledge* are sometimes used interchangeably, the concepts are distinct. **Data** are mere observations or facts (eg, hemoglobin equal to 9 g/dL). A structured collection of data is called a **database. Information** is data placed in meaningful context (eg, hemoglobin equal to 9 g/dL in a breastfed 3-month-old infant). **Knowledge** is the understanding of information and its completeness (eg, hemoglobin equal to 9 g/dL in a breastfed 3-month-old infant may represent a physiological nadir, but may also represent blood loss, increased destruction of red blood cells, or decreased production of red blood cells).

An **information system** is the sum of people, processes, and technology involved in the capture, organization, processing, storage, transmittal, and dissemination of data and information. Depending on the degree to which technology is applied, an information system may be automated or manual but is often both.

A **standard** is a rule that interested parties agree on to ensure uniformity and improve efficiency. For example, the *International Classification of Diseases, Ninth Revision, Clinical Modification* coding system is considered a standard. An **interface** is a special computer program that allows computers to exchange information. This is an important concept in health care because individual patients may be seen in multiple health care settings. If each setting has an information system but cannot exchange information with other information systems, it is difficult to obtain a complete electronic history for the patient. However, the ability to exchange information does not guarantee that the information can be used. **Interoperability** is the ability of information systems to exchange standardized information *and* use the information that has been exchanged. Interoperability is an important goal of **regional health information organizations**: geographically-related networks of interoperable health information systems that are focused on improving the safety, quality, and efficiency of health care by making all of the information about a patient accessible where and when it is needed.

Human-computer interaction is the study of the interactions between people and information technology. Of particular interest here are the ideas of **usefulness** (the degree to which a technology accomplishes its designated task) and **usability** (the ease with which people can control a specific technology).

The ease with which information systems can exchange electronic patient data should not belie the care that must be taken to protect that data. **Protected health information** (PHI) is any information about a patient (such as name or record number) that may be used to identify a patient. **Privacy** is the patient's right to keep this information a secret. **Confidentiality** is the assurance made by health care providers that private information will not be revealed. **Security** involves the policies and technologies that support the assurance of confidentiality. The Health Insurance Portability and Accountability Act defines the measures that must be taken to ensure that PHI is secure and made available only to individuals or organizations with authorization to access the information.

Electronic Health Information Systems

Although all electronic health information systems ultimately deal with managing some aspect of patient care, they are divided here into 4 coarse groupings: electronic records of patient care, administrative systems, ancillary clinical systems, and telemedicine.

Electronic Records of Patient Care

An **electronic medical record** (EMR) represents the clinical documentation and legal record of care provided to a patient by a health care provider or organization. An EMR can usually create and store traditional clinical documentation, such as progress notes and consultations. However, a full-fledged EMR represents more than an "electronic version" of the traditional paper-based record. Important components of an EMR include a clinical data repository (CDR), a clinical decision support system (CDSS), and computerized provider order entry. A **CDR** is a real-time database containing all of the clinically relevant patient data in an institution. A **CDSS** is a special

computer program that applies medical knowledge to clinical data to produce patient-specific recommendations, such as differential diagnoses or clinical recommendations. **Computerized provider order entry** is a special computer program that allows providers to write electronic orders that are directed to the appropriate clinical staff or ancillary department. Computerized provider order entry can decrease errors due to illegible handwriting, decrease delays in the receipt and execution of orders, allow for orders to be entered away from the care setting, and (in conjunction with CDSS) provide for error checking (eg, appropriate weight-based dosing, drug-drug interactions, or drug-allergy interactions).

An EMR generally operates within the functional boundary of a hospital or practice. However, information about a patient's health is not limited to traditional care settings. A **personal health record** (PHR) is a summary of an individual's health history, usually self-maintained, that contains information collected from encounters with different providers, medicolegal documents (eg, living wills or advance directives), and other health information that may be relevant to the patients (eg, regimens for nontraditional remedies or the results of home testing for blood pressure). The concept of a PHR is not new: Patients with multiple medical problems have maintained paper-based PHRs out of necessity—to have at least one reliable and portable source containing a complete medical history. The electronic PHR is an evolving entity. Early versions have consisted of scanned paper documents stored on CD-ROM or a removable hard drive. Newer versions are often Web-based.

The **electronic health record** (EHR) represents the next stage in the evolution of the EMR. An EHR will have all of the desired functionality of a full-fledged EMR, but will capture data from multiple different EMRs to provide the entire longitudinal history of the patient. In addition, the EHR will support functionality related to research and public health, such as identifying patient-appropriate clinical trials, mandatory reporting of notifiable disease, and provision of clinical data (stripped of patient-identifying information) to support clinical and public health research.

Administrative Systems

A **hospital information system** (HIS) encompasses all of the clinical and nonclinical information systems of an institution. An HIS may be a single integrated information system or it may represent multiple information systems that are connected with specially designed interfaces. Hospitals and large practices often have separate information systems to manage individual administrative functions, such as appointment scheduling, insurance eligibility, and billing and reimbursement. A **practice management system** is an information system designed to manage administrative tasks and is considered to be appropriate for small- and medium-sized practices.

Ancillary Clinical Systems

Information systems that support clinical ancillary services focus on a limited set of tasks and data. A **laboratory information system** manages the entry and reporting of laboratory results, often capturing electronic data directly from laboratory analyzers. A **pharmacy**

information system manages patients' prescription information, checks appropriate dosing and drug interactions, and tracks medical insurance. A related concept is e-prescribing (electronic prescribing or eRx), which uses technology to write and transmit prescriptions electronically to a pharmacy information system. A **picture archiving and communication system** (PACS) manages the storage and distribution of patients' electronic medical images; a **radiology information system** incorporates the functionality of a PACS, and also manages radiology service activities, such as reporting, scheduling, and billing. An **immunization information system** (IIS or immunization registry) is used to document and track patient vaccinations. An IIS can send reminder or recall notices, as appropriate, to physicians and parents when vaccinations are due or delinquent. Because these systems are usually maintained regionally by public health entities, they also collect reports on adverse vaccine events and provide summaries of regional vaccination prevalence. These systems are usually able to exchange data with capable EMRs.

Telemedicine

Telemedicine is not an information system, but a related concept of interest in informatics. Telemedicine is the use of information and communication technologies to deliver health care over a distance, often to support patient care in rural or underserved areas. There are many specialties within telemedicine, roughly corresponding to distinct medical specialties, such as teleradiology (the transmission of radiologic images electronically for interpretation) and telesurgery (the use of video and robotic technology to perform surgery). The use of e-mail and Web sites to communicate with patients is also a form of telemedicine.

Drivers

The key health care drivers for the adoption of HIT are the improvement of patient safety, the measurement of health care outcomes, the increased efficiency of workflow in the patient care setting, and the reduction of health care expenditures.

Patient safety, through the reduction of preventable errors, is the primary driver of information technology adoption in many health care organizations. In its report *To Err Is Human*, the Institute of Medicine (IOM) estimated that up to 98,000 US deaths annually are attributable to medical errors. Most errors were noted to be preventable and caused by systems and processes that increase, or fail to prevent, human errors. Computerized provider order entry is an example of information technology that has the potential to improve patient safety—by alerting the physician to errors before an order is submitted.

Changes in the health care marketplace are driving the **measurement of health care outcomes.** Pay-for-performance (relating reimbursement to measures of the quality of care provided) and "medical report cards" that permit comparison of health care plans and providers are 2 examples of market drivers. Information technology is critical to collecting and analyzing data to calculate these measures. In addition, a CDSS may improve health care outcomes through guideline adherence: by reminding physicians and patients about necessary care services that may have been overlooked.

Improvements in **efficiency** are another driver in the adoption of information technology. The automation of highly repetitive, data-intensive activities, such as billing or scheduling, is an example of where efficiency can be improved. However, introduction of information technology into a clinical setting without thorough consideration of workflow may actually decrease efficiency.

Health care spending is approaching 20% of the gross domestic product of the United States and is increasing at a rate nearly twice that of inflation. Information technology is considered to be a potential source of cost savings by reducing duplication of diagnostic studies and decreasing the time spent on administrative tasks. In addition, in the IOM report *Crossing the Quality Chasm*, the use of e-mail was touted as a method for meeting the needs of patients more quickly, and at lower cost than a traditional visit.

Challenges

Despite the significant health care drivers for adopting HIT, there are a number of challenges that prevent the easy implementation of systems.

Appropriate concerns exist about breaches of patient **privacy** when data are stored electronically. Although health information systems often employ sophisticated technical barriers to protect patient data, it is often the case that data breaches are the result of people failing to adhere to policy safeguards. Educating providers and other users of patient data is critical to guaranteeing patient confidentiality.

The **cost** of implementing health information systems can be prohibitive for some practices. The Certification Commission for Healthcare Information Technology provides criteria to evaluate EHRs, helping reduce uncertainty about the functionality of a product.

Change management is an important element to consider when implementing an information system. Introduction of technology inevitably results in changes in the workflow of physicians and nurses and may lead to repurposing of administrative staff. Consequently, resistance to change should be anticipated, and strategies must be developed to mitigate problems.

The **usability** of a technology is important to its acceptance. It is critical to involve physicians and other health care providers in the evaluation and testing of an information system. Effects of technology on the patient-physician interaction must also be considered.

Pediatric Considerations

Although pediatric patients represent approximately one quarter of the US population, pediatric features are often underdeveloped in electronic health information systems. When considering these systems for pediatric settings, particular attention should be focused on the highly specific data, task, and policy needs of pediatric practice.

The presence of functionality to support clinical tasks that are generally, if not uniquely, pediatric should always be examined. Immunization management, including the ability to assess a patient's status or to exchange data with an immunization information system, is highly desirable. Weight-based dosing and the tracking of growth parameters are other functions that are often overlooked. Age-specific documentation and educational materials can be well-managed electronically.

The data and terminology of an information system should suit the highly specific needs of pediatric practice. Units of measure should reflect the requisite data precision. For example, the age of a patient in hours (rather than years, months, or even days) and weight in grams is critical to appropriate care in the neonatal period. Laboratory values should be accompanied by age-appropriate normal ranges. Patient identification must account for the frequent changes in names and numerical identifiers that may occur in infancy or during change of custody. Pediatric terminology, such as developmental milestones, type of cry, or characterization of stool, are often overlooked in information systems designed for adults.

Pediatric policy issues should also be reflected in the design of the information system. Authorization for the child (or the child's parents, guardians, or other legal authority) to view all, none, or parts of a child's medical record should be enforced electronically as it would be for the paper medical record. Likewise, secondary use of patient data for public health, research, or commercial purposes should be allowed or restricted as appropriate.

Pediatricians should be actively involved in the acquisition and development of information technology to ensure that child-specific data and policy needs are addressed. Pediatricians should also be involved in national policy initiatives to ensure that health information systems are certified for pediatric use.

CASE RESOLUTION

In the case history at the beginning of this chapter, the pediatrician speaks with the head of the informatics committee. The pediatrician learns that she has been asked to participate because of her understanding of physician workflow in the office setting and to advocate for the highly specific data needs and policies associated with the pediatric population. Her expertise will help to identify issues that, if addressed, may contribute to successful acceptance of the information system by pediatricians and other physicians.

Selected References

American Academy of Pediatrics Task Force on Medical Informatics. Special requirements for electronic medical record systems in pediatrics. *Pediatrics.* 2001;108:513–515

Gerstle RS, Task Force on Medical Informatics. E-mail communication between pediatricians and their patients. *Pediatrics.* 2004;114:317–321

Kaushal R, Barker KN, Bates DW. How can information technology improve patient safety and reduce medication errors in children's health care? *Arch Pediatr Adolesc Med.* 2001;155:1002–1007

Kemper AR, Uren RL, Clark SJ. Adoption of electronic health records in primary care pediatric practices. *Pediatrics.* 2006;118:e20–e24

Nielsen J. Usability 101: introduction to usability. www.useit.com/alertbox/20030825.html. Accessed December 24, 2006

Shekelle PG, Morton SC, Keeler EB. *Costs and Benefits of Healthcare Information Technology. Evidence Report/Technology Assessment No. 132.* Rockville, MD: Agency for Healthcare Research and Quality; 2006. AHRQ publication 06-E006

Committee on Quality of Health Care in America, Institute of Medicine. *To Err Is Human: Building a Safer Health System.* Kohn LT, Corrigan JM, Donaldson MS, eds. Washington, DC: The National Academies Press; 2000

Shiffman RN, Spooner SA, Kwiatkowski K, Brennan PF. Information technology for children's health and health care. *J Am Med Inform Assoc.* 2000;8:546–550

Spooner SA, Council on Clinical Information Technology. Special requirements for electronic health record systems in pediatrics. *Pediatrics.* 2007;119:631–636

Yasnoff WA, O'Carroll PW, Koo D, Linkins RW, Kilbourne EM. Public health informatics: improving and transforming public health in the information age. *J Public Health Manag Pract.* 2000;6:67–75

Counseling Families About Internet Use

Alan Tomines, MD

CASE STUDY

A 16-year-old girl is accompanied by her mother for a routine visit. The girl is doing well in school, is active in team sports, and has a small circle of friends that are well-known to her mother. The mother describes no new problems at home, nor any changes in behavior, except that she is concerned that her daughter "spends too much time on the computer."

Questions
1. What is the Internet?
2. What are the commonly used Internet services?
3. What are the benefits and risks of the Internet?
4. What strategies may be used to make the Internet safer to use?
5. What signs may indicate that an adolescent is engaging in risky behaviors on the Internet?

The Internet is a worldwide system of interconnected computer networks. At its inception, it was the exclusive domain of the military and academia; today, the Internet is a public gateway to electronic information, communication, and commercial services. The Internet has profoundly changed the way that we learn, work, play, and interact with others. So pervasive is its influence that it has become an integral part of the education and socialization of children—a point of concern for parents who might not be Internet-savvy, or who simply need guidance regarding appropriate Internet use. The impact of the Internet on childhood development is not well studied, nor is its use characterized by developmental milestones. Nevertheless, physicians can provide pragmatic counsel that focuses on Internet benefits and risks, strategies for safer use, and assessing online behavior in adolescents. Physicians should also be prepared to discuss health information that families find on the Internet.

Background

The Internet began in the 1960s as ARPANET (Advanced Research Projects Agency Network): a US Department of Defense project to share government-funded, university-based computer resources across a reliable communications network. Through the 1970s, ARPANET found acceptance with academics and researchers as a conduit for scientific information exchange due in large part to **e-mail** (electronic mail), a technology for sending and receiving messages. However, the network remained largely unknown outside the scientific community.

By 1983 activity on ARPANET had grown beyond its original scope, prompting fundamental changes in its operation and governance, including an update in the technology for transmitting and receiving data; a splitting off of its military components to a separate network, a transition from government-based control to private interests, and a reversal in the long-standing prohibition against commerce. The resulting network, renamed the *Internet,* extended its reach into the business sector and to international researchers but remained relatively inaccessible to the general public.

During the early 1990s, the European Organization for Nuclear Research (CERN) developed protocols to facilitate the sharing of physics research data. These protocols allowed computer files, on different computers and having different formats (such as text and images), to be shared as single documents that could be viewed using a special computer program (browser). This system of linked documents was collectively dubbed the *World Wide Web* (WWW, or simply the Web), with collections of documents referred to as *Web pages* or *Web sites.* In 1993 CERN made their work freely available, leading to the rapid proliferation of commercial and individual Web sites.

Today the most commonly used Internet services are e-mail and the Web. A person actively using an Internet service is said to be **online.** Use of the Web is sometimes referred to as *surfing the Web* or *surfing the Net,* and is facilitated by the use of **search engines** (programs that use keywords or topics to find related documents, images, Web sites, or other services on the Internet). Most people access Internet services using a personal computer or laptop computer, although the use of PDAs and cellular phones for Internet access is increasing. No matter what technology is used, access is usually provided by an **Internet service provider** or ISP (a company that has an Internet connection that it shares with consumers on a subscription basis).

Due to their popularity in the pediatric age group, there are a few specialized Internet services of which physicians should take special note. Web logs (or **blogs**) are Web-based journals. Like a traditional paper-based diary, a blog can be used to express activities, thoughts, or feelings. Blogs may be public (available for anyone to read) or private (having restricted access); the owner of a blog may allow readers to add comments to the blog. **Social networking** Web sites, such as MySpace and Facebook, are similar in content to blogs, with the added dimension that users are encouraged to create a network of online friends by establishing links to other users' Web pages. Blogs and social networking Web sites are examples of **asynchronous** services (the communication between users does not have to take place in real time) whose content may be moderated by the owner of the service to ensure that content is appropriate. In contrast, **chat rooms** are Internet venues that permit the real-time exchange of text messages between multiple simultaneous participants. **Instant messaging** is similar to a chat room, although it is generally limited to one-on-one exchanges of real-time messages. Although sometimes referred to as *text messaging,* instant messaging is a more inclusive term that better reflects the immediacy of interaction and expansion of content to include images and multimedia. Instant messaging is a popular premium service with cellular phone subscriptions, making it possible to have an online presence at all times without a computer. Adolescents have shown an increasing preference for instant messaging—estimated to be used by one-third of all teens.

Internet Benefits and Access

Physicians should be able to identify benefits of Internet use. The Internet provides access to a wealth of educational resources and cultural experiences through the use of text, images, and multimedia (eg, streaming audio and video files). Access to these resources allows children to exercise their reading, writing, information-seeking, and technology skills. The Internet also provides the opportunity to exchange messages frequently with family and friends. In addition, children with common interests, or even common medical conditions, can use e-mail, chat, blogs, or social networking to communicate, commiserate, and encourage.

Physicians may also take a role in reducing disparities to Internet access. Internet use and access is correlated with socioeconomic status. While nearly 90% of adolescents in the United States are regularly online, millions do not have access. Pediatricians may help families gain access to the Internet by identifying institutions that provide safe online environments, such as libraries, community centers, and schools. In addition, Internet-based health interventions are increasingly being studied as a supplement to traditional health care delivery; addressing disparities to Internet access may increase opportunities for these interventions, particularly in underserved communities.

Physicians should also be aware that children with disabilities may have a difficult time using the Internet without **assistive technology** (hardware or software designed to improve the accessibility of computers). Visually impaired or blind children may be aided by the use of special software, including screen magnifiers, Braille embossers, or screen readers (software that uses a computer-generated voice to read e-mail and Web pages); however, it is important to note that many Web sites are not developed to be compatible with screen readers. Hearing-impaired or deaf children may be aided by ensuring that their computers are set to provide visual cues rather than audio prompts; this functionality is usually built into the operating system of a computer. Children with mobility or dexterity challenges may find it difficult to use a traditional keyboard and mouse; alternative keyboards and manual pointing devices, as well as computer touch screens, should be investigated. Pointing devices that employ sound or infrared beams are also available when manual control is not possible.

Internet Threats

While the Internet has many benefits, being online does entail some risks. To understand these risks, it is helpful to understand many of the Internet's neutral properties. The Internet is **interactive:** unlike traditional media, such as newspapers, radio, and television, the Internet user may have real-time interactions with a person or a sophisticated computer program. The Internet has **few restrictions:** anyone can put almost anything on the Internet, without regard to credibility or appropriateness. The Internet is **public and permanent:** although information on a Web site may be removed, it is possible for anyone that visits a Web site to make an electronic copy of what is there. Many Web sites are also archived historically (www.archive.org) and remain publicly retrievable long after they seem to be gone. The Internet is **anonymous:** people are not necessarily who they represent themselves to be. These Internet properties do not encourage, but do enable, the most common threats, which include strangers/predators, interpersonal victimization, and pornography, among others (including gaming, gambling, and shopping).

Strangers/predators are the greatest concern of parents. More than one-half of children online have shared personal information about themselves (including name, address, or phone number) with a stranger. Nearly one-third of children online have "friends" that they have never met in person. Approximately three-fifths of online adolescents have received an instant message or e-mail from a stranger.

Online interpersonal victimization is the receipt of unwanted harassment or sexual attention over the Internet. One fifth of children have reported being victimized, and a high risk factor was talking about sex with someone online. **Cyberbullying** is a specific type of online interpersonal victimization involving the exchange of messages or images that are harmful or threatening. Cyberbullying is believed to be as prevalent online as traditional in-person bullying.

More than 40% of children reported having been exposed to pornography online, and nearly two-thirds of them described this exposure as unwanted. In adolescents between the ages 15 to 17, more than 70% reported accidentally being exposed to online pornography. A high risk factor for exposure to pornography was the downloading of images.

Strategies for Safer Use

The American Academy of Pediatrics (AAP) has provided age-specific guidance for a safer Internet experience: for children through age 14, parents should be actively involved with all online activities, establish rules for safe online behavior, and use Internet safety tools; by age 15, parents may permit Internet access without restriction, but should continue to reinforce rules.

Parents may be actively involved by educating themselves about the Internet and their children's Internet access, sharing time with their children online, and advocating for a safer Internet environment. Parental education can begin with Web-based resources for Internet safety, such as NetSmartz Workshop (www.netsmartz.org) and iKeepSafe.org (http://ikeepsafe.org). Classes may also be available through libraries, community centers, or the local Parent-Teacher Association. Parents should be aware of other venues where their children may access the Internet, such as schools, libraries, and friends' homes, and they should find out what Internet safety policies and technologies have been instituted in these environments.

By sharing time online, parents can promote and model responsible Internet behaviors. Parents should talk about what they see together on the Internet, and encourage children to share what they have experienced when online alone, whether good or bad. Placing the computer in a public location in the home will encourage the idea that the Internet is a shared experience; however, parents should be aware that laptops and cellular telephones can permit covert Internet access. Children should be provided with a separate account to access the Internet, which their parents can also access. Having a separate account will allow parents to directly restrict the software and content that children can access and periodically review Web sites visited and e-mails. Parents should understand that some children may be savvy enough to erase their Web browsing history; absence of a Web browsing history may be a cause for suspicion.

Parents should act as advocates for their children's Internet experience. When a child encounters inappropriate Internet content, or messages that are hurtful or distressing, parents should alert their ISP, as well as the owner of the Web site where the content or messages were discovered. Parents should also contact the appropriate legal authorities and the National Center for Missing and Exploited Children (www.missingkids.com). Commercial Web sites that collect personal information from children younger than 13 are required to follow the Children's Online Privacy Protection Act of 1998, which is enforced by the Federal Trade Commission. According to this law, Internet Web site operators must post their policy indicating what personal information is collected, how that information will be used, and if that information will be shared with a third party. Parents must consent to the collection and use of personal information, and may revoke this consent at any time.

Parents should set and enforce house rules for Internet use. Children should not communicate with nor plan to meet strangers known only to them through the Internet, nor should they respond to unsolicited messages, or any other messages that make them feel uncomfortable. Children should not share personal information or pictures with others on the Internet, nor should they download files from the Internet. Children should be encouraged to be good citizens, including not doing anything that may be hurtful to others or plagiarizing information that they find freely on the Internet. For older children, safety pledges can be used as formal agreements of acceptable use. Time limits should be set and strictly enforced. The AAP recommends not more than 2 hours of total screen time (computer and television) for children older than 2. Any activities that are not allowed should be specifically identified.

Even with house rules in place, physicians should recommend the use of Internet safety tools to protect against inappropriate use and external threats. Although not directly targeted at children, parents should be aware of software to protect against **malware.** Malware generally includes viruses and worms (software programs that can corrupt the information saved on a computer), spyware (software that tracks Internet activity and sends this information to another person), and pop-ups (a new browser window that may contain marketing or other undesired content). Viruses and worms are generally downloaded as attachments in e-mail, whereas spyware and pop-ups are introduced by surfing the Web. Parents should also protect against **spam** (unsolicited e-mail), which may contain undesired content or solicitations.

Filters are special computer programs that allow acceptable Internet content to be presented and block content deemed to be inappropriate. Filtering may use one or more of the following methods: "black lists" of Web sites that are specifically blocked; "white lists" of Web sites that are specifically permitted; the blocking of specific words or terms; and the nascent technology of blocking suspicious image content. Filters are neither perfectly specific nor perfectly sensitive and may require parental adjustment to achieve an acceptable level of filtering. Parents may contact their ISP to enable filtering of content before it enters the home **(server-side filtering).** If server-side filtering is too restrictive for some members in the household, or not restrictive enough for others, parents may acquire filtering software that is installed directly on computers in the home **(client-side filtering).** Client-side filters work with standard Web browsers, although special child-oriented Web browsers may be acquired that have client-side filtering built in.

Monitoring software automates parental tracking of Internet usage by creating a reviewable record of Web sites and images viewed, messages sent and received, and even individual keystrokes entered. The potential benefits of monitoring software should be weighed against the invasiveness to the privacy of the child. Monitoring software often includes **time-limiting software,** which can be set to allow Internet access only during certain hours of the day and can be set to disable access to the Internet after a specified amount of time has elapsed.

Adolescents on the Internet

As with other aspects of their lives, adolescents should feel that they can discuss what they see on the Internet with their parents without imperiling their access to the Internet. Most adolescents have access to the Internet from home, and nearly all have access to the Internet at school or at a friend's house. Parents should be aware that adolescents who have restrictive Internet rules at home are more likely to attempt Internet access outside the home, where their activity may be more difficult to monitor.

Adolescents may engage in risky online behaviors, including communicating with and planning to meet in person strangers met online. From a review of past cases, the Federal Bureau of Investigation has identified specific behaviors that may indicate a child is engaging in risky online behaviors, including spending several hours online, especially at night; having pornographic images on the computer; turning the monitor off, or quickly changing the screen when a parent enters the room; and using unrecognized usernames or accounts. Other non-Internet behaviors that should arouse suspicion include phone calls from unknown adults, outgoing calls to unrecognized phone numbers, gifts or packages received, or unexplained credit card activity.

The physician should consider addressing online activities in the adolescent psychosocial review of systems. Asking adolescents about online activities may unveil risky online behaviors or provide an opportunity to discuss concerns about their health and well-being. Nearly one-third of adolescents have searched the Internet for health information, most often related to sex and sexually transmitted infections, nutrition, and exercise and fitness. Additionally, adolescent girls also search for information on physical abuse, sexual abuse, and dating violence. Online activities worthy of inquiry include health topics searched for on the Internet; maintenance of a social networking (such as MySpace) page; sharing personal information on the Internet; communicating with strangers; meeting people known only via the Internet; and engaging in, or being a victim of, cyberbullying. Adolescents should also be reminded that the Internet is not private, and that colleges and employers may discover information about the adolescent from what adolescents believed to be private social networking pages.

Health Information on the Internet

Patients regard physicians as the preferred and most trusted source for health information; however, patients do seek out health information on the Internet prior to, or sometimes in lieu of, consulting with their physician. It is important to remind families that health information on the Internet may be outdated, incomplete, incorrect, intentionally misleading, or easily misinterpreted. When patients have questions about information that they find on the Internet, physicians should take care not to disregard the information outright. Inquiries should be viewed as opportunities to address points of concern. Most often, patients simply want their physician's opinion of the information, as opposed to a specific treatment.

Providing patients with Web sites that provide reliable information can improve the quality of information seen and reduce the overwhelming quantity of information that parents must sort through. Physicians may help by identifying evidence-based health information resources on the Internet, such as the AAP (www.aap.

org), the National Library of Medicine's MEDLINEPlus (www.medlineplus.gov), and the US Department of Health and Human Services Healthfinder (www.healthfinder.gov). Specialists should be prepared to identify online information sources and support groups, particularly for rare, chronic, or debilitating conditions.

CASE RESOLUTION

In the case history at the beginning of this chapter, the pediatrician finds out that the girl uses the computer for 1 to 2 hours every afternoon to complete her homework assignments and is on the Internet for 2 to 3 hours every evening surfing the Web and checking her MySpace page. The pediatrician advises the girl that, for safety reasons, personal information should never be shared over the Internet, adding that colleges and employers often research prospective candidates using the Internet. With the mother and daughter, the pediatrician discusses the option to have a parent-child contract that clearly establishes the rules for acceptable Internet use in and out of the home, including appropriate time limits. The pediatrician also directs the mother to Internet-based resources for safeguarding the home environment, and to an Internet for beginner's workshop at the local library.

Selected References

Ahmad F, Hudak PL, Bercovitz K, Hollenberg E, Levinson W. Are physicians ready for patients with Internet-based health information? *J Med Internet Res.* 2006;8:e22

Diaz JA, Griffith RA, Ng JJ, Reinert SE, Friedmann PD, Moulton AW. Patients' use of the Internet for medical information. *J Gen Intern Med.* 2002;17:180–185

Federal Bureau of Investigation. *A Parent's Guide to Internet Safety.* www.fbi.gov/publications/pguide/pguidee.htm. Accessed December 24, 2006

Hesse BW, Nelson DE, Kreps GL, et al. Trust and sources of health information: the impact of the Internet and its implications for health care providers: findings from the first Health Information National Trends Survey. *Arch Intern Med.* 2005;165:2618–2624

Lazarus W, Lipper L. *Parents' Guide to the Information Superhighway.* Santa Monica, CA, and Washington, DC: The Children's Partnership; 1998

Lenhart A, Madden M, Hitlin P. Youth are leading the transition to a fully wired and mobile nation. Pew Internet & American Life Project. July 27, 2005. www.pewinternet.org/pdfs/PIP_Teens_Tech_July2005web.pdf. Accessed October 12, 2007

Mandl KD, Feit S, Pena BM, Kohane IS. Growth and determinants of access in patient e-mail and Internet use. *Arch Pediatr Adolesc Med.* 2000;154:508–511

McClung HJ, Murray RD, Heitlinger LA. The Internet as a source for current patient information. *Pediatrics.* 1998;101:e2

Murray E, Lo B, Pollack L, et al. The impact of health information on the Internet on the physician-patient relationship: patient perceptions. *Arch Intern Med.* 2003;163:1727–1734

Sim NZ, Kitteringham L, Spitz L, et al. Information on the World Wide Web—how useful is it for parents? *J Pediatr Surg.* 2007;42:305–312

US Department of Education. *Parents Guide to the Internet.* www.ed.gov/pubs/parents/internet/index.html. Accessed September 26, 2007

Wolak J, Mitchell K, Finkelhor D. Unwanted and wanted exposure to online pornography in a national sample of youth Internet users. *Pediatrics.* 2007;119:247–257

Principles of Pediatric Therapeutics

Elizabeth A. Edgerton, MD, MPH

CASE STUDY

An 18-month-old girl who has had a cough, runny nose, and fever for 2 days is brought to your clinic for evaluation. The previous night she awoke from sleep crying and pulling at her ear. The patient has no other symptoms. Her mother states she has had previous ear infections, the most recent occurred 2 months ago. The last time she took amoxicillin she broke out in hives. Otherwise the patient has no significant medical history.

On physical examination, the patient is febrile to 102°F (38.9°C) and has yellow rhinorrhea. The ear examination reveals a red, bulging, nonmobile tympanic membrane in one ear, while the other ear appears normal. The remainder of the examination is benign.

Questions

1. What are the current practice guidelines for antibiotic treatment of otitis media? How does treatment change with the age and symptoms of the patient?
2. How does the previous reaction to a medication influence the antibiotic choice?
3. How do factors such as child care, work, and family plans affect the choice of medication?
4. What resources are available to obtain information on therapeutic effectiveness, costs, side effects, and drug-drug interactions?

The use of prescription and over-the-counter (OTC) medications is common in pediatrics. The 2004 National Ambulatory Medical Survey reported that 68% of office visits to a pediatrician had a medication prescribed. Phone surveys to families with children reported that more than 50% of all 3-year-old children had taken some OTC medication within the last 30 days. What is concerning is that only one-third of drugs used to treat pediatric patients have adequately been studied in the populations in which they are being used and have appropriate labeling information. This does not mean that the other two-thirds of medications are unsafe for children but that their use in children is extrapolated from adult studies. The consequences of not fully studying the clinical effectiveness and safety profile of therapeutics can lead to potentially harmful outcomes. Examples include aplastic anemia with chloramphenicol use, dental staining with tetracycline, and kernicterus with sulfonamide use in neonates. Differences in pharmacokinetics among infants, children, and adolescents can produce significant differences in drug efficacy and toxicity.

Since 1962 the US Food and Drug Administration (FDA) has required drugs to be proven safe and effective before they can be marketed. The FDA can only regulate the safety, effectiveness, and labeling of medication and is not authorized to regulate a physician's use of a medication. When data are not sufficient for a specific population or age group, it will be specified in the product labeling that use in that population has not been established. Using a medication for a condition or specific population not specified by the product insert is referred to as **off-label prescribing**. Pediatricians commonly prescribe off-label because so few well-studied medications are available for children. They rely on the published literature, adult studies, and knowledge of pediatric physiology and pharmacokinetics for prescribing. While off-label prescribing is not illegal, it does put children at greater risk of unexpected adverse reactions as well as lack of optimal treatments. The FDA has been mandated by Congress to increase the level of pediatric research prior to approval, during the post-marketing phases. Even with increased regulation, implementation of pediatric clinical trials faces critical issues such as the ethics of parental consent, multiple age groups to be tested, and the unknown long-term effects in a developing child.

Principles of Therapeutics

A drug or therapeutic can be defined as any substance that is ingested, absorbed, or injected that alters the body's function. This includes OTC medications, homeopathic substances, illicit substances, and prescription drugs. Each drug has a different safety profile and level of regulation depending on its category. The most regulated and standardized drugs are those requiring a prescription. Homeopathic substances often lack any standardization, safety testing, and regulation, and illicit drugs such as heroin or cocaine receive no quality testing. Choosing the most appropriate therapeutic is a complex process involving a number of factors: patient characteristics, disease epidemiology, safety profile, patient compliance, and cost-effectiveness (Box 9-1).

Box 9-1. Factors in Choosing the Appropriate Therapeutic	
Patient Characteristics	*Patient Compliance*
Age	Taste
Medical history	Purpose of treatment
Allergies	Storage
Use of other medications	Side effects
Diagnosis	*Cost-effectiveness*
Epidemiology	Drug availability
Age-specific factors	Formulary restrictions
Safety Profile	
Therapeutic Index	
Black box warning	

Patient Characteristics

Infants' and children's organs are growing and maturing, which can affect how a medication is absorbed, distributed, and excreted. Neonates have immature liver and kidney function compared with older children and adults. For example, similar microgram per kilogram doses of fentanyl can result in a 2- to 3-fold higher plasma concentration in the neonate compared with an adult. Knowledge of the **age** of the patient is critical to account for developmental pharmacokinetic differences for age-appropriate as well as weight-based dosing.

The choice of an appropriate therapeutic is influenced by a patient **medical history.** Depending on the type of clinical conditions or surgeries a patient has, the absorption, metabolism, or clinical effectiveness of the therapeutic may be altered. Children with short bowel syndrome can potentially have difficulty absorbing oral medications depending on which portion of the bowel was removed. Children with mental retardation who are given central nervous system–altering medications can be difficult to monitor for changes in mental status seen with systemic infection. In addition, children with glucose-6-phosphate dehydrogenase (G6PD) deficiency can suffer from drug-induced hemolytic anemia when given certain drugs such as sulfonamides. Malnourished children are at a greater risk for drug toxicity because low serum albumin levels decrease the amount of bound drug and result in increased levels of unbound drug in circulation. While not an exhaustive list of medical conditions that can alter medication delivery, these demonstrate the need to consider underlying medical conditions in choosing the most appropriate therapeutic.

Before prescribing any medication, physicians need to ask patients and their families about any previous reactions to drugs and obtain detailed information about the symptoms and class of medications involved in these reactions. **Drug allergies** are those reactions that have an immunologic basis. Of the 4 types of immune mechanisms associated with drug allergies, immunoglobulin E–mediated reactions are of greatest concern because they can result in anaphylaxis, a life-threatening condition. **Adverse reactions** can be idiosyncratic or non–immune-mediated. A **side effect** is an expected but undesirable consequence of taking the medication. Families often attribute any symptom the patient suffered while taking the medication to a drug allergy. It is therefore important to know which side effects are associated with a medication to determine whether an allergy is present. Any medication that has been associated with an allergic reaction (eg, skin eruptions, swelling, urticaria, or respiratory difficulty) should not be used again without consulting a specialist.

Finally, knowing what other medications a patient is taking can affect the choice of therapeutic. The mechanism of metabolism of one drug can affect the metabolism of another. Drug metabolism is divided into 2 types: phase I reactions include oxidation, reduction, and hydrolysis; phase II reactions involve adding subgroups to a drug. Other drugs can affect reactions during either phase. For example, the enzyme activity of the P-450 system involved in oxidation can be induced or inhibited depending on the other medications being taken, resulting in an altered rate of metabolism. Common drugs used in pediatrics that inhibit the P-450 system include cimetidine and erythromycin, while phenobarbital and phenytoin induce the system. Drug interactions are not a contraindication to the use of a therapeutic, but the dose and serum levels may need to be closely monitored. Referencing the package insert, the *Physicians' Desk Reference (PDR),* or a pharmacist can aid in determining potential drug-to-drug interactions.

Diagnosis

Choosing the appropriate medication depends on understanding the condition being treated as well as the epidemiology of the disease for a specific age group. Etiologies of pneumonia for an infant, child, and adolescent can be completely different, thus requiring a different type of antibiotic. Even when a potential organism is identified, the profile of the medication needs to be reviewed. For a patient with group A streptococcal pharyngitis, a gram-positive organism, penicillin G, penicillin V, erythromycin, or a first-generation cephalosporin is an acceptable choice. Although tetracycline and sulfonamides can be effective in treating patients with gram-positive infections, tetracycline is contraindicated in young children, and sulfonamides do not eradicate group A streptococcal infection. Treatment duration can also vary depending on the age of the patient. An adult with a simple urinary tract infection may receive only a 1- to 3-day course of treatment, while a child may receive 7 to 10 days of treatment because of the high recurrence of infection that has been observed with a shorter duration of treatment.

Safety Profile

The safety profile of a medication is the balance between its benefits and its potential risks. The risks can be dependent on the duration of treatment, dose, or interactions with other medications. Using the therapeutic index is one way to quantify the risk associated with a specific dose. The therapeutic index is the difference between the dose that provides a desired effect and the dose that provides an undesired effect. For example, a medication with a wide therapeutic index is one in which a desired effect is achieved with a dose much lower than that required to produce a toxic effect. In general, a medication with a wide therapeutic index, such as acetaminophen, is considered safer than a medication with a narrow therapeutic index. The higher the morbidity and mortality associated with a condition the smaller the accepted therapeutic index can be. Food-drug interactions and drug-drug interactions are other risks that can be anticipated. These are best delineated in pharmacologic references. Many handheld clinical decision tools have programs to specifically review these risks. There are also risks that are independent of the dose of the therapeutic called idiosyncratic effects. These are unexpected and usually unavoidable risks associated with the medication.

In the United States, a **black box warning,** also known as a **black label warning,** is a type of warning that appears on prescription drugs that may cause serious adverse effects. Named for the black border that usually surrounds the text of the warning, it means that medical studies indicate that the drug carries a significant risk of serious or even life-threatening adverse effects. The FDA can require a pharmaceutical company to place a black box warning on the labeling of a prescription drug or in literature describing it. It is the strongest warning that the FDA requires. A list of the pediatric medications with a black label warning can be found at www.fda.gov. This warning does not preclude the use of the medication, but requires the physician and family to evaluate the risks and benefits of its use.

Patient Adherence

Patient adherence is dependent on the convenience of administering and taking the medication, the patient's and caregiver's comprehension of the medication's purpose, and the discomfort caused by side effects. Because children are dependent on their caregivers to administer medications, it is crucial that caregivers know why the drug has been prescribed, how it should be dispensed, and why it must be given for a specific length of time. For a child with tinea capitis, a fungal infection of the scalp and hair follicles, parents may think that a topical antifungal is sufficient to treat the infection. Explaining the difference of a fungal skin infection (tinea corpus) versus the fungal scalp infection can facilitate adherence with the treatment. To eliminate the fungal infection in the hair follicles, a systemic medication is needed. Furthermore, because of the slow growing cycle of both the fungus and the hair, patients need to take the medicine for up to 6 weeks. To ensure accurate dosing, a staff member should demonstrate how to dispense the medication and then ask the parent to repeat the process. Such a simple intervention can make an important difference in obtaining adherence and influence the effectiveness of the therapeutic.

The taste and texture of a medication are also important considerations in pediatrics. Children may not be able to understand the importance of taking a medication and refuse to take it because they don't like the taste. Physicians should be familiar with the taste and consistency of medication and be prepared to find alternatives. Prednisone is a commonly used medication for the treatment of acute asthma. It comes in both a pill and suspension form. For children requiring a suspension, a vast difference exists in taste depending on the preparation prescribed. Children are known to vomit the less palatable version. Knowing in advance what is acceptable to children may prevent complications with noncompliance.

Cost-effectiveness

Cost-effectiveness is defined as the best outcome per unit cost. The outcome is the treatment of a condition or alleviation of a symptom; the cost includes the price of the medication and the time spent by the physician and family. For instance, a specific medication may cost less but be less effective, so that in the long run it costs more to the patient in return visits to the doctor. Many physicians practice in settings where the pharmacy has a set inventory or formulary of medications, limiting the selection of medications for each condition. Thus the physician's choice of a cost-effective drug might depend on which are available in the formulary. From the patient perspective, many families may have limited or no health insurance coverage and may have to incur the total cost of a medication. The cost of an antibiotic for a course of otitis media can differ by 10-fold depending on the medication prescribed. Thus an appropriate drug of choice is influenced by the out-of-pocket cost to the family. The perceived cost-effectiveness of a therapeutic is different for each situation and depends on the external factors affecting the physician and the family.

Drug Dosing

Most medications used in the adult population are based on a standard dose for an individual regardless of age or body size. In pediatrics, a patient's size and metabolism vary with age such that dosing is usually based on weight or body surface area. When drug dosing is determined by weight, it represents a proportion of the adult dose; when a child reaches adult weight, the dosing is changed to a standard dose. This usually occurs when the patient approaches 40 to 50 kg. Body surface area is more commonly used for drugs with a narrow therapeutic index, such as chemotherapy medications.

Once a drug is identified, the appropriate dosing schedule must be determined. Dosing guidelines can be presented as a total dose per 24 hours or an amount per dose. Usually a range is given per unit weight, and then the physician must determine the amount of medication based on the concentration of therapeutic agent. An example for dosing acetaminophen for a 1-year-old child is given in **Box 9-2.**

Medication Errors and Adverse Drug Events

Increasing data demonstrate that a significant number of errors can occur in the delivery of medications. Pediatric patients are at greater risk because most of the dosing needs to be calculated based on weight or surface area, and pharmacists may need to prepare solutions or suspensions rather than use manufacturer-produced pills. These medication errors can lead to potential or actual adverse drug events. It is estimated that 5 medication errors occur per 100 dispensed medications, of which 0.21 per 100 go onto non-preventable

---

Box 9-2. Dosing

A 1-year-old is suffering from a fever and the family wants to know how much acetaminophen to give her. She weighs 11.2 kg. The recommended dose of acetaminophen is 10 to 15 mg/kg every 4 to 6 hours. Acetaminophen drops are sold in a concentration of 80 mg/0.8 mL or as a suspension with the concentration of 160 mg/5 mL.

1. Determine the amount of medication needed by multiplying the weight of the child by the recommended dose.

$$11.2 \text{ kg} \times 10 \text{ mg/kg} = 112 \text{ mg acetaminophen}$$

2. Determine the volume of medication based on the concentration of acetaminophen to be used. Either the dropper or the suspension can be used.

Dosing volume =
(amount of medication) ÷ (concentration of medication)

Dropper

$$\begin{aligned} \text{Dosing volume} &= 112 \text{ mg} \div 80 \text{ mg/0.8 mL} \\ &= (112 \times 0.8)/80 \\ &= 1.12 \text{ mL} \end{aligned}$$

(This can be rounded to 1.2 mL because the lower range of 10 mg/kg was used to calculate the dose.)

Suspension

$$\begin{aligned} \text{Dosing volume} &= 112 \text{ mg} \div 160 \text{ mg/5mL} \\ &= (112 \times 5)/160 \\ &= 3.5 \text{ mL} \end{aligned}$$

The family can be instructed to give their daughter either 1.2 mL using the drops or 3.5 mL of the suspension of acetaminophen orally every 4 to 6 hours as needed for fever.

---

adverse drug events. More than half of these errors occur during the prescribing stage, the phase where the medication dose is calculated. Referencing a pediatric drug manual and consulting a pharmacist can be used as steps to reduce medication errors. Many health care systems are developing computerized physician order entry, which provides another layer of error prevention.

Therapeutic References

Various resources provide information on drug uses, dosing, side effects, and costs. The *PDR* is a comprehensive listing of FDA-approved prescription and commonly used OTC drugs that provides a description of the drug, pharmacology, indications and contraindications, adverse reactions, drug interactions, and manufacturer name. The *Medical Letter* is a periodical that reviews drugs, citing current research on risks and benefits as well as cost comparisons of newly released drugs with those already approved for similar indications. Pocket manuals that are specific to pediatrics include the *Pediatric Dosage Handbook* and *Harriet Lane Handbook*. Both of these references provide pediatric-specific dosing guidelines and are updated every few years.

CASE RESOLUTION

After obtaining the history and performing a physical examination, the pediatrician determines that the patient has acute otitis media. Depending on the age of the child and the severity of symptoms, the American Academy of Pediatrics clinical practice guideline* suggests a stratified approach to therapeutics. For children younger than 2 years, pediatricians can treat with antibiotics if the diagnosis is certain or observe the patient without antibiotics if the patient is otherwise healthy. In this case the pediatrician discusses the options with the family and, because of the severity of pain and previous ear infections, chooses to treat the infection. The antibiotic of choice for treatment of otitis media is amoxicillin at a dose of 80 to 90 mg/kg/d. The mother stated that her daughter had hives with amoxicillin, a type I hypersensitivity. Other antibiotic choices would include azithromycin 10 mg/kg on day 1 followed by 5 mg/kg for the remaining 4 days or clindamycin at 30 to 40 mg/kg/d. The treatment of pain is essential with otitis media. The patient can take oral acetaminophen or ibuprofen or use otic benzocaine drops.

If the patient was not allergic to amoxicillin, it would have been the drug of choice. It is inexpensive, has a narrow microbiological spectrum, and is palatable. Amoxicillin does require refrigeration, which would be of concern if the family was traveling. While this case illustrates several obvious constraints, it is important to emphasize that choosing the appropriate medication is dependent on both the intrinsic needs of the patient and the extrinsic factors that can affect adherence and ultimately the effectiveness of treatment.

---

*American Academy of Pediatrics Subcommittee on Management of Acute Otitis Media, American Academy of Family Physicians. Clinical practice guideline: diagnosis and management of acute otitis media. *Pediatrics*. 2004;113:1451–1465.

Selected References

American Academy of Pediatrics Committee on Drugs. Use of drugs not described in the package insert (off-label uses). *Pediatrics*. 2002;110:181–183

Frush KS, Luo X, Hutchinson P, Higgins JN. Evaluation of a method to reduce over-the-counter medication dosing error. *Arch Pediatr Adolesc Med*. 2004;158:620–624

Hughes RG, Edgerton EA. Reducing pediatric medication errors: children are especially at risk for medication errors. *Am J Nurs*. 2005;105:79–80

Kaushal R, Barker KN, Bates DW. How can information technology improve patient safety and reduce medication errors in children's health care? *Arch Pediatr Adolesc Med*. 2001;155:1002–1007

Lasser KE, Allen PD, Woolhandler SJ, Himmelstein DU, Wolfe SM, Bor DH. Timing of new black box warnings and withdrawals for prescription medications. *JAMA*. 2002;287:2215–2220

Leonard MS, Cimino M, Shaha S, McDougal S, Pilliod J, Brodsky L. Risk reduction for adverse drug events through sequential implementation of patient safety initiatives in a children's hospital. *Pediatrics*. 2006;118:e1124–e1129

Pollock M, Bazaldua OV, Dobbie AE. Appropriate prescribing of medications: an eight-step approach. *Am Fam Physician*. 2007;75:231–236

Roberts R, Rodriguez W, Murphy D, Crescenzi T. Pediatric drug labeling. Improving the safety and efficacy of pediatric therapies. *JAMA*. 2003;290:905–911

SECTION II

Health Maintenance and Anticipatory Guidance

10. Neonatal Examination and Nursery Visit 41

11. Newborn Screening 47

12. Caring for Twins and Higher-Order Multiples 51

13. Circumcision 57

14. Nutritional Needs 63

15. Breastfeeding 71

16. Sleep: Normal Patterns and Common Disorders 75

17. Oral Health and Dental Disorders 81

18. Normal Development and Development Surveillance, Screening, and Evaluation 87

19. Language Development: Speech and Hearing Assessment 95

20. Literacy Promotion in Pediatric Practice 101

21. Gifted Children 105

22. Children and School: A Primer for the Practitioner 109

23. Immunizations 115

24. Health Maintenance in Older Children and Adolescents 121

25. Health Care for International Adoptees ... 129

26. Health Care Needs of Children in Foster Care 137

27. Well-Child Care for Children With Trisomy 21 143

28. Well-Child Care for Preterm Infants 149

29. Care of Children With Special Health Care Needs 155

30. Reproductive Health 161

31. Injury Prevention 169

32. Fostering Self-Esteem 175

33. Sibling Rivalry 179

34. Toilet Training 183

35. Crying and Colic 189

36. Discipline 193

37. Temper Tantrums 199

38. Breath-Holding Spells 203

39. Fears, Phobias, and Anxiety 207

40. Thumb Sucking and Other Habits 213

41. Enuresis 219

42. Encopresis 223

Neonatal Examination and Nursery Visit

Julie E. Noble, MD, and Monica Sifuentes, MD

CASE STUDY

You are performing a discharge examination on a 1-day-old infant who was born at 39 weeks' gestation to a 28-year-old healthy primigravida via normal vaginal delivery. There were no complications. The infant weighed 7 lb, 1 oz (3,200 g) and was 19.7 inches (50 cm) long at birth. The mother received prenatal care beginning at 10 weeks' gestation; had no prenatal problems, including infections; and used no drugs, alcohol, or tobacco during the pregnancy. Her blood type is O positive. She is negative for hepatitis B surface antigen, human immunodeficiency virus, and Group B streptococcus and nonreactive for syphilis. The father is also healthy.

On physical examination, the infant is average size for gestational age with a length and head circumference in the 50th percentile. Aside from small bilateral subconjunctival hemorrhages, the rest of the physical examination is entirely normal.

Questions
1. What parts of the maternal history are important to review before performing the infant's physical examination?
2. What aspects of the physical examination of newborns are essential to explain to parents?
3. What physical findings mandate a more extensive workup prior to discharge?
4. What are important points to cover with parents at the time of discharge for a normal term newborn?
5. What laboratory studies, if any, should be performed prior to discharge?

While a key purpose of the newborn examination is to assess the status of the infant and detect any underlying medical problems, the other function is to be able to answer the question foremost in a parent's mind: "Is the baby normal?" By performing a physical examination in the parents' presence during the infant's first 24 hours of life, pediatricians can play a major role in allaying parental anxiety. In addition, medical problems that the newborn may experience in this important transitional period to extrauterine life may be detected. Treatment can be initiated, if necessary, before discharge from the nursery.

Pediatric Prenatal Visit

Ideally, the pediatrician has spoken with the parents at a prenatal visit before meeting them in the hospital. The prenatal meeting provides a time when the parents are able to interview the physician as well as the rest of the office staff regarding general policies and procedures for well-child appointments, sick visits, and contacting the physician after hours. It also is a time to discuss what will take place at the hospital and explain the role of allied health care professionals (eg, lactation specialists) in the overall care of the mother and newborn. For pediatricians and other health care practitioners, the prenatal visit is a time to gather vital medical information regarding the current pregnancy, inquire about any problems with previous deliveries, and review any pertinent family history. In addition, it is important that physicians be sensitive to cultural rituals or ceremonies surrounding the birth of an infant and inquire about any specific familial preferences before delivery. Whether the infant is born at a birthing center or in the more traditional hospital setting, arrangements should be made to accommodate the wishes of the family. The prenatal visit also allows physicians to assess any psychosocial issues that may negatively influence initial maternal-infant bonding, such as maternal drug use, paternal uninvolvement, or the absence of a supportive social network. Other issues such as breastfeeding, circumcision, infant sleep position, and child passenger safety can also be discussed.

Neonatal Nursery Visit

The timing of the newborn visit and its length depend on several factors, including the type of delivery (vaginal delivery or cesarean section), the extent of prenatal care, and the occurrence of any perinatal complications, such as severe, prolonged bradycardia or meconium aspiration. These complications may warrant an early neonatal examination in the nursery. A screening risk assessment should be performed promptly after birth by nursery personnel, and the physician notified of any complicating factors. Other reasons for an early initial visit include suspected congenital anomalies (eg, congenital heart disease, hydronephrosis) as noted on prenatal fetal ultrasound, a history of prematurity, the presence of maternal fever or sepsis, ABO or Rh incompatibility, and any evidence of infant drug withdrawal.

Evaluation

Perinatal History

The prenatal history and results of maternal laboratory tests, such as blood type; rapid plasma reagin status; human immunodeficiency virus status; and chlamydial, gonococcal, and Group B streptococcus cultures, should be noted (Questions Box). Perinatal events should then be reviewed before performing the physical examination of the neonate. This review helps the physician focus the examination on findings suggested by the maternal history. The occurrence of any unusual circumstances surrounding the delivery must also be explained to the parents at this time. They may have been very puzzled by a sudden change in plans such as the need for an emergent cesarean section. It is also important to be prepared to discuss the medical implications of such events and to address any concerns the parents have about the newborn infant.

Questions

Neonatal Examination

- Did the mother receive prenatal care? If so, since what month of gestation?
- Were all prenatal studies normal?
- Does either parent have a history of sexually transmitted infections, such as syphilis, gonorrhea, or herpes?
- Does either parent have a history of alcohol, tobacco, or illicit drug use?
- Did the mother take any prescribed or over-the-counter medications routinely during pregnancy?
- Did the mother have any complications, such as bleeding or decreased fetal movement, during pregnancy?
- Were there any indications of a complicated delivery?
- Is the mother planning to breastfeed?
- Does the neonate have any siblings? If so, what are their ages?
- Is anyone available to help with the new baby or siblings?

Physical Examination

Every attempt should be made to perform the neonatal physical examination at the bedside. This gives the physician an opportunity to meet with parents and gives parents a chance to have all their initial questions answered immediately. In certain circumstances, such as when the infant is premature or when the mother is being treated for a medical complication, an initial bedside examination may be impossible to perform. In any event, the physician or other health care provider should speak to parents about the results once the examination has been completed.

The neonatal examination should be performed with the infant completely unclothed and the infant's body temperature maintained. The infant should be assessed for evidence of birth trauma and congenital malformations, and an assessment of normal physiology of organ systems should be done. The infant's birth weight, length, and head circumference should be plotted; physicians should keep in mind that these measurements are often made in the delivery room and may be subject to error. Temperature, respiratory rate, and heart rate should be reviewed via the nursery record.

The infant's overall appearance should be noted, particularly for the presence of any dysmorphic features. Physicians should determine whether the infant looks normal or has any abnormal facial features such as low-set ears and widely spaced eyes (see Chapter 57).

Skin

The presence and location of any rashes or birthmarks should be carefully described and pointed out to the parents; the particular location of the lesion may aid in its diagnosis. Skin color should also be noted, such as the presence of jaundice suggesting hyperbilirubinemia or plethora suggesting polycythemia.

Head

Head size and shape, including the size of the fontanelles and the position of the sutures, should be evaluated. The head may be significantly molded into a cone deformity secondary to pelvic pressure at the time of delivery. This resolves within days after birth. A cephalohematoma, which is a subperiosteal bleed that does not cross the suture line, appears as a unilateral or bilateral discrete lump on the side of the head. This finding may predispose the infant to hyperbilirubinemia, and resolution may take up to 2 months. A cephalohematoma should be differentiated from a caput succedaneum, which is scalp edema that crosses the midline, and may be ballotable. Edema usually resolves rapidly. All head findings may be a source of concern to parents.

Eyes

The eyes should be evaluated for subconjunctival hemorrhages, colobomas, extraocular movements, and the presence of red reflexes. Difficulty eliciting a red reflex should be pursued because the absence of a red reflex suggests conditions such as congenital cataracts or retinoblastomas.

The placement, size, and shape of the pinnae should be noted as well, along with any preauricular pits or appendages. The presence of a significant auricular abnormality may correlate with hearing loss or suggest a genetic syndrome.

Nose

The nose should be checked carefully for patency of both nares. This can be easily accomplished by occluding airflow from one nare and observing airflow from the other. Choanal atresia is an important condition to rule out because infants are obligate nose breathers until 3 months of age, and choanal atresia may lead to respiratory distress.

Mouth

The oropharynx should be examined closely for any defects in the hard or soft palate. A bifid uvula may indicate a submucosal defect of the soft palate that may be difficult to appreciate without palpation (see Chapter 58). Common normal findings in the oropharynx, including Epstein pearls located at the midline on the hard palate and epithelial cysts along the gum line, should also be noted. Loose natal teeth should be removed to prevent the possibility of aspiration (see Chapter 59). The tongue should be evaluated for macroglossia or a tight lingual frenulum, which may interfere with effective breastfeeding.

Chest

The neck should be palpated for sternocleidomastoid hematomas and the clavicles for fractures, especially in infants who are large for gestational age (LGA). The chest should be inspected for respiratory effort and lungs auscultated to ensure normal breath sounds throughout. Chest wall deformities such as pectus excavatum should be noted. The presence of breast buds and supernumerary nipples are of no clinical consequence, although widely spaced nipples are a minor malformation that may suggest Turner syndrome.

Heart

The heart should be auscultated to ensure that it is in the proper position on the left side of the chest. Cardiac murmurs should be appreciated and documented. The presence of a murmur does not always indicate complex congenital heart disease. In the first 24 hours, a murmur may be a closing ductus, and newborns can also have functional murmurs. Each case should be evaluated on an individual basis. If a murmur is associated with cyanosis, tachypnea, poor feeding, or congenital anomalies there is high suspicion of a pathologic cause. A consult from specialists in pediatric cardiology should be sought as necessary. Equal and symmetrical pulses should also be palpated in all extremities.

Abdomen

The abdomen should be palpated for any masses or organomegaly (eg, polycystic kidneys, hepatosplenomegaly, adrenal hemorrhage) that warrant further investigation.

Genitalia

In female neonates, the labia majora may be swollen, but the urethra and vaginal opening should be visualized to ensure patency. It is not uncommon to see hymenal tags. Clitoral size should be noted. Parents should be told that a physiological vaginal discharge and the presence later of a pink or blood-tinged discharge are a normal neonatal response to maternal estrogen withdrawal. In uncircumcised male infants, it is imperative that the foreskin be retracted sufficiently to reveal the location of the urethral meatus. A testicular examination can rule out hydroceles, inguinal hernias, and cryptorchidism.

Skeleton

The infant hip examination is important to detect developmental dysplasia of the hip seen more commonly after a breech position in utero. The Ortolani test is performed to detect a dislocated hip. The "clunk" felt when performing the examination is the relocation of the femoral head of the affected hip in the joint capsule. In contrast, a "click" may indicate normal perinatal ligament laxity. The Barlow test detects an unstable dislocatable hip. If either test is positive, an ultrasound may be undertaken to assess the position of the femoral head. Orthopedic consultation should also be elicited. The spine should be palpated completely to the sacrum. Sacral defects, deep sacral pits, or sacral tufts of hair warrant an investigation for such conditions as spina bifida occulta. All long bones should be evaluated for a potential fracture secondary to birth trauma. Fingers and toes should be counted. The feet may be turned inward, outward, or up and should be gently moved to a normal position to ensure flexibility. Clubfoot deformations should receive orthopedic evaluation.

Neurologic Examination

Infants' resting positions should be assessed to evaluate tone. They then can be held prone under the shoulder girdle for further evaluation of tone. All extremities should be flexed. Infants should be observed for motor activity, moving arms and legs symmetrically. Response to sensory stimulation and deep tendon reflexes should be elicited. Facial movements should be closely observed for symmetry. Primitive reflexes such as suck, rooting, grasp, stepping, and Moro, are an important part of the newborn neurologic examination. The infant should also respond to sound, fixate on your face, and be capable of attempts at self-consolation.

Normal findings of the nursery physical examination are summarized in Box 10-1. Significant findings that must be addressed immediately when noted at the initial nursery examination include evidence of hydrocephalus, a ductal-dependent cardiac lesion, a diaphragmatic hernia, an abdominal mass, or a possible chromosomal abnormality such as trisomy 13 or trisomy 18. The physical conditions associated with trisomy 21 are rarely life-threatening, although suspicion of the diagnosis does warrant a genetics consultation and evaluation for cardiac and abdominal anomalies (see Chapter 27).

Laboratory Tests

All newborns undergo newborn screening tests prior to discharge from the nursery. Heel stick blood usually is evaluated for inheritable conditions such as phenylketonuria, galactosemia, hypothyroidism, hemoglobinopathies, cystic fibrosis, congenital adrenal hyperplasia, and other inborn errors of metabolism. Mandated neonatal screening varies by state and depends on the prevalence of a particular disease in a given region (see Chapter 11). In most states, hearing screening is also part of the mandated newborn screening. Screening methods may be by automated auditory brain stem response, otoacoustic emission testing, or conventional auditory brain stem response.

Other laboratory tests that are often performed in a newborn include a serum glucose, especially in infants at high risk for hypoglycemia (which includes infants who are small for gestational age or LGA, infants of diabetic mothers, and infants who are symptomatic). A hematocrit is necessary in jaundiced or ruddy-appearing

---

Box 10-1. Common Physical Findings in Newborns

Skin
Milia, erythema toxicum, salmon patch, nevus flammeus, hemangiomas, mongolian spots, lanugo (body hair)

Head
Cephalohematoma, caput succedaneum

Face
Swollen overall appearance

Eyes
Swollen eyelids, subconjunctival hemorrhages

Ears
Preauricular appendages/pits, folded pinnae

Nose
Flattened nose, milia over bridge

Mouth and Throat
Epstein pearls, epithelial pearls, natal teeth, shortened frenulum

Chest
Supernumerary nipples, breast buds, galactorrhea, pectus excavatum or carinatum

Genitalia
Females: swollen labia, hymenal tags, vaginal discharge
Males: hydrocele, undescended testicle (palpated in inguinal canal)

Hips
Click

Extremities
Feet turned up, in, or out, but malleable

Neurologic Examination
Primitive reflexes: Moro, grasp, rooting, stepping

---

newborns and in twins. In cases of ABO or Rh incompatibility, a serum bilirubin and a Coombs test are important to obtain. Screening for hyperbilirubinemia to prevent kernicterus is recommended for all newborns. This can be done by a transcutaneous reading followed by a serum level if the transcutaneous reading is elevated (see Chapter 101).

Imaging Studies

Routine x-rays are not indicated in neonates whose examination is normal or who have minor abnormalities such as pectus excavatum. Vertebral x-rays are appropriate in the neonate with a deep sacral pit or sacral tuft of hair for the diagnosis of spina bifida occulta. Clavicular x-rays are indicated if swelling or pain is located in the clavicular area or if an asymmetrical Moro reflex is elicited. A chest x-ray and electrocardiogram are warranted for a significant murmur. If multiple anomalies are found, a renal ultrasound looking for malformations of the kidneys should be performed. More extensive studies are indicated if an emergent physical finding is discovered.

Management

After stabilization in the delivery room, the infant should be thoroughly dried and given to the mother for breastfeeding and bonding. If mother and baby are healthy, the infant should stay with the mother, receiving an initial bath when the temperature is stable. The administration of intramuscular vitamin K to prevent hemorrhagic disease of the newborn and the application of ophthalmic ointment or silver nitrate in the newborn's eyes to prevent gonorrheal infection is universal. Every hospital should encourage rooming-in of the infant with the mother. The infant should feed within 2 hours of birth and continue to feed every 2 hours to prevent hypoglycemia. The preferred method is breastfeeding, and the mother should receive sufficient postpartum support to ensure success (see Chapter 15). Vital signs should be monitored every 30 minutes until stable, then every 4 hours. Daily weights as well as strict documentation of voiding and stooling are necessary to monitor the infant for adequacy of intake and for dehydration.

If desired, the circumcision is usually performed on the day of discharge (see Chapter 13). Local anesthesia is now universally recommended for the procedure, but its use remains at the discretion of the physician and parents. Following the procedure, the parents are instructed to leave the gauze or Plastibell in place. It will fall off spontaneously. Petroleum ointment may also be placed on the corona of the penis to prevent its sticking to the diaper. The physician should be notified if excessive bleeding or oozing occurs (eg, soaking of the diaper with blood) after discharge from the nursery. Hepatitis B vaccine is also administered prior to discharge.

Discharge Planning and Counseling

Before the infant is discharged home, physicians should discuss normal variants found on the physical examination with parents. Abnormal physical findings and their relevance should also be explained. If studies other than routine neonatal screening were performed, parents should also be informed of the results.

Other topics that should be covered at the bedside include breastfeeding versus bottle-feeding, sleeping and elimination patterns in the newborn, umbilical cord care, bathing the newborn, and safety issues such as car safety seats and sleeping position. In addition, the timing of the first dose of the hepatitis B vaccine should be discussed. It can be administered prior to hospital discharge or at the first follow-up visit. Guidelines regarding symptoms of illness and when to call the office or emergency department should also be addressed. These include a rectal fever of 100.4°F (38.0°C) or greater, respiratory distress, irritability, lethargy, decreased feeding, and evidence of dehydration. If parents have any concerns about their infant, they should be encouraged to call the physician's office. A follow-up visit should be arranged for 1 to 3 weeks after discharge if the infant was delivered by cesarean section or is formula feeding. If the newborn is sent home at less than 48 hours or is breastfeeding, a follow-up visit should be scheduled in 2 days.

CASE RESOLUTION

In the case presented at the beginning of the chapter, the parents should be told that the weight, length, and head circumference are all normal. The subconjunctival hemorrhages should be shown to the parents and their self-limited nature explained. Routine neonatal screening, feeding, sleeping, elimination, bathing, and safety should be reviewed. Prior to discharge, the infant should receive the hepatitis B vaccine and newborn screening tests. A follow-up appointment should be made in 48 hours to follow breastfeeding progress.

Selected References

American Academy of Pediatrics Committee on Fetus and Newborn. Hospital stay for healthy term newborns. *Pediatrics.* 2004;113:1434–1436

American Academy of Pediatrics Committee on Fetus and Newborn. Controversies concerning vitamin K and the newborn. *Pediatrics.* 2003;112:191–192

American Academy of Pediatrics Committee on Psychosocial Aspects of Child and Family Health. The prenatal visit. *Pediatrics.* 1996;97:141–142

American Academy of Pediatrics, The American College of Obstetricians and Gynecologists. *Guidelines for Perinatal Care.* 6th ed. Washington, DC: American College of Obstetricians and Gynecologists; 2008

Coloherty J, Eichenwald E, Stark A, eds. *Manual of Neonatal Care.* 5th ed. Philadelphia, PA: Lippincott Williams & Wilkins; 2004

Irons M, ed. Neonatology part I: neonatal screening. *Pediatr Ann.* 2003; 32:505–550

Kendig J, Howard C. Caring for the normal newborn in an era of managed care. *Pediatr in Rev.* 1998;19(12-CD)

Kessel J, Ward RM. Congenital malformations presenting during the neonatal period. *Clin Perinatol.* 1998;25:351–369

Rademacher R, Kliegman R. Common issues and concerns in the newborn nursery, part II. *Pediatr Clin North Am.* 2004;51:xv–xvi

Newborn Screening

Derek Wong, MD

CASE STUDY

A 1-week-old male infant is brought to his pediatrician's office for a positive newborn screening test for congenital adrenal hyperplasia. The baby was a product of a 38-week gestation and was born by normal spontaneous vaginal delivery to a 30-year-old gravida II para II woman with an unremarkable pregnancy. Birth weight was 3,300 g, and the baby is feeding and acting appropriately. Family history is unremarkable, and the physical examination is normal.

Questions

1. What are the proposed benefits of newborn screening?
2. Which newborn screening tests are most commonly performed?
3. How are the results of newborn screening tests reported to physicians?
4. How should a patient with an abnormal newborn screening result be managed?
5. What are the most common causes of false-positive and false-negative results?
6. What are the ethical issues and future challenges surrounding newborn screening?

Newborn screening programs are designed to identify infants at risk for catastrophic outcomes from treatable illnesses. During the past 40 years, technological advances such as tandem mass spectrometry have made it possible to test for more than 50 metabolic disorders from a single blood spot. New techniques in molecular biology allow for rapid diagnostic testing of conditions such as cystic fibrosis.

From the inception of newborn screening in the 1960s until 2005, each state chose a different set of conditions for their newborn screening programs based on disease prevalence, cost, availability of treatment, and false-positive rate. Recently, the American Academy of Pediatrics and other agencies produced a series of articles that outlined a strategy to move toward a uniform national newborn screening panel. In 2005 an expert panel from the American College of Medical Genetics recommended 29 core disorders for which newborn screening was most effective (Table 11-1), as well as 25 secondary disorders that are in the differential diagnosis of a core disorder. Currently all states offer screening for congenital hypothyroidism, sickle cell disease and related hemoglobinopathies, galactosemia, and phenylketonuria. By the end of 2006, 43 states offered testing for at least 25 of the 29 core disorders. Most infants born in Europe, Japan, and Australia undergo similar screening, and other nations are actively exploring similar technologies.

Primary care physicians have 3 crucial roles in the newborn screening process. First, they provide education to parents about the newborn screening process. Second, they ensure that specimens are drawn under proper circumstances and that the results are promptly followed up. Finally, they provide medical follow-up and referral in positive cases. Providers need to have contact information for state newborn screening programs and local pediatric subspecialists. The following Web sites link to contact information for these groups:

1. State newborn screening programs—http://genes-r-us.uthscsa.edu/
2. Geneticists, metabolic and clinical—The Society for Inherited Metabolic Disorders (www.simd.org) and The American College of Medical Genetics (www.acmg.net)
3. Pediatric endocrinologists—The Lawson Wilkins Pediatric Endocrine Society (www.lwpes.org/)
4. Pediatric hematologists—The American Society of Pediatric Hematology/Oncology (www.aspho.org)
5. Pediatric pulmonologists—The Cystic Fibrosis Foundation (www.cff.org/) (under "Care Center Network")

Epidemiology

More than 4 million infants are screened each year in the United States. Several large studies have estimated that 1 in 3,900 to 1 in 4,600 newborns have a metabolic disorder detected by newborn screening. Approximately 1 in 3,500 infants have congenital hypothyroidism and 1 in 15,000 infants have congenital adrenal hyperplasia. Several disorders are more common in particular ethnic groups: Cystic fibrosis has an incidence of 1 in 2,500 in whites, and sickle cell disease has an incidence of 1 in 400 in African Americans.

Table 11-1. Core Newborn Screening Disorders[a]	
Disorder	*Possible Signs and Symptoms in Neonates[b]*
Organic Acid Disorders	
Glutaric aciduria type I	Macrocephaly
Biotinidase deficiency	
Multiple carboxylase deficiency	
HMG-CoA lyase deficiency	Vomiting, lethargy, tachypnea
Cobalamin A,B deficiency	Seizures, coma, anion gap acidosis
Isovaleric aciduria	Hyperammonemia
Methylmalonic acidemia	Anemia, neutropenia, thrombocytopenia
Propionic acidemia	
3-methylcrotonyl-CoA carboxylase deficiency	
Beta-ketothiolase deficiency	Asymptomatic[c]
Fatty Acid Oxidation Disorders	
Medium-chain acyl-CoA dehydrogenase deficiency	Lethargy, coma, sudden death, hypoketotic hypoglycemia
	Reye-like syndrome
Very long-chain acyl-CoA dehydrogenase deficiency	Lethargy, coma, sudden death, hypoketotic hypoglycemia
Long-chain L-3-OH acyl-CoA dehydrogenase deficiency	Cardiomyopathy, arrhythmias
Trifunctional protein deficiency	Cholestasis, Reye-like syndrome
Carnitine uptake defect	Asymptomatic[c]
Amino Acid Disorders	
Maple syrup urine disease	Poor feeding, vomiting, lethargy, seizures, coma, maple syrup odor
Citrullinemia	Hyperammonemia, vomiting, seizures, lethargy, coma
Argininosuccinic acidemia	
Tyrosinemia type I	Hepatomegaly, increased PT/PTT, liver failure, boiled cabbage odor
Homocystinuria	Asymptomatic[c]
Phenylketonuria	Asymptomatic
Hemoglobinopathies	
Sickle cell disease (Hb SS)	Dactylitis
Sickle beta thalassemia	Asymptomatic[c]
Hemoglobin sickle cell disease	
Other	
Congenital hypothyroidism	Umbilical hernia, enlarged fontanelle, macroglossia, jaundice
Congenital adrenal hypertrophy	Virilization in females; salt wasting crisis
Galactosemia	Cataracts, jaundice, poor feeding, sepsis
Cystic fibrosis	Meconium ileus, intestinal obstruction

Abbreviations: HMG, 3-hydroxy-3-methylglutaryl; CoA, coenzyme A; PT, prothrombin time; PTT, partial thromboplastin time.

[a]Most of these conditions may not be asymptomatic outside of the neonatal period.

[b]Many neonates with these disorders are completely asymptomatic.

[c]"Asymptomatic" covers the first month of life and does not exclude very rare case reports of neonatal presentation.

Clinical Presentation

Most infants with disorders detected by newborn screening are clinically asymptomatic in the first 2 weeks of life, but the remainder may have significant signs and symptoms (see Table 11-1). The presence of such features may lead to a more urgent workup and/or hospitalization. Unfortunately, severe forms of some metabolic disorders may cause coma and encephalopathy by 48 hours of age. In these cases, the newborn screening results are critical, for they will suggest a probable diagnosis and will allow early optimization of therapy.

Differential Diagnosis

While newborn screening techniques are continually improved, both false-positive and false-negative errors occur. Mislabeled specimens, technical errors, and reporting errors can occur in any laboratory. Any specimen collected before 12 hours of age is at risk for a false-negative metabolic result or a false-positive hypothyroidism result. Premature infants have a reduced metabolic capacity and therefore exhibit higher metabolite levels and increased false-positive results compared with term infants. Anemia or polycythemia can affect the amount of serum per blood spot and increase false-negative results, and transfusion may alter galactosemia and hemoglobinopathy testing. Infants on hyperalimentation may have increased amino acid and lipid levels, especially if the newborn screen is drawn from a central line. To ensure accurate and uniform testing, it is imperative to communicate relevant clinical information to the state newborn screening office.

Newborn Screening Practices

Parental Education and Consent

All parents should therefore be informed of the state screening program either at the prenatal visit or during the initial newborn examination. Written materials that explain the screening program are available from the state screening office, and online materials explaining abnormal results are available on fact sheets at Web sites such as www.pediatrics.org/cgi/content/full/118/3/e934. Health care providers are responsible for educating parents regarding the method for obtaining the blood specimen, the risks and benefits of the screening tests, the conditions to be screened, and the implications of positive results.

It is important to tell parents that positive results do not necessarily mean that their infant has a particular disorder; the results must be confirmed by more specific tests. In addition, parents should know that disorders in some children are missed either because of sampling errors, faulty testing, or inadequate accumulation of the abnormal metabolite at the time of testing.

Newborn screening is mandatory in all states, although many states allow exemptions for religious beliefs or other reasons. In most states, parents have given informed consent if practitioners have discussed the state-mandated program with them and they have agreed to participate. A few states require signed consent to opt into the newborn screening program, and several more require consent to disclose identifiable information. Providers should document parental refusal regardless of state laws.

Specimen Collection and Handling

Proper specimen collection and handling are essential components of a successful screening program. All newborns should be screened before discharge from the hospital, ideally between 48 to 96 hours of age. Early screening increases the chance of a false-negative metabolic result or a false-positive hypothyroidism result. For this reason, some states have a mandatory second screen between 1 and 6 weeks of age, while others require a second screen only if the first screen is obtained before a specified time (12–48 hours depending on the state). Late screening increases the sensitivity of metabolic testing, but also increases the chances for a delay in diagnosis of life-threatening conditions such as galactosemia. If possible, blood samples should be obtained prior to any transfusions or dialysis. Otherwise, screening tests should still be performed as outlined previously, and arrangements should be made to have them repeated at an appropriate time.

Only a few drops of blood are needed for each disk on the filter paper, but the sample must saturate the paper evenly. The use of needles and glass capillary tubes for blood collection is discouraged because they may cause hemolysis or microtears in the filter paper. The specimens must be individually air-dried in a horizontal position, thus avoiding contamination and excessive exposure to heat. They should be mailed to the laboratory within 24 hours of collection. Inadequate specimen collection and handling can lead to test inaccuracies, delays in reporting results to physicians, and unnecessary repetition of screening tests. Therefore, all individuals who are involved in the newborn screening process should adhere strictly to the procedures set forth by their state program.

Reporting of Results

In most states, all results of neonatal screening tests, whether normal or abnormal, are reported to the physician of record. Normal results are mailed to the physician for placement in the patient's medical record. Abnormal results are usually reported by telephone or letter, depending on the significance of the abnormality. Results are also sent to the hospital where the infant was born for inclusion in the medical record. The physician of record is responsible for contacting the parents regarding the need for confirmatory testing and, if necessary, referral to an appropriate subspecialist. If a newborn is no longer under the care of this physician or if the family cannot be located, state and local public health departments can be called on to assist in the search for the infant and family.

Diagnostic and Therapeutic Considerations

A health care team consisting of a primary care physician and staff, state newborn screening office personnel, the state newborn screening laboratory, local laboratories, and subspecialty physician is responsible for care and follow-up of patients with positive newborn screening results. All infants with abnormal results, whether borderline or clearly significant, should be evaluated by the primary care physician. A complete history and physical examination as well as a family history should be obtained. Abnormal results for some newborn screening tests, such as very long-chain acyl–coenzyme A (CoA) dehydrogenase deficiency, may normalize with a second screen. Therefore, most follow-up evaluation centers on targeted diagnostic tests. Depending on the nature of the suspected disorder, initiation of treatment before confirmatory laboratory results are known may be appropriate. For example, prophylactic antibiotics should be administered if sickle cell anemia is suspected. After confirmatory results have been received, the treatment can be modified or halted.

Potentially life-threatening conditions in the newborn period such as galactosemia, maple syrup urine disease, and congenital adrenal hyperplasia are particularly important to evaluate and treat emergently. Depending on the clinical picture, the suspected disorder, and the experience of the practitioner, telephone consultation with a specialist or immediate referral to a regional medical center may be necessary.

Nearly all of the diseases in the current newborn screening panels are inherited in an autosomal-recessive manner. Families of affected infants should be offered genetic counseling for future pregnancies, in addition to written information about the newly diagnosed condition. Depending on the condition, older siblings may need to be evaluated. In some conditions, such as 3-methylcrotonyl-CoA carboxylase deficiency, a positive newborn screen may reflect an affected asymptomatic mother whose metabolites have passed to her infant.

Current Issues and Future Challenges

Protecting patient privacy is of the utmost importance; as of 2005, 28 of the 51 programs had laws to protect a patient's personal information and blood spots, and 30 programs had genetic privacy laws to protect a patient's genetic information. There is great concern amongst parents and providers that insurance companies will use newborn screening information to discriminate against children and their families.

There is no dispute that newborn screening saves lives. Additionally, the cost of newborn screening programs is outweighed by the reduction in morbidity and mortality from a purely economic standpoint. However, some diseases under consideration for newborn screening have extremely costly treatments, which may total several million dollars over the lifetime of the patient and produce significant morbidity. Cost-benefit analysis will be crucial to shaping future newborn screening panels. Pediatricians and other health professionals need to advocate for insurance coverage for newborn screening panels because patients may be charged up to $130.

Currently a large percentage of false-positive results occur in premature infants, in part due to the lack of age-specific laboratory values for all metabolites. In several states, a lack of appropriate cutoff values led to a large numbers of babies in neonatal intensive care units that strained the state programs. In the future, careful pilot testing of new tests in infants of all gestational ages will be needed to improve the screening process.

There is debate about the benefit of early detection of disorders such as cystic fibrosis. While recent studies have suggested that patients benefit from early therapy, it is unclear how much early detection improves the long-term pulmonary or nutritional status of affected children. Some disorders, such as short-chain acyl-CoA dehydrogenase deficiency, are asymptomatic in most individuals and have a high rate of false-positive tests due to the presence of common polymorphisms in the population. The lifelong treatment of patients who would otherwise become asymptomatic, the added burden of a genetic diagnosis, and family stress caused by a false- or true-positive result have led several countries to remove this disorder from their newborn screening panels.

Several newborn screening tests detect asymptomatic carrier states in infants. While the knowledge of a patient's carrier status may be of some advantage for childbearing, it has no immediate benefit for the infant and may lead to discrimination and stigmatization. Parents of affected infants (who are usually asymptomatic carriers) face the same dilemma and should be given the option to refuse testing for carrier status.

New challenges will emerge as genetic technology advances toward the ultimate goal of sequencing a patient's entire genome. Practitioners will have to weigh the decision of whether to inform parents about non-treatable or late-onset conditions. Currently the American Academy of Pediatrics Committee on Bioethics advises against screening for such conditions, but the debate may be reopened as more data accumulate. Finally, some conditions that are caused by a complex interaction between genetics and environment, such as celiac disease, may require screening at school age. Pediatricians should be involved in decisions concerning the addition of new disorders to existing newborn screening programs because they are key players in the implementation of these programs.

CASE RESOLUTION

This patient should have a full evaluation, including an electrolyte panel due to the possibility of salt wasting congenital adrenal hyperplasia. Confirmatory testing, including measurement of precursor hormones such as 17-hydroxyprogesterone and subsequent molecular testing, and glucocorticoid therapy should be considered in consultation with a pediatric endocrinologist.

Selected References

Alexander D, van Dyck PC. A vision of the future of newborn screening. *Pediatrics.* 2006;117:S350–S354

American Academy of Pediatrics Committee on Bioethics. Ethical issues with genetic testing in pediatrics. *Pediatrics.* 2001;107:1451–1455

American College of Medical Genetics Newborn Screening Expert Group. Newborn screening: toward a uniform screening panel and system—executive summary. *Pediatrics.* 2006;117:S296–S307. www.acmg.net/resources/policies/NBS/NBS-sections.htm

Hewlett J, Waisbren SE. A review of the psychosocial effects of false-positive results on parents and current communication practices in newborn screening. *J Inherit Metab Dis.* 2006;29:677–682

Kaye CI, American Academy of Pediatrics Committee on Genetics. Introduction to the newborn screening fact sheets. *Pediatrics.* 2006;118:1304–1312

Kaye CI, American Academy of Pediatrics Committee on Genetics. Newborn screening fact sheets. *Pediatrics.* 2006;118:e934–e963. www.pediatrics.org/cgi/content/full/118/3/e934

Marsden D, Larson C, Levy HL. Newborn screening for metabolic disorders. *J Pediatr.* 2006;148:577–584

National NBS Resource Center. http://genes-r-us.uthscsa.edu/

Therrell BL, Johnson A, Williams D. Status of newborn screening programs in the United States. *Pediatrics.* 2006;117:S212–S252

Wagener JS, Sontag MK, Sagel SD, Accurso FJ. Update on newborn screening for cystic fibrosis. *Curr Opin Pulm Med.* 2004;10:500–504

Caring for Twins and Higher-Order Multiples

Lynne M. Smith, MD

CASE STUDY

An expectant mother visits you. She has been advised by her obstetrician that an ultrasound shows she is pregnant with twins. She asks about care of twins and what special considerations she should keep in mind as she looks forward to the delivery. In particular, she is concerned about the feeding schedule and whether she will be able to breastfeed.

Questions

1. What is the incidence of multiple births?
2. What is the difference between fraternal and identical twins?
3. What major medical problems may affect twins and higher-order multiples?
4. What developmental and behavioral problems are associated with raising multiples?

With the advent of artificial reproductive therapy, the incidence of twins and higher-order multiples is increasing. Counseling the parents of multiples provides a unique opportunity for pediatricians. Much of what is known about caring for multiples comes from work with twins. Many societies have been fascinated with twins, and many myths and superstitions surround their birth. Some people believe that a mother of twins must have been unfaithful to her husband because a father cannot sire 2 children. Native Americans of the Iroquois nation believed that one twin was good and the other was evil. To prevent the recurrence of twins, the Khoikhain remove one of the father's testicles.

Parents of multiples often have many questions that concern the care of their children, but they rarely pose them to health care providers. In one study in which 18 out of 29 mothers breastfed their twins, only 3 received information about breastfeeding from their physicians. One mother had been told by her obstetrician that she could not breastfeed her twins. Physicians should become knowledgeable about caring for multiples and the unique challenges they present to parents related to feeding, sleeping, and behavior.

Epidemiology

Since 1980 there has been a 74% increase in twin deliveries, and the number of higher-order multiples has increased 5-fold. A major contributor to the increase in multiple births is that women are starting their families later than in previous generations. Because of the increased risk of infertility with advanced maternal age, more couples are choosing to conceive with assisted reproductive technologies including ovulation-stimulating drugs, in vitro fertilization (IVF), and intracytoplasmic sperm injection. Assisted reproductive technology results in multiple gestations in approximately 50% of pregnancies. In addition, advanced maternal age is associated with increased follicle-stimulating hormone levels and the release by the ovary of multiple eggs, increasing the chance of multiple births.

The overall natural incidence of twin births is about 1 in 87. Twins account for just slightly more than 1% of all births, and 20% of infants born under 30 weeks' gestation are twins. The average incidence of monozygotic or identical twins, which is the same for all women regardless of race and age, is about 1 in 300 births. The incidence of dizygotic or fraternal twins varies among different groups and method of conception. In the United States, African Americans and whites have comparable incidences of live-born twin deliveries and both have significantly higher rates than Hispanic women. A maternal family history of dizygous twins correlates most strongly with an increased incidence of twinning. A family history of monozygous twins or a paternal family history of dizygous twins does not increase the risk of twins.

Pathophysiology

Higher-order multiples, conceived either naturally or via artificial reproductive technology, may be fraternal or a combination of monozygotic twins and fraternal siblings. Monozygotic twins result from the splitting of a single egg. They may share a placenta (monochorionic, Figure 12-1A and 12-1B). When splitting occurs early (after several cell divisions of the zygote), each fetus develops its own

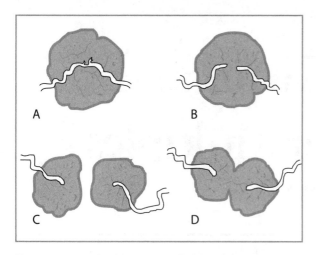

Figure 12-1. Variations in placentas in twin births. A. Monochorionic, monoamniotic placenta, cords close together. B. Monochorionic, monoamniotic placenta, cords farther apart. C. Dichorionic, diamniotic placentas, separate. D. Dichorionic, diamniotic placentas, fused.

chorion and amnion, leading to dichorionic and diamniotic placentas. Dizygotic twins result from 2 eggs, and each egg is fertilized by a different sperm. Dizygotic twins have 2 placentas (Figure 12-1C). Although these placentas may fuse together like 2 pancakes, they are almost always dichorionic and diamniotic (Figure 12-1D).

Following the birth, it is important to determine whether twins are monozygotic or dizygotic. Different sex twins are almost always dizygotic, although monozygotic twins of different sexes have been reported in the literature. This occurs when one twin loses a Y chromosome and becomes a phenotypic female with Turner syndrome (XO). Occasionally the male twin may be XXY and have Klinefelter syndrome.

To determine whether twins are monozygotic or dizygotic, a number of procedures can be undertaken. Visual or pathologic examination of the placenta is helpful. About two-thirds of monozygotic twins have a common chorion and share one placenta. Finding a single chorion usually means the twins are monozygotic, unless the placentas of dizygotic twins have fused together. DNA testing is the preferred method for determining zygosity. Most commercially available testing involves examining DNA obtained from buccal swabs from each child. Identification of short tandem repeats via polymerase chain reaction is typically accurate 99% of the time and is similar to techniques used in forensic medicine. Commercial laboratory charges are approximately $300, though prices vary significantly.

Differential Diagnosis

Diagnosing multiples is not difficult, but physicians should be aware of the problems these newborns may experience.

Perinatal Complications

Multiple births are associated with a significantly higher risk for perinatal complications relative to singleton births. The maternal complication most commonly reported with multiples is pregnancy-induced hypertension. Maternal preeclampsia rates are higher in twins and increased nearly 5-fold with triplets. In addition, mothers of twins who conceived via IVF have a higher rate of preeclampsia than mothers of twins who conceived naturally. Other maternal complications include placenta previa, antepartum hemorrhage, and uterine atony.

Neonatal mortality is 4-fold higher in twins and 15-fold higher in higher-order multiples. Neonatal morbidity is much higher in multiple births because of the increased incidence of prematurity and growth restriction. The risk for these complications increases with the number of fetuses. The perinatal mortality of monozygotic twins is 8 times that of singletons and 4 times that of dizygotic twins.

Monozygotic twins are at greater risk for death and cerebral palsy because of complications such as twin-to-twin transfusion. Twin-to-twin transfusions are seen in 10% to 15% of monochorionic pregnancies and result from vascular anastomosis within the shared placenta. The diagnosis is suspected by ultrasound when one twin is growth restricted with oligohydramnios and the other fetus has evidence of volume overload with polyhydramnios. Until recently the treatment was drainage of amniotic fluid in the twin with polyhydramnios to reduce the risk of preterm delivery. Endoscopic laser ablation of placental anastomoses is emerging as the treatment of choice. Laser ablation addresses the primary pathology and results in an average gestation at delivery of 33 weeks, which is a significant improvement from the average 29 weeks with serial amniotic fluid reductions.

One percent of monozygotic twins are monochorionic-monoamniotic. Monoamniotic twins are at very high risk for cord accidents. Monoamniotic pregnancies are monitored closely, and once the fetuses reach viability, emergent delivery is indicated if fetal distress is noted to avoid fetal death. Because fetal death significantly increases the risk of cerebral palsy and other neurologic disorders in the surviving twin, it is no longer recommended to allow fetal death in one to lengthen the gestation of the non-distressed twin.

Congenital Malformations

Twins and higher-order multiples conceived naturally have an increased risk of cardiac, renal, gastrointestinal, and neurologic anomalies. Multiples conceived via IVF or intracytoplasmic sperm injection have increased risk for anomalies and aneuploidy. Disorders of genetic imprinting (eg, Beckwith-Wiedemann, Angelman syndrome) are also increased with intracytoplasmic sperm injection. These genetic complications are thought to be secondary to the underlying cause of the infertility instead of artificial reproductive technologies. Because the costs associated with infertility treatments are substantial, many couples choose not to obtain a comprehensive chromosomal analysis looking for deletions or translocations on themselves prior to using reproductive technologies.

In addition to the increased risks for malformations, multiples are at risk for deformations secondary to crowding including torticollis, hip dislocation, plagiocephaly, and foot deformities.

Postnatal Complications

Approximately 50% of twins and 90% of triplets are born prematurely, increasing the risk of morbidity and mortality. Though growth in twins tends to be normal until 30 to 34 weeks, growth restriction is commonly associated with multiple births. Smaller twins have an increased incidence of hypoglycemia in the newborn period and have higher rates of targeted learning deficits and school failures during childhood. In addition, children born growth-restricted have an increased risk for obesity and diabetes in later life.

Evaluation

History

A general medical history should be obtained, including a history of the pregnancy. Any specific medical complaints should also be addressed (Questions Box).

Questions

Caring for Twins

- Did the mother have any problems during the pregnancy?
- How long did the pregnancy last?
- Did the mother take any medications, including fertility drugs?
- Did the children have any problem after the delivery or in the newborn nursery?

Physical Examination

The initial evaluation of newly born twins involves assessment of gestational age and determination of the presence of any medical problems or anomalies (see Chapter 10). Older twins should undergo health maintenance visits where routine as well as specific complaints are addressed.

Laboratory Tests

Newborns should be assessed for the presence of anemia or polycythemia with a hemoglobin determination. Hypoglycemia may occur in the newborn period and should be assessed frequently until glucose levels are stable. If the twins are premature, they may have many of the problems seen in preterm infants, such as respiratory distress syndrome and necrotizing enterocolitis.

Older children should receive an appropriate evaluation for age, with a specific focus on any behavioral concerns.

Management

The focus of the management of multiples involves counseling the parents about issues related to routine care and the anticipated stress of caring for more than one newborn simultaneously. Parents often care for 2 or more children at the same time, but multiples present unique issues related to multiple children who are developmentally and chronologically at the same point. Baby care books that specifically deal with birthing and raising multiples are available.

Support groups and Web sites also provide information for families of multiples.

Feeding multiple newborns is often an exhausting challenge for parents, and consultation with a lactation expert is recommended. The physical demands of feeding multiple newborns are often compounded by women recovering from prenatal complications such as preeclampsia. Because prematurity is common, the newborns may have an immature suck reflex, making feeding more challenging. Few multiples are still receiving breast milk by 3 to 4 months of age, and common reasons cited for unsuccessful breastfeeding of multiples include maternal stress, depression, and fatigue. Despite these obstacles, parents should know that breastfeeding is possible even for triplets.

Some options for breastfeeding twins are as follows:

1. Feed both infants *at the same time*, with one on each breast. This method is recommended only after adequate breastfeeding has been established in each twin, typically at at least 1 week of age. It is advised that the baby having fewer problems latching be placed on the breast first so that the milk ejection reflex is already established for the poorer-feeding baby. Because the babies may not drink the same amount, it is important that they feed on the opposite breast for the next feeding to maximize milk production.

   The infants may be put in a number of positions. The mother can be sitting and cradling one infant while holding the other infant like a football. Alternatively, the mother may cradle both infants, so that they are cross-positioned over one another, or she may have both infants under her arms in a football position. Breastfeeding pillows designed for feeding multiples are helpful, and electric breastfeeding pumps are essential.

2. Feed the infants *at different times*. The mother breastfeeds one infant and then the other. The mother starts with the more vigorous feeder. This approach may pose a problem; both infants may be hungry at the same time and maternal fatigue may inhibit success because the chance for sleep is diminished with this method.

3. *Breastfeed one infant and bottle-feed the other*, which gives the mother a free hand. Most parents use a combination of breastfeeding and bottle-feeding. A mother can let the first infant feed on demand but wake up the second one when the first one is done. Eighty percent of parents of twins acknowledge that they prop the bottle instead of holding it, and they should be counseled against this. There are several effective feeding positions that do not require bottle propping, and parents should be encouraged to adopt one of these positions.

   Breastfeeding triplets and higher-order multiples is even more challenging than breastfeeding twins. Mothers of triplets exclusively breastfeeding report they feed 2 children on each breast, and the third follows on both breasts. Because the hindmilk has higher fat content, it is important to rotate the feeding order of the children. Another popular option is to breastfeed 2 and have the third bottle-feed simultaneously.

Feeding twins or higher-order multiples may decrease the amount of sleep a mother gets. Because sleep deprivation is associated with maternal depression and exclusively breastfeeding mothers of multiples report more sleep problems compared with mothers who do not breastfeed or who formula-feed and breastfeed, these factors should be discussed when offering feeding options to the parents.

Sleeping in the same crib is no longer recommended because of concerns regarding cosleeping. It is important to counsel parents about **car safety seats.** Parents who cannot afford the cost of 2 car safety seats may resort to placing one twin in the car safety seat and the other on the seat of the car, a dangerous practice that is illegal throughout the United States. Parents should be advised about the need for car safety seats for both infants.

Bathing should be done separately in the interest of safety until infants can sit up. Toilet training is reportedly easier with some twins because one twin learns from the other via modeling and/or peer pressure.

Maintenance of individuality for multiples may be challenging. Researchers suggest that mothers can bond to only one infant at a time, a concept called *monotropy.* In addition, mothers bond more strongly with the twin who leaves the hospital first. For this reason, twins are often dressed alike and given similar names. This may facilitate the bonding process. To help with individual development, physicians are encouraged to obtain history and examine each child individually. Physicians should attempt to distinguish the children from one another independent of parental reminders. Twins should not be referred to as "the twins" but by their respective names. As multiples get older, issues related to classrooms and birthday parties frequently arise, and they should be consulted concerning their preferences. Individual birthday parties and gifts should be considered. (Some multiples comment on their disappointment at receiving the same present for birthdays and holidays. There is no surprise in opening gifts if the other twin opened a gift first.)

Whether multiples should be placed in the same or different classrooms is unclear. Placement in different classrooms is advocated to support each child's individual development. However, there are no data to support separate classroom placement. It is currently recommended that school districts have a flexible policy regarding school placement of twins. A checklist has been created to assist families and schools determining the best school placement for twins (available at www.twinsandmultiples.org). Families with higher-order multiples are more likely to have children in separate schools because of the higher risk that some of the children will have developmental delays.

Sibling rivalry is common among co-multiples as well as other siblings within a family. Older siblings may resent the attention paid to the new babies, so family and friends should be reminded to shower attention on the older siblings. Because twins often exclude siblings and peers socially, parents are encouraged to schedule times when one twin and sibling are with one parent and the other twin is alone with another family member. Isolating twins (or 2 triplets who exclude the third) fosters more sibling interaction and less

dependency between the twins. These separations are encouraged to begin early in development because the later in development isolation is introduced, the less agreeable they are to the separations.

Developmental differences among multiples may also contribute to sibling rivalry. The smaller or more delayed child may become jealous of their co-multiple. Conversely, normal children may become frustrated when the sibling with special needs receives more attention than they receive.

Until age 3 years, **language development** is delayed in twins relative to singletons. Contributing factors to language delay include less time for individual facilitated play, which is helpful for language development. If twins communicate with a private language they have an increased risk of language and cognitive delays. Language delays usually become much less pronounced by mid-childhood.

The risk for **cerebral palsy** is increased with higher multiples because of the increased rates of prematurity and intrauterine growth restriction. Fetal death of a co-multiple and monochorionic placentas are the biggest risk factors for developing cerebral palsy.

Attention-deficit/hyperactivity disorder is more common in twins. The temper tantrums multiples display can be severe and are understandable given the heightened need to gain parental attention from their sibling. Having twins in the home is a risk factor for **child abuse,** either to a twin or to their siblings.

Prior to delivery, parents should be made aware that **maternal depression** is frequently reported after the birth of multiples. The physical stress of caring for multiple newborns can be overwhelming, and the parents often feel isolated at home. The incidence of depression is higher in mothers of twins than of singletons, with sleep deprivation being a cited contributing factor. It is important to suggest that parents of multiples obtain outside aid, including help from high school students after school and family members to decrease fatigue and increase their ability to experience respite even for short periods.

In addition to exhaustion and isolation, the increased financial demands that accompany multiple newborns can strain the parents' relationship. Mothers often have to leave work earlier in the pregnancy than women with singleton pregnancies, adding financial burden. The medical costs associated with prematurely delivered newborns can be substantial. To cover for the loss of income at a time of increasing family expenses, the father is often required to work more hours. This increased occupational stress comes at a time when child care demands at home have increased significantly. Financial burdens are especially difficult with multiples conceived artificially because of the cost associated prior to birth. This may be a contributing factor to why parents of twins conceived artificially reported less satisfaction than parents of twins conceived naturally.

Grief is another significant contributor to parental depression. Approximately 15% of children from multiple births grow up as a singleton survivor. Birthday celebrations serve as reminders to the parents of the death of the other child. Parents grieving the loss of one of their twins have comparable grief to those grieving the loss of a singleton pregnancy. It is imperative that physicians caring for the family acknowledge the parents' grief because family and friends often do not acknowledge the parents' pain if there is a surviving newborn.

Surviving children born prematurely and/or small for gestation are at increased risk for developmental delays. The stress of raising a child with special needs is also a source of grief because parents mourn the loss of their dreams of having a normal child.

Prognosis

Although multiples have a higher incidence of perinatal problems, appropriate anticipatory guidance and routine health maintenance can help families optimize their children's outcome.

CASE RESOLUTION

The mother in the case scenario is advised that breastfeeding is not only possible but recommended. She is told about the options for timing and positioning of the infants. The issues of family history and child passenger safety are also discussed, and anticipatory guidance regarding the potential stress of raising multiples is given.

Selected References

Physicians

Allen MC, Donohue PK. Neuromaturation of multiples. *Semin Neonatol.* 2002;7:211–221

Brand PLP. Test weighing found to be too imprecise to measure milk intake in newborns. *World Medl Rev Perinatol.* 2006;24:5–6

Cowan JM, Demmer LA. Assisted reproductive technology and preimplantation genetic diagnosis: impact of the fetus and newborn. *NeoReviews.* 2007;8:e127–e132

Grether JK, Nelson BK, Cummings SK. Twinning and cerebral palsy: experience in four northern California counties, births 1983 through 1985. *Pediatrics.* 1993;92:854–858

Hansen M, Kurinczuk JJ, Bower C, Webb S. The risk of major birth defects after intracytoplasmic sperm injection and in vitro fertilization. *N Engl J Med.* 2002;346:725–730

Hay DA, Preedy P. Meeting the educational needs of multiple birth children. *Early Hum Dev.* 2006;82:397–403

Klock SC. Psychological adjustment to twins after infertility. *Best Pract Res Clin Obstet Gynaecol.* 2004;18:645–656

Moore JE. Q&A's about multiple births. *Contemp Pediatr.* 2007;24:39–55

Siegel SJ, Seigal MM. Practical aspects of pediatric management of families with twins. *Pediatr Rev.* 1982;4:8–12

Sutcliffe AG, Derom C. Follow-up of twins: health, behavior, speech, language outcomes and implications for parents. *Early Hum Dev.* 2006;82:379–386

Thorpe K. Twin children's language development. *Early Hum Dev.* 2006;82:387–395

Parents

Center for Loss in Multiple Birth, Inc. (CLIMB). www.climb-support.org

Luke B, Eberlein T. *When You're Expecting Twins, Triplets, or Quads, Revised Edition: Proven Guidelines for a Healthy Multiple Pregnancy.* New York, NY: HarperCollins Publishers Inc.; 2004

Mothers of Supertwins (MOST). http://MOSTonline.org

Neifert M. *Dr. Mom's Guide to Breastfeeding.* New York, NY: Penguin Group; 1998

Circumcision

Lynne M. Smith, MD

CASE STUDY

An expectant mother visits you prenatally. She talks about circumcision in addition to issues relating to breastfeeding and car passenger safety. Her husband is circumcised. She is unclear about the medical indications for circumcision and asks your opinion about circumcision in the newborn period.

Questions
1. What are the benefits of circumcision?
2. What are the indications for circumcision in older children?
3. What are the techniques used to perform circumcision?
4. What are the complications of circumcision?

Male circumcision, a procedure in which the foreskin of the penis is removed, has been performed for more than 4,000 years. It is routinely performed in certain groups, most notably among Jewish and Muslim people. In many other cultures (eg, Abyssinian, Australian [aborigine], Polynesian), circumcision is presumably performed to facilitate intercourse. Circumcision can be viewed as a ritual procedure, but its role as a medical one is open to greater controversy.

The benefits of male circumcision have been debated for years. Over the past 20 years, even the American Academy of Pediatrics (AAP) has changed its official position on the medical indication for circumcision. Disadvantages of routine circumcision in infants concern cost-effectiveness and the risk of complications. The procedure is sometimes viewed as an archaic and maiming ritual. Female circumcision, which may involve clitorectomy or resection and closure of the labia minor or majora, is infrequently practiced in Western culture and is not discussed here. There are no medical benefits attributable to female circumcision.

Circumcision in newborns has been performed in a routine and preventive manner, much the same way immunizations are administered. Primary care physicians should be aware of the risks and benefits of the procedure to be able to counsel parents and make referrals to consultants when certain medical conditions arise.

Epidemiology

The prevalence of neonatal circumcision, a procedure that became increasingly popular in the United States in the 1950s and 1960s, once ranged from 69% to 97% depending on cultural mores. In recent years the prevalence has decreased to about 65%. Changing cultural patterns have resulted in a lower frequency of circumcision. Rates also vary by race, religion, and geographic region. In 1999 the circumcision rate in the western United States was 37% compared with 81% in the Midwest. The higher Hispanic birth rate in the West contributes to these regional differences because Hispanic neonates are less likely to receive a circumcision. The prevalence of neonatal circumcision in Australia is reported to be 10%; in Canada, 35%; and in the United Kingdom, 6%. Circumcision is the second most common surgical procedure after vasectomy in males. It is the most commonly performed operation in children.

A reported 10% of uncircumcised males ultimately require circumcision as adults because of complications of phimosis and balanitis. Uncircumcised males with diabetes are particularly prone to these complications.

Clinical Presentation

Most often parents will query their pediatrician about the advisability of a circumcision and the infant will not have any clinical symptomatology. Older infants and children in need of a circumcision can present with symptoms of phimosis, in which the foreskin balloons out on urination; paraphimosis, in which a retracted foreskin cannot be returned to its normal position; or recurrent problems of infection or inflammation of the foreskin (posthitis), glans (balanitis), or both (balanoposthitis).

Pathophysiology

In uncircumcised males, the foreskin adheres to the glans until about the age of 6 years. This adhesiveness, or crusting, may be controlled by androgens. A gradual, normal lysing of the adhesive bands connecting the foreskin to the under portion of the glans then occurs. Non-physiological phimosis occurs as a result of scarring of the preputial wing. Lysing of adhesions in an effort to treat the phimosis usually leads to further adhesions. If the foreskin is retracted and remains in that position, paraphimosis develops.

Differential Diagnosis

The differential diagnosis relates to conditions that may be managed with a circumcision. Such conditions include phimosis, paraphimosis, and infection and inflammation of the penis. Conditions such as hypospadias may be mistaken for a partially circumcised penis because the condition is associated with absence of the ventral foreskin. A careful history will differentiate hypospadias from a circumcision.

Evaluation

History

In cases involving newborn infants, a history should include the presence of any coagulopathies involving family members, which would preclude the performance of a circumcision. In older infants and children, the history should include problems relating to voiding, such as ballooning of the foreskin or difficulty initiating the urinary stream.

Physical Examination

The physical examination should assess the genitalia, particularly to determine if there is evidence of hypospadias, in which the urethral orifice is not located at the tip of the glans. In such a situation, circumcision should be delayed because the foreskin is used to reconstruct the urethra. In cases of phimosis, the degree of phimosis should also be assessed.

Laboratory Tests

Routine laboratory tests are not indicated, although a urinalysis may be obtained in children with a history of prior urinary tract infection. Coagulation studies would be appropriate if there is a family history of a bleeding disorder.

Imaging Studies

Imaging studies are not indicated in most children undergoing a circumcision. Such studies would be relevant if there was concern that the urogenital anatomy was abnormal.

Prognosis

The prognosis is excellent with complications being exceedingly rare.

Benefits

It has been stated that circumcision facilitates penile hygiene by removing the foreskin, which may serve as a repository for bacteria, smegma, and dirt. Retractability of the foreskin increases with age (Table 13-1) and, thus, penile hygiene is easier to achieve in older children. The term **phimosis** refers to inability to retract the foreskin. In male infants beyond the newborn period, phimosis is the major indication for circumcision. Phimosis is normal in children up to about 6 years of age but is non-physiological if urination results in ballooning of the foreskin, regardless of age. When the retracted

Table 13-1. Retractability of the Foreskin in Boys (by Age)

Age	Percentage With Retractable Foreskin
Birth	4%
6 mo	15%
1 y	50%
3 y	80%
6 y	90%

foreskin acts as a tourniquet in the midshaft of the penis, **paraphimosis** occurs, preventing the return of lymphatic flow. Paraphimosis is commonly related to traumatic retraction of the foreskin, typically during cleaning or by medical personnel during bladder catheterization. Because of this parents are no longer advised to retract the foreskin in an effort to lyse adhesions. The incidence of paraphimosis is increasing in adults secondary to body piercing. Newly placed penile rings can cause enough pain to prevent foreskin retraction.

Balanitis, or inflammation of the glans, is not uncommon in young infants. It is frequently associated with *Candida* infection, and the glans is swollen and erythematous. Posthitis, or inflammation of the foreskin, is also often secondary to *Candida* infection. Other organisms, including gram-negative microbes, may be associated with balanitis. The presence of recurrent balanitis is an indication for circumcision. In older males, indications for circumcision include phimosis, paraphimosis, balanitis, posthitis, and balanoposthitis.

Bacterial colonization of the skin also leads to possible balanitis and posthitis. Group B streptococci, which bind to the foreskin of adults, causing balanitis, may be transmitted sexually. The incidence of sexually transmitted infections (STIs), particularly herpes and condyloma acuminatum, is increased in uncircumcised men.

Penile cancer, which is reported in 0.7 to 0.9 per 100,000 men in the United States, is also thought to be related to lack of circumcision of the penis. Only a few isolated cases of cancer of the penis occur in circumcised men. The lifetime risk of penile cancer is 1 in 500 in uncircumcised males compared with 1 in 50,000 to 1 in 12 million in circumcised males. In the last 45 years, 11,000 men have died from penile cancer. The reported mortality of penile cancer is 25%. Whether lack of circumcision, poor hygiene, or the presence of STIs is responsible for the increased incidence of penile carcinoma is unclear.

Cervical carcinoma among the partners of uncircumcised men has been reported with increased incidence. In addition, current partners of circumcised men with a history of multiple sexual partners have a decreased risk of cervical cancer compared with partners of uncircumcised men. Human papillomavirus (HPV) types 16 and 18 are believed to play a role here. Uncircumcised men are 4 times more likely than circumcised men to carry HPV. Herpes simplex virus type 2 has also been linked with cervical cancer.

Circumcision has been associated with a lower risk of human immunodeficiency virus (HIV) infections in numerous observational studies. In addition, The National

Institutes of Health terminated 2 clinical trials investigating the effects of adult male circumcision in sub-Saharan Africa. An interim analysis of the data concluded circumcision significantly reduces a man's risk of acquiring HIV through heterosexual contact. Thus male circumcision may play an important role in HIV prevention in regions similar to the locations in which the clinical trials were conducted.

Urinary tract infections (UTIs) reportedly occur 10 times more often in uncircumcised (1:100) than in circumcised infants (1:1,000). In young uncircumcised boys, UTIs are directly related to colonization of the foreskin with urotoxic organisms. Pyronephritogenic, fimbriated *Escherichia coli* bind to the inner lining of the foreskin within the first few days of life. Other bacteria preferentially bind to this mucosal surface, including fimbriated strains of *Proteus mirabilis* and non-fimbriated *Pseudomonas, Klebsiella,* and *Serratia* species. The incidence of UTIs has increased as the rate of circumcision has decreased. In addition, complications associated with UTIs, particularly bacteremia, meningitis, and subsequent death, have occurred.

Risks

The risks related to circumcision are related to complications from the procedure. These are listed in Box 13-1 and discussed under Management.

Box 13-1. Complications Associated With Circumcision

- Bleeding
- Infection
- Repeat circumcision
- Phimosis
- Skin bridges
- Urinary retention
- Meatitis
- Inclusion cysts
- Penile lymphedema
- Urethrocutaneous fistulae
- Penile cyanosis
- Penile necrosis
- Wound dehiscence

Parent Counseling

Parents of Newborns

In the newborn period, proper counseling of the parents, including a discussion of the risks and benefits of circumcision, is important. Opponents to neonatal circumcision cite psychological trauma to neonates from so painful a procedure. Local anesthesia minimizes this effect. Parents should be informed about the benefits of circumcision, including a reduction in occurrence of UTIs, STIs, and cancer of the penis and cervix. Problems related to the foreskin itself, such as phimosis, paraphimosis, posthitis, and balanitis, should also be discussed.

It is appropriate to tell parents that boys who are not circumcised in the neonatal period may need to be circumcised later in life. In addition, parents should be told that approximately 10% of circumcised neonates require a second circumcision. Parents should be informed about the risks associated with circumcision in newborns, which are discussed in greater detail in the following text. In older individuals, risks include hemorrhage, infection, and injuries to the penis and urethra.

Research has shown that parents are more influenced by the circumcision status of the father, religion, and race than by physician attitude regarding their ultimate decision about circumcision. Counseling during the second trimester of pregnancy results in no change in parents' decision about circumcision

Parents of Older Infants

The need for circumcision in young male infants who present with UTIs is problematic. The evaluation usually tries to determine the existence of other predisposing conditions that could lead to the UTI. Investigators disagree on the need for circumcision following the initial UTI in uncircumcised boys. No clear-cut evidence indicates that circumcision at this time decreases the incidence of future UTIs, so the decision is parental rather than medical. In older children who present with significant phimosis or paraphimosis, circumcision is usually recommended to prevent recurrences of these problems. Medical management, including the use of topical steroids for phimosis, may obviate the need for surgery in some children. Such treatment involves the daily external application of betamethasone cream from the foreskin tip to the corona glandis for 4 to 6 weeks. A history, including the duration of symptoms and whether the child has had similar episodes in the past, helps formulate the appropriate management.

Management

The medical attitude toward circumcision has changed over the last 40 years, with an initial inclination toward circumcision, followed by a move away from circumcision. The present position on circumcision as described by the AAP Task Force on Circumcision suggests that newborn circumcision has potential medical benefits and advantages as well as disadvantages and risks. When circumcision is considered, the benefits and risks should be explained to the parents, and informed consent should be obtained. Parents should be advised that the frequency with which third-party payers reimburse for circumcisions, particularly for routine circumcisions in the newborn period, has decreased.

Contraindications

Circumcisions should only be performed in completely healthy neonates. Contraindications to circumcision are well defined. Any abnormalities of the penis, such as hypospadias, absence of any portion of the foreskin, or chordee, preclude circumcision. Ambiguous genitalia and prematurity are contraindications. Circumcision should be delayed in premature and ill term newborns until they are ready for discharge. Patients with a personal or family history of bleeding diathesis should not be circumcised. Infants from such families should be assessed for evidence of coagulation problems. If these are present, circumcision should not be carried out. Infants with meningomyelocele should also not be circumcised because it is easier to fit such boys with an external collecting device if they are uncircumcised.

Circumcision Procedure

Numerous techniques are used to perform circumcisions. These procedures may involve clamp techniques with Gomco, Mogen, or Plastibell clamps. Any of these techniques is believed to give comparable results in the hands of trained, experienced operators. Formal surgical excision may also be carried out, usually in older children and adults. Three guidelines should be followed to decrease the incidence of complications: (1) marking of the coronal sulcus in ink, (2) dilation of the preputial wing, and (3) retraction of the foreskin so that the urethral meatus is visualized. This prevents cutting the meatus. Electrocautery should never be used in conjunction with metal clamps because of the danger of extensive injury.

Appropriate anesthesia in newborns undergoing circumcision is now considered the standard of care. The pain and stress of circumcision is evidenced by changes in infant state and behavior. Local anesthesia is the preferred method of pain management. Dorsal penile nerve block, the subcutaneous injections of local anesthetic at the base of the penis, is effective at reducing pain responses during circumcision. Ring block, the subcutaneous circumferential injection of a local anesthetic around the midshaft of the penis, has been shown to be effective and avoids the potential complication of injecting local anesthesia into the dorsal vessels. Topical application of lidocaine/prilocaine cream (EMLA) or oral sucrose solution on a pacifier also reduces pain and its associated stress, but to a lesser extent than local anesthesia. Neonatal circumcision without attention to pain relief is no longer accepted.

Complications

A number of complications are associated with circumcision in newborns (see Box 13-1). The most common complication is **bleeding,** which may occur in 0.2% to 8% of cases. Bleeding can usually be controlled using local pressure. More significant bleeding may require local pressure with 1:1,000 adrenaline-soaked gauze or with the use of other topical agents such as Surgicel. The second most frequently seen complication is **infection,** reported in up to 8% of circumcised infants. Plastibell clamps are associated with a higher incidence of infection than Gomco clamps. Most infections usually respond to local treatment, though intravenous antibiotics should be considered because neonatal sepsis and necrotizing fascitis may occur secondary to infections following circumcision.

Poor cosmetic outcome is also a complication of circumcision. **Phimosis** may occur if removal of the foreskin is insufficient. If the foreskin is inadequately freed up from the inner preputial epithelium, a concealed penis, with the shaft retracted backward into the abdominal wall, may develop. **Skin bridges** may form between the glans and the shaft, leading to accumulation of smegma or the tethering of the erect penis. Most post-circumcision adhesions are reported to resolve at the time of puberty with the onset of masturbation or sexual activity.

In the immediate postsurgical period, urinary retention may occur secondary to tight surgical bandages. This complication can be prevented by applying local pressure rather than tight bandages to obtain hemostasis. Meatitis and meatal ulcers possibly caused by irritation from ammonia or damage to the frenular artery at the time of circumcision are also reported in circumcised males. Inclusion cysts that represent implantation of smegma are also seen. Additional injuries following circumcision may include penile lymphedema, urethrocutaneous fistulae secondary to misplaced sutures, penile cyanosis, and necrosis secondary to tight Plastibell clamps. Wound dehiscence, which involves separation of the penile skin from the mucous membrane, and denudation of the penile shaft may occur more frequently with Gomco than Plastibell clamps.

CASE RESOLUTION

In the case history at the beginning of this chapter, the risks and benefits of circumcision should be discussed with the mother. The father should be encouraged to participate in the decision-making process.

If the parents elect not to have their son circumcised, they should be instructed on the appropriate care of the uncircumcised penis, which involves gentle external washing without retraction of the foreskin.

Selected References

Alanis MC, Lucidi RS. Neonatal circumcision: a review of the world's oldest and most controversial operation. *Obstet Gynecol Surv.* 2004;59:379–395

American Academy of Pediatrics Task Force on Circumcision. Circumcision policy statement. *Pediatrics.* 1999;103:686–693

Anderson JE, Anderson KA. What to tell parents about circumcision. *Contemp Pediatr.* 1999;16:87–103

Auvert B, Taljaard D, Lagarde E, Sobngwi-Tambekou J, Sitta R, Puren A. Randomized, controlled intervention trial of male circumcision for reduction of HIV infection risk: the ANRS 1265 trial. *PLoS Med.* 2005;2:e298

Binner DS, Mastrobattista JM, Day MC, et al. Effect of parental education on decision-making about neonatal circumcision. *South Med J.* 2002;95:457–461

Brady-Fryer B, Wiebe N, Lander JA. Pain relief for neonatal circumcision. *Cochrane Database Syst Rev.* 2004;4:CD004217

Castellsague X, Bosch FX, Munoz N, et al. Male circumcision, penile human papillomavirus infection, and cervical cancer in female partners. *N Engl J Med.* 2002;346:1105–1112

Castellsague X, Peeling RW, Franceschi S, et al. Chlamydia trachomatis infection in female partners of circumcised and uncircumcised adult men. *Am J Epidemiol.* 2005;162:907–916

Fergusson DM, Boden JM, Horwood LJ. Circumcision status and risk of sexually transmitted infection in young adult males: an analysis of a longitudinal birth cohort. *Pediatrics.* 2006;118:1971–1977

Gee WF, Ansell JS. Neonatal circumcision: a ten year overview. With comparison of the Gomco clamp and the plastibell device. *Pediatrics.* 1976;58:824

Langer JC, Coplen DE. Circumcision and pediatric disorders of the penis. *Pediatr Clin North Am.* 1998;45:801–812

National Center for Health Statistics. Trends in circumcision among newborns. Centers for Disease Control and Prevention. www.cdc.gov/nchs/products/pubs/pubd/hestats/circumcisions/circumcisions.htm

Schoen EJ. Ignoring evidence of circumcision benefits. *Pediatrics.* 2006;118:385–387

Wiswell TE, Tencer HL. Circumcision in children beyond the neonatal period. *Pediatrics.* 1993;92:791–793

Nutritional Needs

Wendy T. Hui, MD, and Geeta Grover, MD

CASE STUDY

At a routine health maintenance visit, a mother asks if she may begin giving her 4-month-old daughter solid foods. The infant is taking about 4 to 5 oz of formula every 3 to 4 hours during the day (about 32 oz per day) and sleeps from 12:00 am to 5:00 am without awakening for a feeding. Her birth weight was 7 lbs (3,715 g), and her present weight and height (13 lbs [5,897 g] and 25 in [63.5 cm], respectively) are at the 50th percentile for age. The physical examination, including developmental assessment, is within normal limits.

Questions

1. What are some of the parameters that may be used to decide when infants are ready to begin taking solid foods?
2. Up to what age is breast milk or infant formula alone considered adequate intake for infants?
3. At what age do infants double their birth weight? At what age do they triple their birth weight?
4. What problems are associated with the early introduction of solid foods?

Good nutrition is essential for normal growth and development. The physician plays an important role not only in assessing the growth of children from infancy through adolescence but also in counseling parents regarding the nutritional needs of maturing children. The primary care physician should be knowledgeable about key nutritional concepts in children, including growth patterns and nutritional requirements of normal children and how they vary with age; feeding patterns of infants and children; assessment of nutritional status; and common feeding and nutritional disorders.

Growth Patterns and Nutritional Requirements of Normal Children

Monitoring the growth and nutritional status of infants and children is an integral component of well-child care. The average normal expected increases in weight, height, and head circumference for the first several years of life are listed in Table 14-1.

The energy and nutritional requirements of children vary with age. Postnatal growth is most rapid during the first 6 to 12 months of life. Hence, caloric and protein needs are very high at this time. The average daily energy and protein needs of children from birth to 18 years of age are presented in Table 14-2.

On average, newborns weigh 7.7 lb (3.5 kg), are about 20 in (50 cm) long, and have a head circumference of 14 in (35 cm). They lose about 5% to 10% of their birth weight during the first several days of life and usually regain this weight by the age of 10 to 14 days. During the first several months of life, weight gain serves as an important indicator of children's general well-being. Failure to gain weight during this time may be a clue to a wide variety of problems, ranging from underfeeding to malabsorption. Newborns gain about 30 g/d (roughly 1% of their birth weight per day) for the first 3 months of

Table 14-1. Normal Expected Increase in Weight, Height, and Head Circumference of Infants and Children

Normal Weight Gain in Children	
Age	Expected Weight Increase
0–3 mo	25–35 g/d
3–6 mo	12–21 g/d
6–12 mo	10–13 g/d
1–6 y	5–8 g/d
7–10 y	5–11 g/d
Normal Height Increase in Children	
Age	Expected Height Increase
0–12 mo	10 in/y (25 cm/y)
13–24 mo	5 in/y (12.5 cm/y)
2 y–puberty	2.5 in/y (6.25 cm/y)
Normal Increase in Head Circumference	
Age	Expected Increase in Head Circumference
0–3 mo	2 cm/mo
4–6 mo	1 cm/mo
7–12 mo	.05 cm/mo
Total increase	12 cm in the first year

life, and about 10 to 20 g/d for the rest of the first year. Infants double their birth weight by 6 months of age and triple their birth weight by 12 months of age. On average, children weigh about 10 kg at 1 year of age, 20 kg at 5 years of age, and 30 kg at 10 years of age. A rough

Table 14-2. Energy and Protein Needs of Children

Age (y)	Calories (kcal/kg/d)	Protein (g/kg/d)
0–1	90–120	2.5–3.0
1–7	75–90	1.5–2.5
7–12	60–75	1.5–2.5
12–18	30–60	1.0–1.5

rule of thumb that can be used to estimate the expected weight of a child based on age is 2 × (age in years) + 10 = weight (kg).

Feeding Patterns of Infants and Children

Liquid Foods

Breast milk or one of the several iron-fortified infant formulas provides complete nutrition for infants during the first 4 to 6 months of life. During the first month or two of life, infants take about 2 to 3 oz of formula (approximately 10 minutes on each breast) every 2 to 3 hours.

Because breast milk is more easily digested than formula, it passes out of the stomach in 1½ hours. Formula may take up to 4 hours. Therefore, during the first 4 to 6 weeks of life, breastfed infants want to feed more frequently (8–12 times in 24 hours) than formula-fed infants (6–8 times in 24 hours), with an increased number of nighttime feedings as well. By about 3 to 5 months of age, breastfed and bottle-fed infants do not differ in the number of nighttime feedings, although some breastfed infants continue to awaken out of habit.

Most infants 6 months of age or younger consume about 4 to 5 oz per feeding every 4 to 5 hours. Under routine circumstances, breast milk is preferred to infant formulas because it has emotional,

nutritional, and immunologic advantages. Breastfeeding allows infants and mothers to develop a unique relationship that can be emotionally satisfying (see Chapter 15).

The composition of breast milk varies over time. Colostrum, the first milk produced after delivery, is high in protein, immunoglobulins (Igs), and secretory IgA. Colostrum gradually changes to mature milk 7 to 10 days after delivery. The nutrient content of human milk of mothers who deliver preterm compared with those who deliver at term may vary considerably. Individual assessment may be necessary to determine the appropriateness of breast milk for preterm infants.

Nutritionally, breast milk is uniquely tailored to meet the specific needs of human infants. Human milk provides approximately 20 kcal/oz, the same as routine infant formulas. Table 14-3 compares the composition of human milk and several infant formulas. Human milk has relatively low amounts of protein compared with cow's milk (1% vs 3%), yet the levels are sufficient to provide for satisfactory growth of infants.

Qualitative differences also make human milk more desirable. The casein-whey ratio in human milk is about 40:60, making it easier to digest than most infant formulas, which tend to have higher casein-whey ratios. Lactose is the major carbohydrate of both human and cow's milk, but it is present in higher concentrations in human milk. Fat is the primary source of calories in human milk. The fat in cow's milk, which contains primarily saturated fatty acids, is not as well digested by infants as human milk fat, which is predominantly composed of polyunsaturated fats. Recently, the long-chain polyunsaturated fatty acids docosahexaenoic acid (DHA) and arachidonic acid (ARA) have been added to most infant formulas to simulate the higher levels found in human milk. Although research suggests that DHA and ARA supplementation may enhance visual and

Table 14-3. Composition of Human Milk and Select Infant Formulas (Calories: 20 kcal/oz)

Formula	Protein	Carbohydrate	Fat
Human milk (mature)	40% casein and 60% whey	Lactose	Human milk fat
Cow's milk	80% casein and 20% whey	Lactose	Butterfat
Enfamil Lipil	Nonfat cow's milk and whey	Lactose	Palm olein, soy, coconut, and high-oleic sunflower oils; DHA, ARA
Similac Advance	Nonfat cow's milk and whey	Lactose	High-oleic safflower oil, coconut and soy oils, DHA, ARA
ProSobee Lipil	Soy protein and methionine	Corn syrup solids	Palm olein, soy, coconut, and high-oleic sunflower oils
Isomil Advance	Soy protein and methionine	Corn syrup solids and sucrose	High-oleic safflower oil, soy and coconut oils; DHA, ARA
Nutramigen Lipil	Casein hydrolysate, cystine, tyrosine, tryptophan	Corn syrup solids and cornstarch	Palm olein, soy, coconut, and high-oleic sunflower oils; DHA, ARA
Pregestimil Lipil	Casein hydrolysate, cystine, tyrosine, tryptophan,	Corn syrup solids, modified cornstarch, and dextrose	MCT, high-oleic safflower and soy oils, DHA, ARA
Alimentum Advance	Casein hydrolysate, cystine, tyrosine, tryptophan	Sucrose modified tapioca starch	Safflower oil, MCT, soy oil, DHA, ARA

Abbreviations: DHA, docosahexaenoic acid; ARA, arachidonic acid; MCT, medium-chain triglycerides.

cognitive development in formula-fed infants, the exact degree of effect remains unclear.

Human milk from well-nourished women should provide adequate amounts of all vitamins and other micronutrients. However, vitamin K, vitamin D, iron, and fluoride are not present in sufficient quantities to satisfy all nutritional needs over a prolonged period, and supplementation should be considered. The American Academy of Pediatrics (AAP) recommends that all newborns receive a prophylactic dose of 0.5 to 1 mg of parenteral vitamin K in the immediate newborn period to help prevent bleeding disorders. Even though the vitamin D content of human milk is low compared with cow's milk, infants of healthy mothers have generally not been observed to develop rickets if there is sufficient exposure to sunlight. The newborn requires about 1 minute of exposure to sunlight on the face to produce enough vitamin D. However, adequate sun exposure is difficult to assess, and there are increasing concerns over the harmful effects of sunlight. The most recent AAP recommendation calls for all infants exclusively breastfed and infants taking less than 500 mL (about 17 oz) of vitamin D–fortified formula to receive 200 IU of vitamin D supplementation per day. Although human milk contains less iron than iron-fortified formulas (fortified to about 12 mg/L of iron), the bioavailability of the iron in human milk is greater. Breastfed infants do not need iron supplementation until 6 months of age. Exclusively breastfed infants and infants who are fed ready-to-eat formulas or formulas prepared with bottled water should all receive supplementation with 0.25 mg of fluoride per day starting at 6 months of age (see Chapter 17).

Human milk has several immunologic advantages, which are both allergy-protective and infection-protective, over standard cow's milk–based formulas. Its allergy-protective characteristics are attributed, in part, to the decreased intestinal permeability associated with human milk compared with standard formulas. The host defense factors present in human milk include Igs, complement, and cellular components (eg, macrophages, neutrophils, lymphocytes). Studies have shown that the incidences of both viral and bacterial illnesses are lower in exclusively breastfed infants compared with their formula-fed peers.

Breastfeeding is the recommended method of infant feeding during the first 6 months of life, but it is not always possible and is occasionally contraindicated. Although maternal infection is usually not a contraindication to breastfeeding, maternal human immunodeficiency virus (HIV) infection is one exception to this recommendation in the United States. This is not necessarily true, however, in many developing countries, where the risk of death during the first year of life without breastfeeding is greater than the risk of HIV infection. Antibiotics are generally safe during breastfeeding, but certain other drugs are contraindicated.

Solid Foods

Supplemental foods may be added to infants' diets between the ages of 4 to 6 months. Solid foods should be introduced as soon as infants require the additional calories and are developmentally mature (eg, infant can sit and support the head). Early introduction of solid foods has been associated with an increased incidence of food allergy and may contribute to overeating and obesity. Factors that indicate infants may be ready for solid foods include (1) current weight twice that of birth weight, or about 13 lbs; (2) consumption of more than 32 oz of formula per day; (3) frequent feeding (regularly more than 8–10 times per day or more often than every 3 hours); and (4) persistent dissatisfaction due to hunger.

The quantity of formula should be limited to no more than 32 oz to allow for the introduction of solid foods. An iron-fortified infant cereal, most commonly rice cereal because it does not contain gluten, is usually the first solid food offered to infants. Other single-grained cereals, such as barley cereal or oatmeal, are also appropriate early supplemental foods. Fruits and vegetables may be introduced within a few weeks. The order is not as important as the need to add only one new food at a time—no more than 1 to 2 new foods per week. Meats may be introduced after 6 months of age.

Although commercially prepared infant juices are an important source of vitamin C for infants and may provide a smooth transition to solid foods, excessive juice intake may be associated with diarrhea and growth failure. About 2 oz of apple juice can be given at 4 to 6 months of age. This can be gradually increased to about 4 oz/d. Once infants have accepted the juice, juice can be mixed with a small quantity of cereal and offered to infants with a spoon. Solid foods should not be mixed in the bottle; caregivers should wait until the infant can accept spoon feedings. The vitamin C in the juice increases the bioavailability of the iron in the cereal. It is not unusual for infants to reject their first several spoonfuls of cereal because the tastes and textures are new. If they refuse the feeding, it should be stopped. Solid foods should be reintroduced in 1 week.

Precooked infant cereals, such as rice cereal, can be mixed with a variety of liquids, including breast milk, formula, infant fruit juices, or water. Initially, the cereal should be mixed to a thinner consistency (eg, about 1 tablespoon of cereal to 2 oz of liquid), and once infants have accepted the new taste and texture, the mixture should gradually be worked to a thicker consistency. By about 7 to 8 months of age, infants should be taking 4 to 6 tablespoons of cereal mixed with enough liquid to give the mixture the consistency of mustard. Mixed cereal grains may be introduced to older infants.

A wide variety of commercially prepared baby foods designed to be developmentally appropriate and labeled by stage (ie, first, second, third stage) are available. The jars of different stages contain the amount of food that an infant at a given age should be able to eat at one sitting. This is not always the case, however, and opened jars of baby food may safely be stored in the refrigerator for 2 to 3 days. Infants should not be fed directly from the jar, because saliva on the spoon mixes with the remaining food and digests it, causing it to liquefy. Vegetables and meats may be offered at room temperature but should be warmed slightly for greater palatability. Fruits and desserts may be at room or refrigerator temperature.

First-stage foods, for infants 4 to 6 months of age, include strained infant juices; single-grain cereals; and puréed fruits and vegetables, such as bananas, carrots, and peas. These foods contain no egg, milk, wheat, or citrus, to which some infants may be sensitive. Second-stage foods, for infants from about 6 to 9 months of age, are smooth, mixed-ingredient foods, such as mixed vegetables, or meat dinners, such as chicken noodle. Third-stage foods, or junior foods, are for infants about 9 to 10 months of age who can sit well without support, have some teeth, and have begun self-feeding. These more coarsely textured foods contain a wider variety of nutrients, such as vegetable and meat dinner combinations. Finger foods, such as crackers, cheese wedges, or cookies, can also be introduced by 9 to 10 months of age, once infants have developed a pincer grasp. Most infants are eating the same meals as the rest of the family (table foods) by about 1 year of age. Foods that can easily be aspirated, such as raw carrots, nuts, and hard candies, should be avoided, however, until children are older than 4 years.

Baby foods can be prepared at home as long as they are finely puréed or strained and contain enough liquid to make them easy for infants to swallow. One danger of preparing foods at home is that sugar, salt, or spices can be easily added to make foods palatable to adults. These ingredients are not necessary for infants. In addition, homegrown, home-prepared vegetables may be contaminated with high levels of nitrates (eg, due to contaminated well water) and nitrites (eg, in vegetables such as carrots, beets, and spinach). Nitrates and nitrites have been implicated in the development of methemoglobinemia, especially in infants younger than 6 months. Methemoglobinemia decreases the oxygen-carrying capacity of the blood, leading to anoxic injury and death.

Weaning from the breast or bottle to a cup usually occurs at 6 to 12 months of age but may be delayed up to 18 months of age in some children. Homogenized, vitamin D–fortified cow's milk may be given at 12 months of age. Skim milk or low-fat milk (2% milk fat) should not be given before 2 years of age.

Diet of Children and Adolescents

The caloric and protein needs of children decrease in the second year of life, paralleling the decrease in growth rate during this time. Milk intake also decreases, and may drop to 16 oz/d by 24 to 36 months of age. Except for increased caloric requirements, the diet of school-aged children and adolescents should be similar to that of normal adults. Evidence that foods eaten during childhood may have long-lasting effects on adult health is increasing, and it is important that children develop healthy eating habits early in life. Atherosclerosis, osteoporosis, and obesity are some of the diseases that may have their beginnings during childhood.

A major revision to the US Department of Agriculture's (USDA) dietary guidelines and food pyramid for ages 2 and older was released in 2005. This new pyramid emphasizes physical activity, moderation, gradual improvement, personalization, portionality, and variety in food groups. A child-friendly version of this pyramid has been incorporated in the highly interactive Web site of these new dietary guidelines.

To promote lifelong heart healthy habits, the American Heart Association (AHA) released a statement of dietary recommendations for children and adolescents. It recognizes that children are often offered nutrient-poor foods that are high in fat and sugar and overly processed. The AHA recommendations support the USDA guidelines and include eating fruits and vegetables daily while limiting juice intake, using vegetable oils and soft margarines low in saturated fat and trans-fatty acids instead of butter or other animal fats, eating whole grain rather than refined grain breads and cereals, using nonfat or low-fat milk and dairy products, eating more fish, and reducing salt intake. The AHA also encourages behaviors for parents/caregivers that promote healthy habits for the whole family. These recommendations ask parents/caregivers to choose meal-times, to provide a social context for eating by having regular family meals, to lead by example in their own eating habits, and to allow children to self-regulate food intake and not to force them to finish meals if not hungry.

Children who consume a varied diet do not need routine vitamin supplementation. However, children and teens who are considered "picky eaters," as well as children at nutritional risks, may benefit from supplementation. This includes children and teens who are anorexic or those who follow fad diets, those with chronic diseases, those who consume a vegetarian diet, and those with failure to thrive. A standard pediatric vitamin-mineral supplement should contain no more than the dietary reference intakes of its components. Parents should be counseled to teach their children that the supplements are not candy and to keep them out of reach. Serious overdoses can occur, especially with iron-containing formulations.

Bone health is determined by calcium and vitamin D intake, as well as weight-bearing physical activity. Unfortunately, calcium intake for most US children, and particularly adolescents, is generally below the recommended levels. Barriers to adequate calcium intake may be due to the preference of sweetened juice and soft drinks over milk as well as lactose intolerance in certain populations. Nondairy calcium sources include salmon, white beans, broccoli, and calcium-fortified foods such as orange juice, breakfast cereals, and soy milk. Adequate calcium intake can be achieved by eating 3 (or 4 for adolescents) age-appropriate servings of dairy products or other calcium-rich food per day. In children and adolescents who do not consume adequate amounts of calcium from dietary sources, a calcium supplement is recommended. This can be in the form of a multivitamin in the younger child or in the form of calcium carbonate tablets with or without vitamin D for the adolescent.

Adolescence is a period of tremendous physical and emotional growth, both of which greatly affect nutritional needs and habits. Although their rapid physical growth requires increased energy and nutrients, the common eating habits of teens do not always support their needs. Teens tend to skip meals, eat outside the home, consume fast food and snacks, and experiment with different restrictive diets that are fad diets or various forms of vegetarianism.

Teen athletes also have their own unique nutritional concerns. They want to maximize performance while maintaining the desired physique for their particular sport or weight class. While there are many nutritional supplements such as creatinine, carnitine, various amino acids, and dehydroepiandrosterone that claim to enhance athletic performance, none have thus far been fully evaluated scientifically. Instead, teen athletes should be counseled on the importance of a basic nutrient: water. Proper hydration does enhance performance and prevents heat injury. Approximately 4 to 8 oz of fluid for every 15 minutes of exercise is recommended regardless of actual thirst. Carbohydrate loading before competition is believed to enhance performance; however, this practice has no effects on non-endurance events and may confer only a modest effect for endurance events to prolong time to exhaustion. In counseling a teen athlete, specific questions should also be directed to elicit any unhealthy practices to maintain or lose weight.

Vegetarianism is gaining popularity among adolescents. Reasons for choosing vegetarianism are varied, including health benefits, means for weight loss, animal cruelty concerns, and religious beliefs. It is important to ask the vegetarian their specific restrictions as these relate to their nutritional risks. Semi-vegetarians are those who avoid red meat but eat fish and chicken in moderation. Lacto-ovovegetarians consume animal products such as dairy and eggs but avoid animal flesh. Vegans do not eat any animal products such as dairy, eggs, honey, or gelatin. Those who follow a macrobiotic diet restrict not only animal products but also refined and processed foods, foods with preservatives, and foods that contain caffeine or other stimulants.

A well-planned vegetarian diet can provide for all of the necessary nutrients; however, many teens experiment with vegetarianism in a nonvegetarian household and require guidance. The nutrients that may be deficient in a vegetarian diet are protein, calcium, vitamin D, vitamin B_{12}, iron, and zinc. Protein intake is usually not a concern for lacto-ovovegetarians because eggs and dairy have high-quality proteins. Vegans and macrobiotic followers have a variety of plant-based protein sources from which to choose such as legumes, cereals, nuts, seeds, and fruits. Since vitamin B_{12} is only found in animal-based foods, vegans and macrobiotic followers must ensure adequate intake by taking supplements or consuming vitamin B_{12}-fortified foods such as soy and nut beverages and cereals.

Lastly, familiarity with the latest fad diets is an asset for any primary care practitioner. These diets are usually restrictive in certain nutrients and recommend unusual dietary patterns that are inconsistent with current USDA guidelines. Although there are some suggestions that these diets work for some adults, there are almost no scientific data for children and adolescents. Popular plans include Atkins and other high-fat/low-carbohydrate diets; the Zone Diet, which emphasizes a very specific ratio of protein and carbohydrates; the Ornish diet, which is extremely low fat; the South Beach Diet, which alters the types of carbohydrates for an optimal glycemic index; and the more exotic liquid or detoxification plans. To keep abreast of the latest fads, the reader is referred to the American Dietetic Association's Web site, which maintains an annual review of such popular fad diets.

Evaluation

History

Nutritional assessment begins with a complete dietary history. The dietary assessment should emphasize the quantity, quality, and variety of foods in the diet. Any special or restricted dietary habits should be noted (eg, vegetarian diet). A 3-day food record listing the types and quantities of food eaten throughout the day can be very helpful in evaluating the dietary history.

In addition, the child's routine medical, family, and social history all may influence nutritional status. For example, the economic status of families may affect the variety and type of foods that they may be able to purchase, and the level of education of parents influences their ability to understand the concepts of a healthy diet. Poverty and ignorance regarding nutritional needs are among the most common reasons for malnutrition in children. Family access to food can be estimated by asking parents about how often the family skips meals during the average month. Such information assesses food insecurity within a household. Specific cultural food preferences and feeding practices should also be included in the history.

Physical Examination

Weight, length or height, head circumference, weight for length, and body mass index (BMI) should be measured or calculated routinely and plotted on a longitudinal basis on appropriate growth curves. In addition to the Centers for Disease Control and Prevention charts, charts are available for special populations for which growth is altered such as infants and children with low birth weight and prematurity, Down syndrome, Turner syndrome, and several other chromosomal and genetic disorders. Changes in the rate of growth over time are more useful than a single measurement in time in the assessment of nutritional problems. Calculation of the height age (age for which the child's height is at the 50th percentile), weight age (age for which the child's weight is at the 50th percentile), and ideal weight for actual height may be useful when deviations from normal are noted.

In addition to the overall impression regarding nutritional status, certain findings on physical examination may be characteristic of particular nutritional disorders. The evaluation of the hair, skin, eyes, lips and oral mucosa, dentition, and musculoskeletal system should be emphasized because the examination of these areas is most likely to show the effects of malnutrition. Muscle wasting; hepatosplenomegaly; skeletal deformities; decayed teeth; rough, dry skin; easily pluckable hair; and irritability may all be clues to inadequate nutrition.

Laboratory Tests

Suspected malnutrition or nutrition-related disorders, based on history and physical examination, can be further investigated with laboratory studies. Tests that may be used in the evaluation of anemia, one of the most common nutrition-related disorders seen in children, include a complete blood count, reticulocyte count, serum iron, ferritin, and total iron-binding capacity. Investigation of suspected malnutrition begins with an assessment of protein status, with measures of indicators such as serum albumin, total protein, and prealbumin. Liver function tests and a lipid profile may also be useful in the evaluation of suspected malnutrition. Screening tests that may be used in the evaluation of failure to thrive (FTT) include thyroid function studies, urinalysis, and bone age (see Chapter 117). More specific tests, such as serum vitamin levels (eg, folate or vitamin B_{12} levels in suspected malabsorption) or hormone assays (eg, growth hormone levels in the evaluation of short stature), may be obtained in certain instances.

Common Feeding and Nutritional Problems of Childhood

Several gastrointestinal (GI) problems have been attributed to diet. A small amount of spitting up is seen in most children, especially during the first 6 months of life. However, vomiting can be a sign of several disorders, ranging from viral GI tract infections to more severe illnesses such as pyloric stenosis, urinary tract infection, and GI obstruction (see Chapter 95). Constipation, which is seen more commonly in formula-fed than breastfed infants, may be due to insufficient fluid intake (see Chapter 99). The simple addition of 4 to 6 oz of water to an infant's diet or temporary use of apple or prune juice may solve the problem. Enemas and suppositories should not be recommended routinely.

Chronic nonspecific diarrhea of childhood, or "toddler's diarrhea," may be seen in infants and children 6 months to 5 years of age with low dietary fat intake and excessive fruit juice consumption (see Chapter 98). Failure to absorb sugars, especially sorbitol and fructose, can lead to an osmotic diarrhea.

Underfeeding or a diet that is not nutritionally balanced may result in FTT (see Chapter 117). The opposite problem, obesity, is one of the most common nutritional problems of children in the United States (see Chapter 122). The prevalence of this condition in children 6 to 11 years of age is estimated to be about 20% to 25%. Finally, the eating disorders anorexia nervosa and bulimia nervosa are estimated to affect about 1 in 100 adolescent females 16 to 18 years of age (see Chapter 120).

The "picky eater" is a common parental concern in the primary care setting. For practitioners who work with the Latino population, the child who "no come nada," literally translated as the child "does not eat anything," is a similar common parental concern. Parents can be reassured by their child's normal weight for height or BMI and growth velocity. They should be counseled that it is normal for preschoolers to exert their individuality by limiting food preferences, the fact that it may take up to 10 exposures for a child to accept a new food, the difference between child and adult portion sizes, and the concept that children can self-regulate food intake to sustain normal growth and health.

Nutritional disorders include malnutrition and deficiencies of vitamins and minerals. Iron deficiency anemia is one of the most common nutrition-related problems seen in children and adolescents. Malnutrition is one of the leading causes of childhood morbidity and mortality worldwide. Although primary protein-calorie malnutrition (PCM) is rare in most parts of the United States, surveys conducted on pediatric wards have demonstrated that about one-third of pediatric inpatients with chronic disease have evidence of some degree of PCM. The most common deficits were weight for height below 90% of standard (ie, evidence of acute malnutrition) and height for age below 95% of standard (ie, evidence of chronic malnutrition). The 2 forms of PCM are marasmus (severe caloric depletion) and kwashiorkor (inadequate protein intake). Untreated PCM can result in impaired growth, poor intellectual development, and impaired immune functioning.

CASE RESOLUTION

The infant described in the case history is probably ready to begin some solid foods because she is consuming 32 oz of formula per day and continues to be hungry. In addition, she has reached a weight of 13 lbs and has almost doubled her birth weight. The mother is counseled to begin feeding her daughter a single-grain infant cereal mixed with either formula or juice. (The cereal should be fed by spoon, not given in a bottle.) Within a few weeks, once the infant is taking the cereal well, other first foods such as fruits and vegetables may be introduced.

Selected References

American Academy of Pediatrics. *Pediatric Nutrition Handbook.* 5th ed. Kleinman RE, ed. Elk Grove Village, IL: American Academy of Pediatrics; 2004

American Dietetic Association. Food & Nutrition Information. www.eatright.org/

American Academy of Pediatrics Committee on Drugs. The transfer of drugs and other chemicals into human milk. *Pediatrics.* 2001;108:776–789. http://pediatrics.aappublications.org/cgi/content/full/108/3/776

Balint JP. Physical findings in nutritional deficiencies. *Pediatr Clin North Am.* 1998;45:245–260

Belamarich PE, Ayoob KT. Keeping teenage vegetarians healthy and in the know. *Contemp Pediatr.* 2001;18:89–108

Cahill JB, Wagner CL. Challenges in breastfeeding. *Contemp Pediatr.* 2002;19:94–138

Chandran L. Is there a role for long-chain polyunsaturated fatty acids in infant nutrition? *Contemp Pediatr.* 2003;20:107–124

Chandran L, Gelfer P. Breastfeeding: the essential principles. *Pediatr Rev.* 2006;27:409–417

Fiocchi A, Assa'ad A, Bahna S; Adverse Reactions to Foods Committee; American College of Allergy, Asthma and Immunology. Food allergy and the introduction of solid foods to infants: a consensus document. *Ann Allergy Asthma Immunol.* 2006;97:10–21

Fiorino KN, Cox JM. Nutrition and growth. In: Robertson J, Shilkofski N, eds. *The Harriet Lane Handbook: A Manual for Pediatric House Officers.* 17th ed. St Louis, MO: Mosby; 2005:525–608

Garcia RS. No come nada. *Health Affairs.* 2004;23:215–219

Gartner LM, Greer FR, American Academy of Pediatrics Section on Breastfeeding and Committee on Nutrition. Prevention of rickets and vitamin D deficiency: new guidelines for vitamin D intake. *Pediatrics.* 2003;111:908–910

Gidding SS, Dennison BA, Birch LL, et al. Dietary recommendations for children and adolescents: a guide for practitioners: consensus statement from the American Heart Association. *Circulation.* 2005;112:2061–2075

Greer FR, Krebs MD, American Academy of Pediatrics Committee on Nutrition. Optimizing bone health and calcium intake of infants, children, and adolescents. *Pediatrics.* 2006;117:578–585

Heird WC. Progress in promoting breast-feeding, combating malnutrition, and composition and use of infant formula, 1981–2006. *J Nutr.* 2007;137:499S–502S

Kleinman R. Chronic nonspecific diarrhea of childhood. *Nestle Nutr Workshop Ser Pediatr Program.* 2005;56:73–79, discussion 79–84

Maternal and Child Health Bureau, US Department of Health and Human Services. *Growth Charts Training: Using the CDC Growth Charts for Children With Special Health Care Needs.* http://depts.washington.edu/growth/. Accessed April 11, 2007

Ogden CL, Kuczmarski RJ, Flegal KM, et al. Centers for Disease Control and Prevention 2000 growth charts for the United States: improvements to the 1977 National Center for Health Statistics version. *Pediatrics.* 2002;109:45–60

US Department of Agriculture. Center for Nutrition Policy and Promotion. MyPyramid for kids. www.mypyramid.gov/kids/index.html. Accessed April 10, 2007

Breastfeeding

Julie E. Noble, MD

CASE STUDY

A 25-year-old female, pregnant with her first child, comes into your office with her husband for a prenatal visit. She would like to know what advice you can give her regarding breastfeeding. She expects a normal delivery, has had no breast surgery, is not on any medications, but does smoke cigarettes occasionally. She plans to return to work when the baby is 4 months old.

Questions
1. What is the normal physiology of lactation?
2. What are the benefits of breastfeeding?
3. What are the contraindications to breastfeeding?
4. What management maximizes a mother's success at breastfeeding?
5. How do you manage some of the common problems that may arise during breastfeeding?

Breast milk is the natural food source for human infants. It is a complete nutritional product made specifically for human infants, and all **formulas** are incomplete attempts to try to replicate it. **Breast milk** is made of water, fat, lactose-containing carbohydrates and protein, as well as vitamins, **immunoglobulins,** enzymes, hormones, and even phagocytes and lymphocytes. It is a dynamic fluid that changes in composition as the infant grows. From the early **colostrum,** which is high in lactose and protein and very immunologically active, it matures to a substance with lower protein in the form of whey and casein.

Epidemiology

In previous generations, infants were totally dependent on breastfeeding from their mother or a wet nurse for their survival. When artificial feeding was attempted at foundling hospitals in Europe in the late 18th century, the infant mortality rate was as high as 85%. The first **formulas** of cow's milk came on the market in the late 1800s. With poor mothers in cities working outside the home and upper-class mothers choosing not to breastfeed, the breastfeeding rates declined over the course of the 19th century. **Formula** feeding became the norm. But current scientific understanding of the many benefits of breastfeeding has prompted a push to again promote breastfeeding as the preferred food source for infants.

In the United States today only 68% of mothers begin breastfeeding and 50% of these stop early. The **Healthy People 2010 Initiative** includes a national agenda that calls for an increase in the rate of breastfeeding. The American Academy of Pediatrics, in its policy statement Breastfeeding and the Use of Human Milk (2005), also endorses breastfeeding and delineates the physician responsibility to promote and support it.

Anatomy and Physiology of Lactation

During pregnancy the breast responds to **estrogen, placental lactogen, prolactin,** and **progesterone** by enlarging. There is an increase in breast lobules and alveoli where milk is produced; and the **ductile system** grows, leading to 10 to 15 milk duct openings in the nipple. The nipples develop and the surrounding areolas enlarge. Prolactin from the anterior pituitary is inhibited by progesterone and estrogen. After delivery with the drop in these hormones, the **prolactin** is free to stimulate increased milk production. With the stimulus of suckling, **oxytocin** is released from the posterior pituitary and causes contraction of myoepithelial cells, which squeeze milk from the alveoli. Production of **breast milk** is dependent on infant suckling. The more the infant feeds and the more the breast is effectively emptied, the more milk will be produced.

Benefits of Breastfeeding

For the infant, the benefits to being breastfed are myriad. Studies have demonstrated that breastfed infants have a decreased incidence and severity of **infectious illnesses** including diarrhea, respiratory infections, otitis media, bacterial meningitis, and urinary tract infections. There have also been studies demonstrating better performance on **cognitive testing** among breastfed infants. Breastfeeding in infancy reduces the later incidence of **atopy, allergies, asthma, obesity, diabetes,** and even childhood **cancer.** Decreased rates of **sudden infant death syndrome** (see Chapter 47) have also been documented.

For the mother, an immediate benefit to breastfeeding is oxytocin-induced decreased postpartum blood loss and enhanced infant bonding. Lactation amenorrhea may serve subsequently as birth control. Breastfeeding has also been associated with decreased risk of breast cancer, ovarian cancer, and osteoporosis.

Societal benefits from breastfeeding include decreased annual health care costs. A decreased incidence of illness among infants would enable mothers to miss fewer workdays, benefiting the workplace. In addition there would be a reduction in environmental waste from bottles and **formula** containers.

Contraindications

The true contraindications to breastfeeding are few, but need to be addressed. If an infant has **galactosemia** as detected by newborn screening, and is therefore unable to metabolize lactose or galactose, he may not breastfeed. Infants can also inherit defects in protein metabolism that may call for a special diet, precluding breastfeeding.

Maternal infections prohibiting breastfeeding include active, untreated tuberculosis, human immunodeficiency virus, and human T-cell lymphotropic virus types I and II. If herpetic vesicles are present on the breast, the mother should not breastfeed.

Many medications are safe for a mother to use while breastfeeding, but each should be reviewed for potential contraindications before administering because most medications pass into **breast milk.** Chemotherapeutic agents, antimetabolites, and radioactive isotopes are all contraindicated for breastfeeding. Drugs of abuse are definitely contraindicated in a breastfeeding mother, although a mother with a history of drug use may benefit from breastfeeding as long as her toxicology results are negative and closely monitored.

Breastfeeding Management

The management of breastfeeding should begin in the prenatal period. The pregnant woman should be counseled by her pediatrician or obstetrician regarding the benefits of breastfeeding and her history reviewed for potential contraindications. If she commits to breastfeeding before the baby is born, she is more likely to be successful.

At the time of delivery if there are no complications, the infant should be dried, assigned Apgar scores and, after a screening physical examination, be placed skin-to-skin on the mother's abdomen or chest for warmth and contact. He will find his way to the breast and latch on. This early breastfeeding experience will greatly facilitate further breastfeeding. The infant should not be separated from the mother except for medical reasons.

During the hospital stay, the infant should breastfeed every 1 to 2 hours on both breasts for as long as he wants. Without pacifiers or supplemental feeds, the infant will learn to breastfeed more quickly. The mother should be counseled regarding appropriate latch-on, positioning of the infant, and manual expression of milk. Breastfeeding support should be available. Generally the infant should nurse at least 8 times a day. The infant should be monitored for weight, evidence of jaundice, and urination and stools patterns. A successful breastfeeding infant should urinate 3 to 5 times per day and stool 3 to 4 times per day by 3 to 5 days of age and not lose more than 7% of his birth weight. By day 5 to 7 of life he should urinate 4 to 6 times per day and pass 3 to 6 stools per day.

Vitamin K (1.0 mg intramuscularly) is indicated within the first 6 hours of life to prevent hemorrhagic disease of the newborn. The only supplement to breastfeeding that is needed is Vitamin D 200 IU daily after 2 months of age to prevent rickets.

After hospital discharge the breastfeeding infant should be seen by his physician at day 3 to 5 of life and again at 2 weeks of age to support breastfeeding. Again, weight, feeding schedules, voiding and stooling patterns, and jaundice should be evaluated. The mother's breasts should be examined and feeding observed.

The infant can exclusively breastfeed until he is 6 months of age. At that time an iron source is needed, and iron-fortified cereal can be given with a gradual introduction of other pureed foods. Breastfeeding should continue until at least 1 year of age or as long as the mother and infant are content.

Sometimes pediatricians will be consulted about weaning the breastfed infant. There is no age at which weaning must occur, and in many cultures toddlers nurse until the age of 3 to 4 years. While some infants readily give up the breast, others are more reluctant to do so. There are no easy solutions to dealing with a reluctant toddler, and some suggestions include the adage, "Don't offer and don't refuse." Lactation consultants may be a valuable resource at this time.

Potential Problems

Attachment

Latching-on is the first step that is essential for successful breastfeeding. If an infant is not latching effectively, a medical professional should evaluate the mother-infant dyad for problems. Causes can include inverted nipples, flat nipples, ankyloglossia, small mandible, or nipple confusion. Treatment may consist of help with positioning, nipple shields, frenectomy, or syringe feeding until the infant learns to latch.

Sore Nipples

Breastfeeding should not be painful. If the mother is experiencing pain, the infant is probably not latching correctly. The infant should be positioned on the breast to get as much of the areola in the mouth as possible. Cracked nipples can be treated with lanolin and/or hydrogel pads and repositioning, and/or with expressing milk using a breast pump. Occasionally sore nipples are secondary to a candidal infection and should be treated with an antifungal medications such as nystatin.

Engorgement/Mastitis

When there is milk stasis for any reason, a mother may become **engorged.** The breast will appear full, firm, lumpy, and tender. Treatment is to empty the breast, and the infant is the most effective breast pump. Warm packs before feeding can be helpful. Sometimes an electric breast pump expedites emptying, softens the breast, and facilitates infant latching.

If a mother develops **mastitis,** a breast infection with erythema and fever, she should continue to breastfeed. Again emptying the breast is important. Oral antibiotics and rest are mandatory. There are isolated reports of breastfed infants acquiring a bacterial infection if the mother has mastitis. Mastitis involves cellulitis of the breast, and the organisms are usually not in the ducts or **breast milk.** Infants may refuse to breastfeed on an affected breast if the taste of the milk is affected. The mother may then elect to breastfeed the infant on the unaffected side and pump the affected breast.

Hyperbilirubinemia/Dehydration

If infants lose more than 7% of their birth weight, they are at risk for becoming significantly dehydrated and have a higher likelihood of significant jaundice. Increased intake is necessary, and the frequency of feeds should be increased. If infants are not latching on well, expressed **breast milk** can be given by syringe. Infants should be closely monitored and **formula** can be offered after breastfeeding if supply is insufficient. The mother should be assisted in increasing her milk supply. This may be accomplished using a breast pump because greater demand increases supply. If the infant appears jaundiced, blood levels of bilirubin should be obtained. Physiological jaundice is related to hepatic immaturity with decreased conjugation of bilirubin as well as decreased excretion. Breastfeeding infants tend to have higher levels of unconjugated bilirubin. Increased feeding will frequently resolve the problem as hydration status improves and frequency of stooling increases. The infant should be evaluated for any other causes of jaundice and should be followed closely (see Chapter 101).

Resources for the Breastfeeding Mother

Many hospitals and health care organizations have lactation specialists who can assist nursing mothers and answer questions related to lactation. Health facilities may loan **electric breast pumps** to new mothers to help establish a good supply of milk. Some mothers may choose to purchase such pumps, especially if they are planning to continue to breastfeed after returning to work or to have additional children.

Access to information can also be obtained through community agencies or national organizations such as the **La Leche League** (www.lalecheleague.org) or the Special Supplemental Nutrition Program for Women, Infants, and Children (WIC) program. Such agencies provide a resource to the clinician in assisting mothers with breastfeeding.

CASE RESOLUTION

In the case presented, the mother should be informed of the many benefits of breastfeeding to the baby, herself, and society. She should be encouraged to breastfeed because she has no contraindications. You recommend she stop cigarette smoking completely for her own health as well as the baby's. In the hospital she should request she be given her infant to breastfeed in the delivery room and continue to room-in to breastfeed every 2 hours. Reassure her that both the hospital and your office will give her support and guidance with breastfeeding. Even though she is anticipating going back to work, she should initially breastfeed exclusively. She can begin to introduce the bottle with pumped breast milk at 2 months of age. Her workplace should provide an area for nursing mothers to pump and refrigerate their breast milk. You encourage her to explore the lactation policies at her place of work.

Selected References

American Academy of Pediatrics, American College of Obstetricians and Gynecologists. *Breastfeeding Handbook for Physicians.* Schanler R, Dooley S, Gartner LM, Krebs NF, Mass SB, eds. Elk Grove Village, IL: American Academy of Pediatrics; 2005

American Academy of Pediatrics. Policy statement: breastfeeding and the use of human milk. *Pediatrics.* 2005;115:496–511

Brenner M. You can provide efficient, effective, and reimbursable breastfeeding support—here's how. *Contemp Pediatr.* 2005;22:66–76

Chandran L, Gelfer P. Breastfeeding: the essential principles. *Pediatr Rev.* 2006;27:409–417

Lawrence RA, Lawrence RM. *Breastfeeding: A Guide for the Medical Profession.* Philadelphia, PA: Elsevier; 2005

Schanler R, ed. Breastfeeding 2001. Part I: the evidence for breastfeeding. *Pediatr Clin North Am.* 2001;48:(entire issue)

Schanler R, ed. Breastfeeding 2001. Part II: the management of breastfeeding. *Pediatr Clin North Am.* 2001;48:(entire issue)

Wellstart International. *Lactation Management Self-Study Modules, Level I.* 2nd ed. San Diego, CA: Wellstart International; 2004

Sleep: Normal Patterns and Common Disorders

Geeta Grover, MD

CASE STUDY

During a routine 6-month health maintenance visit, a mother states that although her 6-month-old son falls asleep very easily at about 10 pm every night while breastfeeding, he wakes every 2 to 3 hours and cries until she nurses him back to sleep. A review of the dietary history reveals that the infant is breastfed about every 3 hours and was begun on rice cereal 2 weeks ago. His immunizations are current. The boy has no medical problems, and his physical examination is normal.

Questions

1. How old are most infants when they can begin to sleep through the night (at least 5 hours at a stretch) without a feeding?
2. What factors contribute to frequent nighttime wakings during infancy?
3. What advice can be given to parents to facilitate an infant's sleeping through the night?
4. What are sleep disturbances experienced by older children and adolescents?

Sleep disorders are common during infancy and childhood. Getting children to go to bed, fall asleep, stay asleep, and stay in bed can be no small challenge. Parents frequently ask pediatricians about sleep-related problems at routine health maintenance visits. Age-appropriate suggestions on how to help children sleep well are usually welcomed by parents.

Epidemiology

Sleep problems are one of the most common concerns seen in pediatric practice. Bedtime struggles and frequent night wakings occur in 20% to 25% of children younger than 3 years. In preschool-aged children, nighttime fears (eg, fear of noises, fear of the dark) or separation anxiety often contribute to these problems. Estimates of parent-reported sleep problems in school-aged children range between 11% and 40%. As children get older, nightmares and night terrors may contribute to night wakings. About 5% of individuals experience nightmares, which usually begin before the age of 10 years and are seen more often in girls than in boys. Night terrors are a specific form of partial night waking from deep sleep that may begin during the preschool years. The incidence in children is reported to be between 1% and 4%, with the greatest frequency between 5 and 7 years of age. Such terrors are more common in boys than in girls, and a familial tendency has been reported. Febrile illness and obstructive sleep apnea may be predisposing factors.

In most Western countries, children are expected to sleep in their own beds. However, in many cultures, it is not uncommon for infants and young children to sleep in their parents' bed (the "family bed"). Bedsharing in infants younger than 10 to 12 weeks is associated with a higher incidence of sudden infant death syndrome, especially if the mother smokes. Accidental asphyxia from overlaying or the presence of soft bedding or overheating may contribute to bedsharing-related deaths. Parents should always be advised about safe sleeping practices (see Chapter 47). In older infants and children, cosleeping is not a problem in and of itself, and the decision to cosleep, like the decision to breastfeed or bottle-feed, is an entirely personal one. Most infants who share a bed with their parents have sleep-onset associations. Therefore, parents who share a bed with their young children commonly have to lie down with them for 20 to 30 minutes to get them to fall asleep. Several studies have shown that cosleeping infants are 2 to 3 times more likely to have night awakenings than those who sleep alone. Furthermore, infants who are both breastfeeding and bedsharing sleep the shortest periods prior to awakening. Parents who only plan on cosleeping with their infants for a limited period will need a clear transition plan, such as ending this practice by 5 to 6 months of age, before the infants are old enough to object excessively. For children with sleep problems, bedsharing is not a good solution. However, in the absence of any preexisting sleep problems or psychological concerns, cosleeping, as a lifestyle choice, has not been associated with any long-term developmental, behavioral, or psychological problems in the cosleeping children.

Clinical Presentation

Parents may raise concerns about their child's sleep pattern during a routine health maintenance visit. Because some parents may be reluctant to "bother" their physician with such seemingly minor concerns, the physician should routinely question parents about their children's sleep patterns and offer anticipatory guidance as appropriate.

Pathophysiology

To understand disturbances associated with sleep, the physiology of normal sleep and the development of normal sleep behavior in children must be understood.

Sleep States

Normal sleep has 2 distinct states, **rapid eye movement (REM)** and **non–rapid eye movement (NREM)** sleep. Rapid eye movement sleep develops at about 29 weeks' gestation and then persists throughout life. It is an active, lighter stage of sleep that occurs in association with rapid eye movements. Other features of REM sleep include suppression of muscle tone; rapid, irregular pulse and respiratory rate; and body twitches. Dreams occur during REM sleep. The electroencephalogram (EEG) pattern of REM sleep is very similar to stage 1 NREM sleep.

Non–rapid eye movement sleep begins at about 32 to 35 weeks' gestation. During NREM sleep, pulse and respiratory rates are slower and more regular, and body movements are minimal. Most of the restorative functions of sleep occur during this state. After the first several months of life, NREM sleep may be divided into 4 stages ranging from drowsiness to very deep sleep. Each stage represents a progressively deeper state of sleep and has a characteristic EEG tracing: stage 1 has low-voltage, fast activity; stage 2 is notable for the presence of sleep spindles and K complexes against a low-voltage background; and stages 3 and 4 are identified by varying amounts of high-amplitude, slow waves known as delta waves.

The Sleep Cycle

Rapid eye movement and NREM sleep together make up the sleep cycle. Typically, the deepest sleep takes place during the first several hours of the night, with lighter stages of NREM sleep and REM sleep occurring during most of the rest of the night. Although sleep stages are the same in both infants and adults, several differences concerning the onset and duration of REM and NREM sleep between infants and adults exist. First, the sleep cycle is shorter in infants (50–60 minutes) than in adults (90–100 minutes), which means that infants have more periods of active REM sleep compared with adults. Second, the total amount of time spent in REM sleep decreases with increasing age. Term newborns spend about 50% of their total sleep time in REM sleep (up to 80% in premature infants); this decreases to about 30% by 3 years of age and to 20% by adulthood. Third, infants may have very little REM latency, entering their first REM cycle very shortly after falling asleep. Adults, in comparison, generally enter their first REM period about 90 minutes after the onset of sleep.

Sleep-Wake Patterns

Sleep patterns follow a normal developmental sequence in children; the amount of sleep children need changes with maturation (Figure 16-1). Healthy term newborns sleep 16 to 17 hours per day. Because they are unable to sleep for more than a few hours at a time, sleeping and waking periods are fairly evenly distributed throughout the day and night. Many infants are able to sleep through the night (at least 5 hours uninterrupted) by the age of 3 months; most infants are capable of this by 4 months. Brief arousals are a normal part of the sleep cycle at all ages, but children should be able to return to sleep on their own without requiring parents' attention. Children should definitely be able to fall asleep on their own by the age of 4 to 6 months. Otherwise, parental participation to fall asleep becomes required at every awakening throughout the night.

By 12 months of age, infants sleep about 14 hours per day, divided into 2 naps during the day and a period of about 10 hours at night. During the second year of life, most children stop napping in the

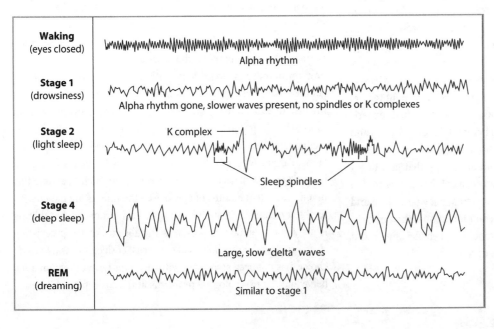

Figure 16-1. Typical sleep patterns in childhood. (Reproduced with permission from Ferber R. *Solve Your Child's Sleep Problems.* New York, NY: Simon & Schuster; 1985:19.)

morning. By 2 years of age, they require about 13 hours of sleep per day (1–2 hours in an afternoon nap and 11–12 hours at night). Most children take an afternoon nap until 3 years of age, and some children continue this until 5 years of age. The amount of nighttime sleep children need gradually continues to decline, decreasing from about 12 hours during the preschool years to about 8 to 9 hours during adolescence.

Sleep Abnormalities

The etiology of sleep disorders can be complex, involving the interaction of children's temperamental characteristics, psychosocial stressors in the home, parental childrearing philosophies, and the developmental nature of normal sleep states and sleep cycles.

Differential Diagnosis

The differential diagnosis of sleep disorders may be distinguished by problems associated with falling asleep or frequent night wakings (Box 16-1). Falling asleep may present 2 types of difficulties: problems associated with settling children to sleep and bedtime refusal.

In infants, **inappropriate sleep-onset associations** are the most common reason for difficulty settling to sleep. These infants require parental participation (eg, holding, rocking, feeding) to fall asleep. They have not learned the critical skills of self-calming and initiating sleep on their own. Because these infants do not have the self-soothing behaviors necessary to fall back asleep after normal nighttime arousals, they may also have nighttime wakings. Brief arousals are a normal component of sleep. Nighttime wakings are different, because parents' participation is needed to resettle children. The difficulty that the children experience falling back to sleep on their own, not the waking itself, is the problem.

An example of an inappropriate sleep-onset association is the child who needs to be breastfed or bottle-fed to fall asleep. The term **trained night feeder** has been coined to describe children who need to be fed before going back to sleep after normal nighttime awakenings. Although they are developmentally old enough to receive all nutrition during the day, they have become conditioned to require nighttime feedings. These children are often breastfed or bottle-fed until they fall asleep and only then placed in the crib. They are conditioned to require feeding to initiate sleep, and when they experience normal nighttime arousals, they require the breast or bottle to go back to sleep.

The term **trained night crier** refers to children who, like trained night feeders, lack the self-comforting and self-initiating skills necessary to fall asleep on their own. Trained night criers awaken, cry, and want to be held, comforted, or entertained before they can go back to sleep.

Acute illness may also be a cause of sleep disturbances. Children with otitis media may awaken at night because of pain. They may continue to experience awakenings after the infection has resolved, however, and require comforting or some sort of attention to fall asleep again.

In children between the ages of 9 and 18 months, **separation** and **separation anxiety** may also affect sleep patterns. Children may cry

Box 16-1. Practical Approach to the Differential Diagnosis of Sleep Disorders in Children
Difficulty Falling Asleep
Circadian and sleep schedule disturbances
• Irregular sleep/wake patterns
• Advanced sleep phase
• Delayed sleep phase
• Regular but inappropriate sleep schedules without phase shifts (eg, late evening naps)
Habits, associations, and expectations
• Inappropriate sleep-onset associations
• Bedtime refusal/bedtime struggles
• Poor or inconsistent limit setting
Overstimulation
Psychosocial
• Separation anxiety
• Nighttime fears (eg, fears of the dark, monsters)
• Family and social stresses
Medical
• Acute illness
• Underlying medical problems
• Medications (eg, antihistamines, stimulants, codeine, anticonvulsants)
Nighttime Waking
Normal variation (eg, breastfed infant)
Habits, associations, and expectations
• Inappropriate sleep-onset associations (eg, age-inappropriate night wakings for feeding)
Psychosocial
• Nighttime fears
• Family and social stresses
Medical
• Acute illness
• Underlying medical problem
• Medications
Nightmares
Arousal disorders (eg, night terrors, sleepwalking, and sleep talking)
Miscellaneous Sleep Disorders
Intrinsic sleep disorders
• Narcolepsy
• Sleep apnea (obstructive or central)
• Restless leg syndrome
• Periodic leg movements
Sleep-wake transition disorders (eg, head banging, rocking)

when parents leave the room and have difficulty settling to sleep. Ability to climb out of the crib or bed can be associated with nighttime wakings in older toddlers. The transition from a crib to a bed is usually made between 2 and 3 years of age. Children who can climb out of their cribs or beds may come out of their rooms repeatedly for drinks of water, trips to the bathroom, or to sleep in the parents' bed.

Such factors as nighttime fears of the dark influence sleep behaviors during the preschool years (3–5 years of age). Children's growing needs for autonomy and control over their environment may lead to bedtime refusals during both the toddler and preschool years.

Disorders of the sleep-wake cycle may contribute to sleep schedule irregularities. Circadian rhythms govern the regularity and degree of wakefulness and sleepiness. The circadian clock inherent in humans is not an exact 24-hour pattern but can be modified or entrained onto one by environmental cues. Regular and consistent structure needs to be provided by parents because development of children's sleep-wake rhythms depends on an interaction of the child's inherent biological rhythms with the environment. Entrainment requires predictable occurrence of time cues such as light and dark, mealtime, and bedtime. A consistent waking time in the morning is one of the most important of these cues.

Irregular sleep-wake cycles may be seen in children living in chaotic environments with irregular mealtimes and sleep-wake schedules. A delayed sleep phase and regular but inappropriate sleep-wake schedule are the most common forms of sleep rhythm disturbance. Children with **delayed sleep phase** have a resetting of their circadian rhythm; they are not sleepy at bedtime and have excessive morning sleepiness. This is a common problem because the inherent circadian clock has a cycle closer to 25, not 24, hours. This clock has not been entrained to a 24-hour schedule in these children.

Examples of **regular but inappropriate sleep-wake schedules** include children who nap at the "wrong" time (eg, a child who regularly naps at 7 pm for 1 hour and then has trouble going to bed at 9 pm) and infants who seem to have day and night confused. These children sleep most of the day and stay up most of the night.

Night terrors (pavor nocturnus), **sleepwalking** (somnambulism), and **sleeptalking** (somniloquy) are all forms of partial awakenings that occur during deep or stage 4 NREM sleep, most often during the transition from stage 4 NREM sleep to the first REM sleep period. Sleepwalking and sleeptalking usually occur during the school-aged years, whereas night terrors begin during the preschool years.

Both nightmares and night terrors may begin during the preschool years and may continue throughout childhood. Night terrors are different from nightmares and occur during a different stage of the sleep cycle (Table 16-1). With night terrors, children usually sit up in bed and cry or scream inconsolably for up to 15 minutes. They may appear dazed and have signs of autonomic arousal such as tachycardia, tachypnea, and sweating. These children cannot be consoled. When they finally go back to sleep, they do not remember the event in the morning. Because parents are often frightened by the experience, they may think the child is having a seizure or is suffering from an emotional disturbance and may seek medical advice. Although attacks may be precipitated by stressful events or fatiguing daytime activities, night terrors do not indicate excessive stress or emotional disturbance in children's lives unless they recur.

Nightmares usually occur during the last third of the night during REM sleep, whereas night terrors more often take place during the early part of the night. Nightmares are scary dreams that

Table 16-1. Nightmares Versus Night Terrors		
Characteristic	*Nightmare*	*Night Terror*
Time of night	Late	Early, usually within 4 hours of bedtime
Sleep stage	Rapid eye movement sleep	Partial arousal from deep non–rapid eye movement sleep
State of child	Scared, but consolable	Disoriented, confused, and inconsolable
Memory of event	Clear recall of dream	Usually none
Return to sleep	Reluctant because of fear	Easily, unless fully awakened
Management	Reassure child	Reassure parents

may awaken children, who can often remember them. Children can usually be consoled by parents but are reluctant to go back to sleep because of their fears.

Excessive daytime sleepiness can be a symptom of medical problems such as depression, sleep apnea, or illness. Viral illness is perhaps the most common medical cause of such sleepiness in children. Inadequate sleep at night may also be a potential cause of sleepiness during the day. Narcolepsy, a disorder of excessive sleepiness, is characterized by an overwhelming desire to sleep during the daytime despite adequate sleep at night. Its symptoms include excessive daytime sleepiness, cataplexy, sleep paralysis, and hypnagogic hallucinations. Cataplexy is an abrupt loss of muscle tone that is usually precipitated by an emotional reaction such as laughter or anger. Sleep paralysis is an inability to move or speak that occurs as patients fall asleep or awaken. Hypnagogic hallucinations, which can be visual or auditory, occur while falling asleep.

Narcolepsy affects about 0.05% to 0.1% of the general population. The prevalence increases to 50% of family members when the family history is positive. The exact genetic basis of inheritance is unknown. The age of onset is usually between 10 and 20 years. The diagnosis is often delayed or missed for months to years in some cases because not all symptoms may be present initially. Diagnosis is important because pharmacologic therapy with central nervous system (CNS) stimulants may provide some symptomatic relief.

Obstructive sleep apnea syndrome (OSAS) in children is a disorder of breathing during sleep. It is characterized by prolonged partial upper airway obstruction and/or intermittent complete obstruction (obstructive apnea) that disrupts normal gas exchange and normal sleep patterns. Risk factors for OSAS include adenotonsillar hypertrophy, obesity, craniofacial anomalies, and neuromuscular disorders. Obstructive sleep apnea syndrome is thought to be secondary to a combination of adenotonsillar hypertrophy and reduced neuromuscular tone of the upper airway during sleep. Large tonsils and adenoids alone do not necessarily indicate that the child has OSAS. Symptoms include nightly snoring (often with intermittent pauses or gasps), disturbed sleep, and daytime neurobehavioral problems. Obstructive sleep apnea syndrome should be distinguished from

primary snoring, which is defined as snoring without obstructive apnea, arousals from sleep, or abnormalities in gas exchange. Obstructive sleep apnea syndrome can not only disturb the quality of sleep but can also cause potentially serious complications such as failure to thrive and, in severe cases, cor pulmonale.

Restless leg syndrome, or periodic leg movements, is a recently described condition characterized by uncomfortable creeping or crawling feelings mainly occurring in the lower extremities, when the child is resting or inactive and relieved by movement. The condition may be attributed to growing pains in younger children (see Chapter 91) and can be associated with delayed sleep onset.

Evaluation

History

Evaluation of children with sleep difficulties begins with a thorough, detailed sleep history taken from both parents and children, if old enough (Questions Box). The use of a specific screening questionnaire, such as the Children's Sleep Habits Questionnaire by Judith Owens, MD, may facilitate the evaluation. It is designed to screen for the most common sleep problems in children aged 4 to 12 years and is available online at www.kidzzzsleep.org. It is not intended to be used to diagnose specific sleep disorders, but rather to identify children possibly needing further evaluation.

Questions

Sleep

- Does the child have regular nap times and bedtimes, or do these depend on changing parental schedules?
- What time does the child go to bed?
- What does the child do in the hour before bedtime? Is there a consistent bedtime routine?
- Where does the child sleep (eg, ask about cosleeping, noise, temperature)?
- Is the child able to fall asleep on his or her own, or does he or she require the parent's participation?
- Does the child require feeding or fluids at night?
- When does the problem occur relative to bedtime and what does the child do (detailed explanation)?
- How often does the problem occur?
- How long has the child been having sleep problems?
- How does the parent respond?
- Does the child snore?
- When does the child wake up in the morning? Is the child difficult to awaken?
- Is the child sleepy during the day?
- How much caffeine does the child consume (eg, in coffee, tea, soda, chocolate)?
- Is the child taking any medications?
- Is there a family history of sleep disturbances?
- Is there any stress within the home due to marital or financial difficulties that may affect the home environment and cause the child to be anxious or stressed?

Evaluation should also include an assessment of children's temperament and psychological well-being. Children's developmental status and level of function should also be evaluated. Children with developmental, neurologic, and psychological concerns have higher rates of sleep disturbances. For example, it is estimated that 25% to 50% of children with attention-deficit/hyperactivity disorder seen in clinical practice will have sleep problems, especially difficulties in initiating and maintaining sleep.

Physical Examination

Physical examination is important to rule out organic causes of sleep difficulties. Special attention should be paid to the airway and nervous system. Acute illness (eg, otitis media), obstructive sleep apnea resulting from adenoidal or tonsillar hypertrophy (most commonly), colic, gastroesophageal reflux, and any CNS disease or abnormality may all alter the sleep-wake cycle.

Laboratory Tests

In most cases, a detailed history and physical examination should be sufficient to establish the reason for the sleep disturbance. Laboratory assessment is usually not necessary. Further evaluation, when warranted, should be tailored to the child's clinical presentation. An EEG may be useful if a central abnormality such as a seizure disorder is suspected. Polysomnography, the simultaneous monitoring of EEG, electrocardiogram, chin muscle tone, eye movements, and respirations during a night of sleep in a sleep laboratory, may be very useful in certain children when significant sleep disturbances such as nocturnal seizures, narcolepsy, or OSAS is suspected. Any child with snoring or abnormal breathing during sleep should be evaluated for OSAS.

Management

The goal of management is to help children develop a healthy pattern of sleeping, not simply eliminate the immediate problem. Healthy sleep associations include providing a consistent schedule of naps and bedtime, along with a pleasant bedtime routine. It is important to put infants in their cribs while they are relaxed and drowsy but not already asleep. This gives them the opportunity to develop skills to put themselves to sleep. If they become accustomed to being fed or rocked until they fall asleep, they will seek the same means of falling asleep every time they normally wake up during the night. In addition, overstimulation in the evening may make settling to sleep difficult for toddlers or young children. Instead, a routine such as a bath followed by a story in the child's bedroom with a clearly defined endpoint when the parent leaves the child in the crib or bed sleepy but awake may help facilitate sleep. Children must learn to fall asleep on their own.

Trained night feeders and trained night criers are infants who have not learned to fall asleep on their own. The basic treatment for these children is to put them in their cribs when they are sleepy but awake and ignore the subsequent crying. Their last memory before falling asleep should not be of their mothers holding or feeding them. If the crying persists, the contact with the infants should be brief and boring. Scheduled awakening is a technique in which infants are slightly aroused by the parent 15 to 60 minutes before an expected spontaneous awakening in an effort to prevent spontaneous awakening. Scheduled awakenings may be an effective treatment alternative for some trained night criers. If infants awaken for a feeding, parents should try to stretch the interval between waking and feeding so that children have an opportunity to practice self-calming techniques. Specific sleep disorders can be addressed individually. Older toddlers and preschoolers who delay going to bed or refuse to stay in their rooms at night need clear, firm limits. It is important that these children have consistent bedtime routines and nighttime interventions for when they awaken. A gate may need to be installed in the bedroom doorway to prevent children who refuse to stay in their rooms at night from moving about the house and potentially hurting themselves or disturbing others. Parents of children who have night terrors may require reassurance that their children are not suffering from significant emotional problems or stressors. A nightlight may help alleviate the anxieties of preschoolers who are unable to sleep at night because of their fears of darkness. Disturbances of the sleep-wake schedule can be corrected over time by gradually shifting children's schedules in the desired direction. For example, children with a delayed sleep phase who go to bed very late can have their morning wake-up time progressively advanced about 15 minutes per day; this is followed by a progressive advancement in their bedtime until the desired schedule is reached.

Implementation of good sleep hygiene practices is an important first step for school-aged children and adolescents who are experiencing sleep problems, especially sleep-onset problems. Sleep hygiene refers to the establishment and maintenance of schedules and conditions conducive to healthy, restorative sleep. Good sleep hygiene practices are outlined in Box 16-2. It is important to remember that

Box 16-2. Good Sleep Hygiene
Environment
• Dark
• Quiet
• Comfortably cool
Schedule
• Regular bedtime
• Regular waking time
• Naps, if needed, should be early in the day with consistent time and duration
General
• No frightening/stimulating television or stories and no vigorous physical activities in the hour before bedtime
• Limit caffeine, especially after lunchtime
• Consistent and calming bedtime routine
• Consistent soothing methods
• Children put to bed drowsy but awake

adolescents require at least as much sleep as they did as preadolescents—about 9 hours of sleep per night. Referral to a sleep specialist may be necessary for some children, especially when significant sleep disturbances such as narcolepsy, nocturnal seizures, or OSAS are suspected.

Prognosis

Unfortunately, infants with sleep problems tend to grow into children with sleep problems. Researchers have found that about 40% of infants with sleep problems at the age of 8 months still had a problem at 3 years. It is to the parents' advantage to help their children develop healthy sleep habits rather than ignore the problems and hope that the children outgrow them.

CASE RESOLUTION

The 6-month-old infant described in the case history has disordered sleep associations. He has been conditioned to nighttime feedings, although he is old enough not to require them for nutrition. The physician suggests several things the mother can do to try to solve her son's sleep problem. She can begin by gradually lengthening the interval between daytime feedings to 4 to 5 hours. When he cries at night, she can wait progressively longer before feeding him and can then eventually eliminate the feedings altogether. He will learn to fall asleep on his own without requiring feeding.

Selected References

American Academy of Pediatrics Section on Pediatric Pulmonology. Clinical practice guideline: diagnosis and management of childhood obstructive sleep apnea syndrome. *Pediatrics.* 2002;109:704–712

Anderson JE. Cosleeping: can we ever put the issue to rest? *Contemp Pediatr.* 2000;17:98–121

Ferber R. *Solve Your Child's Sleep Problems: New Revised and Expanded Edition.* New York, NY: Fireside; 2006

Givan DC. The sleepy child. *Pediatr Clin North Am.* 2004;51:15–31

Howard BJ, Wong J. Sleep disorders. *Pediatr Rev.* 2001;22:327–341

Okami P, Weisner T, Olmstead R. Outcome correlates of parent-child bedsharing: an eighteen-year longitudinal study. *J Dev Behav Pediatr.* 2002;23:244–253

Owens JA. The ADHD and sleep conundrum: a review. *J Dev Behav Pediatr.* 2005;26:312–322

Owens JA, Spirito A, McGuinn M, Nobile C. Sleep habits and sleep disturbance in school-aged children. *J Dev Behav Pediatr.* 2000;21:27–36

Pohl CA, Renwick A. Putting sleep disturbances to rest. *Contemp Pediatr.* 2002;19:74–96

Sheldon SH. Parasomnias in childhood. *Pediatr Clin North Am.* 2004;51:69–88

Oral Health and Dental Disorders

Charlotte W. Lewis, MD, MPH

CASE STUDY

The parents of a 9-month-old girl bring her to the office because they are concerned that their daughter has no teeth yet. Growth and development have proceeded normally, and the physical examination is unremarkable.

Questions

1. What is the mean age and range for the eruption of the first tooth?
2. What is meant by *mixed dentition*?
3. When should oral hygiene using a toothbrush begin?

Dental caries comprises the most common chronic disease of childhood. Pediatricians and other health care providers often see young children multiple times before children have their first dental visit. Primary care providers are thus in a prime position to counsel families on preventive oral health and to identify early signs of dental decay so that timely treatment can occur. In 2003 the American Academy of Pediatrics issued a recommendation that pediatricians and other pediatric health care providers begin regular oral health anticipatory guidance and risk assessment before patients are 6 months old. This recommendation affirms the essential need for clinicians to educate themselves on normal and abnormal patterns of dental eruption and occlusion, early and advanced signs of dental caries and its complications, and appropriate preventive oral hygiene practices. Establishing collaborative partnerships with community dentists is helpful in promoting ongoing clinician and family education and appropriate patient referrals.

Epidemiology

Among 5- to 17-year-olds, dental caries is 5 times more common than asthma and 7 times more common than hay fever. Sixty percent of children have at least one or more filled or decayed primary teeth by the age of 5 years and three-quarters of all 17-year-olds have experienced at least one carious lesion in their permanent dentition. Certain groups are at increased risk for earlier and more severe dental caries. Both individual and population risk factors for caries are listed in Box 17-1. Occlusal abnormalities are also common in children. At least 30% of the population is estimated to have moderate to severe orthodontic needs.

Box 17-1. Population and Individual Risk Factors for Dental Decay

Population Risk Factors

- Low socioeconomic status
- Recent immigrant
- Latino, Native American, and other non-white race/ethnicity
- No dental insurance or limited access to professional dental care

Individual Risk Factors

- Currently active decay or history of decay in patient
- History of high amount of dental decay in mother or siblings
- Frequent and/or prolonged intake of foods containing fermentable carbohydrate (or frequent/ongoing use of liquid medications prepared with sucrose)
- Presence of visible plaque on the teeth
- Exposed root surfaces
- Impaired ability to maintain oral hygiene (eg, developmentally disabled or otherwise handicapped individuals)
- Inadequate exposure to fluoride
- Reduced salivary flow
- History of radiation therapy to head and/or neck
- Wearing of orthodontic appliances or prostheses

Clinical Presentation

Dental development begins in utero. Subsequently, the teeth erupt into the upper or **maxillary** jaw and into the lower or **mandibular** portion of the jaw. Teeth have a crown and root section (Figure 17-1). The **crown** is the visible portion of the tooth above the gumline. The **root** is that part contained within the socket of the

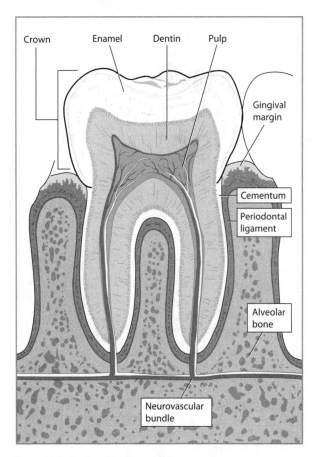

Figure 17-1. Tooth anatomy.

alveolar bone. The outer, hard coating of the crown is the **enamel.** Beneath the enamel is the **dentin,** composed of microtubules for transport of nutrients from the pulp to the outer portions of the tooth. The **pulp** contains nerves and vascular structures critical for the health and viability of the tooth. Teeth are anchored to the jaw through **periodontal ligaments.**

There are 20 **primary or deciduous teeth,** which erupt between approximately 6 and 36 months of age (Figure 17-2). The first primary teeth to erupt typically are the lower **central incisors.** These teeth erupt on average at 6 to 10 months of age. A simple but not always precise rule of thumb is that the first tooth erupts at 6 months of age and then one tooth per month erupts until all primary teeth have erupted by about 24 to 30 months of age. In the normal pattern of primary tooth eruption, the incisors erupt followed by eruption of the first molars, then canines (cuspids), and finally the second molars (hence the helpful mnemonic for primary eruption order in each quadrant of the mouth: forward-forward-back-forward-back for incisor-incisor-first molar-cuspid-second molar). There is variation in the timing of tooth eruption in the population, and normal tooth eruption can vary by 6 to 12 months from average. The eruption process may occasionally be preceded by a bluish discoloration to the gum, called an **eruption hematoma,** a benign process. More often eruption of the primary teeth is associated with more generalized symptoms such as fussiness and drooling. These symptoms are commonly referred to as *teething.* **Teething** does not cause diarrhea, respiratory infections, or true fever, although these entities may be present coincidentally with tooth eruption in infants.

The primary teeth are replaced by the **permanent teeth** (see Figure 17-2), which begin eruption at approximately 6 years of age. Both permanent and primary teeth are present during the **mixed dentition phase,** which occurs between 6 and 13 years of age. Early mixed dentition is sometimes referred to as the "ugly duckling" stage because the permanent dentition looks large and awkward relative to the remaining primary teeth and because there may be transient malpositioning of the teeth. There are 32 permanent teeth; the last to erupt are the **third molars,** commonly known as **wisdom teeth,** at about 17 to 21 years of age.

Variations from the normal in number of teeth are not uncommon. **Hypodontia** refers to fewer than normal teeth. The most

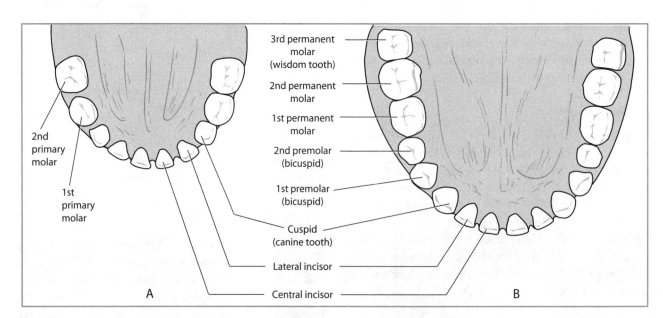

Figure 17-2. A. Primary dentition. B. Permanent dentition. (Used with permission from Zitelli BJ, Davis HW, eds. *Atlas of Pediatric Physical Diagnosis.* 2nd ed. Philadelphia, PA: JB Lippincott; 1992.)

common teeth to be congenitally absent are the third molars, second premolars, or maxillary lateral incisors. Congenital absence of a central incisor is distinctly uncommon and should raise concern for the presence of other midline defects. Several teeth may be missing in disorders such as **Down syndrome** or **ectodermal dysplasia.** **Anodontia** is the congenital absence of teeth. Extra teeth are called **supernumerary teeth.** Children may be born with teeth already erupted, known as **natal teeth.** Teeth that erupt shortly after birth are referred to as **neonatal teeth** if their eruption occurs in the first month of life. These teeth are usually incisors, and at least 90% represent normal dentition, rather than supernumerary teeth. The presence of natal or neonatal teeth may be familial, and on rare occasion may suggest an underlying syndrome. In addition to variations in number of teeth, teeth may also demonstrate variations in color and structure due to abnormalities in the tooth development, trauma, or extrinsic factors.

Caries may occur anytime after eruption of the teeth. **Early childhood caries** (ECC), a more general term referring to what in the past was called *baby bottle tooth decay* or *nursing bottle caries,* affects a substantial portion of children. The pattern of decay seen in ECC is different from that seen in the teeth of older children and adults. Typically ECC first affects the maxillary incisors and spares the lower incisors. This pattern of decay is hypothesized to result from prolonged and frequent exposure of the teeth to sweet liquids, for example, falling asleep with a juice bottle in the mouth, whereby the beverage pools around the upper incisors but the lower teeth are protected by the overlying tongue. The **pit and fissure surfaces** of the molars are more likely sites of decay in older children. Fermentable carbohydrates, particularly those of a sticky nature, become embedded in these surfaces and are not easily reached by the bristles of a toothbrush. This allows for prolonged action of acid-producing bacteria and subsequent caries formation.

In its earliest stages, caries appear on physical examination as white, opaque areas at the gumline **(white spot lesions).** At this early stage the lesion is potentially reversible if remineralization can occur. However, once the decay has eroded the enamel, irreversible damage has occurred. Symptoms differentiate the degree and depth of caries involvement; however, young children often have difficulty localizing dental pain. A cavity into the dentin may produce intermittent pain especially on exposure to temperature change or pressure on the affected tooth. Once cavitation has extended into the pulp, the resulting pulpitis may cause severe, persistent, often throbbing pain in the affected tooth, possibly awakening the child from sleep. Eventually the pulp undergoes necrosis and pain may disappear. However, the infection is still present and may spread around the tooth apex, forming a periapical abscess or fistula. Dental infection can progress to involve the maxilla or mandible and then move into the fascial planes of the head and neck producing facial cellulitis, abscess, and airway obstruction.

The relationship of the maxillary to the mandibular dentition has both functional and esthetic implications. **Malocclusion** is an abnormal relationship between the upper and lower teeth and may be developmental, genetic, or environmental in etiology. Children with craniofacial disorders often have significant occlusal problems and facial asymmetries necessitating early referral for craniofacial team care. Other children may have more mild malocclusion that needs orthodontic care. Normal occlusion occurs when the maxillary incisors are slightly in front of the mandibular incisors and the posterior molars interdigitate (Figure 17-3). This is called **Class I occlusion. Class II occlusion** occurs when the maxillary teeth project too far anteriorly from the mandibular teeth. This may be associated with an **overjet,** commonly known as *buck teeth,* which can predispose to dental injury when children fall. **Class III occlusion** occurs when the mandibular teeth are anterior to the maxillary. This is also commonly referred to as an *underbite.* Other common forms of malocclusion include an **anterior open bite,** whereby the posterior teeth come together but there is an opening between the top and bottom anterior teeth. A **crossbite** occurs when some of the upper teeth are located inside of the lower teeth during occlusion.

Pathophysiology

Hypodontia may be familial or occur secondary to an underlying syndrome. However, failure of one tooth to erupt is also commonly caused by another tooth in the path of eruption or insufficient space in the dental arch. Defects of tooth structure have a variety of causes. Medications, infection, jaundice, metabolic disorders, and irradiation may adversely affect normal tooth formation or mineralization. The permanent teeth begin to develop in utero and mineralize after birth, making them susceptible to both prenatal and postnatal exposures. **Intrauterine infection** with rubella, cytomegalovirus, or syphilis may adversely affect tooth structure. Local oral infection, for example, a periapical abscess involving a primary tooth in early childhood, can damage the developing permanent tooth bud resulting in a malformed permanent tooth.

Discolored teeth may be due to intrinsic or extrinsic factors. Tetracycline given to pregnant or lactating women or children younger than 7 to 8 years can cause intrinsic staining of the permanent teeth. Exposure to high levels of fluoride during early childhood can cause **fluorosis** of the permanent dentition. Fluorosis, when it occurs in the United States, is usually mild, characterized by white striations on the permanent teeth. Children with mild fluorosis have teeth that are less prone to dental decay. Teeth more severely affected by fluorosis may display hypoplastic enamel.

Inherited enamel or dentin defects may cause abnormal color of

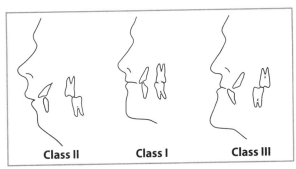

Figure 17-3. Classes of occlusion. Class I (middle) is considered most desirable from a functional and aesthetic perspective.

the teeth. These conditions may be isolated to the teeth, as in the case of **dentinogenesis imperfecta,** or as part of a systemic disorder, such as porphyria or osteogenesis imperfecta. A single dark tooth is usually non-vital or has bled within the tooth structure after dental trauma. Extrinsic staining is superficial and is usually due to poor oral hygiene; smoking; chewing tobacco or betel nuts; certain beverages such as coffee, tea, or wine; or medications such as liquid iron supplements.

Malocclusion can be caused by tooth crowding, an underlying craniofacial condition, abnormal jaw growth relationship, or malpositioning of the teeth, most commonly as the result of digit (usually the thumb) sucking. The most common types of malocclusion associated with digit sucking are **anterior open bite,** overjet, or posterior crossbite.

Dental decay is the most common disorder of the teeth and is a transmissible infectious disease. Caries results from bacterial action on teeth. Bacteria coat the teeth in the form of plaque or biofilm. Cariogenic bacteria are acquired early in life, usually before 2 to 3 years of age, through transmission from caregivers via contact with and transfer of oral fluids. *Streptococcus mutans,* believed to be one of the cariogenic bacteria, produce acid as the end-product of metabolism of carbohydrates. These acids dissolve the calcium-phosphate mineral of the tooth enamel or of the dentin in a process called *demineralization.* If not reversed or halted, this process results in formation of a carious lesion.

Differential Diagnosis

It can be difficult to differentiate tooth staining from a carious lesion, particularly when there are small areas of discoloration on the pit and fissure surfaces. If the lesion disappears with cleaning, staining is the etiology; however, staining is not always readily removed and examination by a dentist and radiographs can help evaluate such lesions. White spots on the teeth also can have multiple etiologies. When the white spot is chalky in appearance and located along the gingival margin, one needs to consider demineralization that could progress to frank decay. On the other hand, small intrinsic defects of the enamel may also appear as white spots; however, these are usually located throughout the crown and not just along the gingival margin and they also reflect light like the rest of the teeth (ie, not chalky).

Evaluation

History

Dental pathology is diagnosed primarily through history and physical examination. Many physicians have not traditionally included the teeth and supporting structures as part of their routine physical examination. However, pediatricians and other health care providers caring for children are generally the first, and often the only, health care providers to examine a child during the early years of life and therefore play a key role in identification of dental pathology. This is particularly true in settings where access to professional dental care is limited. Early diagnosis facilitates timely referral to dental specialists who provide definitive management.

Physical Examination

During each well-child visit, the medical provider should closely assess the mouth and its structures for the pattern of eruption and dental development; the presence of caries, plaque, gingivitis, and other oral lesions (see Chapter 59); and malocclusion. Physicians should examine the gingiva of children, particularly those with dental decay and/or toothache, to assess for evidence of periapical abscess, which may need antibiotic therapy and/or incision and drainage.

The oral cavity of a young child can be examined most easily with the caregiver and examiner in a **knee-to-knee position,** with the child's head in the examiner's lap and the legs wrapped around the caregiver's waist. Older children can be examined on the examination table or while seated in a chair. It is useful to have a disposable mouth mirror and a good light source. A toothbrush can be used to prop the mouth open to allow for examination of the teeth and oral cavity. The toothbrush can later be used to demonstrate good tooth brushing techniques.

A child's occlusion is best examined by looking at the child face from the anterior and lateral perspectives and watching the child's front and back teeth as the child opens and then bites down. Having the child bite down on a tongue depressor placed horizontally between the child's upper and lower teeth will demonstrate if there is a cant or asymmetry of the occlusion. The lateral profile of a child's face can be particularly revealing. Constructing an imaginary line between the bridge of the nose, the base of the nose, and the tip of the chin defines the shape of the lateral profile. In preschool and older children, a slightly convex profile is preferable both from a functional and aesthetic perspective. A concave profile is never normal and may be due to midface underdevelopment or from protrusion of the mandible. These children usually have a class III malocclusion. An overly convex profile may be due to an overjet or to mandibular retrusion. These children usually have a class II malocclusion.

Laboratory Tests

An ill-appearing child with a dental abscess or facial cellulitis of odontogenic etiology should have a complete blood count and a blood culture obtained.

Imaging Studies

Dental x-rays are useful in evaluating for the presence and extent of dental decay. They can also aid in determining whether a tooth that has not erupted as expected is absent or prevented in some way from erupting. Finally, when there is concern for pathology, imaging, particularly a Panorex or computed tomography scan, can be useful in evaluating the facial skeleton.

Management

Much of the definitive management of dental disorders falls to dental professionals. However, physicians play an important role in educating families about prevention, identifying pathology, and in facilitating dental referrals. Some dental conditions commonly fall into the realm of the primary care practitioner. For example, teething symptoms can be alleviated by giving the child a cold teething toy to suck on or with acetaminophen or ibuprofen given orally. Over-the-counter topical anesthetic agents often contain alcohol and are not recommended.

The American Academy of Pediatric Dentistry recommends the first professional dental care visit by 12 months of age. This is particularly important for children at high risk for dental caries. Occasionally, very young infants require a dental consultation. For example, if the natal/neonatal teeth interfere with feeding or are so loose as to pose an aspiration risk, they should be extracted; otherwise they require no intervention. When no teeth have erupted by 18 months of age, a dentist may choose to take x-rays to determine the status of the child's future dentition. If few developing teeth are seen, this can point to other diagnoses where hypodontia or anodontia occur. Most superficial extrinsic tooth stains can be removed during professional cleaning. Intrinsic stains can be treated by a dentist with abrasion and bleach techniques or application of a composite veneer. Malocclusion, when not reversible or self-limited, often is treated with orthodontics. More severe cases may require orthognathic surgery.

In some communities it may be difficult to find a dental provider who will care for a child younger than 3 years, and this further emphasizes the importance of medical providers in monitoring children's teeth and surrounding structures. Publicly insured children may also encounter difficulty accessing professional dental care. Clinicians should be aware of the closest source of specialized pediatric dental care if it is not within their own community. Dental schools or pediatric dental residency training programs generally offer specialized dental care for children, including sedation or anesthesia that may be needed to provide appropriate care.

Particularly in settings of limited access to dental care, physicians play an important role in educating families about the prevention of caries through advice about cariogenic food and beverages, regular tooth cleaning, and appropriate use of fluoride. Although physicians commonly advise parents not to allow their child to take a bottle to bed, it is particularly important that the child not take a bottle with **juice** or other sweetened beverages to bed. The evidence that breast milk, formula, or cow's milk causes caries is equivocal.

Physicians can also actively intervene if early caries lesions or white spots are identified. Application of **fluoride varnish** to the teeth can help to remineralize and reverse early caries lesions. When a child has more advanced caries, prompt referral to a dental provider is indicated. Pulpal involvement and abscess formation may result if a carious lesion is ignored. If dental care is not immediately available, antibiotics (penicillin V or clindamycin) and analgesics (eg, ibuprofen) may alleviate symptoms temporarily; however, more definitive treatment (**root canal** or extraction) is necessary to remove the source of infection and prevent resurgence of symptoms and further complications. When an abscess has spread to involve the cheek, face, or neck, admission to the hospital for intravenous antibiotics and surgical drainage is usually indicated.

Prevention

Prevention of dental disorders and promotion of good oral health are the combined responsibility of the primary physician, child, family, and dentist. Protection against virtually all decay is theoretically possible. Important preventive practices include regular home oral hygiene; access to routine dental care; sound dietary practices including avoiding frequent and/or prolonged exposure to fermentable carbohydrates, especially sucrose; regular use of **fluorides;** and sealant application. Increasing availability of fluoridated water and fluoride-containing toothpaste has dramatically decreased the prevalence of decay in the United States and other developed countries over the last 30 years. Fluoride can reverse or arrest early carious lesions through (1) enhancement of tooth mineralization and (2) reversal of tooth demineralization. The composition of the fluoride-containing enamel, fluoroapatite, is harder and less acid soluble than the original enamel that it replaces. Fluoride works best at remineralizing teeth when it is provided in a topical rather than systemic form (eg, taking fluoride supplements). Topical exposure to fluoride occurs through such means as drinking fluoridated water (which also has a systemic effect), using fluoride toothpaste, and professional applications.

Tooth brushing should begin with first tooth eruption. By the age of about 7 years, most children have developed sufficient fine motor skills to begin flossing and brushing their teeth independently. Until then, parents should help their children brush. Children at high risk for dental decay or who live in communities with non-fluoridated water can begin using a small amount (smaller than a pea) of fluoride toothpaste at first tooth eruption. Children at low risk for caries who live in areas with community water fluoridation can postpone use of fluoride toothpaste until they are 2 to 3 years of age to avoid excessive fluoride intake that can contribute to fluorosis. **Sealants** placed on the pit and fissure surfaces of the permanent molars can also be an important defense against caries in these surfaces. Children should be seen by a dentist for evaluation for sealant placement within 6 to 12 months of eruption of their first permanent molars.

Certain types of malocclusion are preventable. Because caries and trauma can both lead to premature tooth loss and subsequent loss of spacing and overcrowding, prevention of these entities will minimize the need for later orthodontic treatment. Prolonged digit sucking contributes to malocclusion. If children can discontinue these practices before age 4, digit-associated malocclusion is usually reversible. Dentists can employ specific devices and treatment to help stop digit sucking.

Prognosis

Many dental disorders are preventable. Early identification and prompt referral can prevent complications. In the past, edentulism in adulthood resulting from dental decay and periodontitis was common. Fluoride use and increased attention to preventive oral hygiene have reduced this condition as well as the incidence of permanent teeth caries; however, substantial disparities continue to adversely impact the oral health of low-income and minority children and adults in the United States.

CASE RESOLUTION

The parents of the infant in the case history should be reassured that the absence of teeth in their 9-month-old daughter is normal. Her first tooth may not appear until she is 12 months old. As long as she is growing and developing normally, there is no cause for concern.

Selected References

American Academy of Pediatrics. Oral Health Risk Assessment Training for Pediatricians and Other Child Health Professionals. www.aap.org/healthtopics/oralhealth.cfm

Holt R, Roberts G, Scully C. ABC of oral health. Oral health and disease. *BMJ.* 2000;320:1652–1655

Lewis CW, Johnston BD, Linsenmeyar KA, Williams A, Mouradian W. Preventive dental care for children in the United States: a national perspective. *Pediatrics.* 2007;119:e544–e553

Lewis CW, Milgrom P. Fluoride. *Pediatr Rev.* 2003;24:327–336

Recommendations for using fluoride to prevent and control dental caries in the United States. Centers for Disease Control and Prevention. *MMWR Recomm Rep.* 2001;50:1–42

US Department of Health and Human Services. *National Call to Action to Promote Oral Health.* Bethesda, MD: Public Health Service, National Institutes of Health, National Institute of Dental and Craniofacial Research; 2003. NIH Publication No. 03-5303

US Department of Health and Human Services. *Oral Health in America: A Report of the Surgeon General.* Rockville, MD: US Department of Health and Human Services, National Institute of Dental and Craniofacial Research, National Institutes of Health; 2000

Normal Development and Developmental Surveillance, Screening, and Evaluation

Geeta Grover, MD

CASE STUDY

The parents of a 12-month-old child are concerned that she is not walking yet. They report that she sat independently at 7 months and began crawling at 8 months. She can pull herself up to stand while holding on but is not cruising. Her birth and medical history are both unremarkable. The physical examination is within normal limits, and review of your records reveals no concerns on a developmental screening test administered at 9 months of age.

Questions

1. What are the major areas in which development is assessed?
2. What are the gross motor, fine motor, and personal/social milestones for a 12-month-old child?
3. What developmental screening tests could you administer to further assess her development?
4. How is developmental delay in children defined?

Development refers to the acquisition of functional skills during childhood. Monitoring the growth and development of children is an integral part of the assessment of pediatric patients. Recording the acquisition of developmental milestones provides a systematic approach by which to observe the progress of children over time. For ease of monitoring, these developmental milestones may be divided into 5 major domains or areas: gross motor, fine motor/adaptive, personal/social, language, and cognitive. This chapter discusses these major areas of development and the principles that govern them.

Four principles apply to all aspects of development. First, motor development is a continuous process that proceeds in the cephalocaudal direction and parallels neuronal myelination; therefore, developmental milestones reflect the maturation of the nervous system. Second, the sequence of development is the same in all children, but the rate of development may vary from child to child (eg, all children must walk before they run, but the age at which children walk or run varies from child to child). Third, the rate of attainment of milestones in one area may not parallel that in another. Fourth, certain primitive reflexes must be lost before corresponding voluntary movements can be attained (eg, the asymmetrical tonic neck reflex must disappear before children can roll over).

Pathophysiology

Development is influenced by both biological and environmental factors. Biological factors such as prematurity, exposure to drugs in utero, or the presence of chronic disease may place children at increased risk for developmental problems and delays. Environmental factors influencing development include parental attitudes and actions, sociodemographic factors, and cultural and societal influences. The quality of parental stimulation may influence the rate of acquisition of certain skills, especially cognitive and language abilities in preschool-aged children. Poverty and other socioeconomic factors may make it difficult for parents to provide their child with an optimal environment for growth and development.

Development in Newborns and Infants

Normal, full-term newborns enter the world capable of responding to visual, auditory, olfactory, oral, and tactile stimuli. They can be quieted and can even soothe themselves. Newborns can signal needs (eg, crying when hungry or wet), but they have a limited ability to respond to caregivers, primarily exhibiting disorganized and seemingly purposeless movements when stimulated. The newborn's reflexive generalized symmetrical movements (eg, arm waving and kicking) in response to environmental stimuli are eventually replaced by cortically mediated voluntary actions in older infants and children. Additionally, in newborns, certain primitive reflexes can be elicited by appropriate peripheral stimuli. Eventually, primitive reflexes are replaced by reactions that allow children to maintain postural stability in response to a variety of sensory inputs (proprioceptive, visual, and vestibular).

Primitive reflexes are mediated by the brain stem; they are involuntary motor responses that are elicited by appropriate peripheral stimuli. They are present at birth and disappear during the first 6 months of life. Normal motor development seems to be related to the suppression of these reflexes (Figure 18-1). Persistence or reappearance of these reflexes may indicate the presence of brain damage. **Postural reactions,** which are ultimately smoothly integrated into adult motor function (Figure 18-1), appear between 2 and 9 months of age. These reactions help maintain the orientation of the body in space and the interrelationship of one body part to another. The 3 major categories of postural reactions are righting, protection, and equilibrium.

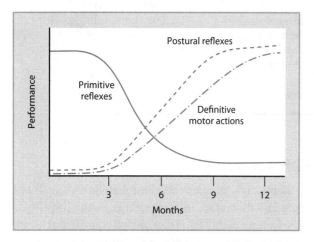

Figure 18-1. **Primitive reflex profile. (Reproduced with permission from Caputi AJ, Accardo PJ, Vining EPG, Rubenstein JE, Harryman S.** *Primitive Reflex Profile.* **Baltimore, MD: University Park Press; 1978:10.)**

The profile generated by combining primitive reflexes and postural reactions can be used to monitor the course of normal development and identify cases of problematic development. Persistence of primitive reflexes or failure of development of postural reactions can signal developmental problems. Authorities estimate that there are more than 70 primitive reflexes and postural reactions. Researchers do not agree on which of these reflexes or reactions are the most useful in the monitoring of development. The 7 most commonly used primitive reflexes are described in Box 18-1, and selected postural reactions are presented in Box 18-2.

Normal Development

A developmental assessment should include an evaluation of milestones in each of the 5 major areas. **Gross motor skills** are overall movements of large muscles (eg, sitting, walking, running). **Fine**

Box 18-1. Selected Primitive Reflexes

Moro Reflex
Allowing the infant's head to drop back suddenly results in abduction and upward movement of the arms followed by adduction and flexion. This reflex disappears by 4 months of age.

Rooting Reflex
Touching the corner of the infant's mouth results in lowering of the lower lip on the same side and movement of the tongue toward the stimulus.

Sucking Reflex
Placing an object in an infant's mouth causes vigorous sucking.

Grasp Reflex
Placing a finger in an infant's palm causes the infant to grasp it; the infant reinforces the grip as the finger is drawn upward. A similar response is seen in the foot grasp. Both of these reflexes disappear by 2 to 3 months of age.

Placing Reflex
Stroking the anterior aspect of the tibia against the edge of a table results in the lifting of the infant's leg to step onto the table.

Stepping Reflex
Holding the infant upright and slightly leaning forward produces alternating flexion and extension movements of the legs that simulate walking. This reflex disappears by 5 to 6 weeks of age.

Asymmetrical Tonic Neck Reflex
With the infant lying supine, turning the head to one side results in extension of the extremities on that side and flexion of the opposite extremities (fencer position). This reflex disappears by 3 to 4 months of age.

Box 18-2. Selected Postural Reactions

Righting Reactions
These allow the body to maintain normal postural relationships of the head, trunk, and extremities during all activities. The different reactions appear at different ages, beginning shortly after birth and ranging up to 12 months of age.

Protection and Equilibrium Reactions
Protective Equilibrium Response
When gently pushed toward one side while in a sitting position, infants increase trunk flexor tone toward that side to regain their center of gravity and extend the arm on the same side to protect against falling. This response usually emerges at about 4 to 6 months of age.
Parachute Reactions
When held in ventral suspension and suddenly lowered (downward parachute), infants extend their arms as if to protect themselves from a fall; similar reactions are seen with forward and backward stimulation. These reactions appear at 8 to 9 months of age.

---

motor-adaptive skills involve use of the small muscles of the hands, the ability to manipulate small objects, problem-solving skills, and eye-hand coordination. **Language skills** include hearing, understanding, and use of language. **Personal-social skills** involve socialization and ability to care for personal needs. **Cognitive skills** involve the ability to use higher mental processes including comprehension, memory, and logical reasoning.

Table 18-1 outlines the normal pattern of development with regard to each of these skills. The table lists the average age of attainment of these skills as well as the normal ranges where available. Development is an orderly and sequential process, and children must proceed through several stages before any given milestone is attained. Therefore, the physician should document not only *what* children can do but *how* they do it. For example, to sit without support, children first achieve head control. Several stages later they are able to sit in a "tripod" position with arms extended in front for support, and finally sit with the head steady and back straight without support (Figure 18-2).

Figure 18-2. **Stages in the development of sitting. A. Head control. B. "Tripod sitting." C. Head steady and back straight without support.**

Gross Motor Skills

During the first year of life, the ultimate goal of gross motor development is walking. The first step toward this goal is head control. By 6 months of age, children are able to sit without support for a few seconds. At 9 to 10 months children are able to pull themselves to a standing position, and by 12 to 17 months of age they are able to walk. Children then learn to run, negotiate stairs, hop on one foot, and skip—in that order.

Fine Motor Skills

Development of the 2-finger pincer grasp is the major goal of fine motor development during the first year (Figure 18-3). The hands primarily remain in a fisted position until 3 months of age. Infants

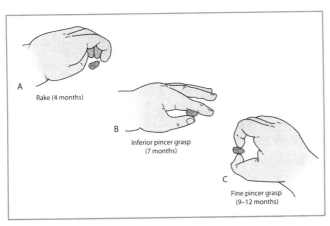

Figure 18-3. **Development of the pincer grasp. A. Rake (4 months). B. Inferior pincer grasp (7 months). C. Fine pincer grasp (9–12 months).**

also discover the midline at this age, and shortly thereafter they may play with the hands in the midline. Four-month-old children begin reaching for desired objects; by 6 months of age they are able to transfer objects from one hand to the other. By 7 months they have a 3-finger pincer grasp, and by 9 to 10 months they have developed the 2-finger grasp, which allows them to manipulate small objects such as raisins and pencils. By 14 months they begin to scribble, and by 3 to 5 years they are able to copy geometric shapes. Children with early preference for the use of one hand over another, especially prior to about 18 months of age, should be assessed for the presence of paresis or other neuromuscular problems. Handedness may develop by 3 years but often is not firmly established until the age of 4 to 5 years.

Language Skills

The development of normal speech and language skills is discussed in Chapter 19.

Personal-Social Skills

These skills enable children to interact and respond to the surrounding world. Deficits in the development of age-appropriate social skills/social relatedness (eg, social orienting, social referencing, joint attention, and pretend play) are a defining feature of the autism spectrum disorders (ASDs). For children within this spectrum, the development of social skills is characteristically "out of sync" with their overall level of functioning. Joint attention is the inclination to share enjoyment, interests, or achievement with other people, and like other developmental skills, seems to develop in graduated stages (early skills include reciprocal smiling at the sight of a familiar person followed by later emerging skills like the ability to isolate one's index finger and point by 12–15 months of age). Lack of joint attention seems to be a core deficit in ASDs; it also seems to be specific to ASDs. (ASDs are discussed fully in Chapter 112.)

Cognitive Skills

These abilities allow children to think, reason, problem-solve, and understand the surrounding environment. The concept of object permanence or object constancy, the realization that objects may exist even if they cannot be seen, develops at approximately 7 to 9 months of age. The understanding of time comes much later. Children develop the concept of "today" at 24 months of age, "tomorrow" at 30 months, and "yesterday" at 36 months. It is extremely important that health care providers realize that children's perception and understanding of pain, disease, and illness are guided by their stage of cognitive development. The psychologist Jean Piaget generated complex generalizations by observing what children did and how they did it; his theories are the cornerstone of knowledge in this area. Piaget's 4 stages of cognitive development are presented in Box 18-3.

Developmental Delay

Children are said to be developmentally delayed if they fail to reach developmental milestones at the expected age. This age ranges widely because of the wide variation among normal children.

Table 18-1. Normal Pattern of Development[a]

Skill	Mean Age	Normal Range
Gross Motor Skills		
Reflex head turn; moves head side to side	Newborn	0–3 mo
Lifts head when prone	1 mo	1–4 mo
Lifts shoulders up when prone	2 mo	1–4 mo
Lifts up on elbows; head steady when upright	3 mo	2–5 mo
Lifts up on extended hands; rolls front to back; no head lag when pulled to sitting from supine position	4 mo	3–6 mo
Rolls back to front	5 mo	4–7 mo
Sits independently (≥30 s)	6 mo	5–9 mo
Crawls on hands and knees	8 mo	6–11 mo
Pulls to stand	9 mo	6–12 mo
Cruises	11 mo	9–14 mo
Walks	12 mo	9–17 mo
Walks backward	15 mo	13–17 mo
Runs	15 mo	13–20 mo
Kicks a ball	24 mo	18–30 mo
Walks up and down stairs (taking one step at a time and holding on)	24 mo	
Stands on one foot	30 mo	
Walks up stairs alternating steps	30 mo	28–36 mo
Peddles a tricycle	3 y	30–48 mo
Walks down stairs alternating steps/hops on one foot	4 y	
Skips	5 y	
Fine Motor-Adaptive Skills		
Tracks horizontally to midline	1 mo	
Tracks past midline/tracks vertically	2 mo	1–3 mo
Unfisted for >50% of the time; tracks 180 degrees; visual threat; discovers midline	3 mo	3–4 mo
Reaches for bright object; brings object to mouth	4 mo	
Transfers object from one hand to the other	6 mo	4–7 mo
3-finger pincer grasp	7 mo	6–10 mo
Neat pincer grasp	9 mo	7–10 mo
Bangs cubes in midline	9 mo	7–11 mo
Tower of 2 cubes; scribbles spontaneously	14 mo	14–20 mo
Tower of 4 cubes	18 mo	17–24 mo
Copies vertical and horizontal line; tower of 6 cubes	2 y	
Copies circle	3 y	
Copies cross (†)	4 y	
Copies square; draws person with 3 parts	5 y	
Copies triangle; draws person with 6 parts	6 y	
Personal-Social Skills		
Regards face	Newborn	
Spontaneous social smile	6 wk	1–3 mo
Discriminates social smile; relates to parent with real joy	6 mo	
Displays stranger anxiety; plays peek-a-boo	7 mo	7–9 mo

Table 18-1. Normal Pattern of Development[a], continued		
Skill	*Mean Age*	*Normal Range*
Personal-Social Skills, continued		
Orients to name, uses gestures to get needs met	12 mo	
Drinks from a cup	15 mo	10–18 mo
Uses a spoon, spilling a little	15 mo	12–18 mo
Uses sounds, pointing, or other "showing" gestures to draw attention to object of interest	15 mo	12–15 mo
Simple pretend play (eg, feeding doll)	18 mo	
Imitates housework	18 mo	14–24 mo
Helps with undressing	2 y	22–30 mo
Washes and dries hands	2 y	
Parallel play; enjoys being next to other kids	2 y	12–30 mo
Undresses self	3 y	30–40 mo
Toilet training		24–36 mo
Imagines self as different characters	3 y	
Cooperative play	3 y	24–48 mo
Dresses without assistance	5 y	
Language Skills		
Alerts to bell	Newborn	
Searches with eyes for sound	2 mo	
Cooing	3 mo	1–4 mo
Turns head to voice or bell; laughs	4 mo	3–6 mo
Babbles	6 mo	5–9 mo
Mama/Dada nonspecific	8 mo	6–10 mo
Understands the word "no"	10 mo	
Mama/Dada specific	10 mo	9–14 mo
Follows 1-step command with gesture; 3–5-word vocabulary	12 mo	10–16 mo
Follows 1-step command without gesture	15 mo	12–20 mo
Can point to several body parts	18 mo	12–24 mo
50-word vocabulary	2 y	
Two-word sentences; pronouns indiscriminately	2 y	20–30 mo
States first name	34 mo	30–40 mo
250-word vocabulary; 3-word sentences; speech intelligible to strangers 75% of time	3 y	
Uses pronouns appropriately	3 y	30–42 mo
Cognitive Skills		
Sensorimotor		Newborn–2 y
Preoperational		2–6 y
Concrete operational		6–11 y
Formal operations		>11 y
Miscellaneous Cognitive Milestones		
Concept of today	24 mo	
Concept of tomorrow	30 mo	
Concept of yesterday	36 mo	
Concept of right and left	7 y	

[a]Detailed language milestones are presented in Chapter 19, Table 19-1.

Box 18-3. Stages of Development of Piaget

Sensorimotor (Birth–2 Years)

Children approach the world through sensations and motor actions. They develop a sense of object permanence, spatial relationships, and causality.

Preoperational (2–6 Years)

Children's mental processes are linked to their own perception of reality. They do not separate internal and external reality.

Concrete Operational (6–11 Years)

Children can perform mental operations in their heads if they relate to real objects. They develop concepts of conservation of mass, volume, and number.

Formal Operations (>11 Years)

Children develop the capacity for abstract thought.

Individual children may be delayed in one area or several areas of development.

Differential Diagnosis

Three factors are involved in the differential diagnosis of children with developmental delays: (1) determination of the area or areas of development in which delay is apparent; (2) if motor delay is evident, determination of whether the condition is progressive or nonprogressive; and (3) assessment to see if developmental milestones previously achieved are lost or if age-appropriate milestones were achieved at all.

Children with an early history of normal development who subsequently experience a slowing of developmental progression, often associated with cognitive delays or seizures, may have a metabolic defect. Children who attain developmental milestones and subsequently lose them may have a neurodegenerative disease (eg, multiple sclerosis, adrenoleukodystrophy) or a lesion of the spinal cord or brain. The presence of habitual rhythmic body movements (eg, body rocking, head banging) may be a sign of a pervasive developmental disorder such as autism.

Cerebral palsy, the classic example of nonprogressive motor abnormality, is a form of static encephalopathy characterized by abnormal movement and posture. The type of cerebral palsy depends on which area of the brain is injured. Spastic cerebral palsy, seen most commonly, is secondary to upper motor neuron injury. The ataxic form of the disease is related to lesions of the cerebellum or its pathways. Dyskinetic cerebral palsy manifests as uncontrolled and purposeless movements that often result from a basal ganglia lesion (eg, athetosis following bilirubin deposition in the basal ganglia [kernicterus]). The onset of symptoms is either in infancy or early childhood. The key factor in making the diagnosis is establishing that the motor deficits are static and nonprogressing.

Evaluation

When evaluating children for possible delays in development, it is important to remember that there is a great deal of variation in the age of attainment of milestones. In addition, the rate of acquisition of milestones in one area of development may not parallel that in another. Routine and ongoing assessment of a child's level of development at all periodic health maintenance visits through observation, history, physical examination, and screening tests allows the physician to form a longitudinal view of the child. The physician is thus able to identify and differentiate true deficits and delays from temporary setbacks.

History

Evaluation of children for suspected delays in development includes a complete history (Questions Box). Family history is important because other family members may have relatively delayed attainment of milestones. Perinatal factors that place children at high risk for developmental difficulties include a history of maternal drug or alcohol use during pregnancy, prematurity in the infant, and congenital infections. Other historical risk factors for developmental delay include history of seizures, sepsis or meningitis, exposure to lead or other toxins, and poor feeding or growth. Environmental factors such as stressful home conditions, history of abuse or neglect, and lack of stimulation may also contribute to delayed development.

Physical Examination

Both height and weight should be checked. Abnormal growth (ie, height or weight <5th percentile or head circumference either <5th percentile or >90th percentile) may be a marker for developmental delay. The presence of congenital anomalies (eg, cataracts, hypertelorism, spina bifida) or neurocutaneous lesions (eg, café-au-lait spots) may be suggestive of chromosomal anomalies or other genetic diseases. Neuromuscular examination should emphasize age-appropriate milestones. Abnormalities in muscle tone (eg, hypotonia, hypertonia), bulk, or strength may be clues to the presence of neuromuscular disease (eg, muscular dystrophy), cerebral palsy, or Down syndrome.

Laboratory Tests

Age-appropriate assessment of the child's vision and hearing should be performed if signs of motor, cognitive, or language delays are apparent. Chromosomal studies may be conducted if dysmorphic features are noted on the physical examination. Evidence of

---

Questions

Normal Development

- Has anyone in the child's family had developmental problems or delays?
- Did the mother use any drugs or alcohol during pregnancy?
- Was the child premature?
- Does the child have a history of seizures?
- Has the child had meningitis or sepsis?
- Does the child have any history of not feeding well or poor growth?
- Is the child's home environment characterized by any stresses (eg, divorce, limited financial resources)?

cognitive or motor delays may warrant metabolic studies (eg, organic and amino acids).

Imaging studies of the head such as magnetic resonance imaging scans or electroencephalograms may be necessary if the child has a history of seizures or an abnormal neurologic examination.

Developmental Surveillance, Screening, and Evaluation

Early detection of developmental delays is a responsibility of all pediatric health care professionals. Unfortunately current detection rates of developmental disorders are lower than their actual prevalence. About 20% of children between the ages of 3 to 17 years will have one or more developmental, learning, or emotional disorders, with 4% to 5% having developmental delays. Without the use of specific developmental screening tools, only about 30% of developmental disabilities are identified, but with the use of tools this identification rate increases to 70% to 80%.

Developmental surveillance, the ongoing process of monitoring individual children's developmental status, should be incorporated at each health maintenance visit. Surveillance involves eliciting and attending to parental concerns about their children's development and usually involves age-specific queries such as whether the child is walking, talking, or pointing. Surveillance has been referred to as a kind of developmental growth chart. Recognition of children who may be at risk of developmental delays is the goal of developmental surveillance.

Developmental screening is the administration of a brief standardized tool to identify children at risk of a developmental disorder. Box 18-4 lists frequently used developmental screening tools. A formal developmental screening should be performed when developmental surveillance elicits a risk factor for developmental delay; in the absence of established risk factors or parental concerns, the administration of a general developmental screening tool is recommended by the American Academy of Pediatrics (AAP) at the 9-, 18-, and 30-month (or 24-month) health maintenance visits (AAP, 2006). The AAP further recommends that in addition to a general developmental screening tool, an autism-specific screening tool should also be administered at the 18-month visit. (See Chapter 112 for a listing of autism-specific screening tools.) Periodic screening is necessary to detect emerging disabilities as children grow. Screening instruments should have a broad developmental focus and should be brief, inexpensive, valid, and reliable. Screening tests are not diagnostic. A failed screening test should lead to a referral for a further developmental evaluation.

Developmental evaluation (developmental assessment) is performed when surveillance or screening identifies a child as being at high risk of a developmental disorder. The aim is to identify the specific developmental disorder or disorders affecting the child. Developmental evaluation is performed by trained examiners. Unlike developmental screening, which is not diagnostic, developmental evaluation is diagnostic.

The Bayley Scales of Infant Development II, first published in 1933 by Nancy Bayley, is one of the most commonly used developmental

---

Box 18-4. Frequently Used Developmental Screening Instruments

Developmental Screening Instruments Relying on Information From Parents
- Child Development Inventories
- Child Development Review—Parent Questionnaire (CDR-PQ)
- Infant Development Inventory
- Ages and Stages Questionnaire (ASQ)
- Parent's Evaluation of Developmental Status (PEDS)

Screens Relying on Eliciting Skills Directly From Children
- Bayley Infant Neurodevelopmental Screen (BINS)
- Batelle Developmental Inventory Screening Tool, 2nd Edition
- Brigance Screens—II
- Denver Developmental Screening Test II (Denver II)

---

evaluation tools used today. It has 3 sections: mental, psychomotor, and a behavior rating scale. The Bayley II may be used for children 1 to 42 months of age. Developmental tests, like the Bayley II (emphasizing sensorimotor-based skills), have a poor correlation with later measures of intelligence (emphasizing language and abstract reasoning), especially before 24 to 30 months of age. As such, developmental tests are best used as measures of current developmental functioning, rather than as predictors of future functioning. Intelligence tests, achievement tests, personality tests, or behavior rating scales may be used for preschool and school-aged children having behavioral or emotional concerns, learning disabilities, or developmental disabilities.

Management

Children with identified developmental delays in one or more areas should be referred to the appropriate specialist, agency, or state program for further testing and assessment. Detailed neurologic examination may be necessary if gross motor delays are identified. Language delays may warrant formal hearing and speech assessment by an audiologist or speech pathologist. Cognitive impairment requires formal psychometric assessment, which in some cases can be performed through the child's school.

Prognosis

The early identification of children with developmental delays is critical. Early identification of developmental problems allows for early intervention, thereby making it possible for individual children to reach their maximum potential. Identification and treatment of underlying disease (eg, hypothyroidism or infection) prevents further damage. Removal of children from adverse home environments or placement of children from impoverished home environments in early intervention programs can greatly stimulate their developmental potential. The prognosis for children with mild developmental delays can sometimes be improved greatly from participation in such infant stimulation programs.

CASE RESOLUTION

The parents of the child described in the case history may be reassured that their child is developing normally for her age. Although most children begin walking at about 12 months of age, commencement of walking anywhere up to the age of 17 months is considered to be within normal limits. The American Academy of Pediatrics recommends that standardized developmental screening should be performed when developmental surveillance identifies high risk factors, and routinely at the 9-, 18-, and 30-month health maintenance visits. Administration of a formal screening tool is probably not necessary at this visit, but can be considered again at the 15-month visit if there is a lack of progression in her gross motor skills or if any other risk factor is identified at that time.

Selected References

American Academy of Pediatrics Committee on Children With Disabilities. Developmental surveillance and screening of infants and young children. *Pediatrics.* 2001;108:192–195

American Academy of Pediatrics Committee on Children With Disabilities. Technical report: the pediatrician's role in the diagnosis and management of autistic spectrum disorder in children. *Pediatrics.* 2001;107:e85

American Academy of Pediatrics Council on Children With Disabilities, Section on Developmental Behavioral Pediatrics, Bright Futures Steering Committee, Medical Home Initiatives for Children With Special Needs Project Advisory Committee. Identifying infants and young children with developmental disorders in the medical home: an algorithm for developmental surveillance and screening. *Pediatrics.* 2006;118:405–420

Glascoe FP, Macias MM. How you can implement the AAP's new policy on developmental and behavioral screening. *Contemp Pediatr.* 2003;20:85–102

Glascoe FP. Early detection of developmental and behavioral problems. *Pediatr Rev.* 2000;21:272–279

Roberts G, Palfrey J, Bridgemohan C. A rational approach to the medical evaluation of a child with developmental delay. *Contemp Pediatr.* 2004;21:76–100

Shevell M, Aswal S, Donley, et al. Practice parameter: evaluation of the child with global developmental delay: report of the Quality Standards Subcommittee of the American Academy of Neurology and the Practice Committee of the Child Neurology Society. *Neurology.* 2003;60:367–380

Sices L, Feudtner C, McLaughlin J, Drotar D, Williams M. How do primary care physicians manage children with possible developmental delays? A national survey with an experimental design. *Pediatrics.* 2004;113:274–282

Language Development: Speech and Hearing Assessment

Geeta Grover, MD

CASE STUDY

The parents of a 3-year-old girl bring her to see you. They are concerned because their daughter has only an 8- to 10-word vocabulary, and she does not put words together into phrases or sentences. They report that she seems to have no hearing problems; she responds to her name and follows directions well.

In general, she has been in good health. Her development, aside from delayed speech, is normal. During the physical examination, which is also normal, the girl does not speak.

Questions

1. What language skills should children have at 1, 2, and 3 years?
2. Approximately how many words should 3-year-olds have in their vocabulary?
3. By what age should children's speech be intelligible to strangers at least 75% of the time?
4. What factors may be associated with delayed speech development?
5. What tests are used to assess children's hearing, speech, and language development?

The ability to communicate through language is a uniquely human skill. Speech refers to the production of sounds, whereas language involves both comprehension and expression; it is the use of words, phrases, and gestures to convey intent. Normal hearing is essential for the development of speech and language.

The development of normal speech and language skills is an extremely important developmental milestone that is eagerly awaited by parents. Normal patterns of language development should be as familiar to pediatricians as all other aspects of child development (see Chapter 18). It is important that children with suspected language delays be referred to specialists as early as possible. Children with delayed speech or language development should be suspected of having a hearing deficit. Diminished hearing is an important cause of delayed language development. Delays in language development can also be associated with autism spectrum disorders (ASDs).

Epidemiology

Significant hearing loss is estimated to affect approximately 1 to 6 per 1,000 newborns. Many more infants are born with less severe hearing impairments, and still others develop hearing impairments during childhood. The prevalence of moderate to severe bilateral hearing loss is 1.5 to 2 in 1,000 in children younger than 6 years. If less severe hearing losses and transient losses secondary to middle ear effusions are included, the prevalence increases significantly.

Language disorders may affect 5% to 10% of all children; they are one of the most common childhood disabilities. Although speech and hearing problems are common, they are often missed or minimized, and referral for evaluation and remediation is delayed significantly. Some researchers have estimated that the time from parents' first suspicion that their child may have a hearing loss to referral by the pediatrician to an audiologist for evaluation is as much as 12 months. The proliferation of universal newborn hearing screening programs is decreasing the average age of identification of profound congenital hearing loss in the United States, which until recently had been approximately 30 months. This is encouraging because the critical period for language development is within the first 3 years of life.

When evaluating children with delayed language development, the practitioner is faced with the task of differentiating the children who are "late bloomers," and will eventually catch up to their peers without formal interventions or services, from those children with persistent language impairments who will benefit from early interventions services. Whereas 10% to 15% of 2-year-old children may show language delays, only 4% to 5% will remain delayed beyond 3 years of age. The rate of future language development depends not only on the presence of risk factors, such as family history of language disorders and various perinatal risk factors, but also on positive prognostic indicators such as age-appropriate imitation, symbolic thinking, receptive language, and social and nonverbal communication skills.

Clinical Presentation

Lack of response to sound at any age, failure to achieve age-appropriate expressive language skills, and parental concern regarding a child's hearing are the most important signs of hearing or language impairment. Deaf infants coo normally and may even babble; therefore, an infant's vocalizing does not preclude a hearing loss.

Pathophysiology

The left hemisphere of the brain is responsible for language skills in 94% of right-handed adults and approximately 75% of left-handed adults. Peripheral auditory stimuli are transmitted to the primary auditory areas in both temporal lobes. Sounds then undergo a series of analyses, primarily in 3 main areas in the left cerebral cortex: Wernicke area (or auditory association area), which is responsible for the comprehension of language; Broca area (or motor encoding area), which is responsible for the preliminary conversion of language into motor activity; and the primary motor cortex and supplementary motor cortex, which control the movements necessary for speech. This complex process is responsible for the comprehension and production of language.

Speech and language develop in a predictable, orderly sequence. Language skills can be either receptive or expressive. Early receptive milestones refer to ability to hear and respond to sound, whereas later milestones reflect ability to understand spoken words. Early expressive milestones relate to speech production; later, children use language to convey their intent to others. In the first year of life, receptive skills are more advanced than expressive skills.

Knowledge of normal receptive and expressive language skills (Table 19-1) is essential to recognition and identification of developmental delays. Box 19-1 lists "danger signals" that indicate possible delays and serves as a guide for referral to specialists. It is most important to remember that by the age of 3 years, 75% of children's speech should be intelligible to strangers.

Differential Diagnosis

The various causes of delayed language development include hearing loss, disorders of central nervous system (CNS) processing, anatomical abnormalities, and environmental deprivation (Box 19-2). Although birth order (eg, the belief that younger children speak later than first-born children because older siblings speak for them), laziness (eg, "Don't give him what he wants when he points. Make him ask for it"), and bilingualism are commonly believed to lead to speech and language delay, their contributory role has never been proved.

Hearing loss (see Chapter 61), which may lead to language delays, is either congenital or acquired. Most cases of congenital deafness are the result of genetic factors. The TORCHS infections (toxoplasmosis, rubella, cytomegalovirus [CMV], herpes simplex, syphilis), especially CMV and rubella, are the most common nongenetic causes of hearing loss in the newborn period. Factors associated with high risk for infant hearing loss are outlined in Box 19-3. The leading cause of acquired hearing loss in older infants and children is meningitis.

Table 19-1. Receptive and Expressive Language Milestones (Birth to 3 years)

Skill	Mean Age	Normal Range
Receptive Milestones		
Alerts to sound	Newborn	
Orients to sound/turns to voice	4 mo	3–6 mo
Responds to name	4 mo	4–9 mo
Understands "no"	10 mo	9–18 mo
Follows 1-step command with gesture	12 mo	10–16 mo
Follows 1-step command without gesture	15 mo	12–20 mo
Points to several body parts	18 mo	12–24 mo
Follows 2-step command with gesture	24 mo	22–30 mo
Expressive Milestones		
Cooing (vowel sounds)	3 mo	1–4 mo
Laughs	4 mo	3–6 mo
Babbling (consonants added to vowel sounds)	6 mo	5–9 mo
Dada/Mama nonspecifically	8 mo	6–10 mo
Dada/Mama specifically	10 mo	9–14 mo
3–5 word vocabulary	12 mo	
Immature jargoning (gibberish with inflection)	13 mo	10–18 mo
Mature jargoning (gibberish with occasional word)	18 mo	16–24 mo
50-word vocabulary	24 mo	
2-word phrases	24 mo	20–30 mo
Uses pronouns indiscriminately	24 mo	22–30 mo
States first name	34 mo	30–40 mo
Uses pronouns appropriately	36 mo	30–42 mo
250-word vocabulary	36 mo	
75% of speech intelligible to strangers	36 mo	

Box 19-1. Danger Signals in Language Development

- Inconsistent or lack of response to auditory stimuli at any age
- No babbling by 9 months
- No intelligible speech by 18 months
- Inability to respond to simple directions or commands (eg, "sit down," "come here") by 24 months
- Speech predominantly unintelligible at 36 months
- Dysfluency (stuttering) of speech noticeable after 5 years
- Hypernasality, inappropriate vocal quality, pitch, or intensity at any age

---

Box 19-2. Causes of Delayed Language Development

- Hearing impairment
- Perinatal risk factors leading to hearing impairment
- Disorders of central nervous system processing
  — Global developmental delay
  — Mental retardation
  — Autism spectrum disorders
- Developmental language disorders
- Disorders of language production
  — Articulation disorder
  — Dysarthria
  — Verbal apraxia
- Presence of anatomical abnormalities (eg, cleft lip, cleft palate)
- Environmental deprivation

Box 19-3. High-Risk Indicators for Hearing Loss in Children (Birth to 24 months)[a]

Neonatal Period (Birth–28 days)
- Family history of sensorineural hearing loss (SNHL)
- In utero infection associated with SNHL (eg, TORCHS infections [toxoplasmosis, rubella, cytomegalovirus, herpes simplex, syphilis])
- Anatomical malformations of the head and neck region
- Hyperbilirubinemia at a level requiring exchange transfusion
- Low birth weight (<1500 g)
- Bacterial meningitis
- Low Apgar scores
- Respiratory distress (eg, meconium aspiration)
- Mechanical ventilation for 10 days or more
- Exposure to ototoxic medications (eg, aminoglycoside antibiotics) for more than 5 days or in combination with loop diuretics
- Stigmata of syndromes known to be associated with hearing loss (eg, Down syndrome)

Infants and Children (29 days–24 months)
- Parental concern about hearing, speech, language, or developmental delay
- Recurrent or persistent otitis media with effusion for at least 3 months
- Severe head trauma (associated with fracture of the temporal bone)
- Infections associated with SNHL (eg, bacterial meningitis, mumps, measles)
- Neurodegenerative disorders or demyelinating diseases
- Any of the newborn risk factors listed above

[a]Adapted with permission from Joint Committee on Infant Hearing, American Academy of Audiology, American Academy of Pediatrics, American Speech-Language-Hearing Association, Directors of Speech and Hearing Programs in State Health and Welfare Agencies. Year 2000 position statement: principles and guidelines for early hearing detection and intervention programs. *Pediatrics.* 2000;106:798–817 and Cunningham M, Cox EO, American Academy of Pediatrics Committee on Practice and Ambulatory Medicine and Section on Otolaryngology and Bronchoesophagology. Hearing assessment in infants and children: recommendations beyond neonatal screening. *Pediatrics.* 2003;111:436–440.

On the basis of etiology, hearing loss can be divided into 2 categories: central (cortical hearing impairment) and peripheral. Peripheral causes are further subdivided into 2 broad groups: conductive (problems with transmission of sound through the external or middle ear) and sensorineural (inadequate transduction of sound waves into neural activity at the level of the inner ear or cranial nerve VIII).

Otitis media with effusion is the most common cause of conductive hearing loss in children (see Chapter 60). Fluid in the middle ear can decrease sound conduction by an average of 25 decibels. Other conditions that may result in conductive hearing loss include impaction of cerumen in the external ear canal, perforation of the tympanic membrane, atresia or stenosis of the ear canal, otosclerosis, abnormalities of the ossicles, and cholesteatoma. Injury to cranial nerve VIII or damage or maldevelopment of inner ear structures due to ototoxic agents, noise, cochlear agenesis, or perilymphatic fistula of the round or oval window membrane may lead to sensorineural hearing loss. Mixed hearing loss, a combination of conductive and sensorineural loss, may be seen in some children with developmental abnormalities.

Disorders of CNS processing include global developmental delay, mental retardation, ASDs (see Chapter 112), and developmental language problems. Developmental language disorders produce speech or language delays in children in the absence of hearing loss, anatomical abnormalities of the vocal tract, mental retardation, or global developmental delay. "Late talkers," or children who have normal comprehension but simply begin speaking late, have mild developmental language problems. Children who are completely nonverbal have more severe problems.

Anatomical abnormalities may also result in both speech and language delays. Cleft palate is the abnormality most commonly associated with difficulties in speech production. Children with cleft palate characteristically have hypernasal speech secondary to velopharyngeal incompetence (eg, dysfunction of the soft palate). In addition, conductive hearing losses may result from chronic serous otitis media, which is common in these children. The presence of a submucous cleft palate, characterized by a bifid uvula, diastasis of the muscles in the midline of the soft palate with intact mucosa, and notching of the posterior border of the hard palate, should be considered in children without an overt cleft palate who have recurrent symptomatic serous otitis media and phonation difficulties.

Environmental deprivation is another cause of delayed language development, especially in families where children are not spoken or read to. Sometimes there is additional historical or physical evidence of deprivation (eg, profound failure to thrive, physical or sexual abuse) or emotional trauma (eg, domestic violence).

Evaluation

History

At present, an estimated 70% of children with acquired hearing loss are initially identified by their parents. Therefore, parental suspicion that their children do not hear should be sufficient reason to initiate a formal hearing evaluation. When evaluating children younger than 3 years, pediatricians must rely primarily on parental reports of children's language capabilities (Questions Box). Children who are 3 years of age and older can usually be engaged in

Questions

Language Development

- Are the child's language capabilities appropriate for age?
- Do the parents feel that their child has difficulty hearing?
- Is there any family history of childhood deafness?
- Has the child been exposed to any ototoxic agents (eg, aminoglycoside antibiotics)?
- Is there a history of neonatal asphyxia, hyperbilirubinemia, or low birth weight?
- Has the child ever had bacterial meningitis?
- Did the mother have a TORCHS infection (toxoplasmosis, rubella, cytomegalovirus, herpes simplex, syphilis) during pregnancy?

conversation during the visit, but younger children are more likely to be uncooperative or remain silent when confronted by strangers or new situations.

Historical factors such as a family history of childhood deafness, exposure to ototoxic agents (eg, aminoglycoside antibiotics), neonatal asphyxia, hyperbilirubinemia, maternal cocaine abuse, or low birth weight provide valuable information in the identification of high-risk infants (see Boxes 19-1 and 19-3).

Physical Examination

Examination should include a thorough assessment of the head and neck region. Microcephaly may indicate the presence of mental retardation or structural abnormalities. Abnormalities of the external ear (eg, microtia) may be associated with sensorineural hearing loss. Otoscopic examination of the ear is essential. Presence of a middle ear effusion may be associated with a conductive hearing loss. The tympanic membrane should be examined for evidence of scarring or perforation, often secondary to recurrent otitis media. Pneumatic otoscopy provides subjective assessment of tympanic membrane mobility (compliance) when it is subjected to a pulse of air. Tympanometry (impedance audiometry) performed in the office can provide objective information regarding the mobility of the tympanic membrane and the presence of middle ear effusions (Figure 19-1). Tympanometry is not a hearing test but rather an assessment of middle ear functioning that uses sound energy to determine the compliance of the tympanic membrane and pressure in the middle ear. Physical stigmata of any syndromes that may be associated with deafness (Box 19-4) should be noted.

Laboratory Tests

The advantages of early identification of hearing loss cannot be overemphasized. The Joint Committee on Infant Hearing's Year 2000 Position Statement, which was endorsed by the American Academy of Pediatrics, endorses universal hearing evaluation of all infants prior to 3 months of age. High-risk indicators for hearing loss (see Box 19-3) serve 2 purposes. First, they help identify infants, living in areas where universal newborn hearing screening is not yet available, who should receive an audiological evaluation.

Figure 19-1. **Basic tympanometry curves. The Type A curve indicates a normally compliant tympanic membrane (TM). The Type B curve indicates little or no motion of the TM and can be seen with middle ear effusion, a scarred TM, or a cholesteatoma. The Type C curve indicates negative middle ear pressure and may be seen with a resolving middle ear effusion or eustachian tube dysfunction. Other variations can occur in these basic curves that are not illustrated here.**

Box 19-4. Syndromes Commonly Associated With Hearing Impairment

Autosomal-Dominant Conditions
- Brachio-otorenal syndrome
- Goldenhar syndrome (facioauriculovertebral dysplasia)
- Stickler syndrome
- Treacher Collins syndrome
- Waardenburg syndrome

Autosomal-Recessive Conditions
- Alport syndrome
- Jervell and Lange-Nielsen syndrome
- Pendred syndrome
- Usher syndrome

Chromosomal Disorders
- Trisomy 13 syndrome
- Trisomy 18q syndrome

Miscellaneous Disorders
- CHARGE association (coloboma, congenital heart disease, choanal atresia, growth and mental retardation, genitourinary anomalies, ear anomalies, and genital hypoplasia)
- TORCHS syndrome (toxoplasmosis, rubella, cytomegalovirus, herpes simplex, syphilis)

Second, these risk indicators help identify infants who require ongoing medical and audiological monitoring because normal hearing at birth in these children may not preclude the development of later hearing loss (eg, delayed onset).

The evaluation of any child with delayed language development or suspected hearing loss begins with a hearing assessment. Various techniques are available, depending on the child's age and the degree of sophistication required. (A detailed discussion of the various tests used to evaluate children's hearing is presented in Chapter 61.)

In addition to a hearing evaluation, a full speech, language, and communication assessment (eg, assessment of pragmatic language skills) should be performed on children with suspected language delays. Language assessment may be aided by the use of screening tests such as the Denver Developmental Screening Test II or the Early Language Milestone Scale. These tests are used to supplement the clinical history of a child's language abilities.

Management

The first 3 years of life are extremely important to language development. Hearing impairment is one of the most common causes of delayed language development in young children. The history, physical examination, and initial screening can be used to suggest referral to various specialists (eg, audiologists, speech pathologists, child psychologists, otolaryngologists) for further clarification of hearing, speech, or language deficits and treatment. Early identification of hearing impairment and its degree of severity allow for early intervention in the form of amplification of sound, special education for children, and counseling and support services for the families with affected children.

As soon as a diagnosis of significant hearing loss is made, **hearing aids** may be provided. **Cochlear implants** are experimental at present, but they may be useful in children with acquired hearing loss, such as toddlers with meningitis. With severe hearing loss, training in **sign language** and **lip reading,** which are most helpful for those children who already know a language, may be begun as early as possible. Special education is of prime importance in the management of children with language difficulties. The Education for All Handicapped Persons Act, federal legislation passed in 1975, requires that public schools provide individualized and appropriate education for all children with disabilities. Knowledge of available community resources (eg, special schools) can aid pediatricians in providing **support services** such as special community agencies and support groups for disabled children and their parents.

CASE RESOLUTION

The child described in the case history has delayed development of expressive language skills. At the age of 3 years, she should have a 250-word vocabulary and speak in 3-word sentences; in addition, her speech should be primarily intelligible to strangers. Because of the delay, she should be referred immediately for a hearing assessment and speech and language evaluation. Hearing loss is an important diagnosis to rule out. Simply because her parents report no hearing problems does not mean she does not have a deficit. She may have learned to respond to nonverbal cues, or she may hear only some things.

Selected References

Bachmann KR, Arvedson JC. Early identification and intervention for children who are hearing impaired. *Pediatr Rev.*1998;19:155–165

Cunningham M, Cox EO, American Academy of Pediatrics Committee on Practice and Ambulatory Medicine and Section on Otolaryngology and Bronchoesophagology. Hearing assessment in infants and children: recommendations beyond neonatal screening. *Pediatrics.* 2003;111:436–440

Fierro-Cobas V, Chan E. Language development in bilingual children: a primer for pediatricians. *Contemp Pediatr.* 2001;18:79–98

Joint Committee on Infant Hearing, American Academy of Audiology, American Academy of Pediatrics, American Speech-Language-Hearing Association, Directors of Speech and Hearing Programs in State Health and Welfare Agencies. Year 2000 position statement: principles and guidelines for early hearing detection and intervention. *Pediatrics.* 2000;106:798–817

Zebrowski PM. Developmental stuttering. *Pediatr Ann.* 2003;32:453–458

Literacy Promotion in Pediatric Practice

Lynn Hunt, MD

CASE STUDY

You are seeing a 6-month-old boy for the first time for a well-child check. The child has a completely negative history and seems to be thriving. The patient's mother works part-time as a housekeeper and his father is a seasonal worker in agriculture. The infant is up to date on his immunizations and is due for his 6-month shots. The family history is negative, but the mother mentions that the 6-year-old sister needs to repeat kindergarten. The teachers advised the mother that though her oldest daughter is cooperative, she has not mastered letters and early reading yet. They feel with "a little more time" she will be fine. The mother does not seem terribly concerned.

Questions

1. What is the single most important activity parents can do to prepare a child for kindergarten?
2. Should you be worried that the 6-month-old patient may have trouble in school too?
3. What are risk factors for school failure?
4. What can you do as a health care provider to help this infant succeed when he gets to school?

Early literacy promotion in the office setting is now recognized as an essential part of pediatric primary care. Both the American Academy of Pediatrics and the Canadian Paediatric Society encourage providers to include literacy promotion in the routine clinical care of young children.

Literacy promotion does not mean teaching a child to read. Eventual mastery of reading depends on skills such as language ability, imagination, and familiarity with books and the reading process. Children develop many of these skills in the first few years of life before they go to school or even to preschool. In fact, a child's language at 2 years of age is strongly correlated with later cognitive performance. Literacy promotion should begin before a child learns to speak and depends heavily on the parent-child interaction.

Reading aloud to children on a regular basis is one of the most effective ways to promote early literacy and language development. Language skills are the foundation for later reading ability and are dependent largely on the amount and quality of language exposure. These early experiences can actually affect the architecture of the child's brain. A developing brain is physically altered by activities during infancy. At birth a baby's brain contains 100 billion neurons, which go on to form trillions more connections. Not all of these connections will endure. Synapses that are stimulated by frequent use will persist, and less-used connections will be eliminated by a process called pruning as the brain matures. Reading aloud and book sharing will help ensure the preservation of brain connections associated with skills such as memory, creativity, comprehension, and language.

Consequences of Low Literacy

There are significant consequences to low literacy as children get older. Poor academic skills are consistently linked with higher dropout rates, entrance into the juvenile justice system, and unemployment. One-third of all juvenile offenders are reported to read below the fourth-grade level and more than 80% of inmates are high school dropouts.

Literacy level and health outcomes are also intimately related. Health literacy is defined as the degree to which individuals can obtain, process, and understand the basic information they need to make appropriate health decisions.

Multiple studies have demonstrated that low literacy impacts health and well-being negatively. Individuals with limited health literacy are more likely to engage in risky behavior and less likely to receive the care they need. Adolescents with low reading ability were more likely to smoke, use alcohol, carry a weapon, and be in a physical fight requiring medical treatment. Conversely, higher levels of literacy were associated with breastfeeding as mothers and appropriate use of inhaled asthma medication in adults.

Promoting literacy is good medicine not only for the individual but also for society. Low literacy is common in the United States and affects millions of adults. Besides the societal impact of school failure, individuals with limited literacy incur medical expenses that are up to 4 times greater than patients with adequate literacy skills. Low literacy costs the health care system billions of dollars every year in preventable visits and hospital stays.

Literacy Promotion in the Medical Office

Reading aloud exposes children to vocabulary they don't hear in daily conversations (3 bears, beanstalks, etc). Reading aloud also stimulates the imagination (cows jumping over the moon). Over time children learn that the abstract letters on the page represent words, and they become aware of different smaller sounds making up words. All of these experiences lead to reading readiness.

Reach Out and Read (ROR) is the most widespread model for promoting literacy in the pediatric setting. The ROR model has 3 main components.

1. Anticipatory guidance: Health care providers encourage parents to read aloud to their young children during regular health supervision visits. The advice is age-appropriate, and concrete examples are provided.

2. Books: A new developmentally and culturally appropriate book is given by the doctor at each well-child visit so that parents have the tools to follow their provider's advice.

3. Waiting rooms: When possible, community volunteers read aloud in the waiting rooms, modeling for parents the pleasures and techniques of reading aloud to very young children.

Reach Out and Read had its origins in an urban clinic serving a high proportion of needy families. Reach Out and Read has always had a special focus on children growing up in poverty. For complex reasons, poverty is a powerful predictor of children's exposure to language. Children in low-income homes are 40% less likely to be read to on a daily basis than other children. Studies estimate that by age 4, a child living below the poverty line will hear only one-third as many words in total as those growing up in middle-income households.

Advice to parents is easiest and most effective when the book is brought in at the beginning of the visit. That way, physicians can naturally weave in guidance that is appropriate to the age of the child (see Box 20-1 and Table 20-1). Advice should be brief and to the point, supportive and nonthreatening, and part of a general conversation about the child's development and behavior.

Another advantage of presenting the book early in the visit is the amount of developmental and relationship information that can be garnered. The book is a tool that can speed the developmental assessment. If a 2-year-old says "doggie says wow-wow!" there is no doubt about using 2 words together. If a 1-year-old uses an index finger to point and looks to see if his mother is watching, the provider will know information about fine motor ability and the child's social interaction in only a few moments.

Ideally books should be in the family's preferred language or bilingual. If no book is available in the right language or the parents are not confident with their own reading skills, the primary care provider should encourage parents to look at books, name pictures, and talk about what is going on in the pictures with their children. Children benefit from storytelling and book time in whatever fashion is most comfortable for the parent. This activity is supposed to be fun for the parent and the child. Providers should be aware of adult literacy and English as a second language programs in their area

---

Box 20-1. Talking With Parents About Books[a]

Here are suggestions for brief anticipatory guidance, combining information about the child's emerging literacy with other developmental and behavioral issues.

6–12 Months
- She's really looking and moving her arms with excitement. Even infants love picture books.
- You can make story time part of your baby's routine, before bed or naps.
- You're teaching your baby that looking at books feels good.
- Babies love rhymes and songs.

12–18 Months
- When you ask, "What's that?" and name the picture in a book, it teaches your baby that things have names.
- Some babies will want to be up and around during a story. That's OK.
- Offer stories each day, but let your child be in charge of how long you read.
- When your child grabs the book, he is showing a healthy drive for independence. He's not being bad.

18–36 Months
- If your toddler listens to a story for 5 minutes, that's a long time. Stories are a good way to help toddlers increase their attention spans.
- You don't have to read what's actually written in the book. You can just talk about the pictures instead.
- Your toddler will want to pick the book, the time, and the person to do the reading.
- Children learn by imitating. Does she ever read to her teddy bears or dolls?

3 Years and Older
- One way children learn to read is by hearing the same story over and over. It might be boring to you, but it isn't to her.
- Your child might want to tell you a story, and it may be a very different one from the one you thought you were reading! Each time she retells the story, she is practicing using language in a very important way.
- Play writing is the first step toward learning how to spell. Does she ever pretend to write or ask you to show her her name?

[a] Adapted from 2005 Reach Out and Read Program Manual.

---

because parents may ask for resources when literacy is discussed in the examination room.

Primary Care Providers Can Make a Difference

The primary care setting is the ideal venue for literacy promotion for several reasons. First, almost all parents will bring in their child for immunizations, so there is an opportunity to reach a broad group, not just those seeking learning experiences for their children. Second, each child is seen for multiple visits from a very young age, providing repeat opportunities to discuss reading aloud during the critical first years. Further, suggestions supporting literacy-focused activities are a logical extension of the advice about growth and development parents are already receiving at these visits. And, hopefully,

Motor	Cognitive	What Parents Can Do
Table 20-1. Developmental Milestones of Early Literacy[a]		
6–12 Months		
• Reaches for books • Book to mouth • Sits in lap, head steady • Turns pages with adult help	• Looks at pictures • Vocalizes, pats pictures • Prefers pictures of faces	• Hold child comfortably; face-to-face gaze • Follow baby's cues for "more" and "stop" • Point and name pictures
12–18 Months		
• Sits without support • May carry book • Holds book with help • Turns board pages, several at a time	• No longer mouths right away • Points at picture with one finger • May make same sound for particular picture (labels) • Points when asked, "where's…?" • Turns book right side up • Gives book to adult to read	• Respond to child's prompting to read • Let child control the book • Be comfortable with toddler's short attention span • Ask "where's the …?" and let child point
18–24 Months		
• Turns board pages easily, one at a time • Carries book around the house • May use book as a transitional object	• Names familiar pictures • Fills in words and familiar stories • "Reads" to dolls or stuffed animals • Recites parts of well-known stories • Attention span highly variable	• Relate books to child's experiences • Use books in routines, bedtimes • Ask child "what's that?" and let child answer • Pause and let child complete the sentence
24–36 Months		
• Learns to handle paper pages • Goes back and forth in books to find favorite pictures	• Recites whole phrases, sometimes whole stories • Coordinates text with picture • Protests when adult gets a word wrong in a familiar story • Reads familiar books to self	• Keep using books in routines • Read at bedtime • Be willing to read the same story over and over • Ask "what's that?" • Relate books to child's experiences • Provide crayons and paper
3 Years and Older		
• Competent book handling • Turns paper pages one at a time	• Listens to longer stories • Can retell familiar story • Moves finger along text • "Writes" name • Moves toward letter recognition	• Ask "what's happening?" • Encourage writing and drawing • Let child tell story

[a]Adapted from www.reachoutandread.org/FileRepository/RORmilestones_English.pdf.

parents trust and value the advice from their primary care provider, giving credibility to the early literacy message.

The effectiveness of a primary care intervention to promote reading aloud to young children has been demonstrated in multiple research studies. Parents who received even one book were much more likely to read aloud to their children and report reading as a favorite activity of their child. The effect was greatest for the poorest families, an important finding for children who may need this intervention the most. The outcome was similar for non–English-speaking families, and the findings held even if the book was given in English. There is also a "dose response" effect: The more a family is exposed to literacy promotion in the pediatric setting, the greater the home literacy environment. Finally, and most encouraging, toddlers who had received care in clinics applying the ROR model had higher scores on language and vocabulary assessments than children not involved with ROR.

Literacy promotion and the ROR model of giving books along with advice provide benefits for all concerned. Medical providers have a tool to assess development and parent-child interactions and a way to build stronger bonds with families. Parents receive important information about reading aloud and advice tailored to the age of their child. And most importantly, children receive the benefits of reading aloud as well as beautiful, developmentally appropriate books.

CASE RESOLUTION

You speak to the mother about the value of reading aloud to her children. You find 2 age-appropriate books that you can give her. You demonstrate, showing how the 6-month-old is interested in the pictures and follows the story as you turn the pages.

Selected References

AMA Foundation—Health Literacy
www.ama-assn.org/ama/pub/category/8115.html

Developmental Milestones of Early Literacy
www.reachoutandread.org/FileRepository/RORmilestones_English.pdf

Reach Out and Read
www.reachoutandread.org

Summary of studies of relationship between health services, outcomes, costs, or disparities and literacy
www.ncbi.nlm.nih.gov/books/bv.fcgi?rid=hstat1a.table.32324

What Children Like in Books
www.reachoutandread.org/FileRepository/WhatChildrenLikeinBooks.pdf

Gifted Children

Iris Wagman Borowsky, MD, PhD, and Rachel S. Darling, MD

CASE STUDY

A 3-year-old girl is brought to your office for well-child care. Her parents believe that she may be gifted because she is much more advanced than her sister was when she was the same age. The parents report that their younger daughter walked at 11 months of age and was speaking in 2-word sentences by 18 months. She is very "verbal," has a precocious vocabulary, and constantly asks difficult questions such as, "How do voices come over a radio?" The girl stays at home with her mother during the day but recently began going to a preschool program 2 mornings a week. She enjoys preschool and plays well with children her own age. She also likes to play with her sister's friends from school.

The girl is engaging and talkative. She asks questions about what you are doing during the examination and demonstrates impressive knowledge of anatomy. The physical examination is normal.

Questions
1. How are gifted children identified?
2. What characteristics are associated with giftedness?
3. What are the best approaches for dealing with the education of gifted children?
4. What is the role of the pediatrician in the management of gifted children?

Giftedness has been defined in several ways. The psychometric definition of giftedness is based on scores obtained on standardized intelligence tests. The 2 most frequently used cutoff points are 2 standard deviations above the mean (IQ = 130–135) and 3 standard deviations above the mean (IQ = 145–150). Children with these scores are in the upper 2% and 0.1% of the IQ distribution, respectively. IQ, which is considered to be fairly stable after the age of 3 or 4 years, is the best single predictor of scholastic achievement at all levels, from elementary school to college.

A second definition of giftedness is based on real-life achievements or performance of exceptional skills rather than on test scores. Children with special talents (other than general intelligence) in areas such as music, mathematics, ice skating, chess, or drama fit this description. Other definitions of giftedness recognize motivation, commitment, perseverance, high self-esteem, and creativity as personality traits that allow children with above-average ability to develop exceptional talents.

Epidemiology

The prevalence of giftedness depends on the somewhat arbitrary definitions of giftedness and the varied approaches for identification of gifted children. Traditional screening systems identify 3% to 5% of students for participation in gifted programs in schools. Some schools use an alternative system, where 10% to 15% of children are recognized as above average. In an effort to foster giftedness in these children, schools offer them enriched programs.

Intellectual giftedness in children has been associated with the social, economic, and educational background of their families. Factors that correlate with higher IQ scores in children are more years of parental education, higher IQ scores of mothers, increased family income, smaller family size, and longer intervals between siblings. Children from low-income and minority backgrounds are less likely to be identified as gifted than other children. African American, Hispanic, and Native American students are underrepresented by 30% to 70% in gifted programs in the United States.

Larger head size at 1 year of age and greater height and weight at 4 years of age have also been reported in children with high IQs. Although researchers have found that academically gifted children, as a group, begin to walk, verbalize, and read earlier, such factors are not useful for predicting giftedness in individual children.

Evaluation

One of the primary goals of child health promotion is **developmental monitoring.** The early identification of developmental delays, which allows for prompt intervention, is one of the primary purposes of such monitoring. Techniques for developmental assessment include **review of developmental milestones** with parents and discussion of parental concerns, **informal observation** of children in the office, and **formal screening with standardized tests** such as the Denver II.

Identification of Gifted Children

Although parents' first concern is usually to confirm that their child is developing normally, it is not uncommon for parents to ask if their child is gifted. Such questions are typically motivated by parents' desire to optimally encourage their child's development. Sharing information and observations with parents during developmental monitoring may facilitate parent-child interaction and child development. In a competitive society, the pediatric provider should look for signs that above-average abilities are the result of undue pressures placed on children, such as incessant teaching or over-scheduling of time.

Infancy and early childhood may not be the best time to determine whether a child is gifted. Age of attainment of developmental milestones and performance on standardized tests (eg, Bayley Scales of Infant Development) during the first 2 years of life are both unreliable predictors of intellectual giftedness. Reasons for this lack of reliability may include weaknesses in the tests and variable rates of child development that result in transient precocity or delay. Tests that focus on visual memory tasks in infants may be better predictors of later academic intelligence; this possibility requires more research. In addition, many special talents that comprise giftedness, such as creativity or artistic or musical ability, may not manifest themselves until children are older.

The determination of giftedness in older children may involve several factors (Box 21-1). The early identification of giftedness allows for the development of an appropriate educational program that is optimally matched to a particular child's ability to learn. Without early identification and intervention, intellectually gifted children may become disillusioned with school, lose interest in learning, fail to develop study skills because they are never challenged to think and work hard, and develop a pattern of underachievement that may be difficult to reverse by the middle grades.

Box 21-1. Factors Used in the Identification of Giftedness in Children

- Intelligence tests
- Standardized achievement tests
- Grades
- Classroom observations
- Parent and teacher rating scales
- Evaluation of creative work in a specific field (eg, poems, drawings, science projects)

Special Groups of Gifted Children

Giftedness is harder to identify in some children. In **physically disabled children,** giftedness is often obscured by their obvious physical disability, which demands attention. These children may participate in special programs where their physical needs are the major concern at the expense of their academic or artistic potential. In addition, poor self-esteem associated with the disability may prevent these children from realizing their potential. To identify giftedness in physically disabled children, parents and teachers must make a concerted effort to search for potential and encourage its development. Strengthening a child's capacities may involve training in the use of a wheelchair or computer or taking frequent breaks to prevent fatigue.

Giftedness also commonly goes unnoticed in children who are **learning disabled.** It is quite possible for exceptional and poor abilities to coexist in a given child. In fact, an estimated 10% of gifted children have a reading problem, reading 2 or more years below grade level. Albert Einstein, Auguste Rodin, and John D. Rockefeller are famous examples of brilliant individuals who had reading and writing problems. An extreme example of the occurrence of both extraordinary and deficient abilities together in one individual is the child savant. Affected children possess amazing abilities in one area (eg, music, drawing, mathematics, memory), but they are delayed in other respects. In addition, they have behavioral problems that resemble autism, such as repetitive behavior, little use of language, and social withdrawal.

Learning disabilities may obscure children's talents, thus preventing awareness of their potential. Conversely, children's giftedness may mask their weaknesses, depriving them of needed help. Worst of all, gifted children who are learning disabled may manage to barely "get by" in the regular classroom setting and fail to receive recognition for strengths or weaknesses. Large differences on intelligence and achievement tests between scores in different areas, such as language and spatial abilities, may indicate both giftedness and a learning disability. Attention should be given to both weaknesses and strengths. Research suggests that programs that focus on strengths, not deficits, however, enhance self-esteem in gifted children who are learning disabled and can be extremely beneficial in their academic development.

The identification of giftedness is also difficult in **underachieving children.** Parents may approach the pediatrician with the following frustrating problem: their child is doing poorly at school, although they believe that the child is bright because of the child's abilities and participation in advanced activities at home. Underachievement may result from a learning disability; poor self-esteem; lack of motivation; or the absence of rewards, either at home or at school, for succeeding in academics.

As previously stated, giftedness is less likely to be recognized in children from low-income or ethnically diverse families. Many of the tests used to identify giftedness have been "normed" on white, English-speaking, middle-class children. In the absence of tests that are sensitive to socioeconomic differences, other means for identifying giftedness, such as assessment of creative work and teacher and student nominations, should be stressed. Schools with students from low-income or minority backgrounds tend to use their limited resources to help students who are doing poorly in school, rather than gifted students. Research has shown that programs for gifted children from such backgrounds benefit all students by creating positive role models and promoting the school as a place for the cultivation of excellence.

Management

At Home

Loving, responsive, stimulating parenting should be encouraged for all children, including gifted children. Parents of gifted children may feel inadequate, fearing that their child is smarter than they are. The pediatrician can provide **parental reassurance** by telling parents, "You must have been doing something right for your child to have been identified as gifted." Children's librarians, periodicals written for parents and teachers of gifted children (eg, *The Gifted Child Today*), and the local chapter of the National Association for Gifted Children are good resources for parents.

Parents are often overwhelmed with complex questions from their precocious preschool children about issues ranging from homelessness and world hunger to theology and the creation of the universe. The pediatrician should tell parents that they (1) should not be afraid to admit that they do not know all the answers and (2) should work together with their child to find the answers.

The pediatrician may need to warn parents about putting too much pressure on their gifted children. For example, enrolling children in multiple classes often leaves little free time for unstructured play. Play affords many opportunities for self-learning, interaction with peers, and development of creativity and initiative. Parents of infants, toddlers, and preschoolers should be encouraged to take cues from their children. If children have a rich environment with plenty of objects and books to explore, diverse experiences, and stimulating interactions, they will develop their own interests. Other educational materials and special instruction can then be provided in a particular area of interest.

Gifted children are often mistakenly considered to fit the stereotype of troubled, socially awkward "nerds." With the exception of children at the genius extreme (IQ>180), gifted children are generally more sociable, well-liked, trustworthy, and emotionally stable than their peers, with lower rates of mental illness and delinquency. Nevertheless, they have the same emotional needs as other children. Gifted children may prefer to play with older children whose interests and abilities are closer to their own. This should be allowed as long as these relationships are healthy.

Parents should be encouraged to treat gifted children the same way they do their other children. Siblings of gifted children may become resentful if attention is centered on their brother or sister. They may feel inferior, particularly if gifted children surpass them in school. Tensions may be magnified if gifted children become friends with their older sibling's friends. To preserve a sense of self-worth and competence in siblings, the pediatrician should recommend to parents that they set aside special time to spend with each of their children. Parents should encourage other talents (eg, musical or athletic abilities) in siblings. Older siblings should receive the special privileges and responsibilities that come with age, such as staying up later or doing different chores. Any tensions within the family should be openly discussed and addressed.

At School

Parents often seek advice from their pediatrician about educational planning for gifted children. A learning environment with the optimal degree of challenge—hard enough to require new learning and stave off boredom, but not so hard as to be discouraging—is the goal for all children. Parents of young children should look for preschools with flexible programs and capable teachers to accommodate children with precocious skills. Parents of school-aged children must decide whether **acceleration** (starting school earlier or skipping grades) or **enrichment** (staying in the same grade but supplementing the regular curriculum) is more appropriate (Table 21-1). The choice depends on the particular child.

Parents and teachers of gifted children are usually concerned that children in accelerated programs may have problems with social adjustment if their classmates are older. Existing evidence, however, suggests that gifted children benefit socially from acceleration. Gifted children in accelerated programs participate in school activities (except contact sports) more often than gifted children placed with classmates of the same age. Even when gifted children are placed with children their own age, they tend to make friends with older children with whom they share more interests. Gifted children also make up any curricular content missed by grade skipping. Because the process may be difficult to reverse, acceleration may not be the best option when the decision is a borderline one.

Enrichment involves keeping gifted children with same-age classmates, but supplementing the regular curriculum. Regular class placement with a teacher who is willing to offer extra work (eg,

Table 21-1. Acceleration Versus Enrichment in Gifted Education		
	Advantages	*Disadvantages*
Acceleration	May provide suitable academic challenge	Difficult to reverse
	May have social benefits	May have to skip more than one grade to be properly challenged
	Can be offered by all schools	
	Inexpensive	
Enrichment	Classmates are same age	May be expensive
	May expose children to subjects they would not otherwise learn	Inadequate for highly gifted children
	Appropriate for mildly gifted children	May isolate gifted from non-gifted children and encourage "elite" label
		May lead to excessive homework if children have to make up work of regular class

special projects) in addition to grade-level assignments, part-time programs to supplement regular class work (eg, field trips, foreign language classes), honors classes that group bright children together for their basic curriculum, and independent study by the family at home are all examples of enrichment programs. These programs may work well for some gifted children, depending in large part on the resources and funding available and the experience, creativity, and enthusiasm of the teachers involved.

Some enrichment programs may isolate gifted from non-gifted children, however, and encourage labeling of the gifted students as elite. If children are required to make up the regular class work that they miss when they are involved in the enrichment program, they may find themselves overloaded with homework.

Often a **combination of acceleration and enrichment** programs is the best option. Either acceleration or enrichment alone may not be enough for the brightest children. Acceleration may not be sufficient for markedly advanced children who would have to skip 2 or 3 grades to be appropriately challenged. The pediatrician should recommend that parents work closely with teachers to achieve the best learning environment for their children. Some factors that should be considered are age, physical size, motor coordination, emotional maturity, personality, and particular areas and degrees of giftedness of the child. Acceleration may be a better option for a large, outgoing child than for a small one. Gifted children should be asked what they would like to do.

When evaluating the suitability of an educational situation for their gifted child, parents should watch for some warning signs. Excessive homework should neither be expected nor tolerated because it cuts into the child's time to play and develop socially. The emphasis in gifted education should be on broadening perspectives, not increasing busy work. If gifted children are developing a sense of elitism or peer animosity, the nature and philosophy of the program should be questioned. Boredom with schoolwork, not needing to study, signs of depression, or symptoms suggestive of school phobia, such as recurrent abdominal pain or headaches on school mornings, should prompt investigation into the suitability of the child's program.

Prognosis

Gifted children are a diverse group, comprising children with exceptional academic, artistic, or other abilities, combined with the creativity and commitment to achieve their potential. Gifted children may be gifted in one area and average or even below average in another area. The purpose of identifying gifted children is to provide them with an educational environment to help maximize their potential. The prognosis for gifted children is excellent. Pediatricians can serve as a resource for parents in raising their gifted child, and help the child and family to obtain appropriate evaluation, educational programs, and supportive resources.

CASE RESOLUTION

In the case presented, the physician should reaffirm the parents' observations that their child is gifted. The parents should be encouraged to explore programs in which their daughter's talents may be fostered, but at the same time, they should understand that even gifted children need time for play and unstructured activities.

Selected References

Colangelo N, Davis GA, eds. *Handbook of Gifted Education.* 3rd ed. Needham Heights, MA: Allyn & Bacon; 2002

Jaffe A. The gifted child. *Pediatr Rev.* 2000;21:240–242

Liu YH, Lien J, Kafka T, Stein MT. Discovering gifted children in pediatric practice. *J Dev Behav Pediatr.* 2005;26:366–369

Lovett BJ, Lewandowski LJ. Gifted students with learning disabilities: who are they? *J Learn Disabil.* 2006;39:515–527

Robinson A, Clinkenbeard PR. Giftedness: an exceptionality examined. *Annu Rev Psychol.* 1998;49:117–139

Robinson NM, Olszewski-Kubilius PM. Gifted and talented children: issues for pediatricians. *Pediatr Rev.* 1996;17:427–434

Shaunessy E, Karnes FA, Cobb Y. Assessing potentially gifted students from lower socioeconomic status with nonverbal measures of intelligence. *Percept Mot Skills.* 2004;98:1129–1138

Winner E. The origins and ends of giftedness. *Am Psychol.* 2000;55:159–169

Children and School: A Primer for the Practitioner

Martin Baren, MD, and Geeta Grover, MD

CASE STUDY

An 8-year-old boy is brought in by his parents in early April because his third-grade teacher informed them that he is currently failing in school and may not be promoted to the fourth grade. Review of his medical, developmental, and school histories reveals that he was a very colicky infant and continued to be difficult as a toddler. His language skills were somewhat delayed, although not enough to warrant a full evaluation. His preschool teacher felt that he was easily distracted when doing seat work. In kindergarten he had some difficulty learning all of his letters, numbers, and sounds. Early reading was difficult in kindergarten and first grade, but improved by the end of the year. Second grade was fairly good except for continued concerns regarding inattention and distractibility. By third grade he was struggling more, especially with writing, and not reaching grade level in several areas. He also continued to be inattentive and distractible in his classroom.

Examination reveals a well-developed and well-nourished boy whose growth parameters are within normal limits for his age. He appears somewhat anxious in the examination room, and when asked about school he tells you that he feels he is just not as smart as the other children in his class.

Questions

1. Should grade retention be considered when a child is failing in school?
2. What are the advantages and/or disadvantages of grade retention?
3. What is the differential diagnosis of school failure?
4. What steps should be taken at this time by the parents and the school for the boy in the opening scenario?

Pediatricians, because of their routine contact with young children and their families, are often the professionals most knowledgeable about child development. Pediatricians' longitudinal perspective on their patients' lives places them in a unique position to evaluate, diagnose, and manage not only children's medical needs, but also their developmental, social-emotional, behavioral, and educational ones. Traditionally, the 5-year-old health maintenance visit has been regarded as the "school readiness" visit. However, waiting until this date to address concerns regarding educational readiness is too late. **School readiness** must be promoted from infancy through early childhood.

During the school-aged years, pediatricians should continue to monitor children's school progression by inquiring about academic, social-emotional, and behavioral development. Parents often turn to pediatricians for advice regarding their children's behavioral or academic difficulties at school, which may be leading to **school failure.** The evaluation and management of school failure requires a multidisciplinary approach under the guidance, support, and advocacy provided by pediatricians. It is important that pediatricians have an understanding of the evaluation and management of both children's school readiness needs and school difficulties, should such arise.

Epidemiology

School readiness is the term used to describe those qualities and traits that are considered prerequisites for a child to be ready to be successful in school. According to national surveys of kindergarten teachers, about one-third of children are not ready for school when they enter, and of these children, 25% will repeat either kindergarten or first grade. Language deficiencies and problems with emotional maturity are cited most often as the factors that most restrict school readiness.

School failure is a multifaceted issue and epidemiologically complex. Overall, about 20% of children have one or more developmental, learning, behavioral, or emotional disorders. Only 10% to 15% of children in the United States are receiving special education services because of difficulties with school performance. Finally, we know that children with concerns such as these are 2 to 3 times more likely to drop out of school than children without any of these concerns.

Given that the average child in the United States spends nearly 50% of his or her waking day in a school or a similar learning situation for approximately 12 or 13 years, it follows that a lack of success in these settings will lead to difficulties for much, or all, of adult life.

Undetected school difficulties can create a lifelong pattern of frustration and failure. Children with **attention-deficit/hyperactivity disorder (ADHD)** are 2 to 3 times more likely to drop out of high school than their peers without ADHD; children with ADHD who attend college are less likely to graduate than their non-ADHD peers (see Chapter 113). About 40% of all juvenile offenders have learning disabilities; many have never received any help for their disabilities. Even more alarming is that 85% of juvenile delinquents and 75% of adult prisoners are functionally illiterate—somehow these children slipped through the cracks of our educational system.

Clinical Presentation

Defining **school readiness** is not an easy task because the intellectual, physical, social, and emotional development among kindergarten-aged children varies tremendously. Generally school readiness means that children are adequately prepared to participate in formal schooling. It is the term used to describe those traits that are considered prerequisites for a child to be ready to succeed in school (Box 22-1). Readiness implies not only adequate pre-academic skills, but also adequate physical, developmental, language, social-emotional, and behavioral skills to allow children to be successful in the formal schooling environment.

With regard to **school failure,** the non-specificity of children's presenting signs and symptoms and of parental complaints make it challenging to determine a specific etiology. For instance, parental concern regarding a child's inability to focus could suggest an attention disorder, learning disability, mood disorder or perhaps all 3. Parental concerns can be categorized into 3 broad areas: learning

---

Box 22-1. Kindergarten Readiness Skills

Academic
- Counts to at least 10
- Recognizes some printed letters and perhaps a few words (eg, name)
- Beginning to understand connection between oral and written language (evidence of phonological skills)
- Recognizes and matches shapes and colors that are the same/different, etc

Personal, Social, Emotional, and Developmental
- Able to separate from parents for several hours at a time
- Takes care of personal hygiene and toileting
- Verbally communicates personal needs
- Able to relate personal experiences, ideas, thoughts, and feelings with words
- Sustains attention to task for 10 to 15 minutes
- Able to understand and follow directions with 2 or 3 steps
- Able to communicate and play cooperatively with other children (eg, shares and takes turns)
- Copes with anger and frustration

Motor
- Uses pencil, crayon, and scissors
- Runs, jumps, hops, skips, and throws ball
- Draws a person and basic shape

(eg, learning disability or problems with higher-order cognition including mental retardation), attention (eg, ADHD), and emotional/behavioral (eg, anxiety, depression, or serious emotional disturbance). Signs of school failure are presented in Box 22-2. It is important to look not only at academic skills, but also at other components of the educational experience such as social and emotional experiences. Finally, it is important to ascertain the basis for the perception that a child is failing. Does the problem exist in the eyes of the student, parent, teachers, or everyone?

Box 22-2. Signs of School Difficulties

- Grade retention
- Loss of self-esteem
- Short attention span/hyperactivity
- Not able to follow directions, pay attention, or finish a task
- History of speech-language problems
- Not able to carry thoughts or ideas to paper
- Not able to read, write, or spell appropriate to age and educational level
- Requires excessive time to complete homework/excessive parental involvement with homework
- Previously tested but not eligible for special education (eg, child may be a "slow learner")
- Child hates school/psychosomatic symptoms
- Child has few, if any, friends or change of friends
- Sudden change in behavior
- Depression
- Substance use

Academic achievement across subjects must be assessed, especially in the areas of reading, mathematics, and writing. In addition, it is also important to evaluate students who have good skills but fail to perform satisfactorily in the areas of writing, planning, organization, project completion, test taking, or classroom participation. Difficulty with academic performance may lead to school failure in spite of satisfactory academic skills.

In addition to academic skills and performance, the development of good social skills and peer relations is equally important. Some students have difficulties "fitting in," which leads to a disappointing educational experience in spite of academic excellence.

Pathophysiology

Developmentally there is support for the concept of promoting **school readiness** from a young age. The developing brain continues to make new synaptic connections and "prune" away underused connections from birth to about age 5—well before formal schooling begins. For example, we know that children who grow up without being read to and with little exposure to books or printed language during the first 5 years of life are at an increased risk of developing reading failure and subsequent school failure (see Chapter 20). School readiness must be promoted from infancy throughout early childhood—waiting for the 4- to 5-year-old well visit is too late.

Most children with learning disabilities experience language, motor skills, or behavior problems well before they encounter difficulties in the classroom.

School failure is a complex issue with a wide variety of causes. Both intrinsic, or child-related causes, and extrinsic, or environmental-related causes, relating either to the home or the school setting must be considered (Box 22-3). In most cases, school failure is the result of a complex interaction between child, family, and school-related variables, and not simply the result of a single factor (eg, ADHD). Before looking for specific learning disabilities or disorders or intellectual problems, investigate any type of external situation that may be causing the problem. Medical problems should always be considered. Neurologic, psycho-emotional, and behavioral disorders based in the central nervous system may be responsible for school failure.

Unrecognized ADHD, learning disorders, and learning disabilities are common causes of school failure. Learning disorders are defined problems within the central nervous system that prevent children from learning to their full potential. The brain has difficulty handling information (processing skills), which therefore affects the child's ability to learn and/or perform in school. Some of these processes include memory, language, attention, and coordination. A specific learning disability is a particular type of learning disorder

---

Box 22-3. Causes of School Failure

Intrinsic

- Low cognitive skills (intellect)
- Learning disorders
- Specific learning disabilities
- Attention-deficit/hyperactivity disorders
- Speech and language disorders
- Mood and anxiety disorders
- Low self-esteem
- Social-emotional difficulties
- Neurodevelopmental delays
- Motor coordination disorders
- Chronic or serious medical illness (eg, seizure disorders, cystic fibrosis, asthma)
- Vision, hearing, or speech difficulties
- Poor nutrition
- Sleep problems
- Substance use/abuse
- Genetic history (eg, family history of school problems)

Extrinsic

- Language/cultural differences
- Serious psychosocial concerns: parental depression, history of abuse or neglect
- Disruption in the family (eg, many moves)
- Poor school readiness/absence of enrichment prior to school entry (eg, early book exposure)
- Parental or school expectations not commensurate with child's abilities
- School, classroom placement (poor "fit" or poor teaching)

---

that is defined as a significant difference between a child's natural ability (intelligence—IQ) and his level of achievement, as defined by federal and state laws. This difference is determined by psycho-educational testing performed by psychologists and educators.

Federal law (Public Law 101-476: Individuals with Disabilities Education Act [IDEA]) defines specific learning disability as "a disorder in one or more of the basic psychological processes involved in understanding or in using language, spoken or written, that may manifest itself in an imperfect ability to listen, think, speak, read, write, or to do mathematical calculations, including conditions such as perceptual disabilities, brain injury, minimal brain dysfunction, dyslexia, and developmental aphasia." Operationally, specific learning disabilities are characterized by a discrepancy between ability (as measured by intelligence tests) and actual academic achievement (as measured by school performance). However, specific learning disability does not include children who have "learning problems that are primarily the result of visual, hearing, or motor disabilities, mental retardation, emotional disturbance, or environmental, cultural, or economic disadvantage."

Another important reason for school failure is an unsatisfactory student/teacher relationship. A poor "fit" with either teacher or classroom placement may cause major damage to a child's program.

Finally, there are students who are labeled "lazy" by school personnel. These students are usually found to have one or more of the previously mentioned school difficulties but have never been properly diagnosed. Rarely a student is found who has no major identifiable problem but just isn't motivated to take part in the educational experience. Alternative placement or home schooling may be an answer for these students.

Evaluation

History

In the past, pediatricians assessed **school readiness** during the 5-year-old health maintenance visit. Clinical approaches to early identification of children at risk for school failure include risk assessments and developmental surveillance and screening. Children most at risk for school problems are those from economically and socially disadvantaged backgrounds. Developmental surveillance and screening (see Chapter 18) allows pediatricians to identify children with developmental, behavioral, and emotional delays, and to provide appropriate anticipatory guidance, as well as referral to early intervention programs.

Historical factors associated with an increased risk of school-related problems include **prematurity; low birth weight; small for gestational age;** and **maternal history of tobacco, alcohol, or illicit substance abuse** during pregnancy (Questions Box: School Readiness). Developmental risk factors especially include delays in the acquisition of language skills. Medical factors that may impact school readiness include lead poisoning, iron deficiency anemia, and failure to thrive. The presence of chronic medical conditions (eg, asthma, diabetes mellitus, and seizure disorders) may impact school readiness either directly or indirectly via absenteeism, medication effects, or self-esteem issues. Environmental risk factors include poverty and lower socioeconomic status, parental depression, domestic violence, substance abuse, or a family history of school problems or learning disabilities.

School Readiness · Questions

- Has the child had any preschool or group child care experience and how has the child responded in these settings?
- Were any behavioral, developmental, or emotional concerns raised during those group care experiences?
- Does the child play well with age-appropriate peers or does the child seem to consistently prefer to play with younger or older children/adults?
- Is the child's speech understandable to strangers and can the child hold a conversation about everyday topics of interest?
- Can the child sit and listen to stories or sustain attention to a quiet activity for 10 to 15 minutes?
- Can the child identify colors, shapes, and some letters and numbers?

School Failure

When evaluating for **school failure,** historical information should be sought from parents, schools, teachers, and the children themselves (Questions Box: School Failure). A review of present and past report cards not only provides information regarding academic progress, but also the behavioral and social-emotional assessments. Teacher behavior rating forms and evaluations and results of any psycho-educational evaluations should also be reviewed.

School Failure · Questions

- How many days of school has the child missed?
- Have any behavioral or attentional concerns been raised by the classroom teacher?
- Is the child having problems in all academic areas or are there particular subjects that are especially difficult for the child?
- Has any testing (eg, psycho-educational evaluation) been performed either by the school district or privately?
- Is the child receiving any special services (eg, speech therapy) or accommodations at school?

Physical Examination

With regard to **school readiness,** the most important aspect of the 5-year-old health maintenance physical examination includes careful hearing, vision, speech, and language assessments.

The physical examination in the evaluation of **school failure** has a limited but important role. Signs of short attention span, distractibility, overactivity, sadness, or anxiety should all be noted. Special attention should be paid to head circumference, minor congenital anomalies, abnormal facies, and skin lesions suggestive of neurocuta-

neous disorders (eg, multiple café-au-lait spots or ash leaf spots). The pediatrician should assess for vision, hearing, speech and language, and other appropriate evaluations as suggested by the history.

Neurodevelopmental Assessment

School readiness assessment begins with routine pediatric surveillance and screening (see Chapter 18). Several brief school readiness tests have been developed for use by pediatricians (eg, The Pediatric Examination of Educational Readiness). However, because their reliability and ability to detect subtle learning disabilities or arrive at more complicated diagnoses is not established, it is difficult to recommend any of them for routine use. If a specific school readiness evaluation is warranted, it is best to make a referral either to the school district or to an independent specialist (eg, developmental and behavioral pediatrician or educational psychologist) for a full evaluation.

Neurodevelopmental assessment can help identify the etiology of **school failure.** Neurodevelopmental assessment surveys a child's abilities across the different areas of development (eg, fine motor, language, visual-spatial, and memory skills) and helps to identify areas of strength and weakness. Such an assessment can be performed by professionals such as a developmental and behavioral pediatrician or a psychologist. Psycho-educational assessment is also critical in the evaluation of children with school failure. Such an assessment includes an evaluation of the children's cognitive abilities, academic achievement across subjects (eg, reading, writing, and mathematics), and assessments of perceptual strengths and weaknesses and social and emotional functioning. This can be accomplished either through the public school system via the **Individualized Education Plan (IEP)** process, as mandated by federal law (**IDEA**) or privately by an educational psychologist.

Management

The first aspect of management is the counseling or demystification of parents and children. Empowering parents with knowledge gives them the confidence to interact positively with their children's schools and allows them to advocate effectively for their children's educational needs. For children, the process of demystification should begin with the assurance that all people have strengths and weaknesses—mentioning one's own weaknesses or citing famous or successful people that have dealt effectively with their own learning concerns helps "humanize" and destigmatize the situation for children. It is important to use an optimistic tone. In addition to addressing the needs of families and children, the physician also serves an important advisory role for the school regarding behavioral consequences of a child's disorder (eg, Should this child have a seizure or a behavioral outburst in the classroom, how should the situation be managed?) or the educational implications of chronic medical conditions.

Early intervention is the key to success with regard to children's **school readiness.** For many at-risk children, early childhood education programs such as Head Start and other preschool compensatory programs may come too late. Programs for younger children and their families (eg, Early Head Start) that promote good parenting, language stimulation, and learning through play are valuable and available in some communities.

Reading aloud to children is one of the most important parental interventions that physicians can promote, and it builds the child's skills required for eventual success in reading (see Chapter 20). Reading promotes language mastery, and language mastery, in turn, is one of the keys to school readiness.

The pediatrician can assist families with children who have clear developmental disabilities, such as mental retardation, cerebral palsy, or autism, to access special education services as mandated by the **IDEA of 1990 and the Amendments of 1997** and **2004.** These laws require public schools to provide a free and appropriate education in "the least restrictive environment" for all children with a disability and require schools to use the IEP process (or Individualized Family Service Plan [IFSP] for children <3 years of age) to identify and evaluate the educational needs of children in order to develop an appropriate educational program to meet each child's needs. Pediatricians should be familiar with their local laws so that they can advocate for these children at the time of school entry if needed.

Children who are at increased risk for school readiness problems because of medical, social-emotional, behavioral, or environmental concerns should be monitored carefully. If these children do not appear to demonstrate age-appropriate skills, they should be referred for further evaluation. Despite early intervention, some children may still not be ready for school at the age-appropriate time. Options for these children include delaying school entry or special educational programs. Delaying school entry may not be the best solution if children remain in the same environment that failed to produce readiness in the first place. In addition, studies have shown that students who are older than their classmates because of delayed school entry have higher rates of behavior problems, substance abuse, and other health risk behaviors in adolescence. An alternative is for these children to enter school along with their same-aged peers, and provide special classrooms or programs for those having difficulties.

The management of school failure requires a multidisciplinary approach. Information from the school, including school reports, teacher conferences and notes, testing that has been completed, and input from other school officials, if appropriate, should be requested. The primary care physician can assist the child and family to work with the school system to obtain the appropriate services. The primary physician may also refer to appropriate resources in the community (eg, educational psychologist or developmental and behavioral pediatrician).

Not infrequently, external factors such as social, family, and school-based issues may be very difficult to alter. Knowledge of the educational laws and community services, as well as ongoing developmental surveillance and screening by the primary care physician, is necessary to build a base from which the prevention of failure in school is possible

Grade retention is often suggested as the treatment for school failure. At the end of each school year, from kindergarten through 12th grade, the question of promotion is addressed. Though school personnel may regard this decision as "business as usual," the impact of this decision can be far-reaching. Evidence that retention in kindergarten or first grade is helpful in affording mastery of critical reading and other skills is lacking. Retention in higher grades has not been shown to be effective because educational gaps (eg, lack of mastery of first-grade skills) are not readdressed by retention in a higher grade. It is unlikely that "more of the same" will ensure mastery of needed skills.

In fact, data suggest the effect of grade retention on most students is adverse. Most retained students do not improve and many are worse after retention. Self-esteem problems, evident in many cases, often lead to self-destructive behavior and, in later grades, problems such as substance abuse, behavior difficulties, sexual promiscuity, and early drop out from school. In addition, children characterize retention as as bad as losing a parent.

To minimize the adverse effects of grade retention, each child's needs and strengths should be addressed and educational programs individualized.

Educational alternatives to retention include extra support in the form of classroom accommodations (**section 504 of the Rehabilitation Act of 1973** and also the **Americans with Disabilities Act**) or special education services (**IDEA**). In addition, educational therapy, counseling, or one-on-one tutoring may be beneficial for some children. Equally as important as remediating the areas of weakness is recognizing the child's areas of strength (eg, the idea of using a child's strengths to leverage his weaknesses).

Finally, the pediatrician's role in advocacy can never be underestimated. Examples of advocacy roles for physicians include involvement with the assessment team processes at children's schools, consulting with local school districts, and participation in local or state early intervention interagency councils.

Prognosis

In most cases, most children who show signs of school failure fall into the group of mild to moderate learning and/or neurobehavioral disorders with average cognitive skills. With proper support from educational, medical, family, and psychological sources, most of these students should be able to overcome their particular problems and enjoy successful school careers. Students who may have endured major socioeconomic upheavals will often continue to struggle unless changes in their entire support system are instituted early in their lives. The progress of children who have significant cognitive and/or neurobehavioral or psychological processing problems depends on the severity of their problems and the intensity and timing of the interventions they receive.

CASE RESOLUTION

The pediatrician should advise the family to request in writing a psycho-educational evaluation from the school. The pediatrician can also institute an evaluation for attention-deficit/hyperactivity disorder by gathering information from both the family and the school. All of this information should then be discussed with the parents so that formal diagnostic procedures and interventions may be instituted. Ideally the pediatrician will have the time, interest, and training to guide the family through this entire process. However, if this is not possible, referral to an appropriate professional is indicated. With the data from the educational evaluation and the medical workup, an appropriate plan of treatment can be developed.

Selected References

Byrd RS. School readiness: more than a summer's work. *Contemp Pediatr.* 1998;15:39–53

Byrd RS, Weitzman M, Auinger P. Increased behavior problems associated with delayed school entry and delayed school progress. *Pediatrics.* 1997;100:654–661

Dworkin PH. School failure. In: Parker S, Zuckerman B, Augustyn M, eds. *Developmental and Behavioral Pediatrics: A Handbook for Primary Care.* 2nd ed. Philadelphia, PA: Lippincott, Williams & Wilkins: 2005:280–284

Green M, Sullivan P, Eichberg C. Helping academic underachievers become achievers in their own right. *Contemp Pediatr.* 2005;22:29–36

Levine M. *A Mind at a Time.* New York, NY: Simon and Schuster; 2002

McInerny TK. Children who have difficulty in school: a primary pediatrician's approach. *Pediatr Rev.* 1995;16:325–332

Reiff MI. Adolescent school failure: failure to thrive in adolescence. *Pediatr Rev.* 1998;19:199–207

Rief SF. *Ready-Start-School! Nurturing and Guiding Your Child Through Preschool and Kindergarten.* Paramus, NJ: Prentice Hall Press; 2001

Robinson NM, Olszewski-Kubilius PM. Gifted and talented children: issues for pediatricians. *Pediatr Rev.* 1996;17:427–434

Shaywitz SE, Shaywitz BA. Dyslexia (specific reading disability). *Pediatr Rev.* 2003;24:147–152

Immunizations

ChrisAnna M. Mink, MD

CASE STUDY

A 20-month-old boy who emigrated with his family from Botswana is brought in for a checkup. He has his World Health Organization Expanded Immunization Programme card from his homeland showing that he received a bacille Calmette-Guérin vaccine at birth; 3 diphtheria, tetanus, and pertussis vaccines; 3 doses of live oral poliovirus vaccine at 2, 3, and 4 months of age; 3 doses of hepatitis B vaccine at birth and 2 and 9 months of age; and a monovalent measles vaccine at 9 months of age. It is August and his parents plan to enroll him in child care and have brought him for a checkup. His parents report that he is a healthy boy with no immune problems. They report that his uncle, who is infected with the human immunodeficiency virus, lives with them. The boy has had a 3-day history of a runny nose, cough, and tactile fever. His examination is normal other than mild clear coryza and a rectal temperature of 37.9°C (100.3°F). What immunizations may be given?

Questions

1. What are the different kinds of vaccines?
2. What are the mechanisms of action for live and inactivated vaccines?
3. What are the routinely recommended immunizations for *healthy* pediatric populations?
4. What are the considerations for immunizing selected pediatric populations such as preterm infants, immunocompromised children, immigrants, international adoptees, and travelers?
5. What are reliable resources for up-to-date information about immunizations?

The Centers for Disease Control and Prevention (CDC) considered immunizations among the top 10 greatest health accomplishments of the 20th century, and vaccines continue to play a major role in the improvement of the health of the world's population. In the United States, all of the pathogens for which there are routine vaccinations have decreased in incidence by 95% to 100% since the early 1900s. The only exception to this is pertussis, which has had approximately an 80% reduction. In 2004 the immunization rates for children in the United States were at their highest, with nearly 81% of children aged 19 to 35 months immunized for the 4:3:1:3:3 series (4 diphtheria, tetanus, and acellular pertussis [DTaP]: 3 polio: 1 measles, mumps, and rubella [MMR]: 3 *Haemophilus influenzae* type b [Hib]: 3 hepatitis B virus [HBV]). Worldwide, the percentage of children immunized with 3 doses of diphtheria, tetanus, and pertussis (DTP) and oral polio vaccines and a measles-containing vaccine is approaching 70%, which is nearly a 3-fold increase in the past 20 years. Generally, immunizations are safe, well tolerated, and cost-effective, with range of $5 to $16.50 saved for every dollar spent.

Another less recognized benefit of vaccinations is that the schedule has essentially provided the backbone for routine pediatric care in the United States, with regular visits scheduled around the recommended intervals for immunizations. These visits have afforded health care providers opportunities for serial evaluation of infants and young children, as well as education and anticipatory guidance for parents. Increasing availability of new vaccines targeted for older children and adolescents should permit opportunities for improved health care delivery to these older age groups, who have often been medically underserved. Additionally, health care practitioners for adults have growing appreciation of the critical role of vaccinations for protecting their patients, as well as all members of the family.

General Principles

When considering providing immunizations for an individual, 2 important factors to consider are the health status of the recipient and the type of immunization to be given. The risks and benefits of using the vaccine in the specific host should be weighed carefully. Vaccines are intended for a host who is capable of mounting an appropriate immune response, who will likely benefit from the protection provided and ideally incur little or no risks.

Vaccination Schedule

Factors for developing the schedule include

- Host ability to respond (eg, lost maternal antibody)
- Need for multiple doses (eg, inactivated poliovirus vaccine [IPV])
- Minimal intervals needed between serial doses
- Available products (eg, combination vaccines)

A synchronized immunization schedule is posted annually from the American Academy of Pediatrics (AAP) Committee on Infectious Diseases (*Red Book: 2006 Report of the Committee on Infectious Diseases*), American Academy of Family Practitioners, and the Advisory Committee for Immunization Practices of the CDC. In 2007, 2 immunization schedules were posted for the pediatric age groups: one for children younger than 7 years and one for individuals 7 through 18 years of age. A separate schedule was prepared for adults older than 18 years. The US schedules are posted each January at www.cdc.gov/nip/recs/child-schedule.htm. Schedules for countries worldwide are available at www.who.int/immunization_monitoring/en/globalsummary/scheduleselect.cfm.

Vaccine Recipients

Healthy Pediatric Populations

Routine immunizations on the synchronized schedule are targeted for healthy infants, children, and adolescents. All licensed vaccines have undergone review by the US Food and Drug Administration (FDA) and have proven safety and immunogenicity and/or efficacy for the targeted population. However, no vaccine is completely free of adverse events nor will provide 100% protection for every recipient. Every effort should be made to provide immunizations when the recipient is healthy and has the best chance to mount an optimal immune response without delaying vaccination or risking a "missed opportunity."

Special-Risk Pediatric Populations

Although immune responses to vaccinations are likely most favorable in healthy recipients, a growing segment of the pediatric population has underlying health problems. Because of congenital or acquired immune dysfunctions, some individuals should not receive immunizations as directed by the routine schedules. Special accommodations need to be made for immunizing these individuals, such as adjusting the schedule or possibly not administering some agents. There are no indications for giving decreased or partial doses of vaccines. Some of the selected populations for whom special consideration is indicated are discussed below.

Immunocompromised Child

The plan for vaccination of an **immunocompromised** child should be determined by the nature and degree of immunosuppression. The health care practitioner should weigh risk and benefits for each child individually, keeping some general principles in mind. For example, live vaccines should not be given to severely compromised individuals because of the possible risks. Generally inactivated vaccines and immunoglobulin (Ig) may be safely administered to nearly all recipients; however, immunocompromised individuals may not mount an optimal immune response. In this setting, try to adjust timing of vaccination to optimize the chance of a good immune response. Guidelines include waiting for 3 to 4 weeks post-chemotherapy and white blood cells greater than 1,000 cells/mm^3 for chemotherapy patients, 4 weeks after stopping high-dose steroids (dose equivalent $\geq$2 mg/kg/d of prednisone for $\geq$14 days), and sufficient time after receipt of Ig (see AAP *Red Book*).

Types of Immunodeficiency

Infants and children may have abnormalities of any arm of the immune system, which may affect their ability to receive vaccinations. Weighing the risks (of the disease, as well as vaccine) and benefits of protection is essential. A reasonable approach to developing a vaccination plan for children with immune abnormalities is to consider the pathogenesis of immune defense against the vaccine agents and if the needed defense mechanism is deficient, then immunizing with that agent may not be appropriate. For example, **cellular immunity** is essential in defending against **viral agents.** Thus children with abnormalities of their cell-mediated immunity (primary or acquired) may not be candidates for receipt of live viral vaccines.

Primary immunodeficiencies are generally inherited and secondary ones are acquired, such as infection with human immunodeficiency virus, malignancy, illnesses (such as malnutrition and uremia), or related to medications (eg, chemotherapy or immunosuppressive agents), among others. For primary humoral immunity abnormalities (not able to make antibodies), oral poliovirus vaccine (OPV) is contraindicated but MMR vaccine may be indicated for some individuals. For cell-mediated abnormalities, generally live viral vaccines should not be used. With complement abnormalities, receipt of live viral vaccines is acceptable for most individuals. For abnormal phagocytic function, live bacterial vaccines should not be given. For individuals with asplenia (traumatic or surgical), vaccination with pneumococcal, meningococcal, and Hib vaccines is indicated and should be considered emergently in the case of trauma. Chemoprophylaxis may also have a role in protection for compromised individuals.

For immunocompromised household contacts of pediatric vaccinees, it is generally acceptable to give MMR, varicella-zoster virus (VZV), and oral rotavirus vaccines. Some live vaccines should not be given, including OPV and live-attenuated influenza vaccine (LAIV). Additionally, use of some vaccines, such as trivalent influenza vaccine (TIV), is encouraged to protect the vaccinee, as well as the compromised contacts.

Pregnancy

Pregnancy is associated with **some impairment of cell-mediated immunity.** With this decreased immunity, pregnant women may not have protective immune responses to some infectious agents. With this in mind, generally no live vaccines should be administered to pregnant women, though the risks and benefits should be weighed for individual cases. Rubella vaccine should not be given to pregnant women, though there have been no reported cases of rubella embryopathy following inadvertent immunization of a pregnant woman.

Some immunizations are recommended during the second or third trimester to provide protection for the mother (ie, TIV) and possibly the infant (eg, tetanus and diphtheria toxoids [Td]). Residing with a pregnant household contact is generally not a contraindication for a child to receive live viral vaccines, a question often asked of pediatricians.

Preterm (<37 Weeks) and Low Birth Weight (<2,500 g) Infants

In general, medically stable premature and low birth weight infants may be immunized at the same dose, schedule, and postnatal age as full-term infants.

Special consideration should be given to use of hepatitis B vaccine in infants that weigh less than 2,000 g as follows:

- Hepatitis B surface antigen (HbsAg)-positive or unknown status in mom→Give vaccine and hepatitis B immunoglobulin (HBIG), then give 3 additional vaccine doses.
- HBsAg-negative mom→Give hepatitis B vaccine at 30 days (sooner if the infant is stable for discharge), and then follow the usual schedule, such that the infant receives a total of 3 doses.

Other Conditions Affecting Immunization Schedule

Egg-Allergic Child

For children with known anaphylactic reactions to eggs or egg components, special consideration is warranted for use of vaccines prepared using egg products. Current measles and mumps vaccines are prepared using chick-derived cell lines, but do not contain significant amounts of proteins that cross-react with egg proteins. Children with egg allergies, including severe hypersensitivity, are at low risk of anaphylaxis from measles- or mumps-containing vaccines. Additionally, skin testing against these antigens is not predictive of an adverse reaction. Thus egg-allergic children may be immunized with measles and mumps vaccines alone or in combination preparations (eg, MMR, MMR and varicella [MMRV]) without skin testing. Influenza (TIV, LAIV) and yellow fever (YF) vaccines are prepared in eggs and may contain egg proteins, and may rarely induce an immediate allergic reaction. For children with a history of anaphylaxis to eggs or egg components, both TIV and LAIV are generally contraindicated because of the risk of an adverse event and the need for annual immunization. For YF vaccine, skin testing before use is recommended in children with a history of anaphylaxis to eggs.

International Adoptees, Travelers, Immigrants, and Refugees

It is important to remember that travelers are from all socioeconomic strata, so inquiries about foreign travel should be included in routine visits in all clinical settings. First, the health care practitioner should review the child's record to ensure that all routine vaccines are up to date for age. The child should receive vaccinations and other preventive measures (eg, malaria prophylaxis) targeted for his or her destination. There may be a need for accelerated schedule (eg, early MMR for infants 6–12 months of age traveling to a measles-endemic area). Use of Ig prophylaxis should be considered for individuals susceptible to hepatitis A (eg, not previously immunized). The health care practitioner should check the current recommendations to ensure healthy travel at www.cdc.gov/travel and www.who.int.

Immigrants, refugees, and international adoptees may present with additional health concerns. Many of these children have been in poor living conditions and exposed to health hazards of environments like refugee camps and orphanages. Their health status, possible intercurrent illnesses, and need for immunizations should all be evaluated soon after arrival. The United States requires proof of the first dose of vaccines for entry into the country, though there are exemptions for adoptees younger than 10 years and refugees at entry. These high-risk children often have not been immunized or have missing records. Written, dated, and appropriate records (eg, age, dates, interval, and number of doses) may be considered valid, and subsequent immunization may resume according to the US schedule. Another option, especially when documentation is questionable, is to perform serologic studies for vaccine-induced antibodies.

Adolescents

Although the AAP has recommended a routine health visit at 11 to 12 years of age, compliance with this visit has been low. Until recently, no immunizations were routinely recommended in this age group. In the late 1990s, hepatitis B catch-up immunization was the first vaccine encouraged at this age and became required for middle-school entry in several states. Now several vaccines are available for protecting teens. One of these vaccines is tetanus, diphtheria, and pertussis (Tdap) for use as a single booster dose in adolescents 11 to 18 years of age who have previously received a series of DTP–containing vaccines.

Two meningococcal vaccines are available for use routinely at age 11 to 12 years, as well as catch-up dosing for students entering high school, college freshmen planning to live in dormitories, and others at increased risk of meningococcal diseases. The 2 meningococcal vaccines are the capsular polysaccharide (CPS) vaccine (MPSV4, Menomune) and the CPS-protein conjugate vaccine (MCV4, Menactra), with the latter formulation being preferred by the AAP. Both vaccines contain 4 serotypes (A, C, Y, and W135).

The human papillomavirus (HPV) vaccine is also available for immunizing females from ages 9 through 26 years, preferably before their sexual debut. The currently licensed vaccine (Gardasil, Merck & Co., Inc.) contains 4 serotypes (6, 11, 16, and 18) protecting against about 70% of strains related to cervical cancer. It is administered in a 3-dose regimen at day 0, 2 months, and 6 months.

Additionally, at the adolescent visits (including precollege visits), the provider should review the teen's records to ensure that he or she has received all recommended vaccines, inquire about household contacts of infant or compromised host, and provide anticipatory guidance for safe and healthy living for the teen and the parent.

Types of Immunizations

The 2 major types of immunizations are active and passive.

Passive Immunization

Passive immunization refers to the deliver of preformed antibodies, usually as Ig. Immunoglobulin may be a general formulation or hyperimmune Ig developed with high concentrations of antibodies against a specific disease, such as HBIG.

Delivery of Ig may be useful in 3 settings:

1. A host is not able to make antibodies (eg, congenital immunodeficiency).
2. Preventive (pre-exposure or postexposure) especially when there is not sufficient time for the host to mount an antibody response (eg, acute exposure to hepatitis A).
3. Treatment—Ig may be used to ameliorate symptoms when disease is already present (eg, intravenous Ig for Kawasaki disease).

Active Immunization

With **active immunization,** all, part, or a modified product (eg, toxoid or purified antigen) of a microorganism is given to the host to elicit an immune response. The intact organisms may be inactivated (killed) or live-attenuated (weakened). The elicited immune response usually mimics the response to natural infection and, ideally, this occurs with little or no risks to the recipient.

Inactivated Vaccines

Inactivated vaccines may contain **inactivated or killed organisms,** purified components (subunit), or inactivated toxins (toxoids) of the organism. These vaccines are not capable of replication in the host. Most inactivated vaccines are delivered by the intramuscular (IM) injection. Generally, inactivated vaccines may be administered simultaneously with other inactivated vaccines, as well as live viral vaccines.

A few viral vaccines are inactivated, including TIV, hepatitis A (HAV), HBV, IPV, HPV, and rabies vaccines. Toxoid vaccines that are used routinely include tetanus and diphtheria toxoids alone or in combinations with whole-cell or acellular pertussis components (eg, DTaP, DTP, Td, and Tdap). The acellular pertussis vaccines are composed of one or more purified antigens of *Bordetella pertussis,* in contrast to the whole-cell pertussis vaccines, which are made with killed, whole *B pertussis* organisms. Diphtheria and tetanus toxoids combined with whole-cell pertussis (DTP) vaccines are no longer marketed in the United States, but are used in most developing areas of the world. Other inactivated bacterial vaccines include CPS vaccines, such as the 23-valent pneumococcal vaccine and tetravalent meningococcal CPS vaccine.

Conjugate Vaccines

Capsular polysaccharide antigens have been chemically linked to a protein carrier, which converts the T-cell independent polysaccharides to T-cell dependent antigen that can trigger an immune response, even in young infants. The first CPS-protein conjugate vaccine available was for Hib. The Hib bacterium is covered with a CPS, polyribitol-phosphate (PRP). Children younger than 2 years are not efficient at mounting antibodies to the PRP CPS, but with linkage to a protein carrier, the CPS is immunogenic. Since licensure for infants of the Hib conjugate vaccines in 1991, there has been a more than 95% reduction in Hib disease. With the success of the Hib CPS-protein conjugate vaccines, conjugation techniques have been used for other CPS pathogens including *Streptococcus pneumoniae* and *Neisseria meningitidis.*

Live-Attenuated Vaccines

Live-attenuated vaccines are infectious agents that replicate in the host to elicit an immune response. The administration is generally not IM but by other delivery routes such as oral, intranasal, or subcutaneous. The live vaccines are often viral, including MMR, VZV, rotavirus, LAIV (FluMist), OPV, and YF vaccines. Two live bacterial vaccines are available including oral typhoid (Ty21) and bacille Calmette-Guérin used against *Mycobacterium tuberculosis.*

Following measles vaccination, there is a transient suppression of T-cell immunity in the 2 to 4 week postvaccination period. Because of this, for vaccination with live viral vaccines, give 2 or more live vaccines at the same time or wait 4 weeks between vaccines. This principle is also true for tuberculosis skin testing; place the purified protein derivative at the same time as a live viral vaccine or wait at least 4 weeks to avoid a false-negative skin test because of the T-cell suppression. Although this has not been extensively studied with live viral vaccines other than measles, following the same guidelines with other live viral vaccines is recommended.

Immunizations Received in Other Countries

Most vaccines used worldwide are produced with adequate quality control and may be considered reliable. Healthy individuals immunized in countries outside of the United States should receive vaccines according to the recommended schedule for healthy infants, children, and adolescents in the United States. In most cases, only written documentation should be accepted as proof of previous vaccination. Written, dated, and appropriate records (eg, correct age, dates, interval, and number of doses, etc) may be considered as valid, and immunizations may resume according to the US schedule.

Although most vaccines are acceptable, there may be some concerns for vaccine potency due to unsuitable storage and handling. Other concerns include inaccurate documentation and possibly inadequate response in some children due to other factors (eg, malnutrition or underlying illnesses). If vaccination status is uncertain, the options include vaccinating or checking serologic testing against the vaccine antigen, if testing is available. Generally, receipt of additional doses of diphtheria and tetanus toxoids alone or in combination with a pertussis-containing vaccine (ie, DTP, DTaP, Td, and Tdap) may lead to an increase in reactions (especially injection site reactions), and checking antibody titers against diphtheria and tetanus toxoids is encouraged. At this time, no FDA-approved assays for pertussis antibodies are available, and testing for pertussis antibodies is not recommended. For other vaccines, if the status is unknown, vaccination should be performed because extra doses are generally well tolerated. Most developing countries do not have VZV, conjugated pneumococcal, or Hib vaccines, and these should be given as indicated per the US schedule.

Adverse Events and Vaccine Information

Adverse Events

As noted previously, no vaccine is completely free of adverse events, and the known adverse events should be discussed with vaccinees (non-minors) and/or parents/legal guardians. In addition to discussing the risks and benefits of vaccination, the health care practitioner should include education about the risks associated with the natural disease. This is especially important in current times, when many individuals have not seen the diseases for which vaccines have been successful in controlling or eradicating.

In addition to safety information from the AAP and CDC, the manufacturer's package insert provides information about the rates of adverse events and contraindications for the specific vaccine. Most adverse events observed following routine immunizations are local injection site reactions such as erythema, swelling, and pain, and systemic reactions such as fever or fussiness. Although most of these adverse events are mild and self-limiting, some may be associated with significant dysfunction for the child (eg, not using a limb due to pain).

Rarely, serious adverse events may occur following immunization, and these may be associated with permanent disability or life-threatening illness. The occurrence of an adverse event after immunization does not prove a cause-and-effect relationship of the vaccine and the event, but a temporal relationship. If a vaccine recipient experiences a serious adverse event, a complete evaluation for all plausible causes, including the role of the vaccine antigen, should be performed. Additionally, all clinically significant adverse events should be reported to the Vaccine Adverse Event Reporting System (VAERS) at http://vaers.hhs.gov/, which is maintained by the CDC and FDA. Adverse event reporting is important because it helps identify possible unexpected events that were not observed in the prelicensure clinical trials.

Precautions and Contraindications

The Vaccine Information Statement (VIS) and package insert provide information for health care practitioner, vaccinees (non-minors), and parents/legal guardians about the precautions and contraindications for specific products.

A precaution suggests that careful analysis of risks and benefits of the vaccine should be done, and if benefits outweigh risks, the vaccine may be given. A contraindication means that a vaccine should not be administered. An example of a contraindication is known anaphylaxis to any component of the vaccine. Breastfeeding does not interfere with oral immunization with rotavirus or OPV vaccines and is not a contraindication.

Minor illness without fever (temperature ≤38°C [100.4°F]) should not be considered a contraindication to vaccination. Fever above 38°C (100.4°F) may not be a contraindication, depending on the physician's assessment of the child, the illness, and the vaccine to be given. If the child is early in the disease and the course is not predictable or the illness is moderate to severe, delaying immunization is reasonable. Deferring immunization without appropriate justification can cause a missed opportunity and may lead to inadequate immunization of the child.

Informing Vaccine Recipients and Parents

Vaccine recipients and parents should be informed about the risks and benefits of vaccination and about the disease for which the vaccine is designed. The National Childhood Vaccine Injury Act of 1986 requires that parents receive a VIS each time a child receives a vaccine covered under this legislation, whether the vaccine was purchased with public or private funds. The VISs are available from the CDC at the National Immunization Program site at www.cdc.gov/VIS/default.htm. The health care practitioner should document in the patient's chart the vaccine manufacturer, lot number, and date of administration and that VISs were provided and discussed with the vaccinee (non-minor) and parent/legal guardian.

Vaccine Information

Information about current immunizations for health care practitioners and for laypersons is available from many resources including the CDC, AAP, FDA, and the World Health Organization, among others. A list of Web sites is provided in Table 23-1.

Table 23-1. Internet Sources of Vaccine Information	
Source	**Web Site**
American Academy of Pediatrics (AAP)	www.aap.org
Centers for Disease Control and Prevention (CDC)	www.cdc.gov
National Immunization Program	www.cdc.gov/vaccines/pubs/ACIP-list.htm
Morbidity and Mortality Weekly Reports (MMWR)	www.cdc.gov/mmwr/preview/mmwrhtml/rr5102a1.htm
Food and Drug Administration (FDA)	www.fda.gov/cber/vaccine/lic-vacc.htm
Vaccine Adverse Event Reporting System (VAERS)	http://vaers.hhs.gov/
American Society for Tropical Medicine and Hygiene (ASTMH)	www.astmh.org
World Health Organization	www.who.int
Global Alliance for Vaccines and Immunization (GAVI)	www.gavialliance.org

CASE RESOLUTION

The boy was appropriately immunized for Botswana recommendations through the age of 9 months, though now his immunization would be considered delayed for age on the US schedule. He is past due for the fourth dose of diphtheria, tetanus, and acellular pertussis (DTaP); measles, mumps, and rubella (MMR); and varicella-zoster virus vaccines. Additionally he has not received any conjugate vaccines or hepatitis A vaccine. The dose of monovalent measles vaccine does not change his need to receive 2 doses of MMR and varicella (MMRV) vaccines after the age of 12 months as listed on the US schedule. His uncle's immune status does not affect the use of MMRV. His current respiratory illness is considered mild, and he does not have significant fever (<38°C [100.4°F]), so this is not problematic for receiving the needed immunizations.

During this visit, he may receive DTaP, MMRV #1, one dose of *Haemophilus influenzae* type b conjugate vaccine, dose 1 of 2 of conjugate pneumococcal vaccine (2 months apart), and dose 1 of 2 of hepatitis A (at least 6 months apart). All Vaccine Information Statements should be provided. He is scheduled to return in 2 months in October for his next dose of conjugate pneumococcal vaccine and dose 1 of 2 of inactivated influenza vaccine. He may not receive the live-attenuated influenza vaccine (LAIV) because of his young age (LAIV is licensed for children ≥24 months of age), as well as his uncle's immunocompromised status. He will need a fourth dose of inactivated poliovirus vaccine before school age. He is too old to receive the oral rotavirus vaccine.

Selected References

American Academy of Pediatrics. Vaccine information. In: Pickering LK, Baker CJ, Long SS, McMillan JA, eds. *Red Book: 2006 Report of the Committee on Infectious Diseases.* 27th ed. Elk Grove Village, IL: American Academy of Pediatrics; 2006:2–103

Centers for Disease Control and Prevention. Recommended Immunization Schedules for Persons Aged 0–18 Years—United States, 2007. *MMWR Morb Mortal Wkly Rep.* 2007;55:Q1–Q4

Centers for Disease Control and Prevention. 2007 NIP Annual Report. *A Global Commitment to Lifelong Protection through Immunization.* www.cdc.gov/nip/webutil/about/annual-rpts/ar2007/2007annual-rpt.htm

Dennehey PH, Peter G. Active immunizing agents. In: Feigin RD, Cherry JD, eds. *Textbook of Pediatric Infectious Diseases.* 5th ed. Philadelphia, PA: W. B. Saunders; 2004

James JM, Burks AW, Roberson PK, Sampson HA. Safe administration of measles vaccine to children allergic to eggs. *N Engl J Med.* 1995;332:1262–1265

Kroger AT, Atkinson WL, Marcuse EK, Pickering LK, Advisory Committee on Immunization Practices Centers for Disease Control and Prevention. General recommendations on immunization: recommendations of the Advisory Committee on Immunization Practices (ACIP). *MMWR Recomm Rep.* 2006;55:1–48

Losonsky GA, Wasserman SS, Stephens I, et al. Hepatitis B vaccination of premature infants: a reassessment of current recommendations for delayed immunization. *Pediatrics.* 1999;103:e14

Markowitz LE, Dunne EF, Saraiya M, et al. Quadrivalent human papillomavirus vaccine. *MMWR Recomm Rep.* 2007;56:1–24

Health Maintenance in Older Children and Adolescents

Hali Sherman, MD, and Monica Sifuentes, MD

CASE STUDY

Before a 13-year-old girl enters a new school, she is required to have a physical examination. She has not seen a physician in 5 years and has been healthy. Currently she has no medical complaints. Her examination is completely normal.

Questions

1. What are the important components of the history and physical examination in healthy older children and adolescents?
2. What immunizations are recommended for older children and adolescents?
3. What laboratory tests should be performed at health maintenance visits? Why?
4. What are the results of screening tests likely to show?

Older children and adolescents are generally healthy individuals who infrequently visit physicians. Visits are often for acute complaints such as upper respiratory infections or sports-related injuries and are therefore very problem-oriented. Statistics regarding health maintenance visits in this age group are not readily available because patients go to several different sites for health care and often do not receive comprehensive care at any of these places. Older children and adolescents seek treatment for both acute and chronic conditions in private offices, public health clinics, public hospitals, and emergency departments. It is estimated that less than 15% of adolescents go to pediatricians for health care in general, and the same percentage probably applies to older children as well.

This all too common practice contributes to missed opportunities for anticipatory guidance, health education, and screening for preventable conditions. Screening tests also can be used to identify treatable conditions such as hypertension, anemia, and tuberculosis. Ideally, older children and adolescents should receive recommended immunizations; counseling concerning sexual activity, contraception, and sexually transmitted infections (STIs), including human immunodeficiency virus (HIV); guidelines for adequate nutrition; education about tobacco, drugs, and alcohol; and information about physical fitness and exercise.

Guidelines for preventive child and adolescent health care have been published by the American Academy of Pediatrics (AAP) Committee on Practice and Ambulatory Medicine, the federal Child Health and Disability Prevention Program, the AAP Section on Adolescent Health, and the American Medical Association. Box 24-1 is a brief summary of these guidelines.

The Health Maintenance Visit

The purpose of the health maintenance visit is to assess the general health and well-being of the child or adolescent. Questions asked during this visit should initially be simple and focus on how the patient feels in general. More specific questions can then be formulated from the initial responses. In healthy patients, the medical history can be obtained using a questionnaire that parents and children complete in the waiting room. If this method is used, a separate form should be given to adolescents if he or she is accompanied by one or both parents. The information is then reviewed at the start of the interview. Chronic medical conditions also should be addressed at this time.

Medical History

Older children and adolescents should always be questioned directly about their medical history (Questions Box: Screening in Older Children and Adolescents). Parents should be encouraged to participate only after their children have responded to questions or if invited by children or adolescents themselves. The degree of parental participation also is influenced by the current cognitive and developmental stage of patients.

Psychosocial History

The psychosocial component of the interview should be conducted with older children or adolescents alone as well as together with parents (Questions Box: Screening in Older Children and Adolescents). General questions about school, outside activities or

Box 24-1. Guidelines for Adolescent Health Maintenance Evaluation

Screening History	Physical Exam	Labs/Studies	Anticipatory Guidance and Counseling
Eating disorders	Body mass index	Cholesterol	Parenting/communication
Sexual activity	Blood pressure	• If the patient is obese or there is a significant	Pubertal development
Tobacco use	Comprehensive exam	family history of hyperlipidemia	Diet/nutrition
Alcohol use/abuse	Pelvic exam[a]	Urine NAAT for GC/chlamydia, HIV, RPR, viral	Exercise
Drug use/abuse (CRAFFT		hepatitis	Injury prevention
questionnaire[b])		• If the patient is sexually active	Lifestyle modifications
School performance		Pap smear[a]	• Abstinence
Depression			• Safe sexual activity
Risk for suicide			• Contraception
			• Avoidance of tobacco, alcohol, and drugs

Abbreviations: NAAT, nucleic acid amplification testing; GC, gonorrhea; HIV, human immunodeficiency virus; RPR, rapid plasma reagin.

[a]A pelvic examination with a Pap smear is recommended within 3 years of the onset of sexual activity or age 21.

[b]See Chapter 119 for CRAFFT questionaire.

Questions

Screening in Older Children and Adolescents

Questions for both the patient and parent

- How has the child or adolescent been doing lately? Does the parent have any complaints or concerns?
- How does the child or adolescent like school? How are they doing academically?
- What activities does the child or adolescent currently participate in?
- Does he or she have any hobbies?
- With whom does the child or adolescent live?
- Are there any significant illnesses in the immediate or extended family, such as hypertension, diabetes, or cancer?
- Does the child or adolescent take any medications, herbs, or supplements (prescribed or over the counter) regularly?

Questions for the child or adolescent alone

- Do you have any questions or concerns?
- How are things at home? Are there any problems with parents or siblings? Do you feel safe at home?
- Are you attending school?
- Do you like school?
- Have you ever been truant, suspended, or expelled?
- Do you have friends?
- What do you do for fun?
- Do you or your friends use tobacco, drugs, or alcohol?
- Are you or your friends members of a gang?
- Are you or your friends sexually active? With men, women, or both? Do you engage in oral, anal, or vaginal intercourse?
- Do you or any of your friends use contraception? If so, what method?
- Are you ever really sad?
- Have you ever thought of, or tried to commit, suicide?
- Do you have access to a gun?
- Do you or your friends diet or use performance-enhancing steroids?
- Are you using medications, exercise, or self-induced vomiting to control your weight?

hobbies, and family are often less threatening than inquiries about friends and tobacco or drug use. More sensitive topics relating to sexuality and sexual activity should be addressed after parents have left the room. Subjects initially discussed with parents should be reviewed once again with the teenager alone.

A useful tool for conducting the psychosocial interview has been developed and refined by physicians who specialize in pediatrics and adolescent medicine. Known by the acronym **HEADDSSS**, it reviews the essential components of the psychosocial history: home, education or employment, activities, diet, drugs, sexual activity, suicide or depression, and safety (see Chapter 5).

Dietary History

A general dietary history should be obtained, with particular focus on eating habits, level of physical activity, and body image. Dietary restrictions, if any, should be investigated. Daily calcium and iron intake also should be reviewed, especially in adolescent females.

Family History

Significant illnesses such as hypertension, hyperlipidemia, obesity, and diabetes in first- and second-degree family members should be reviewed. Family use of alcohol, tobacco, and illegal substances also should be determined. Age and cause of death in immediate family members should be recorded.

Medications and Allergies

Prescription as well as nonprescription (over-the-counter) medications, herbs, and supplements should be reviewed along with the indications and frequency of usage.

Physical Examination

The height and weight of patients should be plotted on a growth curve, with particular attention paid to the velocity of growth and the body mass index ($BMI = weight (kg) /[height (m)]^2$). The blood pressure also should be noted and compared to age- and height-related normative values.

Aspects of the physical examination that are influenced by puberty should be emphasized. The skin should be carefully inspected for acne, and clinicians should offer treatment whether or not patients acknowledge that they have skin problems. The oropharynx should be examined for any evidence of gingivitis or other signs of poor dental hygiene or malocclusion. The neck should be palpated for adenopathy and the thyroid gland for hypertrophy or nodules, especially in adolescent females. The back should be examined for any evidence of scoliosis, which is important to diagnose during this time of rapid growth.

Assessment of the pubertal development of the breasts and genitalia in preadolescent or adolescent females and the genitalia, including presence of pubic hair, in adolescent males is essential. The sexual maturity rating (SMR) (Tanner stage) can then be correlated with other signs of puberty, such as the appearance of acne and body odor. For example, the adolescent female with SMR 4 breasts and immature pubic hair distribution may have an underlying problem such as testicular feminization syndrome.

The abdomen should be palpated for organomegaly and the testicles for masses. The external female genitalia should be inspected for lesions. A speculum examination should be performed in females who have been sexually active for 3 years or who complain of vaginal discharge or unexplained vaginal bleeding. (See Chapter 30 for additional indications for a pelvic examination.) In general, virginal girls do not require a speculum examination; gentle inspection of the external genitalia is adequate in most cases. A rectal examination is generally reserved for patients with chronic abdominal pain or other specific acute complaints.

Immunizations

Many recent additions have been made to the preadolescent/adolescent vaccination schedule (Table 24-1). As always, practitioners should verify that patients have completed the primary immunization series. If not, they should be given catch-up doses according to the Centers for Disease Control and Prevention (CDC) recommendations. The newest vaccines, tetanus and diphtheria toxoids and acellular pertussis (Tdap) (Adacel, Boostrix), human papillomavirus (HPV) (Gardasil), and meningococcal conjugate vaccine (MCV4) (Menactra) should be given to preteens at the 11- to 12-year visit. The Tdap vaccine replaces the tetanus/diphtheria booster previously given at this age. Pertussis was added to the booster because immunity to pertussis has been noted to wane 5 to 8 years after vaccination, and there has been an increasing prevalence of pertussis detected in adolescents and adults with chronic cough. A conjugate vaccine against *Neisseria meningitidis* (MCV4 or Menactra) was also approved by the US Food and Drug Administration in 2005. The Advisory Committee on Immunization Practices now recommends that MCV4 be given to all 11- to 18-year-olds. Finally, a vaccine against the major cancer-causing types of HPV was approved in 2006 (Gardasil). While there has been some controversy surrounding this vaccine, the current recommendations state that the 3-dose series of the quadrivalent vaccine should be given routinely at 11 to 12 years of age and to all young women and girls between the ages

Table 24-1. Recent Changes to the Recommended Immunization Schedule Affecting Adolescents[a]

	Recommended Age (y)			
	11–12	*13–14*	*15*	*16–18*
Tetanus, diphtheria, pertussis	Tdap	Tdap	Tdap	Tdap
Human papillomavirus	HPV (3 doses)	HPV (3 doses)	HPV (3 doses)	HPV (3 doses)
Meningococcal	MCV4	MCV4	MCV4	MCV4
Varicella	Varicella 2-dose series			

Abbreviations: Tdap, tetanus and diphtheria toxoids and acellular pertussis; HPV, human papillomavirus; MCV4, meningococcal conjugate vaccine.

[a]Modified from Centers for Disease Control and Prevention table available at www.cdc.gov/nip/recs/child-schedule.htm.

of 13 and 26. Ideally the vaccine should be administered before the initiation of sexual activity, but it also may be given to young girls who are already sexually active.

Recommendations regarding some of the older vaccines have changed as well. A second dose of the varicella vaccine is now part of the primary vaccine schedule, so if an adolescent has only received one dose, a second dose should be administered. Similarly, if the adolescent has not had the disease or been vaccinated, he or she should receive the 2-dose series. Routine vaccination against hepatitis B also is recommended, regardless of sexual activity, if it has not been administered previously. The 2-dose hepatitis A series should be given to all teenagers not previously vaccinated if they reside in high-incidence communities. Influenza vaccine should be given annually to adolescents with high-risk conditions and to those who come into close contact with individuals with high-risk conditions. Pneumococcal vaccine should be offered to high-risk groups as well. In addition, a Mantoux skin test for tuberculosis should be placed. (For complete recommendations, please refer to Chapter 23.)

Laboratory Tests

A hemoglobin level should be obtained to check for anemia and a urinalysis performed to assess for protein, blood, and pyuria. Other suggested screening tests include hearing and vision tests, and a cholesterol and lipid profile. Although cholesterol screening remains controversial, it is important to consider in patients who are morbidly obese or have a positive family history for hyperlipidemia or premature atherosclerotic heart disease.

In addition to the above laboratory tests, sexually active adolescents should be screened for STIs. If a pelvic examination is performed, an endocervical specimen should be obtained for nucleic acid amplification testing (NAAT) for gonorrhea and chlamydia. However, if a pelvic examination is not done, routine screening for gonorrhea and chlamydia may be performed with a urine sample alone using NAAT methods. The 2006 recommendations from the CDC state that all sexually active women younger than 26 years should be screened annually. Males should be screened if they are symptomatic or have a history of multiple partners and unprotected intercourse. In addition, a rapid plasma reagin test for syphilis and an HIV test should be obtained, especially if another STI is suspected. All of the above tests should be offered in the clinically appropriate setting after patients have received pretest counseling with a follow-up visit scheduled to discuss the results.

Patient Education

At the conclusion of the health maintenance visit, positive as well as negative findings should be reviewed with patients and their parents. Depending on the nature of these findings and the age of the patient, practitioners may initially choose to address these findings with the patient alone. All recommended screening laboratory studies and immunizations also should be reviewed before their administration, including the need for further follow-up. Subsequent vaccine doses must be outlined for patients and parents. The timing of the next visit and reasons for this visit should be discussed.

The remainder of the visit should be spent addressing any specific concerns of patients and parents, highlighting health care problems (eg, obesity, high blood pressure), and identifying any factors that may be related to high-risk behavior such as drug or alcohol use. Older children or adolescents who are not participating in any deleterious activities should be praised for their positive behavior as well as provided with information regarding injury prevention.

Preparticipation Physical Evaluation for School-aged and Adolescent Athletes

The preparticipation physical evaluation (PPE) is essentially the "sports physical" that many schools require for participation in organized athletic programs. The primary objective of the PPE is to assess the young athlete's readiness to compete safely and effectively in a given sport. Ideally, it also should identify athletes at risk for injury or sudden death, as well as those with an underlying medical condition that may affect athletic participation.

Controversy exists about the appropriate location for performance of the PPE. Community physicians are often asked to perform limited en masse examinations at schools, or a group of clinicians is asked to perform the examinations in the gymnasium using "stations." Either way, the patient does not truly receive a complete physical examination or assessment, and neither approach lends itself to privacy. In addition, parents have a false sense of security and believe that their children have received adequate medical care. Ideally, primary care physicians should perform the PPE annually in their office during a scheduled visit at least 4 to 6 weeks before the beginning of the athletic season. Pediatricians can use this required visit as an opportunity to perform an annual comprehensive health maintenance examination on older children and adolescents, including the various screening tests.

History

The medical history for the PPE should primarily focus on previous athletic participation and any injuries that may have occurred (Questions Box: Preparticipation Physical Evaluation). A standard

Questions

Preparticipation Physical Evaluation

- What sport(s) does the child or adolescent wish to participate in?
- Has the child or adolescent ever experienced a sports injury? If so, how much time did the athlete miss doing sports activities as a result of this injury?
- Has the athlete ever suffered a concussion?
- Does the child or adolescent have a significant underlying health problem?
- Is the child or adolescent taking any prescribed or over-the-counter medications?
- Does the child or adolescent have any allergies?
- Has the child or adolescent ever had syncope, palpitations, or angina during exercise?
- Does the child or adolescent have a family history of sudden, early, non-traumatic deaths?

questionnaire codeveloped by the AAP for this purpose may be used in the office setting. In addition, many practitioners record the results of the physical examination as well as their recommendations regarding the degree of athletic participation on this standard form (Figure 24-1).

Physical Examination

A complete physical examination should be performed when possible. If circumstances preclude this, specific attention should be paid to the eyes, heart, abdomen, skin, and musculoskeletal system. Height, weight, blood pressure, and visual acuity also should be measured. Examination of the eyes is essential to document physiological anisocoria (different papillary diameters). A thorough cardiac evaluation should be performed for murmurs, abnormal heart sounds, or arrhythmias. The abdomen should be palpated for an enlarged liver or spleen, especially in the adolescent with a recent viral illness that could suggest mononucleosis. In males, the genitalia should be examined for sexual maturity in addition to assessing for abnormalities such as atrophy, absence of a testis, or presence of a mass. The skin should be inspected for lesions such as tinea corporis, impetigo, or herpes simplex infection.

The 2-minute orthopedic examination consists of a head-to-toe assessment of all muscle groups and joints; any deformities, anomalies, or evidence of previous injuries should be noted (Table 24-2). Recent studies suggest expanding this examination to include a more detailed evaluation of high-risk areas for injury such as the knee, ankle, and shoulder.

Laboratory Tests

Routine laboratory screening tests, except for those performed during the general health maintenance visit, are not recommended for the PPE. Screening young athletes for anemia or proteinuria has not been found to be particularly helpful. Such screening may be useful with highly competitive professional athletes, however. Although

This evaluation is only to determine readiness for sports participation. It should not be used as a substitute for regular health maintenance examinations.

NAME _____ AGE _____ (YRS) GRADE DATE _____

ADDRESS _____ PHONE _____

SPORTS _____

The Health History (Part A) and Physical Examination (Part C) sections must both be completed, at least every 24 months, before sports participation. The Interim Health History section (Part B) needs to be completed at least annually.

PART A—HEALTH HISTORY

To be completed by athlete and parent

	YES	NO
1. Have you ever had an illness that:		
a. required you to stay in the hospital?	_____	_____
b. lasted longer than a week?	_____	_____
c. caused you to miss 3 days of practice or a competition?	_____	_____
d. is related to allergies (eg, hay fever, hives, asthma, insect stings)?	_____	_____
e. required an operation?	_____	_____
f. is chronic (eg, asthma, diabetes)?	_____	_____
2. Have you ever had an injury that:		
a. required you to go to an emergency department or see a doctor?	_____	_____
b. required you to stay in the hospital?	_____	_____
c. required x-rays?	_____	_____
d. caused you to miss 3 days of practice or a competition?	_____	_____
e. required an operation?	_____	_____
3. Do you take any medication or pills?	_____	_____
4. Have any members of your family younger than 50 years had a heart attack, heart problem, or died unexpectedly?	_____	_____
5. Have you ever:		
a. been dizzy or passed out during or after exercise?	_____	_____
b. been unconscious or had a concussion?	_____	_____
6. Are you unable to run ½ mile (2 times around the track) without stopping?	_____	_____
7. Do you:		
a. wear glasses or contacts?	_____	
b. wear dental bridges, plates, or braces?	_____	
8. Have you ever had a heart murmur, high blood pressure, or a heart abnormality?	_____	_____
9. Do you have any allergies to any medicine?	_____	
10. Are you missing a kidney?	_____	_____
11. When was your last tetanus booster? _____		
12. For Women		
a. At what age did you experience your first menstrual period? _____		
b. In the last year, what is the longest time you have gone between periods? _____		

EXPLAIN ANY "YES" ANSWERS _____

_____

_____

_____

I hereby state that, to the best of my knowledge, my answers to the above questions are correct.

Date _____

Signature of athlete _____

Signature of parent _____

PART B—INTERIM HEALTH HISTORY:

This form should be used during the interval between preparticipation evaluations.

Positive responses should prompt a medical evaluation.

1. Over the next 12 months, I wish to participate in the following sports:

   a. _____

   b. _____

   c. _____

   d. _____

2. Have you missed more than 3 consecutive days of participation in usual activities because of an injury this past year?

   Yes _____ No _____

   If yes, please indicate:

   a. Site of injury _____

   b. Type of injury_____

3. Have you missed more than 5 consecutive days of participation in usual activities because of an illness, or have you had a medical illness diagnosed that has not been resolved in this past year?

   Yes _____ No _____

   If yes, please indicate:

   a. Type of illness _____

4. Have you had a seizure, concussion or been unconscious for any reason in the last year?

   Yes _____ No _____

5. Have you had surgery or been hospitalized in this past year?

   Yes _____ No _____

   If yes, please indicate:

   a. Reason for hospitalization _____

   b. Type of surgery_____

6. List all medications you are presently taking and what condition the medication is for.

   a. _____

   b. _____

   c. _____

7. Are you worried about any problem or condition at this time?

   Yes _____ No _____

   If yes, please explain: _____

   _____

   _____

   _____

   _____

   _____

I hereby state that, to the best of my knowledge, my answers to the above questions are correct.

Date _____

Signature of athlete _____

Signature of parent _____

Figure 24-1. Sports Participation Health Record

PART C: PHYSICAL EXAMINATION RECORD

NAME _____ DATE _____ AGE _____ BIRTHDATE _____

Height _____   Vision: R _____ / _____ , corrected _____ , uncorrected _____

Weight _____   L _____ / _____ , corrected _____ , uncorrected _____

Pulse _____ Blood Pressure _____ Percent Body Fat (optional) _____ Body Mass Index (BMI) _____

	Normal	Abnormal Findings	Initials
1. Eyes			
2. Ears, nose, throat			
3. Mouth and teeth			
4. Neck			
5. Cardiovascular			
6. Chest and lungs			
7. Abdomen			
8. Skin			
9. Genitalia—hernia (male)			
10. Musculoskeletal: range of motion, strength, etc			
a. neck			
b. spine			
c. shoulders			
d. arms/hands			
e. hips			
f. thighs			
g. knees			
h. ankles			
i. feet			
11. Neuromuscular			
12. Sexual maturity (Tanner stage)		1. 2. 3. 4. 5.	

Comments re: Abnormal Findings: _____

_____

_____

_____

_____

_____

PARTICIPATION RECOMMENDATIONS:

1. No participation in: _____

_____

2. Limited participation in: _____

3. Requires: _____

_____

4. Full participation in: _____

Physician Signature _____

Telephone Number _____

Address _____

Figure 24-1. **Sports Participation Health Record, continued**

Table 24-2. The 2-Minute Orthopedic Examination	
Instructions	*Points of Observation*
Stand facing examiner	Acromioclavicular joints, general habitus
Look at ceiling, floor, over both shoulders; touch ears to shoulders	Cervical spinal motion
Shrug shoulders (examiner resists)	Trapezius strength
Abduct shoulders 90 degrees	Deltoid strength
Full external rotation of arms	Shoulder motion
Flex and extend elbows	Elbow motion
Arms at sides, elbows 90 degrees flexed; pronate and supinate wrists	Elbow and wrist motion
Spread fingers; make fist	Hand or finger motion and deformities
Tighten (contract) quadriceps; relax quadriceps	Symmetry and knee effusion; ankle effusion
"Duck walk" 4 steps (away from examiner with buttocks on heels)	Hip, knee, and ankle motion
Back to examiner	Shoulder symmetry, scoliosis
Knees straight, touch toes	Scoliosis, hip motion, hamstring tightness
Raise up on toes, raise heels	Calf symmetry, leg strength

controversial, some groups believe that an electrocardiogram should be a routine part of the PPE as well.

Exclusion Criteria

The most common causes of unexpected death during athletics include cardiomyopathies, anomalous coronary arteries, heart valve defects, primary cardiac rhythm disorders, and pulmonary hypertension, and part of the PPE is geared toward determining if a patient has risk factors for any of these conditions. Medical exclusion criteria for athletic participation are based on information obtained in the medical as well as family history. Significant historical clues include a family history of sudden, non-traumatic death; premature coronary artery disease in a first- or second-degree relative; a history of palpitations, angina, or syncope during exercise; and recent, documented infection with the Epstein-Barr virus. Controversy exists regarding when athletes can return to collision sports after infectious mononucleosis. A history of a recent concussion or multiple concussions in the past also requires close consideration regarding whether the athlete is cleared to participate in a given sport.

Findings discovered during the physical examination such as stature consistent with Marfan syndrome, a cardiac arrhythmia, or the midsystolic click of mitral valve prolapse could preclude the adolescent from participation in a particular sport. Specific conditions, such as the athlete with one eye or one kidney, should be evaluated on an individual basis by a physician qualified to assess the safety of the particular sport for the athlete (contact/collision versus limited contact).

Special circumstances to consider during the PPE are menstrual disorders and the female athlete; exercise-induced bronchospasm; anabolic steroid use; and eating disorders that may be associated with certain activities such as gymnastics, ballet, and wrestling.

CASE RESOLUTION

The young adolescent described in the case history should first be interviewed with the parent and then alone. Her medical and psychosocial history should be reviewed. A complete physical examination should be performed as well as a pelvic examination if she is sexually active and has a history of abnormal vaginal bleeding or discharge. General laboratory screening tests should be performed and the results reviewed with the patient. The remainder of the visit should be spent discussing issues such as nutrition, exercise, illicit substance abuse, sexuality and sexual activity, and safety. Results of the physical examination and screening tests should then be discussed with the parent who accompanied her to the office. If necessary, a follow-up visit should be scheduled. Otherwise, the adolescent should be seen annually.

Selected References

American Academy of Pediatrics Committee on Infectious Diseases. Prevention of human papillomavirus infection: provisional recommendations for immunization of girls and women with quadrivalent human papillomavirus vaccine. *Pediatrics.* 2007;120:666–668

American Academy of Pediatrics Committee on Infectious Diseases. Prevention of pertussis among adolescents: recommendations for use of tetanus toxoid, reduced diphtheria toxoid, and acellular pertussis (Tdap) vaccine. *Pediatrics.* 2006;117:965–978

American Academy of Pediatrics Committee on Infectious Diseases. Recommended childhood and adolescent immunization schedule—United States, 2006. *Pediatrics.* 2006;114:239–240

American Academy of Pediatrics Committee on Sports Medicine and Fitness. Medical conditions affecting sports participation. *Pediatrics.* 2001;107:1205–1209

American Academy of Family Physicians, American Academy of Pediatrics, American College of Sports Medicine, American Medical Society for Sports Medicine, American Orthopaedic Society for Sports Medicine, American Osteopathic Academy of Sports Medicine. *Preparticipation Physical Evaluation.* 3rd ed. McGraw-Hill Co; 2004

Elster A, ed. *American Medical Association Guidelines for Adolescent Preventive Services (GAPS): Recommendations and Rationale.* Baltimore, MD: Williams & Wilkins; 1994

Greydanus DE, Patel DR, Luckstead EF, Pratt HD. Value of sports pre-participation examination in health care for adolescents. *Med Sci Monit.* 2004;10:RA204–RA214

Hergenroeder AC. The preparticipation sports examination. *Pediatr Clin North Am.* 1997;44:1525–1540

Jenkins RR, Saxena SB. Keeping adolescents healthy. *Contemp Pediatr.* 1995;12:76–89

Laos C, Metzl JD. Performance-enhancing drug use in young athletes. *Adolesc Med Clin.* 2006;17:719–731

McCrindle BW. Cardiovascular risk factors in adolescents: relevance, detection, and intervention. *Adolesc Med.* 2001;12:147–162

Mentzl JD. The adolescent preparticipation physical examination. Is it helpful? *Clin Sports Med.* 2000;19:577–592

Metzl J. Preparticipation examination of the adolescent athlete: part 1. *Pediatr Rev.* 2001;22:199–203

Middleman AB. Immunization update: pertussis, meningococcus, and human papillomavirus. *Adolesc Med Clin.* 2006;17:547–563

Richamond TK, Freed GL, Clark SJ, Cabana MD. Guidelines for adolescent well care: is there consensus? *Curr Opin Pediatr.* 2006;18:365–370

Rupp RE, Rosenthal SL. New immunization strategies for adolescent patients. *Adolesc Health Update.* 2006;19:1–8

Health Care for International Adoptees

ChrisAnna M. Mink, MD

CASE STUDY

Jaxon is a 14-month-old boy adopted from Thailand. His biological mother was a 26-year-old commercial sex worker who entered a maternity house during her pregnancy to receive care and to relinquish the baby for adoption. His mom reported that she was physically and sexually abused as a child and became a street child when she was 14 years old. She used illicit drugs 5 years ago, but none since. She identifies the father as a European customer, but has no other information. Jaxon was born at 32 weeks' gestation and was placed in an incubator but did not have any respiratory problems. He has been in foster care in a Thai family's home with his care supervised by an internationally respected adoption organization. He was selected by his parents at the age of 4 months, and they have received monthly progress reports on his growth, development, and medical status. Reportedly he has had several "colds" and one ear infection but otherwise has been growing and developing well. Before departure to pick up Jaxon, his adoptive parents met with you to prepare for his arrival.

From the Bangkok airport, the parents placed a call to you because Jaxon would not stop crying. They report that on the morning that his foster mom left him with them, he cried quite a bit but had settled by bedtime and seemed to be adjusting well during the week. However, over the past 12 hours he hasn't stopped crying and refuses to eat. They question if his discomfort is related to teething because he has been drooling, but they have not noticed any other symptoms. They are gravely concerned that he doesn't like them and is having attachment difficulties.

Questions

1. What factors influence the prevalence of international adoption?
2. What are some of the potential health problems of international adoptees?
3. What is an appropriate medical evaluation for international adoptees?
4. What is the pediatrician's role in caring for the child and the newly formed family?

Annually approximately 20,000 children are adopted internationally by parents in the United States, and the number of adoptees has increased approximately 10% each year since 1992. Although these children come from a wide range of birth countries, many of their health-related issues are similar. Many of the children have lived in orphanages in impoverished areas of the developing world and have incurred the maladies associated with poverty and deprivation.

Epidemiology

From 1971 to 2001 a total 265,677 children were adopted internationally into the United States. Most of these children (90%) are from Asia (China and South Korea most commonly), Eastern Europe, and South America (Guatemala and Colombia). Many factors influence adoptive parents to choose international adoption. In the United States, delays in childbearing and associated infertility have increased the demand for adoptable children. At the same time, more readily available birth control has decreased the number of US infants available

for adoption. In addition to the shortage of **adoptable** children in the United States, additional factors for the increase in international adoptions include real and perceived risks of domestic adoption (eg, failure of birth parents to relinquish rights), fear of adopting a special needs child from the domestic system, and limited availability of children with desired traits (age and ethnicity). Also, prompt termination of rights of birth parents in international adoption is cited as a factor in the choice.

The advent of **intercountry adoption (ICA)** in the United States occurred with World War II and the large number of orphaned children in Europe, many of whom were fathered by American soldiers. The second, and more formalized, wave of ICA occurred with the Korean War. Because of the need to care for unwanted orphans, primarily of mixed ethnicities also fathered by American soldiers, South Korea established a foster care system and the children became available for adoption to Americans. War and political turmoil are still factors for children becoming available for adoption. For example, the fall of Communism was a significant factor for Russia and other states of the former Soviet Union becoming common birth countries for adoptees in the 1990s and the early part of this century. Recently, with worsening poverty and political strife, more children are being adopted from African countries.

Societal values are also factors for influencing adoption practices. China is often the leading birth country for **adoptees** because of the population control initiatives of the government mandating that families have only one child. With this practice and the desire to have a male heir, some newborn girl infants are abandoned and subsequently become available for adoption. In some countries, local laws and/or cultural practices are prohibitive for adoption, especially for foreigners and, thus, these countries are infrequent birth countries. The United States is the birth country for about 500 children adopted into other countries. Absolute statistics for children adopted out of the United States are not available because the government does not track the number of exit visas issued for adopted children. These US children are often males of African American or mixed ethnicity and are adopted by families in Canada and Western Europe. The children are available purportedly due to the low desire for these infants by adoptive parents in the United States.

The status of the country of origin (ie, war, turmoil, poverty, and societal values) aside, there is significant overlap in the reasons that children from foreign countries and from the United States become available for adoption (eg, parental substance use, abandonment, chronic neglect, abuse, and domestic violence).

Until the 1990s, most international **adoptees** were from South Korea, which had in place an excellent **foster care** system and health care. Since the 1990s, nearly two-thirds of **adoptees** come from institutions in poor nations without a developed foster care system, resulting in a significant decline in the health and well-being of the **adoptees.**

Clinical Presentation

Most internationally adopted children are female (64%), in part reflecting the adoption of girls from China, as well as a preference among some adoptive parents (especially single women) to adopt a girl. International adoptees are young, with approximately 46% being younger than 1 year and 43% between 1 and 4 years of age.

Pre-Adoption

Some **adoptees** become known to the US health care provider **"only on paper"** during the **pre-adoption stage.** Adoptive parents may ask their health care provider for help in assessing the child's medical status. Often parents receive a written health report (varying in the quantity and the quality of information) and photos or videos of the child they are considering adopting. The written documents may be in a foreign language or not translated by an experienced medical translator. Some countries prohibit international adoption of healthy children, so diagnoses may be embellished to improve the child's chances for adoption. Additionally, some medical records contain diagnoses that are nonsensical in US medicine but represent terms used in the country of origin. For example, **adoptees** from Russia often have neurologic diagnoses such as **perinatal encephalopathy,** which suggests serious brain injury and would carry a grave prognosis in Western medicine; in Russia this term may reflect a minor deprivation or a lack of prenatal care and not a specific neurologic injury. However, at other times, a term may have the same meaning and intent to Russian physicians as to US physicians. These inconsistencies are therefore quite challenging when trying to evaluate the medical records of potential **adoptees.** Many physicians may not feel comfortable with reviewing medical records given so many limitations; however, even with all of the caveats, review of the records may still provide insight into the health status of the potential adoptee.

Also during the **pre-adoption stage,** the health care provider may provide information for parents and families for preventive health measures to prepare for travel to a developing area of the world. The Centers for Disease Control and Prevention traveler's information Web site (www.cdc.gov/travel) is a good resource for health care providers and the parents. Up-to-date information may also be obtained from the World Health Organization and the US State Department (Table 25-1). Additionally, parents should be informed about the possible infections seen in international adoptees, and they should receive appropriate education and vaccinations (eg, hepatitis B because of the increased risk of the child being positive for hepatitis B surface antigen (HbsAg), seen in 1%–5% of adoptees).

Table 25-1. Web Sites for International Health, Travel, and Adoption Information

Resource	Information	Web Site
Centers for Disease Control and Prevention	• Up-to-date information for travelers' health	www.cdc.gov/travel
US State Department	• Up-to-date information for travelers' risk (eg, civil unrest) • Intercountry adoption statistics • Intercountry adoption procedures	www.travel.state.gov www.state.gov www.travel.state.gov/family/adoption/adoption_485.html
World Health Organization	• Health status and recommendations for immunizations for each country	www.who.int/en/
US Child Welfare	• Adoption information and procedures	www.childwelfare.gov

During the Adoption Trip

All internationally adopted children are required by the US State Department to have a **physical examination** before admission into the country; however, this examination is quite limited in scope and performed primarily to rule out severe impairments or certain communicable diseases that may pose a public health threat. This examination should not be considered as a complete medical evaluation for an individual child. Some health care providers are able to provide support for families during travel via e-mail or telephone, similar to telephone consultations performed in general practice.

Post-Adoption

After the adoption, the health status of the children on presentation to the American health care provider is quite variable ranging from well (eg, infants from Korean foster care) to severely ill with acute infections or chronic diseases (eg, malnutrition and tuberculosis). The adopted child should be seen by the physician within 2 to 3 weeks of arrival in the United States, or sooner if he or she has an acute illness. This 2-week period allows for the child (and parents) to recover from jet lag and to become more familiar with each other, permitting a better assessment at the visit. If an acute illness visit is required, a separate appointment for a comprehensive evaluation should be scheduled.

Health Care Issues

In addition to the problems commonly related to **poverty** and **deprivations,** many health issues are specific to the country of origin (eg, increased risk of **fetal alcohol spectrum disorder [FASD]** in children from Russia, malaria from Africa, etc). Published data regarding health care issues are limited for children from more recent countries of origins (eg, China and Russia) (Figure 25-1).

Generally, the health care issues for **adoptees** are extensive including acute illnesses (eg, respiratory infections), chronic illnesses (eg, anemia, malnutrition, poor dental hygiene, tuberculosis, asthma, and parasite infestation), delayed or unknown immunizations, and impaired growth and development.

Some children have assigned birth dates (eg, **abandoned infants** and **street children** for whom the birth dates are not known), and they may have small growth parameters, making it difficult to know their true age and expected development. **Developmental delay,** most commonly language delay, is frequently identified. Assessment of development may be even more difficult in infants and young children who are nonverbal and older children who speak their native language.

Growth delay is common for **adoptees.** Many children are malnourished or have failure to thrive (FTT), and these afflictions are often multifactorial in origin, including poor prenatal environment (maternal stress, malnutrition, drug and alcohol abuse) inadequate calories, inadequate nurturing, unrecognized genetic or congenital disorders (eg, FASD), and untreated chronic illnesses (eg, rickets). Institutionalized children may suffer from **psychosocial dwarfism,** and may lose 1 month of linear growth for every 3 to 4 months spent in the orphanage. Delay in puberty may be observed in adolescents from deprived environments such as **orphanages.**

Immunization records may not be available, may be incomplete, or may be in a foreign language, which hinders assessing the vaccination status of adoptees. Additionally, many vaccines available in the United States are not available in the developing world (eg, *Haemophilus influenzae* type b [Hib] and pneumococcal conjugate vaccines) and, thus, children will not have had them. Adopted children immigrating to the United States who are younger than 10 years are exempt from the Immigration and Nationality Act regulations requiring proof of immunizations before arrival; however,

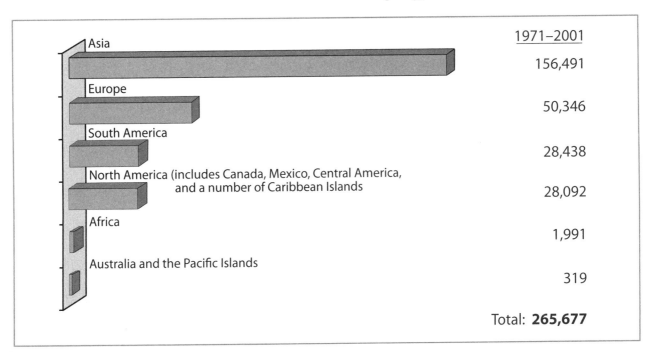

	1971–2001
Asia	156,491
Europe	50,346
South America	28,438
North America (includes Canada, Mexico, Central America, and a number of Caribbean Islands	28,092
Africa	1,991
Australia and the Pacific Islands	319
	Total: **265,677**

Figure 25-1. **Countries of origin for children adopted by parents in the United States.**

adoptive parents are required to sign a waiver that they will comply with US recommended immunizations after arrival.

Psychosocial, emotional, and **mental health problems** are some of the more challenging problems to assess. The spectrum of mental health problems is related to age and previous life experiences for the child. Children may have suffered from physical and/or sexual abuse prior to placement in an institution, where the potential for such abuse also exists. This may be inflicted by adult caretakers or bigger children when supervision is inadequate. Attachment disorders are some of the most concerning abnormalities for adoptive parents, adoption professionals, and health care providers. Because the fundamentals for learning healthy attachments are greatly influenced by early infant-caretaker relationships, many international adoptees have difficulties bonding, in part because they have not had secure caretaker relationships. Issues for attachment and bonding may be especially problematic for children who have resided in an orphanage and/or had multiple caretakers from an early age. Because the children have had multiple caretakers, they may be indiscriminately friendly, which poses risks for their safety. Other common mental health problems include depression, attention-deficit/hyperactivity disorder (ADHD), post-traumatic stress disorder, abnormal behaviors (eg, self-stimulating behaviors, hoarding food, sleep disturbances), and oppositional-defiant disorder. As mentioned previously, communication with the child may be difficult due to language barriers, causing another obstacle to assessing the mental health of the child.

Sensory integration difficulties are increasingly recognized in adoptees. The children may have adverse responses to touch (including new clothing, hugs and kisses, bathing, etc) or textures (such as new foods). Individual or all of the senses (hearing, vision, taste, or smell) may be notably increased or decreased, and some children have decreased sensation to physical pain leading to an increased risk for injuries. Dyskinesia (clumsiness or injury prone) has also been observed.

The most common identified medical issues are **infectious diseases.** These include acute illnesses (eg, upper respiratory infection, bronchitis, otitis, and infectious diarrhea, among others), as well as longer-term infections such as tuberculosis and parasite infestations (scabies and *Giardia* are common). Because of their biological mother's lifestyle and their time residing in institutions, many adoptees are at increased risk of exposure to infectious diseases such as syphilis, human immunodeficiency virus (HIV), and hepatitis B and C.

Preventive care considered "routine" in the United States is unlikely to have been part of the child's care and needs to be performed as appropriate for age. This includes newborn screening laboratory studies and assessments of hearing, vision, dental, and mental health. Anticipatory guidance for the new parents should be incorporated into the initial, and all, visits.

Evaluation

The initial office visit with the physician should be scheduled for an extended period because of the complexity of the evaluation and the additional time needed for parental education. If the physician's schedule does not permit extended visits, ancillary staff (eg, nursing, dietitian, and therapists) may perform parts of the evaluation and education.

Observation of the child's behavior, development, and interactions with the adoptive parents and health care provider is a critical element of the evaluation. Most health care providers include such observations in their visits routinely, but particular attention is necessary for new adoptees. Things to notice include the child's behavior. Are they easily engaged or withdrawn? Do they make eye contact with the parent or health care provider? Do they make any vocalizations or words, depending on the child's age? Do they play with toys? Are they too friendly or afraid of strangers? Do they seek comfort from the new parents?

History

Limited medical information is available from most birth countries, though there are some exceptions (eg, from foster care in Korea or Guatemala). Family history and birth history are rarely obtainable for adoptees. Immunization histories are becoming increasingly available. Previously, vaccine records were considered unreliable; however, in recent years, data have emerged to suggest that well-documented immunizations may be considered valid. Written records showing the age of the child when vaccinated, the date of administration, dose given, and proper intervals between dosing that are consistent with the World Health Organization schedules or are comparable to US schedules may be considered acceptable for proof of immunization. (See under Management for guidelines when vaccine records are not available.)

Dietary history is important for assessing the child's nutritional status. Questions to ask include: What food and formula/milk is the child receiving? Has he or she received adequate calories? Is there known or suspected food intolerance (eg, lactose intolerance is more common in Asian ethnicities)? Are there abnormal behaviors associated with food or eating (eg, preoccupation with food, hoarding, food refusal, or gorging)?

An interim medical history may be available because many children are selected by their adoptive parents several months before immigrating to the United States. The interim medical history may be provided from the orphanage or foster care provider through the adoption agency. Parents should be encouraged to solicit as much information as possible from the caretakers of the child. At a minimum, this history should include serial growth parameters, known illnesses, hospitalizations, surgeries, allergies, and immunizations given while the child was under their care. Parents should also ask the caretakers about any food preferences, special fears, toys, or friends from the current placement. If the child has a special "lovey," the parents should request to bring it with the child for a transitional object.

Physical Examination

A complete unclothed physical examination should be performed on infants and children of all ages. However, due to previous trauma such as sexual abuse, some parts of the examination may have to be done over a series of visits to minimize the possibility of additional trauma from an examination. All aspects of the physical examination are absolutely essential. Accurate measurements of height, weight and, depending on age and size, head circumference should be obtained. Plotting of parameters on the growth curves for the United States (compared with birth country) should be used, with few exceptions. The child should be closely inspected for unusual scars or bruises, evidence of fractures (old or recent), rachitic changes, and genital or rectal scars. The skin should be examined for rashes, lesions, and a bacille Calmette-Guérin (BCG) scar (typically on the upper deltoid). A developmental screen should be performed, and a more complete developmental assessment should be scheduled at a separate visit (when the child is not distressed or acutely ill). A dental examination should be included and referral for a formal dental evaluation will likely be necessary. Screening evaluations of hearing and vision should be performed, and formal testing may be needed depending on the age of the child and ability to cooperate.

Laboratory Testing

Laboratory testing should include complete blood count, lead levels, and thyroid function testing (iodine is not in many diets in Asia). Additionally, testing for illnesses associated with specific countries of origin, findings on examination (eg, comprehensive metabolic panel for malnourished child), and as directed by the child's age (eg, newborn screening for metabolic disorders in infants) should be performed.

Because of the **increased risks of exposures,** laboratory screening for infectious diseases should be undertaken. Serum samples should be tested for syphilis (non-treponemal and treponemal antibodies), hepatitis B panel (HBsAg, hepatitis B surface antigen antibody (HbsAb), hepatitis B core antibody), hepatitis C antibody, and HIV 1 and 2 antibodies. Human immunodeficiency virus polymerase chain reaction may be indicated in some children. Stool samples should be sent for ova and parasite examination (at least 2 times) and *Giardia* and *Cryptosporidium* antigen testing. Stool for bacterial pathogens (eg, *Salmonella* and *Shigella)* should be sent from children from some regions such as the Indian subcontinent. Because cytomegalovirus infection is ubiquitous, routine testing is not recommended. Routine testing for hepatitis A antibodies is also not recommended because most children in the developing world acquire hepatitis A at an early age. Administering hepatitis A vaccine, as recommended in the United States, is not problematic for children who may have had previous hepatitis A infection.

Tuberculosis (TB) skin testing (ie, purified protein derivative [PPD]) should be performed on all children; history of receipt of BCG is not a contraindication to skin testing. Bacille Calmette-Guérin vaccinations are usually given at birth in most developing nations, and its influence on skin test status is controversial. Generally, BCG

given within the previous 1 to 2 years may contribute to a positive PPD skin test; however, a positive PPD test is more likely reflective of true infection with *Mycobacterium* with or without active disease and merits further evaluation. Latent TB infection has been reported from 0.6% to 30% of international adoptees, which is not surprising because most adoptees come from TB-endemic areas.

Management

Counseling for the Transition

Education and **preparation** for the parents and all family members is a priority. Parents should provide firm structure and boundaries in a loving milieu for the adoptees. A scheduled regimen may be especially important to previously institutionalized children because it has been their way of life, but even noninstitutionalized children benefit from a predictable routine. Parents should maximize their one-on-one interactions with the adoptee, while still allowing time for themselves and other family members (not an easy task with multiple children). Touching and affection may initially need to be tempered as directed by the child's tolerance. Parents should try to enhance bonding and attachment by frequently identifying themselves as "Mom" or "Dad." Other strategies to enhance attachment include initially limiting contact with individuals outside of the family and not "handing" the child to others, including non-household family members because these are strangers to the child. Frequent verbal reassurances and talking to the child about the people and the new world around them should be encouraged. In caring for the child, parents should be encouraged to "meet the child" at his or her developmental level and not the chronological age.

Growth and Nutrition

When children are identified as malnourished or FTT, a multidisciplinary treatment plan is recommended, including parents, physician, nutritionist, and therapists (eg, occupational therapist for feeding difficulties). The child should be offered familiar foods, if that is his or her preference, and each meal may include a new more nutritional offering. Children should be offered frequent meals and snacks because they may not be able to eat much at one sitting. Foods should be calorie-dense (eg, added butter, cheese, avocado, or peanut butter, depending on age and previous dietary history). Dietary supplements, such as PediaSure, may be indicated.

Precocious puberty has been observed in female international adoptees, more than males, and is thought to be related to the rapid improvement of nutrition. If signs of precocious puberty are observed, evaluation by a pediatric endocrinologist is recommended.

Development

Because developmental delays are so common, most adoptees should have a developmental assessment. Language delays, especially expressive, are frequent and, when identified, formal audiology testing should be part of the assessment.

Mental Health

Mental and emotional health problems are common and may manifest early or late, or occur as relapses. Initial problems seen may include sleep disorders, fears and phobias, bizarre behaviors, and self-stimulating behaviors. Unless the behaviors pose a safety risk, the parents should tolerate them because most dissipate with time in a secure environment. At times of emotional distress, parents may observe a relapse of behavior problems. The health care provider may provide guidance for parents for the milder disorders; however, moderate and severe disorders merit prompt referral to a mental health professional, ideally someone with expertise in adoption.

Immunizations

If vaccinations are considered valid, as described previously, resuming immunizations per the US schedule (see Chapter 23) is appropriate. If immunization status is unknown or incomplete, repeating immunizations or checking antibody concentrations to vaccine antigens is an acceptable option. Most areas of the world routinely administer BCG, polio (oral), and diphtheria and tetanus toxoids and acellular pertussis vaccines. Receipt of additional diphtheria, tetanus, and possible pertussis antigens may be associated with an increase in adverse events; measuring antibodies to diphtheria and tetanus is warranted to minimize adverse events. There are no US Food and Drug Administration–approved antibody tests available commercially for pertussis antibodies. Receipt of additional doses of inactivated polio vaccine is not usually associated with adverse events. Testing for HbsAb should be performed on all adoptees, and the results will guide the plan for further immunizations. Hepatitis B vaccine will only elicit HBsAb; the presence of other antibodies suggests natural infection. For measles, mumps, and rubella (MMR), various formulations and combinations (1- and 2-component more commonly than 3-component) vaccines are available worldwide. Checking antibodies to these antigens is possible, but likely administering a US-licensed combination (eg, MMR or MMRV) may be necessary to ensure protection against all antigens. Most of the other vaccines available in the United States are not available in the developing world (eg, Hib and pneumococcal conjugates, varicella, hepatitis A, etc), and the child should receive these vaccines as recommended for age per the US schedule.

Infectious Diseases

Any acute identified infectious disease (eg, scabies, otitis) should be treated following standard practice, keeping in mind the possibility that different antibiotic resistance patterns exist in other parts of the world. Thus, if the child does not have the predicted response to treatment, consultation with a pediatric infectious diseases specialist should be considered. For other infectious diseases screening noted previously, additional evaluation and possible treatment should be initiated promptly (eg, penicillin therapy for syphilis) and pediatric infectious diseases consultation may be considered.

For TB evaluation, any positive skin testing merits further investigation for true infection with TB. A compounding problem is that some children may be anergic due to malnutrition, giving a false-negative skin test. If malnutrition is suspected, consider a chest radiograph even if the PPD is negative, and consider repeating the PPD when the child's nutritional status has improved. Routinely repeating the PPD 6 months later is advisable if the child is from an endemic area, because late exposure to an infected individual is possible.

Prognosis

Being prepared for the complex needs related to international adoption has been identified as the best determinant for parents to consider the adoption experience as positive, regardless of the number or severity of the medical needs of the adoptee.

With improved nutrition and environment, most children have significant catch-up growth; however, up to one-third of adoptees may have unrecoverable loss in linear growth. For intellectual development, by 1 year of age, nearly all children in orphanages have one or more areas of delay. However, their prognosis is generally good with an increase in 2 developmental quotient points per month after arrival in the United States. After 3 years of age in an orphanage, the length of time institutionalized and delays noted at age 11 months correlate negatively with IQ (8 months in orphanage, average IQ = 90; 2 or more years in orphanage, average IQ = 69).

Many children have ongoing mental and psychosocial problems, and some disorders do not manifest until the children are older (eg, ADHD or learning disorders when the child is school-aged). Ongoing attachment disorders seem to occur with greater frequency in children with lower IQs, more behavior problems, and adoptive families with a lower socioeconomic status.

Assessment of the overall outcome for children who spent 8 or more months in institutional care in Eastern Europe, when evaluated at least 3 years after adoption, showed about one-third had multiple serious problems (including IQ ≤85, insecure attachment, and severe behavior problems), about one-third had a few serious problems but were thought to be making progress, and about one-third had progressed very well. The best predictors of major problems were (1) greater length of time in the orphanage, (2) increased number of children adopted at same time, (3) younger adoptive mother, (3) lower socioeconomic status of mother, and (4) father alone selected the child. Although the impact of these risk factors may not be identical for all birth countries, they do provide some insight. Reviewing these risk factors with adoptive parents during the pre-adoption period may aid in their decision-making.

Pediatrician's Role

The pediatrician's role is not to tell the adoptive parent whom to adopt; the parents are essentially choosing life partners, which is an individual decision. Pediatricians, however, can assist the parents in reviewing the available medical information, which may aid them in making an informed decision about proceeding with an adoption.

During the adoption process, the health care provider must assume an active role as a child advocate, as well as parental advocate and educator. This may be the first parenting experience for the adoptive parents and, thus, they need the "basics" for child care, no matter what the age of the adoptee. This might include feeding and routine care (eg, estimate the number of diapers needed if traveling to an area with no access to supplies), as well as discipline techniques for a traumatized child. Preparation for caring for illnesses is needed because many adoptees are ill at the time of the adoption and travel. The pediatrician can facilitate emotional preparation because the parents may be isolated from their usual support systems while embarking on the new role of parent.

After returning home, the pediatrician has a role as primary care provider, as well as serving as a referral source for other needed specialists (eg, subspecialists, mental health providers, post-adoption support services, developmental interventions, and nutritionists, among others).

Counseling Adoptive Parents About the Expectations

Parents should be informed that it is unlikely that an institutionalized child will emerge unscathed. With this in mind, parents may make preliminary preparations for treatments and rehabilitation for the child. Families should be counseled that it is OK to say "no" to a potential adoptee. No one has benefited from adoption of children by families that do not have the resources needed to care for them. Most importantly, parents should be reassured that optimism is appropriate. Being prepared matters!

CASE RESOLUTION

In talking with the parents, they report that they have not observed any injuries and no areas seem tender when they examine Jaxon, as you have suggested. They elect to give him some diphenhydramine and take the flight home with the plan to come see you on arrival. Although they are exhausted, they come directly to your office for an acute visit. They report that he remained inconsolable and that the flight home was miserable for him (and everyone around them). On entering the examination room, Jaxon was screaming and noticeably uncomfortable but trying to find comfort in his dad's arms.

His temperature was 38.9°C (102°F) axillary; pulse rate, 144/min; and respiratory rate, 30/min. His examination was notable for extensive oral and pharyngeal vesicular lesions with erythema, but there were not labial lesions. He had multiple shotty cervical nodes, and the rest of the examination was noncontributory. A diagnosis of herpangina was made. He was given a dose of ibuprofen, and 15 minutes later he was quiet, able to swallow electrolyte solution, and was cuddling in his dad's arms. His parents were given reassurance that this was an acute infection and not an indication of poor bonding; in fact he was already seeking comfort from them. Additional testing for infections included obtaining antibodies to human immunodeficiency virus, rapid plasma reagin for syphilis, hepatitis C and a hepatitis B panel, especially with his biological mother's history of being a commercial sex worker. Other testing included complete blood count, lead level, and thyroid function tests. He was given an appointment in 2 weeks to complete the assessment, including a developmental assessment, because this was deferred since he was acutely ill.

Selected References

Albers L, Barnett E, Jenista J, Johnson D. International adoption: medical and developmental issues. *Pediatr Clin North Am.* 2005;52:xiii–xv

Ames E. *The Development of Romanian Orphanage Children Adopted to Canada: Final Report.* Burnaby, British Columbia, Canada: Simon Fraser University; 1997

American Academy of Pediatrics. Medical evaluation of internationally adopted children for infectious diseases. In: Pickering LK, Baker CJ, Long SS, McMillan JA, eds. *Red Book: 2006 Report of the Committee on Infectious Diseases.* 27th ed. Elk Grove Village, IL: American Academy of Pediatrics; 2006:182–191

Barnett ED. Immunizations and infectious disease screening for internationally adopted children. *Pediatr Clin North Am.* 2005;52:1287–1309

Cederbald M, Hook B, Irhammar M, Mercke AM. Mental health in international adoptees as teenagers and young adults. An epidemiological study. *J Child Psychol Psychiatry.* 1999;40:1239–1248

Centers for Disease Control and Prevention. Elevated blood lead levels among internationally adopted children—United States, 1998. *MMWR Morb Mortal Wkly Rep.* 2000;11:97–100

Evan B. Donaldson Adoption Institute. *International Adoption Facts.* www.adoptioninstitute.org/FactOverview/international_print.html

Johnson DE. *International Adoption: New Kids, New Challenges.* www.med. umn.edu/peds/iac/preadoption.htm

Lieberthal JK. Adoption in the Absence of National Boundaries. Paper presented at: 25th Conference of the North American Council on Adoptable Children; 1999, 2003; Vancouver British Columbia, Canada. www.adoptioninstitute.org/policy

Miller LC, Hendrie NW. Health of children adopted from China. *Pediatrics.* 2000;105:e76

Peterson K. Preparing to meet foreign bugs. Travel, immigration, and international adoptions require special precautions. *Postgrad Med.* 2001;110:67–70, 73–74, 77

Saiman L, Aronson J, Zhou J, et al. Prevalence of infectious diseases among internationally adopted children. *Pediatrics.* 2001;108:608–612

Selman P, ed. *Intercountry Adoption: Developments, Trends and Perspectives.* London, England: British Agencies for Adoption and Fostering; 2000:545

Sloutsky V. Institutional care and developmental outcomes of 6- and 7-year-old children: a contextualist perspective. *Int J Behav Dev.* 1997;20:131–151

US Department of State. Immediate Relative Visas Issued. http://travel.state.gov/family/adoption/info/info_458.html

Weitzman C, Albers L. Long-term developmental, behavioral, and attachment outcomes after international adoption. *Pediatr Clin North Am.* 2005;52:1395–1419

Health Care Needs of Children in Foster Care

Sara T. Stewart, MD, and ChrisAnna M. Mink, MD

CASE STUDY

A 7-year-old girl is brought to your office by her foster parent for a general physical. The foster parent states that the girl has been living in her home for the past week. When she was initially brought by the social worker, her skin was dirty, and she was wearing dirty clothes. There are no medical records and no immunization records available for your review, and the child states that she saw a doctor "a long time ago." The girl states that she used to go to school, but that she did not return when her friends did at the end of the last school break. She gets tearful when she is asked about her family, and states that she misses her brothers and sisters, but that she does not want to return to live with her mother and father right now. The only history known by the foster parent is that the child required some type of special services in school, and that the social worker found drug paraphernalia in her home at the time of her removal. The foster parent also states that 2 nights ago, the patient accidentally broke a dish and responded by running to the corner of the room, crying that she didn't want to get hit.

On physical examination, the patient is alert, quiet, and cooperative. Her weight and height are in the 10th to 25th percentiles for her age. She has poor dentition with multiple dental caries, a thin upper lip, and a flat philtrum. She has a few basilar wheezes on lung examination and has scattered bruises on her anterior shins.

Questions

1. What are the medical, psychological, and behavioral issues that commonly affect children in the foster care system?
2. What is the role of the primary care provider in providing a medical home for the child in foster care?
3. How does a child's legal status as a child in foster care affect how medical care can be delivered?
4. What are the appropriate health care referrals and community resources to access for a patient who is in foster care?

The term **foster care** refers to the **temporary placement** of a child in the home of another caretaker or **foster parent** due to a threat to the child's safety or well-being in the original home environment. Placement of a child in foster care results from an investigation of the child's home environment by **child protective services (CPS)** and may be arranged via voluntary agreement of the parent or through court sanction. The foster parent may be related to the child or may be a nonrelative. For those children in voluntary placement, the biological parent retains the right to terminate the placement at any time. For those placed by **legal sanction,** a series of court hearings gives parents, the child, and the **CPS** agency the opportunity to present their perspective on the circumstances surrounding the allegations and their respective views on interventions to ensure the child has access to the best home environment.

Children in **foster care** may present to the primary care provider soon after placement in foster care, or may present after having been with a foster parent for a long time. In either scenario, it is recognized that as a subpopulation of pediatric patients, children in foster care have a significant number of **unmet medical** and **mental health** needs and should be considered to be a **"special needs"** patient population. At the time of initial removal, the CPS worker may not be able to obtain a medical history or essential information about medications for the child. Changes in foster care placement may interrupt continuity of care with a health care provider, and frequent changes in the assigned social services caseworker can create barriers to consistent communication among foster parents, health care providers, and caseworkers. These children have rates of medical and mental health disorders that are higher than those of children from equivalent socioeconomic backgrounds who are not in foster care. There has traditionally been a lack of appreciation within the general medical community as to the complexity of the needs of this patient population, and due to low reimbursement rates, there has been difficulty allotting the amount of time necessary in an office visit to complete the level of evaluation needed by these children. For those children with mental health needs, there is often a paucity of available resources. This is particularly true for children younger than 5 years.

These unmet needs have long-lasting effects on the well-being of children, even after exiting the foster care system. Because of their complex health care issues and vulnerability to fragmented care, these children merit a medical home, providing comprehensive, multidisciplinary services and medical case management.

Epidemiology

At any point during a given year, between 500,000 and 600,000 children nationwide are in the foster care system. Approximately 300,000 children enter the system annually, and reasons for placement, in descending order of prevalence, include neglect, parental incapacity, physical abuse, abandonment, and sexual abuse.

Foster children are of all ethnicities, but there is disproportionate representation of children of color within the foster care population. The age distribution is bimodal, with children younger than 5 years and older adolescents comprising most of the population. Over the past several decades an increasing percentage of new entrants into foster care are children in the youngest age bracket, particularly infants younger than 1 year. Many of these infants are prenatally substance exposed and are placed in foster care due to a combination of factors related to the maternal drug use.

Approximately 60% of children leave foster care within 2 years of placement, and more than half of them are reunited with their biological parent or primary caretaker. Fifteen percent to 20% remain in foster care for more than 5 years, and approximately 10% of all children leaving foster care reenter the system due to a new report within a year. The number of adoptions from foster care has increased since the late 1990s to account for 18% of those leaving the child welfare system, and an additional 9% of those leaving foster care are emancipating out of the system by reaching 18 years of age. Almost half of the children in foster care will experience 3 or more placements, which leads to further fragmentation of their health care and education. Multiple foster care placements are more common for those children with behavioral, emotional, or coping problems.

As a population, children in the foster care system come from home environments that experience high rates of poverty, parental mental illness, parental substance abuse, low levels of education, high rates of unemployment, and frequent involvement with the criminal justice system. These children have high rates of exposure to domestic violence, and many are victims themselves of physical abuse, sexual abuse, and neglect. Their biological parents often have limited parenting skills, and the children experience inconsistent parenting behaviors along with minimal developmental stimulation and emotional support. All of these factors combine to cause unpredictable, stressful, and unsafe home environments for these children, prompting their removal and placement into foster care.

Clinical Presentation

Medical Issues

Children in the foster care system have been shown to have high rates of both **acute and chronic illness** at the time of their initial medical evaluations after placement (Dx Box). In one study in Maryland, 90% of children had at least one medical problem at the time of entrance into foster care. Common maladies include **neurologic disorders** (~30%), **vision or hearing problems** (20%), **gastrointestinal diseases** (20%), **dental caries** (~40%), and other inadequately treated chronic illnesses such as **asthma and anemia.** Acute infections are also common, including respiratory tract infections, skin infections, otitis media, sexually transmitted infections (STIs), and intestinal infestations with parasites. Low immunization rates are also a frequent occurrence.

Dx

Common Issues of Children in Foster Care

- Acute infection
- Undiagnosed or inadequately treated chronic illnesses
- Dental caries
- Growth delay and failure to thrive
- Incomplete immunization histories
- Prenatal or perinatal exposure to sexually transmitted infections
- Effects of prenatal substance exposure
- Physical sequelae of physical and sexual abuse
- Developmental delay
- Attention-deficit/hyperactivity disorder
- Post-traumatic stress disorder
- Anxiety
- Depression
- Conduct and oppositional defiant disorders
- Attachment disorders
- Educational disabilities

Nearly one-quarter of children entering foster care have growth delay with a weight, height, or head circumference measurement less than the 5th percentile for age. This may be due to a combination of factors, including inadequate nutrition, environmental deprivation, prenatal alcohol exposure, genetic predisposition, or underlying illness such as human immunodeficiency virus (HIV) infection. Environments that are chronically stressful or that lack the necessary stimulation and support for a child may also lead to behaviors such as rumination and social withdrawal. (For further discussion of failure to thrive, see Chapter 117.)

Many children placed in foster care have a history of **prenatal exposure** to illicit drugs, alcohol, and tobacco. These children have high rates of premature birth and of prenatal or perinatal exposure to infections such as **hepatitis C, hepatitis B, HIV, syphilis,** and

herpes simplex. This risk of exposure to infectious agents is related to maternal drug use and its frequent association with prostitution, needle sharing, and drug use in sexual partners.

Children who have been placed in foster care may present with physical sequelae of prior physical and sexual abuse. Physical abuse may result in skin trauma, skeletal fractures, head trauma, abdominal trauma, and chest trauma. Sexual abuse may result in genital trauma or symptoms of STIs.

Developmental and Mental Health Issues

A high prevalence of developmental delay, behavioral disorders, and educational difficulties has been noted in foster children of all age groups. These disorders are more common in children with a history of neglect or abandonment than in those who have suffered other forms of child maltreatment. Of children younger than 6 years entering foster care, 23% to 61% have significant developmental delays and 25% to 40% have behavioral difficulties. Speech and language difficulties, delayed fine motor skills, and poor social-adaptive skills are common, and up to one-fifth of school-aged children entering foster care had been receiving special education services prior to the time of placement.

Common mental health issues in the foster care population include attention-deficit/hyperactivity disorder, depression, anxiety, and suicidal ideation. **Post-traumatic stress disorder** is common and is more prevalent in those who have experienced or witnessed family violence. Adolescents in foster care may "act out" as a manifestation of mental health difficulties, resulting in sexual promiscuity, substance abuse, and truancy, as well as in rates of conduct and oppositional defiant disorders that are higher than those in the general adolescent population.

Attachment disorders are seen more frequently in the foster care population and account for a portion of the behavioral difficulties in these children. A secure attachment to a primary caretaker is necessary to the development of emotional security and the sense that one's needs are important. Children who are removed from violent homes, or who may have suffered child abuse or neglect, are likely to have never developed a secure attachment to a primary caretaker in that home environment, and may therefore have difficulty bonding with a foster parent. This problem is then compounded if the same child is moved among multiple foster homes, never allowing time for the development of a healthy attachment to a caretaker. In addition to their lack of emotional reciprocity, these children may exhibit self-stimulatory behaviors or sleep disturbances.

The behavioral difficulties that children in the foster care system manifest are often due to multiple factors. These children may be predisposed to behavioral disorders by a history of prenatal drug or alcohol exposure or by a history of abuse or neglect. It can also be difficult to determine whether a child's behaviors predate placement in foster care, or whether they are a response to the removal from his or her home. As a result of placement in foster care, children often experience fear, sadness, and a feeling of guilt or responsibility for the family discord that resulted in their removal. Foster placements are invariably sudden and unexpected, involve the loss of a familiar caretaker, and are traumatic for children of all ages.

Evaluation

It is important for a provider to be familiar with the **medical consent legalities** concerning foster children in his or her geographic locale. While specifics vary by locality, generally foster parents have the authority to provide consent for routine medical care. The placement of a child in foster care does not supersede the right of a biological parent to participate in the medical decision-making for his or her child, and many do retain the authority to consent for medical tests and procedures. Any medical procedure or test that requires specific written consent is likely to require **authorization** by the **legally recognized parent** (eg, child welfare agency, the courts, or the biological parent). Two common clinical scenarios that frequently require consent beyond the foster parent's authority are HIV testing and the administration of psychotropic medications.

History

Children in foster care may be brought for medical evaluation by a foster parent, a relative of the foster parent, or by the social service caseworker. Often the biological parent is absent from the visit, and the child's medical records are not available at the time of the evaluation. Obtaining past medical records can be difficult, but the caseworker can be of assistance in this process. It is important to ascertain the circumstances that prompted a child's placement in foster care, as this may modify portions of the evaluation.

The biological family history is useful to evaluate for the presence of genetic disorders and communicable diseases. A maternal history regarding drug use or STIs will assist in identifying those children who may have had prenatal exposures to infectious agents.

Birth history should include any history of prenatal care and complications such as prematurity or drug withdrawal. The results of routine newborn screening (eg, hearing, inborn errors of metabolism, thyroid function, hemoglobinopathies, etc) should also be obtained.

A complete medical and surgical history should be gathered, including the identification of a regular health care provider if the child has one. Older, verbal children may be able to provide some of their own histories. Known medications and allergies should be documented, and all available immunization records should be obtained. Documentation of a child's immunization history is frequently unavailable, so all possible sources of records, such as biological parents or school districts, should be identified. Feeding history and nutritional assessments should include the type and amount of formula or breast milk for infants, and types and quantities of foods for older children.

The psychosocial history includes a history of a child's current and prior foster placements or living arrangements, and whether there was exposure to domestic violence, physical abuse, or sexual abuse

(Questions Box). Verbal children may also be able to discuss their feelings about their current foster placement. Adolescents should have a confidential screening (eg, HEADDSSS [home, education and employment, activities, drugs, sexuality, safety, suicide and depression] examination) (see Chapter 5) to address drug, alcohol, and tobacco use; issues related to the home and school; sexual activity; violence; and gang involvement.

Questions

Psychosocial

- When was the child placed in foster care?
- Why was the child placed in foster care?
- Has the child had prior foster placements? If so, when? Why did placement change?
- Was there prior exposure to domestic violence? Physical or sexual abuse?
- Does the child have siblings in foster care?
- How does the child feel about the current foster placement?
- How has the child integrated into the foster family?
- Has the child previously received mental health services? Therapeutic services for developmental delay or educational difficulties?
- What is the child's social service plan? Parental visits? Reunification? Termination of parental rights?

The **developmental history** should include the results of prior developmental assessments, as well as a listing of therapeutic or early intervention services received. The behavioral history should also include results of prior assessments, mental health services used, and any psychotropic medications prescribed. The foster parent, biological parent, or CPS caseworker may be able to provide useful observations regarding the child's developmental capabilities, behavioral patterns, and social interactions. The biological parent or CPS caseworker may also be able to assist in collecting records from prior assessments.

Educational history is often not available at the time of the medical evaluation. It is helpful, however, to know a child's history of prior evaluations by the school system, special education services provided, or prior therapeutic services (eg, physical therapy, occupational therapy, speech therapy) received through the school district.

Physical Examination

A complete, unclothed physical examination should be performed on each child. Growth parameters, including height, weight, and occipitofrontal head circumference, should be plotted on a reference chart, and a close inspection should be performed for signs of prior trauma. The child should be assessed for **dysmorphic features** consistent with prenatal alcohol exposure or other genetic syndromes. The physical examination should include a **genital examination** to also assess for signs of trauma in children of all ages, and sexually active females should have a pelvic examination within 3 years of

the onset of sexual activity. (See Chapters 115 through 118, for further descriptions of physical findings.)

Additional Assessments

All children should undergo both mental health and developmental screenings and should be referred for comprehensive testing if abnormalities are noted. Vision and hearing screenings should also be performed on all children old enough to cooperate. A referral for expert vision or hearing evaluation should be made if it is indicated by history or physical examination, or the patient is unable to perform the screening procedure (eg, infant or toddler with speech delay).

Laboratory Tests

Routine screening laboratory tests should be performed on foster children just as they are indicated for the general pediatric population. For example, hemoglobin level should be checked annually in all infants, toddlers, and preschool-aged children. Serum lead levels should be checked according to local guidelines but should be checked at least once for a child during the toddler years. A urinalysis should also be recorded at least once in all children at the time of entry into kindergarten and once during adolescence.

For infants with a history of prenatal drug exposure or other known risks for maternal STI, at least a rapid plasma reagin, hepatitis C antibody, hepatitis B surface antigen and surface antibody, and HIV test should be performed.

Adolescents who are considered to have at-risk sexual behaviors, patients with signs or symptoms consistent with an STI, and children with a history of sexual abuse that could result in the transmission of infection should be tested for STIs. Often adolescents are able to sign their own consent forms for evaluations and treatment related to STIs; however, local statutes should be consulted.

Imaging Studies

If a child has a history or physical findings concerning for physical abuse, imaging such as a radiographic skeletal survey, computed tomography and magnetic resonance imaging of the head, or radionucleotide bone scan may be indicated. (For more specific recommendations, see Chapter 115.)

Management

Given the breadth of health-related needs for this patient population, and given the frequency with which they change foster homes, **close case management** is an essential component of health care delivery to this population. There should be consistent communication with the child's caseworker to ensure that medical and mental health recommendations are incorporated into the child's social service plan. Ideally, a child should have a medical home and continuity with a health care provider over time, but changes in home placements often make this difficult. If continuity of care is broken, incorporation of the health care plan into a child's broader social service plan should ensure that medical history and medical and mental health recommendations are not lost. The use of **electronic health records** is a growing practice in many foster care systems and promotes continuity of care.

Children in foster care often need referral to medical subspecialists, dentists, dietitians, speech therapists, occupational therapists, mental health providers, and other service providers. Case management is necessary to track these referrals and to contact the foster family and/or caseworker if an appointment is missed.

Immunizations should be given as appropriate for age, and if immunization records cannot be located, the child should be considered to be unimmunized. In this situation, the options include restarting the vaccination series or checking the antibody titers for selected vaccine antigens (see Chapter 23 for further information). All children should also receive a purified protein derivative to screen for tuberculosis. Anticipatory guidance should be provided to the foster parent, and age-appropriate issues should be discussed with older children and adolescents.

Prognosis

The population of children in foster care has a spectrum of mental health and medical needs, spanning from the needs of a newborn to those of an adolescent emancipating from the child welfare system. Preliminary studies have documented improved physical health status, improved school performance, and improved adaptive functioning of young children after placement in foster care; however, these studies require replication. The strength of the bond between the foster parent and the child, as well as the consistency and predictability of the foster home environment, are significant to the development of that child's sense of safety and well-being.

To date, much of the research on the health status of children in foster care has focused on the delineation and description of the health-related issues that these children face. There has been more limited evaluation of the different models of health service delivery to the foster care population, as well as of the subsequent medical, developmental, and emotional outcomes for the children in these different models.

While there is a need for continued study of health care delivery to the foster care population, it is widely accepted that children in the foster care system benefit from the establishment of medical homes with case management capabilities and providers who are well-versed in the complex medical and mental health issues that affect this vulnerable population.

CASE RESOLUTION

This case illustrates many of the common issues that affect children when they are placed in foster care. Medical and immunization records are frequently unavailable to the medical examiner, and chronic medical needs have often gone unmet. This child exhibits behaviors that are concerning for a history of prior physical abuse, her prior lack of personal hygiene points to a history of parental neglect, and given the presence of drug paraphernalia, her parents are likely involved with substance abuse. The presence of a thin upper lip and flat philtrum on examination may be markers for prenatal alcohol exposure, and based on that suspicion, this child should have a thorough assessment for behavioral problems, developmental delays, and education-related disabilities. The child is able to clearly state that she does not want to return to her parents' care, but she still misses her family members. This may be remedied through her child welfare plan, by arranging for her to remain in contact with her siblings throughout their foster placement. Given her experiences in her prior home environment, she is likely to have multiple emotional needs that will require mental health services. She will also require evaluation by her new school system to determine her specific educational needs and appropriate grade placement.

Her growth parameters are appropriate for age, but poor dentition is a common finding in the foster care population and requires referral for dental care. The presence of mild wheezing in a child who otherwise states that she feels fine is a likely marker for untreated reactive airway disease, and may be a reflection of poor continuity of medical care for the girl prior to her placement.

Selected References

American Academy of Pediatrics Committee on Early Childhood, Adoption, and Dependent Care. Developmental issues for young children in foster care. *Pediatrics.* 2000;106:1145–1150

American Academy of Pediatrics Committee on Early Childhood, Adoption, and Dependent Care. Health care of young children in foster care. *Pediatrics.* 2002;109:536–541

American Academy of Pediatrics Committee on Practice and Ambulatory Medicine. Recommendations for preventative health care. *Pediatrics.* 2000;105:645–646

American Academy of Pediatrics Task Force on Health Care for Children in Foster Care, American Academy of Pediatrics District II. *Fostering Health: Health Care for Children in Foster Care.* 2nd ed. Elk Grove Village, IL: American Academy of Pediatrics; 2005

Jee SH, Simms MD. Health and well-being of children in foster care placement. *Pediatr Rev.* 2006;27:34–36

Horowitz SM, Owens P, Simms MD. Specialized assessments for children in foster care. *Pediatrics.* 2000;106:59–66

Racusin R, Maerlender AC Jr, Senqupta A, Isquith PK, Straus MB. Psychosocial treatment of children in foster care: a review. *Community Ment Health J.* 2005;41:199–221

Simms MD. Foster children and the foster care system, part I: history and legal structure. *Curr Probl Pediatr.* 1991;21:297–321

Simms MD, Dubowitz H, Szilagyi MA. Health care needs of children in the foster care system. *Pediatrics.* 2000;106:909–918

Takayama JI, Wolfe E, Coulter KP. Relationship between reason for placement and medical findings among children in foster care. *Pediatrics.* 1998;101:201–207

Well-Child Care for Children With Trisomy 21

Derek Wong, MD

CASE STUDY

A 6-month-old girl with trisomy 21 whom you have known since birth is brought to your office for well-child care. She and her parents have been doing well, although she has had several episodes of upper respiratory infections. Her medical history is significant for a small ventricular septal defect, which has since closed spontaneously, and one episode of otitis media at 5 months of age. Her weight gain has been good—along the 25th percentile on the trisomy 21 growth chart. She now sleeps through the night and has a bowel movement once a day. She has received all of the recommended immunizations for her age without any problems.

The infant smiles appropriately, grasps and shakes hand toys, and has some head control, but is unable to roll from supine to prone position. Since she was 1 month old, she has been enrolled in an early intervention program. An occupational therapist visits her at home twice a month.

On physical examination, she has typical facial features consistent with trisomy 21, a single palmar crease on each hand, and mild diffuse hypotonia. Her eyes have symmetrical movement, and her tympanic membranes are clear. She has no cardiac murmurs.

Questions

1. What is the prevalence of trisomy 21 (Down syndrome) in the general population? What is the association of maternal age with trisomy 21?
2. What are the clinical manifestations of this syndrome?
3. What medical conditions are associated with trisomy 21 in the newborn period, during childhood, and in adolescence? When should screening tests for these conditions be performed?
4. What is the role of early intervention services for these patients and their families?
5. What specific psychosocial issues should be included in your anticipatory guidance and health education?
6. What is the prognosis for children with trisomy 21?

Trisomy 21, or Down syndrome, is the most commonly known genetic cause of mental retardation in children. The primary care provider is in a unique position to offer affected children routine health care maintenance and anticipatory guidance, follow-up of intercurrent illness and chronic problems, and information on the latest recommendations for screening for conditions associated with trisomy 21. In addition, the general pediatrician has the opportunity to develop rapport with children and families that is particularly important when considering the complex medical and social implications of raising these children. An important goal of the well-child visit is to provide children with trisomy 21 and their families with counseling about educational, social, and financial resources and support to ensure a healthy and productive transition into adulthood.

Epidemiology

The prevalence of trisomy 21 is approximately 1 in 800 to 1,000 live births. It is estimated that trisomy 21 is responsible for up to one-third of all cases of moderate to severe mental retardation. Trisomy 21 has a male to female ratio of 1.3:1.

Ninety-five percent of all cases of Down syndrome are caused by chromosomal nondisjunction, and most of these events occur in the mother. The chance of nondisjunction is determined by maternal age. A 25-year-old woman has a 1 in 1,240 risk of having a live baby with Down syndrome, and the risk increases to 1 in 340 at age 35 and 1 in 98 at age 40. It is estimated that approximately one-half of trisomy 21 embryos abort spontaneously. The risk of recurrence of nondisjunction Down syndrome in subsequent pregnancies is 1 in 100 until age 35, after which the risk determined by age takes precedence. Other family members are generally not at increased risk of bearing children with this type of Down syndrome.

Approximately 3% to 4% of Down syndrome cases are caused by Robertsonian translocations with another acrocentric chromosome (14/21, 15/21, or 21/21). Parental karyotypes should be obtained because balanced translocation carriers have an increased risk of Down syndrome in future children. Approximately 1% to 2% of Down syndrome cases are mosaic. These children are often less severely affected than those with "full" Down syndrome. A small percentage of affected children have a chromosomal rearrangement resulting in 3 copies of a portion of chromosome 21.

Recent advances in first and second trimester screening allow prenatal diagnosis of Down syndrome with a sensitivity of 80% to 90%. If a prenatal diagnosis of Down syndrome is made, and the general pediatrician is asked to participate in counseling the family, the points listed in Box 27-1 should be covered.

Dx   Trisomy 21

- Microcephaly, with flattening of both occiput and face
- Upward slant to the eyes with epicanthal folds
- Brushfield spots in eyes
- Small ears and mouth (therefore, tongue appears large)
- Low-set ears
- Flat nasal bridge
- Broad, stocky neck, with loose skin folds at the nape
- Funnel-shaped or pigeon-breasted chest
- Small, stubby feet, hands, and digits, with brachyclinodactyly of the fifth digits
- Single transverse palmar crease on each hand
- Wide space between first and second toes
- Fair, mottled skin in newborns; dry skin in older children
- Hypotonia

Box 27-1. Counseling the Family After a Prenatal Diagnosis of Down Syndrome

- Review the data that established the diagnosis in the fetus.
- Explain the mechanism of occurrence and risks for recurrence.
- Review the manifestations of trisomy 21, commonly associated conditions, and the variable prognosis based on the presence of these conditions.
- Discuss other modalities that confirm the presence of associated anomalies such as a fetal echocardiogram in the case of congenital heart disease.
- Explore treatment options and interventions for associated conditions.
- Offer resources to assist the family with decisions related to completing or terminating the pregnancy.
- Refer the family to a clinical geneticist or genetics counselor.

Clinical Presentation

Infants and children with trisomy 21 have a characteristic appearance (Dx Box). They may be microcephalic, with flattening of both the occiput and face. The eyes have an upward slant, with prominent epicanthal folds, the ears are low set and small, the nasal bridge is flattened, and the tongue appears large. The feet, hands, and digits are small and stubby, and the fifth digit is slightly turned in (clinodactyly). A single palmar crease and a wide spacing between the first and second toes may be evident. After the newborn period, diffuse hypotonia and developmental delay are universally seen.

Pathophysiology

Approximately 95% of cases of Down syndrome are caused by trisomy 21 resulting from meiotic nondisjunction. The remaining cases are translocations (3%–4%) and mosaics (1%–2%). The translocations are unbalanced and usually occur with another acrocentric chromosome, usually 14/21 or 15/21. Approximately 75% of these are new mutations, and 25% are the result of a familial translocation. Therefore, if a child has a translocation, the parents must be evaluated

for a balanced translocation. Mosaicism implies the presence of 2 cell lines: one normal and one with trisomy 21. As might be expected, children with mosaic Down syndrome are usually affected less severely than children with other types of Down syndrome.

Evaluation

Routine health care maintenance for infants, children, or adolescents with trisomy 21 should cover the same issues in health education, prevention, and counseling that are discussed with other healthy patients and their families. The schedule of health maintenance visits for infants and young children with trisomy 21 is essentially the same as that recommended by the American Academy of Pediatrics for other children, while older children with Down syndrome should be evaluated annually. The following sections will emphasize additional medical and psychosocial conditions often seen in patients with trisomy 21.

Newborn Period

Verification of the diagnosis of trisomy 21 is perhaps the single most important focus of the initial family visit. Sometimes the diagnosis has been suspected prenatally due to abnormal biochemical markers and ultrasound, and verified by chorionic villus sampling or amniocentesis (see Box 27-1). If there is no prenatal testing and the diagnosis is suspected due to clinical findings, a karyotype must be sent from the nursery and reviewed at the 1- to 2-week visit.

Several conditions that are associated with trisomy 21 are important to identify in the newborn period. They include hearing loss, congenital heart disease (most commonly endocardial cushion defect), duodenal atresia, Hirschsprung disease, congenital hypothyroidism, and ocular anomalies (cataracts, strabismus, and nystagmus). Hematologic abnormalities include polycythemia, leukemoid reactions that resemble leukemia but resolve during the first month of life and, rarely, leukemia.

History

A feeding history is critical because hypotonia often leads to swallowing difficulties (Table 27-1). A history of vomiting may be indicative of gastroesophageal reflux, or less commonly a gastrointestinal malformation. Constipation may be the first indication of Hirschsprung disease or hypothyroidism. A detailed family and social history should also be obtained if this was not done in the hospital.

Physical Examination

A detailed physical examination should reveal some common features of newborns with Down syndrome (see Dx box). All growth parameters should be recorded and compared with those obtained at birth. The size of the fontanelles should be evaluated because of the increased incidence of congenital hypothyroidism. Bilateral red reflexes and conjugate gaze should be documented to exclude congenital cataracts or strabismus. A careful cardiac examination must be performed, noting any cyanosis, murmurs, irregular heart rates, abnormal heart sounds, or asymmetry of pulses. The abdomen should be palpated for organomegaly or any masses, and patency of the anus should be verified. An Ortolani and Barlow test should also be performed for hip laxity. Finally, the infant should be evaluated for hypotonia.

Laboratory Tests

A karyotype is an important tool to verify the diagnosis and to assess recurrence risk. Newborn screening laboratory tests must be reviewed, especially hearing evaluations and thyroid screens. In addition, a cardiac evaluation for congenital heart disease should be performed, which may include an electrocardiogram, chest x-ray, echocardiogram, and formal cardiology referral. A complete blood count is indicated to look for hematologic abnormalities including leukemoid reaction, transient myeloproliferative disorder (pancytopenia, hepatosplenomegaly, and immature white blood cells), and neonatal thrombocytopenia.

Management

The primary care physician should discuss the increased propensity for respiratory infections in children with Down syndrome. Other important issues to address include those pertaining to available resources for children and families such as early intervention programs and Down syndrome support groups in the community. Educational materials such as pamphlets and books may also be supplied at this time. Upcoming appointments with other physicians and allied health professionals should be reviewed.

Infancy and Early Childhood

History

Some additional historical issues to address include a detailed developmental assessment focusing on progress made since the last visit because most affected children have motor and speech delays (see Table 27-1). It is important to review any ancillary services such as physical, occupational, and speech therapy in anticipation of school entry. The parents should provide their assessment of the child's vision and hearing. A history of recurrent respiratory infections should raise concern about otitis media. Many children at this age develop constipation. A history of snoring and restless sleep may indicate obstructive sleep apnea and require a sleep study. Finally, it is extremely important to document any history of neck pain, gait changes, increased clumsiness, or other neurologic symptoms that would indicate spinal cord compression from atlantoaxial dislocation.

Physical Examination

All growth parameters should be plotted on growth charts for children with Down syndrome (Figures 27-1 through 27-4). Children with trisomy 21 are shorter than other children and may have poor weight gain in their first year. Later in life, obesity unrelated to the syndrome may become a problem, however. As with routine well-child visits in other infants and children, a complete physical examination

Table 27-1. Health Supervision for Children With Down Syndrome		
	Initial Evaluation	*Subsequent Evaluations*
History and Physical		
Developmental assessment	Newborn	Same as regular well-child care schedule until age 5, then annual evaluation
Visual and hearing assessment (subjective)		
Laboratory Assessment		
Karyotype	Newborn	None
Thyroid screen	Newborn screen	6 months, 12 months, then annually
Complete blood count	Newborn	Same schedule as other children
Celiac screen	2–3 years	Every 5 years[a]
Echocardiogram	Newborn	Depends on condition
Neck radiographs	Age 3–5 years	Sports activities or Special Olympics entry[a]
Audiological evaluation	Newborn	12 months, then annually (if no ear, nose, throat problems)
Consultation		
Genetics	Newborn	As needed[b]
Cardiology	Newborn	Depends on condition
Ophthalmology	6 months	Every 2 years until age 5, then annually
Ear-nose-throat	As needed	As needed
Dental	By 3 years of age	Twice per year

[a]Lack of expert consensus on evaluation.
[b]Depending on experience and comfort level of primary care physician.

Figure 27-1.   Growth chart for boys with Down syndrome: 1–36 months. (Reproduced with permission from Cronk C, Crocker AC, Pueschel SM, et al. Growth charts for children with Down syndrome: 1 month to 18 years of age. *Pediatrics.* 1988;81:102–110.)

Figure 27-2.   Growth chart for boys with Down syndrome: 2–18 years. (Reproduced with permission from Cronk C, Crocker AC, Pueschel SM, et al. Growth charts for children with Down syndrome: 1 month to 18 years of age. *Pediatrics.* 1988;81:102–110.)

Figure 27-3.   Growth chart for girls with Down syndrome: 1–36 months. (Reproduced with permission from Cronk C, Crocker AC, Pueschel SM, et al. Growth charts for children with Down syndrome: 1 month to 18 years of age. *Pediatrics.* 1988;81:102–110.)

Figure 27-4.   Growth chart for girls with Down syndrome: 2–18 years. (Reproduced with permission from Cronk C, Crocker AC, Pueschel SM, et al. Growth charts for children with Down syndrome: 1 month to 18 years of age. *Pediatrics.* 1988;81:102–110.)

should be performed at each patient encounter. Noteworthy aspects of the examination in infants and children with trisomy 21 are given in Box 27-2. In particular, the ear canals of these children are easily collapsed, making the tympanic membrane difficult to visualize. In some cases, an otolaryngology referral may be necessary for an adequate otoscopic examination. A complete neurologic examination should be performed at each visit, including an assessment of the degree of hypotonia.

Box 27-2. Physical Examination of Children With Trisomy 21

- Look for dry, sensitive skin and alopecia, which develops in approximately 10% of children and resolves spontaneously.
- Monitor the size of the anterior and posterior fontanelles because delayed closure may indicate hypothyroidism.
- Check for visual abnormalities, such as strabismus, nystagmus, cataracts, refractive errors, and blepharitis.
- Document recurrent serous otitis media. It is estimated that 40% to 60% of children with trisomy 21 have significant conductive hearing loss and 20% to 30% have some degree of neurosensory loss.
- Examine the oropharynx carefully for delayed dentition, malocclusion, and caries.
- Perform a thorough cardiac examination and note any evidence of previously unrecognized congenital heart disease.
- Palpate the abdomen for distention or organomegaly. Children with trisomy 21 have a slightly increased risk of developing acute non-lymphoblastic or acute lymphoblastic leukemia.
- Perform a rectal examination in infants or children with a history of constipation.
- Evaluate any musculoskeletal abnormalities such as overall hypotonia and joint laxity (most commonly in the knees and hips) that might contribute to overall gross motor delay.

Laboratory Tests

Hearing evaluation should be performed annually, starting with the newborn hearing screen. Developmentally appropriate gross visual screening should be performed in infants between 6 and 12 months of age at each visit, and a formal ophthalmology examination is recommended at 6 months and every 2 years thereafter. Thyroid screening tests should be repeated at 6 and 12 months and then annually.

Children with congenital heart disease should be given antibiotic endocarditis prophylaxis for dental or other procedures. In addition, these children should be considered for monoclonal antibody therapy against respiratory syncytial virus in the winter.

Children with Down syndrome have an increased risk for autoimmune disorders such as celiac disease, Grave disease, and type 1 diabetes. Because the signs of celiac disease may be subtle, most pediatric gastroenterologists recommend measuring tissue transglutaminase immunoglobulin (Ig) A antibodies, as well as an IgA level, at 2 to 3 years of age. Rescreening for celiac disease is currently a topic of debate, but several experts suggest that retesting approximately every 5 years during childhood may be appropriate.

Children with Down syndrome have an increased incidence of atlantoaxial instability when screened with routine lateral cervical radiographs with flexion and extension views. Any patient with signs or symptoms of cord compression should be evaluated by computed tomography or magnetic resonance imaging and referred to an orthopedic surgeon or neurosurgeon. Symptomatic children should be kept out of any sports that involve contact or neck extension, such as swimming, gymnastics, and soccer. Experts have debated the value of routine x-rays, and most agree that careful neurologic screening at health supervision visits is a much better predictor of serious injury. However, at this time routine x-rays are still recommended at age 3 to 5 years and are required prior to participation in events such as the Special Olympics.

Management

Infants with trisomy 21 should have all routine screening tests and immunizations. Growth and developmental progress should be reviewed with parents at the end of each visit, and any concerns or unmet expectations should be addressed at this time. Often the developmental delay associated with trisomy 21 is not apparent to families until infants are 4 to 6 months of age and not achieving the expected milestones of rolling over or sitting. It should also be emphasized to families that the degree of mental retardation in trisomy 21 is quite variable, ranging from mild to severe. However, social function is not necessarily related to IQ. If the child is not already enrolled in an early intervention program, the positive role of such an experience should be addressed. The availability of support groups for parents and other family members should also be discussed.

In the early childhood years, plans for preschool attendance and future educational opportunities should be reviewed with families. The role of discipline and the presence of common behavioral problems such as temper tantrums and biting should be assessed in preparation for school entry and socialization. Nutrition should be reviewed because children with Down syndrome have a reduced metabolic rate and are at increased risk for obesity.

A dental referral should be made by the age of 1 year in accordance with the latest recommendation for all children.

Older Childhood and Adolescence

History

School-aged children with Down syndrome should continue to visit their primary care physician at least annually. Educational issues should be discussed, including individual education plans and the transition from school. Specific medical issues to address during the history include visual or hearing deficits, evidence for hypothyroidism (decreased activity, coarse and dry hair, and constipation), skin problems including eczema, and dental problems. A careful nutritional history should also be taken because of the propensity for obesity, and the children should be closely monitored for signs of obstructive sleep apnea.

Physical Examination

Height and weight should continue to be plotted. The skin should be examined closely for xerosis, acne, or syringomas (multiple papules often present on the eyelids and upper cheeks) during adolescence. A cardiac examination is important because of an increased risk of mitral valve prolapse and valvular dysfunction. The sexual maturity rating (Tanner stage) of both males and females should be noted and discussed with the parents. A pelvic examination is not indicated as a part of the routine visit unless there is concern about sexual abuse or a sexually transmitted infection, but a testicular examination is important due to the increased risk of testicular cancer. A complete neurologic examination should also be performed in the patient participating in sports activities to look for signs indicating impending atlantoaxial dislocation.

Laboratory Tests

Annual thyroid screening (thyroid-stimulating hormone, thyroxine) is recommended for all school-aged children and adolescents with trisomy 21, in addition to other routine screening tests. An audiological evaluation should also occur at least once in older children and then annually thereafter. Because of the risk of keratoconus, an annual ophthalmology consultation should be arranged after the age of 10 years. In addition, children with trisomy 21 should be encouraged to continue biannual dental visits because gingivitis, periodontal disease, and bruxism (teeth grinding) are common in these individuals.

Management

The major part of the visit with school-aged and adolescent children should be spent on developmental, educational, and vocational anticipatory guidance. Educational placement and future goals should be both developmentally appropriate for the child and acceptable for the parent. Activities requiring socialization and the development of responsibility should continue to be encouraged; however, these events can be very stressful for parents and other family members. Injury prevention should be highlighted as well, especially because older children are becoming more independent. In early adolescence, prevocational and vocational training within the school curriculum should be reviewed. In addition, brief discussions regarding independent living, group homes, and financial resources (eg, community-supported employment for young adults) should begin during adolescence.

Puberty, fertility, and contraception are extremely important to address with adolescents and their parents. The patient's psychosocial development and physical sexual maturation should be discussed, including menstrual hygiene and any foreseeable problems with its management. Contraception and the potential for victimization must be addressed as well, particularly with female patients. Males with trisomy 21 are usually sterile, but females have an approximately 50% chance of having children with Down syndrome.

Prognosis

Individuals with trisomy 21 can often live well past the age of 50 unless they are born with a congenital heart lesion, which may limit life expectancy. One major cause of morbidity and mortality is the development of symptomatic Alzheimer disease, which occurs in approximately 15% of adults after the fourth decade. Fortunately, most adults with Down syndrome remain asymptomatic, despite histopathologic evidence of the disease.

CASE RESOLUTION

In the case described at the beginning of the chapter, the family should be encouraged by the healthy progress of their daughter. For this visit, anticipatory guidance should consist of a review of early intervention services, available resources, and general support services for the patient and her family. The increased risk for both upper respiratory infections and otitis media should be reviewed. Medical screening should include thyroid screening, subjective hearing screening, and a formal evaluation by a pediatric ophthalmologist. If the results are normal, the next visit should take place in 3 months.

Selected References

American Academy of Pediatrics Committee on Genetics. Health supervision for children with Down syndrome. *Pediatrics.* 2001;107:442–449

Braganza SF. Atlantoaxial dislocation. *Pediatr Rev.* 2003;24:106–107

Cassidy SB, Allanson JE, eds. *Management of Genetic Syndromes.* 2nd ed. New York, NY: Wiley-Liss; 2004

Cohen WI. Current dilemmas in Down syndrome clinical care: celiac disease, thyroid disorders, and atlanto-axial instability. *Am J Med Genet C Semin Med Genet.* 2006;142:141–148

Cohen WI, Nadel L, Madnick M, eds. *Down Syndrome: Visions for the 21st Century.* New York, NY: Wiley-Liss; 2002

Van Cleve SN, Cohen WI. Part I: clinical practice guidelines for children with Down syndrome from birth to 12 years. *J Pediatr Health Care.* 2006;20:47–54

Van Cleve SN, Cannon S, Cohen WI. Part II: clinical practice guidelines for adolescents and young adults with Down syndrome: 12 to 21 years. *J Pediatr Health Care.* 2006;20:198–205

Venail F, Gardiner Q, Mondain M. ENT and speech disorders in children with Down's syndrome: an overview of pathophysiology, clinical features, treatments, and current management. *Clin Pediatr (Phila).* 2004;43:783–791

Well-Child Care for Preterm Infants

Lynne M. Smith, MD

CASE STUDY

A 2½-month-old infant girl was discharged from the neonatal intensive care unit 2 weeks ago, where she had been since birth. She was the 780-g product of a 26-week gestation born via spontaneous vaginal delivery to a 32-year-old primigravida. The perinatal course was complicated by premature rupture of membranes and maternal amnionitis. Several aspects of the neonatal course were significant, including respiratory distress that required surfactant therapy and 2 weeks of endotracheal intubation; a grade II intraventricular hemorrhage on head ultrasound at 1 week of life; hyperbilirubinemia, which was treated with phototherapy; several episodes of apnea, presumably associated with the prematurity; and a history of poor oral intake with slow weight gain.

The infant's parents have a few questions about her feeding schedule and discontinuing the apnea monitor, but they feel relatively comfortable caring for their daughter at home. She is feeding well (2 oz of 22 cal/oz post-discharge formula for premature newborns every 2–3 hours)

and is becoming progressively more alert according to the family. She sleeps on her back in a crib.

The infant's weight gain has averaged 25 g/d. The rest of the physical examination is normal, except for dolichocephaly and a left esotropia.

Questions

1. What constitutes well-child care in preterm infants?
2. What are the nutritional requirements of preterm infants in the months following discharge from the hospital?
3. What information must be considered in the developmental screening of preterm infants?
4. What immunization schedule is appropriate for preterm infants? Do they require any special immunizations?
5. What specific conditions or illnesses are more likely to affect preterm infants than term infants?

Premature infants are born at less than 37 completed weeks' gestation and often weigh less than 2,500 g. Providing primary care for these infants is an important and challenging task and often requires coordination of medical, developmental, and social services for multiple chronic conditions. Because preterm infants are at increased risk for both impaired growth and developmental delay, longer visits may be necessary to evaluate the infants' nutritional and developmental progress and to assess how families have adjusted to caring for them at home. Primary care physicians must learn to manage these and many other complex issues while providing families with comprehensive anticipatory guidance.

Though most preterm newborns are delivered between 34 and 36 weeks' gestation, these neonates are at increased risk for morbidity and mortality relative to infants born at term. In addition, many neonatologists routinely resuscitate neonates born at 23 weeks' gestation, a gestation that has a survival rate of approximately 25%. Given that very low birth weight (VLBW, <1,500 g) and extremely low birth weight (ELBW, <1,000 g) newborns are at risk for cerebral palsy, hearing and vision problems, and mental retardation, the post-hospital care for these children is complex for the primary care pediatrician. The Institute of Medicine estimates the annual societal cost of prematurity is $26 billion.

Epidemiology

In the United States, 1 in 8 newborns is born prematurely, a 30% increase since 1981. The preterm delivery rate is highest for African American women (17.8%) and lowest for white (11.5%) and Asian and Pacific Islander (10.5%) women. Reasons for the increased premature delivery rates include an increased use of artificial reproductive technologies (see Chapter 12) and increased maternal age.

Evaluation

The purpose of the health maintenance visit for preterm infants is the same as for other healthy children: to provide consistent preventive health care and education for patients and their parents. Prematurity, however, places children at risk for additional medical and neurodevelopmental conditions.

History

At the initial visit, it is imperative to review the entire medical history and hospital course with the family. Ideally, the neonatal intensive care unit (NICU) should provide a discharge summary that includes the following information:

1. Birth weight and significant prenatal and perinatal information
2. An overview of the hospital course, including significant illnesses, events, surgical procedures, and pertinent radiographic studies
3. Nutrition information and present feeding regimen
4. A list of current medications, including dosing intervals and, if appropriate, serum drug levels
5. Immunizations given during the hospitalization
6. Pertinent laboratory data, such as most recent hemoglobin, newborn screening results, ophthalmologic and hearing screening information, neurosonogram results, and highest serum bilirubin level
7. Discharge physical examination including most recent height, weight, and head circumference
8. Problems remaining at discharge
9. Follow-up appointments

Any significant complications or concerns should be discussed with the parents as soon as possible to assess their understanding of these issues as well as expectations for improvement.

Specifically, growth, nutrition, and developmental issues should be addressed at each visit (Questions Box). Adequate or desirable weight gain should be explained to the caregivers in terms of the infant's current weight versus the discharge weight. Infants younger than 6 months should gain, on average, 20 to 40 g/d. To ensure continued weight gain, many preterm infants are discharged from the NICU on a 24-hour feeding schedule, which requires that parents feed infants at least every 3 hours. The necessity for this practice should be reevaluated during the first few weeks following discharge after infants have demonstrated adequate weight gain.

A critical component of the health maintenance visit is the developmental history. Parental expectations and observations should be noted, and any developmental concerns should be evaluated. The adjusted developmental age should be calculated by subtracting the number of weeks the infant was born prematurely from the current chronological age in weeks. The adjusted age should then be used for all formal and informal developmental assessments. The importance of correcting for prematurity until children are approximately 2½ years of age must be emphasized when discussing developmental progress and giving anticipatory guidance to parents.

Physical Examination

A complete physical examination should be performed at each visit to monitor the status of associated medical conditions. All growth parameters (weight, height, and head circumference) should be plotted on the growth chart for premature newborns until approximately 50 weeks' postmenstrual age and adjusted for

> ### Questions
>
> **Well-Child Care for Preterm Infants**
>
> - How much did the infant weigh when discharged from the hospital?
> - Is the infant breastfed or formula-fed? Is the infant on any special formula?
> - How often and how much does the infant feed? How long do feedings take?
> - Does the infant have any feeding problems (eg, pain, vomiting, gastroesophageal reflux)?
> - Does the infant take dietary supplementation of vitamins and minerals?
> - What developmental milestones has the infant reached? Does the infant roll over? Smile? Sit up?
> - Does the infant seem to hear and see?
> - Who cares for the infant?
> - Where and in what position does the child sleep?
> - Do the parents have any concerns regarding growth, development, or nutrition?
> - Is the infant on an apnea monitor? Have there been any apneic episodes?

prematurity on standard growth charts until age 2. Because catch-up head growth generally precedes catch-up weight and length, preterm infants may appear to have disproportionally large heads. The onset of accelerated head growth may begin within a few weeks after birth (36 weeks' postconception) or as late as 8 months adjusted age. Average daily weight gain in grams per day should also be calculated.

The size and shape of the head must be evaluated, especially if the infant has a history of intraventricular or intracranial hemorrhage or hydrocephalus. An increase in head circumference of more than 2 cm per week should be cause for concern in these infants. In infants who have been treated neurosurgically for hydrocephalus, ventriculoperitoneal shunt and tubing may be palpated. Visual abnormalities such as strabismus must be carefully ruled out by examination as well as by history because up to 20% of preterm infants may have an ophthalmologic problem (see Chapter 64). Oropharyngeal abnormalities such as a palatal groove, high-arched palate, or abnormal tooth formation may occur as a result of prolonged endotracheal intubation. Baseline intercostal, substernal, or subcostal retractions; wheezing; stridor; and tachypnea in former premature babies with moderate-to-severe bronchopulmonary dysplasia (BPD) should be documented.

Chest scars secondary to the placement of chest tubes should be noted. Adult female breasts may be affected if scarring occurs on or close to breast tissue. The umbilicus may appear hypoplastic as a result of umbilical catheter placement and suturing. Multiple scars on the heels from blood sampling or on the distal extremities from intravenous catheters and cutdowns may be evident.

The genitalia of both male and female preterm infants should be examined closely for inguinal hernias. The incidence of inguinal hernias in preterm newborns is 26% in males and 7% in females. If hernias are surgically repaired under general anesthesia, infants should be monitored for apnea for up to 24 hours postoperatively. The male scrotum should be examined for cryptorchidism because only 25% of testes are in the scrotum of prematurely delivered males at term gestation. By 1 year of age, more than 90% of testes are intrascrotal. A careful evaluation for developmental dysplasia of the hip should be performed until children are ambulatory (see Chapter 88).

A thorough neuromuscular examination is essential in these children. Increased muscular tone, asymmetry, and decreased bulk should be noted along with the presence of any clonus or asymmetry of deep tendon reflexes. Inappropriate reflexes such as a persistent Moro or fisting beyond 4 months of age should also be documented. Other abnormalities (eg, scissoring or sustained clonus) in the neurologic examination may become more apparent as infants become older. The detection of subtle early findings is important so appropriate intervention services can begin as soon as possible.

Laboratory Tests

In addition to the standard screening tests performed on all healthy infants and children during health maintenance visits, several laboratory studies are important in preterm infants. Such tests include a complete blood count and reticulocyte count to check for anemia; electrolytes in infants with BPD on diuretics to detect electrolyte abnormalities; and serum calcium, phosphorus, and alkaline phosphatase levels in infants with documented rickets.

Pulse oximetry is indicated for oxygen-dependent infants as well as those presenting with respiratory symptoms greater than baseline. Results from newborn screening tests including auditory and ophthalmologic examinations should be reviewed and repeated as indicated. Cranial ultrasound studies should be reviewed with caution because nearly 30% of infants born weighing less than 1,000 g with normal head ultrasound findings develop cerebral palsy or developmental delay. In addition, infants with a grade I or II intracranial hemorrhage have an increased risk for developmental delay. Brain magnetic resonance imaging scans should be considered in infants with a concerning abnormal neurologic examination or an abnormal rate of head growth.

Management

Well-child care in relatively healthy preterm infants has 2 components. One is the provision of routine health care maintenance for infants and appropriate developmental anticipatory guidance for parents. The other component involves the incorporation of treatment for chronic conditions into each visit. Health care maintenance should include nutrition counseling, developmental surveillance, immunizations, and assessment of vision and hearing in addition to standard screening tests discussed previously. Outside resources concerning developmental delay can be reviewed with parents (Box 28-1). Care related to chronic conditions includes adjusting medication doses such as diuretic therapy, weaning from supplemental oxygen, and discontinuing the apnea monitor.

Box 28-1. Physician Support and Education of Parents With Preterm Infants

- Understand parental expectations.
- Legitimize parental fears.
- Be a source of support and encouragement.
- Provide consistent, honest information.
- Assume the role of the overall coordinator of care.
- Provide referrals to outside resources, including respite care.

Parents should be given anticipatory guidance prior to discharge that caring for a NICU graduate is challenging. Premature newborns have poorly organized sleep-wake cycles resulting in more frequent awakening than term newborns. In addition, premature newborns have immature suck-swallow coordination, causing them to feed more frequently and for longer periods. Colic is reported twice as frequently in VLBW infants relative to term newborns, and many are described as having difficult temperament until past their first birthdays.

The medical costs associated with the care of premature newborns often strain the family finances at a time when many women decrease their work schedules. Additional stressors include uncertainty about the long-term outcome of the child, guilt many women feel after delivering prematurely, and anxiety about future pregnancies. The difficulty of caring for these complicated, challenging children results in significant parental stress and can interfere with their ability to properly bond to their newborn.

Nutrition

According to the American Academy of Pediatrics (AAP) Committee on Nutrition, the average daily energy requirement for most hospitalized healthy preterm infants is 105 to 130 kcal/kg/d to achieve adequate growth. Energy requirements vary with individual infants depending on associated chronic conditions such as BPD or malabsorption. Growth is considered adequate in the newborn weighing more than 2,000 g if weight gain is more than 20 g/d and length and head circumference increase 0.7 to 1.0 cm/wk.

At 40 weeks' corrected age, preterm newborns are usually smaller than term newborns. Adequate nutrition in the first year of life is critical because catch-up weight gain is unlikely to occur after age 3. Children born at 32 weeks or less and/or weighing less than 1,500 g are usually discharged home on a nutritionally enhanced post-discharge formula (Similac NeoSure Advance, Enfamil EnfaCare LIPIL). These formulas are 22 cal/oz and have a higher vitamin and mineral content relative to term formulas. Because breast milk is insufficient for providing adequate protein and micronutrients to preterm newborns, human milk fortifier is added to breast milk in the NICU. Human milk fortifier is not covered by insurance in the outpatient setting, so fortifying breast milk is not a practical option for most parents. For ELBW infants receiving breast milk, 2 to 3 feedings of enriched formula may be required the first few weeks after discharge to maintain adequate growth.

Infants continue to receive post-discharge formula until they are approximately 4.5 kg or 9 to 12 months' corrected age. Formula-fed infants require multivitamin supplementation until 750 mL/d of formula is consumed. Breastfed premature newborns may benefit from continuing multivitamin solution as long as breast milk is the predominant source of nutrition. Vitamin D supplementation is recommended for all breastfed infants. Because premature newborns are at increased risk for osteopenia of prematurity, soy formulas are to be avoided because of the low phosphate content.

The introduction of solid foods is appropriate once infants have developed acceptable oral-motor skills for swallowing solids.

Developmental Assessment

Both informal and formal developmental surveillance should include referral to an early intervention program, particularly in ELBW infants because routine screening tests are not sensitive enough to pick up subtle neurodevelopmental abnormalities (Box 28-2; see Chapter 18). Because many developmental issues do not manifest until school age, frequent developmental assessments and enrollment in preschool are especially important for infants born prematurely.

Immunizations

Routine immunization schedules recommended by the AAP Committee on Immunization Practices should be followed. The administration of any vaccine is determined by the chronological or postnatal age, not the gestational age. Standard doses and intervals should also be used (see Chapter 23). Several studies have shown an adequate serologic response despite a history of prematurity. Absolute and relative contraindications to specific vaccine components or to live vaccines for preterm infants are identical to published guidelines for term infants and children. In addition to following the recommendation that all infants 6 to 23 months of age be vaccinated against influenza, all household contacts of premature newborns should also be strongly urged to be vaccinated.

If adequate weight gain has been established, it is safe to administer hepatitis B vaccine to medically stable neonates weighing less than 2,000 g as early as 30 days of age or at discharge, whichever comes first. All neonates born to mothers who are hepatitis B surface antigen (HBsAg) positive should receive hepatitis B vaccine and hepatitis B immune globulin (HBIG) within 12 hours of delivery. When maternal HBsAg status is unknown, neonates weighing less than 2,000 g should receive HBIG within 12 hours, neonates weighing more than 2,000 g should receive HBIG within 7 days, and all should be vaccinated for hepatitis B within 12 hours.

Because respiratory syncytial virus (RSV) causes an increased morbidity and mortality in NICU graduates, the following infants are recommended to receive RSV-specific immunoglobulin every month from October to April: younger than 24 months with chronic lung disease requiring treatment (eg, oxygen, diuretics) within 6 months of the start of RSV season, younger than 24 months with hemodynamically significant congenital heart disease, less than 32 weeks' gestation and younger than 6 months at the start of RSV season, less than 28 weeks' gestation and younger than 12 months, and

born at 32 to 35 weeks' gestation and younger than 6 months with 2 or more risk factors (risk factors: cigarette exposure, attendance at group child care, school-aged siblings, exposure to environmental air pollutants, congenital anomalies of the airways, or severe neuromuscular disease).

Box 28-2. Guidelines for Developmental Surveillance[a]

For pediatricians using developmental screening tests, the yielded score should be used to determine when to refer. For those who choose not to use standardized tests, the following guidelines are suggested. Be concerned if

At 6 months' adjusted age, the infant
- Is not sitting, even with support
- Makes no effort to reach or bat at objects
- Does not localize sound
- Only momentarily grasps
- Keeps hands fisted
- Does not mouth objects

At 12 months' adjusted age, the infant
- Is sitting but not crawling
- Does not search for hidden objects
- Does not vocalize consonant and vowel combinations
- Does not attend to books
- Does not respond to simple, familiar directions such as "pat-a-cake"
- Does not respond to their name

At 18 months' adjusted age, the child
- Does not walk
- Does not imitate sounds or motor actions
- Cannot build a tower with blocks
- Is most interested in putting toys in mouth at play
- Knows fewer than 8 words

At 24 months' adjusted age, the child
- Does not put 2 words together in speech
- Has play skills that remain primarily imitative
- Has gross motor skills that are lacking in balance and control
- Cannot complete a simple puzzle or shape sorter
- Cannot identify basic body parts

At 36 months' chronological age, the child
- Does not follow simple commands, including "give me"
- Does not use prepositions in speech
- Cannot copy a circle
- Has such poor articulation that it is impossible for others to understand
- Does not jump with both feet off the ground

At 4 years, the child
- Still uses phrases instead of sentences
- Does not know color names
- Cannot give first and last name
- Cannot pedal a tricycle

[a]Modified with permission from Bernbaum JC, Hoffman-Williamson M. *Primary Care of the Preterm Infant.* St Louis, MO: Mosby-Year Book; 1991:71.

Assessment of Vision and Hearing

Follow-up visits for visual and auditory sequelae of prematurity must be arranged at the health maintenance visit. An initial ophthalmologic screening examination should have been performed between 5 and 9 weeks of age in infants weighing less than 1,500 g or less than 32 weeks' gestation, irrespective of oxygen exposure. Infants between 1,500 g and 2,000 g or greater than 32 weeks' gestation with an unstable clinical course should also be screened. The frequency and need for repeat examinations are determined based on the initial findings. Preterm infants, regardless of the presence of retinopathy of prematurity, are at increased risk for the development of strabismus, myopia, amblyopia, and glaucoma and need an ophthalmologic examination beginning at 6 months of age.

The AAP recommends universal hearing screening for all newborns. Neonatal intensive care unit graduates account for approximately 50% of all newborn hearing screening failures, and severe sensorineural hearing loss occurs in up to 10% of ELBW infants. Screening is recommended immediately prior to discharge.

Other Possible Problems

Preterm infants with chronic lung disease are at increased risk for respiratory illness, especially during the winter. Parents should be informed of this risk and counseled about symptoms such as tachypnea and wheezing associated with a simple upper respiratory infection. Practitioners should have a low threshold for considering a diagnosis of pneumonia in these infants in the appropriate clinical setting.

Primary care providers should also keep in mind that preterm infants are at increased risk for sudden infant death syndrome (SIDS) (Chapter 47). The AAP recommends that all infants sleep in the supine position. In the NICU, neonates are often placed on their stomachs if they have respiratory difficulties and on their sides if they have symptomatic gastroesophageal reflux. Neonatal intensive care unit personnel need to begin placing these babies on their backs in anticipation of discharge. Parents should also be reminded that co-sleeping is not recommended.

Home apnea monitors are not associated with the prevention of SIDS and should be reserved for infants who are considered to have extreme cardiorespiratory instability. Discontinuation of home monitoring may be considered at 42 weeks' postmenstrual age and when significant apneic events have ceased, whichever comes later.

Preterm survivors who were critically ill can be particularly at risk for developing **vulnerable child syndrome** because their parents often perceive them as fragile and vulnerable. Features of this syndrome include abnormal separation difficulties for both the mother and child, sleep difficulties, parental overprotectiveness and over-indulgence, lack of appropriate discipline, and excessive preoccupation with the infant's health. Serious behavioral problems may arise as a result of such parent-child interactions. Primary care providers must be cognizant of early signs of this syndrome and should try to prevent its occurrence by reassuring parents about the infant's well-being. Every effort should be made to normalize the family's schedule once the infant is stable and to encourage parent-infant interactions unrelated to health care.

Prognosis

Neurodevelopmental impairment is a concern for physicians who care for preterm infants. Risk factors for developmental delay include postnatal steroid exposure, BPD, and small for gestational age. Chorioamnionitis is a risk factor for cerebral palsy in term infants and possibly in infants born prematurely. Extremely low birth weight infants and those born between 20 to 25 weeks' gestation have significant risk for developmental issues. At 18 to 30 months of age, approximately 30% to 50% of infants born from 23 to 25 weeks' gestation or weighing less than 750 g have moderate or severe neurodevelopmental disability. By age 6, 43% of children born at 20 to 25 weeks' gestation have IQs lower than 82.

During adolescence, 50% of former VLBW infants will have an IQ in an abnormally low range, and 30% will have attention-deficit/hyperactivity disorder. Though former premature newborns report more health-related and learning difficulties in adolescence relative to their normal birth weight peers, the VLBW teens rated their quality of life higher than their peers. Parents should also understand that long-term follow-up information may not accurately reflect the outcome for their child because these adolescents were managed prior to advances in prenatal and neonatal care.

CASE RESOLUTION

In the case presented at the beginning of the chapter, the infant's current feeding schedule should be continued because appropriate weight gain has occurred. Iron and multivitamin supplementation is recommended until 750 mL/d of formula is consumed. Discontinuation of the apnea monitor can be considered after the infant reaches term gestation and has been event-free. The first set of immunizations should be administered at this visit, and any questions that the family has should be answered. A follow-up visit should be scheduled in 3 to 4 weeks. Formal developmental testing should be arranged in 1 to 2 months, and the parents should be encouraged to continue having the child sleep on her back.

Selected References

American Academy of Pediatrics. Pickering LK, Baker CJ, Long SS, McMillan JA, eds. *Red Book: 2006 Report of the Committee on Infectious Diseases.* 27th ed. Elk Grove Village, IL: American Academy of Pediatrics; 2006

American Academy of Pediatrics Task Force on Sudden Infant Death Syndrome. The changing concept of sudden infant death syndrome: diagnostic coding shifts, controversies regarding the sleeping environment, and new variables to consider in reducing risk. *Pediatrics.* 2005;116:1245–1255

Bernstein S, Heimler R, Sasidharan P. Approaching the management of the neonatal intensive care unit graduate through history and physical assessment. *Pediatr Clin North Am.* 1998;45:79–105

Carver JD, Wu PY, Hall RT, et al. Growth of preterm infants fed nutrient-enriched or term formula after hospital discharge. *Pediatrics.* 2001;107:683–689

Hack M, Flannery DJ, Schluchter M, Cartar L, Borawski E, Klein N. Outcomes in young adulthood for very-low-birth-weight infants. *N Engl J Med.* 2002;346:149–157

Institute of Medicine. Preterm birth: causes, consequences and prevention. 2006

Kelly MM. Primary care issues for the healthy premature infant. *J Pediatr Health Care.* 2006;20:293–299

Kelly MM. The medically complex premature infant in primary care. *J Pediatr Health Care.* 2006;20:368–373

MacDonald H, American Academy of Pediatrics Committee on Fetus and Newborn. Perinatal care at the threshold of viability. *Pediatrics.* 2002;110:1024–1027

Martin JA, Hamilton BE, Sutton PD, Ventura SJ, Menacker F, Kirmeyer S. Births: final data for 2004. *Natl Vital Stat Rep.* 2006;55:1–3

Trachtenbarg DE, Golemon TB. Care of the premature infant: part I. Monitoring growth and development. *Am Fam Physician.* 1998;57:2123–2130

Trachtenbarg DE, Golemon TB. Office care of the premature infant: part II. Common medical and surgical problems. *Am Fam Physician.* 1998;57:2383–2390, 2400–2402

Verma RP, Sridhar S, Spitzer AR. Continuing care of NICU graduates. *Clin Pediatr (Phila).* 2003;42:299–315

Care of Children With Special Health Care Needs

Julie E. Noble, MD, and Monica Sifuentes, MD

CASE STUDY

A 5-year-old physically disabled girl is brought to your office for her first visit for a routine physical examination for school entrance. The girl was the full-term product of a pregnancy complicated by an elevated screening alpha fetoprotein and a subsequent fetal ultrasound that demonstrated a lumbar myelomeningocele and no hydrocephalus. Delivery was elective cesarean section with Apgar scores of 9 at 1 minute and 9 at 5 minutes, to a 25-year-old gravida I para 0–I female. The mother used no illicit drugs, alcohol, or any other medications during pregnancy, but was not on vitamins or folate supplementation at the time of conception. At delivery, a low lumbar spinal malformation was noted without other malformations. The quadriceps muscles were strong but the feet demonstrated a rocker bottom deformity.

Shortly after birth the myelomeningocele malformation was closed by neurosurgery. She has had orthopedic surgical release of Achilles tendon contractions but is ambulatory with ankle-foot orthotics. She has a neurogenic bladder and requires intermittent catheterization.

She has chronic constipation treated with a bowel regimen. Her cognitive function is age-appropriate.

She will be entering a school program for the first time since moving to this community and has not established care with any specialists.

Questions

1. Why is early identification and intervention important for infants and children with special health care needs (SHCN)?
2. What are the unique needs of infants and children with SHCN?
3. What role do primary care practitioners play in the care of children with SHCN?
4. What are the appropriate referrals and resources for families of children with SHCN?
5. What specific psychosocial issues should be addressed whenever children with SHCN visit their primary care practitioners?

Children with special health care needs (SHCN) have disabilities that are defined as abnormalities in body function or structure that interfere with the activities of normal daily life. These disabilities can include physical, sensory, developmental, behavioral, or emotional conditions. They can range from mild to moderate, depending on the nature and extent of the condition. Frequently the care requirements of both families and medical providers for children diagnosed with a disability are dramatically increased. For parents, the diagnosis of a disability in their child can be overwhelming and disappointing. Support of the parents is essential as they transition from this disappointment to acceptance and facilitator of their child's treatment plans.

Early identification of a disabling condition by physicians can lead to appropriate, definitive treatment for many disabilities. Early intervention can sometimes even prevent secondary conditions, such as early management of hearing loss with hearing aids may minimize speech abnormalities. Even when such treatment is not available, prompt identification improves children's long-term outcome and allows families to obtain appropriate resources for their children. Through early intervention, infants and children with irreversible conditions can be introduced to medical, educational, and psychosocial services available in the community that serve to help each child maximize and reach full potential.

Epidemiology

The prevalence of children in the United States with SHCN is difficult to assess. Studies report that approximately 17% of children younger than 17 years have at least one disability, including deafness or hearing loss, blindness, cerebral palsy, physical malformations, speech impediments, and other learning problems. Comorbid conditions such as epilepsy and secondary conditions such as behavior problems have a very high incidence. An estimated 30% of disabled children have more than one disability. A single sensory disability such as deafness affects approximately 3.5% of children, and blindness occurs in 1% of children. The prevalence of cerebral palsy is 1.5 to 2 per 1,000 live births. Advances in medical technology, improving survival of low birth weight infants and children with malformations, have increased the number of children living with such disabilities.

The presence of any disabling condition has a profound impact on the health and education of affected children. Studies show that children with disabilities have 1.5 times more doctor visits and spend 3.5 more days in the hospital than children without these conditions. Children with disabilities miss twice the number of school days and are twice as likely to repeat a grade compared with children without disabilities.

In addition, numerous associated conditions occur more commonly in children with disabilities. These include mental retardation, growth failure, and nutrition problems. Problems with dentition, respiratory infections, and bowel and bladder continence may also develop. Significant emotional disturbances may occur as the child adapts to his disability.

Clinical Presentation

Children with disabilities can present in a variety of ways depending on their diagnosis. Many physical disabilities may be readily apparent at birth on the newborn examination or through newborn screening. Some diagnoses, such as cerebral palsy, may be detected later, as the motor impairment becomes more evident. Following development at routine health maintenance visits is essential to early detection of developmental delay. Children with disabilities can also present with specific complaints, such as poor vision or hearing, or with more general concerns, such as growth failure (Dx Box). Behavioral problems or difficulties in school may be the reason for the initial visit.

Dx **Children With Physical and Sensory Disabilities**[a]

- Growth failure
- Microcephaly
- Abnormal neurologic examination, including hypertonicity, spastic diplegia or quadriplegia, and brisk deep tendon reflexes
- Developmental delay
- Speech or hearing deficit
- Visual deficit
- Physical malformations

[a]May not be present in all children.

Pathophysiology

The pathophysiology of disabilities is totally dependent on the disabling condition. Conditions may be secondary to an embryological defect such as myelomeningocele or an infection such as congenital cytomegalovirus (CMV), which interferes with cochlear development and leads to hearing loss. Etiologies are often multifactorial. For some conditions, autism being an example, the pathophysiology is unknown.

Disabilities may be classified as acquired or congenital, and static or progressive. **Cerebral palsy,** for example, is a group of nonprogressive neuromotor disorders resulting from a central nervous system insult prenatally or in the first 2 years of life. It is characterized by abnormal motor movements and posturing and may be accompanied by other problems. Causes of cerebral palsy include prematurity, low birth weight, asphyxia, prenatal abnormalities (eg, placental insufficiency), congenital infections (eg, toxoplasmosis, CMV), and biochemical abnormalities (eg, severe hyperbilirubinemia). Other causes are environmental (eg, alcohol [maternal alcoholism]) and genetic (eg, inborn errors of metabolism). Severe postnatal injuries or infections can also lead to cerebral palsy (eg, shaken baby syndrome and meningitis). However, an estimated 25% to 50% of cases of cerebral palsy have no discernible cause.

Differential Diagnosis

The term *special health care needs* is used in a broad sense to include conditions that require additional medical care and supervision. Children may have significant physical, sensory, or developmental disabilities that may result from prematurity, congenital infections such as CMV, or exposure in utero to alcohol or illicit substances. Some children are born with inborn errors of metabolism that mandate special diets and occupational or physical therapy. Other children with SHCN include those with chronic medical conditions such as asthma and sickle cell anemia.

Evaluation

History

When initially evaluating children with newly diagnosed disabilities, practitioners should first determine any specific parental concerns. A complete medical history should then be obtained, including information about the pregnancy and birth. The history should also include any possible exposures as well as significant infections. General screening questions about development are also important to ask (Questions Box) so that the child's developmental progress can be assessed. Specific questioning is warranted if parents are concerned about delayed development or if any of their responses indicate that their children are not attaining age-appropriate developmental milestones.

In cases of children with known sensory or physical disabilities, families should be asked directly at each visit about daily activities and the child's ability for self-help skills. Because many children with disabilities are also on daily medication for either seizures or other chronic conditions, it is also important to ask about the presence of any side effects of drugs.

Behavioral or emotional problems that the child might be having should be identified. In addition, an overall assessment of family dynamics should be made. It is important to inquire about the relationships between children with disabilities and their siblings, as well as the impact these children have on the parents' marriage.

Questions

Children With Special Health Care Needs

- Were there any perinatal complications, such as premature rupture of membranes or fetal distress?
- Was the infant born prematurely? If so, how long did the infant remain in the hospital and for what reasons?
- Was the infant exposed to any toxins (eg, alcohol, illicit drugs) in utero?
- Is there any history of infection during the perinatal period or infancy?
- What developmental milestones has the infant or child mastered?
- Is the child attending school or some type of early intervention program?
- How does the child get there?
- What does the child do on returning from school?
- Who feeds and bathes the child?
- Can the older child use the toilet without assistance?
- How is the child sleeping? Does the child take naps at school and at home?
- Has respite care been arranged for the family?
- Does the caregiver seem overwhelmed or excessively tired, especially one who is caring for a child with multiple disabilities?
- Do other family members help care for the child?
- Is the extended family available to help with the siblings?
- Are there any other disabled people in the family?
- Does the family receive any financial assistance for care of the child?

Physical Examination

In general, a complete physical examination, including a neurologic assessment and neuromotor examination, should be performed at each visit. The height, weight, and head circumference should be plotted on the growth chart and compared with previous measurements. A failure of adequate growth as measured by any of these parameters should be examined closely. For example, microcephaly, nutritional problems, and growth failure are not uncommon in children with cerebral palsy. Depending on the disability, the examination should then focus on physical findings associated with the particular condition. For children with physical disabilities such as congenital or acquired amputations, for instance, assessment of the skin that comes in contact with prosthetic devices is a pertinent aspect of the physical examination. Pressure sores may be found in non-ambulatory children with cerebral palsy. In children with sensory disabilities such as unilateral hearing loss, the evaluation of a middle ear effusion or infection in the unaffected ear should be a priority.

Overall, for most children with disabilities, the neurologic examination is extremely important. The following questions should be addressed: Are normal primitive reflexes such as the Moro and rooting reflexes present in neonates? Have all primitive reflexes been extinguished in older children? Do infants appear to visualize and track objects appropriately? Are there any abnormal movements of the trunk or extremities at rest? Is the muscle tone normal? Is any hypertonicity or hypotonicity evident? Is any asymmetry of the upper and lower extremities apparent? Are the deep tendon reflexes normal and symmetrical? Is the gait appropriate for age?

An age-appropriate developmental assessment is also an essential part of the examination at all health maintenance visits.

Laboratory Tests

The laboratory evaluation of infants or children with physical or sensory disabilities depends on the specific condition. Not all patients need a costly array of diagnostic procedures. A **chromosomal karyotype** using peripheral blood is helpful in children with suspected genetic disorders (eg, abnormal facies or a major anomaly and developmental delay). Routine testing for fragile X syndrome in all mentally retarded boys and in girls with a family history should be strongly considered. Other testing should be specific, relating to the suspected diagnosis (see Chapter 57).

Metabolic screening for inborn errors of metabolism should be performed on children with mental retardation and any of the following symptoms: intermittent vomiting or lethargy, loss of developmental milestones, or seizures. Such screening is not needed in the routine evaluation of children with developmental delay and no other symptoms.

A screening test for visual acuity (Snellen test) and hearing (audiogram) should be performed in all children suspected of having sensory deficits, even mild ones. For infants or toddlers, a brain stem auditory evoked response or behavioral audiogram is a more appropriate screening test for hearing. A visual evoked response can be performed to test vision.

Psychometric testing may be helpful in certain school-aged children to assess intellectual function.

An electroencephalogram is indicated in all patients who have a history of seizures or seizure-like episodes.

Imaging Studies

Brain imaging studies, such as magnetic resonance imaging scans of the head, can be informative when intrauterine infection, intraventricular hemorrhage, or genetic disorders with associated developmental delay and even isolated global developmental delay are suspected. An electromyogram can be used to differentiate cerebral palsy from a congenital myopathy.

Management

Caring for children with either a single disability or multiple disabilities can be both a rewarding and challenging task for primary care pediatricians. Although all cases should be handled individually, general guidelines have been developed for the provision of pediatric services for infants and children with SHCN. They include recommendations for establishing a medical home with the primary care provider, medical services, suggestions for parental involvement, assistance from community agencies, and fulfillment of specific federal requirements for educational opportunities for children with disabilities. Pediatricians who care for children with SHCN should be familiar with the principles of care, published by the American Academy of Pediatrics (AAP), and should incorporate these principles into the overall treatment plan. Pediatricians should also be knowledgeable about the rights of such individuals as established by various legislation, including the Americans with Disabilities Act. Coordination of intervention services and the use of adaptive or assistive technology are essential components of management.

General Considerations

The major role of primary care pediatricians who care for children with disabilities is 4-fold: (1) provide primary medical care, (2) serve as the patient and family advocate in evaluating therapeutic options, (3) inform families of available community resources and, most importantly (4) serve as a proactive coordinator of care. The first task of the pediatrician is to establish the diagnosis and recognize comorbid conditions. Whether the diagnosis is an obvious physical malformation or one that is not readily apparent, physicians are placed in the challenging position of breaking the news to families. Parents should be informed of the diagnosis as soon as possible, but care should be taken to refrain from discussing the prognosis, especially if it is still unknown. The cause of any disability and the possible complications of the condition should be reviewed with the parents. *The primary goal is to help children with disabilities reach their full potential.*

Health care providers are in a unique position to establish a treatment plan with families that includes medical, psychosocial, and educational services. A multidisciplinary team that includes the pediatrician, a member of the school system, a social worker, and a representative of an early intervention program should be identified. Federally funded, nonprofit, regional centers can provide an organized treatment plan and entry into an early intervention program to some children with disabilities. To qualify, children must be diagnosed with certain disorders such as cerebral palsy, epilepsy, autism, or global developmental delay. In addition, infants considered at risk for developing disabilities qualify for assistance (eg, premature infants with bronchopulmonary dysplasia and intraventricular hemorrhage). For children who do not qualify, similar services can be coordinated on an individual basis by the physician's office or the school district.

Children with severe physical and sensory disabilities are often cared for by many medical subspecialists in addition to primary care pediatricians. Referrals to pediatric orthopedic surgeons, plastic surgeons, geneticists, ophthalmologists, otolaryngologists, child neurologists, and psychologists may be necessary. Special comprehensive clinics, such as craniofacial or spina bifida, are established in some children's referral centers to facilitate care of patients, with multiple subspecialists forming a multidisciplinary team in the same clinic setting. In addition, speech and language therapists, occupational therapists, and physical therapists are often an integral part of the medical team. Initial and ongoing therapeutic services provided by each of these individuals must be monitored periodically to assess the progress and overall effectiveness of the treatment plan. Ideally, services should be coordinated so that children as well as

parents miss a minimum number of school days and workdays (eg, Saturday and after-school appointments, visits to several providers on one day). All information from diagnostic studies and initial evaluations should be shared among each of the health care providers. The AAP has published a Care Coordination Toolkit, which can be very helpful to the primary provider.

The family has a vital role in caring for the disabled child, though this can frequently be stressful and emotionally draining. Family support and counseling should be readily available. Sociocultural factors in the family should be addressed.

As the child with a disability matures, the transition into adult services can be challenging. Preparation for this transition should begin as early as 11 years of age to ensure success. The family and child should be evaluated to determine whether the child is capable of independent living, a group home, an institution, or remaining with the family. A successful transition to adult health care providers must be ensured and financial issues such as insurance coverage should be addressed.

Economic Concerns

The cost of care for children with disabilities places a significant financial burden for as many as 40% of these families in the United States. Families with an affected child are more likely to have a single income, have a single parent, live in poverty, and have poor-quality housing. Economic evaluation should be performed by the caseworker to determine the eligibility of individual children for special services such as Supplemental Security Income and Medicaid. The caseworker can then assist families to apply for the appropriate assistance or to other programs such as food stamps and the Low Income Home Energy Assistance Program, which can help extend a families resources.

Specific Medical Conditions

A number of medical conditions commonly occur in children with moderate to severe disabilities. While providing children with comprehensive well-child care, general pediatricians can also address and treat these conditions.

Problems with adequate nutrition, which usually result from insufficient caloric intake, are manifested by growth failure. Depending on the degree of disability and amount of oropharyngeal dysfunction, the placement of a nasogastric or gastrostomy tube may be necessary. Caloric needs are 10% to 50% higher than normal basal needs to ensure growth.

Respiratory illness is not uncommon among these children. Close observation and conservative treatment of viral illnesses are often necessary. Aspiration pneumonia is likely to occur, especially in children with severe developmental delay because of poor handling of oral secretions or severe oral dyspraxia. To help minimize respiratory infections, influenza vaccine should also be administered during the winter months.

Maintaining good oral hygiene is another challenge because some children with disabilities do not clear oral secretions well and retain food in their mouths, predisposing to cavity development. In addition, many children are treated with anticonvulsants and antibiotics that can cause gingival and enamel dysplasias. Abnormal oromotor coordination, tone, and posturing also contribute to the development of oropharyngeal deformities such as high-arched palate and overcrowded teeth. As with other children, fluoride supplementation and consistent preventive dental care are recommended.

Bowel and bladder continence is important to attain for several reasons. It allows children to function in a socially acceptable fashion, provides independence, and prevents the development of complications such as recurrent urinary tract infections, diaper dermatitis, and decubitus pressure sores. Behavior modification techniques coupled with positive reinforcement are associated with complete or partial success for bowel training.

Community Resources

Optimal care for children with developmental disabilities depends on maximum use of community agencies and resources. An assessment of parental and patient needs should first be performed and prioritized. The appropriate resources should then be identified for individual children. Early intervention services should be used. Primary care physicians may need to help determine the appropriateness of specific services for patients and families. Emphasis should be placed on integrating each child into support services. Parent-to-parent support and support groups can be very helpful in relieving stress, helping parents to understand the disability, and avoiding feelings of isolation. Support groups for siblings as well as parents are available. Respite care to give parents a break from caregiving, and in-home health service programs should also be investigated. Physicians should act as liaisons between all agencies. Case conferences are occasionally necessary to review the progress of individual children with each member of the health care team.

Education

By federal law, every child with a disability is entitled to an education. Every effort should be made to enroll children with disabilities in conventional schools and to provide opportunities for socialization at an early age. The concept of structured independence and mainstreaming, the placement of disabled children in classes with nondisabled children, can be a very productive setting for the child and schoolmates.

Mainstreaming may not be available in some areas, and the severity of some disabilities may not allow attendance on a regular school campus. Then several other educational possibilities can be considered, and each case should be evaluated on an individual basis. Options include special education classes in designated schools (full- or part-time), special education classes in regular schools (full- or part-time), part-time special education classes and part-time regular classes, or home education. The decision can be facilitated through the development of an Individualized Education Plan (IEP) by a multidisciplinary team at the school. Parents and primary physicians are encouraged to participate in this evaluation (see Chapter 22).

Prognosis

The prognosis for children with SHCN is dependent on the diagnosis, the severity and extent of any disability, medical and supportive intervention, and the environment of the child. It may be impossible to establish a prognosis at the time of diagnosis. Children can adapt differently to the same disability. It is important to establish realistic goals to determine the best intervention. Most affected children are able to lead productive, independent lives when they receive adequate early intervention and education.

CASE RESOLUTION

Although the girl's medical condition of low lumbar spina bifida seems stable, the physician should inquire about any ongoing problems or concerns. A complete examination should be done. Routine screening laboratory tests and immunizations required for school entry should be performed. The family should be evaluated for financial stability and support services. The mother should be placed on folate supplementation for prevention of recurrence in future children. The patient should be referred to the local spina bifida clinic for comprehensive specialist care by orthopedics, urology, and physical therapy. Integration into the regular classroom should be recommended. The school should be contacted to arrange for adaptive physical education and school nursing intermittent catheterization. A follow-up visit is scheduled with the primary care physician in 2 months to review the child's integration into services.

Selected References

American Academy of Pediatrics Council on Children With Disabilities. Care coordination in the medical home: integrating health and related systems of care for children with special health care needs. *Pediatrics.* 2005;116:1238–1244

American Academy of Pediatrics, American Academy of Family Physicians, American College of Physicians-American Society of Internal Medicine. A consensus statement on health care transitions for young adults with special health care needs. *Pediatrics.* 2002;110:1304–1306

Anderson D, Dumont S, Jacobs P, Azzaria L. The personal costs of caring for a child with a disability: a review of the literature. *Public Health Rep.* 2007;122:3–16

Boyle CA, Decoufle P, Yeargin-Allsopp M. Prevalence and impact of developmental disabilities in US children. *Pediatrics.* 1994;93:399–403

Cooley W, American Academy of Pediatrics Committee on Children With Disabilities. Providing a primary care medical home for children and youth with cerebral palsy. *Pediatrics.* 2004;114:1106–1113

Davies S, Hall D. "Contact a Family": professionals and parents in partnership. *Arch Dis Child.* 2005;90:1053–1057

Dias MS. Neurosurgical management of myelomeningocele (spina bifida). *Pediatr Rev.* 2005;26:50–60

Liptak GS, Accerdo P. Health and social outcomes of children with cerebral palsy. *J Pediatr.* 2004;145:S36–S41

Liptak GS. The pediatrician's role in caring for the developmentally disabled child. *Pediatr Rev.* 1996;17:203–210

McPherson M, Arango P, Fox H, et al. A new definition of children with special health care needs. *Pediatrics.* 1998;102:137–140

Michaud JL, American Academy of Pediatrics Committee on Children With Disabilities. Prescribing therapy services for children with motor disabilities. *Pediatrics.* 2004;113:1836–1838

Taft LT. Cerebral palsy. *Pediatr Rev.* 1995;16:411–418

Reproductive Health*

Monica Sifuentes, MD

CASE STUDY

An 18-year-old female college student in good health comes in for a routine health maintenance visit during her spring break. She is unaccompanied by her parents and has no complaints, stating that she just needs a checkup. She enjoys college, passed all of her fall and winter classes, and has some new friends. She denies tobacco use but says most of her friends smoke. She occasionally drinks alcohol and has tried marijuana once. Although she is not sexually active, she is interested in discussing oral contraception. Her last menstrual period, which occurred 2 weeks ago, was normal. She is taking no medications. Her physical examination is entirely normal.

Questions

1. What issues are important to discuss with adolescents at reproductive health maintenance visits?
2. What are the indications for a complete pelvic examination?
3. When is a Pap smear indicated, and how often should it be performed?
4. What methods of contraception are most successful in adolescent patients? What factors regarding each method should be considered?
5. What are the legal issues involved in prescribing contraception to minors in the absence of parental consent?

Adolescent visits to primary care physicians are relatively infrequent by the time teenagers reach puberty. At most, healthy adolescent patients are seen once or twice during high school for preparticipation sports or camp physicals. If adolescents are not involved in athletics or if their schools do not require periodic assessments, these teenagers will probably never visit their health care providers again while in high school. Therefore, it is extremely important to use any interaction with an adolescent as a unique opportunity for anticipatory guidance and health education, particularly reproductive health education.

Reproductive health can be defined as sexuality-related services, screening, and counseling. Such services should be included as a part of the routine health maintenance examination for both male and female adolescents for several reasons. The high incidence of sexually transmitted infections (STIs) in this age group, the risk of acquiring human immunodeficiency virus (HIV), and the reality of an unplanned pregnancy make reproductive health issues increasingly important for teenagers. In addition, adolescents rarely schedule appointments with health care providers prior to the initiation of coitus. Experimentation with drugs and alcohol at this time in their lives also contributes to early, unplanned sexual experiences (Box 30-1).

Aside from issues of sexual activity, adolescents also may have questions about their progression through puberty. Normal variants in body habitus or certain physical characteristics can be a source of unnecessary anxiety for uninformed teenagers. Health education to alleviate these fears is ideal. Adolescents who come for physical examinations should be allotted extra time so that topics such as puberty, abstinence, sexual activity, STIs, and contraception can be discussed. In addition, during more acute, problem-oriented visits, adolescents should be encouraged to voice any other concerns they may have. Depending on the nature of these issues, follow-up appointments can be scheduled.

Normal Secondary Sexual Development

Puberty begins during early adolescence with the development of secondary sexual characteristics. Because there can be tremendous variation with regard to the age, duration between pubertal stages, and somatic growth of adolescents, a sexual maturity rating (SMR) scale (Tanner staging) is used to describe breast and pubic hair development in females and genital development and pubic hair growth in males (Figures 30-1, 30-2, and 30-3). The average age of menarche in the United States is 12.5 years and for most females occurs during SMR 3 and 4. In contrast, spermarche occurs early in pubertal development in boys, at approximately 13 years of age, with little to no pubic hair development. Full fertility is generally achieved by age 15 years, or mid-adolescence, in most boys and girls.

---

*This chapter is largely devoted to a discussion of the reproductive health of adolescent females. However, Evaluation is divided into 2 sections— one for females and one for males. The reader is referred to Chapter 85 for more information regarding male reproductive health.

Box 30-1. Reproductive Health: Sexual Activity

Statistics regarding sexual activity among adolescents in the United States are startling. One in 4 females and 1 in 3 males have had sexual intercourse by 15 years of age. Among adolescents from 15 to 19 years of age, more than half are sexually active, and only one-third of these teenagers use contraception. As a result, nearly 1 million adolescent females younger than 20 years, or 1 out of every 10, become pregnant each year. Most of these pregnancies are unintended and occur premaritally, especially among certain racial and ethnic minority groups. The outcome of these pregnancies in 15- to 19-year-olds varies. An estimated 50% to 60% of these pregnancies result in live births, 30% end in abortion, and 10% to 15% are miscarried or stillborn.

Unprotected sexual activity among adolescents has several adverse health consequences, the most obvious being teenage pregnancy. Of the adolescents who continue their pregnancies, prematurity (<37 weeks' gestation) and low birth weight (<2,500 g) are 2 of the most frequently reported neonatal complications. Long-term maternal psychosocial sequelae of adolescent pregnancy include undereducation/school failure, limited vocational training and skills, economic dependency on public assistance, subsequent unwanted births, social isolation, depression, and high rates of separation and divorce among teenaged couples.

In addition to unintended pregnancy, the risk of contracting a sexually transmitted infection (STI) such as chlamydia, human papillomavirus, herpes, and human immunodeficiency virus (HIV) is increased. In cases of pelvic inflammatory disease from gonorrhea or chlamydia, future problems with fertility and an increased risk of ectopic pregnancy can occur. Human papillomavirus, which is associated with the development of genital warts, cervical dysplasia, and cancer, has a prevalence of up to 40% in adolescents. The prevalence rates of other STIs such as chlamydia and gonorrhea are still highest among 15- to 19-year-old females compared with older age groups in the United States. More alarming, however, is the relationship between acquired immunodeficiency syndrome in young adults aged 20 to 29 and probable exposure to HIV during adolescence.

Many factors have been associated with the initiation of early coitus in adolescents. They include male gender; race/ethnicity; poverty; a large, single-parent family; previous teen pregnancy in the household (either mother or sibling); poor academic achievement; discrepancy between the onset of physical puberty and cognitive development; peer group encouragement; and problem behaviors such as drug use. In addition, religious affiliation and cultural norms probably influence this decision. The role of hormonal changes during puberty and their influence on behavior is yet to be determined.

An estimated 6% of adolescents have limited typical functioning because of a chronic illness. However, most of these adolescents experience normal pubertal development and fertility because of advances in medical treatment for conditions such as diabetes and sickle cell disease. Like their healthy peers, many of these adolescents begin sexual intercourse at an early age. Pregnancy and childbirth can exacerbate some illnesses and increase risks significantly for both adolescents and fetuses. The genetic implications and specific patterns of inheritance of certain chronic conditions must also be considered. For this reason, attention to sexual issues is essential for adolescents with chronic medical illness.

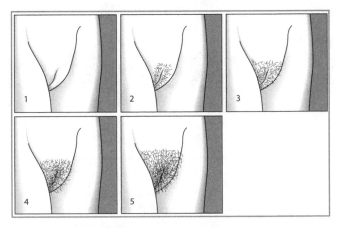

Figure 30-1. Female pubic hair development. Sexual maturity rating 1: prepubertal, no pubic hair. Sexual maturity rating 2: straight hair is extending along the labia and between ratings 2 and 3, begins on the symphysis pubis. Sexual maturity rating 3: pubic hair is increased in quantity; is darker, coarser, and curlier; and is present in the typical female triangle. Sexual maturity rating 4: pubic hair is more dense, curled, and adult in distribution but is less abundant. Sexual maturity rating 5: abundant, adult-type pattern; hair may extend on the medial aspect of the thighs.

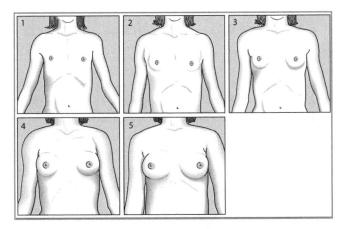

Figure 30-2. Female breast development. Sexual maturity rating 1: prepubertal, elevations of papilla only. Sexual maturity rating 2: breast buds appear, areola is slightly widened and projects as small mound. Sexual maturity rating 3: enlargement of the entire breast with no protrusion of the papilla or of the nipple. Sexual maturity rating 4: enlargement of the breast and projection of areola and papilla as a secondary mound. Sexual maturity rating 5: adult configuration of the breast with protrusion of the nipple, areola no longer projects separately from remainder of breast.

Evaluation

History

The history obtained at a reproductive health visit should include 2 parts: the medical history, which focuses primarily on the gynecologic history in females, and the psychosocial interview. Regardless of the type of visit scheduled, practitioners should take a few moments at the beginning of the interview to address routine health maintenance issues with the adolescent (Questions Box: Reproductive Health). The provider should find out whether the female adolescent

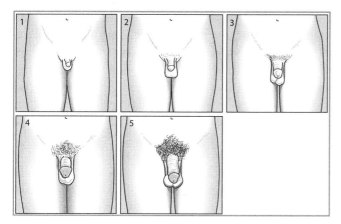

Figure 30-3. Male genital and pubic hair development. Sexual maturity rating 1: prepubertal, no pubic hair, genitalia unchanged from early childhood. Sexual maturity rating 2: light, downy hair develops laterally and later becomes dark, penis and testes may be slightly larger, scrotum becomes more textured. Sexual maturity rating 3: pubic hair is extended across pubis, testes and scrotum are further enlarged, penis is larger, especially in length. Sexual maturity rating 4: more abundant pubic hair with curling, genitalia resemble those of an adult, glans has become darker. Sexual maturity rating 5: adult quantity and pattern of pubic hair, with hair present along the inner borders of the thighs. The testes and scrotum are adult in size.

has ever had a pelvic examination. In addition, current methods of contraceptive use, if any, should be reviewed (Questions Box: Contraceptive Use). If the adolescent female takes oral contraceptives, a review of the more emergent complications of birth control pills is warranted, especially at an initial visit. **ACHES** (abdominal pain, chest pain, headaches, eye problems, severe leg pain) is a useful acronym to remember life-threatening reactions that can be associated with hormonal contraceptive use (Box 30-2).

Box 30-2. Danger Signs Associated With Oral Contraceptive Use	
A	**A**bdominal pain (severe)
C	**C**hest pain (severe), shortness of breath
H	**H**eadaches
E	**E**ye problems (visual loss or blur)
S	**S**evere leg pain (calf/thigh)

The rest of the psychosocial history, otherwise known as the **HEADDSSS** interview (home, employment and education, activities, diet, drugs, sexual activity/sexuality, suicide and depression, safety), should be completed whether or not the adolescent is currently sexually active (see Chapter 5). Risk factors for teenage pregnancy or multiple exposures to STIs should be kept in mind when formulating health care plans with the teenager.

Physical Examination

A complete physical examination should be performed on all adolescents, with particular attention paid to their SMR.

Questions

Reproductive Health

For males and females
- How is the adolescent feeling overall?
- Has the adolescent had any recent illnesses or conditions that the health care provider should know about?
- When was the last physical examination performed? Did it include a pelvic examination?
- Is the adolescent sexually active?
  — If so, when was the last episode of vaginal intercourse?
  — Was the last episode of sexual intercourse protected or unprotected?
  — Does the adolescent have anal or oral sex?
  — How old was the adolescent when he or she initiated coitus? Was it consensual?
  — How many sexual partners does the patient have currently? How many sexual partners have they had in their lifetime? What gender are they (all contacts may not be heterosexual)?
- Is there any history of physical or sexual abuse?
- Has the adolescent or any of his or her partners ever been treated for a sexually transmitted infection or tested for human immunodeficiency virus?

For females only
- What was the age at menarche?
- What was the date of the last menstrual period and the duration and amount of flow?
  — Are any symptoms such as cramping, bloating, or vomiting associated with menses?
  — Are any of these symptoms incapacitating? Do they cause the adolescent to miss school or work?
  — Does the mother or siblings have similar problems? If so, how do they manage them, if at all?

Questions

Contraceptive Use

- Does the adolescent use condoms: never, sometimes, or always?
- Is any other method, such as spermicidal foam or jelly, also used?
- Is the adolescent female currently using oral contraceptives?
  — If so, what particular type is she taking, and how long has she been using this method of contraception?
  — How often does she forget to take the pill? or What does she do when she forgets to take the pill?
  — Does she experience common minor side effects such as breakthrough bleeding or nausea?
  — Is the adolescent female using a long-acting progestin, such as Depo-Provera? If so, has she experienced irregular bleeding, weight gain, hair loss, headache, or acne?
  — Is there another method of contraception that the adolescent has used or might be interested in starting?
  — What does the adolescent know about emergency contraception?

Males

The genitalia should be examined closely for penile and testicular size, distribution of pubic hair, and presence of any ulcerative, vesicular, or wart-like lesions. Any urethral erythema or discharge should be noted. Clinicians can use this opportunity to teach male adolescents how to perform a testicular self-examination.

Females

Prior to performing the physical examination, the physician should determine whether a full-speculum examination is indicated (Box 30-3). This decision should be based on the details of the individual case and not solely on the basis of sexual activity. With the advent of noninvasive screening methods for STIs, a routine pelvic examination may be unnecessary. Most experts now recommend the use of urine-based nuclei-acid amplification tests (NAATs) to screen for gonorrhea or chlamydia instead of endocervical swabs. However, if a Pap smear or speculum examination is indicated, proper preparation of the adolescent is imperative. This should include an explanation of the procedure and the physical sensations felt while the endocervical specimen is being obtained. The choice of who should be present during the examination (eg, parent or friend who may have accompanied the patient), and a discussion of the desired positioning (ie, supine vs semisitting) are also important points to review. In addition, the speculum, specimen swabs, and other equipment should be shown to the adolescent before she is draped. The goal is to minimize the adolescent's fears, anxieties, misconceptions, and discomfort regarding the examination.

Box 30-3. Indications for a Complete Pelvic Examination

- Contraceptive management
- Pregnancy
- Request by adolescent
- Sexual activity
- Partner with sexually transmitted infection (STI)
- Previous history of STI
- History of hepatitis B
- Unexplained lower abdominal pain
- Abnormal vaginal discharge
- Unexplained vaginal bleeding
- External genital warts
- Urinary symptoms

A breast examination should be performed on female adolescents, and any breast tenderness, nodularity, or masses should be noted. Again, this portion of the examination can be used to educate patients about the purpose and importance of breast self-examinations.

The external genitalia should be examined in all adolescent females whether or not they are sexually active. The SMR and any congenital anomalies such as an imperforate hymen should be noted.

In sexually active adolescents, the external genitalia must be carefully examined for warts, ulcers, and vesicular lesions. Any urethral erythema, edema, or discharge that may indicate an otherwise asymptomatic chlamydial infection should be noted. A vaginal discharge may be appreciated prior to inserting the speculum but, ideally, the cervix should be examined for cervical ectopy, friability, and any lesions or discharge from the os. The vaginal mucosa should also be inspected as the speculum is withdrawn.

During the bimanual examination, the cervix should be palpated for any cervical motion tenderness. Uterine size and position should be appreciated, and adnexal tenderness or masses should be noted. Because normal ovaries are approximately the size of almonds, they are often not palpated by many clinicians. A rectovaginal examination is necessary to rule out fistulas, especially in postpartum adolescents. If the practitioner is unable to perform a vaginal bimanual examination, a rectoabdominal examination can be done to assess uterine size and position and the presence of adnexal masses.

Laboratory Tests

Because most *Chlamydia trachomatis* and *Neisseria gonorrhoeae* infections in adolescents are asymptomatic, noninvasive urine-based NAATs should be sent in all sexually active adolescents who have a history of unprotected intercourse. If the adolescent has vaginal discharge or cervical friability noted on speculum examination, the specimen should be obtained directly from the cervix and sent for NAAT. A saline and KOH wet mount should also be collected in symptomatic patients. A Pap smear should be performed in females who are sexually active, have external genital warts, or have persistent vaginal discharge. The Pap smear can also help detect *Trichomonas vaginalis* or the cytological changes associated with human papillomavirus (HPV). A culture for herpes simplex virus (HSV) should be performed if painful vesicles are noted on examination.

Other laboratory tests include a rapid plasma reagin test for syphilis and an HIV test (after appropriate pretest counseling). Baseline complete blood count, liver function tests, cholesterol, and fasting glucose may be indicated before starting oral contraceptives but certainly are not mandatory. A pregnancy test is warranted in sexually active females if the practitioner chooses to begin oral contraceptives mid-cycle.

Management

Reproductive Health Education

All management plans during reproductive health visits should include a frank **discussion of puberty, sexuality, and STIs** regardless of current sexual activity. The adolescent should be counseled about abstinence as an acceptable choice. Ideally, preventive health care measures such as **breast and testicular self-examinations** have been reviewed during the physical examination. It is hoped that by encouraging adolescents' familiarity with these self-examinations, they will continue to perform them throughout their adult lives. The use of posters, plastic models, and written materials to support the discussion is greatly encouraged. The goal of education should be to assist adolescents in identifying and communicating their thoughts and feelings about sexual abstinence as well as sexual activity and to aid in the prevention of unintended pregnancies, parenthood, and STIs. Prevention programs offered by schools must be supplemented by open parental communication in the home about sexuality.

Legal Issues

The issue of **confidentiality** is important to consider when providing reproductive health care for adolescents. Parental involvement should be strongly encouraged, but health care practitioners are not required to disclose any information to parents except in cases of suicidal ideation, harmful intent to others, and sexual or physical abuse. In most states, contraceptive services can be provided to adolescents of any age without specific parental knowledge or consent. The complex issue of parental consent and pregnancy termination varies from state to state.

Pap Smear

The current recommendation of the American Cancer Society and the American College of Obstetricians and Gynecologists is that cervical cancer screening should begin approximately 3 years after the onset of vaginal intercourse and no later than 21 years of age. After the initiation of screening, a Pap smear should be performed annually with conventional cervical cytology smears or every 2 years using liquid-based cytology. After age 30, low-risk women who fulfill specific criteria may be screened every 2 to 3 years. The rationale for these recommendations is that there seems to be little risk in missing an important cervical lesion until 3 to 5 years after initial exposure to HPV, and screening prematurely may result in an overdiagnosis and treatment of cervical lesions that will most likely regress spontaneously in the adolescent.

Management of an abnormal Pap smear depends on the presence of atypia versus low-grade or high-grade squamous intraepithelial lesions. Further evaluation with colposcopy and cervical biopsy may be warranted. This decision should be made in consultation with the cytopathologist who reviewed the specimen and a gynecologist familiar with the management of cervical dysplasia in young women.

Contraceptive Methods

The appropriate method of contraception should be individualized. Barrier methods include condoms (male and female), diaphragms, and cervical caps. Vaginal spermicides such as nonoxynol 9 are available in a variety of forms (foams, gels, creams, and suppositories) and can be used alone or can provide extra protection if used with a barrier method. Hormonal methods include oral contraceptives, long-acting progestin agents, transdermal methods, and the intravaginal ring. Intrauterine devices generally are not recommended for teenagers because of the increased prevalence of STIs and pelvic inflammatory disease in this age group. The withdrawal method, or coitus interruptus, and natural family planning are ineffective methods for adolescents for protection against pregnancy.

Hormonal Contraception

Combined low-dose oral contraceptives are an effective means of birth control for adolescents. Monophasic pills contain a fixed dose of estrogen and progestin throughout the 21-day pill cycle. Biphasic preparations contain a lower dose of the progestin component during the first 10 days of the cycle. In triphasic pills, the doses of both estrogen and progestin or the progestin component alone is varied 3 times throughout the cycle. This contraceptive was created to decrease the overall progestin-related side effects such as hypertension, acne, and lipid abnormalities. Most recently, lower-dose estrogen (20 μg) pills have been developed to minimize estrogen-related side effects and decrease discontinuation rates. In addition, 3-month continuous hormonal therapy has been advocated followed by 1 week of withdrawal bleeding for young women who prefer to menstruate only 4 times a year. Clear benefits associated with oral contraceptive use include prevention of pregnancy, protection against ovarian and endometrial cancers, decreased risk of functional ovarian cysts, and decreased menstrual symptoms such as dysmenorrhea. The potential risks, which include thromboembolic phenomena, hypertension, and changes in the lipid profile, are minimal in most adolescents compared with the morbidity and mortality associated with teenage pregnancy and childbirth.

The long-acting progestin depot medroxyprogesterone acetate (Depo-Provera) is given intramuscularly every 3 months to inhibit ovulation for at least 14 weeks. The most common side effect is irregular menstrual bleeding, especially in the first few months, and eventual amenorrhea with prolonged use. Weight gain remains a significant issue for some patients and clinicians, particularly in obese adolescents where exaggerated increases in weight can be seen. In 2004 the US Food and Drug Administration (FDA) issued a black box warning for medroxyprogesterone acetate regarding its use and a potential reduction in bone mineral density, especially during adolescence when peak bone mass occurs. Bone loss is greater with increasing duration of medroxyprogesterone acetate use and may not be completely reversible. As a result, many physicians who prescribe depot medroxyprogesterone acetate are recommending a change in contraceptive method after approximately 2 years.

A new subdermal implant (Implanon) has received recent approval by the FDA and is available for young women. It is designed to deliver a low, steady dose of continuous progestin for 3 years via a single plastic polymer rod placed below the skin. Formal instruction for insertion and removal is required for the health care professional interested in providing this form of contraception.

Emergency Postcoital Contraception

Emergency contraception, or the "morning-after pill," is an effective way to prevent unintended pregnancy in adolescents. It requires, however, that the physician educate teens about its availability and usage and that teens feel comfortable contacting their health care provider within 72 to 120 hours of unprotected or inadequately protected intercourse. Although not meant to be used repeatedly as the sole method of contraception, emergency contraception is useful for the "unplanned" sexual encounter, which is often the case with adolescents. The morning-after pill contains a high dose of hormone that is thought to inhibit ovulation, disrupt follicular development, and/or interfere with the maturation of the corpus luteum. Emergency contraception does not interrupt or disrupt an already-established pregnancy, and is not an abortifacient.

The original regimen was a combination of high-dose estrogen and progestin, known as the Yuzpe method; however, nausea and vomiting occurred in about 25% to 30% of patients. Plan B is the progestin-only method of emergency contraception that is currently available by prescription for adolescents younger than 18 years. It consists of 2 doses of 0.75 mg of levonorgestrel, which should be taken 12 hours apart within 3 days of unprotected intercourse. Based on recent data reported by the World Health Organization, this regimen has been modified to *take both pills at once up to 5 days after unprotected or inadequately protected intercourse*. Plan B is most highly effective when used within the first 24 hours after unprotected coitus. Although less common than with the Yuzpe method, side effects of Plan B include nausea, vomiting, breast tenderness, and irregular bleeding patterns such as spotting, shortened interval to menses, and lighter or heavier menses. Because emergency contraception is both safe and highly effective in preventing pregnancy, physicians should consider providing the sexually active teen with a prescription or advance supply of Plan B at the health maintenance visit.

The patient should be given a follow-up office or clinic appointment 2 to 3 weeks after using emergency contraception so that a pregnancy test can be performed, treatment failures can be identified early, STI screening can occur, and issues of contraception can be discussed.

Nonhormonal Contraception

Numerous studies and clinical experience have shown that nonhormonal methods are less effective in adolescents. However, latex condoms in conjunction with a spermicide have become crucial as a method of contraception since the emergence of acquired immunodeficiency syndrome. Although they help prevent transmission of some STIs such as gonorrhea, chlamydia, trichomonas, and HIV, condoms do not protect against HPV and HSV infection overall because the genital area is not completely covered. A few moments, therefore, should be taken during the visit to explain these details and demonstrate proper use of condoms. Risks of condom use are minimal, except for allergic reactions to the spermicide, latex, or lubricants. Although available, the female condom is not widely used by adolescents but may be helpful in situations where a male partner refuses to wear a condom. The inner ring is inserted into the vagina up to 8 hours prior to intercourse, and a prescription or physician visit is not necessary to obtain a female condom. Some teenagers, however, may be uncomfortable with its insertion and the fact that the outer ring remains on the vulva during vaginal intercourse. Similar issues are encountered when considering the diaphragm as a contraceptive method for teens, therefore, it is not recommended as a

first-line contraceptive method for most adolescents. Other nonhormonal methods should be reviewed with adolescents as they become available.

Sexually Transmitted Infections

All STIs should be treated according to specific guidelines published by the Centers for Disease Control and Prevention based on current epidemiology. See Chapter 85 for details regarding the diagnosis and management of STIs in adolescents.

CASE RESOLUTION

In the case scenario presented at the beginning of the chapter, a more detailed history should be obtained regarding the adolescent's menstrual history and daily activities (eg, With whom does she spend most of her time? What does she like to do in her spare time?). In addition, the indications for a pelvic examination should be reviewed. If they do not apply, the pelvic examination can be deferred until the next visit or within 3 years of the adolescent becoming sexually active. A discussion should then follow regarding both barrier and hormonal methods of contraception and their role in the prevention of pregnancy and sexually transmitted infections. Emergency contraception should also be reviewed with the teen.

Selected References

American Academy of Pediatrics Committee on Adolescence. Condom use by adolescents. *Pediatrics.* 2001;107:1463–1469

American Academy of Pediatrics Committee on Adolescence. Contraception and adolescents. *Pediatrics.* 1999;104:1161–1166

American Academy of Pediatrics Committee on Adolescence. Emergency contraception. *Pediatrics.* 2005;116:1026–1035

American Academy of Pediatrics Task Force on Pediatric AIDS. Adolescent and human immunodeficiency virus infection: the role of the pediatrician in prevention and intervention. *Pediatrics.* 1993;92:626–629

Bonny AE, Harkness LS, Cromer BA. Depot medroxyprogesterone acetate: implications for weight status and bone mineral density in the adolescent female. *Adolesc Med Clin.* 2005;16:569–584

Boonstra H, Nash E. Minors and the right to consent to health care. *Issues Brief (Alan Guttmacher Inst).* 2000;2:4–8

Burkett AM, Hewitt GD. Progestin only contraceptives and their use in adolescents: clinical options and medical indications. *Adolesc Med Clin.* 2005;16:553–567

Calderoni ME, Coupey SM. Combined hormonal contraception. *Adolesc Med Clin.* 2005;16:517–537

Eaton DK, Kann L, Kinchen S, et al. Youth risk behavior surveillance—United States, 2005. *MMWR Surveill Summ.* 2006;55:1–108

English A. Reproductive health services for adolescents: critical legal issues. *Obstet Gynecol Clin North Am.* 2000;27:195–221

Greydanus DE, Patel DR, Rimsza ME. Contraception in the adolescent: an update. *Pediatrics.* 2001;107:562–573

Gupta N. Advances in hormonal contraception. *Adolesc Med Clin.* 2006;17:653–671

Hillard PJ. Overview of contraception. *Adolesc Med Clin.* 2005;16:485–493

Klein JD, American Academy of Pediatrics Committee on Adolescence. Adolescent pregnancy: current trends and issues. *Pediatrics.* 2005;116:281–286

Mulchachey KM. Practical approaches to prescribing contraception in the office setting. *Adolesc Med Clin.* 2005;16:665–674

Murphy NA, Elias ER. Sexuality of children and adolescents with developmental disabilities. *Pediatrics.* 2006;118:398–403

Rimsza M. Counseling the adolescent about contraception. *Pediatr Rev.* 2003;24:162–170

Saslow D, Runowicz CD, Solomon D, et al. American Cancer Society guideline for the early detection of cervical neoplasia and cancer. *CA Cancer J Clin.* 2002;52:342–362

Sieving RE, Oliphant JA, Blum RW. Adolescent sexual behavior and sexual health. *Pediatr Rev.* 2002;23:407–416

Westhoff C. Emergency contraception. *N Engl J Med.* 2003;349:1830–1835

Injury Prevention

Allison Golnik, MD, MPH, and Iris Wagman Borowsky, MD, PhD

CASE STUDY

A 3-year-old girl was brought to the emergency department with a BB in her right eye. The girl's 10-year-old brother inadvertently fired his BB gun, and a BB lodged in her right eye. The BB was surgically removed, but as a result of the injury, the girl is legally blind in that eye.

Questions

1. How extensive is the injury problem in children?
2. What are the different methods for injury prevention? How could this particular injury have been prevented?
3. What injury prevention program has been developed by the American Academy of Pediatrics?
4. What are some general guidelines for effective injury prevention counseling?

Traditionally, unintentional injuries have been called accidents. The problem with the term *accident,* however, is that it implies unpredictability, carrying with it connotations of chance, fate, and unexpectedness. The perception that injuries are random, chance occurrences that cannot be predicted or prevented has been a major barrier to progress in injury prevention and the study and control of injury as a scientific discipline. According to the modern view of injury, accidents must be anticipated in order to be prevented. Specialists in injury prevention have tried to replace the word *accident* with *injury* and have developed the idea of "reducing injury risk." Thus injuries are not random events at all; rather, they occur in predictable patterns determined by identifiable risk factors. For example, if a 10-year-old boy plays unsupervised with a "toy" BB gun, which is capable of expelling projectiles at velocities much greater than those required to penetrate the eye, the resulting injury can hardly be called an accident. On the contrary, the injury is entirely predictable.

Epidemiology

Unintentional injuries are the leading cause of death among people aged 1 to 44 in the United States. In 2004 unintentional injuries claimed the lives of 12,184 Americans younger than 20 years. Of unintentional injury–related deaths, motor vehicle crashes are the leading cause in people aged 1 to 64. The second most common cause of unintentional injury–related deaths is drowning for ages 1 to 4 and 10 to 14, burns for ages 5 to 9, and poisonings for ages 15 to 64. Intentional injuries are also a major cause of mortality in young people. Among all causes of death, homicide ranks fourth for ages 1 to 14 and second for ages 15 to 24, and suicide ranks third for ages 10 to 24.

In addition to deaths, nonfatal injuries lead to more than 10 million emergency department (ED) and 10 million primary care office visits each year. In 2005, 8.9 million nonfatal unintentional injuries occurred in persons younger than 20 years in the United States. The most common causes of nonfatal unintentional injuries in people aged 1 to 24 are falls, being struck by or against something, bites, cuttings/piercings, overexertion, and motor vehicle occupancy. Traumatic injuries are the leading cause of hospital admission, with more than 300,000 hospitalizations each year. Overall, 1 of every 5 children in the United States receives medical attention for an injury each year.

Several epidemiological factors are associated with higher rates of pediatric injuries. These include male gender, low income, and family stressors (eg, death in the family, new residence, birth of a sibling). There is a bimodal distribution of injuries, with infants and adolescents at greatest risk. Females are most likely to experience rape or assault. Geography influences injury rates; for example, drowning deaths tend to be higher in coastline states (Alaska and California) or states with a higher number of swimming pools (Texas), injury-related deaths are higher in rural areas and may be related to decreased access to emergency medical care, and homicide occurs more frequently in urban areas. Rates of fatal injuries are higher for those of minority and low-income status.

Strategies for Injury Prevention

During this century, efforts to prevent injuries have shifted from changing the behavior of individuals to modifying the environments in which injuries occur. William Haddon, a medical epidemiologist, devised 2 useful frameworks for developing injury prevention strategies.

Haddon Matrix

This matrix relates 3 factors (host, vector, and environment) to the 3 phases of an injury-producing event (pre-event, event, and post-event). The 3 factors interact over time to produce injury. Table 31-1 shows a Haddon matrix of motor vehicle crash injuries. The precrash phase describes elements that determine whether a crash will occur, the crash phase describes the variables that influence the nature and severity of the resultant injury, and the postcrash phase describes the factors that determine the degree to which the injury is limited and repaired after the crash occurs. By describing the "anatomy" of an injury, the Haddon matrix illustrates the numerous characteristics that determine an injury and the many corresponding strategies for interfering with the production of an injury.

Table 31-1. The Haddon Matrix[a]			
Phase	*Host (Human)*	*Vector (Vehicle)*	*Environment*
Precrash	Driver vision Alcohol consumption	Brakes Tires Speed	Speed limit Road curvature Road signs
Crash	Use of safety belts Osteoporosis	Vehicle size	Median barriers Laws about use of car seats and safety belts
Post-crash	Age Physical condition	Fuel system integrity	EMS personnel training

Abbreviation: EMS, emergency medical service.
[a]From *The American Journal of Preventive Medicine* 5(3) Supplement 1: p. 8 (1989). Originally adapted from Haddon, Suchman, and Klein. *Accident Research: Methods and Approaches.* New York, NY: Harper and Row; 1964.

Haddon also developed a list of **10 countermeasures to prevent injuries** or reduce the severity of their effects.

1. Prevent creation of the hazard (eg, stop producing poisons, toys with small parts, and non-powder firearms; do not participate in dangerous sports).
2. Reduce the amount of the hazard (eg, package drugs in smaller, nonlethal amounts; reduce speed limits).
3. Prevent the release of the hazard (eg, use child-resistant caps for medications, toilet locks, and safety latches on cabinets and drawers).
4. Modify the rate or spatial distribution of release of the hazard (eg, require air bags in cars, use child safety seats and seat belts, make poisons taste bad).
5. Separate people from the hazard in space or time (eg, make sidewalks for pedestrians, bikeways for bicyclists, and recreation areas separated from vehicles).
6. Separate people from hazards with material barriers (eg, use bicycle helmets and protective equipment for athletes, install fences around swimming pools, build window guards).
7. Modify relevant basic qualities of the hazard (eg, place padded carpets under cribs, require guns to have safety locks).
8. Increase resistance to damage from the hazard (eg, train and condition athletes, make structures more earthquake-proof, use flame-retardant sleepwear).
9. Limit the damage that has already begun (eg, use fire extinguisher, begin cardiopulmonary resuscitation).

10. Stabilize, repair, and rehabilitate injured individuals (eg, develop pediatric trauma centers and physical rehabilitation programs).

Haddon's work served as a practical guide for thinking about ways to prevent injury. It emphasized the importance of considering injuries as a result of a sequence of events, with many opportunities for prevention. The shift of emphasis away from changing human behavior to preventing injury is particularly appropriate with regard to injuries in children because inhibiting children's curiosity is impractical as well as undesirable.

Passive and Active Interventions

Interventions to prevent injuries can also be categorized as passive or active. **Passive or automatic strategies** protect whenever they are needed, **without the action of parents or children.** An example is the automobile air bag that automatically inflates to cushion the occupants during a crash. Other examples of automatic strategies are water heater temperatures set to 120°F or lower, not having guns in the home, and energy-absorbing surfaces under playground equipment. In contrast, **active interventions require action to become effective.** For example, nonautomatic safety belts are active strategies; every time protection is needed, individuals must "buckle up." Watching children continuously is another example of an injury prevention strategy that requires constant activity.

Some strategies are partially automatic, requiring some action by individuals. Smoke detectors can be very effective in preventing injury and death in house fires, but roughly one-third of smoke detectors do not have working batteries. Batteries should be changed once a year and, ideally, tested once a month. As might be expected, the greater the effort required for children to be protected, the smaller the chance that protection occurs. Therefore, whenever possible, passive measures are preferable because they are the most effective.

Several approaches have been used successfully to prevent childhood injuries, including engineering, education, legislation, and enforcement. An engineering intervention, the car seat, is extremely effective when used correctly (see Table 31-2). Child safety seats in passenger cars reduce the risk of death by 71% for infants and 54% for toddlers aged 1 to 4 years. Booster seats reduce injury risk by 59% for children aged 4 to 7 years compared with safety belts alone. Unfortunately, studies indicate that between one-third and two-thirds of car seats are used incorrectly. To address this, newborn care units often have car seat education programs. Police departments

Table 31-2. General Pediatric Car Seat Guidelines		
Type of Car Seat	*Start At*	*Continue Until At Least*
Rear-facing (infant or convertible)	Term infant	1 year and 20 pounds (both criteria must be met)
Forward-facing car seat	1 year and 20 pounds	4 years and usually 40 pounds and 40 inches tall[a]
Booster seat	Usually 40 pounds and 40 inches tall[a]	Usually 80 pounds and 57 inches tall[a]

[a]See Biagioli citation under Selected References for detailed guidelines.

and private motor companies hold free public events to teach and manually check appropriate car seat use. In addition to education, passage and strict enforcement of child restraint laws are essential to compliance. Since 2001, 26 states and the District of Columbia updated their child passenger safety laws. Nevertheless, some loopholes still exist, such as car seat exemptions when feeding, changing, or rocking a child to sleep; when an automobile has an out-of-state registration; or when an automobile is driven by someone other than a parent or legal guardian. Such exemptions reinforce parental misconceptions, particularly that the lap of an occupant (the "child crusher" position) is a safe position.

Counseling by Pediatricians

Although the existence of significant gaps in parental knowledge about injury prevention has been clearly established, studies have shown that pediatricians spend surprisingly little time counseling parents about childhood safety. One survey found that only 40% of caregivers of children younger than 15 years who had a medical visit in the past year recalled receiving injury prevention information. Another survey found that while 55% of pediatricians responded that they provided injury prevention information, only 19% of their patients recalled receiving this information. Reasons for limited discussion of safety issues may include lack of emphasis on preventive medical care in medical schools and pediatric training programs, inadequate time or reimbursement, and lack of perceived self-efficacy or effectiveness. Research, however, has shown that injury prevention counseling in primary care settings is effective, resulting in

increased knowledge and improved safety practices. Parents report that they would listen to physicians much more than any other group regarding child safety.

The Injury Prevention Program (TIPP) was developed in 1983 by the American Academy of Pediatrics (AAP) to firmly establish injury prevention as a standard of care for pediatricians. TIPP has been shown to be cost-effective. The AAP suggests that providers focus their safety counseling on a few topics targeted to individual risk factors (eg, age, gender, location, season of the year, socioeconomic status of family). Table 31-3 shows the age-specific counseling schedule of TIPP, which indicates the minimum topics to cover at each visit. Topics are scheduled for discussion before children reach a particular developmental milestone. For example, a discussion of falls is scheduled for the 2- or 4-week visit, before infants normally begin to roll over, and a discussion of choking is scheduled for 4 months, before they can grasp and put things in their mouths. Specific preventive measures should be reinforced at each visit. Areas of injury prevention guidance recommended for adolescents include (1) traffic safety (eg, seat belts, alcohol use, motorcycle and bicycle helmets), (2) water safety (eg, alcohol use and diving injuries), (3) sports safety, and (4) firearm safety.

Health care professionals should involve parents and patients in educational efforts (eg, have a bicycle helmet in the office for children to try on). Advice should be well-defined and practical rather than general information (eg, write the poison control center number on the phone, never leave children unattended in a bathtub, wear a bicycle helmet). Safety counseling probably will not be especially effective

Table 31-3. The Injury Prevention Program (TIPP) Safety Counseling Schedule for Early and Middle Childhood[a]		
Visit	*Introduce*	*Reinforce*
Prenatal/newborn	Infant car seat, smoke detector, crib safety	
2 d–4 wk	Falls	Car safety seat
2 mo	Burns—hot liquids, choking/suffocation	Car safety seat, falls
4 mo	Water safety—bathtubs	Car safety seat, falls, burns, choking/suffocation
6 mo	Poisonings, burns—hot surfaces	Falls, burns, choking
9 mo	Water/pool safety, toddler car safety seat, firearms	Poisonings, falls, burns
1 y		Water/pool safety, falls, burns
15 mo		Car safety seat, poisonings, falls, burns
18 mo		Car safety seat, poisonings, falls, burns, firearm hazards
2 y	Falls—play equipment, tricycles, pedestrian safety	Car safety seat, water/pool safety, burns, firearm hazards
3 y		Car safety seat, pedestrian safety, falls, burns, firearm hazards
4 y	Booster seat use	Pedestrian safety, falls—play equipment, firearm hazards
5 y	Water/pool safety, bicycle safety	Firearm hazards, pedestrian safety, booster seat
6 y	Fire safety	Bicycle, booster seat, pedestrian, and firearm hazards
8 y	Sports safety, seat belt use	Bicycle
10 y	Firearm hazards	Sports, seat belt use, bicycle safety

[a]Adapted and reproduced with permission from the American Academy of Pediatrics Committee and Section on Injury and Poison Prevention. *TIPP: The Injury Prevention Program, Implementing Safety Counseling in Office Practice.* Elk Grove Village, IL: American Academy of Pediatrics; 2001.

if parents are given a long list of hazards; 2 or 3 topics should be discussed per visit. Whenever possible, pediatricians should coordinate their educational efforts with current injury prevention efforts (eg, bicycle helmet campaigns, handgun regulation) in the community.

Recent Recommendations

The AAP has multiple safety recommendations. The following are a few of the newer and revised recommendations. Research failed to show benefit for children who were treated with ipecac and, therefore, pediatricians should now advise parents to discard and not use ipecac in the home (2003). Shopping carts with child seats should provide restraints (seat belts), and children should be supervised while in them. Alternatives to shopping carts include strollers, wagons, front/backpack child carriers, or having the child walk (2006). The AAP recommends a ban on the manufacture and sale of mobile infant walkers. Stationary activity centers should be promoted as a safer alternative (2001). The AAP recommends that 2- and 4-wheeled off-road vehicles and snowmobiles only be operated by children older than 16 years who have undergone a licensing program (2000). Additionally, snowmobiles should never tow others in tubes or sleds (2000). Children should not play around lawn mowers and, if younger than 6 years, should stay inside while a mower is being operated. Children should display appropriate judgment prior to operating a lawn mower (typically at least 12 years for a push mower and 16 years for a riding mower). Children should never be allowed to ride as passengers on riding mowers or be towed behind in carts or wagons (2001). Swimming pools should have 4-sided fences around them, and children should always be supervised around water (2003). The AAP recommends that restraints be used for all children riding on an aircraft (2001). When children use skateboards and non-powered scooters, they should not ride in traffic, should wear protective gear, and should be supervised by an adult when younger than 10 years for skateboards and 8 years old for non-powered scooters (2002). Trampolines should never be used at home, in physical education classes, or in outdoor playgrounds (1999). Among teenagers who are killed, 63% are drivers and 37% are passengers of motor vehicles. The AAP recommends that pediatricians know their state laws regarding teenage drivers, encourage seat belt use, discourage distractions when driving, encourage restrictions on nighttime driving and limits on the number of passengers, and counsel teenagers about the dangers of driving while impaired (2006). Additional guidelines can be found at http://aappolicy.aappublications.org/ using keywords "injury prevention."

Pediatricians as Advocates

Pediatricians can play a major role in injury prevention outside of the clinical setting. As advocates for child safety, health care professionals can contribute to community efforts in injury prevention either by starting a program or by providing support to ongoing programs. Safe Kids (www.safekids.org) is a worldwide organization made up of safety experts, educators, corporations, foundations, governments, and volunteers whose mission is to prevent childhood injury through education and advocacy. Health care professionals can advocate through legislation and regulatory interventions. States have enacted laws covering many aspects of injury prevention, including car safety seats, poison control centers, cribs, playgrounds, amusement parks, protective gear for sports, swimming pools, and school buses. Dramatic reductions in injuries often follow safety legislation. For example, infant walker-related injuries have decreased by 76% since the introduction of the American Society for Testing and Materials F977 voluntary infant walker standard in 1997 and the introduction of stationary activity centers as alternatives to mobile infant walkers. Pediatrics practitioners can heighten awareness about the magnitude of childhood injuries among policy makers (eg, telephoning or writing letters to legislators, testifying about the benefits of specific safety legislation). They can initiate injury prevention legislation individually or collectively (eg, through the AAP). Pediatricians can also direct attention to hazardous products on the market; they can help initiate changes in the design of products and enact appropriate regulations (eg, federal crib standards of 1974 mandating close spacing of vertical slats to reduce the risk of entrapment; the Child Safety Protection Act of 1995 requiring that any small ball, with a diameter less than 1 3/4 inches (4.44 cm), must contain a toy safety label; window blinds manufactured with tassels instead of loops and children's clothing without drawstrings to prevent strangulation; and toy boxes manufactured with safer lids and air holes in case of a trapped child).

CASE RESOLUTION

Some of the factors that influenced the injury suffered by the girl in the case history are the ease with which BB guns are purchased, the marketing of BB guns as toys, the design of the guns, the recreational activities available to children in the community, and the availability of emergency ophthalmologic services. Health care professionals have the opportunity to teach injury prevention to children and their parents as well as to influence the individuals who manufacture the products and pass the laws that affect children's risk of injury.

Selected References

Agran PF, Anderson C, Winn D, Trent R, Walton-Haynes L, Thayer S. Rates of pediatrics injuries by 3-month intervals for children 0 to 3 years of age. *Pediatrics.* 2003;111:e683–e692

Biagioli F. Child safety seat counseling: three keys to safety. *Am Fam Physicians.* 2005;72:473–478

DiGuiseppi C, Roberts IG. Individual-level injury prevention strategies in the clinical setting. *Future Child.* 2000;10:53–82

Dowd MD, Keenan HT, Bratton SL. Epidemiology and prevention of childhood injuries. *Crit Care Med.* 2002;30(suppl):S385–S392

Gardner HG, American Academy of Pediatrics Committee on Injury, Violence, and Poison Prevention. Office-based counseling for unintentional injury prevention. *Pediatrics.* 2007;119:202–206

Hambridge SJ, Davidson AJ, Gonzales R, Steiner JF. Epidemiology of pediatric injury-related primary care office visits in the United States. *Pediatrics.* 2002;109:559–565

Hunter WM, Helou S, Saluja G, Runyan CW, Coyne-Beasley T. Injury prevention advice in top-selling parenting books. *Pediatrics*. 2005;116:1080–1088

National Center for Injury Prevention and Control, Centers for Disease Control and Prevention. Web-Based Inquiry Statistics Query and Reporting System [database]. www.cdc.gov/ncipc/wisqars/

Spady DW, Saunders DL, Schopflocher DP, Svenson LW. Patterns of injury in children: a population-based approach. *Pediatrics*. 2004;113:522–529

United States Department of Health and Human Services, Centers for Disease Control and Prevention. *Injury Fact Book*. www.cdc.gov/ncipc

Fostering Self-Esteem

Rick Goldstein, MD

CASE STUDY

A 4-year-old girl is brought to the office for a physical examination for preschool. Except for an episode of bronchiolitis at 8 months of age, she has been healthy. Her mother expresses concern that her daughter is shy and does not always play well with other children. She has never participated in a child care program or group activities out of the home. She spends most of her time with her mother, grandmother, and 7-year-old sister, with whom she gets along fairly well. Both parents work outside the home, her father full time and her mother part-time.

The girl's medical history is unremarkable. She has reached all of her developmental milestones at appropriate ages, currently speaks well in sentences, is able to dress herself without supervision, and can balance on one foot with no difficulty.

The physical examination is entirely normal. However, numerous times during the visit, the mother tells her daughter to "sit up straight," "stop fidgeting," and "act your age." The mother rolls her eyes as she tells you "she doesn't know how to act."

Questions

1. What is self-esteem?
2. How do parents or other caregivers affect the development of their children's self-esteem both positively and negatively?
3. What observable warning signs in parent-child relationships negatively affect normal development of self-esteem?
4. What role does discipline play in the development of self-esteem?
5. What suggestions can primary practitioners give parents and other caregivers to help foster positive self-esteem in children?

The concept of self-esteem resonates deeply in contemporary American culture. Self-esteem can be defined simply as how one feels about oneself but is much larger than that, incorporating not only a sense of self-worth, but a child's confidence that they can successfully affect their world, the buoyancy of their hope, and their resilience. It is grounded in the fact that success with other people is fundamental to this sense of who they are. Self-esteem is essential to children's health and well-being, and influences the development of relationships during both childhood and adulthood.

While self-esteem is a concept in action throughout our lives, it first comes into clear view in the developing internal self-concept of the 4-year-old. Through the language of a 4-year-old, the pediatrician or allied health professional can find a child who is learning to know herself and appreciate her abilities. The joy in autonomy and initiative are suffused with a need to live up to expectations—the big girl needs to know if she is a good girl. The first stirrings of conscience and the confidence to manage measured responsibility can be seen. The complex interaction of temperament, developmental stage, the family's security, the parental style of discipline, sibling and peer interactions, and school experiences coalesce in the experience of a uniquely competent child. For her caregivers, the desire to encourage a kind of fearlessness is balanced by the very real need to keep the child safe and appropriate. The synthesis of these elements is self-esteem.

All parents hope that their children will develop a positive self-concept that will aid them throughout their lives. Unfortunately, discussions related to self-esteem are usually held as a result of a crisis or an observation noted by worried parents or teachers. Primary care practitioners should bring the parents' focus to this important outcome as a normal part of anticipatory guidance. Pediatricians and child health practitioners are in a unique position to offer specific recommendations for fostering self-esteem that may have a major impact on their patients' lives. In their time during health maintenance visits with the child, they should model respect for the child's self-concept and the fostering of the child's self-esteem in their interactions.

Self-Esteem and Growth and Development

While the appearance of what is understood as self-esteem requires the development of certain cognitive abilities, it springs from an accumulated experience created by parents and other caregivers beginning with the responsiveness of the infant's environment and continuing onward. Crying newborns quickly adapt to the calming influence of a maternal figure. Infants who are 3 to 4 months of age often smile at all individuals for social interaction and protest being left alone. As infants become more verbal and develop more advanced motor skills, they begin to respond consistently to verbal and nonverbal cues from parents (eg, laugh with parents, follow simple commands, are taken aback by a stern voice). If parental figures are warm and loving as well as supportive and consistent, infants learn to trust and enjoy these interactions.

By the time children are toddlers, they have developed a specific relationship with their caregivers and the rest of their environment. Presumably they are learning to live within consistently set limits and have been corrected when they go beyond them in their attempts at exploration. All children, regardless of temperament, exhibit negative behaviors such as temper tantrums and selfish behavior, which elicits some type of response from parents.

Preschool children become much more independent, and they spend more time away from primary caregivers. This newly acquired independence, however, does not remove the need for attention, interest, and approval from their parents. Opportunities to demonstrate the competence of children can be seen in the autonomy that appropriate parenting affords, and heard as a source of pride in parents taking note of it. Preschoolers also enjoy playing alongside other children, although not necessarily in cooperative play (eg, helping each other in addition to playing together).

Much of a child's concept of self-worth and competence is established and reinforced by those around them, especially their primary caregivers. This continues into the school years, with peers and teachers eventually assuming a more influential role in the continued development and reinforcement of self-esteem. The development of self-esteem is transactional, built by the responses children receive to their increasing initiative and abilities, resting on a foundation of security.

Encouragement Versus Pressure

Parents should understand the difference between encouragement and pressure, and should be introduced to the concept of positive communication. To build positive self-esteem, children need encouragement at all levels of their development (Box 32-1). This is communicated both verbally and nonverbally and should be distinguished from overt pressure. For example, a first grader learning to spell should be praised for his early, if flawed, application of phonemes when he spells "winter" as "wntur," and may not need correction at that point. In general, children should be allowed to develop at their

own rate and be neither coaxed into activities before they are ready nor judged too harshly for earnest, early attempts.

Successful parenting creates opportunities for the child to safely extend their boundaries while assuring the child's feeling of personal control. An overly critical or controlling style of parenting constrains the emergence of a child's young sense of competence and, by extension, affects their self-esteem. Being handed a scribble drawing by a preschooler and told what it represents is emblematic. An appreciative, interested, positive response to the disordered marks is sustaining; disinterest or criticism undermines.

When pressure occurs, it is often from parents' having unrealistic expectations of how the child learns and develops, or a false sense of how little development has occurred and how the child has to work harder. Inadvertent pressure can be detrimental and cause tremendous frustration when, for example, parents try to lead a toddler into toilet training when the child has shown few signs of readiness, even if most of the children in his preschool class are out of diapers. Pressuring young children to give up pacifiers or another security object without giving thought to the child's readiness may also be quite anxiety provoking to them.

Well-intentioned pressure may be equally harmful later in childhood. Forcing children to participate in rigid, structured play, and sometimes classes or lessons, does not foster individual creativity or independence. Children are merely doing what the parents have arranged. Ideally, children should be encouraged to explore and occasionally take risks. They should be helped to build on their "islands of competence." Mistakes should be put into the context of a sincere effort and seen in terms of what can be learned rather than as a humiliation. Pressuring children to do things "right" or "perfectly" discourages normal, healthy, risk-taking behavior and interferes with future efforts by children to participate in activities unless they are certain they can succeed.

A variation on this theme is overprotection, where the parent controls the child's environment so as to reduce any risk of failure or discomfort to the child. This generally comes at the cost of sacrificing the experience of novel achievement and developing the competence to work through frustrations and disappointments. This has been shown to have a negative impact on self-esteem.

Communication That Builds Self-Esteem

Specific ways to communicate that build self-esteem include active listening, use of positive language, discarding "labels," use of encouragement rather than pressure, and the use of the "I" method of communication (Box 32-2). The pediatrician should coach parents that this is not a rigid code to be followed at all times and at great hazard, but rather that the goal is a "good enough" environment where well-intended parents put up a fairly consistent effort to be mindful of how they deal with their children. A useful way to set the correct tone with parents and caregivers is the use of strength-based counseling, where advice grows out of a focus on what parents are doing right.

Box 32-1. Encouraging Self-Esteem
Don'ts
Have negative expectations.
Focus on mistakes.
Expect perfection.
Overly protect children.
Dos
Show confidence in children's abilities.
Build on children's strengths.
Value children as they are.
Stimulate independence.

Box 32-2. Communication That Builds Self-Esteem
Active listening
Use of positive language
Discarding "labels"
Use of encouragement
Use of the "I" method of communication

The purpose of active listening is to hear the child's message and understand its meaning. Its success rests on a centered approach to important parenting moments: Parents must be attentive, stop what they are doing, and look directly at children. Nonverbal cues such as body posture and facial expression should be appreciated. If children are having trouble understanding their feelings, the parent should repeat what they hear them saying ("It sounds like…").

A nonjudgmental response, validating and non-dismissive, should be the goal of communication between primary caregivers and children. The basic message should be stated simply, clearly, and at a level that respects the maturity of the child. Words should be easily understood and spoken in a moderate tone, especially when discipline is necessary. Facial expression and body language should also be consistent with the message parents or caregivers are trying to convey.

The importance of positive language should be emphasized, even when disciplining children. For instance, when children are playing kick ball in the house, most parents initially reprimand children by yelling, "Don't play ball in the house!" or "Haven't I told you before? No ball playing inside!" While emotionally honest parenting in a loving context is the best parenting, there should be some awareness of when the parent is speaking in a reprimanding and negative fashion. Parents or other adults should tell children what they can do, what the limits are, and the reason for these rules. For example, caregivers should say: "You have to stop this right now. If you kick it inside, you may break a window or hurt yourself or someone else. You may kick the ball outside in the backyard." Communicating in a clear manner changes the tone of the interaction from a reprimand for being bad to one where rules are clarified to a child who wants to do the right thing.

Parents should praise their children for successes and achievements. Failures should be put into context whenever possible, although the acknowledgment of mistakes can be important. For example, correcting a child's homework assignment for errors should be done in a nonthreatening manner. Parents should involve the child in the review process rather than simply marking up the paper with a red pen and telling the child to redo the assignment. Negative labels have no helpful role. If children hear themselves referred to as "dumb-dumb" or "turkey" by their primary caregivers, not only are they having an undesirable behavior modeled, but they will feel undermined and wonder about the truth of such statements, no matter how innocuous they may initially seem to parents.

At the other extreme, parents should be cautioned against always speaking in the superlative to their child and staying blind to any shortcomings. Children are adept at seeing the world as it is. A failure

to see themselves reflected realistically by parents or caregivers may feed a kind of insecurity where despite the glowing language of the parents, the child feels insecure of their actual worth.

Talents and abilities should be recognized and highlighted. Children should know that parents have confidence in their abilities and that any display of effort is appreciated. Even small successes should be noted and not overshadowed by the large ones or the failures. Children thrive on the joy and pride they see in the eyes of their parents. Lack of encouragement can limit their optimism for continued success.

Many parenting courses teach primary caregivers to use the "I" method of communication, which requires that parents explain their feelings to children rather than blame them for their actions. This approach is believed to be less threatening and demeaning for children, especially in situations requiring discipline. The "I" method has 4 recommended steps.

1. Statement of behavior or situation to be addressed (eg, "When you…")
2. Statement in specific terms how one feels about the effect of the situation on oneself (eg, "I feel…")
3. Statement of reason (eg, "because…")
4. Statement of expectations (eg, "I would like…" or "I want…")

Using this approach, a parent's statement might be: "When you speak so unkindly, I feel upset because I would never speak with you in that way. It makes you seem like the kind of person that you are not. I would like you to speak with me in the way we all try to speak with you, no matter how angry you feel."

Vulnerable Times in a Child's Life

There are certain instances when a child's self-esteem can be particularly vulnerable. The primary care provider should be especially cognizant of circumstances where a child may feel shame, confusion, or guilt for problems occurring in them or their family. Problems with self-esteem may be found in overweight children and in those with conditions such as enuresis or encopresis. Negative experiences in school and at home can predispose a child to feelings of shame and worthlessness. Marital conflict, divorce, or the abuse of a parent may negatively influence the self-esteem of children who may feel responsible for the problem. In such circumstances, parents are often concerned about the impact on the child, which provides an opportunity to work together to minimize negative effects. Honest, open communication with parents can reinforce the need for sensitive support of the child and help them set priorities or rehearse how they will talk with the child about the matters at hand (see Chapter 123).

Discipline and Self-Esteem

Parents should consider their understanding of the complex relationship between discipline and self-esteem, and they should be questioned about their impressions of their child's independence and competence. As children grow, so does their ability to act responsibly and their ability to maintain greater self-control. This central insight is an important way to help parents see beyond discipline in simply punitive terms. Several different approaches to discipline have been adapted by various ethnic, cultural, religious, and socioeconomic groups. While a discussion of each of these methods is beyond the scope of this chapter (see Chapter 36), it is important to explore strategies with parents and caregivers. Regarding self-esteem, however, children do best when they are provided with clear, consistent guidelines for their behavior while at the same time being encouraged to do well, pursue their interests, and increase their abilities. They do this even better when they see this modeled in the adults around them. Parents and other caregivers should remember that certain methods of discipline, particularly if harsh or shame provoking, can be very destructive to a child's self-esteem. For instance, making an enuretic child sleep in wet bed sheets or reprimanding a child with physical punishment (eg, spanking) in public places can be demeaning.

CASE RESOLUTION

In the case history, the health maintenance visit provides the perfect opportunity for promoting parental support of their child's self-esteem. The shy child should be approached by giving sincere general compliments (eg, "My goodness, you are so big." or to a girl dressed in all pink, "What a beautiful pink outfit!") and, in the interview, inviting her to tell you some things about herself (eg, "What are your favorite things?" "What is your favorite color?"), while employing humor and enthusiasm to engage her in some details. This models interactions, which allow the child to demonstrate her autonomy, with the hope that this approach will be repeated by the parent at home. The health care provider can reassure the girl and her mother that the child's overall health and development are normal. In addition, once the careful, protective experience the parents have managed for their child is appreciated, the practitioner should attempt to normalize the child's behavior for the parent. Concrete suggestions should be offered for positive communication, such as minimizing "don't" and "no" phrases and being cognizant of how one speaks about the daughter. The parents should be encouraged to think about the child's temperament when considering involvement in multiple school activities but reminded that they have not yet seen her in an independent setting, where she may negotiate very well and show a sociability not yet evident at home.

Selected References

American Academy of Pediatrics Committee on Psychosocial Aspects of Child and Family Health. Guidance for effective discipline. *Pediatrics.* 1998;101:723–728

Berman BD, Winkleby M, Chesterman E, Boyce WT. After-school child care and self-esteem in school-age children. *Pediatrics.* 1992;89:654–659

Briggs DC. *Your Child's Self-Esteem.* New York, NY: Doubleday; 1970

Brooks RB. Self-esteem during the school years: its normal development and hazardous decline. *Pediatr Clin North Am.* 1992;39:537–550

Brooks RB. *The Self-Esteem Teacher.* Circle Pines, MN: American Guidance Service; 1981

Coleman WL, Lindsay RL. Making friends: helping children develop interpersonal skills. *Contemp Pediatr.* 1998;15:111–129

Howard BJ. Discipline in early childhood. *Pediatr Clin North Am.* 1991;38:1351–1369

Sieving RE, Zirbel-Donish ST. Development and enhancement of self-esteem in children. *J Pediatr Health Care.* 1990;4:290–296

Sibling Rivalry

Carol D. Berkowitz, MD

CASE STUDY

An 8-year-old boy is brought to the office for an annual checkup. During the course of the evaluation, his mother complains that her son and his 6-year-old sister are always fighting. She says her son hits his sister and pulls her hair, and nothing she does prevents them from fighting. The boy is a B+ student and has no behavior problems in school. The medical history and the physical examination are completely normal.

Questions

1. What is sibling rivalry?
2. What is the physician's role in counseling a family about sibling rivalry?
3. What is the role of anticipatory guidance in preparing older children for the birth of a new sister or brother?
4. What are some practical suggestions to share with parents about sibling rivalry?

Sibling rivalry refers to the rivalry between siblings based on the need for **parental love** and **esteem.** Historical examples of sibling rivalry include relationships between the biblical figures Cain and Abel, Joseph and his brothers, and Jacob and Esau. Sibling rivalry is also noteworthy in pairs of celebrities, such as actresses Joan Fontaine (Academy Award winner for *Suspicion)* and her older sister, Olivia de Havilland (Academy Award winner for *To Each His Own* and *The Heiress*). Their relationship was termed one of the most dysfunctional sibling relationships in Hollywood, and may have had its roots in their simultaneous nomination for an Academy Award in 1942. By 1975 the sisters were no longer in communication with each other.

Sibling rivalry is a **universal phenomenon** occurring even in the animal kingdom. For instance, the firstborn eaglet pushes the other eaglets out of the nest as soon as they are hatched as a way of ensuring an adequate food supply. In humans, the fear of displacement, dethronement, and loss of love occurs with the birth of a new brother or sister, leading to sibling rivalry. Older children fear they are not good enough and need to be replaced. Such feelings lead to a **fear of abandonment.** Jealousy also plays a role, and older children may be angry with younger siblings for displacing them within the family.

Sibling rivalry frequently has a negative effect on parents because it is hard for them to see one of their children hurt, even if it is by a sister or a brother. The challenge for parents is to know when, and when not, to intervene and what strategies to use to minimize conflicts. Physicians can help by offering **anticipatory guidance** to all parents and specific recommendations to parents who are experiencing such individual problems.

Epidemiology

Sibling rivalry is a universal phenomenon, and a number of factors influence its development. Time interval between children affects the degree of rivalry, as does the age of the older children. Toddlers who are entering the "**terrible twos**" may have a particularly hard time mastering independence and tolerating the presence of their younger sibling. Close spacing results in more problems, particularly when the children are fewer than 2 years apart. In such situations, older children still have dependency needs, often feel less secure, and experience a need for maternal attention. They stay closer to mothers, are less playful, and are more tense. Closely spaced children engage in less spontaneous play, seem more angry, and issue sterner commands to their playmates.

Position in the family also influences sibling rivalry. Middle children experience what is referred to as "**middle-child syndrome**"; they lack the prestige of older children or the privileges of younger ones. These children are often least secure and strive hardest to gain affection. Special difficulties may develop if middle children are the same gender as older ones. Middle children grow up to be flexible, adaptable, and good negotiators. In myths and folklore, youngest children are "favorites." They are often the ones defended by parents when there are bouts of fighting.

Twins rarely present a problem of sibling rivalry; instead they have a problem maintaining their individuality. However, sets of twins create problems for older siblings because they are not as unique as the pair of twins.

Step-siblings also present a unique problem in sibling rivalry. Children of divorce frequently feel abandoned by one parent and in competition for the time and love of the custodial parent (see Chapter 123). Competition with step-siblings is especially difficult if the step-siblings are in the same home.

Issues of sibling conflict change over time. Toddlers are protective of their toys and belongings and are particularly upset when a younger sibling touches their possessions. Sharing is a challenging theme of the toddler years. Children during their school-aged years are concerned about equity and fairness. They may be upset by what they construe as preferential treatment, for instance when a 1-year-old sibling is not expected to put their toys away. Adolescents with their additional responsibilities including minding younger siblings may resent the siblings for imposing on their time.

Clinical Presentation

Parental complaints related to sibling rivalry consist of fighting between siblings, including physical violence and verbal abuse, bickering, and regression to immature behavioral patterns. Although such immature behavior occurs most often following the birth of a new baby, it may also be apparent if one sibling is receiving more attention, such as during an illness or after a major accomplishment. Regressive behavior includes bedwetting, drinking from a bottle, and wanting to be carried to bed. Substitution behavior, such as nail-biting, in place of biting the new sibling, may occur after the birth of a new baby.

Before the birth of a new baby, parents may complain that their children exhibit temper tantrums, irritability, and solemnness. They may mimic the pregnancy by eating a lot and putting a pillow under their clothes. In addition, children may have psychosomatic complaints such as stomachaches or headaches. Risk factors for maladjustment following the addition of a sibling include family discord, physical or emotional exhaustion in parents, and housing insecurity. Conversely, a good marital relationship and family support facilitates the adjustment to new siblings.

Differential Diagnosis

Dilemmas concerning the correct diagnosis of sibling rivalry most often relate to the appearance of behavioral changes such as regressive or aggressive patterns after the birth of a new sibling. For example, a child who was previously toilet trained may become incontinent of urine. Although urinary tract infection may be considered in the diagnosis, a careful history concerning the birth of the sibling reveals the correct etiology.

Evaluation

The evaluation of children with suspected sibling rivalry involves a history of the problem and parental strategies for dealing with the difficulties. The parent should be particularly queried about one-on-one opportunities between parents and individual children. The physical examination and laboratory assessment are noncontributory.

Management

The focus of management is to allow the parents to recognize the normalcy of sibling rivalry while helping them define the behaviors that are acceptable and not acceptable within the family context. Parents may not appreciate their child's fear of loss of parental love.

They should be told that many children think, "If I am so good, why do I have to be replaced?" Parents should be asked to empathize by imagining how they would feel if their spouse brought home another mate, even if they were reassured about being loved. Physicians can also help parents deal with sibling rivalry by having them consider their treatment of children in terms of uniqueness versus uniformity and quality versus inequality. In general, parents should be advised to set the ground rules for acceptable behavior. Such rules include no hitting, punching, hair pulling, name-calling, cursing, or door slamming. There may be a neutral area in the home that can be set aside for arbitration should disagreements arise. Moving to a neutral area also allows for some time to cool off.

Birth of New Siblings

Parents may notice the behavioral changes in their children before the birth of the new sibling. These changes depend on the age of the children and the presence of other siblings. Children should be told about the upcoming birth. The timing depends on the children's age; younger children do not need much lead time. Some studies have evaluated the inclusion of older children in the birthing process. The results of these studies vary, but they suggest that children younger than 4 years need their mother for emotional support and are concerned about her physical exertion during the birthing process. Some older children may also want to distance themselves from the actual events.

Physicians should suggest that older children be involved in planning for the arrival of the new baby as a means of minimizing their feelings of exclusion. For example, they can help purchase clothes or prepare the baby's room. Physicians should also suggest that parents purchase a gift for older children that represents a present from the new baby such as tee shirts that announce the older sibling's new status, such as "big sister" or "big brother." In addition, older siblings may be given a doll to serve as a baby they can care for. Parents should point out the advantages of being older with comments such as, "You can stay up later" or "You can walk and play with all these toys." Frequently, the birth of a new baby is met with regressive behavior in older siblings. Regressive behavior should be handled with tolerance and a realization that symptoms resolve with time.

Once the mother goes to the hospital, she should be advised to maintain contact with older children by telephoning. Many hospitals now allow for visitation by siblings. At present, hospital stays are so brief that this period of separation is much shorter than previously. Household changes that may be necessitated by the birth of the new baby, such as room changes, the substitution of a bed for a crib, and entrance into nursery school, should be made before the arrival of the new baby.

Rivalry Between Older Children

Physicians need to consider individual parenting techniques when counseling parents of older children. Parents who compare one child with the other may foster contentious behavior, and those who strive to treat all children equally may inadvertently perpetuate rivalry.

Children need to feel that they are unique rather than ordinary. For example, parents who buy both children the same presents may think they are preventing rivalry from developing, but they are actually depriving each child of a sense of uniqueness. The harder parents try to be uniform, the more vigilantly the children may look for inequality. Each child needs a parent's undivided attention, time alone together. Siblings also need time apart from each other, and they should be encouraged to hold separate play dates and individual activities. Not all children in a family need piano lessons and soccer practice. Individuality and uniqueness are important. The more agreeable a parent-child relationship, the more agreeable a sibling-sibling relationship, because each child has good self-esteem. Practitioners should recommend uniqueness and quality in each parent-child relationship.

Parents sometimes have to deal with sibling rivalry between older children. Physicians should reassure parents that these older children should be allowed to vent their negative feelings toward each other. For example, if a girl refers to her brother by saying "I hate him," the parents should respond by validating these emotions and saying something like, "It sounds as if he's done something to really annoy you." Parents should also be advised not to take sides. They should examine how they usually respond to squabbling between siblings. Is one child's name always called first during a fight? Do they perpetuate sibling rivalry by using certain nicknames (eg, "turkey brain") or other derogatory terms? Parents should assume that both parties are at least partially guilty and should not allow themselves to be drawn into the fight as referees. Parents can respond to a request for arbitration with a statement such as, "I wasn't here when things started, so I don't know who is right or wrong." The parents should also advise siblings that they do not have to be friends with one another, but they should not hurt each other's feelings.

Anticipatory guidance helps parents anticipate conflictual situations such as who sits where during long car rides and who holds the remote control device. Children should be allowed to work out a solution by themselves, with the stipulation that the parents will solve the problem if the children do not reach an agreement. If fights between siblings have recurrent themes (eg, which television shows to watch [who controls the remote] or video games to play), parents can devise a weekly schedule. Failure to abide by the schedule means both children forfeit the activity. Box 33-1 lists suggestions for parents who are seeking advice about fighting between children.

Prognosis

Although sibling rivalry may last for years, most siblings become good friends as adults. Rarely, mental health services are needed especially if the sibling conflict has lead to marital discord, there is concern about physical or severe emotional harm, or there is evidence of another psychiatric disorder such as depression. Learning how to negotiate with one's siblings enables children to develop skills to collaborate with peers and colleagues as adolescents and adults.

Box 33-1. Coping With Rivalry Between Siblings: Physicians' Advice to Parents

Dos
- Allow children to vent negative feelings.
- Encourage children to develop solutions.
- Anticipate problem situations.
- Foster individuality in each child.
- Spend time with children individually.
- Compliment children when they are playing together.
- Tell children about the conflicts you had with your siblings when you were children.
- Define acceptable and unacceptable behavior.

Don'ts
- Take sides.
- Serve as a referee.
- Foster rivalry.
- Use derogatory names.
- Permit physical or verbal abuse between siblings.

CASE RESOLUTION

In the case history presented at the beginning of the chapter, the mother should be advised not to serve as a referee. She should learn how to validate each child's feelings about the other. The physician can help her by talking to her son about his feelings. She should be advised to have a discussion with her children during which each child has the opportunity to define areas of conflict and the means to resolve them. The mother has the right and responsibility to prohibit physical fighting and encourage verbal dialogue.

Selected References

Adams MM. *Sister for Sale*. Grand Rapids, MI: ZonderKidz; 2002

Anderson JE. Sibling rivalry: when the family circle becomes a boxing ring. *Contemp Pediatr*. 2006;23:72–90

Dunn J. Annotation: sibling influences on childhood development. *J Child Psychol Psychiatry*. 1988;29:119–127

Goldenthal P. *Beyond Sibling Rivalry: How to Help Your Child Become Cooperative, Caring and Compassionate*. New York, NY: Henry Holt and Company; 2000

Hass E, Light P. Talking about the new baby. *Parents Magazine*. 1983;58:68–70

Leung AK, Robson WL. Sibling rivalry. *Clin Pediatr (Phila)*. 1991;30:314–317

Pakula LC. Sibling rivalry. *Pediatr Rev*. 1992;13:72–73

Samalin N, McCormick P. How to cure sibling fights. *Parents Magazine*. 1993;68:147–150

Schmitt BD. Sibling rivalry toward a new baby. *Contemp Pediatr*. 1990;7:111–112

Schmitt BD. When siblings quarrel. *Contemp Pediatr*. 1991;8:73–74

Toilet Training

Lynne M. Smith, MD

CASE STUDY

A 2-year-old boy is brought to the office for a well-child visit. His mother, who is about to begin toilet training her son, asks your advice. The mother says that by the time her daughter was 2 she was already toilet trained, and she wants to know if training her son will be any different. The boy was the product of a full-term pregnancy and a normal delivery. He has been in good health, and his immunizations are up to date. He is developmentally normal, uses some 2-word phrases, and has been walking since the age of 13 months. His physical examination is normal.

Questions

1. When should physicians begin discussing toilet training with parents?
2. What factors help determine children's readiness to begin toilet training?
3. Is toilet training in boys different from toilet training in girls?
4. What are some of the methods used to toilet train children?

The age at which toilet training is carried out is culturally determined. Some cultures train children at a very early age. For example, in the East African Digo culture, some children between 2 to 3 months of age are conditioned to urinate or defecate when placed in certain positions. Similar conditioning practices are carried out in China. Chinese children are kept without diapers, and when caregivers who are holding them sense a change in their bodies in response to a need to eliminate, they place their children in an appropriate position. In addition, children are dressed in clothing that facilitates toileting. Split pants, with the back and bottom portion missing, are used so that children can squat and eliminate without removing complicated clothing.

American culture has emphasized the learning aspects of toilet training as opposed to the conditioning aspects. This training focuses on the cognitive development of children and children's readiness to learn the complexity of the task. It has been demonstrated that infants as young as 6 months can be trained to signal the need to urinate or defecate and suppress emptying for brief periods.

Toilet training is potentially both a rewarding and frustrating experience for children and parents. Parents may have unrealistic expectations of their children's capability or may be very intolerant of normal accidents that occur in the training process. It is important for physicians to introduce the topic of toilet training early on to prevent these unrealistic expectations. Children's refusal to toilet train or accidents related to toilet training are often cited as a precipitating event for child physical abuse. It is recommended that the issue of toilet training be introduced and anticipatory guidance provided by the age of 9 months.

Epidemiology

The age at which children are toilet trained varies depending on social considerations and social pressures. Prior to the 1920s, the American approach to toilet training was permissive. This attitude then changed, and the methods became more rigorous, requiring that children be trained at an earlier age. In 1947 only 5% of children were not trained by 33 months of age, but by 1975, this figure had increased to 42%. Currently approximately 25% of American children are toilet trained at 24 months and 98% by 36 months. Cultural and socioeconomic factors also influence parental beliefs about toilet training. Horn and colleagues found that white race and higher family income were associated with parents favoring later initiation of toilet training. There has been a renewed interest in earlier toilet training in the United States. This has been attributed to 3 societal factors: the lower cost and increased options for child care and schooling associated with children once toilet trained, concerns about contagious illnesses such as hepatitis and infectious diarrhea in child care facilities where diapers are changed, and the adverse environmental effects of nonbiodegradable disposable diapers. There may be some reversal in these trends related to the development of highly absorbent, biodegradable disposable diapers that are also flushable, and the marketing of pull-ups to children as old as 4 years of age.

As a general rule, girls are trained a bit earlier than boys, but only by a matter of a few months. Most children (80%) are trained simultaneously for bladder and bowel control. Approximately 12% are trained first for bowel control and about 8% for bladder control. Girls achieve nighttime continence at a younger age than boys.

Pathophysiology

Toilet training involves the ability both to inhibit a normal reflex release action and then relax the inhibition of the involved muscles. For the process to be successful, a certain degree of neurologic and biological development is essential. Myelinization of the pyramidal tracts and conditioned reflex sphincter control are necessary. Voluntary control is evidenced by myelinization of the pyramidal tracts by the age of 12 to 18 months. Conditioned reflex sphincter control occurs by 9 months of age and voluntary cooperation between 12 to 15 months of age. In assessing the neurologic development of children, walking is viewed as one of the milestones that indicates motor readiness for toilet training.

Toilet training depends on both physiological and psychological readiness. Cognitive development is assessed by a child's ability to follow certain instructions.

Two years of age has been suggested as the appropriate age to initiate toilet training in most children. Toilet training usually takes 2 weeks to 2 months to learn, although training may occur in less time using more intense conditioning methods.

Differential Diagnosis

The differential diagnosis of toilet-training difficulties focuses on factors that contribute to a delay in acquisition of skills. Physicians should look for associated symptoms, such as dysuria, a weak urinary stream, constantly wet underwear, or fecal soiling, when assessing children who continue to manifest signs of either urinary or stool incontinence. In addition, it is important to determine if children are essentially toilet trained but are having intermittent accidents.

The most common cause of isolated daytime wetting in previously trained children is urinary tract infection (**UTI**) (see Chapter 41). **Chemical urethritis** may also be associated with urinary incontinence. **Stress incontinence,** which has also been called *giggle incontinence,* may result in wetting. **Urgency incontinence** occurs when children delay going to the bathroom and then are unable to hold urine any longer. Some children have ectopic ureters, which can empty into the lower portion of the bladder, vagina, or urethra and cause a constant dribble of urine. **Labial fusion** may also be associated with daytime wetting. Urine pools behind the fused labia during voiding, and when children stand up, the urine exits. Children with **neurogenic bladders** may also have symptoms of daytime enuresis.

Stooling accidents may be associated with chronic constipation and overflow incontinence or with Hirschsprung disease (See Chapter 42).

Evaluation

History

Typically developing toddlers should be assessed for both their physiological and psychological readiness to initiate toilet training, as well as any underlying medical conditions that may affect their ability to learn toileting skills at the customary age. Physicians should provide anticipatory guidance to parents about toileting readiness. Affirmative answers should be obtained to the following 3 questions:

1. Do children exhibit bladder control as evidenced by (1) periods of dryness that last up to 2 hours and (2) facial expressions that show their physiological response to the elimination process?
2. Do children have the motor skills necessary to get around? This essentially involves the children's ability to walk and remove their clothing.
3. Do children have the cognitive ability to understand the task at hand?

Cognitive ability can be assessed by giving children 10 one-step tasks and seeing if they are able to carry out at least 8 of the 10 tasks (Box 34-1). The ability to carry out these tasks does not ensure a willingness to be toilet trained.

Box 34-1. Requests or Imperatives Used to Help Assess Toilet-Training Readiness	
Bring me the ball.	Give the pen to your Mom.
Go to the door.	Put the ball on the table.
Sit on the chair.	Put the doll on the floor.
Pick up the doll.	Take off your shoes.
Open the door.	Open the book.

Stress in the home may negatively affect a toddler's ability to master the task of toilet training. The physician might counsel a family to delay toilet training if the family has moved recently, the birth of a new baby is expected, or there has been a major family crisis such as a death or serious illness.

Children who have had difficulties with toilet training need to undergo a similar assessment.

Physical Examination

A physical examination to rule out underlying problems such as spina bifida occulta, which may be associated with a neurogenic bladder, should be performed. A careful examination of the genitalia is important in children who are having urinary incontinence to determine if conditions such as labial fusion are evident. In children who are having stooling problems, physicians should check for an abdomen with feces-filled intestines, a sign of obstipation. In addition, a rectal examination should be considered to determine the presence of hard or impacted stools or any other abnormalities in the anal area.

Laboratory Tests

Although a laboratory assessment is not indicated in normal toddlers who are being toilet trained, diagnostic studies may be appropriate in children who are having problems with training. In older children, urinalysis may show evidence of a UTI.

Management

Physicians should help parents understand the appropriate approach to the toilet-training process. Unfortunately, most parents do not obtain the necessary advice from physicians. In one report, no parents attending a clinic and only 7% of parents in a private practice received advice about toilet training from their physicians. Therefore, it is important for physicians to initiate the discussion early enough to prevent the development of any problems.

There are 2 contrasting styles of toilet training. The first method described by Azrin and Foxx uses intense conditioning methods. The 4 components of the method include increasing the amount of fluids consumed, regularly scheduled times for toileting, positive reinforcement when successful, and time-out from positive reinforcement/cleanliness training following accidents. Though this method has been effective in training normal children as well as individuals with mental disabilities, it is not recommended for training typically developing children.

The second method, endorsed by the American Academy of Pediatrics, is a child-oriented approach that stresses the child's physiological and psychological readiness to toilet train. This method involves gradual training and emphasizes the use of **rewards,** not punishments. Children with autism who do not understand the social reward system advocated by this method may benefit from the intense conditioning methods described by Azrin and Foxx.

When toilet training typically developing children, parents should be advised to take the following approach:

1. Teach children the **appropriate vocabulary** related to the toilet-training process. This could include words such as "pee," "poop," "dry," "wet," "clean," "messy," and "potty."

2. Tell children what the **purpose of the potty** is. Placing the contents of a soiled diaper into the toilet can educate them on the purpose of the potty. In general, a child potty chair should be purchased. The potty chair has a number of advantages over the toilet. Parents can encourage children to decorate the potty and put their names on it. The potty can be kept in a place where children spend much of their time, not necessarily in the bathroom. Children can sit on the potty and have their feet on the floor, which is more physiologically sound and gives them a greater sense of security. Children should be allowed to sit on the potty with their clothes on for about a week before the process of toilet training begins. Then children should sit on the potty without their clothes on, but no attempt to catch either stool or urine should be made. Boys should learn to urinate in the seated position because they may resist sitting for defecation.

   When away from home the potty chair should be packed to maintain the established routine. It is important that all individuals caring for the child (grandparents, babysitters) understand the parents' plans for toilet training.

   Toilet adapter rings can be used if the family is resistant to using a potty chair, or if the transition from a potty chair to the toilet is likely to be stressful as is true for many children with autism. Adapter rings fit directly onto the toilet and do not require emptying as do separate potty chairs. They require that the toddler climb up on the toilet, and they need to be removed for others to use the toilet. A stool should be used to aid in climbing onto the toilet as well as to provide more leverage while defecating.

3. Encourage cleanliness and dryness by **changing children frequently.** Parents should ask their children whether they need to be changed using the appropriate vocabulary. This phase is important to continue as the toilet-training process proceeds. Some parents mistakenly do not change their soiled children as a means of punishing them for having accidents. This gives children a confusing message about the need for cleanliness.

4. Explain the **connection between dry pants and going to the potty** to children. Children should understand that dry pants feel good and that they can keep their pants dry by going to the potty.

5. Help children understand the **physiological signals** for using the toilet. Parents can facilitate this by observing children's behavior around the time of elimination and making comments such as, "When you jump up and down like that, Mommy knows you have to go to the bathroom."

6. Children must have the physiological ability to postpone the "urge to go." This usually occurs when children have the ability to delay voiding for at least 2 hours. Parents then can initiate toilet training by taking children to the bathroom at 2-hour intervals. In addition, children should sit on the toilet immediately after naps and 20 minutes after meals. Children should not be left on the toilet for more than 5 minutes and should be permitted to get up if they want. While sitting on the potty, they can be entertained with reading a story or playing games. It is helpful to have designated toys or books enjoyed only when the child is sitting on the potty. Parents are encouraged to rotate the toys so potty training continues to be interesting to the child.

Additional suggestions involve allowing children to have their clothes off and keeping the potty chair near them during play. This facilitates using the potty and is reminiscent of the practice of using split pants in China.

Children who use the potty successfully should be rewarded. Rewards can be in the form of verbal comments such as "Mommy is so proud of you"; hand clapping; or the use of star charts that can be redeemed for rewards. Children can be consulted about what rewards they like. Punishment should not be used, particularly physical punishment. One report indicates that 15% of parents of clinic patients believe that spanking their children for accidents is acceptable. Parental disapproval of accidents can be articulated; however, parents should understand that accidents may continue to occur for months. Regression in a toilet-trained child may also occur with stressors such as a recent move, new sibling, or divorce.

If children are trained on a potty chair, they can generally begin using a toilet between 2½ to 3½ years of age. Children should wash their hands following sessions sitting on the toilet. Children can also use training pants, which are thickened underwear, or pull-ups, which are diaper-like underwear, rather than diapers. Pull-ups are now marketed to children as old as 4 to 5 years of age, and there is anecdotal evidence to suggest that the age of completion of toilet training may be delayed by the use of pull-ups. Regular underwear is promoted as advantageous because it feels different from diapers and encourages the use of the potty. Using a bigger size or snipping the waistband facilitates children's ability to remove their underpants and can be recommended.

If children demonstrate resistance to toilet training, the process should be delayed for 1 to 2 months. Children who learn how to withhold need additional time to learn how to relax their sphincter when sitting on a potty. It is important for parents to avoid an aggressiveness/resistance struggle, because this then may become the source of future bowel problems, including constipation. Children who are regular, particularly those who have a bowel movement at the same time every day, are more easily toilet trained. Children who prefer to stand in a corner to defecate should be commended for recognizing their physiological urge. However, parents should be aware that children who hide while stooling in their diaper are more likely to be constipated, which contributes to toileting refusal. Successful treatment of constipation may decrease the incidence of toileting refusal.

Some children seem fearful of certain aspects of the toilet-training process. These include fear of falling into the toilet (this is circumvented with the use of a potty) or fear of the loud noise of the flush. Allowing the child to flush the toilet without using it may dispel the fear. Some children become fascinated with flushing or rolling toilet paper, and parents have to prevent children from wasting water or paper.

Parents should suggest that children stand fully clothed in the bathroom as an initial step in encouraging their use of a potty.

One of the major components of toilet training children is **modeling.** Children should be allowed to enter the bathroom with the parents and even sit on the potty as one or the other parent sits on the toilet. Some children who are very strong-willed and independent, coupled with perfectionist parents, may have problems with toilet training.

Special considerations have to be made for children attending child care. Their teachers should be advised about the toilet training. Children should have "open bathroom privileges," which means that they should be permitted to leave the room to go to the bathroom without raising their hands or other reminders. Child care offers the advantage of peer modeling and peer pressure during the toilet-training process. Potty chairs should not be used in child care settings because of the risk of infectious diseases.

Medications have a limited role in toilet training. Some physicians recommend the use of drugs to increase bladder capacity. Although oxybutynin (Ditropan) increases bladder capacity and decreases the frequency of bladder contraction, it should not be used because it does not actually assist children with the toilet-training process. However, children who are constipated may require stool softeners such as mineral oil or the addition of fiber bulk to their diet to facilitate the stooling process. Physicians should see children who seem to have toilet-training problems on a weekly or biweekly basis until they show improvement.

Parents can also be referred to the many books on toilet training, particularly if problems develop. Many books are geared for children to help them understand their body and the elimination process. Videotapes are also available to help children with toilet training. Children may also have the opportunity to practice with dolls designed to wet or poop after being fed.

Prognosis

All normal children are eventually toilet trained. The age when this occurs varies and is significant only if it restricts children from participating in school.

CASE RESOLUTION

The mother in the case history should be advised that this is a good time to initiate the toilet-training process. She should be told that boys, as a group, are successfully toilet trained at a later age than girls. Her son can be assessed to see if he can follow at least 8 out of 10 instructions (see Box 34-1). If he can, the mother should be given the stepwise approach to initiating the toilet-training process. The mother should be informed that nighttime continence can take months to years after daytime continence is achieved.

Selected References

Physicians

Azrin NH, Foxx RM. *Toilet Training in Less Than a Day.* New York, NY: Simon & Schuster; 1974

Blum NJ, Taubman B, Nemeth N. During toilet training, constipation occurs before stool toileting refusal. *Pediatrics.* 2004;113:e520–e522

Blum NJ, Taubman B, Nemeth N. Why is toilet training occurring at older ages? A study of factors associated with later training. *J Pediatr.* 2004;145:107–111

Brazelton TB, Christophersen ER, Frauman AC, et al. Instruction, timeliness, and medical influences affecting toilet training. *Pediatrics.* 1999;103:1353–1358

Horn IB, Brenner R, Rao M, Cheng TL. Beliefs about the appropriate age for initiating toilet training: are there racial and socioeconomic differences? *J Pediatr.* 2006;149:165–168

Luxam M, Christophersen E. Behavioral toilet training in early childhood: research, practice, and implications. *Dev Behav Pediatr.* 1994;15:370–378

Macias MM, Roberts KM, Saylor CF, Fussell JJ. Toilet concerns, parenting stress, and behavior problems in children with special health care needs. *Clin Pediatr (Phila).* 2006;45:415–422

Michel RS. Toilet training. *Pediatr Rev.* 1999;20:240–245

Schonwald A, Sherritt L, Stadtler A, Bridgemohan C. Factors associated with difficult toilet training. *Pediatrics.* 2004;113:1753–1757

Schum TR, Kolb TM, McAulffe TL, et al. Sequential acquisition of toilet training skills: a descriptive study of gender and age differences in normal children. *Pediatrics.* 2002;109:e48

Stadtler AC, Gorski PA, Brazelton TB. Toilet training methods, clinical interventions, and recommendations. *Pediatrics.* 1999;103:1359–1368

Taubman B, Blum N, Nemeth N. Children who hide while defecating before they have completed toilet training. A prospective study. *Arch Pediatr Adolesc Med.* 2003;157:1190–1192

Taubman B, Blum NJ, Nemeth N. Stool toileting refusal. A prospective intervention targeting parental behavior. *Arch Pediatr Adolesc Med.* 2003;157:1193–1196

Toilet training guidelines: clinicians—the role of the clinician in toilet training. *Pediatrics.* 1999;103:1364–1366

Toilet training guidelines: day care providers—the role of the day care provider in toilet training. *Pediatrics.* 1999;103:1367–1368

Toilet training guidelines: parents—the role of the parents in toilet training. *Pediatrics.* 1999;103:1362–1363

Parents and Children

American Academy of Pediatrics. *Guide to Toilet Training.* Wolraich ML, ed. Elk Grove Village, IL: American Academy of Pediatrics; 2003

Brooks JG. *I'm a Big Kid Now.* Neenah, WI: Kimberly-Clark Corporation; 1990

Frankel A. *Once Upon a Potty.* Hauppauge, NY: Barron's Educational Series, Inc.; 1980

Mack A. *Toilet Learning: The Picture Book Technique for Children and Parents.* Boston, MA: Little, Brown and Company; 1978

Mayer G, Mayer M. *The New Potty.* New York, NY: Golden Book Publishing Company, Inc; 1992

Miller V. *On Your Potty.* Cambridge, MA: Candlewick Press; 1994

Rogers F. *Going to the Potty.* New York, NY: Penguin Putnam Books for Young Readers; 1986

Smith DC, McClure D. *Monkey Learns to Potty.* Knoxville, TN: PottyMD LLC; 2004

Crying and Colic

Geeta Grover, MD

CASE STUDY

The parents of a 2-week-old infant bring their son to the emergency department because he has been crying persistently for the past 4 hours. He has no history of fever, vomiting, diarrhea, upper respiratory tract infection, or change in feeding. The infant is breastfed.

On physical examination, the infant appears well developed and well nourished. His weight is 7 lb, 7 oz—7 oz more than when he was born. Although he is fussy and crying, he is afebrile with normal vital signs. The remainder of the physical examination is within normal limits.

Questions

1. What is the normal crying pattern in young infants?
2. What is colic?
3. What conditions are associated with prolonged crying in young infants?
4. What are key factors in the history of crying infants?
5. What laboratory tests are indicated in crying infants?
6. List a few of the management strategies that can be used by parents to soothe their crying or colicky infants.

Crying, an important method of communication between infants and caregivers, is nonspecific, and many stimuli can produce the same response (eg, hunger, fatigue, pain). Parents report that they can discriminate among various types of cries in their infants. Crying can be divided into 3 categories: (1) normal or physiological crying, (2) excessive crying secondary to distress (eg, hunger) or disease, and (3) excessive crying without an apparent cause.

The difference between normal and excessive crying may be more qualitative than quantitative. Deciding whether crying is excessive varies with parents' expectations and thresholds. Expressed parental concern about extreme crying or fussiness requires attention. If parents complain that infants cry inconsolably or continuously as well as excessively, the crying may have an underlying organic etiology.

Colic, a poorly understood, benign, self-limited condition, falls into the third category. It manifests as unexplained crying or fussing in infants that usually occurs in the late afternoon or evening. During an episode of colic, infants cry and may either draw the knees up to the chest or rigidly stiffen the legs, flex the elbows, clench the fists, and turn red (Figure 35-1). Although infants may appear to be totally miserable during an episode of colic, they are otherwise healthy, eat well, and demonstrate good weight gain.

Epidemiology

Qualitatively, **excessive crying** is any amount of crying that concerns or worries parents. Quantitatively, definitions of excessive crying have been based on the results of Brazelton's study of normal infants. Excessive crying begins at 2 weeks of age (median daily crying time about 2 hours per day), peaks at 6 weeks of age (median daily crying time about 3 hours per day), and then decreases to less than 1 hour per day by 12 weeks of age. Apparently, more crying occurs during the evening hours, especially between the ages of 3 and 6 weeks.

Figure 35-1. **Colicky infant.**

Although many infants exhibit a fairly similar pattern of fussiness that peaks at about 6 weeks of age, infants with colic tend to be inconsolable for longer periods and cry with more intensity. **Colic** affects 10% to 20% of infants younger than 3 months. There is no seasonal variation in its occurrence, and breastfed and formula-fed infants are affected equally. Colic usually begins at 2 to 3 weeks, peaks at 6 to 8 weeks, and resolves by 3 to 4 months of age. In studies of infant colic, the definition of colic that is cited most frequently is the Wessel definition (Wessel MA, et al, 1954), which describes colicky infants as having unexplained paroxysmal bouts of fussing and crying that last for more than 3 hours a day, for more than 3 days a week, and for more than 3 weeks' duration ("rule of threes").

Clinical Presentation

Colicky infants are otherwise healthy infants younger than 3 months who cry or fuss inconsolably for extended periods, usually during the afternoon or evening. The crying usually resolves within a few hours.

Pathophysiology

Crying is a complex vocalization that changes during the first year of life as infants develop. In the first few weeks of life, crying is a signal that infants are experiencing a disturbance in homeostatic regulation (eg, hunger, discomfort). As infants mature and begin to differentiate internal from external stimuli, crying may also be an indication of too little or too much environmental stimulation. During the second half of the first year, as infants mature neurologically and gain voluntary control over vocalizations, crying can be an expression of different affects (eg, frustration, fear).

A variety of explanations for the etiology of **colic** have been proposed. Some authorities believe that colic may not be a pathologic entity but simply an extreme variant of normal crying. The condition may result from an allergy, cow's milk intolerance, abnormal intestinal peristalsis, or increased intestinal gas, which are some of the more frequently associated factors. Others have proposed that colic is caused by problems in the interaction between infants and their environment, specifically their parents. This interactional theory requires not only excessive crying on the part of the infant, but also an inability of the parents to soothe the crying infant. The "missing fourth trimester" theory of colic posits that infants cry because they are born "three months too soon" (ie, human gestation should last 3 months longer). There is no scientific evidence to support this hypothesis. Whether maternal anxiety has any role in colic remains a controversial issue. More than one of these factors may contribute to the pathogenesis of colic.

Differential Diagnosis

An acute episode of excessive crying may be secondary to disease (eg, fever, otitis media). An organic etiology should be suspected in infants who present with inconsolable crying of acute onset. Box 35-1 lists the most common causes. Some conditions occur in a more chronic or recurrent pattern, particularly if the condition is not treated.

The differential diagnosis of infants who experience recurrent episodes of excessive crying focuses more on behavior and temperament. Colic, persistent night awakening, or difficult infant temperament (eg, extreme fussiness, neonatal drug withdrawal) may cause recurrent crying. Persistent night awakening and difficult infant temperament are discussed in Chapters 16 and 37, respectively.

Box 35-1. Most Common Causes of Acute Unexplained, Excessive Crying in Infants

Idiopathic[a]
Colic[a]
Infectious
Otitis media
Urinary tract infection
Stomatitis
Meningitis
Gastrointestinal[a]
Constipation
Anal fissure
Gaseous distention
Peristalsis problems
Reflux
Intussusception
Trauma
Corneal abrasion
Foreign body in the eye
Hair tourniquet syndrome
Behavioral[a]
Overstimulation
Persistent night awakening
Drug Reactions
Immunization reactions (previously common: with diphtheria-tetanus-pertussis vaccine)
Neonatal drug withdrawal (narcotics)
Child Abuse
Long bone fractures
Retinal hemorrhage
Intracranial hemorrhage
Hematologic[a]
Sickle cell crisis
Cardiovascular
Arrhythmia (supraventricular tachycardia)
Congestive heart failure
Anomalous left coronary artery

[a]May present as acute or recurrent episodes of excessive crying.

Evaluation

A thorough history and physical examination usually provide clues to the diagnosis in instances of acute onset of crying.

History

The focus of the history should be on determining the presence of any associated symptoms. In addition, the circumstances surrounding the crying (eg, occurrence during day or night) should be ascertained (Questions Box).

Crying and Colic — **Questions**

- Is this the first time the infant has cried inconsolably or does this happen on a recurring basis?
- Has the infant had a fever?
- Does the infant have any cold symptoms, vomiting, or diarrhea?
- Is the infant having any difficulty feeding? Is the infant formula-fed or breastfed?
- Has the infant had a recent fall or accident?

Physical Examination

A thorough physical examination is required for accurate diagnosis. Particular attention should be given to the following aspects of the examination:

1. Careful inspection of the skin after all clothing has been removed to look for any suspicious bruises or marks
2. Palpation of all long bones to detect fractures
3. Examination of all digits and the penis to check for hair tourniquets (single strands of hair wrapped around digits or the penis)
4. Examination of the retina to look for retinal hemorrhages (a sign of intracranial hemorrhage)
5. Eversion of the eyelids to check for foreign bodies
6. Fluorescein staining of the cornea to look for corneal abrasion

Laboratory Tests

Except for urinalysis, most screening laboratory tests are probably not useful. Test selection can be guided by the history and physical examination (eg, infants with fever without an apparent cause should have a septic workup, with an examination of blood, urine, and cerebrospinal fluid). Urinalysis, which may provide clues to an underlying metabolic deficiency, is sometimes helpful. Even when the initial history and physical examination are non-diagnostic, infants who persist in crying inconsolably should be suspected of having a serious underlying condition (eg, intracranial hemorrhage, drug ingestion). Such infants may warrant an extended period of observation or a more extensive workup that includes laboratory assessment.

Imaging Studies

Roentgenographic studies such as long bone x-rays may be necessary in some situations (eg, infants with long bone pain on palpation, suspicion of child abuse). Infants with retinal hemorrhages should have a computed tomography scan.

Management

Management and treatment depend on identification of the cause of the crying. Underlying organic conditions (eg, urinary tract infection, fractures) should be treated. Management of colic depends on presumptions regarding its etiology. It is important for practitioners to **reassure** parents regarding the benign nature of colic and its resolution over time. Physicians should provide a caring and supportive

environment in which the parents may express their concerns and frustrations. Reassurance along with practical suggestions regarding infant feeding and handling techniques (eg, cuddling, swaddling, or rocking) may often suffice.

Management suggestions for colic should be customized for infants and families. The more common management techniques are listed in Box 35-2.

Box 35-2. Management of Colic
Parental reassurance
Alteration in techniques of infant feeding and handling
Alteration of sensory input to infant
Prevention of swallowed air from passing through pylorus
Dietary alterations
Medication
Folk remedies
Increase carrying
Respond quickly to crying

Changes in sensory input (eg, soothing sounds or motions) may resolve crying and soothe colicky infants. According to the "missing fourth trimester" theory of colic, recreating the sensory environment of the womb calms infants by triggering a soothing response—the calming reflex—and promotes relaxation. Five maneuvers (swaddling, side or stomach position, shushing, swinging, and sucking—"the 5 S's") that mimic uterine sensations are noted to activate this calming reflex. It is further recommended by proponents of this theory that 3 to 5 of these maneuvers should be performed simultaneously and vigorously to activate the calming reflex.

Prophylactic measures to prevent the passage of swallowed air through the pylorus can also be useful. Such techniques include feeding in an upright position and limiting the period of sucking at the breast or bottle to about 10 minutes (after this time, greater amounts of air are swallowed relative to the amount of milk ingested). Some infants eat very fast and swallow a lot of air. Burping these infants every 5 to 10 minutes during feeds may help alleviate discomfort due to excessive air swallowing (aerophagia).

Methods to decrease intestinal spasm (eg, abdominal massage, warm baths, avoidance of overfeeding) may be helpful. The use of suppositories or rectal thermometers to break up rectal spasm and thereby release retained gas should be discouraged.

Data regarding **dietary changes,** such as the use of hypoallergenic diets by breastfeeding mothers, have been inconclusive, but suggest that there may be some therapeutic benefits. Similarly, the use of soy-based or hypoallergenic infant formulas also seem to have beneficial effects on the symptoms of colic. Generally, these dietary modifications should be reserved for infants with additional symptoms of allergy (eg, wheezing, rash) or intolerance (eg, vomiting, diarrhea, hematochezia, or weight loss).

Various drugs, including anticholinergics, motility-enhancing agents, barbiturates, laxatives, and anti-flatulents, have limited success and are best avoided. Currently, anti-flatulents (eg, simethicone) are prescribed most commonly. Despite lack of scientific evidence to support their efficacy, parents indicate that they are effective.

As long as no adverse effects are evident, limited amounts (eg, 1–2 oz per day) of **folk remedies** (eg, chamomile tea) can be supported if parents report satisfaction. Over-the-counter homeopathic preparations are also innocuous but may be advocated as efficacious by some parents.

Finally, the practitioner should encourage parents to respond to the infant's cries quickly and carry the infant as much as possible (eg, at least 3–4 hours daily). Parents should be advised that they cannot "spoil" infants younger than 4 months and that they might actually improve behavior by their own increased responsiveness.

Presently, the best evidence-based approaches to the management of colic include a trial of dietary modifications, limited amounts of herbal teas, and attempting to minimize infants' environmental stimulation levels.

Prognosis

Fortunately, the natural history of persistent crying during infancy is resolution over time. Long-term sequelae of infantile colic that have been identified include possible relationships with irritable bowel syndrome and increased levels of externalizing behavior problems (eg, hyperactivity, conduct concerns, and decreased adaptability) in childhood.

CASE RESOLUTION

The infant described in the case history is experiencing an acute episode of unexplained crying. Despite a normal physical examination, he was observed for 1 hour in the emergency department because his crying persisted. Subsequently, a septic workup was initiated, which revealed that a urinary tract infection was the source of the irritability.

Selected References

Barr RG, Paterson JA, Macmartin LM, Lehtonen L, Young SN. Prolonged and unsoothable crying bouts in infants with and without colic. *J Dev Behav Pediatr.* 2005;26:14–23

Brazelton TB. Crying in infancy. *Pediatrics.* 1962;29:579–588

Garrison MM, Christakis DA. A systematic review of treatments for infant colic. *Pediatrics.* 2000;106:184–190

Karp H. The "fourth trimester": a framework and strategy for understanding and resolving colic. *Contemp Pediatr.* 2004;21:94–116

Wessel MA, Cobb JC, Jackson EB, Harris GS, Detwiler AC. Paroxysmal fussing in infancy, sometimes called "colic." *Pediatrics.* 1954;14:421–434

Wolke D, Rizzo P, Woods S. Persistent infant crying and hyperactivity problems in middle childhood. *Pediatrics.* 2002;109:1054–1060

Discipline

Carol D. Berkowitz, MD

CASE STUDY

A 3-year-old boy is being threatened with expulsion from preschool because he is biting the other children. His mother states that he is very active and aggressive toward other children. In addition, his language development is delayed. She is at her wit's end about what to do. The birth history is normal, and the mother denies the use of drugs or cigarettes, but she drank socially before she realized she was pregnant. The medical and family histories are noncontributory, and the physical examination is normal.

Questions

1. What is the definition of discipline?
2. What are the 3 key components of discipline?
3. What strategies can parents use to discipline children?
4. What are the guidelines for using time-out?
5. What is the relationship between corporal punishment and child abuse?

Discipline can be defined as an educational process in which children learn how to behave in a socially acceptable manner. The word is derived from *disciplinare,* meaning to teach or instruct. It involves a complex set of interactions of attitudes, models, instructions, rewards, and punishments. Discipline is not synonymous with punishment. The goal is to help children gain self-control and respect for others and to learn behavior that is appropriate for given situations. It is also to ensure a child's safety in the environment. Proactive discipline is action taken by parents to encourage good behavior, and reactive discipline is parental action following misbehavior. To be effective, child discipline must have 3 components: a learning environment with a positive supportive parent-child relationship, a refined strategy for teaching and reinforcing desired behaviors, and a defined strategy for decreasing or extinguishing undesired behaviors. Children thrive in a supportive environment in which they are praised for socially appropriate behavior and are able to participate in the responsibilities and activities of the household. Parents, however, are more often interested in eliminating unwanted behaviors and may bring these specific concerns to their pediatrician.

Physician-Parent Interactions Concerning Discipline

Practitioners can assist parents by giving them guidelines for appropriate childhood discipline related to both routine and problem development. The age and temperament of the child are important factors to consider. In addition, pediatricians can discourage corporal punishment as the major method of discipline. Pediatricians may also have a role in advising against corporal punishment in schools. While most states have banned corporal punishment in the school setting, some states still permit it.

It is important to encourage parents to establish a positive interactive environment with verbal communication, monitoring children's behavior and commending desirable behavior, ignoring trivial problems, and consistently applying predetermined consequences for misbehavior. Rules should be simple, clear, and established ahead of time. Frequently physicians fail to inquire about children's behavior. Unless parents bring up the topic, it is not discussed during the physician visit. On average, physicians spend only 90 seconds per visit on anticipatory guidance and counseling. However, one survey of mothers in a physician waiting room showed that up to 90% were concerned about one aspect of behavior. Sixty percent of mothers surveyed found physician intervention quite helpful. The American Academy of Pediatrics recommends anticipatory guidance about discipline at each health maintenance visit between 9 months and 5 years. Such counseling is especially important to help parents understand the value of appropriate discipline in shaping their children's self-esteem. Information about discipline in the media may be confusing and contradictory, and often supports the unfounded approaches of nonprofessionals.

Early in the physician-parent relationship, physicians may express their interest in behavioral problems by saying, "I am interested not only in your child's physical well-being, but also in his (or her) growth and development and how he (or she) gets along with friends and family." They may then question parents about how children spend their days. During subsequent visits, pediatricians may say, "Parents of children of (child's name)'s age frequently worry about discipline. I wonder if you have any concerns." In making these inquiries, the physician may establish what factors, such as religious or ethnic beliefs, or family influences are shaping parents' decisions about discipline.

Problem Behaviors

Behavioral problems can be placed in 5 major categories.

1. **Problems of daily routine.** Such problems refer to the refusal of children to go about their daily activities, such as eating, going to bed, awakening at a certain time, and toilet training.

2. **Aggressive-resistant behavior.** This behavior is characterized by negativism and includes temper tantrums and aggressive responses to siblings and peers. Some undesirable behavior can place children or those around them in danger or at risk for injury.

3. **Overdependent or withdrawal behavior.** Such behavior is typical of children who are very attached to their mothers. These clingy children find separation difficult, especially in a preschool setting.

4. **Hyperactivity or excessive restlessness.**

5. **Undesirable habits,** which include thumb sucking, nail biting, throat clearing, and playing with genitals (see Chapter 40).

Some of the behaviors listed above are age-appropriate, and physicians can help parents by counseling them about stage-related behavior, such as oppositional behavior in a 2-year-old and independence-dependence problems in a 3- to 5-year-old. Parents may be more tolerant of a particular behavior if they understand what is normal at a given age. Just because something is normal, however, does not mean that it should be tolerated. Physicians can suggest to the parents ways of dealing with age-appropriate behavior (eg, placing breakable objects out of reach of toddlers).

Certain behavioral problems reflect differences in childhood temperaments. Temperament is the biological predisposition to a style of behavior. Carey has compiled a series of temperament scales to assess children and adolescents of different ages. For example, some children are shy and have a hard time adjusting to new situations. If parents anticipate such problems, they are often less angry when difficulties arise. Parental expectations can vary with a child's gender. Boys may be permitted to act a certain way ("He's all boy!") that would be disapproved of in girls. Physicians can discuss such expectations at health maintenance visits.

Physicians can also be particularly helpful in detecting and advising parents about disparities in the achievement of different developmental skills. Some children acquire motor skills before verbal skills, yet parents expect their children to be equally versatile in speech and movement.

Psychophysiology

All behaviors are modified by the responses and reactions of other individuals. The basic premise of discipline is to discourage unwanted behavior and to encourage desired behavior. This is accomplished by using techniques that are based on conditioning modalities.

Several factors contribute to an increased incidence of behavioral problems in children. Ten percent to 15% of all preschool children are raised in grossly disrupted family situations. These homes are impacted by divorce, death, separation, parental substance abuse, mental illness, or extreme poverty. Parental insecurity may also be a factor. In addition, families may have fewer social contacts than they once did because of greater mobility within society. As a result, families face greater social isolation.

Differential Diagnosis

In addition to providing anticipatory guidance about discipline, physicians must make 2 diagnostic decisions. First, they must determine whether a specific behavioral problem represents normal childhood behavior or an abnormality in behavior that warrants more specific intervention. Between 8% and 18% of behavioral disturbances may deserve physician intervention. More intensive management may be necessary for problems related to aggressive-resistant behavior and hyperactivity. Hyperactive behavior, which may exist as part of attention-deficit/hyperactivity disorder (ADHD), may be a sign of a significant underlying problem that warrants one-on-one intervention or the use of neuropharmacologic agents (see Chapter 113).

Second, physicians must differentiate between acceptable corporal punishment and child abuse. Some individuals feel that any form of corporal punishment is unacceptable. The use of physical punishment is widely accepted in our society, however, and it is legally condoned in the home setting. Fractures and bruises are not acceptable, and physical abuse should be suspected in children who present with such injuries.

Evaluation

History

The key component in the evaluation process is the assessment of the means parents use to discipline children (Questions Box). To obtain this information, physicians may simply ask parents, "How do you get your child to mind you?" This question is designed to lead to a discussion of how parents interact with their children. If parents have specific complaints, such as oppositional behavior, they should be questioned about the strategies they have used in their effort to discipline their children.

Physical Examination

Children's behavior should be assessed during the office visit. A general physical examination is useful to check for any signs of physical abuse as well as to evaluate children's well-being. A developmental assessment is also helpful because it may delineate disparities in the

---

Questions

Discipline

- What does the child do that the parents wish he or she would not do?
- What do the parents do to stop unwanted behavior?
- Does the child usually obey the parents?
- When and where does most of the unwanted behavior occur? Does it occur mainly if a child is tired?
- Which parent is responsible for disciplining the child?

achievement of certain skills. Some hyperactive children may warrant a more extensive psychodevelopmental assessment to look for findings consistent with ADHD. Behavioral checklists may be used to evaluate children's temperament.

Laboratory Tests

No specific laboratory or imaging studies are indicated for children with discipline problems. Such studies are indicated if child abuse is suspected (see Chapter 115).

Management

Physicians should assist parents in establishing appropriate guidelines for disciplining their children and reinforce the role of parents as the source of authority (Box 36-1). It is important for parents to realize that total freedom results in uncontrollable anxiety. Children mimic behavior, and **parents should act as role models.** If parents have temper tantrums when they are frustrated, their children may act in a similar manner. **Consistency** is also important. A system with a limited number of enforced rules is better than one with many different rules. In families where both parents are working, especially if they have overlapping time schedules, consistency is sometimes difficult to attain.

Box 36-1. Advice for Parents About Discipline
Set rules
Set limits
Define consequences
Be consistent
Ignore trivial problems
Compliment desirable behavior
Take time-out when angry

Physicians should emphasize to parents that it is best to **avoid power struggles.** Children engaged in a struggle often win because they have final control (eg, refusing to eat). Children should always be given the opportunity to graciously back out of a situation and save face. It is easier to avoid situations that lead to head-on confrontations than to get out of them once the confrontation has occurred. Parents should be the source of information for physicians. This helps strengthen parents' egos and validates their ability to handle their children appropriately.

In the past, specific methods of dealing with children with discipline problems concerned the issues of permissiveness versus overpermissiveness and accommodation versus strict punishment. Over-permissiveness refers to the allowing of undesirable acts and may exacerbate anxiety and increase demands for privilege.

Physicians should remind parents that preventing many behavioral disorders is easier than treating them. Reasoning is a useful modality, but it is unrealistic to expect infants and toddlers to have the cognitive skills to understand adult reasoning or to consistently respond to verbal commands or reprimands. Discipline should not only discourage bad behavior but also reinforce good behavior. Following are 5 examples of reactive discipline.

Redirection

Redirection is a simple and effective method in which the parent removes the problem and distracts the child with an alternative. This technique is frequently used to remove some object (such as a valued nicknack) from the hands of an infant, replacing it with a toy. Parental patience, ingenuity, and enthusiasm facilitate this approach. This approach is also important in teaching children what is acceptable behavior. For instance, one cannot draw on the wall but can draw on a piece of paper. Children also respond to making tedious routines into a game. For instance, children can be challenged to see who can get their clothes on faster or who can brush their teeth first. Parental creativity and energy often avert confrontations.

Spanking

Spanking involves inflicting physical pain, which is usually successful in bringing about the immediate cessation or a decrease in problem behavior. Spanking is highly prevalent as a form of discipline, with between 70% and 94% of parents reporting using the practice. Spanking is used more often for younger children and for boys and correlates with parental attributes such as age, education, socioeconomic status, and religious orientation. Spanking is often employed when other methods of discipline have failed to abort the unwanted behavior. Spanking tends to clear the air and get the punishment over with rather than producing a lingering guilt. To be truly effective, however, physical punishment must immediately follow the act. The "wait until Daddy comes home" approach is less effective because of the lack of temporal association. In addition, spanking tends to become situation-specific so that children associate a particular action with being spanked. This learning does not generalize to other situations. Spanking can teach children to be afraid of adults rather than to respect them.

Spanking may actually be damaging to the parent-child relationship and have a long-term effect on a child's self-esteem. Many parents feel remorseful after having spanked a child, and some acknowledge that they spank out of anger and question the efficacy of this modality. Most pediatricians discourage spanking as a means of disciplining children. Differentiation of physical punishment from child abuse is often difficult. In general, punishment with the hands is acceptable, but punishment with objects and spanking on parts of the body other than the buttocks or thighs is unacceptable. Spanking may be an early precursor of later physical violence and subsequent abuse. Again, parents act as role models. Children should never be allowed to hit their parents. This makes children feel extremely insecure.

Devices that are marketed for child discipline and inflict physical pain on a child, such as a sudden sting (modified stun gun), are never appropriate.

Scolding

Scolding involves the excess use of reasoning and explanations and is used by most parents as part of the discipline process. In families where communication or interaction is minimal, scolding or verbal reprimands may result in an initial increase in inappropriate behavior because this is the only way children receive any attention. Verbal reprimands are more effective if used infrequently. Verbal reprimands should not be used during time-outs because they reinforce undesirable behavior.

Scolding, because of its negative focus, can be damaging to children's self-esteem.

Ignoring

Ignoring represents the opposite of explaining and reasoning. This form of discipline is difficult to use successfully because parents must totally ignore children's behavior. If even the least flicker of recognition occurs, then activity increases. A brief initial increase in unwanted behavior, a so-called response burst, may occur with ignoring. This disciplinary method works better in younger children.

Time-out and Removal of Privileges

Time-out, the form of discipline most recommended, refers to time out from positive reinforcement. In sports, teams call a time-out to rethink what they are doing and to replan their strategies. Children are placed in a neutral or boring environment whenever they engage in inappropriate behavior. The time-out technique can be used to discourage undesired habits. For example, parents may say, "You can suck your thumb, but you may only do it in such and such a room." This type of discipline is better than ignoring, especially if "ignored" children are receiving attention from siblings and peers. Children should understand the rules ahead of time and why the behavior is unacceptable. Once this is accomplished, time-out may occur without any warning.

A timer should be used, and children should stay in the time-out area for 1 minute per 1 year of age. An appropriate area must be selected. This area should be fairly boring, so children's rooms are often not appropriate. A laundry room, a corner, or a specific chair may be better. If children act unacceptably during the time-out, the timer should be reset. If children have to go to the bathroom during the time-out, they are allowed one trip. After they return from the bathroom, the timer is reset.

The use of the time-out method is sometimes difficult. If the inappropriate behavior occurs in the morning when children are getting ready for school, time-out just encourages children's desire to delay. "Beat the buzzer" is another idea that may be used in such situations. With "beat the buzzer," the timer is set. If children are dressed before the timer goes off, they may be rewarded for the behavior by being allowed to go to bed half an hour later. If the buzzer "beats" them, then they have to go to bed half an hour earlier.

Inappropriate behavior away from home presents the greatest difficulty. These situations can be dealt with in numerous ways, particularly if the behavior problem involves temper tantrums. When children are crying or screaming uncontrollably, it is best to remove them from the embarrassment of the situation. This "manual guidance" often occurs in a supermarket, where children select something that parents do not wish to buy. Parents can often circumvent this problem easily by walking into the supermarket and saying, "If you are a good boy (or girl) during the whole trip, then I will get you something at the checkout counter." If children still have temper tantrums, then they should be removed from the area and brought to a neutral place such as the automobile or a restroom and allowed to finish their crying and screaming. It has been said that a glass of cold water splashed in a child's face is sometimes beneficial because it rapidly aborts the behavior. If the inappropriate behavior does not develop into a temper tantrum, then "marking" time-out is helpful. This consists of putting a mark with a colored water-soluble marker on the child's hand every time he or she engages in an inappropriate behavior. When the child returns home, the marks are totaled, and the time-out method is used.

Removal of privileges is a strategy applied in older children. Classically this involves grounding a child, prohibiting television or video games, or loss of driving privileges. The privilege must be something of value to the child for this method to be effective.

Parents who complain about inappropriate behavior should be asked to keep a record of children's behavior for 1 to 2 weeks. This helps determine if the behavior is really inappropriate and what is motivating it. Parents should be encouraged to talk to their children in a reasonable manner and to verbalize what they think children are feeling. They might say something like this, "It's terrible to be three years old and get so upset. You feel that you can't get the things you want, but some day you will grow up and then you will be in charge. I am really sorry it is so hard for you right now." Physicians should tell parents that it is important to set limits for children and to avoid threatening, judging, and constantly criticizing children. Parents should ask themselves, "If someone said this to me, how would I feel?" Many parents have themselves been disciplined only with spanking and know no other means, and the advice that physicians offer is valuable.

Prognosis

Children raised in a supportive environment that teaches respect for others and self-control grow up as caring adults. Children who have been exposed to excessive corporal punishment show aggressive behavior later.

CASE RESOLUTION

In the case presented at the beginning of the chapter, further history should be elicited about the mother's disciplining techniques. It is also significant that the child's speech is delayed. The boy's ability to articulate his feelings may be limited, and a formal speech and hearing assessment is warranted. The preschool should be advised that the evaluation is underway. A report from the preschool concerning the boy's behavior would be appreciated.

Selected References

American Academy of Pediatrics Committee on Psychosocial Aspects of Child and Family Health. Guidance for effective discipline. *Pediatrics.* 1998;101:723–728

American Academy of Pediatrics Committee on School Health. Corporal punishment in schools. *Pediatrics.* 2000;106:343

Barkley RA. *Defiant Children: A Clinician's Manual for Assessment and Parent Training.* 2nd ed. New York, NY: The Guilford Press; 1997

Burke MG. Is a 12-month-old too young to be disciplined? *Contemp Pediatr.* 2006;23:109–110

Carey WB. Pediatric assessment of behavioral adjustment and behavioral style. In: Levine MD, Carey WB, Crocker AC, eds. *Developmental-Behavioral Pediatrics.* 2nd ed. Philadelphia, PA: W. B. Saunders; 1992:609–612

Corwin DG. The fine art of the time-out. *Parenting.* 1996;November:171–172

Regalado M, Sareen H, Inkelas M, Wissow LS, Halfon N. Parents' discipline of young children: results from the National Survey of Early Childhood Health. *Pediatrics.* 2004;113:1952–1958

Schmitt BD. Discipline: rules and consequences. *Contemp Pediatr.* 1991;8:65–69

Schmitt BD. Time-out: intervention of choice for the irrational years. *Contemp Pediatr.* 1993;10:64–71

Schmitt BD. When a child hurts other children. *Contemp Pediatr.* 1990;7:81–82

Socolar RRS, Stein REK. Maternal discipline of young children: context, belief, and practice. *J Dev Behav Pediatr.* 1996;17:1–8

Straus MA, Sugarman DB, Giles-Sims J. Spanking by parents and subsequent antisocial behavior of children. *Arch Pediatr Adolesc Med.* 1997;151:761–767

Trumbull DA, Larzelere RE, Wolraich M. To spank or not to spank. *Pediatrics.* 1999;103:696–698

Vittrup B, Holden GW, Buck J. Attitudes predict the use of physical punishment: a prospective study of the emergence of disciplinary practices. *Pediatrics.* 2006;117:2055–2064

Waterson T. Giving guidance on child discipline. *BMJ.* 2000;320:261–262

Temper Tantrums

Geeta Grover, MD

CASE STUDY

During a routine office visit, the parents of a 3-year-old boy express concern about his recent behavior. They report that whenever he is asked to do something he does not want to do, he throws a "fit." He cries fiercely, falls to the floor, bangs his hands, and kicks his feet until his parents give in. He often displays such behavior at bedtime or mealtime if he is asked to turn off the television or eat foods that he does not want. He has 2 to 3 such episodes per week. The parents state that their home life has not changed, and the boy's teacher reports that he displays no such behaviors at preschool.

Questions

1. At what age are temper tantrums common in children?
2. How do parents' reactions encourage or discourage temper tantrums?
3. What appropriate management strategies may help control such oppositional behavior?
4. What factors or aspects of such oppositional behavior indicate underlying pathology?

Temper tantrums are common, normal, age-related behaviors in young children. To a certain degree, oppositional behaviors such as negativism, defiance, and tantrums are part of the normal progression toward self-reliance and independence. Toddlers need to assert their freedom and explore their environment, which often puts them at odds with the limitations imposed by society and well-meaning parents. Young children cannot appreciate that rules and limitations have been established in the interest of their own safety and well-being. They see only that their own desires have been thwarted, and they may react to this disappointment with intense emotions. Children are not simply upset because they cannot have their way. They are angry and frustrated, and they lose control over their emotions. During tantrums children cry and scream uncontrollably. They may fall to the floor, bang their heads, kick their feet, pound their hands, and thrash about wildly. Some children may throw things, try to hit one another, or destroy property.

Such intense displays of anger may be a terrifying experience for both children and parents. Some children use tantrums to gain attention, whereas others use them to achieve something or to avoid doing something. Recurrent temper tantrums may strain relationships among parents, children, and other family members.

Epidemiology

Temper tantrums are noted most often in children who are 2 to 3 years of age, but they may occur any time between the ages of 12 months and 5 years. Parental surveys reveal that about 20% of 2-year-olds, 18% of 3-year-olds, and 10% of 4-year-olds have at least one tantrum per day. Most children are able to express their feeling verbally by 3 to 4 years of age, so temper tantrums begin to taper off. Children who are not able to express their feelings well with words

(eg, children with developmental delays—especially children with speech and language delays or children with autism spectrum disorders [ASDs]) are more likely to continue to have tantrums. Boys and girls are affected equally. Although temper tantrums are unusual in school-aged children, they often reappear in the form of verbal tantrums during adolescence, when autonomy and independence once again become developmental issues.

Pathophysiology

Appreciation of children's level of maturity and the developmental tasks normally associated with the toddler and preschool years, when temper tantrums occur most often, facilitates an understanding of tantrum behavior. Young children who are exploring the world and developing a sense of autonomy think primarily in egocentric terms. They view reality from their own perspective and are unable to appreciate the perspective of other individuals. Only as they mature and enter school do they learn to recognize the position of others and begin to develop a sense of morality, of right and wrong. Toddlers may become frustrated or angry because of their lack of control over the world, inability to communicate, or limitations of their cognitive and motor abilities, which do not allow them to accomplish desired tasks. Unlike adults who have the ability to verbalize frustrations or simply walk away from unpleasant situations, young children have neither the sophisticated ability to articulate their feelings nor the freedom to walk away. Therefore, they may react to disappointments with temper tantrums.

Temper tantrums may be classified as normal or problematic based on their cause, frequency, and characteristics. Normal tantrums can simply be demands for attention or signs of frustration, anger, or protest. In the interval between tantrums, the child's disposition and mood are normal. The well-behaved 3-year-old boy who has an occasional tantrum following the birth of a sibling, the 2½-year-old girl who throws a tantrum to express frustration because no one understands what she is trying to say, and the 2-year-old boy who cries uncontrollably because he cannot complete the puzzle he has started or run fast enough to keep up with his 4-year-old brother are all examples of normal tantrums. A typical reason for an avoidance-type tantrum is not wanting to go to bed at bedtime. All types of tantrums are more common when children are tired, ill, or hungry, because their ability to cope with disappointment and frustration is limited under these circumstances.

Frequent tantrums (>5 per day) or tantrums that result in destruction of property or physical harm to the child or others are signs of problematic tantrums (Box 37-1). These tantrums result from factors that are beyond the child's control such as parental problems, school difficulties, or health-related conditions (Box 37-2). For example, the child with unrecognized hearing loss may be performing poorly at school and resort to tantrum behavior in frustration. Marital discord or domestic violence may create anxiety for a child, which may manifest as frequent or destructive tantrums.

Box 37-1. Features of Problematic Tantrums
- Tantrums that persist or get worse beyond 5 years of age
- Frequent tantrums (>5 per day)
- Persistent negative mood or behavior in intervals between tantrums
- Recurrent tantrums at school
- Destruction of property during tantrums
- Harm to self or others during tantrums
- Other behavioral problems (eg, sleep disorders, aggressive behaviors, enuresis)

Box 37-2. Underlying Causes of Problematic Tantrums
Parent-Related Factors
- Marital discord
- Abusive behavior toward children
- Domestic violence
- Substance abuse
- Depression
- Inappropriate parental expectations

Child-Related Factors
- Developmental and/or learning disabilities
  — Hearing loss
  — Speech and language delays
  — Autism spectrum disorders
- Mood disorders (eg, depression)
- Attention-deficit/hyperactivity disorder
- Temperament (eg, high persistence and intensity of response and slow adaptability)
- Illness
  — Unrecognized illness (eg, otitis media, sinusitis)
  — Chronic or recurrent illness

Differential Diagnosis

Temper tantrums are readily recognizable because of their classic pattern where a toddler-aged child becomes frustrated, reacts physically, and cries or screams. Sometimes temper tantrums are indicative of more significant problems such as speech or language delays or ASDs (see Chapter 112).

Evaluation

History

Thorough history taking is essential (Questions Box). The frequency of the temper tantrums, circumstances that provoke them, a description of actual tantrums, and parental reaction must be ascertained. In some instances, this reaction may provide insight as to why the tantrums recur. In addition, parental expectations should be assessed. Expectations that are inappropriate for children's age and developmental maturity may create unnecessary tensions between parents and children and lead to tantrum behavior. Factors associated with problematic tantrums should also be assessed (see Box 37-2).

Questions
Temper Tantrums
- How often does the child have temper tantrums?
- What circumstances provoke the tantrums?
- How does the child behave during the tantrums? What does the child do?
- How does the child behave in the interval between tantrums?
- How do the parents react to the child during the tantrums? What do they do or say?
- Are parental expectations consistent with the child's developmental stage?
- Have there been any changes at home or school (eg, birth of a sibling, new school)?
- Is the child having any other behavioral or development-related problems (eg, enuresis, sleep difficulties)?

Tantrums that are frequent (>5 per day), severe, or persist after the age of 5 years may be a sign of underlying conditions such as depression or low self-esteem. Frequent tantrums may also be associated with attention-deficit/hyperactivity disorder (ADHD). Children with a history of impulsivity, hyperactivity, and inattention that are inappropriate for age should be evaluated for ADHD. Children who hurt themselves or others or destroy property during tantrums may have significant emotional problems. Peer pressure may inhibit tantrum behavior; if tantrums occur frequently at school, the presence of learning disabilities or speech and hearing deficits should be considered.

It is important to remember that physicians usually see children whose tantrums are frequent, severe, or cannot be controlled by parents. First, pediatricians must determine whether any underlying pathology may be contributing to the behavior and, if so, what parental or child factors may be provoking it. Second, they must differentiate between normal tantrums and problematic tantrums. Identification and remediation of the cause of problematic tantrums are the first steps toward cure. Children with suspected underlying conditions such as ADHD or mood disturbances should be referred to the appropriate specialist for further evaluation.

Physical Examination

A thorough physical examination is appropriate as is a developmental assessment to determine if there are findings such as speech delay or behavioral signs consistent with ASDs. Most often, the physical examination is normal.

Laboratory Tests

There are no laboratory tests indicated in the assessment of the child with temper tantrums. Routine tests that are age-appropriate and suggested as part of health maintenance are appropriate.

Management

Punishment is not the solution to temper tantrums (see Chapter 36). Health maintenance visits are an ideal time to provide **anticipatory guidance** regarding tantrums and discuss strategies to prevent or minimize this behavior. Parents typically report that their children become defiant and difficult to manage during the "terrible twos." At the 12- and 15-month visits, physicians should alert parents that this period is approaching and remind them that it is a normal part of development. Preventive strategies such as **childproofing** the home to minimize unnecessary conflicts should be discussed. In addition, parents can give young children **frequent opportunities to make choices** (eg, which color shirt to wear or which of 2 foods to have for lunch). These opportunities allow children to exercise independence and autonomy in a positive rather than a negative manner. Physicians can provide **reassurance** that this unpleasant stage will pass; children will eventually become more cooperative and agreeable.

Parents should be told that helping children learn self-control and how to handle anger are keys to management. To expect that children will never get angry is unrealistic. Children should be taught how to **vent their anger and frustration in an acceptable manner** (eg, articulating their feelings or hitting a designated punching bag or pillow). As children mature, their ability to verbalize their feelings increases, but even young toddlers can say "me angry." Physicians should emphasize that it is **important for parents to remain calm** during children's temper tantrums. Shouting and spanking indicate to children that parents are also out of control. Children feel more secure if the adults around them are calm and in control.

Different types of temper tantrums may require specific treatment and management strategies. Parents should **be supportive** of children who are having tantrums resulting from frustration or fatigue by letting the children know that they understand. Children's energy should be redirected into activities they can do well. Parents should be encouraged to **praise positive behavior** (eg, completing tasks properly, handling anger in an acceptable fashion). They should **ignore some tantrums,** such as those for purposes of attention seeking or wanting something. If children have no audience, they have no need to perform. **Time-outs** may also be used in such situations (see Chapter 36). Parents should not give in to children's wishes; this may reinforce tantrum behavior. **Physical movement** of children to where they belong may be necessary if they are refusing to do something (eg, bed for the child who is refusing to go to sleep at bedtime) or in danger of hurting themselves. **Holding children** who are raging may give them a sense of security and help calm them. If temper tantrums occur outside the home, it may be necessary to accompany children to a **quiet, private place** such as an automobile until they calm down.

CASE RESOLUTION

The child in the case scenario seems to be having normal, age-appropriate tantrums. The boy's tantrums occur when he is asked to do something that he does not want to do. In these situations the parents should try to ignore the tantrums as much as possible and not give in to the child's wishes.

Selected References

Beers NS, Howard B. Managing temper tantrums. *Pediatr Rev.* 2003;24:70–71

Needlman R, Howard B, Zuckerman B. Temper tantrums: when to worry. *Contemp Pediatr.* 1989;6:12–34

Potegal M, Davidson RJ. Temper tantrums in young children: behavioral composition. *J Dev Behav Pediatr.* 2003;24:140–147

Potegal M, Kosorok MR, Davidson RJ. Temper tantrums in young children: tantrum duration and temporal organization. *J Dev Behav Pediatr.* 2003;24:148–154

Breath-Holding Spells

Geeta Grover, MD

CASE STUDY

A 15-month-old girl is brought to the office because of parental concern about seizures. In the last month she has passed out momentarily 3 times. Each episode seems to be precipitated by anger or frustration on her part. Typically she cries, holds her breath, turns blue, and passes out. Each time she awakens within a few seconds and seems fine. The medical history and family history are unremarkable, and the physical examination is entirely within normal limits.

Questions

1. What are breath-holding spells (BHS)?
2. What is the differential diagnosis of BHS?
3. What, if any, laboratory studies are indicated in the evaluation of BHS?
4. What measures can be taken to prevent BHS? Are anticonvulsants necessary?
5. What, if any, are the long-term sequelae of BHS?

Breath-holding spells (BHS) are a benign, recurring condition of childhood in which anger or pain produce crying that culminates in noiseless expiration and apnea. The frequency of BHS, an involuntary phenomenon, is variable and ranges from several episodes a day to only several episodes per year. Although the spells are innocuous, they usually provoke parental fear and anxiety because children often turn blue and become limp. The diagnosis can usually be made on the basis of a characteristic history and description of the episode, but the possibility of seizures should be considered.

Epidemiology

Breath-holding spells occur in about 5% of all children between the ages of 6 months and 6 years, but they are most common in children between 12 and 18 months of age. Most children have experienced their first episode by 18 months and virtually all by 2 years of age. Although BHS have been described in children younger than 6 months, occurrence in such young infants is uncommon. Boys and girls are affected equally. A positive family history is found in about 25% of cases.

Clinical Presentation

The typical clinical sequence of the major types of BHS is described later in the chapter (see Pathophysiology and Dx Box). After the spells, children may experience a short period of drowsiness.

Pathophysiology

Breath-holding spells may be classified as one of the non-epileptic paroxysmal disorders of childhood. These recurrent conditions, which have a sudden onset and no epileptiform focus, resolve spontaneously. Other disorders in this heterogeneous group include syncope, migraine, cyclic vomiting, benign paroxysmal vertigo,

Dx **Breath-Holding Spells**

- Identifiable precipitating event or emotion
- Brief duration
- Color change, if present, prior to loss of consciousness and rhythmic jerking of extremities
- Rapid restoration of full activity
- Normal neurologic examination

paroxysmal torticollis, sleep disorders (narcolepsy, night terrors, somnambulism), and shudder attacks.

Types of BHS

The 2 major types of BHS are **cyanotic** and **pallid.** The cyanotic type is more common. Approximately 60% of children with BHS have cyanotic spells, 20% have pallid spells, and 20% of affected children have both types. Most commonly, affected children experience several spells per week. Approximately 15% of children with BHS have complicated features. Complicated BHS are defined as typical BHS followed by seizure-like activity or rigid posturing of the body.

Cyanotic episodes are more often provoked by an upsetting event, anger, frustration, or scolding rather than by injury or fear. Children usually cry or scream loudly. The cries become noiseless as children open their mouths and hold their breath in expiration. After approximately 30 seconds of apnea, a color change is apparent as children become cyanotic. The spell may terminate at this point, or children may proceed to lose consciousness and become limp. Rarely, loss of consciousness may be followed by a few seconds of rhythmic clonic jerking of the extremities, mimicking seizure-like activity, or rigid opisthotonic posturing of the body. The entire attack lasts less than 1 minute. Children generally resume full activity within a few minutes.

Unlike the postictal period of epileptic seizures, prolonged periods of lethargy or drowsiness following spells are uncommon.

Pallid spells are similar to cyanotic BHS with some exceptions. Pallid episodes are more commonly provoked by minor injury, pain, or fear rather than frustration or anger; the initial cry is minimal prior to apnea and loss of consciousness; and children become pale rather than cyanotic. In pallid BHS, children often lose consciousness or tone after only a single gasp or cry, whereas in the cyanotic form, the period of apnea prior to loss of consciousness is much longer.

Etiology

Although the spells are triggered by identifiable stimuli, they are involuntary phenomena. It is believed that loss of consciousness in both the cyanotic and pallid forms is caused by cerebral anoxia. The actual mechanisms of the 2 types of BHS are different. The processes involved in cyanotic BHS are not clear. Proposed mechanisms include centrally mediated inhibition of respiratory effort and altered lung mechanics, which may inappropriately stimulate pulmonary reflexes, thus resulting in apnea and hypoxia. In the pallid form, the pale coloration and loss of tone are thought to result from vagally mediated severe bradycardia or asystole. Pallid spells have been spontaneously induced in the electroencephalogram (EEG) laboratory using ocular compression to trigger the oculocardiac reflex. Vagally mediated bradycardia or asystole lasting more than 2 seconds has been produced by this maneuver.

An association between iron deficiency anemia and BHS has been recognized for many years but is poorly understood. It may be related to iron's importance in the function of various enzymes and neurotransmitters in the central nervous system, or may be because children with anemia have decreased cerebral oxygenation—making them more susceptible to BHS.

Differential Diagnosis

The differential diagnosis primarily includes seizures and syncope secondary to cardiac arrhythmia or a vasovagal episode. Although vasovagal syncope, like BHS, may be provoked by fear or pain, it is uncommon in children younger than 12 years. Three factors may help differentiate BHS from true epileptic seizure activity. First, spells are usually provoked by some upsetting event or emotion, unlike seizures, which generally do not have a recognizable precipitating event. Second, episodes are brief in duration and followed by rapid restoration of full activity. Third, color change precedes loss of consciousness and rhythmic jerking of the extremities, whereas in the typical epileptic seizure, convulsive activity and loss of muscular tone usually precede change in color. See Box 38-1 for the differential diagnosis of BHS.

Evaluation

History

The history alone may be diagnostic (Questions Box). A family history of BHS should be obtained. It is essential to record a detailed history of the suspected breath-holding episode. The sequence in

Box 38-1. Differential Diagnosis of Breath-Holding Spells
Central Nervous System
Seizures (epilepsy)
Occult or overt brain stem lesions (causing dysfunction within the pontomedullary area)
Benign paroxysmal vertigo
Cardiovascular
Cardiac arrhythmia (eg, prolonged QT syndrome)
Syncope (orthostatic or vasovagal)
Miscellaneous
Gastroesophageal reflux/Sandifer syndrome
Cataplexy (transient loss of muscle tone associated with narcolepsy; rare before adolescence)
Central or obstructive apnea
Munchausen syndrome by proxy

which the events occurred may help differentiate BHS from epileptic seizures.

> **Questions**
>
> **Breath-Holding Spells**
>
> - What happened before the episode?
> - Was the child crying?
> - What was the child's color before and during the episode?
> - Was the child lethargic after the episode?
> - Does the family have a history of breath-holding spells?

Physical Examination

Children should have a complete physical examination, including a thorough neurologic evaluation. Focal neurologic signs or evidence of structural lesions such as meningomyelocele or hydrocephalus may lead the physician away from a diagnosis of BHS.

Laboratory Tests

If the history is consistent with BHS and the physical examination is normal, laboratory evaluation is usually unnecessary. Because of the association of BHS with iron deficiency anemia in some children, it is appropriate to determine a hemoglobin level. An EEG may be performed if the physician is concerned about the possibility of epileptic seizures. In both forms of BHS, the EEG shows generalized slowing followed by flattening (a pattern characteristic of cerebral anoxia) during attacks, although it is unusual to record the EEG during BHS. Simultaneous EEG and video recordings can be very useful in helping to distinguish BHS from seizures, especially in children having frequent episodes. The interictal EEG is normal in children with BHS, whereas it may often be abnormal in children with epilepsy. An electrocardiogram may be obtained if there is any question about cardiac arrhythmia (eg, prolonged QT syndrome).

Management

Management of BHS includes **parental support and reassurance.** Breath-holding spells may be extremely frightening for parents to witness, especially if the episodes are routinely associated with loss of consciousness or seizure-like activity. Parents should be told about the involuntary nature of the attacks and be cautioned against reinforcing the spells by giving in to the child's wishes. They should be advised to avoid unnecessary confrontations with the child. Similarly, it is impossible to ensure that the child will never be frustrated or injured. Instead, parents should be encouraged to handle the episodes in a "matter-of-fact" manner and continue age-appropriate discipline. They should be reassured that the long-term prognosis is excellent.

Pharmacologic therapy is usually not necessary, but atropine sulfate may be considered in the management of children with frequent pallid BHS because of atropine's anticholinergic action. Anticonvulsants are not effective. A recent clinical trial showed that iron therapy was effective in the treatment of both cyanotic and pallid BHS, especially in children who were iron deficient. Referral to a neurologist or psychiatrist may be considered at the family's request if the episodes are frequent and associated with loss of consciousness or if there is uncertainty regarding the diagnosis or management.

Prognosis

Breath-holding spells resolve spontaneously in most children by 5 to 6 years of age. About 50% of cases resolve by 4 years of age, and 90% resolve by 6 years of age. Neither pallid nor cyanotic BHS are associated with an increased risk of development of epilepsy, although children with pallid BHS do have an increased incidence of developing syncopal attacks during adulthood.

CASE RESOLUTION

The child presented in the opening case scenario has a history and physical examination suggestive of breath-holding spells (BHS). The girl's episodes are consistent with cyanotic BHS. The episodes are preceded by an identifiable emotion, are brief in duration, and are followed by a rapid recovery of normal consciousness and activity. Assessment of the hemoglobin level revealed mild iron deficiency anemia. The child received iron therapy, and the parents were reassured about the benign nature of BHS.

Selected References

Anderson JE, Bluestone D. Breath-holding spells: scary but not serious. *Contemp Pediatr.* 2000;17:61–72

Daoud AS, Batieha A, al-Sheyyab M, Abuekteish F, Hijazi S. Effectiveness of iron therapy on breath-holding spells. *J Pediatr.* 1997;130:547–550

DiMario FJ. Prospective study of children with cyanotic and pallid breath-holding spells. *Pediatrics.* 2001;107:265–269

Kelly AM, Porter CJ, McGoon MD, Espinosa RE, Osborn MJ, Hayes DL. Breath-holding spells associated with significant bradycardia: successful treatment with permanent pacemaker implantation. *Pediatrics.* 2001;108:698–702

Mocan H, Yildiran A, Orhan F, Erduran E. Breath holding spells in 91 children and response to treatment with iron. *Arch Dis Child.* 1999;81:261–262

CHAPTER 39

Fears, Phobias, and Anxiety

Carol D. Berkowitz, MD

CASE STUDY

A 5-year-old girl is brought into the office by her mother, who complains that her daughter has been frightened of sleeping alone since the occurrence of an earthquake. The house did not sustain any significant damage, but the entire family was awakened. The mother says that the girl has become more timid. As nighttime approaches, she becomes particularly fearful. She will not stay in her bed, and she is comforted only by sleeping with her parents. In addition, the girl has begun bed-wetting since the earthquake, and the mother wonders whether she should put her daughter in diapers. The physical examination, including the vital signs, is normal, except for the observation that the child is very clingy and whiny.

Questions

1. What are normal childhood fears?
2. When do these fears commonly occur?
3. What strategies are used to deal with these fears?
4. What are simple phobias? What are social phobias?
5. What is school phobia, and how is it best handled?
6. What are common anxiety disorders in children and adolescents?
7. How can families deal with childhood disturbances that emerge after natural and man-made disasters?

Fears are normal feelings that cause emotional, behavioral, and physiological changes that are essential for survival. Fears are associated with psychological discomforts such as a negative, unpleasant feeling. Children may develop fears in response to actual events (eg, earthquakes) or as a result of the temporal association of 2 events (eg, seeing a scary movie on a rainy day and then becoming afraid of rain). Some fears seem to be innate, and others seem to be developmental. Children fear different things at different ages. For example, school phobia is sometimes particularly problematic in young, school-aged children.

Phobias are overwhelming, intense, highly specific, and often irrational fears. Social phobias are specific to social situations that arouse intense concerns about humiliation or embarrassment. Fear of speaking in public may represent a social phobia. Selective mutism involves children who are able to speak but are unable to do so in certain settings, such as school. This probably represents one form of a social phobia. When these fears are combined with avoidance behavior, they may be incapacitating. Anxiety refers to fear without a definable source. It is a vague feeling of uneasiness, apprehension, and foreboding of impending doom. A child may experience an anxiety **problem** where there is significant but not severe distress and an anxiety **disorder** when the distress is excessive or functioning is impaired. Up to 8% of children and adolescents have anxiety disorders. These may be referred to as generalized anxiety disorders.

Different strategies are useful for dealing with different fears. It is important for parents not to trivialize these fears, nor to reinforce them, but to empower children to deal with them.

It is also important to realize that parents sometimes foster fears by using threats with children such as "the doctor will give you a shot unless you eat your spinach" or "the boogie man will get you." By fostering fears, the parents are also fostering dependency. Parents lack the imagination that children have and find it difficult to understand the degree of fear that children experience.

The opportunities for primary care providers to counsel families about childhood fears has increased over the past 10 years, related to a number of catastrophic events such as the terrorist attacks of 9/11, the tsunami in Asia, and hurricane Katrina. Acts of violence such as the shootings at Columbine High School and Virginia Tech also create fear and anxiety in children who witness these events on the television. It is important to recognize the pervasiveness of mental health sequelae following disasters, and the factors that influence the prevalence of these disturbances. One percent of children in New York City lost a relative on 9/11. There is a greater risk of mental health sequelae if there are poor social supports, a prior history of psychopathology, or the child is fearful or shy by nature. Natural disasters have less of an impact than intentional ones. While many of the recent disasters have been acute and unexpected, there are children who are continuously exposed to what has been called "process trauma" in the form of war and child abuse.

Epidemiology

Fears follow a developmental pattern. Neonates are believed to have no fear, although young infants whose faces are covered with a blanket struggle to toss off the blanket. Infants who are 6 months of

207

age exhibit what is known as **stranger anxiety** in response to unfamiliar persons, places, or objects. To combat this anxiety, infants seek refuge with a parent. Stranger anxiety becomes equated with separation anxiety and reaches a peak at 2 years of age. Children between 6 months and 2 years of age are also frightened by loud noises and falling or quickly moving objects.

Children between the ages of 2 and 5 years are in what is termed the **age of anxiety.** They fear many things, including animals, abandonment, loud noises, and darkness. Children in this age group are particularly fearful of physicians, hospitals, and getting hurt. Young children are afraid of the physically disabled, who represent bodily injury, and monsters and scary movies. They sometimes displace their anger onto monsters and witches and attribute to these imaginary characters the bad feelings they are experiencing. Children in this age group have strong imaginations, which makes it difficult for them to differentiate fantasy from reality.

School-aged children between 6 years of age and adolescence tend to have more abstract thoughts, and their fears are less relevant to physical immediacy. These children are afraid of the death of their parents or the burning of their home. They also fear war, growing up (expressed as "How will I know what to do?"), going into the next grade, being alone or being kidnapped, and the divorce of their parents. Children in this age group are often reluctant to bother their parents with their fears, and they can easily misinterpret parental concerns when they overhear parental conversations.

Separation anxiety, which may manifest as school phobia and may be referred to as separation anxiety disorder, may occur in school-aged children. The prevalence is estimated at 3.2% to 4.1%, though up to 50% of third graders report separation anxiety symptoms. Separation anxiety disorder is defined as developmentally inappropriate, excessive anxiety precipitated by actual or anticipated separation from home or family. Affected children develop physical complaints (eg, stomachaches) on school days. The mother-child relationship is often disturbed, and the child is fearful of leaving the parent alone. Childhood school phobia and parental history of panic attacks and agoraphobia may be associated.

Fears during adolescence relate to social functioning such as public speaking or talking to members of the opposite sex. Older children are also concerned about school failure and physical injury. They have many of the same fears expressed by younger school-aged children, although phobias are uncommon. Phobias, which occur in less than 1.7% of the general population, are reported in 13% of disturbed children.

Anxiety disorders are rare in childhood, but more common during adolescence. They may include panic attacks, which involve the sudden onset of intense fear or discomfort associated with physiological symptoms such as palpitations and shortness of breath. Fear about a panic attack may lead to agoraphobia, the avoidance of going away from home. Post-traumatic stress disorder (PTSD) involves a set of symptoms that recurs after a person has experienced a traumatic event. Symptoms include intense fear, helplessness, or a sense of horror. The person reexperiences the trauma,

avoids circumstances that are reminiscent of the trauma, and is in a state of hyperarousal. It is estimated that 5% of men and 10% of women have a lifetime prevalence of PTSD.

Pathophysiology

Fear has its basis in a series of psychophysiological reactions, which are mediated through a series of neurotransmitters. Elevated levels of certain transmitters such as γ-aminobutyric acid and norepinephrine are associated with feelings of anxiety. Excess serotonin has also been related to anxiety disorders. Patients with panic attacks and anxiety disorders have disturbances in neurotransmitter regulation.

Differential Diagnosis

The challenge for physicians is to assess the etiology of the fear and to differentiate normal fears from those that may be signs of unusual stresses or signs of psychopathology. Appropriate fears represent a real reaction to a real danger. As a rule, children are more resilient than adults and recover more rapidly from traumatic events. On the other hand, children are prone to inappropriate fears, which may develop for a number of reasons.

Inappropriate fears may occur because of operant conditioning, in which a conditioned stimulus becomes associated with another object. Fear of the other object becomes reinforced through this association. Inappropriate fears may also develop in a child whose parent has the fear (modeling) or through witnessing a fearful event in the media (informational). True phobias represent neuroses and may occur in more than one family member.

School phobia, also called school refusal, may occur under 3 distinct conditions. Not uncommonly, young children who are entering school for the first time are frightened. This fear is a normal component of separation anxiety, which usually resolves within a few days of starting school. In contrast, older children may experience school phobia because they are truly afraid of a school situation. They may fear a teacher, violence, or a bully. To avoid the problem, children may actually request to change classrooms or schools. It is important to talk to children to find out what is behind their fear of school.

On the other hand, some children who seem fearful of school are actually concerned about parental separation (ie, separation anxiety). Frequently these children enjoy school and miss attending it. Absences occur when feelings of separation from parents are so intense that they do not allow children to function well in school settings. This separation anxiety disorder may result from parental illness or parents' fostering dependency in children. Children then see parents as vulnerable and are uncomfortable about leaving them alone.

School refusal is the third leading cause of school absenteeism after transient illness and truancy. Fifty percent of children with school refusal have other problems, including depression (28%), tantrums (18%), sleep disturbances (17%), obsessive-compulsive behavior (11%), other fears (10%), enuresis (3%), and learning disabilities (3%). Overall, school refusal has a good prognosis, although adolescents do not do as well as younger children, and individuals with a higher IQ have a poorer outcome. Twenty percent of parents of children with school refusal have a diagnosable psychiatric disorder. Issues of mother-child dependency are often a concern.

Another type of childhood fear concerns physicians and hospitals. Children have many concerns about what happens to them at the doctor's office. They are particularly fearful of needles. To children, needles represent possible mutilation. When asked to represent needles in drawings, children often portray needles as larger than themselves and very pointed. They comment that needles are sharp (eg, "Needles can make you pop, just like a balloon." "Needles can also take out all your blood until you die."). In addition, children are preoccupied with what happens to their blood. One youngster commented, "They check out your blood to see if it's good or bad, and if your blood is bad, then it means that you need to have more tests." Another youngster thought that physicians were doing a "blood taste" rather than a blood test.

Hospitalization raises other issues concerning parental separation as well as painful procedures. As children adjust to hospitalization, they progress through 3 stages: protest, during which they complain about the hospital and cry; despair, during which they have given up hope that their parents will return; and detachment, during which they seem to be adjusting but actually have distanced themselves from their parents.

Evaluation

Physicians should explore the area of childhood fears and phobias at routine health maintenance visits, even if parents do not have specific concerns. Sometimes parents are embarrassed by children's fears (eg, the fear of an older child to sleep without a night light). Parents may not report children's fears unless these fears seem to be unusually intense. Practitioners may ask children, "What is the scariest thing you can think of?" If children are having difficulty providing details, physicians may ask them to name things that other children fear or to complete the sentence, "I feel afraid when…." Alternatively, practitioners may suggest things that other children may fear: "Do the kids you know seem to be worried about kidnapping?"

There are a number of instruments that have been used to assess the level of anxiety in children. These include the Multidimensional Anxiety Scale for Children, Spence Children's Anxiety Scale, and Screen for Child Anxiety Related Disorders. The latter instrument is in the public domain and readily available.

History

The evaluation of children with specific fears demands a careful history that provides information about situations in which children are fearful (Questions Box). Physicians should consider fears within a developmental context because many childhood fears are normal and experienced by all children. It is also important to look at changes in the family situation. Children sometimes develop what seem to be fears but in fact are behaviors designed to manipulate other family members. For instance, young children who sense marital discord

may insist on sleeping with their parents as a way of ensuring that the parents are together rather than separate.

Fears and Phobias — Questions

- What fear does the child have? Exactly what does the child fear?
- Under what circumstances was the fear originally expressed? Did any changes in the child's life occur around the time that the fear appeared?
- Under what conditions is the fear currently expressed?
- How long has the child had the fear?
- How does the fear affect the daily living of the child and family?

Physical Examination

A routine examination is warranted, but findings are usually normal. Such an evaluation, however, is particularly important if presenting complaints include symptoms such as abdominal pain, headache, or palpitations.

Laboratory Tests

As a rule, laboratory tests are not required unless the symptoms suggest an organic etiology such as hyperthyroidism as the cause of palpitations.

Management

The management of the fear or phobia is determined by the degree to which children are incapacitated. As a general rule, **children should be empowered to conquer their fears.** Children's books that address the issues of certain fears can help achieve this empowerment. Books such as *The Berenstain Bears in the Dark* (Random House, 1982) discuss specific worries such as fear of lightning and thunder. These books often explain the basis of such natural phenomena in easy-to-understand terms. The books also normalize particular fears and show how one character is fearful. Parents can also re-create some of the sounds that children fear. For example, children who are afraid of the noise the wind makes are shown a teakettle where the hot steam blows through the whistle, creating the same noise as the wind. For fears about nuclear war, empowering children to become active, such as joining a nuclear protest group, may be useful.

Parents may feel helpless because they do not know how to deal with children's fears. Physicians should give them the necessary information. Children's fears should not be trivialized. Even if the **fears** are unfounded, they **should be validated.** In general, children should be questioned about whether they are fearful about a situation. The following 2 examples illustrate the proper handling of fears in children.

If children are visiting the dentist for the first time, it is appropriate for parents to ask, "Are you afraid?" If children reply, "Yes, a little bit," parents can say, "Almost everybody is afraid. Tell me what it is you're afraid of. Fear is a normal emotion, and I'm glad you told me about it."

Parents of children who express fear of imaginary characters can reassure children that they do not exist. In addition, parents can tell children what the parents would do if such characters did exist. For instance, the father of a little girl who was afraid of witches told her, "There are no such things as witches. But if there were, and they came into your room, I would punch them in the nose and punch them in the stomach and beat them up, and then there would be no more witches to hurt you." By doing this, parents establish the reality of the situation and then also create a plan to deal with the problem should it actually happen.

Parents can also help to limit or reduce children's fears by **minimizing** their **exposure to fear-provoking situations** such as television shows or scary movies. These programs can be particularly frightening for some children, who should not watch them without adult supervision. Minimizing exposure to television is particularly important following a disastrous event. The recurrent images of planes flying into buildings on 9/11 were interpreted by children as repeated different attacks.

When dealing with children who have school phobia because of problems in school, it is important to determine if a change in school would be appropriate to facilitate their school attendance. This may be particularly appropriate in children whose schools are plagued with violence.

Cognitive-behavioral therapy (CBT) is reported to have the highest rate of success for dealing with anxiety-related conditions. Cognitive-behavioral therapy includes psychoeducation, somatic management (eg, relaxation techniques), cognitive restructuring (modifying negative thoughts), and exposure methods including desensitization.

When school refusal is linked to separation anxiety, then a program of **desensitization or habituation (graded exposure)** is recommended. Desensitization may involve the participation of mothers in the classroom for a time. When children acclimate and can tolerate some separation, mothers move to another area in the school such as the principal's office. Next they go outside the school grounds. As children reestablish a sense of well-being in spite of the separation, the mothers gradually move farther and farther away. This solution is somewhat problematic for mothers who work outside the home. There is some research to suggest that children adjust more readily if they resume school immediately without the gradual withdrawal of their parent. Children with significant school refusal may need the assistance of child psychologists or psychiatrists.

Phobias may be treated using the concept of **flooding,** which consists of rapid, prolonged exposure to the feared item. For example, a child who is afraid of dogs is exposed to a friendly, docile, small dog while in the company of his or her parents. Alternatively, systematic desensitization, during which children are exposed to the feared objects over a series of weeks, coupled with relaxation techniques, is also used. Phobias usually require the help of mental health specialists. Selective serotonin reuptake inhibitors (see Chapter 114) have been found to be beneficial in the management of certain anxiety disorders in children and adolescents. They are noted to be effective for

panic disorders, social phobia, generalized anxiety disorder, obsessive-compulsive disorder, and PTSD. Benzodiazepines are safe and generally used on a short-term basis. Sedation is a frequent side effect, and there is the potential for abuse, tolerance, and drug dependence. Propranolol lessens the peripheral autonomic nervous system symptoms of social phobias and may be used for specific instances. Combined therapy involving CBT and medication is beneficial in some patients.

Children who must undergo hospitalization benefit from a prehospital visit, when possible. This visit familiarizes the child with the facilities and explains proposed procedures. Many hospitals have child life specialists who ease the adjustment of children as well as their parents to the hospital stay.

Prognosis

Most childhood fears resolve with time, nurturing, and reassurance. Most fears last only several weeks, and then new fears develop. As a rule, specific fears should not last longer than 2 years, and the younger the child, the shorter the duration of the fear.

Prognosis is good for children with true phobias, with 100% resolution of monosymptomatic phobias. More significant anxiety disorders may persist into adulthood, where similar management involving CBT and medications may be indicated.

CASE RESOLUTION

In the case scenario, the girl's fear of sleeping in her bed was triggered by a significant environmental event. Although earthquakes are uncontrollable, the girl can be empowered to deal with manageable aspects of an earthquake as much as possible. She should be assured that in the same situation, many adults probably would also fear sleeping alone. The parents should stock a box with shoes, flashlight, radio, and water and place the box under the child's bed. In addition, they may also have their daughter get into her bed and then shake it, simulating the jiggling that she would experience during an earthquake. The girl should also practice getting out of bed and standing in the doorway. To combat the child's fear of separation during times of natural disaster, the parents should reassure their daughter that they will all be together.

Selected References

Physicians

American Psychiatric Association. *Diagnostic and Statistical Manual of Mental Disorders.* 4th ed. Washington, DC: American Psychiatric Association; 1994

Bothe D, Olness K. Worried sick. Anxiety among youth. *Contemp Pediatr.* 2007;24:58–63

Brown EJ. Clinical characteristics and efficacious treatment of posttraumatic stress disorder in children and adolescents. *Pediatr Ann.* 2005;34:138–146

Emotions and moods. In: Wolraich ML, ed. *The Classification of Child and Adolescent Mental Diagnoses in Primary Care: Diagnostic and Statistical Manual for Primary Care (DSM-PC) Child and Adolescent Version.* Elk Grove Village, IL: American Academy of Pediatrics; 1996:145–149

Jurbergs N, Ledley DR. Separation anxiety disorders. *Pediatr Ann.* 2005;34:108–115

Kendall PC, Chu BC, Pimentel SS, Choudhury M. Treating anxiety disorders in youth. In: Kendall PC, ed. *Child and Adolescent Therapy: Cognitive Behavioral Procedures*. 2nd ed. New York, NY: The Guilford Press; 2000

Klein RG, Last CG. *Anxiety Disorders in Children*. Newbury Park, CA: Sage Publications; 1989

Sarafino EP. *The Fears of Childhood*. New York, NY: Human Sciences Press; 1986

Williams TP, Miller BD. Pharmacologic management of anxiety disorders in children and adolescents. *Curr Opin Pediatr*. 2003;15:483–490

Compton SN, March JS, Brent D, et al. Cognitive-behavioral psychotherapy for anxiety and depressive disorders in children and adolescents: an evidence-based medicine review. *J Am Acad Child Adolesc Psychiatry*. 2004;43:930–959

Hanna GL, Fischer DJ, Fluent TE. Separation anxiety disorder and school refusal in children and adolescents. *Pediatr Rev*. 2006;27:56–62

Walsh KH. Welcome advances in treating youth anxiety disorders. *Contemp Pediatr*. 2002;19:66–82

Parents and Children

Berenstain S, Berenstain J. *The Berenstain Bears and the Bully*. New York, NY: Random House; 1993

Berenstain S, Berenstain J. *The Berenstain Bears in the Dark*. New York, NY: Random House; 1982

Berenstain S, Berenstain J. *The Berenstain Bears Visit the Dentist*. New York, NY: Random House; 1981

Mayer M. *There's a Nightmare in My Closet*. New York, NY: Penguin Books; 1992

Ziefert H. *Nicky's Noisy Night*. New York, NY: Penguin Books; 1986

Thumb Sucking and Other Habits

Carol D. Berkowitz, MD

CASE STUDY

A 5-year-old boy is brought to the office because of thumb sucking. His mother claims that she has tried nearly everything, including tying his hands at night and using aversive treatments on his thumbs, but nothing has worked. She reports that her son has been teased at school and has few friends. He is in good general health, and his immunizations are up to date.

His growth parameters are at the 50th percentile. Except for a callus on the right thumb, the physical examination is normal.

Questions

1. What are common habits in children?
2. What is the significance of transitional objects?
3. What are the consequences of the common habits in children?
4. What are strategies used to break children of habits?
5. How does one differentiate benign habits from self-injurious behaviors?

Habits are defined as somewhat complicated, repetitive behaviors that become automatized, fixed, and carried out easily and effortlessly. They are different from tics, which are rapid, repetitive muscle twitches involving the head, face, or shoulders. Tics are also referred to as habit spasms (see Chapter 105). Children have many socially unacceptable habits, including thumb sucking, nail biting, skin picking, nose picking, hair pulling (trichotillomania), rocking, biting other children, and teeth grinding (bruxism). Some habits, such as pica, are potentially harmful. Children engage in most of these habits because of their soothing potential. In recent years, "cutting," a form of self-injury in adolescents, has received attention. While not a habit in a traditional sense, cutting is described by teens as a way of dealing with stress and alleviating anxiety. One-third of children use transitional objects for comfort. Blankets or favorite toys are traditional transitional objects that represent an age-appropriate coping strategy. Most transitional objects are strokable, and the stroking often occurs in association with thumb sucking. Transitional objects sometimes present a problem because children experience distress if these objects are lost, misplaced, or need cleaning.

Epidemiology

Thumb sucking probably represents the most common habit of children. A reported 50% to 87% of children engage in this habit. The median age for the onset of hand sucking is 54 minutes of life, and 90% of newborns show hand-sucking behavior by the age of 2 hours. Forty percent of children between the ages of 1 and 3 years, 33% of children between the ages of 3 and 5, and 25% of children at the age of 5 still suck their thumbs. Some children suck their fingers rather than thumbs. Other oral behavior may involve lip sucking, lip biting, and toe sucking. Lip sucking and biting begin at about 5 to 6 months of age and occur in about 90% of infants. It is unusual for these actions to persist as habits. Toe sucking is noted in infants who are 6 to 7 months of age, and it is reported in 80% of normal infants.

Trichotillomania is a disorder once believed to be uncommon but now thought to affect 8 million Americans (about 5 in 1,000). The term, first coined in 1889 by French dermatologist Hallopeau, is derived from the Greek *thrix* (hair), *tillein* (pull), and *mania* (madness). The condition is an impulse control disorder in which alopecia develops from compulsive hair pulling. Hair pulling may involve hair from the head, eyebrows, eyelashes, or pubic area. Although trichotillomania seems to peak during early childhood and adolescence, the disorder is reported from infancy to adolescence. In young children, boys and girls are equally affected, but in older children and adolescents, females outnumber males. The disorder is not associated with comorbid psychopathology, but there may be some association with mood disorders or attention-deficit/hyperactivity disorder. There is a condition in infants, called *baby trichs,* in which infants pull their mother's hair when they are being held or nursed. This is considered normal exploratory behavior.

Rhythmic habits are stereotypical, repetitive behaviors that usually occur in infants younger than 1 year. These habits are reported in 15% to 20% of the population. Rhythmic habits include rocking (about 19% of infants), when infants rock back and forth; jouncing (5%–10%), when they move up-and-down on their hands and knees so that the whole crib rocks; head rolling (8%); and head banging (5%). Rhythmic habits are seen more commonly in boys; the male-female ratio is 3:1. These habits usually occur with a frequency of 60 to 80 movements per minute, often when infants are tired, and last for less than 15 minutes before they fall sleep.

Rhythmic movements have been equated with **sleep tics.** These tics are reported in 20% of children, most often between the ages of 6 and 10 years. As a rule, tics are 3 times more common in boys than in girls. They tend to be noted with increased frequency in children who are shy, are overly self-conscious, or have obsessive-compulsive tendencies. Tics usually occur when children are under stress.

Biting, an aggressive habit noted in toddlers, may be related to teething. It occurs more often in children with slow verbal skills.

Nail biting (onychophagia) is usually believed to be a sign of internal tension. The disorder affects 10% to 40% of children. Nail biting begins between the ages of 3 and 6, and the peak age is 13 years. One-third of adolescents bite their nails, but 50% of these adolescents break the habit by the time they reach adulthood. Nail biting in adults is regarded as a sign of emotional and social immaturity and regression. The family history for nail biting is often positive. Identical twins are concordant for the condition in 66% of cases. In contrast, the incidence in dizygotic twins is 34%.

Nose picking, noted in children and adults, is reported in more than 90% of individuals. In general, adults and older children limit nose picking to when they are unobserved, but younger children will pick their noses in public. There are no gender-based differences in the incidence of nose picking. Epistaxis is the most common complication of nose picking.

Pica, which is not a normal behavior, is defined as the ingestion of nonfood products. The peak incidence of pica is between the ages of 1 and 3 years. The incidence is increased in children from lower socioeconomic levels, and the behavior occurs in 10% of children who present with lead poisoning.

Teeth grinding (bruxism) is reported in 5% to 15% of children. Boys are more commonly affected than girls, and the disorder seems to regress later in life. It is reported with increased incidence among developmentally delayed children including those with autism spectrum disorder. The cause is unknown, although it may be associated with malocclusion in some children. The disorder may contribute to temporomandibular joint dysfunction and pain.

Self-injury has been reported in up to 20% of mentally retarded adults. Autism and the absence of speech are the highest associated risk factors. Nail biting, head banging, and self-biting are frequently described associated behaviors. Severe self-injury related to biting is seen in Lesch-Nyhan syndrome.

Clinical Presentation

Children with common habits, such as thumb sucking or rhythmic movements, may be brought to the physician with these particular complaints because the parent wants advice about stopping the

behavior. Other children may present with consequences of habits, such as alopecia (trichotillomania), paronychia (nail biting), or lead intoxication (pica) (Dx Box).

Dx **Childhood Habits**

- History of a habit
- Callus on thumb or fingers
- Short, chewed nails
- Alopecia
- Lead intoxication
- Iron deficiency anemia

Pathophysiology

Children engage in habits to reduce stress and provide comfort. Thumb sucking is related to nonnutritive sucking. Although the initial purpose of sucking is nutritional, the pleasure associated with sucking reinforces the behavior. Infants who are served from a cup from birth develop no interest in sucking. Humans and other primates spend more time in nonnutritive than in nutritive sucking. Monkeys use a 5-point hold, with 2 hands, 2 feet, and mouth (holding on to their mother's nipple) for attachment. Universal thumb sucking is noted even in orphan monkeys, and sucking is thought to be an important aspect of environmental adaptation. Nonnutritive sucking occurs even in the absence of fatigue, hunger, or discomfort, and has a purpose in itself—to provide comfort and be self-soothing. The maximum intensity of sucking occurs at 7 months. For older children (>3 years), sucking is also a way of dealing with boredom.

In bottle-fed infants, thumb sucking seems to commence when feeding stops. Some infants, described as "type A," seem to be satisfied only when their thumb is in their mouth. As infants spend more time engaged in motor activity, they spend less time thumb sucking. Placid infants who cry less also do less sucking. Some studies have shown that thumb sucking is less common in breastfed infants, and that thumb suckers as a group feed less frequently (every 4 hours rather than 3 and for 10 minutes rather than 20).

Nail biting is related to thumb sucking, a form of oral gratification, and children may progress from thumb sucking to nail biting. The pattern of nail biting usually involves placement of the hand in the vicinity of the mouth, tapping of the fingers along the teeth, quick spasmodic bites with the fingers around the central incisors, and the removal and inspection of the hands. Other oral habits, such as pencil gnawing, gum chewing, lip biting, and nail picking, are related activities, as is nose picking. The cause of teeth grinding is unclear.

Rocking habits are believed to be kinesthetically pleasing and soothing and a means of autostimulation. The etiology of hair pulling is less apparent. In recent years, investigators have linked trichotillomania to disorders of serotonin reuptake and placed it in the category of obsessive-compulsive behavior. Some individuals who engage in trichotillomania have abnormal head positron emission tomography. Although the etiology of trichotillomania is unclear, affected children share certain features, which have been characterized as fiddling SHEEP (sensation, hands, emotion, environment, perfectionism). The overriding factor is a need for tactile stimulation. Pica, which is also considered abnormal, may be associated with mental retardation, environmental deprivation, or inadequate nutrition, particularly iron deficiency.

Differential Diagnosis

The differential diagnosis of most habits is not difficult. Tics or habit spasms should be differentiated from Tourette syndrome. This syndrome, which is reported in 1 in 3,000 children, is a neurologic disorder characterized by severe, frequent, and multiple tics. These tics are also often vocal and consist of sounds such as hissing, barking, grunting, or coprolalia (repeating profanities). Some of the rhythmic habits may be mistaken for seizures but can be easily distinguished because of the stereotypical, repetitive nature of the behavior.

Trichotillomania usually has a classic physical appearance that has been referred to as *tonsure Friar Tuck* pattern baldness, with baldness around the vertex of the head. Unilateral temporal baldness is also a consequence of trichotillomania. The differential diagnosis of trichotillomania includes alopecia areata, tinea capitis, syphilitic alopecia, and androgenic alopecia (see Chapter 107). Broken hairs of variable length usually characterize alopecia secondary to trichotillomania. Other disorders in the differential diagnosis include traction alopecia, related to tight braids or hair brushing; atopic eczema; seborrheic dermatitis; hypothyroidism; systemic lupus erythematosus; and dermatomyositis.

Cutting is not a benign habit, but it can provide stress relief, a feature of many benign childhood habits. It is usually associated with a wide range of psychopathology including depression; anxiety; eating disorders, especially bulimia nervosa; a history of prior sexual abuse; and obsessive-compulsive symptoms. The mechanism by which cutting alleviates stress and anxiety has not been elucidated, but the role of endogenous endorphins has been suggested. Cutting is felt not to represent suicidal behavior, but some studies differentiate the site of cutting as predictive of suicidality: wrist cutters as opposed to arm cutters have a higher rate of suicide ideation and attempts. All cutters are at greater risk for suicide than the general population. Management generally involves referral to a mental health specialist and the use of psychotherapy. Other forms of self-injury are reported with increased frequency among children with developmental disabilities including autism spectrum disorder (see Chapter 112).

Evaluation

History

Children who present with thumb sucking, nail biting, and teeth grinding usually do not require an assessment other than a routine health maintenance history and physical examination. The history should determine the specific circumstances when the habit is manifest. Is the habit more likely to emerge when the child is tired or stressed? Habits must also be evaluated in the context of the child's developmental level and home situation. Understanding the impact of the habit on the child and the family is important. Children who present with movements that resemble tics should be carefully questioned about the frequency and duration of the tics, the effect of the tics on their behavior, and whether coughing is associated with the tics (sign of Tourette syndrome). The occurrence of obsessive-compulsive mannerisms should also be noted (Questions Box).

> ## Questions
> ### Childhood Habits
> - What about your child's habit concerns you?
> - Is your child experiencing any adverse consequences (eg, being teased at school) as a result of the habit?
> - Does the habit interfere with your child's routine activities?
> - Can you identify stressors in your child's life?
> - Is your child comforted by the habit?

Physical Examination

A routine physical examination should be performed. The physical examination may reveal the sequelae of the habit such as thumb calluses, candidal infection of the nails, or evidence of malocclusion with an overbite (Figure 40-1). Children with suspected trichotillomania should have a thorough assessment of their scalp in an effort to differentiate other causes of alopecia (Chapter 107). A careful neurologic examination should be performed in children with tics, and referral to a child neurologist may be indicated in children with suspected neurologic disorders.

Laboratory Studies

Routine laboratory studies are not needed in children diagnosed with habit disorders.

Figure 40-1. Anterior open bite associated with thumb sucking.

Children with trichotillomania should be evaluated for the disorders listed previously. An easy evaluation process for trichotillomania involves shaving the hair in the middle of the area of baldness. The growth of these small hairs is uniform because children are unable to pull them out. Head shaving may not be acceptable, however, to the parent or the child. Disorders such as syphilis and collagen vascular diseases can be ruled out using appropriate laboratory studies. Fungal infections can be differentiated by the use of appropriate cultures. A Wood light examination may reveal fluorescence noted with certain fungal infections.

Children who present with pica should be evaluated for the presence of iron deficiency anemia and lead poisoning.

Management

The management of childhood habits should be directed at the specific symptoms. For older children, self-monitoring and relaxation training may be helpful as alternative means for dealing with stress. The issue of thumb sucking versus the use of pacifiers can be addressed by anticipatory guidance. **Pacifiers,** which were previously discouraged, are now believed to have some advantages over thumb sucking. A recent report from the American Academy of Pediatrics noted a decrease in the incidence of sudden infant death syndrome in infants who used a pacifier. With pacifiers, the risk for dental disturbances is lower because the pacifiers are softer and are accompanied by a plastic shield that puts counter pressure on the teeth. Pacifiers are also detachable and cleanable.

Pacifiers can be lost, however. Parents should be advised not to attach a pacifier to the child's shirt with a string because of risk of strangulation. For children who are pacifier-dependent and are unable to go back to sleep if they lose their pacifier at night, multiple pacifiers can be placed in the crib to make finding one easier. For infants who desire pacifiers because they complete their feeding in less than 20 minutes, a nipple with a smaller hole can be used or the cap can be screwed on the bottle more tightly to prolong the time spent in nutritive sucking. Dental problems may develop when pacifiers are used upside down, all day long, or after the eruption of permanent dentition.

It is suggested that parents do not try to stop thumb-sucking behavior until children have reached the age of 4 years. Dental problems in late thumb suckers include anterior open bite, increased overjet (protruding upper incisors), intruded and flared upper incisors, lingually flipped lower incisors, and warped alveolar ridge. When thumb sucking persists to school age, tongue thrust is noted, as are articulation problems, specifically with consonants s, t, d, n, z, l, and r. The physician should reassure parents that children who stop sucking their thumbs prior to the onset of the secondary dentition are not at risk for poor dentition.

Numerous devices have been proposed to help with the cessation of thumb sucking, but reported success has been variable. The use of arm restraints, particularly at night, is not recommended and may result in rumination. Bitter paints such as Stop Zit seek to reduce thumb sucking by subjecting children to a bitter, aversive taste. This

medication consists of 49% toluene, 19% isopropyl alcohol, 18% butyl acetate, 11% ethylcellulose, and 0.3% denatonium benzoate. A three-quarter–ounce bottle is toxic if ingested in its entirety. Nocturnal application is needed if children suck their thumbs during the night. The principle of retraining, where thumb sucking becomes a duty and children are required to suck all 10 fingers one at a time, has also been recommended. Some recommend that elastic bandages be put on the hand of nocturnal thumb suckers. Problems associated with thumb sucking include sore thumbs, calluses, and candidal infections. Dentists may fashion a reminder appliance, called a palatal crib, making it difficult for children to suck their thumbs.

Encouragement works better than nagging, as a rule, and a **reward system** is particularly useful in children who are 5 to 6 years of age. Parents may be referred to books such as *Danny and His Thumb* (Ernst KF. Englewood Cliffs, NJ: Prentice-Hall; 1973) and encouraged to talk to their children about how good it feels not to suck their thumbs. A star chart and diary are also useful. Sometimes telling children something like, "Mommy would be so proud of you if you didn't suck your thumb now that you're such a big girl or a big boy" is effective. In addition, the pressure to stop thumb sucking becomes greater during the school years. Children who suck their thumbs are regarded by their peers in first grade as less intelligent, less happy, less likable, and less desirable as friends.

In children who suck their thumbs and twirl their hair at the same time, the hair twirling stops once the thumb sucking ends. The phenomenon is referred to as *habit covariance.* Hair pulling in young children seems to often resolve spontaneously but is more problematic in adolescents and adults. Management of trichotillomania usually involves non-pharmacologic treatments. In children, behavior modification, including putting socks on the hands and the use of time out for hair pulling, in addition to extra attention for not pulling the hair, is recommended. Substituting behavior is also encouraged. For instance, children should be advised to sit on their hands, wear gloves, pull rubber bands, or squeeze a ball whenever they have an urge to pull their hair. In older individuals, hair pulling may be related to obsessive-compulsive disorders. Trichotillomania may lead to the presence of bezoars (hairballs) from swallowed hair. Hairballs can be mechanically removed or dissolved with the installation of Coca Cola through a nasogastric tube. Pharmacologic therapy for trichotillomania is not routinely recommended for the management of affected children. In adults, selective serotonin reuptake inhibitors, bupropion, and risperidone have been used. Children whose symptoms have not improved with behavioral interventions should be referred to a mental health worker for additional management.

Nail biting also often responds to behavior modification. Olive oil may be put on the nails to make them soft so there are fewer jagged edges to bite. In the children's book, *The Berenstain Bears and the Bad Habit,* collecting pennies is suggested as a habit substitution for nail biting.

Rhythmic habits are less easy to modify. For the most part, reassurance is all that is available. The use of metronome-like devices has had no demonstrable effect. Children older than 3 years who disturb the family's sleep with their rhythmic habits may be given mild sedatives such as diphenhydramine. Medications to reduce head banging include transdermal clonidine and thioridazine (Mellaril). Other maneuvers involve placing the crib or bed on carpeting to decrease the amount of noise from movement.

Children who engage in biting behavior should be managed with behavior modification, including praising of good behavior and time out for inappropriate behavior. Aversive conditioning involves the placement of some non-palatable food such as a lemon or onion on a necklace, and having the child bite on that object rather than biting another child. Biting behavior is reported to be extinguished with this technique. Another option is the placement of a whistle. The child blows the whistle rather than biting the other child.

Nose picking is a common habit in both children and adults. One suggestion to extinguish or minimize this habit involves letting children look in a mirror and pick their nose. Their reaction is that nose picking looks "gross" and the habit may decrease in frequency.

Iron deficiency resulting from pica requires iron supplementation. Lead intoxication should be managed with chelation and environmental manipulation.

Prognosis

Most habits are not harmful to children's health. The major problem is social acceptability. Parents should be encouraged to stop a habit before it becomes ingrained. This can often be done by praising good behavior and encouraging activities during which the unwanted behavior does not appear. Habits that do not respond to parental influence often resolve spontaneously under peer pressure.

CASE RESOLUTION

In the case history presented at the beginning of the chapter, it is important for the physician and the mother to empower the boy to stop thumb sucking before he finds himself ridiculed by his classmates. He might be allowed to suck his thumb at certain times and in certain places (eg, "You can suck in your room after school for fifteen minutes."). Books geared at children and parents to help stop the thumb sucking are recommended, and the boy is rewarded for times when he is not sucking his thumb.

Selected References

Blum NJ, Barone VJ, Friman PC. A simplified behavioral treatment for trichotillomania: report of two cases. *Pediatrics.* 1993;91:993–995

Brazelton TB. Sucking in infancy. *Pediatrics.* 1956;17:400–404

Collacott RA, Cooper SA, Branford D, McGrother C. Epidemiology of self-injurious behaviour in adults with learning disabilities. *Br J Psychiatry.* 1998;173:428–432

Dimino-Emme L, Camisa C. Trichotillomania associated with the "Friar Tuck sign" and nail biting. *Cutis.* 1991;47:107–110

Friman PC, Schmitt B. Thumb sucking in childhood: guidelines for the pediatrician. *Clin Pediatr.* 1989;28:438–440

Friman PC, Barone VJ, Christopherson ER. Aversive taste treatment of finger and thumb sucking. *Pediatrics.* 1986;78:174–176

Friman PC, McPherson KM, Warzak WJ, Evans J. Influence of thumb sucking on peer social acceptance in first-grade children. *Pediatrics.* 1993;91:784–786

Golomb RG, Vavrichek SM. *The Hair Pulling "Habit" and You: How to Solve the Trichotillomania Puzzle.* Silver Spring, MD: Writers' Cooperative of Greater Washington; 2000

Johnson ED, Larson BE. Thumb-sucking: literature review. *ASDC J Dent Child.* 1993;60:385–391

Peterson JE, Schneider PE. Oral habits: a behavioral approach. *Pediatr Clin North Am.* 1991;38:1289–1307

Repetitive behavioral patterns. In: Wolraich ML, ed. *The Classification of Child and Adolescent Mental Diagnoses in Primary Care: Diagnostic and Statistical Manual for Primary Care (DSM-PC) Child and Adolescent Version.* Elk Grove Village, IL: American Academy of Pediatrics; 1996:269–275

Rosenberg MD. Thumbsucking. *Pediatr Rev.* 1995;16:73–74

Schmitt B. Helping the child with tics (twitches). *Contemp Pediatr.* 1991;8:31–32

Tay YK, Levy ML, Metry DW. Trichotillomania in childhood: case series and review. *Pediatrics.* 2004;113:e494–e498

Enuresis

Carol D. Berkowitz, MD

CASE STUDY

A 9-year-old boy who is in good general health is evaluated for a history of bedwetting. He is the product of a normal pregnancy and delivery, and he achieved his developmental milestones at the appropriate time. The boy was toilet trained by the age of 3 years, but he has never been dry at night for more than several days at a time. Enuresis occurs at least 3 to 4 times a week even if he is fluid-restricted after 6 pm. The boy never wets himself during the day, has normal stools, and is an average student. His father had enuresis that resolved by the time he was 12 years old.

The boy's physical examination is entirely normal.

Questions

1. What conditions account for the symptoms of enuresis?
2. What is the appropriate evaluation of children with enuresis?
3. What is the relationship between enuresis and emotional stresses or psychosocial disorders?
4. What management plans are available for enuresis?
5. How do physicians decide which management technique is appropriate for which patients?

Enuresis is defined as involuntary or intentional urination in children whose age and development suggest achievement of bladder control. Voiding into the bed or clothing occurs repeatedly (at least twice a week for at least 3 consecutive months). Urinary continence is reached earlier in girls than in boys, and the diagnosis of enuresis is reserved for girls older than 5 years and boys older than 6 years. Diurnal enuresis is wetting that occurs during the day. Nocturnal or sleep enuresis refers to involuntary urination that occurs during the night. The term **primary enuresis** is used when children have never achieved sustained dryness, and **secondary enuresis** is used when urinary incontinence recurs after 3 to 6 months of dryness. Monosymptomatic nocturnal enuresis means that nighttime wetting is the only complaint. Children who experience urgency, frequency, dribbling, or other symptoms have polysymptomatic enuresis.

Physicians can be particularly helpful by routinely questioning parents about bedwetting during health maintenance visits. Many families are otherwise reluctant to bring up this embarrassing complaint because enuresis is viewed as socially unacceptable. It poses particular difficulties if children wish to sleep away from home. In addition, enuresis may be a marker for other behavioral or developmental problems.

Epidemiology

Enuresis affects 5 to 7 million patients in the United States. It is one of the most common conditions of childhood, affecting 10% to 20% of first-grade boys and 8% to 17% of first-grade girls. By age 10 years, 5% to 10% of boys have enuresis (1% of army recruits are enuretic). Seventy-four percent of affected children have nocturnal enuresis, 10% diurnal enuresis, and 16% both. Primary enuresis affects the majority (75%–80%) of children with enuresis, and 80% to 85% of these children have monosymptomatic nocturnal enuresis. Although the overall incidence of secondary enuresis is lower (20%–25%), it increases with age; secondary enuresis makes up 50% of cases of enuresis in children 12 years of age.

Several epidemiological factors have been associated with enuresis, including low socioeconomic level, large family size, single-parent family, low birth weight, short height at 11 to 15 years of age, immature behavior, relatively low IQ, poor speech and coordination, and encopresis (fecal incontinence; 5%–15% of cases). Enuresis occurs more often in institutionalized children. Enuresis has a familial basis, and as many as 77% of children are enuretic if both parents were similarly affected. Concordance for enuresis is reported in up to 68% of monozygotic twins and up to 48% of dizygotic twins.

Clinical Presentation

A history of enuresis may be obtained as a presenting complaint or elicited by physicians during a health maintenance visit. Medical complaints such as encopresis or attention-deficit/hyperactivity disorder may be associated with the enuresis (Dx Box). The physical examination is usually normal.

Dx Enuresis

- Bedwetting
- Old enough to be toilet trained
- Precipitating problem such as diabetes or urinary tract infection
- Encopresis
- Attention-deficit/hyperactivity disorder
- Family history of enuresis

Pathophysiology

Delayed control of micturition has several possible causes (Box 41-1).

Box 41-1. Causes of Enuresis

Primary Enuresis
- Faulty toilet training
- Maturational delay
- Small bladder capacity
- Sleep disorder/impaired arousal
- Allergens
- Nocturnal polyuria/relative vasopressin deficiency
- Dysfunctional bladder contraction

Secondary Enuresis
- Urinary tract infection
- Diabetes mellitus
- Diabetes insipidus
- Nocturnal seizures
- Genitourinary anomalies
- Sickle cell anemia
- Medication use
- Emotional stress

---

1. **Faulty toilet training.** Faulty toilet training may perpetuate both diurnal and nocturnal enuresis but is not expected to selectively perpetuate the latter. Parental expectations are believed to play a role in the toilet training experience. Parents who allow children to sleep in diapers may be delaying the achievement of nighttime dryness, but it is unlikely that the use of diapers causes nocturnal enuresis. Poor toilet habits, particularly infrequent voiding or constipation, may be associated with urinary tract infections (UTIs).

2. **Maturational delay.** The development of the inhibitory reflex of voiding may be delayed in some children, which may contribute to enuresis until the age of 5 years. This is similar to the range with which children achieve other developmental milestones. It is unlikely that maturational delay persists as a cause of enuresis beyond this age. Experts believe that maturational delay is not a reasonable explanation if children can achieve dryness in the daytime but not at night.

3. **Small bladder capacity.** Evidence suggests that some children with enuresis have smaller bladder capacities. Bladder capacity in ounces is estimated as the age in years plus 2. For example, 5-year-old children have a bladder capacity of 7 ounces (210 mL). Adult bladder capacity is 12 to 16 ounces (360–480 mL). Small bladder capacity is associated with diurnal frequency or incontinence.

4. **Sleep disorder/impaired arousal.** It has been suggested that children with enuresis are in "deep sleep" and do not sense a full bladder. This is often the parent's perception of their child's sleep pattern. However, studies have shown that enuresis occurs during all stages of sleep, particularly in the first one-third of sleep and in transition from non–rapid eye movement (REM) stage 4 to REM sleep. During this period body tone, respiratory rate, and heart rate increase, and erection and micturition occur. Studies suggest that the arousal center in the brain fails to respond (ie, the child does not awaken) to full bladder sensation. Children with enuresis do not seem to sleep more deeply than other children. However, enuretic children may have diminished arousal during sleep. In one study, 40% of enuretic children, compared with only 8.5% of non-enuretic children, failed to awaken to an 80-decibel noise.

5. **Allergens.** No evidence confirms the notion that exposure to certain foods (eg, food additives, sugar) contributes to enuresis. However, some parents believe that bedwetting is decreased if certain foods such as sodas and sweets are eliminated from the diet. The ingestion of caffeine-containing beverages may exacerbate nocturnal enuresis.

6. **Nocturnal polyuria/relative vasopressin deficiency.** Research has shown that although non-enuretic children exhibit a diurnal variation in vasopressin secretion, this rhythm is disturbed in some children with enuresis, resulting in nocturnal polyuria.

7. **Dysfunctional bladder contraction.** In cases of diurnal enuresis, contractile disturbances of the bladder affect normal voiding. Children with an "uninhibited bladder" have not learned to inhibit bladder contraction. They may assume a certain posture, called Vincent curtsy, in an effort to prevent micturition. Some children exhibit discoordinated, incomplete voiding and the urine exits the urethra in a staccato stream. Trabeculations or bladder wall thickening may be noted on imaging studies.

Differential Diagnosis

Primary nocturnal enuresis is usually related to the conditions discussed in Pathophysiology. An organic problem is rarely the cause. However, secondary enuresis frequently results from an organic problem, such as UTI, diabetes mellitus, diabetes insipidus, nocturnal seizures, genitourinary anomalies (eg, ectopic ureter), sickle cell anemia, medication (eg, diuretics, theophylline), or emotional stress. When primary enuresis is both diurnal and nocturnal, some of these conditions should also be considered. Additional diagnoses include neurogenic bladder, which may occur in association with cerebral palsy, sacral agenesis, or myelomeningocele.

Evaluation

History

A thorough history should be obtained when evaluating children with enuresis (Questions Box).

Questions

Enuresis

- Is the enuresis primary or secondary?
- Is the enuresis diurnal, nocturnal, or both?
- How old was the child when he or she was toilet trained?
- How old was the child when he or she achieved daytime and nighttime dryness?
- How often does the child urinate and defecate during the average day?
- Is the child's urinary stream forceful or dribbling?
- Does the child dribble before or after voiding?
- Does the child experience symptoms such as polydipsia, polyuria, dysuria, urgency, frequency, or problems with stooling?
- Who changes the bed and who washes the bedclothes after bedwetting occurs?
- Does the child wear diapers or pull-ups, or use incontinence pads?
- Does the child seem to delay using the toilet?
- Does the child assume any unusual or distinct postures to avoid being incontinent?
- What is the attitude of the family toward the child with enuresis? Are family members accepting or ashamed?
- Has the family tried any treatments yet?
- Is there a family history of enuresis?
- Does the child have other symptoms such as encopresis or attention-deficit/hyperactivity disorder?

Physical Examination

A general physical examination should be performed, with particular attention to certain areas. The pattern of growth should be plotted. Blood pressure should be obtained. The abdomen should be assessed for evidence of organomegaly, bladder size, and fecal impaction. An anal examination should be performed to evaluate rectal tone.

If possible, physicians should watch children void. Practitioners should determine whether children can start and stop micturition and whether the stream is forceful. Dribbling in girls may indicate an ectopic ureter. The appearance of the genitalia should be assessed. A rash in the genital area may be secondary to wetness from urinary incontinence. Labial fusion in girls may trap urine, allow reflux into the vagina, and lead to dribbling. Meatal stenosis, epispadias, hypospadias, or cryptorchidism may be present in boys. Any of these conditions suggests a possible underlying genitourinary anomaly.

The neuromuscular integrity of the lower extremities should be evaluated. This may provide a clue to a disorder such as spina bifida occulta. The presence of some anomaly in the sacral area, such as a sacral dimple or a tuft of hair, may also be a sign of this condition.

Laboratory Tests

Only a minimal laboratory evaluation is indicated in most children with primary enuresis. Urinalysis, including specific gravity, is usually indicated. A complete blood count, hemoglobin electrophoresis, serum electrolytes, and blood urea nitrogen should also be considered. Studies such as urine culture and blood glucose are more often indicated in cases of secondary enuresis.

Imaging Studies

In cases in which the urinalysis is abnormal, the culture is positive, or genitourinary anomalies are apparent on physical examination, a renal ultrasound and vesicoureterogram may be warranted. Vertebral x-rays or magnetic resonance imaging is appropriate in the diagnosis of spina bifida. An electroencephalogram is indicated if nocturnal epilepsy is suspected. Urodynamic studies to evaluate bladder contractility are controversial but are recommended by some urologists.

Management

Primary Enuresis

Family counseling about enuresis should be part of all management plans. Issues related to psychosocial stress should be explored, particularly in cases of secondary enuresis. Families should be advised that the wetting is not intentional and that punishing children for accidents is inappropriate. However, children may take some responsibility for the consequences of their actions, such as removing soiled bedding or helping with the laundry. They should be rewarded for dry nights. Star charts, in which a sticker or gold star is applied to a calendar for each dry night, have traditionally been used. The exclusive use of these charts without other interventions has limited success, however, and suggests that the enuresis may have a volitional component. Star charts should be used in conjunction with other management strategies.

Two treatment modalities are acceptable for managing enuresis. Most studies do not support the use of fluid restriction as a reliable isolated means of controlling enuresis.

Conditioning therapy involves the use of an alarm that is triggered when children void during the night. Children are awakened by the sounding of the alarm, and further urination is inhibited. Eventually bladder distention is associated with inhibition of the urge to urinate. When conditioning therapy is used for 4 to 6 months, it is associated with a success rate of 70%. If the alarm is used for 4 more weeks with sustained dryness, relapses are uncommon.

Because patient cooperation is needed with the alarm system, its use is reserved for children older than 7 years. A newer system is a transistorized version of the original device that contains a small sensor in the underwear and an alarm on the wrist or collar. Some systems use vibrations so other family members are not disturbed by loud alarms.

Overall, conditioning devices have a cure rate of 70% to 85%, and a relapse rate of 10% to 15%. They incur a one-time cost of $50 to $75. Conditioning devices may be covered by insurance companies if the alarm is prescribed by a physician as a medical device. Conditioning without the use of auxiliary alarms may also be undertaken. One proposed method involves instituting a self-awakening program. Older school-aged children practice lying in bed during the daytime and simulating the experience of awakening, sensing a full bladder, and going to the toilet. Another dry bed training program involves parents' awakening their children first hourly, and then at longer intervals over the period of about 1 week. Children eventually learn to self-awaken. A 92% success rate with a relapse rate of 20% is reported with this program.

Pharmacologic agents include tricyclic antidepressants and desmopressin (DDAVP). Tricyclic antidepressants, especially imipramine, have been successfully used to treat nocturnal enuresis, although the mechanism of action is uncertain. The antidepressant action of the drug, its effect on sleep and arousal, and its anticholinergic properties may all play a role. The bladder capacity of individuals with enuresis may be increased by 34%, which indicates that the anticholinergic effects of the drug may be the most significant.

Imipramine should not be prescribed for children younger than 6 or 7 years because of potential adverse effects. The recommended dosage is 0.9 to 1.5 mg/kg/d. In general, children younger than 8 years are given 25 mg 1 to 2 hours before bedtime, and older children are given 50 to 75 mg. Beneficial results usually occur within the first few weeks of therapy. Medication is usually continued for 3 to 6 months to prevent relapses, which are reported in up to 75% of cases. The drug should be tapered by reducing the dose or using an alternate-night regimen. Side effects are rare and include insomnia, nightmares, and personality changes. Acute overdoses are potentially fatal secondary to cardiac complications. The initial cure rate is 10% to 60% with a relapse rate of 90%. The monthly cost of imipramine is about $5.

Desmopressin, an analog of vasopressin, the antidiuretic hormone, is another pharmacologic agent used for enuresis. Desmopressin probably works to decrease nocturnal urine production. Most patients respond rapidly to desmopressin and become dry within 1 to 2 weeks of the initiation of therapy. The medication is taken orally as 0.2 mg/tablet 1 hour before bedtime. The dose may be increased by 1 tablet at weekly intervals (maximum dose: 0.6 mg). Desmopressin in nasal spray is no longer recommended for the treatment of enuresis because of the risk of severe hyponatremia, seizures, and even death. Hyponatremia has also been reported with oral desmopressin in the face of high fluid intake sometimes associated with habit polydipsia. Fluid restriction is recommended from 1 hour before until 8 hours after desmopressin administration. If patients achieve a 2-week period of dryness, the dose can be tapered at 2-week

intervals. The cure rate is 40% to 50% with a relapse rate of 90% off medication. Desmopressin is expensive, with an average monthly cost of $150 to $250.

Oxybutynin is an antispasmodic, anticholinergic agent used in the management of diurnal or polysymptomatic nocturnal enuresis. The dosage is 5 mg at bedtime for children 6 to 12 years and 10 mg at bedtime for children older than 12 years. The response rate is 33%, and the major side effects include drowsiness, flushing, dry mouth, constipation, and hyperthermia. Hyoscyamine sulfate and flavoxate hydrochloride are 2 other medications used for diurnal enuresis.

Treatment of enuresis in children with small bladder capacities includes bladder retention training. Such children are fluid loaded and asked to delay voiding for 5 to 10 minutes. This strategy is generally reserved for children with diurnal enuresis.

Secondary Enuresis

The management of secondary enuresis should focus on the treatment of the causal disorder, such as a UTI or diabetes mellitus.

Prognosis

The prognosis for children with enuresis is good. The spontaneous cure rate is 15% per year. Medical management results in a reduction in symptoms in more than 70% of affected children.

CASE RESOLUTION

The boy in the case scenario has primary nocturnal enuresis. The history of childhood enuresis in the father is significant. Two management options, behavior modification and treatment with desmopressin or imipramine, can be discussed with the family. The child's symptoms will probably spontaneously improve over time.

Selected References

Bennett HJ. *Waking Up Dry.* Elk Grove Village, IL: American Academy of Pediatrics; 2005

Joinson C, Heron J, von Gontard A, ALSPAC Study Team. Psychological problems of children with daytime wetting. *Pediatrics.* 2006;118:1985–1993

Lawless MR, McElderry DH. Nocturnal enuresis: current concepts. *Pediatr Rev.* 2001;22:399–407

Mercer R. *Seven Steps to Nighttime Dryness: A Practical Guide for Parents of Children with Bedwetting.* Ashton, MD: Brookeville Media; 2004

Robson WL, Leung AKC, VanHowe R. Primary and secondary enuresis: similarities in presentation. *Pediatrics.* 2005;115:956–959

Robson WL. Enuresis. *Adv Pediatr.* 2001;48:409–438

Robson WL, Leung AK. An approach to daytime wetting in children. *Adv Pediatr.* 2006;53:323–365

Treatment of childhood enuresis. *Clin Pediatr (Phila).* 1993;32:(entire issue)

Encopresis

Carol D. Berkowitz, MD

CASE STUDY

A 7-year-old boy presents with the complaint of soiling his underpants. His mother states that he has never been completely toilet trained, and that stooling accidents occur at least 2 to 3 times a week, mainly during the day. The boy rarely has a spontaneous bowel movement without assistance. He sits on the toilet for just a few minutes and has small, pellet-like stools. His mother has never sought medical care before for this problem.

The boy is very fidgety during the physical examination. The vital signs are normal and the child's height and weight are at the 25th percentile. His abdomen is soft but distended, with palpable loops of stool-filled bowel. A small amount of stool is present around the anus and in the boy's underpants. Digital examination of the rectum reveals hard stool. The rectal tone is normal as is the rest of the physical examination.

Questions

1. What is the definition of encopresis?
2. What is the difference between retentive and non-retentive encopresis?
3. What are some physiological conditions that contribute to encopresis?
4. What conditions may be mistaken for encopresis?

Encopresis is the repeated passage of stool into inappropriate places (eg, clothing), either voluntary or involuntary, in children who should be toilet trained on the basis of age (usually at least 4 years, the age at which 95% of children have achieved stool continence) and developmental level and who have no primary organic pathology. One such encopretic event occurs each month for at least 3 months. The term *encopresis,* which was originally used for children with psychogenic soiling, is similar to enuresis. Unlike enuresis, encopresis rarely occurs at night. Now encopresis is used in a broader sense to refer to all types of fecal incontinence.

Retentive encopresis, also referred to as functional fecal retention with encopresis, occurs in the face of constipation (obstipation), in which chronic rectal distention leads to the seepage of liquid stool around hard, retained feces. Sometimes this is called overflow or fecal soiling. The onset of symptoms is usually about 4 years of age. Approximately 95% of cases of encopresis are retentive. **Non-retentive encopresis** is characterized by the passage of soft stool without colonic distention or retention of stool. Some have recognized 2 categories of children with non-retentive encopresis: those who can control defecation but stool in inappropriate places, and those who have true failure to achieve bowel control. Primary encopresis occurs when children have never been completely toilet trained. Secondary encopresis occurs in children who have had a period of complete continence of stool. Most encopretic children have secondary encopresis.

Epidemiology

Encopresis is reported in approximately 1.5% of school-aged children, and boys are reported to be affected 2 to 6 times more often than girls. This gender ratio reverses in the elderly, in which the prevalence of encopresis is twice as high in females as in males. An association between encopresis, enuresis, and attention-deficit/hyperactivity disorder is sometimes present. About 15% of children with enuresis also have encopresis. Family history for encopresis may also be positive; 16% of affected children have one affected parent, usually the father. An association between encopresis and child sexual abuse has been reported in a small number of children.

Clinical Presentation

Children with encopresis have a history of staining of the underpants, which may be hidden in drawers or under beds by embarrassed children. Occasionally parents are unaware of the problem.

Dx Encopresis

- Incontinence of stool
- Constipation
- Hyperactivity
- Distended abdomen
- Stool-filled loops of bowel
- Lax rectal tone
- Soiled clothing or bedding
- Fecal odor

Stooling accidents occur more frequently at home than in school. Some children have a history of constipation. Parents may complain that their children exude a fecal odor, but children are unaware they are malodorous (Dx Box).

Pathophysiology

A history of constipation, often with painful defecation, is associated with retentive encopresis. With time, the colon distends and liquid feces seep around impacted stool (Figure 42-1). In 30% to 50% of children, anal spasm, referred to as animus, occurs and contraction rather than relaxation occurs during evacuation of feces. In another 40%, rectal hyposensitivity is apparent so that the children are unaware of the presence of the stool. Some children have an evacuation release disorder, in which the presence of the stool does not result in relaxation and stool evacuation. In such cases, the rectum is chronically distended by stool. Water is absorbed and the stool becomes harder and drier. The distended rectum fails to sense the presence of the stool. When evacuation is attempted, the process is painful, leading to further retention (see Chapter 99).

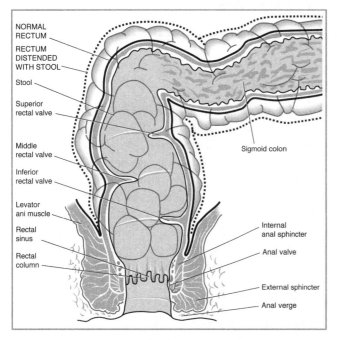

NORMAL RECTUM

RECTUM DISTENDED WITH STOOL

Stool

Superior rectal valve

Middle rectal valve

Inferior rectal valve

Levator ani muscle

Rectal sinus

Rectal column

Sigmoid colon

Internal anal sphincter

Anal valve

External sphincter

Anal verge

Figure 42-1. Diagram of the rectum, anal canal, and sigmoid colon distended with stool.

Encopresis has been associated with a short attention span and a high level of motor activity. Affected children are unable to sit on a toilet for more than a few minutes and do not adequately attend to the task of stool evacuation. As a result, they get off the toilet after the incomplete evacuation of only small amounts of stool. In some toddlers, constipation is related to the struggle of toilet training and an unwillingness to sit on the toilet (see Chapter 34).

The pathophysiology of non-retentive encopresis seems to be psychogenic. Some children who have been chronically sexually abused have lax anal tone, which may contribute to the fecal incontinence. Animus, abnormal anal sphincter contraction, has been reported in up to 30% of children with constipation.

Differential Diagnosis

The differential diagnosis of encopresis focuses on organic conditions associated with chronic constipation. These conditions include Hirschsprung disease, disorders of intestinal motility (eg, pseudo-obstruction), disorders of anal tone and anal anatomy (eg, imperforate anus with fistula), disorders of the lumbosacral spine (eg, meningomyelocele), and previous surgeries (eg, repair of imperforate anus). Neurofibromatosis, lead poisoning, and hypothyroidism are also associated with constipation. Congenital anorectal anomalies, which are reported in 1 in 5,000 live births, are rare.

Most of these conditions can be ruled out on the basis of a careful history and physical examination. In some cases, specific testing such as anal manometry or rectal biopsy may be necessary to exclude a particular disorder.

Evaluation

History

The age of onset of the problem, as well as the age of initiation of toilet training, should be determined. In general, affected children are 4 years of age and older. A detailed history of the stooling pattern should be obtained (Questions Box). The frequency and consistency of stools as well as quantity of stools should also be noted. In addition, the presence of nocturnal episodes of encopresis should be determined. In cases of secondary encopresis, the duration of fecal continence and the occurrence of any events such as the birth of a sibling or the start of school that may have precipitated the episodes of encopresis should be noted. Some children experience the onset of encopresis when they start school. Because of "toilet phobia," they are unwilling to use the public toilet in the school setting.

Questions

Encopresis

- At what age was the child toilet trained?
- Does the child have spontaneous bowel movements (without enemas or suppositories)? If so, how frequently?
- Does the child have large, dry, hard stools that clog the toilet?
- Is the child taking any medications such as aspirin, iron, Ritalin, imipramine, or anticholinergics?
- Does the child seem to resist the urge to defecate (eg, squeeze legs together and rock back and forth)?
- Does the child have a history of enuresis or attention-deficit/hyperactivity disorder?
- What is the pattern of encopresis (ie, is the encopresis primary or secondary)?
- When and where does the child soil (eg, nocturnal, at home)?
- Have there been changes or stresses in the home or family?
- What happens to the child's stained underwear?
- What has the family done to manage the problem?

Physical Examination

The next step involves the performance of a comprehensive physical examination, paying particular attention to the abdomen to check for the presence of distended, stool-filled loops of bowel. The rectal area should be assessed for rectal tone, an anal wink, and the presence of hard stool. Location of the anus should also be noted, and anterior displacement may suggest incomplete forms of imperforate anus. Children with retentive encopresis have normal or tight anal tone on rectal examination because they are frequently contracting their external anal sphincter to prevent the seepage of the liquid stool.

Dysmorphic features should be noted and may suggest a syndrome in which constipation is a feature. Abnormalities around the anus such as fistulas should also be noted. Fistulas are found in Crohn disease. The underpants should be evaluated for the presence of stool, mucus, or pus. A sensory and motor examination of the lower extremities helps determine if any signs of spinal cord dysfunction are evident. An evaluation of the skin over the spinal area may reveal abnormalities such as sacral dimples or tufts of hair.

Children who do not exhibit abdominal distention may have soft stool on rectal examination, which indicates non-retentive encopresis. If patulous anal tone is noted, spinal cord abnormalities or prior child sexual abuse should be suspected.

Laboratory Tests

Most children with encopresis require few laboratory studies. Urinalysis and urine culture are recommended in children with fecal impactions to exclude urinary tract infection. Anorectal manometry, which may be used to measure the pressure generated by the anal sphincter, may also reveal abnormalities of anal tone or evidence of aganglionosis. The Child Behavioral Checklist is useful to determine if certain behavior problems exist. Such problems may either potentiate the encopresis or result from it.

Imaging Studies

In most encopretic children, imaging studies are not necessary. If x-rays of the abdomen are taken in children with retentive encopresis, distended, stool-filled bowel may be noted. A barium enema is useful if Hirschsprung disease is to be ruled out. Strictures, which may occur following necrotizing enterocolitis, will also be detected. Electromyogram to determine whether the innervation of the external anal sphincter is intact is recommended for children with encopresis who fail to respond to routine treatment.

Management

The management of encopresis focuses on complete rectal evacuation and patient and parent education and counseling. Regaining muscle tone of the anal canal usually requires 2 to 6 months.

Rectal evacuation requires **pharmacologic management** to ensure an adequate clean-out of retained stools. The decision about which laxatives to use depends on the degree of constipation. If the degree of fecal retention is mild, a high-fiber diet and stool-bulking agents or oral laxatives, such as senna derivatives, bisacodyl, or lactulose syrup, may be used in association with stool softeners or lubricants, such as mineral oil. The amount of mineral oil may be titrated up to ensure success. Some practitioners recommend that mineral oil be given until it oozes from the rectum. The amount may then be titrated back to a lower level. Magnesium sulfate is also recommended to relieve constipation. Magnesium citrate can be used, but should be administered cautiously and with the admonition to drink plenty of fluids to prevent dehydration. Polyethylene glycol 3350, although costly, has a very high success rate in the management of constipation and encopresis.

If the degree of retention is more severe, suppositories or enemas may be needed. Occasionally, children have to be disimpacted manually. Alternative methods to manual disimpaction include 2 to 3 sodium phosphate enemas over 1 to 2 days or 8 oz of mineral oil a day for 4 days. Pulsed irrigation–enhanced evacuation involves the insertion of a rectal tube and the installation of pulses of warm irrigating solution, simultaneously draining rectal contents. If the above modalities are not successful, children may need to be admitted to the hospital for oral lavage using polyethylene glycol-electrolyte solution at 30 to 40 mL/kg per hour until successful evacuation has occurred. This procedure often requires insertion of a nasogastric tube and 6 to 8 hours of treatment. Once the fecal accumulation has been relieved, every effort should be made to keep children regular. This can be accomplished with the combined use of toilet retraining, stool softeners or laxatives, and enemas or suppositories. Prokinetic agents such as metoclopramide may also be used.

Dietary manipulation is important to ensure sustained regular stooling. Parents should be told that children require a high-fiber diet with fruit juices such as pear or peach juice and decreased milk (≤16 oz/d). It has been suggested that a "team and coach" approach is the most successful route, and that bowel training be likened to fitness training.

The toilet retraining process, sometimes referred to as enhanced toilet training, requires that children sit on the toilet at least 2 or 3 times a day, usually after meals, for about 10 minutes or until they have had a bowel movement. Some practitioners recommend the use of an egg timer to ensure that children spend the appropriate amount of time on the toilet. Children should be requested to maintain a diary of their evacuation, which may take the form of a star chart. Stars or other rewards are given for successful bowel movements in the toilet.

If children skip a day between bowel movements, they may be treated with a suppository, such as a glycerin or bisacodyl suppository. If they still have not succeeded in having a bowel movement, then an enema may be appropriate. This sequence should be maintained until children are having bowel movements in the toilet and not soiling for at least 1 month. In general, stool softeners are required for at least 3 to 6 months. The regimen may have to be modified, particularly in younger children.

Behavior modification and biofeedback, such as using external anal sphincter electromyography, are 2 other modalities that can be used to help manage encopresis. Consultation with specialists such as pediatric gastroenterologists may be required.

Thirty percent of children with encopresis may need psychological consultation. Psychological intervention in the form of interactive parent-child family guidance has been reported successful when standard gastroenterologic intervention has failed. Children with evidence of child sexual abuse or non-retentive encopresis should be referred to a psychologist early in the course of therapy. The underlying psychosocial problems of children with non-retentive encopresis must be adequately addressed before their condition can improve.

Prognosis

The prognosis for children with retentive encopresis is reportedly good with appropriate intervention. In one study, children who were able to defecate a rectal balloon filled with 100 mL of water within 5 minutes were twice as likely to recover from constipation and encopresis. It is estimated that about 30% to 50% of affected children experience long-lasting remission after 1 year and up to 75% are in remission by 5 years.

The prognosis for children with non-retentive encopresis is less predictable and highly dependent on the underlying psychopathology.

CASE RESOLUTION

In the case scenario, the boy exhibits typical manifestations of retentive encopresis. His condition should be managed with the use of laxatives, stool softeners, and toilet retraining with a star chart. The possible attention-deficit/hyperactivity disorder should be addressed separately but may be contributing to his inability to attend to the task of toileting.

Selected References

Abi-Hanna A, Lake AM. Constipation and encopresis in childhood. *Pediatr Rev.* 1998;19:23–31

Borowitz SM, Cox DJ, Sutphen JL, Kovatchev B. Treatment of childhood encopresis: a randomized trial comparing three treatment protocols. *J Pediatr Gastroenterol Nutr.* 2002;34:378–384

Burket RC, Cox DJ, Tam AP, et al. Are constipated kids just being stubborn? *Develop Behav Pediatr.* 2006;27:106–111

Fishman L, Rappaport L, Cousineau D, Nurko S. Early constipation and toilet training in children with encopresis. *J Pediatr Gastroenterol Nutr.* 2002;34:385–388

Fishman L, Rappaport L, Schonwald A, Nurko S. Trends in referral to a single encopresis clinic over 20 years. *Pediatrics.* 2003;111:e604–e607

Loenig-Baucke V. Encopresis. *Curr Opin Pediatr.* 2002;14:570–575

Loenig-Baucke V. Functional fecal retention with encopresis in childhood. *J Pediatr Gastroenterol Nutr.* 2004;38:79–84

Pashankar DS, Bishop WP, Loenig Baucke V. Longterm efficacy of polyethylene glycol 3350 for the treatment of chronic constipation in children with and without encopresis. *Clin Pediatr.* 2003;42:815–819

Reid H, Bahar RJ. Treatment of encopresis and chronic constipation in young children: clinical results from interactive parent-child guidance. *Clin Pediatr.* 2006;45:157–164

Setty R, Wershil BK. Fecal overflow incontinence. *Pediatr Rev.* 2006;27: e54–e55

SECTION III

Acute and Emergent Problems

43. Fever and Bacteremia 229

44. Febrile Seizures 237

45. Respiratory Distress... 241

46. Stridor and Croup 247

47. Sudden Infant Death Syndrome and
    Apparent Life-Threatening Events... 253

48. Syncope.. 259

49. Shock 265

50. Approach to the Traumatized Child 271

51. Abdominal Trauma 277

52. Head Trauma 281

53. Increased Intracranial Pressure 287

54. Fluid and Electrolyte Disturbances 293

55. Acute Renal Failure/Acute Kidney Injury 303

56. Ingestions: Diagnosis and Management 309

Fever and Bacteremia

Paul Bryan, MD

CASE STUDY

An 8-month-old girl is brought to the emergency department with a 2-day history of fever and increased fussiness. She is irritable but consolable by parents. Her parents believe that her immunizations are up to date, but they do not have the immunization record with them. On examination, she has a rectal temperature of 39.5°C (103.1°F). The rest of the physical examination is within normal limits, and no source for the fever is apparent.

Questions

1. What are serious bacterial infections in young febrile infants?
2. What has been the impact of conjugated vaccines against *Haemophilus influenzae* and *Streptococcus pneumoniae* on the incidence of bacteremia and meningitis in febrile infants?
3. What are the challenges in differentiating between serious and benign febrile illnesses in young children?
4. What diagnostic studies are recommended in the evaluation of febrile infants and children?
5. When should febrile infants be hospitalized?

Fever is one of the most common chief complaints among pediatric patients seeking medical attention in physician offices, urgent care centers, and emergency departments and accounts for up to 20% to 30% of these visits. Most of these patients will have a benign, self-limited viral illness. Some patients, however, will have a **serious bacterial infection** (SBI), defined as meningitis, urinary tract infection (UTI)/pyelonephritis, bacteremia, septic arthritis, osteomyelitis, cellulitis, or deep tissue infection. **Bacteremia** is a bacterial infection within the bloodstream. **Occult bacteremia** occurs when there is a bacterial infection in the blood without any apparent source of infection after a thorough physical examination in an otherwise healthy-appearing child.

Epidemiology

Historically, management decisions regarding febrile children have been largely dictated by age. Children have been broken down into age-defined categories: (1) young infants younger than 90 days, (2) infants and young children 3 to 36 months, and (3) children older than 3 years. Young febrile infants (ie, <90 days) have higher rates of SBIs than older children and often represent a diagnostic challenge. They have relatively immature immune systems rendering them particularly susceptible to bacterial infections, have not yet received most of their immunizations, and often have limited responses in the face of bacterial infections and, therefore, exhibit relatively nonspecific signs and symptoms. In addition, young infants have different bacterial pathogens that can cause these serious infections including *Escherichia coli*, *Streptococcus agalactiae* (group B streptococci or GBS), *Listeria monocytogenes*, and other gram-negative organisms (Box 43-1). The prevalence of an SBI amongst young febrile infants

with a fever of 38.0°C (100.4°F) is about 10%, and most bacterial infections are UTIs. A smaller percentage has bacteremia and/or meningitis. Recently, some studies have demonstrated that young febrile infants with diagnosed viral infections have lower rates of SBI than those without (4% vs 12%). None of the young febrile infants with viral infections by diagnostic testing had meningitis, but some did have UTIs and, rarely, some were bacteremic.

Febrile children aged 3 to 36 months are at a higher risk for bacteremia than older children, but less so than young febrile infants. The physical examination, while more reliable than in younger infants, can often be normal without any localizing source of infection. These individuals may in turn have occult bacteremia. In the

---

Box 43-1. Organisms Implicated in Serious Bacterial Infection/Occult Bacteremia in Children

Infants Younger Than 3 Months

- Group B streptococcus
- *Escherichia coli*
- *Listeria monocytogenes*
- *Salmonella* species (infants >1 month)
- *Haemophilus influenzae* type b[a] (infants >1 month)

Children Between 3 and 36 Months of Age

- *Streptococcus pneumoniae*
- *Neisseria meningitidis*
- *Salmonella* species
- *Staphylococcus aureus*
- *H influenzae* type b (Hib)[a]

---
[a]Hib disease has been virtually eliminated with the routine use of Hib conjugate vaccines.

post-*Haemophilus influenzae* type b but pre-pneumococcal conjugate vaccine era, the rates of occult bacteremia ranged from 1.6% to 1.9% in children in this age group with a temperature 39.0°C (102.1°F) or higher and no obvious source of infection. More than 90% of the cases of occult bacteremia in this age group were caused by *Streptococcus pneumoniae*, with the remainder being caused by *Salmonella*, *Neisseria meningitides*, *Staphylococcus aureus*, and a few other rare organisms. Most cases of occult pneumococcal bacteremia resolved spontaneously without any intervention. If untreated, a small percentage (3%–5%) went on to develop pneumococcal meningitis, which has the most serious complication and fatality rate. In 2000 the heptavalent pneumococcal conjugate vaccine was licensed by the US Food and Drug Administration for use within the United States. Following an initial shortage, the vaccine became widely distributed. It is currently recommended by the American Academy of Pediatrics and the Advisory Committee on Immunization Practices for all infants in a 4-dose regimen to be given at 2, 4, 6, and 12 to 15 months. This vaccine provides coverage against the 7 main serotypes of *S pneumoniae* responsible for approximately 80% of the cases of invasive pneumococcal disease in the United States and Canada. Following the introduction of this vaccine, the rate of invasive pneumococcal disease (including bacteremia) and carriage for the serotypes covered by the vaccine dropped considerably. In addition, there is evidence suggestive of herd immunity in that there has been a decline in invasive pneumococcal disease amongst older individuals who have not received the vaccine. What remains to be seen is what effect the widespread immunization of most children will have on the epidemiology of bacteremia. There is some concern that there may be a selective pressure increasing the prevalence of invasive pneumococcal disease caused by strains not covered in the heptavalent vaccine or that other organisms might become more prevalent. Continued surveillance of invasive disease is necessary to ascertain what, if any, impact this change in epidemiology may have on the diagnosis and management of bacteremia in young febrile children.

Clinical Presentation

In many febrile children, fever is the only complaint or manifestation of disease. These children may look fine and behave normally. Young children, especially infants younger than 3 months, have fewer and subtler behavioral signs with bacterial infections. Physicians must, therefore, maintain a high index of suspicion for the presence of an SBI even in the absence of localizing signs (Dx Box). Occult bacteremia, by definition, has no abnormal physical manifestations aside from fever.

Pathophysiology

Fever is an elevation in the thermoregulatory set point of the body. The thermoregulatory center is located in the preoptic region of the anterior hypothalamus, and an elevation in the hypothalamic set point above the normal body temperature initiates the physiological changes that lead to fever. Exogenous pyrogens (eg, bacteria, viruses, antigen-antibody complexes) stimulate host inflammatory cells (eg,

Dx Serious Bacterial Illness

- Lethargy, irritability, or change in mental status
- Tachycardia disproportionate to the degree of temperature elevation
- Tachypnea or labored respirations
- Bulging or depressed anterior fontanelle
- Nuchal rigidity
- Petechiae
- Localized erythema, pain, or swelling
- Abdominal or flank pain
- Fever

macrophages, polymorphonuclear cells) to produce endogenous pyrogens (EPs). Interleukin-1 is currently regarded as the prototypical EP. Endogenous pyrogens cause the hypothalamic endothelium to increase intermediary substances such as prostaglandins and neurotransmitters, which then act on the preoptic neurons of the anterior hypothalamus to produce an elevated set point. The body uses physiological mechanisms (eg, peripheral vasoconstriction, shivering) and behavioral actions (eg, bundling up, drinking hot tea) to increase body temperature to reach and maintain this higher set point, thus producing fever (Figure 43-1).

In contrast, the thermoregulatory set point of the body is normal in hyperthermia. Due to abnormal physiological processes, heat gain

Figure 43-1. Pathophysiology of fever production. Antipyretics work by blocking the synthesis of prostaglandin E₂ (PGE₂).

exceeds heat loss, and the body temperature rises in spite of efforts to return to the control set point.

Differential Diagnosis

In most cases, the duration of fever in children is short, and signs and symptoms are localized. Fever without a source involves an acute episode of fever that lasts 1 week or less in children in whom history, physical examination, and preliminary laboratory tests fail to reveal a source. Most affected children are eventually diagnosed with an acute, generally self-limited, infectious illness. Occult bacteremia has been a major concern in young children, primarily in infants younger than 36 months. High risk factors for occult bacteremia are presented in Box 43-2. Fever of unknown origin (FUO) is fever of at least 8 days' duration in infants or children in whom routine history, physical examination, and laboratory assessment fail to reveal a source.

The differential diagnosis of children with an acute febrile illness is primarily infectious (Box 43-3), including both benign, generally self-limited illness such as upper respiratory infection, and less common, more serious illness such as meningitis and osteomyelitis. Occasionally a child with a fever without a source turns out to have a noninfectious illness such as a collagen vascular disease or neoplasia. By comparison, the differential diagnosis of children with FUO is quite broad (Box 43-4) and contains both infectious and noninfectious disorders.

Evaluation

History

The medical history can provide a great deal of valuable information in the evaluation of children with fever (Questions Box). The history should focus on the duration and severity of the fever. The presence of associated symptoms that may be signs of specific organ system involvement should also be noted.

Physical Examination

Rectal temperatures should be performed in all young infants and children. An elevation in rectal temperature in an infant should not be attributed to overbundling. Vital signs in addition to temperature may provide important diagnostic clues. Tachycardia disproportionate to the degree of temperature elevation may suggest dehydration or sepsis. Tachypnea, which is often the only sign of a respiratory infection, also occurs in response to metabolic acidosis secondary to sepsis or shock. These changes may suggest an occult focus of infection. Response of the temperature and other vital signs to antipyretics should be noted. The physician must remain cautious because a clinical improvement in response to antipyretics can be seen in younger children and infants even in the face of an SBI. Young infants with recorded fevers at home, but who are afebrile on physician evaluation, should be managed as if they have a fever present.

Observation of the overall hydration and activity of infants and children is extremely important. An attempt should be made to

---

Box 43-2. Risk Factors for Occult Bacteremia

- Age 36 months or younger
- Temperature 103.1°F (39.5°C) or higher
- White blood cells 15,000/μL or higher or 5,000/μL or lower
- Total band cells 500/μL or higher
- Erythrocyte sedimentation rate 30 mm/h or higher
- Underlying chronic disease (malignancy, immunodeficiency, sickle cell disease, malnutrition)
- Clinical appearance (irritability, lethargy, toxic appearance)

Box 43-3. Common Infectious Causes of an Acute Episode of Fever in Children

Upper Respiratory Tract
- Upper respiratory infection (common cold)
- Otitis media
- Sinusitis

Pulmonary
- Bronchiolitis
- Pneumonia

Oral Cavity
- Gingivostomatitis
- Pharyngitis
- Dental abscess

Gastrointestinal Tract
- Acute gastroenteritis (bacterial or viral)
- Appendicitis

Genitourinary Tract
- Urinary tract infection
- Pyelonephritis

Musculoskeletal
- Septic arthritis
- Osteomyelitis

Central Nervous System
- Meningitis

Miscellaneous (including noninfectious causes)
- Bacteremia
- Immunization reaction
- Viral exanthems (eg, chickenpox, measles)
- Neoplasia
- Collagen vascular disease

---

determine whether they are behaving and responding in an age-appropriate fashion. Physicians should look for eye contact, spontaneous motor movements, negative responses to adverse stimuli, and positive responses to pleasant stimuli.

All febrile children should receive a complete physical examination. This is important even when the history may suggest involvement of one organ system. For example, in young children, vomiting and fever may be the only signs of viral illness, or possibly a more

---

Box 43-4. Common Causes of Fever of Unknown Origin in Children[a]

Infectious Diseases
Bacterial
- Localized infection: mastoiditis, sinusitis, pneumonia, osteomyelitis, pyelonephritis, abscess (eg, abdominal, pelvic)
- Systemic disease: tuberculosis, brucellosis, salmonellosis, leptospirosis, tularemia

Viral
- Hepatitis viruses
- Cytomegalovirus
- Epstein-Barr virus (infectious mononucleosis)
- Human immunodeficiency virus

Fungal
- Disseminated coccidioidomycosis
- Disseminated histoplasmosis

Miscellaneous
- Malaria
- Rocky Mountain spotted fever
- Syphilis
- Lyme disease

Neoplasia
- Leukemia
- Lymphoma
- Hodgkin disease
- Neuroblastoma

Collagen Vascular Diseases
- Juvenile rheumatoid arthritis
- Systemic lupus erythematosus
- Rheumatic fever

Miscellaneous
- Inflammatory bowel diseases
- Kawasaki disease
- Thyroiditis
- Drugs
- Factitious fever

[a]For a complete discussion of fever of unknown origin, the reader is referred to Lorin MI, Feigin RD. Fever without localizing signs and fever of unknown origin. In: Feigin RD, Cherry JD, eds. *Textbook of Pediatric Infectious Diseases.* 4th ed. Philadelphia, PA: W.B. Saunders; 1998:820–830

Questions

Fever and Bacteremia

- How long has the child had fever? How high has the temperature been?
- Does the child have any other symptoms, such as rash, vomiting, diarrhea, abdominal pain, or dysuria; cough, rhinorrhea, or other respiratory symptoms; or lethargy, irritability or change in mental status?
- Is anyone sick at home?
- Has the child's activity level changed (eg, more sleepy than usual) or is the child more irritable?
- What immunizations has the child received?
- Is the child taking any medications?
- Do any pets live in the house?
- Has there been any history of recent travel, especially outside the country?
- Has the child ever been hospitalized for an infectious illness?
- Does the child have any medical problems, especially asthma, sickle cell anemia, congenital heart disease, or immunodeficiency?

---

inflamed, or exudative tonsils may signal the presence of a viral infection or group A streptococcal infection in older children. Respiratory symptoms such as retractions, nasal flaring, grunting, stridor, rales, rhonchi, or wheezing may all be clues to respiratory tract infections. Enanthems on the buccal mucosa, or exanthems on the skin, are often signs of viral infections. The presence of petechiae in association with fever may indicate serious underlying infection, such as meningococcemia. The capillary refill time, quality of peripheral pulses, and the general temperature of the extremities assess perfusion. Localized areas of pain, erythema, swelling, induration, or fluctuance may point to cellulitis, septic arthritis, osteomyelitis, or the presence of an abscess. Nuchal rigidity can be an important clue to the presence of meningitis. This is rarely present in infants younger than 15 to 18 months, however, and physicians must maintain an index of suspicion for meningitis in febrile children of this age.

Laboratory Tests

Infants 90 Days or Younger

Because the physical examination alone cannot reliably identify an SBI in all febrile infants 90 days of age or younger with a temperature of 38.0°C (100.4°F) or higher, a thorough evaluation for a bacterial source of infection is required. This evaluation includes a complete blood count (CBC) with differential; urinalysis with microscopic evaluation; cerebrospinal fluid (CSF) studies; as well as blood, urine, and CSF cultures. Peripheral white blood cell (WBC) counts, while possibly helpful in older infants and children, do no reliably predict UTIs, bacteremia, or meningitis in young febrile infants. Decisions about whether to send blood and urine cultures, or to perform a lumbar puncture, should not be based solely on the screening peripheral WBC count in this age group. In addition, the standard urinalysis has a sensitivity of only around 85% in this age group and should not be

---

serious infection, such as a UTI or central nervous system (CNS) infection. The underlying condition may go undiagnosed unless a thorough examination and diagnostic evaluation are performed.

The anterior fontanelle should be palpated. It may be normal, bulging as a result of CNS infection, or depressed secondary to dehydration. The ears should be examined carefully and pneumatic otoscopy performed. Careful inspection may reveal otitis media as the source of fever, especially in children younger than 3 years. The occurrence of otitis media should not preclude further workup for invasive bacterial disease in children who do not appear well (see Chapter 60). The oropharynx should also be examined carefully. Dry mucous membranes may indicate dehydration. Enlarged, used to determine the need for urine culture. Rapid viral diagnostic techniques that can reliably identify several of the more common viral pathogens (eg, respiratory syncytial virus, influenza, adenovirus, parainfluenza) have recently become available. The presence of a positive viral test result, however, does not preclude further diagnostic testing, specifically blood and urine cultures. In addition, most young febrile infants warrant lumbar punctures, particularly those younger than 8 weeks. If empiric antibiotics are to be dispensed, a lumbar puncture must be performed so as not to obscure the possibility of partially treated meningitis should pleocytosis be discovered on a subsequent CSF specimen. Stool analysis and culture should be reserved for those young febrile infants with diarrhea. Routine diagnostic radiographic studies (eg, chest x-ray) are not necessary, and should be reserved for infants with respiratory symptoms (eg, tachypnea, hypoxia, rales, wheezes, increased work of breathing).

Infants 3 to 36 Months

The diagnostic approach to older infants and young children has changed following the introduction of pneumococcal conjugate vaccine. Prior to widespread vaccine use, the standard of care involved an aggressive diagnostic approach looking for occult bacteremia in febrile children 3 to 24 months with temperature higher than 39.0°C (102.2°F), and in those 2 to 3 years with temperature higher than 39.5°C (103.1°F) without any apparent source of infection. The workup included a screening CBC, blood cultures, and empirically treating infants and children with an elevated WBC count greater than 15,000/mm³ or an absolute neutrophil count (ANC) greater than 10,000/mm³ because they were at higher risk for occult bacteremia. The ANC is generally considered to be the best predictor of risk for occult bacteremia. Acute phase reactants such as erythrocyte sedimentation rate and C-reactive protein, while commonly elevated in serious infections, have not been shown to be better predictors for occult bacteremia than the peripheral WBC count or ANC. Other laboratory tests, including antigen testing, serum cytokine measurements, and polymerase chain reaction, are not particularly useful because of their limited availability, relatively high false-positive rates, and cost. Currently there is no single test that has been able to reliably identify all young febrile children with occult bacteremia.

With the declining prevalence of invasive pneumococcal disease post-licensure of the heptavalent conjugate vaccine, the need for routine screening, culturing, and selective antibiotic use for occult bacteremia has been challenged. Given the declining rates of bacteremia, infants and children who have received at least 2 to 3 doses of the vaccine can be safely managed without blood tests because this is no longer a cost-effective strategy. Individuals who are unimmunized, whose vaccine status is uncertain, or who have received only 1 dose of the vaccine may need screening evaluation with CBC, blood and urine cultures, and expectant antibiotics if they are found to have an elevated WBC count or ANC. The change in epidemiology of bacteremia following the widespread use of the pneumococcal vaccine may warrant reconsideration of this in the future following long-term surveillance of invasive disease. Infants with fever higher than 39.0°C warrant urine testing, especially in girls younger than 2 years, uncircumcised boys younger than 12 months, and circumcised boys younger than 6 months. Chest x-ray should be considered in infants with significant respiratory symptoms or auscultatory findings suggestive of pneumonia. In infants with temperatures higher than 39.5°C and WBC counts greater than 20,000/mm³, chest x-rays should be obtained to detect occult pneumonias, reported in up to 25% of patients, even in the absence of significant respiratory symptoms or auscultatory findings.

Children Older Than 3 Years

The laboratory evaluation of children older than 3 years is individualized and influenced by the history and physical examination. Healthy children in this age group are not at high risk for occult bacteremia. In addition their physical examination is more reliable and they are better able to communicate their symptoms than younger children. Routine screening tests are not generally indicated in healthy individuals and should be reserved for those who look toxic or have an underlying disease that puts them at increased risk for bacterial infections (eg, sickle cell disease, cancer, immunodeficiency, nephrotic syndrome).

Imaging Studies

As noted previously, chest x-rays are the most common imaging study done in the routine evaluation of an infant or child with fever and symptoms consistent with lower respiratory infection or with fever and no apparent source, especially in infants younger than 3 months.

Other imaging studies such as bone scans, gallium scans, magnetic resonance imaging, and computed tomography scans are indicated if there are suspected infections such as occult abscesses or osteomyelitis.

Management

Management of children with fever includes both controlling the fever and treating the underlying process causing the fever. There is no evidence that fever itself is harmful. To the contrary, animal studies have suggested that fever may have some survival advantage. Despite the possible beneficial effects of fever, febrile children may still feel uncomfortable. Fever should be reduced to relieve the associated discomfort and malaise. **Antipyretics** such as acetaminophen and ibuprofen can be used. Aspirin should be avoided in children because of the association with Reye syndrome and viral illnesses. **Sponging** or **bathing** with tepid water and **unbundling** children aid in fever reduction. Ice water or alcohol baths should be avoided.

All toxic-appearing febrile infants and children, regardless of age, require hospitalization and administration of broad-spectrum antibiotics. Hospitalization and the initiation of empiric intravenous (IV) antibiotics are recommended for all febrile infants 28 days or younger pending culture results. Ampicillin and gentamicin are the most commonly used initial antibiotics within this age group. Careful consideration must be made to resistance patterns within a particular region. With the onset of standard GBS surveillance during pregnancy and the use of intrapartum antibiotics, more gram-negative organisms and increased gentamicin resistance have been reported, necessitating the use of a third-generation cephalosporin, such as cefotaxime, for initial empiric coverage. Ceftriaxone is generally avoided in this age group, particularly amongst jaundiced newborns, because of its ability to displace bilirubin from albumen, thereby increasing the risk of kernicterus.

Well-appearing febrile infants aged 29 to 90 days can be managed safely as outpatients either with antibiotics (ceftriaxone 50 mg/kg intravenously or intramuscularly) or close observation provided they meet established low risk for SBI criteria (Box 43-5). In addition, parents must have a reliable means of communication and transportation in the event of a positive culture result so that they can be notified to return the infant for reevaluation and possible admission. All febrile infants aged 29 to 90 days need very close follow-up, typically within 24 hours. Most pathogens will be isolated from cultures within the first 24 hours, and hospitalization with IV antibiotics is generally warranted for any young infant with a culture result consistent with a pathogen and not a contaminant. The addition of vancomycin must be considered if resistant pneumococcus is a possibility.

> ## Box 43-5. Low-Risk Criteria for Serious Bacterial Infection in Young Febrile Infants
>
> 1. Well-appearing
> 2. No focal bacterial infection on examination
> 3. Previously healthy term infant with unremarkable neonatal course
> 4. White blood cell count between 5,000 to 15,000/mm^3
> 5. Absolute band cell count less than 1,500/mm^3 or a band-to-neutrophil ratio of 0.2
> 6. Normal cerebrospinal fluid examination with less than 8 white blood cells (WBCs) per high-power field and negative gram stain
> 7. Normal urinalysis with less than 10 WBCs per high-power field
> 8. Stool studies with less than 5 WBC per high-power field (if diarrhea present)
> 9. Normal chest x-ray (if respiratory signs/symptoms present)

The management of well-appearing febrile infants and children between 3 to 36 months of age is based on the results of any diagnostic studies. Antibiotics should be administered for any bacterial infection identified. Those well-appearing infants who are tolerating oral fluids well and have no significant respiratory distress or hypoxia can be managed as outpatients even if they have a UTI or pneumonia. Clinicians may administer a dose of ceftriaxone for the first 24 hours and transition to an oral antibiotic thereafter. Continued close follow-up is necessary usually within 24 to 48 hours. Infants who have received one dose or less of the pneumococcal vaccine can receive a dose of ceftriaxone pending culture results if the WBC count is greater than 15,000/mm^3 or the ANC is greater than 10,000/mm^3.

Healthy well-appearing febrile children older than 3 years can be managed as outpatients if they are well hydrated and have no respiratory distress or hypoxia. Children with underlying medical conditions and at risk for bacterial infections may also need hospitalization and IV antibiotics regardless of age.

Children with occult pneumococcal bacteremia who are afebrile and well-appearing at follow-up can probably continue to be managed as outpatients. Additional dosing of ceftriaxone may be necessary or transition to an oral antibiotic can be considered if sensitivity testing has been performed. Repeat blood cultures are probably not necessary if the child is afebrile because of the likelihood persistent bacteremia is low. Those who are younger than 90 days, still febrile at follow-up, or who have clinically worsened warrant hospitalization and IV antibiotics. In addition, a lumbar puncture should be considered if not previously performed in a child with a positive blood culture. All individuals with occult *N meningitides* bacteremia warrant hospitalization and IV antibiotics. A lumbar puncture should also strongly be considered if not previously performed given the substantial risk for meningitis. In general, most other cases of occult bacteremia warrant hospitalization and IV antibiotics. Consultation with an infectious disease specialist may be indicated to determine appropriate antibiotic selection and duration of therapy.

Prognosis

Occult bacteremia may resolve without therapy and have no sequelae, but it may persist or produce localized infections such as meningitis or septic arthritis. In children with bacteremia who do not receive antimicrobial therapy, the risk of persistent bacteremia is approximately 20% and the risk of meningitis is about 5% to 10%. These risks vary depending on which organism is isolated from the blood. In general, the risk of developing serious sequelae is greater with bacteremia caused by *H influenzae* than by *S pneumoniae* (25% vs 5%). Concern about serious bacterial infection related to either of these organisms is now significantly diminished.

> ## CASE RESOLUTION
>
> The infant presented in the case history is irritable and has a high fever of unknown source. Her vaccine status is uncertain. Her physical examination fails to reveal a source of her infection. Because her fever is 39.5°C, she is irritable, and her immune status is uncertain, a complete laboratory assessment, including a lumbar puncture, should be performed. Management should be determined after all laboratory data are available. If laboratory assessment reveals a focus of infection such as a urinary tract infection, she should be managed with antibiotics. If laboratory assessment fails to reveal a source for the fever, and her white blood cell count is greater than 15,000/mm^3 or her absolute neutrophil count is greater than 10,000/mm^3, she can receive an intramuscular injection of ceftriaxone as expectant management for occult bacteremia and be reevaluated in 24 hours or be managed without antibiotics.

Selected References

Alpern ER, Alessandrini EA, McGowan KL, et al. Serotype prevalence of occult pneumococcal bacteremia. *Pediatrics.* 2001;108:23–25

American College of Emergency Physicians Clinical Policies Committee and the Clinical Policies Subcommittee on Pediatric Fever. Clinical policy for children younger than three years presenting to the emergency department with fever. *Ann Emerg Med.* 2003;42:530–545

Bachur RG, Harper MB. Predictive model for serious bacterial infections among infants younger than 3 months of age. *Pediatrics.* 2001;108:311–316

Baker MD, Bell LM, Avner JR. Outpatient management without antibiotics of fever in selected infants. *N Engl J Med.* 1993;329:1437–1441

Baraff LJ. Management of fever without source in infants and children. *Ann Emerg Med.* 2000;36:602–614

Bonsu BK, Harper MB. Identifying febrile young infants with bacteremia: is the peripheral white blood cell count an accurate screen? *Ann Emerg Med.* 2003;42:216–225

Brik R, Hamissah R, Shehada N, et al. Evaluation of febrile infants under 3 months of age: is routine lumbar puncture warranted? *Isr J Med Sci.* 1997;33:93–97

Byington CL, Enriquez R, Hoff C, et al. Serious bacterial infections in febrile infants 1 to 90 days old with and without viral infections. *Pediatrics.* 2004;113:1662–1666

Centers for Disease Control and Prevention. Direct and indirect effects of routine vaccination of children with 7-valent pneumococcal conjugate vaccine on incidence of invasive pneumococcal disease—United States, 1998–2003. *MMWR Morb Mortal Wkly Rep.* 2005;54:893–897

Gajdos V, Foix L'Helias L, Mollet-Boudjemline A, Perreaux F, Trioche P, Labrune P. Factors predicting serious bacterial infections in febrile infants less than three months old: multivariate analysis [in French]. *Arch Pediatr.* 2005;12:397–403

Grijalva CG, Poehling KA, Nuorti JP, et al. National impact of universal childhood immunization with pneumococcal conjugate vaccine on outpatient medical care visits in the United States. *Pediatrics.* 2006:118:865–873

Isaacman DJ, Burke BL. Utility of serum C-reactive protein for detection of occult bacterial infection in children. *Arch Pediatr Adolesc Med.* 2002;156:905–909

Isaacman DJ, Zhang Y, Reynolds EA, et al. Accuracy of a polymerase chain reaction–based assay for detection of pneumococcal bacteremia in children. *Pediatrics.* 1998;101:813–816

Kaplan RL, Harper MB, Baskin MN, Macone AB, Mandl KD. Time to detection of positive cultures in 28- to 90-day-old febrile infants. *Pediatrics.* 2000;106:e74

Kaplan SL, Mason EO Jr, Wald ER, et al. Decrease of invasive pneumococcal infections in children among 8 children's hospitals in the United States after the introduction of the 7-valent pneumococcal conjugate vaccine. *Pediatrics.* 2004;113:443–449

Kuppermann N. Occult bacteremia in young febrile children. *Pediatr Clin North Am.* 1999;46:1073–1109

Lee GM, Fleisher GR, Harper MB. Management of febrile children in the age of the conjugate pneumococcal vaccine: a cost-effectiveness analysis. *Pediatrics.* 2001;108:835–844

Levine DA, Platt SL, Dayan PS, et al. Risk of serious bacterial infection in young febrile infants with respiratory syncytial virus infections. *Pediatrics.* 2004;113:1728–1734

Newman TB, Bernzweig JA, Takayama JI, et al. Urine testing and urinary tract infections in febrile infants seen in office settings: The Pediatric Research in Office Settings Febrile Infant Study. *Arch Pediatr Adolesc Med.* 2002;156:44–54

Pulliam PN, Attia MW, Cronan KM. C-reactive protein in febrile children 1 to 36 months of age with clinically undetectable serious bacterial infection. *Pediatrics.* 2001;108:1275–1279

Singleton R, Hammitt L, Hennessy T, et al. The Alaska *Haemophilus influenzae* type b experience: lessons in controlling a vaccine-preventable disease. *Pediatrics.* 2006;118:421–429

Strait RT, Kelly KJ, Kurup VP. Tumor necrosis factor-alpha, interleukin-1 beta, and interleukin-6 levels in febrile, young children with and without occult bacteremia. *Pediatrics.* 1999;104:1321–1326

Febrile Seizures

Kenneth R. Huff, MD

CASE STUDY

A 12-month-old girl is brought to the emergency department by paramedics because she is having a seizure. She is unresponsive and hypertonic, with arched trunk and extended arms and legs that are jerking rhythmically. Her eyes are open, but her gaze is directed upward. She has bubbles of saliva around her lips as well as circumoral cyanosis. Her vital signs are a respiratory rate of 60/min, heart rate of 125/min, blood pressure of 130/78 mm Hg, and temperature of 105.8°F (41.0°C). An assessment of her respiratory status discloses that she is moving air in all lung fields, and there is no evidence of upper airway obstruction.

The paramedics inform you that the girl has been convulsing for approximately 6 minutes. Glucometer testing reveals a normal serum glucose. Blood samples for other tests are sent to the laboratory, and urine is collected. An intravenous (IV) line is started, and the girl is given lorazepam by IV push. Within 2 minutes, the movements cease, and her respirations become slow and even. Her physical examination shows no signs of trauma. Her only abnormality other than her unresponsive mental status is an inflamed and bulging right tympanic membrane.

The girl's parents tell you that she has had a mildly stuffy nose for 2 days but has been afebrile and has seemed to be her usual self. While she was playing, she became cranky, and her parents put her in her crib for her nap. Thirty minutes later they heard grunting noises, found her in the midst of a seizure, and called the paramedics. The girl has never had a seizure before. Her father recalls that his mother once told him that he had several "fever seizures" as an infant.

Questions

1. What are the characteristics of simple febrile seizures?
2. What is the appropriate evaluation of children with febrile seizures, whether it is the first one or a recurrence?
3. What is the recurrence risk for febrile seizures and the risk of developing unprovoked seizures following a febrile seizure?
4. What are the treatment options for children with febrile seizures?

Febrile seizures are easily recognized, dramatic, generalized convulsions. These seizures are defined by the presence of a fever (often sudden) from a source outside the nervous system; patient age of 5 years or younger; absence (for simple febrile seizures) of chronic brain pathology, including developmental delay; and absence of metabolic or structural abnormalities of the brain. Frequently, familial predisposition to similar seizures plays a role. Despite the relatively uniform presentation of the seizure, genetic abnormalities in channels or neurotransmitter receptor or preexisting hippocampal damage may influence prognosis, and individual clinical variables and social factors may play a part in the treatment.

Epidemiology

Febrile seizures occur in children between the ages of 6 months and 5 years but are more common in those who are younger than 3 years. Some studies indicate that as many as 5% of all children experience at least one febrile seizure. The recurrence rate is 30% to 50% in children younger than 1 year, but drops to 25% between 1 and 3 years, and is only 12% after 3 years. Seizures usually occur with the rise in temperature and often so suddenly that the febrile illness is not

recognized by the family prior to the seizure. Frequently, the febrile illness is eventually diagnosed as an upper respiratory tract or influenza infection. Febrile seizures are seen often in children who have a first-degree relative who experienced the problem at the same age.

Clinical Presentation

Simple febrile seizures are characterized by a single episode of generalized, symmetric, tonic posturing and clonic movements of a few minutes' duration that occur suddenly in children whose developmental progress is generally normal. Fever is present, although it may not have been recognized before the seizure, and its source is

Dx Febrile Seizures

- Sudden unresponsiveness, tonic posturing, and generalized rhythmic jerking
- Fever source outside nervous system
- Age 6 months to 5 years
- Normal neurodevelopmental history

outside the nervous system. A short time after the seizure (after usually 1–2 hours of postictal sleepiness), children become neurologically normal again (Dx Box).

Recently described generalized epilepsy with febrile seizures plus (GEFS+) is characterized by the association of generalized febrile seizures beyond the age of 6 years and afebrile generalized convulsions, a positive family history of epilepsy with variable phenotypes, and a benign prognosis in most cases. The same families may have simple febrile seizures, febrile seizures beyond the age of 6 years, febrile seizures and absences, atonic or myoclonic seizures, and myoclonic-astatic epilepsy.

Pathophysiology

The susceptibility of young children to febrile seizures may be related to an increased incidence of sudden high fevers in this age group, a developmental genetic factor that may lower the seizure threshold, or both. Animal models indicate that the immature brain has a lower seizure threshold than the adult, and seizures in the immature brain are more likely to occur by a different mechanism than those in the adult. A sudden increase in temperature to a sufficiently high level can provoke seizures regardless of age. Seizures occur more frequently with fever in many seizure-prone patients who have seizures of different etiologies, including epilepsy. Perhaps circulating pyrogens interact with a brain cellular circuitry mechanism, causing hypersynchronous depolarization and a seizure. The multigenerational familial history that is often seen suggests an autosomal-dominant form of genetic transmission.

Both the precise definition of the genetic markers and the mechanisms of generalized seizures in all cases are not yet fully understood. Recent work suggests a possible mechanism. Recently mutations in either γ-aminobutyric acid (GABA) A receptor or sodium channel genes have been found to be associated with febrile seizures and GEFS+ pedigrees. GABA A receptors receive inhibitory transmission and are composed of combinations of 5 subunits. The γ-2 subunit is critical for receptor trafficking, clustering, and synaptic maintenance, and mutations in this subunit have been associated with febrile seizure families. It has also been found that the trafficking of mutant receptors with gamma 2 subunit mutations was more highly temperature dependent than mutations of other subunits, and impaired membrane insertion or accelerated receptor endocytosis with brief increases of 37 to 40 degrees occurred. Thus in these families, the febrile seizures may be caused by a fever-induced change in the dynamic membrane state producing reduced numbers of available mutant GABA A receptors.

In other families with GEFS+, it has been found that missense mutations in SCN1A gene, which encodes for the α-1 subunit of the neuronal voltage gated sodium channel, have occurred. However, these mutations have not occurred in sequences that encode for the "pore" region of the subunit protein that participates in ion selectivity and result in a more severe phenotype with early prolonged resistant seizures, Dravet syndrome, which later results in severe myoclonic epilepsy of infancy and mental retardation. Perhaps the less severe GEFS+ phenotype is correlated with a less functionally critical position of the missense mutation in the SCN1A gene.

Differential Diagnosis

When a young child presents with a fever and a seizure, the possibility that the seizure is symptomatic of meningitis, encephalitis, or brain abscess must be considered. Signs of meningeal irritation may not be reliable in children younger than 18 months, and these and other signs of the illness may be obscured in the postictal period. If there is a history of lethargy or persistent vomiting, or the seizure was focal in onset, prolonged, or multiple, an examination of the cerebrospinal fluid (CSF) must be done. The fever also could be coincidental to a seizure of different etiology such as trauma, toxic ingestion, metabolic derangement, degenerative or neurocutaneous disorder, or stroke.

A useful concept for the physician caring for a child with a seizure with fever is the differentiation of simple febrile seizures from complex febrile seizures (Table 44-1). A question that has prognostic implications is whether children in the appropriate age range have had a true febrile seizure or a seizure with fever, which may be an early fever-provoked episode of a nonfebrile seizure disorder. The factors defining a complex febrile seizure also predict an increased likelihood of later unprovoked nonfebrile seizures. The length of a complex febrile seizure is longer than 15 minutes. Most febrile seizures last fewer than 90 seconds, although a significant number present in status epilepticus. More than one febrile seizure during the same infectious illness or 24-hour period makes these recurrent seizures complex febrile seizures. The history of a focal or partial onset or the presence of postictal focal neurologic signs makes the febrile seizure complex. The presence of an abnormal neurodevelopmental history prior to the febrile seizure or abnormal neurologic examination or brain imaging study before or after the seizure also increases the likelihood of later unprovoked seizures.

Table 44-1. Simple Versus Complex Febrile Seizures		
Feature	*Simple*	*Complex*
Onset of clonic movements	Generalized	Focal
Length	<15 minutes (usually <90 seconds)	>15 minutes
Number of seizures per 24 h febrile illness	1	Recurrent
Neurodevelopmental history	Normal	Abnormal
Parent-sibling history of a febrile seizure	Positive	Negative

Evaluation

History

After the seizure has been controlled and the child has been stabilized, a more detailed history relating to the circumstances of the seizure (the child's state leading up to the seizure; prenatal, birth, and developmental histories; and family seizure history) should be obtained (Questions Box).

> ### Febrile Seizures — **Questions**
> - What were the child's symptoms for the few days before the seizure?
> - Where was the child and what was he or she doing immediately before the seizure?
> - Were there any pregnancy-related or perinatal complications?
> - Has the child's development been normal or similar to that of siblings?
> - Have any other family members had seizures of any kind, including during infancy?

Physical Examination

Children should be examined completely after stabilization, noting the possibility that the fever may be coincidental. Physicians should look for bruises, fractures, retinal hemorrhages, or other signs of trauma. The presence of dysmorphic features, enlarged organs, or bony changes should be noted. The skin should be examined for abnormal, pigmented, or textured spots. Lateralized signs of tone or strength should be assessed. An appropriate evaluation to determine the etiology of the fever should be performed (see Chapter 43).

Laboratory Tests

If the seizure is prolonged, focal, or multiple; if there is a history of lethargy, stupor, or persistent vomiting before the seizure; or if the patient still appears ill after the postictal period, cultures should be obtained and metabolic and toxicological blood and urine studies sent. A spinal tap for CSF examination should be done unless there are signs of increased intracranial pressure or a lateralized neurologic examination, in which case antibiotics should be given and an imaging study obtained prior to the spinal tap.

If the seizure is a simple febrile seizure, an electroencephalogram (EEG) has limited usefulness. There is a high rate of abnormality that is nonspecific, and many believe non-predictive of either future simple febrile seizures or unprovoked seizures. If the patient does not fully recover after the postictal period, the EEG may be useful to help define the nature of the encephalopathy.

Imaging Studies

Computed tomography and magnetic resonance imaging scans have a low yield of abnormal results in children with simple febrile seizures. Children who have had an abnormal neurodevelopmental history or who have had a focal or partial onset to their seizure should have an imaging study to detect a structural lesion that may be the source of the seizure provoked by the fever or serve as a nidus for future seizures provoked or unprovoked by fever.

Management

If children are still convulsing on presentation and have been for at least 5 minutes, they should be managed as for status epilepticus (see Chapter 132). The airway must be secure, blood tests drawn and sent to the laboratory, an intravenous line started, and lorazepam administered in the appropriate dose to stop the seizure.

If children are not in status epilepticus, management decisions are made on a more long-term basis (Box 44-1). Whether to recommend **anticonvulsant prophylaxis** for children who have experienced febrile seizures is **controversial.** Factors that must be considered include (1) the benign, age-limited nature of the condition; (2) the morbidity of the anticonvulsant treatment; (3) the chance of recurrence of febrile or nonfebrile seizures; (4) the risk of overmedication during an acute recurrence; and (5) the family's reaction and social disruption caused by the seizures.

> **Box 44-1. Treatment Options for Febrile Seizures**
>
> Cooling measures during febrile illness (antipyretics or bathing in tepid water)
> Family reassurance and education
> Diazepam, 0.3 mg/kg orally or 5–10 mg rectal gel (Diastat) every 8 h (during febrile illness only)
> Phenobarbital, 3–5 mg/kg orally daily, for prophylaxis
> Valproic acid (divalproex), 30 mg/kg orally divided twice daily, for prophylaxis

Daily doses of phenobarbital or valproic acid are effective prophylactic anticonvulsants. The most commonly used regimen is daily phenobarbital, but its potential side effects include hyperactive behavior disorder and depressed cognition. Valproic acid can produce thrombocytopenia and may have the potential of provoking acute liver dysfunction in the patient younger than 2 years who is taking other medications. Fever control measures should be instituted to make the patient more comfortable but have not been found effective as prevention for seizures. Intermittent anticonvulsant therapy has the advantage of reducing side effects but relies on recognizing the fever prior to the seizure and mandates greater vigilance for compliance during each fever. Diazepam administered intermittently is effective within this sometimes considerable limitation. Because prolonged febrile seizures tend to recur as prolonged rather than febrile seizures, this group may benefit by having rectal diazepam to administer at home for recurrence.

Recommendations for prophylactic anticonvulsant treatment are often individualized. Anticonvulsants are usually not recommended unless the child has presented in status epilepticus, has experienced marked respiratory compromise (perhaps needing ventilatory support) during the seizure, or has had complex febrile seizures. There is no definitive evidence yet that anticonvulsant prophylaxis for simple febrile seizures prevents the development of unprovoked sei-zures. Children who have had frequently recurring seizures that are extremely disruptive for the family and deleterious to parent-child interactions despite educational efforts by the medical caretakers may also be candidates for prophylactic anticonvulsant treatment.

Prognosis

Febrile seizures are a common age-limited problem. The progno-sis for children with simple febrile seizures is generally good; the incidence of seizure episodes later in life is 3 to 6 times higher than in the general population at the same age but is still low: 2% to 3%. Those who have a complex presentation have a higher likelihood of developing a nonfebrile seizure disorder, but this risk is only 6% if 2 of the first 3 factors (see Table 44-1) are present or 17% if they are neurodevelopmentally abnormal. Overall, one-third of children with febrile seizures experience a recurrence. The risk of febrile seizure recurrence is most dependent on age: 50% of infants younger than 1 year at the time of their first seizure will have a recurrence, but only 20% of children older than 3 years will have a recurrence. Other fac-tors that have a lesser influence on the recurrence risk include fam-ily history of seizures, temperature at the initial seizure, time since the previous seizure, and history of previous recurrences.

Animal models suggest that seizures, even status epilepticus epi-sodes, in the immature brain are less often associated with neu-ronal death, but that seizures, particularly hyperthermic seizures, can modify brain development by altering the expression of ion chan-nels regulating neuronal excitability, and epileptogenic mechanisms may be more robust than in the adult.

Among patients who had surgery for intractable temporal lobe epilepsy, mesial temporal sclerosis (MTS) was the most frequent pathology, and 30% of these patients had antecedents of prolonged complex febrile seizures compared with 6% in those who did not have MTS. It is possible that MTS is the etiologic consequence of a prolonged seizure when the hippocampus is developmentally vul-nerable. Mesial temporal sclerosis is frequently unilateral, however, although focal complex febrile seizures can actually originate in the temporal lobe in some children. Alternatively, some preexisting dam-age or genetic predisposition may be present in patients with hip-pocampal sclerosis after prolonged febrile seizures, and the complex febrile seizure is an epiphenomenon.

A small percentage of infants with febrile seizures may develop Dravet syndrome.

CASE RESOLUTION

In the case history presented at the beginning of this chapter, the girl had a some-what prolonged simple febrile seizure, a diagnosis supported by a family history positive for febrile seizures. Her family is educated about treatment options. They become comfortable with a decision to use intermittent therapy with diazepam for her subsequent febrile illnesses, realizing that a fever may not be recognized before the seizure occurs.

Selected References

American Academy of Pediatrics Provisional Committee on Quality Improvement and Subcommittee on Febrile Seizures. Practice parameter: the neurodiag-nostic evaluation of the child with a first simple febrile seizure. *Pediatrics.* 1996;97:769–772

Baram T, Shinnar S, eds. *Febrile Seizures.* San Diego, CA: Academic Press; 2002

Cendes F. Febrile seizures and mesial temporal sclerosis. *Curr Opin Neurol.* 2004;17:161–164

Duchowny M. Febrile seizures in childhood. In: Wyllie E, ed. *The Treatment of Epilepsy: Principles and Practice.* Philadelphia, PA: Lea & Febiger; 1993:647–653

Jensen F. Pediatric epilepsy models. *Epilepsy Res.* 2006;8:28–31

Kanai K, Hirose S, Oguni H. Effect of localization of missense mutations in SCN1A on epilepsy phenotype severity. *Neurology.* 2004;63:329–334

Kang J, Shen W, Macdonald RL. Why does fever trigger seizures? GABA-A receptor gamma 2 subunit mutations associated with idiopathic generalized epilepsies have temperature-dependent trafficking deficiencies. *J Neurosci.* 2006;26:2590–2597

Korff C, Nordli D. Epilepsy syndromes in infancy. *Pediatr Neurol.* 2006;34:253–263

Nelson KB, Ellenberg JH. *Febrile Seizures.* New York, NY: Raven Press; 1981

Respiratory Distress

David B. Burbulys, MD

CASE STUDY

A 6-month-old boy has been coughing and breathing fast for the past day. This morning he refused feeding and has been irritable. On examination, the infant is fussy. He has a respiratory rate of 60/min, a pulse of 140/min, and a normal blood pressure and temperature. In addition, he has nasal flaring, intercostal and supraclavicular retractions, and occasional grunting.

Questions

1. What are the causes of respiratory distress in infants and children?
2. What are the signs and symptoms of respiratory distress in infants and children?
3. What are the signs and symptoms of impending respiratory failure in infants and children?
4. What are the critical interventions for infants and children in respiratory distress?

Respiratory distress and respiratory failure may cause significant morbidity and mortality in infants and children. The signs and symptoms of respiratory compromise may be subtle, particularly in small infants. Decompensation may occur rapidly if ventilation or oxygenation is inadequate but may be prevented by prompt recognition and treatment. **Respiratory distress** is defined as increased work of breathing, and it usually precedes respiratory failure. **Respiratory failure** occurs when ventilation or oxygenation is not sufficient to meet the metabolic demands of the tissues. Thus oxygenation of the blood is inadequate or carbon dioxide is not eliminated. This may be caused by diseases of the airway, inadequate gas exchange in the lungs, or poor respiratory effort (Box 45-1).

Epidemiology

Primary care physicians frequently care for children in respiratory distress in both offices and emergency departments. Respiratory distress continues to be the most common reason for hospital admission. Such admissions usually involve young infants with acute infections. Reactive airway disease (asthma) accounts for respiratory distress–related admission, particularly in older children.

Clinical Presentation

Increases in respiratory rate and work of breathing are the most common signs of respiratory disease. Effortless tachypnea may be a sign of respiratory compensation for metabolic acidosis rather than an indication of pulmonary pathology. Tachycardia is often present, although bradycardia, if present, may be an ominous sign of impending cardiopulmonary failure. Signs of poor oxygenation include alterations in mental status, head bobbing, and change in skin color. Pallor, mottling, and cyanosis are often late signs indicating respiratory failure and shock. Children may first appear dusky or pale. If children are anemic, cyanosis may not be evident, although the oxygen saturation is low (Box 45-2).

Pathophysiology

The adequacy of respiration depends on effective gas exchange of carbon dioxide and oxygen and the ability to move an adequate volume of gas in and out of the airways. Infants and children generally

Box 45-1. Causes of Respiratory Distress in Infants and Children	
• Infection	• Submersion injuries
• Bronchiolitis	• Pneumothorax or hemothorax
• Pneumonia	• Pulmonary contusion
• Croup	• Smoke inhalation
• Epiglottitis	• Toxin exposure
• Congenital anomalies	• Cardiac disease
• Foreign body aspiration	• Metabolic disease with acidosis
• Reactive airway disease (asthma)	• Neuromuscular disease
• Allergic reactions	

Box 45-2. Respiratory Distress	
• Increased respiratory rate	• Production of sounds with respiration (eg, gurgling, stridor, rhonchi, grunting)
• Changes in tidal volume or minute ventilation	
• Presence of retractions: intercostal, substernal, diaphragmatic, or supraclavicular	• Diaphoresis
	• Alterations in mental status
	• Poor feeding
• Nasal flaring	• Inability to speak in sentences
• Decreased or absent breath sounds	• Presence of pale or cyanotic skin
• Changes in inspiratory-expiratory ratio	• Presence of central cyanosis

breathe with minimal effort. In very young children, the **diaphragm** and abdominal musculature are primarily used for ventilation, and the tidal volume is approximately 6 to 8 mL/kg. If the tidal volume is decreased because of obstruction, children compensate by increasing the respiratory rate, thus attempting to maintain adequate **minute ventilation** (minute ventilation = rate × tidal volume). If the minute ventilation is still insufficient for adequate gas exchange, or the child can no longer sustain the increased work of breathing, then respiratory failure ensues. Respiratory failure may then lead to acidosis, myocardial dysfunction, and shock and may progress to complete cardiopulmonary arrest.

Infants and children are more prone than adults to respiratory distress because of the differences between their respiratory systems (Box 45-3).

Box 45-3. Comparison of Respiratory Systems in Children and Adults

- The head in children is proportionally larger and has less muscular support.
- The tongue in children is larger in relation to the mouth, is poorly controlled, and can cause airway obstruction.
- The airway diameter is smaller in children and collapses easily. Reductions in size due to secretions or inflammation cause greater resistance to air flow (resistance is proportional to $1/radius^4$).
- The larynx is higher and more anterior in children and the epiglottis is floppy, which makes visualization of the vocal cords more difficult.
- The narrowest part of the airway in children is at the cricoid ring, unlike in adults, where the narrowest point is at the vocal cords.
- The trachea in children is short. In newborns it is 4-cm long, in 18-month-old infants 7-cm long, and in adults 12-cm long.
- The major muscle of respiration in children is the diaphragm. Any interference with diaphragmatic motion in young children impedes respiratory function. Intercostal muscles are immature in children and fatigue easily.
- Children have less pulmonary reserve and higher metabolic demands.
- Normal respiratory rates are higher in children and vary by age.

Differential Diagnosis

The differential diagnosis of children with respiratory distress can include abnormalities with the pulmonary, cardiovascular, or metabolic systems or be related to a reduction in the central nervous system drive. It is also important to make an initial differentiation between upper and lower airway disease based on the presence or absence of stridor on examination. Many common causes are shown in Box 45-1.

Evaluation

History

A brief history should be taken (Questions Box) while physical examination proceeds and initial treatment is begun.

Questions

Respiratory Distress

- For how long has this problem been occurring? Has a similar problem ever occurred before?
- Did the problem begin while the child was eating or playing?
- Has the child had any recent infections?
- Are any members of the household ill?
- Is the child taking any medications?

Physical Examination

Before a complete assessment can proceed, critical interventions that may change children's clinical status should be made. Children should be placed in a position of comfort and oxygen should be applied. Both **ventilation** and **oxygenation** should be assessed.

Respiratory and heart rates should be determined for a period of at least 30 seconds. In infants, abdominal excursions should be counted and, in older children, chest excursions should be counted. **Respiratory rates** in children are higher than in adults; infants may breathe 40 times per minute, 1-year-olds 25 times per minute, and 10-year-olds 18 times per minute (Table 45-1). These rates vary with age and changes of activity, emotion, and illness. Abnormal respiratory rates are defined as being faster than normal (tachypnea), slower than normal (bradypnea), or absent (apnea). Neonates may exhibit **periodic breathing,** with periods of regular respirations alternating with irregular breathing. This is a normal variant for age. True apnea (cessation of respiration) is accompanied by change in skin color or tone or altered level of consciousness.

Table 45-1. Vital Signs by Age

Age	Respiration (breaths/min)	Pulse (beats/min)	Systolic Blood Pressure (mm Hg)
Newborn	30–60	100–160	50–70
1–6 wk	30–60	100–160	70–95
6 mo	25–40	90–120	80–100
1 y	20–40	90–120	80–100
3 y	20–30	80–120	80–110
6 y	12–25	70–110	80–110
10 y	12–20	60–90	90–120

The depth of respiration should be noted. Whether breaths are deep, gasping, or shallow should be determined. Rapid, shallow respirations may not provide enough **inspiratory time** for adequate gas exchange. The heart rate may also reflect respiratory compromise. Breath sounds should first be listened to in the axillae and then at the bases and apices. The absence of breath sounds may be an ominous sign. Children's breath sounds are usually well transmitted across the thorax because of the thin chest wall. It is common to hear upper airway noises when auscultating the lungs.

Abnormal sounds are caused by turbulent air passing through a narrowed airway. Resistance to flow through a hollow tube increases exponentially. Thus the smaller the airway, the greater the resistance to flow generated by even small changes in the radius (eg, as with edema, secretions, or foreign bodies). The nature of the sounds produced depends on the location of the narrowing in the airway. **Gurgling, snoring,** and **stridor** come from the upper airway, and **rales, rhonchi,** and **wheezing** from the lower airway. If no abnormal sounds are evident and breath sounds are absent or decreased, the airways may be totally obstructed. **Grunting** is caused by turbulent air coming in contact with a partially closed glottis. Children who grunt are generating their own partial obstruction of the upper airway and positive end-expiratory pressure to increase oxygenation.

The physician should also observe the effort children expend in breathing. Increased work of breathing occurs when intercostal, subcostal, or supraclavicular **retractions** are present, the **accessory muscles** of respiration are used, breathing is abnormally noisy, or **nasal flaring** is seen. The normal work of breathing consumes 2% to 3% of total oxygen consumption. The increased work of breathing in children with severe respiratory distress can potentially increase total oxygen consumption to 50%. Increased work of breathing can also be demonstrated by feeding difficulties and diaphoresis in young infants.

In addition, the physician should observe the inspiratory-expiratory ratio while assessing the work of breathing. The ratio is approximately 1:1 in most patients. Prolonged expirations are most often seen with reactive airway disease.

Oxygen saturation should be measured by pulse oximetry. Levels less than 93% indicate significant hypoxemia.

Laboratory Tests

Although the physical examination is the most important tool for assessing children in respiratory distress, laboratory tests such as complete and differential blood counts and blood cultures may help in the diagnosis of infection. It should be remembered that meningitis and metabolic derangement may present with effortless tachypnea not associated with increased work of breathing. Arterial blood gases may be beneficial in this situation but in general should be reserved for patients in impending respiratory failure.

Peak expiratory flow or forced expiratory volume in 1-second determinations (FEV_1) can be helpful in assessing compliant children with reactive airway disease. Oxygen saturation measurements can also be helpful in these children because reduced levels below 100% often correlate with the severity of disease.

Imaging Studies

Chest radiographs can aid in assessing children in respiratory distress but should not be routinely performed in patients with known reactive airway disease unless children have a fever or are in status asthmaticus. A patient with significant respiratory distress should not be moved from a monitored setting to the radiology suite but rather portable x-rays should be obtained if needed.

Management

All infants or children in respiratory distress should be managed emergently. As stated earlier, in such situations, assessment and intervention often occur simultaneously. All children in respiratory distress should be reassessed frequently. The highest possible oxygen concentration should be delivered. Children who are able to maintain their own airway should never be forced to use an airway adjunct because this may cause increased anxiety and distress. Patients with clear airways can be maintained with simple interventions such as **oxygen** blown by the face or given by mask or nasal prongs. More advanced airway management such as bag-valve-mask ventilation or endotracheal intubation may be necessary for children who need assisted ventilation, airway protection, or hyperventilation.

Position

Children in respiratory distress who are alert and breathing spontaneously should be allowed to choose a **position of comfort**. Small infants who are incapable of positioning themselves are best placed upright with care taken not to flex or extend the neck. Children and their caregivers should be kept together to reduce anxiety.

The proper position for unconscious children is the "sniffing position," with the neck slightly flexed and the head extended to open the airway. This can be facilitated by placing a towel under the occiput of the head or the shoulders. If simple positioning does not relieve an obstruction, then the airway should be opened using the chin lift or jaw thrust. If spinal trauma is a possibility, only the jaw thrust should be used. If this fails, then **airway adjuncts,** such as nasopharyngeal or oropharyngeal airways, can be placed to help prevent the soft tissue of the oropharynx from collapsing against the posterior pharyngeal wall.

Monitoring

All infants and children in respiratory distress should be carefully monitored. Pulse oximetry will assist the clinician in determining the degree of oxygen saturation and, if available, a cardiac and respiratory monitor will provide constant readings of respirations and heart rate. Frequent assessments of the patient are critical to ensure a good outcome.

Oxygen Administration

Oxygen should be delivered by any method tolerated by children. **Nasal prongs** have 2 advantages: They are noninvasive and allow maintenance of a constant gas flow even when talking and eating. The concentration of oxygen delivered is limited, however, and irritation and drying of the mucous membranes may result.

Oxygen masks deliver a higher concentration of humidified oxygen. Disadvantages include obstruction of children's visual field, potential for carbon dioxide retention, and anxiety because the face is covered. Various types of masks are available.

The **simple mask** can deliver 30% to 60% oxygen concentration at flow rates of 6 to 10 L/min. Room air is drawn into the mask through the exhalation ports in the side of the mask.

A **partial rebreathing mask** is desirable when higher concentrations of oxygen (50%–60%) are required. During exhalation, oxygen flows into the reservoir bag along with one-third of the exhaled gas. Entrapment of room air is minimized when patients breathe oxygen from the reservoir bag.

A **non-rebreathing mask** has valves that allow only oxygen (85%–95%) to flow from the reservoir bag to the patient on inhalation and additional valves on the exhalation ports of the mask that prevent entrapment of room air (Figure 45-1).

Figure 45-1. A non-rebreathing mask can deliver a high concentration of oxygen to a patient in respiratory distress.

The **face tent** is a soft plastic bucket shaped to the chin that is well tolerated by children. The face tent allows up to 40% oxygen to be delivered, and it has the advantage of allowing access to the face and mouth (Figure 45-2).

Figure 45-2. Use of a face tent.

A **venturi mask** is rarely used in children but has the advantage of precisely titrating the oxygen concentration to be delivered from 24% to 60%.

Children with potential respiratory failure require **assisted ventilation** with **bag-valve-mask** devices or **endotracheal intubation.** Masks of the proper size should be used. The upper edge of the mask should fit snugly over the bridge of the nose without touching the eyes. The lower edge should rest directly on or just above the mandible. An oropharyngeal airway should be inserted in unconscious children to prevent the tongue from obstructing the upper airway. If a bag-valve-mask is not available, assisted ventilation can be given with a **pocket mask** with a one-way valve. Oxygen can be attached to the mask at the side port (Figure 45-3). Endotracheal intubation is indicated in those children who require control of the airway, who need airway protection, or who require hyperventilation.

Figure 45-3. A pocket mask with a one-way valve and side oxygen port that can be used for assisted ventilation in the office setting.

Prognosis

Respiratory failure and resulting cardiopulmonary arrest are preventable in most infants and children if their condition is carefully assessed and appropriate critical interventions are made. Careful attention to ventilation and oxygenation of patients usually results in a good outcome.

CASE RESOLUTION

The fussy infant discussed in the case history has obvious signs of respiratory distress, including tachypnea, tachycardia, grunting, nasal flaring, and retractions. The differential diagnosis includes foreign body, infection, and reactive airway disease. It is important to place the infant in a position of comfort and provide supplemental oxygen before any diagnostic studies, such as chest x-ray, are performed. Pulse oximetry should be monitored. The clinical status of the infant should be reassessed periodically to prevent further deterioration.

Selected References

American Heart Association. 2005 American Heart Association (AHA) guidelines for cardiopulmonary resuscitation (CPR) and emergency cardiovascular care (ECC) of pediatric and neonatal patients: pediatric basic life support. *Pediatrics.* 2006;117:e989–e1004

American Heart Association. 2005 American Heart Association (AHA) guidelines for cardiopulmonary resuscitation (CPR) and emergency cardiovascular care (ECC) of pediatric and neonatal patients: pediatric advanced life support. *Pediatrics.* 2006;117:e1005–e1028

Baren JM, Seidel JS. Emergency management of respiratory distress and failure. In: Barkin R, ed. *Pediatric Emergency Medicine: Concepts and Clinical Practice.* St Louis, MO: Mosby-Year Book; 1997:95–103

Losek JD. Office preparedness for pediatric emergencies. *J S C Med Assoc.* 2004; 100:337–341

Stridor and Croup

David B. Burbulys, MD

CASE STUDY

A 2-year-old boy has been breathing noisily for 1 day. For the past 3 days he has had a "cold," with a runny nose, fever (temperature: up to 100.4°F [38°C]), and a slight cough. The cough has gradually become worse and now has a barking quality.

On examination, the child is sitting up and has a respiratory rate of 48/min with marked inspiratory stridor and an occasional barking cough. His other vital signs include a heart rate of 100/min and temperature of 101.2°F (38.4°C). He has intercostal retractions, his breath sounds are slightly decreased bilaterally, and his skin is pale. The remainder of the examination is normal.

Questions

1. What is stridor?
2. What are the common causes of stridor?
3. What is the pathophysiology of viral croup?
4. How are children with stridor managed?

Noisy breathing is a common symptom that often accompanies respiratory infections in children. The presence of **stridor,** a high-pitched crowing sound, often concerns children's caregivers. Some parents try home remedies to alleviate the symptoms, whereas many others immediately seek help in the office or emergency department setting. **Croup,** a type of noisy breathing, is an inflammation of the larynx, trachea, and upper bronchioles (laryngotracheobronchitis). It is one of the most common causes of a seal-like barking cough and stridor in children.

Epidemiology

Croup most commonly affects children between 6 months and 3 years of age, generally in the fall or early winter. Children younger than 1 year make up 26% of cases. The condition is more common in boys than girls; two-thirds of all hospitalized children with croup are boys.

Stridor, which may be indicative of croup, may also be a sign of epiglottitis. The incidence of epiglottitis in children has dramatically decreased since 1988 following the development and widespread use of the Hib vaccine against *Haemophilus influenzae* type b. Many young children may be incompletely immunized and there are other bacteria that may cause epiglottitis; therefore, epiglottitis should still be considered in toxic-appearing children with rapid onset of symptoms of upper airway obstruction. Prior to *H influenzae* type b immunization, the ratio of cases of epiglottitis to croup was 1:100. Today, epiglottitis in children is exceedingly rare.

Pathophysiology

Stridor

Stridor is generally caused by obstruction of the airway between the nose and the larger bronchi. Obstruction at the level of the nose or pharynx may produce snoring or gurgling sounds. Turbulence of airflow in the laryngeal area or upper trachea causes the high-pitched crowing sound characteristic of stridor. Edema and inflammation at the vocal cords and subglottic areas result in **inspiratory stridor,** whereas obstruction below the cricoid cartilage may lead to both inspiratory and **expiratory stridor.**

Some of the more common causes of stridor are listed in Box 46-1.

The sounds produced at various levels of obstruction can give the primary care provider clues as to the etiology of the problem. The most common cause of stridor that begins shortly after birth is tracheomalacia, a condition secondary to the immaturity of the cartilage of the trachea. Laryngomalacia, which is caused by floppy supraglottic structures, resolves after several months.

The upper airway of infants and children is more susceptible to obstruction as a result of anatomical differences between children and adults. The tongues of children are relatively large and the epiglottis is floppy and shaped somewhat like the Greek letter omega (Ω). The angle between the epiglottis and the glottis is more acute in children, which makes direct visualization of the airway more difficult. Cartilaginous structures are less rigid in infants. During inspiration, negative intraluminal pressure is generated below the level of obstruction, which leads to narrowing of the airway and turbulence

Box 46-1. Causes of Stridor	
Congenital Anomalies	**Trauma**
Tracheomalacia	Direct trauma to the upper airway
Laryngomalacia	Post-intubation subglottic stenosis
Choanal atresia	**Neurogenic**
Laryngeal web	Laryngeal paralysis
Laryngocele	Poor pharyngeal muscle tone
Subglottic stenosis	**Caustic or Thermal Injury**
Vascular ring	Lye or caustic ingestion
Macroglossia (Beckwith syndrome)	Hot gas or liquid
Tracheal web or cyst	**Foreign Body**
Inflammatory/Infectious Lesions	Neoplasm
Viral croup	
Epiglottitis	
Abscess (retropharyngeal, peritonsillar, parapharyngeal)	
Tracheitis	
Bronchitis	
Severe tonsillitis	
Angioneurotic edema	
Infectious mononucleosis	
Diphtheria	

of the airflow. This occurs more often in children because the tracheal rings are not well formed. In addition, the smaller size of the airway in children makes resistance to airflow greater when obstruction is present.

The smaller the airway, the greater the resistance to flow (resistance increases exponentially). Alterations in the diameter of the airway are most often caused by edema and inflammation from a variety of conditions, including congenital anomalies, infection, allergic and anaphylactic reactions, cysts, tumors, and trauma. Even small localized areas of airway narrowing in infants and children can lead to respiratory distress because the airway is so small, particularly at the cricoid ring, which is the narrowest portion of the airway in children.

Croup

Croup is most often caused by an infection with **parainfluenza virus** (type I or II). Several other causes include respiratory syncytial virus, influenza virus A or B, adenovirus, rhinovirus, coxsackievirus, measles, and herpes simplex virus. Metapneumovirus and a novel coronavirus, which more commonly cause bronchiolitis, are also implicated. Particularly severe disease may be associated with influenza A, respiratory syncytial virus, or adenovirus infection. Infection occurs via respiratory droplets spread from other infected individuals.

The virus first attacks the nasopharynx and subsequently spreads to the larynx and upper trachea. The infection causes inflammation and edema of the airway that often involves the vocal cords producing the typical barking cough, hoarseness, and inspiratory stridor. Uncommonly, in severe cases, the lower airways also may be involved, leading to impaired alveolar ventilation and wheezing. In some children, secondary bacterial superinfection may rarely occur with bacterial tracheitis or extension of infection to the lower airway producing pneumonia. Airways of infants are small and particularly susceptible to obstruction because of the narrow subglottic region and the laxity of the cartilaginous structures.

Spasmodic croup, an entirely different disease, is common, frequently occurs at night, and may be recurrent. It is characterized by the sudden onset of hoarseness, barking cough, and stridor. This condition may resolve when children are exposed to humid air. The etiology is unknown but is probably either a reaction to a viral infection or an allergic phenomenon. There may be a family history of recurrent stridor in children with spasmodic croup.

Differential Diagnosis

The differential diagnosis of stridor is presented in Table 46-1.

Evaluation

History

A complete history should be obtained (Questions Box).

Table 46-1. Differential Diagnosis of Stridor				
Data	*Viral Croup*	*Spasmodic Croup*	*Epiglottitis*	*Foreign Body*
Age	3–36 mo	3–36 mo	1–8 y	All ages
Prodrome	Upper respiratory infection symptoms; onset over 2–5 d	None; sudden onset at night	Usually none; rapid onset over several hours	None; sudden onset
Fever	Low grade	None	Usually above 102.2°F (39°C)	None
Cough	Barking	Barking	None or dry	May or may not be present
Respiratory distress	Present	Present	Present and severe	Usually present
White blood cell count	Normal or slightly elevated	Normal	Elevated	Normal
Blood culture	No growth	No growth	*Haemophilus influenzae*	No growth
Radiograph	Subglottic narrowing; steeple sign	(±) Subglottic narrowing	Swollen epiglottis	Air trapping; may show a foreign body

Stridor and Croup

- Did the child have an antecedent respiratory infection?
- Does the child have a fever? If so, how high is the temperature?
- Was the onset of stridor abrupt?
- Is there stridor at rest/sleep or only with agitation?
- Does the child have any ill contacts?
- Does the child have any associated symptoms such as vomiting, diarrhea, or rash?
- Is the child feeding normally?
- Is the child drooling?

Physical Examination

It is important to assess the degree of respiratory distress and to place children in a position of comfort; monitor heart rate, ventilation, and oxygenation; and deliver oxygen (see Chapter 45). The stridorous sounds produced are usually inspiratory but may be inspiratory and expiratory if the disease progresses to the lower airway. The presence of stridor at rest or with sleep should be assessed as well as the severity of retractions with breathing. Breath sounds may be decreased bilaterally, and severe tachypnea, with respiratory rates from 40/min to 80/min, may occur. Peripheral or central cyanosis and alterations in mental status associated with severe disease should be noted. Assessment of the croup score may be helpful to direct initial therapy in mild, moderate, or severe cases (Table 46-2).

Laboratory Tests

Investigations, such as a complete blood count and cultures, are rarely helpful unless the physician is concerned about secondary bacterial infection. The white blood cell count may be normal or mildly elevated, and the differential count may show a predominance of polymorphonuclear cells. If epiglottitis is being considered, no blood should be drawn until the airway has been visualized and secured.

Imaging Studies

Radiographs of the soft tissues of the upper airway are often helpful. In children with croup, lateral neck films may reveal ballooning of the hypopharynx, a normal epiglottis, and narrowing of the subglottic area (Figure 46-1). The frontal view shows the classic "steeple sign" of the subglottic area where the airway narrows like a church steeple or pencil tip. Radiographic studies should not delay the management of children with suspected epiglottitis nor should children with respiratory compromise be taken from a monitored area for radiographs. Thickening of the epiglottis (thumbprint-shaped) and obliteration of the vallecular space may be seen on lateral neck films in patients with epiglottitis if radiographs are obtained.

Other imaging studies, such as a barium swallow or computed tomography scan of the thorax, are helpful in diagnosing congenital anomalies (eg, vascular ring).

Table 46-2. Croup Score[a]				
	0	**1**	**2**	**3**
Stridor	None	Only with agitation	Mild at rest	Severe at rest
Retraction	None	Mild	Moderate	Severe
Air entry	Normal	Mild decrease	Moderate decrease	Marked decrease
Color	Normal	Normal	Normal	Cyanotic
Level of consciousness	Normal	Restless when disturbed	Restless when undisturbed	Lethargic
Disease Category by Score				
Score	**Degree**	**Management**		
≤4	Mild	Outpatient—mist therapy		
5–6	Mild to moderate	Outpatient dexamethasone 0.6 mg/kg orally, if child improves in emergency department after mist, is >6 months, and has a reliable family		
7–8	Moderate	Dexamethasone 0.6 mg/kg orally or intramuscularly, consider admission—racemic epinephrine		
≥9	Severe	Admit—racemic epinephrine, oxygen, intensive care unit		

[a]Modified with permission from Taussig LM, Castro O, Beaudry PH, Fox WW, Bureau M. Treatment of laryngotracheobronchitis (croup). Use of intermittent positive-pressure breathing and racemic epinephrine. *Am J Dis Child.* 1975;129:790.

Figure 46-1. Lateral neck radiograph of viral croup. Note the ballooning of the hypopharynx and the narrowing in the subglottic area. (Courtesy of Dr J. S. Seidel, Division of General and Emergency Pediatrics, Harbor-UCLA Medical Center.)

Management

Most children with croup and stridor can be managed as outpatients. Caregivers should be given careful instructions so that they understand the course of the illness, know what to expect, and realize when emergency care is needed. Children with a prolonged or recurrent history of stridor may require consultation with a head and neck specialist. If a specific cause of stridor, such as a foreign body, is identified, appropriate management should be instituted.

Children with croup should be treated with gentleness and should not be upset. Agitation and crying increase respiratory distress and oxygen demand. Procedures should be kept to a minimum. The heart rate, respiratory status, and oxygen saturation should be continuously monitored while the patient is being treated and observed. Airway adjuncts that cause increased agitation should not be used.

Cool mist may be provided by blow-by or mask. **Humidified oxygen or air,** which is thought to decrease the viscosity of secretions and reduces the edema of the airway, has been the mainstay of therapy for croup for quite some time. Several recent randomized, controlled trials have questioned this practice demonstrating no benefit of cool humidified mist therapy. Many find it difficult not to continue this treatment practice at this time though. Symptoms of spasmodic croup usually resolve within 6 hours of the onset without treatment but cool, humidified mist is often employed as the sole therapy in this disorder.

Treatment of croup with **corticosteroids** is less controversial. A number of studies have demonstrated that dexamethasone given as a single dose of 0.6 mg/kg is effective in shortening the course and severity of mild, moderate, or severe croup if given in the first 3 days. Several smaller randomized trials have also suggested that half the dose of dexamethasone may be equally effective. It should be given orally but may be given as an intramuscular injection for children who are unable to take oral medication. Use of the tablet preparation ground up in applesauce is recommended because the liquid preparation does not taste good and is not well tolerated. Recent studies using nebulized budesonide also demonstrate the same efficacy in reducing respiratory distress and lowering of the croup score but at considerably more cost. Continuous or long-term therapy with steroids does not seem to alter the clinical course of the disease or the period of hospitalization and is not recommended. Treatment with antibiotics is not indicated unless infection with bacteria is evident.

Use of **racemic epinephrine** has also been somewhat controversial. Several older studies have shown that there was no difference in the long-term outcome between those children who were treated with epinephrine and those who received a placebo. Other studies have clearly demonstrated an acute effect of the drug when given via nebulizer. This effect lasts a few hours, and repeat respiratory distress after the drug effects have worn off has been reported in the literature. It is therefore prudent that racemic epinephrine only be used on patients who are going to be discharged if they can be observed for 3 to 4 hours after treatment. The anti-inflammatory effects of dexamethasone take several hours for onset, and racemic epinephrine may have more benefit in reducing symptoms during this period.

Hospitalization should be considered for children in severe respiratory distress or with significant stridor at rest who are unable to eat, and those whose parents are unable to cope with the tasks required to manage children at home. It is always indicated for children with a bacterial infection such as epiglottitis or tracheitis.

About 10% of infants and children with croup may need **controlled ventilation with endotracheal intubation.** The indications for intubation include severe respiratory distress, altered mental status, hypoxia, and hypercapnia. A major complication of endotracheal intubation in children with croup is subglottic stenosis, which develops because the endotracheal tube may traumatize the inflamed airway, leading to permanent damage. Patients should be extubated as soon as possible.

Direct laryngoscopy may be necessary in some children where the etiology of the stridor is not clear. This procedure should be done by a practitioner who is experienced in managing the airway.

Prognosis

Stridor is a serious sign, which is indicative of upper airway obstruction and potential respiratory compromise. Although it has many causes, the prognosis is usually determined by the rapidity of diagnosis and the institution of appropriate therapeutic measures, particularly stabilizing the patient and ensuring patency of the airway. Certain conditions such as croup often resolve spontaneously within a few days, although some children require hospitalization and, rarely, assisted ventilation. Other conditions, such as foreign bodies or tumors, necessitate aggressive intervention to prevent death from airway obstruction.

CASE RESOLUTION

In the case history at the beginning of this chapter, the 2-year-old with the antecedent infection and stridor has the classic signs of croup and a croup score of 6. First, adequate ventilation and oxygenation should be ensured. As soon as the assessment and management of airway, breathing, and circulation are completed, other diagnostic studies and specific therapy, such as dexamethasone or racemic epinephrine, or both, can be considered.

Selected References

Bjornson CL, Johnson DW. Croup—treatment update. *Pediatr Emerg Care.* 2005;21:863–870

Cherry JD. Croup (laryngitis, laryngotracheobronchitis, bacterial tracheitis, and laryngotracheobronchopneumonitis). In: Feigin RD, Cherry JD, eds. *Textbook of Pediatric Infectious Diseases.* 5th ed. Philadelphia, PA: W. B. Saunders; 2004:250–265

Colletti JE. Myth: cool mist is an effective therapy in the management of croup. *CJEM.* 2004;6:357–358

Donaldson D, Poleski D, Knipple E, et al. Intramuscular versus oral dexamethasone for the treatment of moderate-to-severe croup: a randomized, double-blind trial. *Acad Emerg Med.* 2003;10:16–21

Geelhoed GC, Macdonald WB. Oral dexamethasone in the treatment of croup: 0.15 mg/kg versus 0.3 mg/kg versus 0.6 mg/kg. *Pediatr Pulmonol.* 1995;20:362–368

Klassen TP, Craig WR, Moher D, et al. Nebulized budesonide and oral dexamethasone for the treatment of croup: a randomized controlled trial. *JAMA*. 1998;279:1629–1632

Scolnik D, Coates AL, Stephens D, Da Silva Z, Lavine E, Schuh S. Controlled delivery of high vs low humidity vs mist therapy for croup in emergency departments: a randomized controlled trial. *JAMA*. 2006;295:1274–1280

Sudden Infant Death Syndrome and Apparent Life-Threatening Events

Lynne M. Smith, MD

CASE STUDY

A 4-month-old male infant is brought to the emergency department by paramedics after being found blue and not breathing by his mother. He had previously been well except for a mild upper respiratory infection. His mother fed him at 2:00 am, and when she checked on him at 6:00 am she found him blue and lifeless. Although the mother smoked cigarettes during pregnancy, the pregnancy and delivery were otherwise normal. The infant received the appropriate immunizations at 2 months of age.

Questions

1. What factors are associated with sudden infant death syndrome (SIDS)?
2. Are SIDS and apparent life-threatening events (ALTEs) related?
3. What is the appropriate evaluation of infants who present with an ALTE?
4. What services are available to families who have lost infants to SIDS?

Sudden infant death syndrome (SIDS), previously referred to as **crib death,** is defined as the sudden, **unexplained death** of an apparently well infant younger than 1 year that is not adequately explained by a comprehensive medical history of the infant and family, a thorough postmortem examination, and a death scene investigation. The syndrome has been known since biblical times; parents were advised not to lie with their children for fear of suffocating them. In the United States, SIDS is the most common cause of death in children younger than 1 year beyond the neonatal period. Research suggests that infants who died of SIDS have **serotonin-mediated dysregulation** of the autonomic nervous system, which increases their vulnerability to exogenous stressors such as prone sleep position.

Sudden infant death syndrome–like events associated with successful resuscitation were once described as **near-miss SIDS** or **aborted crib death.** The term that is now used is **apparent life-threatening event (ALTE).** Apparent life-threatening events are characterized by some combination of **apnea, color change, marked change in muscle tone,** and **choking** or **gagging.** Though some have theorized ALTEs are precursors to SIDS, only approximately 5% to 10% of SIDS victims experienced a previous ALTE. In an attempt to establish the efficacy of home monitoring the **Collaborative Home Infant Monitoring Evaluation (CHIME)** study followed more than 1,000 healthy term infants as well as infants at varying risks for SIDS.

The CHIME study found 43% of term infants experienced apnea/bradycardia episodes indicating these cardiorespiratory events are common in all infants and unlikely to be precursors to SIDS. Thus SIDS and ALTE should not be considered varying manifestations of a similar disease process.

Sudden unexplained death in childhood (SUDC) occurs in children older than 12 months. Sudden unexplained death in childhood is rare, with a reported incidence in the United States in 2002 of 1.3 deaths per 100,000 children, compared with 57 deaths per 100,000 live births for SIDS. Similar to SIDS, the cause of SUDC is unclear.

Epidemiology

Sudden infant death syndrome accounts 2,000 to 3,000 deaths per year in the United States, with an overall incidence of 0.57 per 1,000. These figures were dramatically higher prior to the campaign of the American Academy of Pediatrics (AAP) to place babies in the supine position for sleep. Prior to the institution of the **Back to Sleep** campaign, the annual death rate from SIDS was approximately 5,000 to 8,000 with an incidence of approximately 2 per 1,000. Sudden infant death syndrome affects boys more commonly than girls and occurs more often in the winter months. This seasonality may be related to infection with respiratory syncytial virus (RSV). The highest incidence of SIDS occurs at 2 to 3 months of age, with 90% occurring before the age of 6 months.

The frequency of SIDS differs in different populations in both the United States and other countries. Though the incidence of SIDS is decreasing among all groups, SIDS rates in African American and American Indian/Alaska Native children is 2 to 3 times the national average. One factor contributing to the higher SIDS rate is the higher incidence of non-supine sleeping in African American infants. In 2001 the prevalence of prone positioning was 11% for white infants and 21% for African American infants.

Numerous epidemiological, maternal, and infant factors have been associated with SIDS, including **prematurity** and **intrauterine growth restriction** (Box 47-1). Mothers of children with SIDS are frequently young and unwed, smoke cigarettes, and have had fewer doctor visits during the prenatal and postpartum periods. Despite initial reports and significant research efforts, no clear data have established a causal relationship of ALTEs, apnea, immunizations, or repeated episodes of cyanosis with SIDS.

Box 47-1. Risk Factors for Sudden Infant Death Syndrome

- Male gender
- Maternal youth
- Maternal smoking
- Prematurity
- Low birth weight
- Poor prenatal care
- Sleeping in prone or side position
- Soft bedding
- Overheating
- Bed sharing

Clinical Presentation

Victims of SIDS present in **cardiopulmonary arrest,** with a history of previous good health or antecedent upper respiratory infection. They often present in the early morning hours, having succumbed during sleep.

Infants who have experienced an ALTE may appear pale, cyanotic, hypotonic, lethargic, and have bradycardia. They often present during the day between the hours of 8:00 am and 8:00 pm. If resuscitation is successful, infants may look normal and be fully alert.

Pathophysiology and Risk Factors for SIDS

Despite extensive research efforts, the cause of SIDS is unclear. It is likely SIDS occurs in infants with an underlying vulnerability when they are exposed to known risk factors such as sleeping in a non-supine position. The AAP recommends only the supine sleep position because side sleeping increases the risk of SIDS 2-fold relative to back sleeping.

Sleeping on a firm crib mattress covered by a sheet is the recommended sleep surface for infants. Soft bedding such as waterbeds, couches, stuffed toys, pillows, quilts, and comforters are to be avoided. Though **bed sharing** has been shown to enhance breastfeeding, **accidental suffocation** and unexplained infant deaths suggest bed sharing is dangerous for the infant. The AAP recommends parents sleep in a separate but proximate sleeping environment from their infant. The importance of a safe sleep environment is underscored by the work of Kemp and colleagues who investigated 119 SIDS cases over a 4-year period following the initiation of the Back to Sleep campaign. Only 8.4% of these SIDS victims were found in a non-prone position, alone in their bed, without any potential obstructions of the external airway by bedding.

Because approximately 20% of SIDS cases in the United States occur while in the care of someone other than the parent, there is a critical need to educate secondary caregivers and child care centers regarding the need for babies to sleep on their backs. A 1996 study found that 43% of licensed child care centers were unaware of the relationship between SIDS and infant sleep position. Another group of infants likely to sleep in a non-supine position are infants born weighing less than 1,500 g. These infants are twice as likely to be placed to sleep in the prone position at home than infants weighing 1,500 to 2,500 g. During the first weeks of hospitalization, premature newborns are often placed in a non-supine position because of respiratory complications and gastroesophageal reflux. The children become accustomed to this position, and the parents learn from the hospital staff's modeling to place them in these unsafe positions. The AAP Task Force on SIDS encourages neonatologist and nurses to begin placing premature newborns on their backs "significantly before the infant's anticipated discharge."

One unintended consequence of supine sleep positioning is the increased incidence of **positional plagiocephaly.** To minimize the risk for head deformities and to foster appropriate motor development, parents are encouraged to vary the head position at sleep times and encourage adult observed **tummy time** during waking hours.

In addition to being exposed to an environment that increases the infant's risk for SIDS, most theories suggest that there is an underlying vulnerability in SIDS victims. The brain stems of infants who died of SIDS have significantly higher **serotonergic neuron** counts, decreased **serotonin 1A receptor** binding, and reduced **serotonin transporter** binding in the medulla. These findings suggest that abnormalities in serotonin synthesis, release, and clearance impair the infant's ability to appropriately regulate arousal and respiratory drive in response to potential life-threatening challenges during sleep.

Numerous other associations with SIDS have been reported including altered polymorphisms of pro-inflammatory cytokines, small mandibular size, and the prolonged QT interval syndrome. The AAP does not currently recommend universal electrocardiogram screening at birth to identify potential SIDS victims.

The association between SIDS and **fatal child abuse** has also received attention. The evaluation of the home environment of SIDS victims, referred to as *death scene investigations,* may reveal accidental causes of death for some of these children. Alternatively, such investigations may reveal that children died from inflicted injuries.

A comprehensive autopsy should include an assessment for long bone fractures as well as intracranial hemorrhage, which establish inflicted trauma as the cause of the sudden death. In some municipalities, child fatality boards review each case of reputed SIDS to determine whether an etiology other than SIDS is present. Infants with parents who have Munchausen syndrome by proxy (MSBP) may present with SIDS or ALTE. Such infants are suffocated by the parents until they become apneic or die. Because distinguishing between SIDS and intentional suffocation is very difficult pathologically, the AAP Committee on Child Abuse and Neglect has cited factors that should heighten the clinician's suspicion for possible child abuse (Box 47-2). The use of in-hospital covert video surveillance has facilitated the recognition of apnea secondary to MSBP.

Differential Diagnosis

The major challenge for physicians who care for children with SIDS or an ALTE is to determine if any underlying condition may have caused the episode (Box 47-3). In most cases, no etiology for an ALTE episode can be determined.

Sepsis, respiratory infections, seizures, gastroesophageal reflux, inborn errors of metabolism, infantile botulism, cardiac anomalies, and child abuse should all be considered. The circumstances surrounding ALTEs suggest which of these conditions is suspect. A sepsis evaluation is particularly warranted in children who have symptoms such as fever, vomiting, or diarrhea. Infants with respiratory symptoms such as tachypnea and wheezing may have **RSV** infection, which is associated with apneic episodes, particularly during the first week of illness in infants younger than 3 months who had been premature and experienced apnea of prematurity. Young infants with pertussis do not exhibit the classic cough with whoop and may

present with respiratory distress and apnea. Infants with abnormal movements or ALTEs when awake may be experiencing seizures. The apnea may represent the seizure or a postictal event. Infantile botulism causes decreased muscle tone and weakness. Apnea may also accompany gastroesophageal reflux. In general, affected infants have a history of eating, regurgitating, and then developing apnea. As previously noted, child abuse, particularly with intracranial hemorrhage or MSBP, may result in apnea or SIDS.

Inborn errors of metabolism are reported in 4% to 8% of cases of ALTE. Inborn errors of metabolism should be considered in infants with other symptoms, such as vomiting or failure to thrive, or in the context of a positive family history. Symptoms may first appear when a previously well infant is metabolically stressed as by an acute infectious illness. Rarely cardiac arrhythmias, most notably long QT interval, are associated with apnea or sudden episodes of bradycardia.

Evaluation

History

The history may provide the clue to the etiology of SIDS or ALTE (Questions Box).

Box 47-2. Circumstances Where the Clinician Should Be Alert About the Possibilities of Child Abuse

- Previous recurrent cyanosis, apnea, or apparent life-threatening event (ALTE) while in the care of the same person
- Age at death older than 6 months
- Previous unexpected or unexplained deaths of one or more siblings
- Simultaneous or nearly simultaneous deaths of twins
- Previous death of infants under the care of the same unrelated person
- Discovery of blood on the infants nose or mouth in association with ALTE

Box 47-3. Differential Diagnosis of an Apparent Life-Threatening Event

• Sepsis	• Inborn errors of metabolism
• Pertussis	• Child abuse
• Respiratory syncytial virus	• Intracranial hemorrhage
• Infantile botulism	• Airway anomalies
• Seizures	• Aspiration
• Cardiac arrhythmias/anomalies	• Breath-holding spell
• Gastroesophageal reflux	

Questions

Sudden Infant Death Syndrome (SIDS) and Apparent Life-Threatening Event (ALTE)

- What were the events leading up to the episode?
- Was the child awake and eating, indicating that gastroesophageal reflux should be considered?
- Was the child awake and did the eyes roll back or the body stiffen or jerk, suggesting that a seizure may have occurred?
- How serious was the event? Did breathing resume spontaneously or did cardiopulmonary resuscitation have to be initiated?
- Have similar events occurred in the past?
- Is the infant basically well? Has the infant been ill recently?
- Has the child had respiratory symptoms such as wheezing or cough?
- Do the siblings have a history of SIDS or ALTE that would suggest the presence of a familial disorder or child abuse?
- Were there any problems with the pregnancy or delivery?
- Is there a history of maternal smoking?
- Does the infant sleep in a supine, prone, or side-down position?

Physical Examination

A complete examination should be conducted. If infants are floppy and have poor color or have required either mouth-to-mouth resuscitation or vigorous stimulation, significant events are likely. Physicians should check for the presence of bruises, retinal hemorrhages, dysmorphic features, growth impairment, and abnormal neurologic or developmental findings, which may suggest an alternative etiology. The presence of tachypnea, retractions, wheezing, or cough is consistent with a respiratory infection such as RSV or pertussis.

Laboratory Tests

In general, the laboratory workup is guided by the findings of the history and physical examination (Box 47-4). A sepsis evaluation, including a complete blood count, blood culture, lumbar puncture, and urine culture, is appropriate to rule out sepsis in toxic-appearing infants. Serum electrolytes and glucose are important to check because they may indicate an inborn error of metabolism or other abnormalities (eg, hypoglycemia), which may be associated with apnea with or without the presence of a seizure. When a metabolic etiology is suspected, a test for serum ammonia level should be performed. Hypotonic infants should be evaluated for infantile botulism by sending a stool specimen for testing. All infants with a history of apnea or ALTE should be admitted to the hospital for observation, workup, and monitoring. A pilot study has identified a subset of well-appearing, low-risk patients presenting with ALTE episodes that may be safe to discharge home after a thorough evaluation. However, these data need to be validated in a large study that includes children of all ethnicities.

Box 47-4. Laboratory Studies to Consider in Evaluating Infants With Apparent Life-Threatening Event

Often Indicated	*Sometimes Indicated*
• Complete blood count	• Electroencephalogram
• Blood culture	• Computed tomographic scan
• Lumbar puncture	• Barium swallow
• Urine culture	• Electrocardiogram
• Chest x-ray	• Skeletal survey
• Serum electrolytes	
• Blood sugar	
• Serum ammonia	

Imaging Studies

A chest x-ray should be performed to rule out pneumonia if sepsis is suspected. If the history and physical examination suggest other etiologies, computed tomography, and barium swallow may also be ordered.

Diagnostic Studies

An electroencephalogram should be obtained if a seizure disorder is suspected. In-hospital covert video surveillance is a complex procedure that may be undertaken if MSBP is suspected. Multichannel pneumograms detect apnea and bradycardia, but are not able to identify infants at risk for SIDS.

Management

Infants who have not been fully resuscitated in the field should be resuscitated, stabilized, and admitted. Any identifiable conditions such as sepsis, seizures, and reflux should be appropriately managed. In general, infants who experienced an ALTE but do not have an identifiable precipitating condition are also admitted for monitoring and observation. Recent evidence suggests that infants older than 30 days who have not had multiple ALTEs and have no identifiable medical condition may be safely discharged from the emergency department. Prior to discharge from the hospital, the parents of infants who experienced an ALTE should receive cardiopulmonary resuscitation training and be advised to eliminate tobacco smoke exposure.

Many clinicians prescribe a home apnea monitor for at-risk newborns to avoid SIDS. Based on studies conducted to date, the AAP does not recommend home apnea monitors be prescribed for the prevention of SIDS. Home apnea monitoring may be indicated for premature infants at risk for repeated episodes of apnea of prematurity on discharge from the hospital. Discontinuation should be considered at approximately 43 weeks' gestation.

Home monitoring may be indicated for individuals who are technology-dependent (home ventilators, tracheostomy) or those with ALTEs if the physician wants to monitor episodes of apnea or respiratory failure. The family of an infant who experienced an ALTE should clearly be informed that a home apnea monitor has not been shown to prevent SIDS and is not indicated for that purpose.

Pacifier use has been associated with a lower incidence of SIDS. The AAP recommends that caregivers consider offering a pacifier at nap time and bedtime throughout the first year of life. The pacifier should not be reinserted once the infant falls asleep or coated in any sweet solution. The pacifier should be cleaned often and replaced regularly. Breastfed infants should have pacifier introduction delayed until 1 month of age to ensure that breastfeeding is well established.

In addition to managing infants with ALTE, physicians must provide care to families whose infants have succumbed to SIDS. In most jurisdictions, cases of SIDS must be reported to the coroner's office. The AAP recommends a prompt death scene investigation, appropriate use of available medical specialists by medical examiners and coroners including pediatricians, and a postmortem examination within 24 hours of death including radiographic skeletal surveys and toxicological and metabolic screening. A complete review of the medical records of the victim is essential. It is important for physicians to tell families when they think the cause of death is probable SIDS even before definitive autopsy results are available. A timely information session with parents is recommended when the results of the investigation conclude SIDS or a medical causation for death.

Parents of children who have succumbed to SIDS should be referred to support groups and agencies to help them deal with the loss of their children. Information about these organizations can be obtained from the First Candle (formerly SIDS Alliance) (800/221-SIDS; www.firstcandle.org).

Prognosis

Prevention of SIDS has become a focus of public health measures. Improving maternal risk factors involves smoking cessation and access to prenatal care. Parents must be instructed to avoid soft bedding for their infants, not to bed-share with their infants, and to place their infants in the supine position for sleep. The prognosis for children who have experienced an ALTE varies and depends on predisposing conditions. Abnormal neurodevelopmental conditions are generally associated with a poor prognosis.

CASE RESOLUTION

The infant presented in the case history succumbed to SIDS. In spite of resuscitative efforts by the paramedics, he could not be revived. The mother is advised of the diagnosis of suspected SIDS and referred to appropriate agencies and support groups. The coroner is notified about the case and the presence of any associated physical findings such as bruises.

Selected References

American Academy of Pediatrics Committee on Fetus and Newborn. Apnea, sudden infant death syndrome, and home monitoring. *Pediatrics.* 2003;111:914–917

American Academy of Pediatrics Task Force on Infant Sleep Position and Sudden Infant Death Syndrome. Changing concepts of sudden infant death syndrome: implications for infant sleeping environment and sleep position. *Pediatrics.* 2000;105:650–656

American Academy of Pediatrics Task Force on Infant Sleep Position and Sudden Infant Death Syndrome. The changing concept of sudden infant death syndrome: diagnostic coding shifts, controversies regarding the sleeping environment, and new variables to consider in reducing risk. *Pediatrics.* 2005;116:1245–1255

Claudius I, Keens T. Do all infants with apparent life-threatening events need to be admitted? *Pediatrics.* 2007;119:679–683

Farrell PA, Weiner GM, Lemons JA. SIDS, ALTE, apnea, and the use of home monitors. *Pediatr Rev.* 2002;23:3–9

Horn MH, Kinnamon DD, Ferraro N, Curley MAQ. Smaller mandibular size in infants with a history of an apparent life-threatening event. *J Pediatr.* 2006;149:499–504

Paterson DS, Trachtenberg FL, Thompson EG, et al. Multiple serotonergic brainstem abnormalities in sudden infant death syndrome. *JAMA.* 2006;296:2124–2132

Ramanathan R, Corwin MJ, Hunt CE, et al. Cardiorespiratory events recorded on home monitors: comparison of healthy infants with those at increased risk for SIDS. *JAMA.* 2001;285:2199–2207

Sahni R, Fifer WP, Myers MM. Identifying infants at risk for sudden infant death syndrome. *Curr Opin Pediatr.* 2007;19:145–149

Schwartz PJ, Stramba-Badiale M, Segantini A, et al. Prolongation of the QT interval and the sudden infant death syndrome. *N Engl J Med.* 1998;338:1709–1714

Syncope

David Atkinson, MD, and Elizabeth A. Edgerton, MD, MPH

CASE STUDY

A 16-year-old girl comes to your office complaining of fainting during cheerleading practice after school yesterday. She states that this is the first time she has ever fainted, but that she sometimes feels dizzy for a few seconds after standing up. She reports that prior to the event, she was sitting in the stands watching the marching band play. When her coach called her to come onto the field, she stood up quickly and began to feel dizzy. The next thing she recalls, she was lying on the ground with her coach and teammates around her. Her coach told her she passed out for about 15 seconds. Witnesses report no unusual movements. She denies taking any medications or using any illicit drugs. There is no family history of sudden death or seizures, though her mother reports that once, when the patient was about 18 months old, she fell about 12 inches off the bed onto a carpeted floor, she cried, gasped, stopped breathing, became pale, and passed out for about 30 seconds. Her mother took her to the emergency department where she was told that this was a breath-holding spell and was nothing to worry about. The patient states

that she did not eat lunch, nor did she have anything to drink that day after leaving home for school that morning. Her mother has read that fainting may be associated with sudden death and wishes to know if her daughter should continue to participate in physical activities.

Her physical examination is unrevealing, and her vital signs are all normal. Urine pregnancy test is negative and her electrocardiogram shows normal sinus rhythm with normal intervals and axis for age.

Questions

1. What are the causes of syncope?
2. What type of workup is done primarily to evaluate for syncope?
3. When should patients who experience syncope be referred to a subspecialist?
4. Which pediatric subspecialists assist in the evaluation of a patient with syncope?
5. Which patients presenting with syncope are at the greatest risk for sudden death?

Syncope, or **fainting,** is a transient loss of consciousness and is a very common clinical problem in pediatrics, particularly in pubescent and adolescent patients. The most common causes of syncope in pediatrics are benign neurocardiogenic events; however, syncope may rarely be a harbinger of sudden death due to arrhythmia, obstruction of aortic outflow, or other serious cardiovascular events.

There are 3 general categories of syncope: **neurocardiogenic** (also called vasovagal syncope), **cardiac syncope,** and **noncardiac syncope** (Box 48-1). The workup for syncope can easily become expensive and time-consuming, and may provide little information beyond that gleaned by the initial history and physical examination. It is the role of the pediatrician to appropriately direct the evaluation for syncope so that a cost-effective evaluation may occur without missing the patient who may be at risk for a sudden death event.

Epidemiology

Syncope is defined as a temporary, transient loss of consciousness, usually associated with a rapid recovery. It is the result of a decrease in cerebral blood flow that can occur through many different mechanisms. Syncopal events are very common in the pediatric population; up to 50% of college undergraduates have reported experiencing

syncope or near syncope, and it accounts for 1% to 3% of all pediatric emergency department visits. Many cases of syncope resolve quickly and medical attention is not sought, so the true incidence of syncope is almost certainly underestimated.

Clinical Presentation

The clinical presentation of syncope varies with the etiology. In **vasovagal syncope** there is often a prodrome of symptoms including lightheadedness, visual disturbances, nausea, and diaphoresis. The patient has usually been standing for a long period or has suddenly gone from the supine or sitting position to standing. Other forms of **neurally mediated syncope** include **hair-grooming syncope,** which occurs mostly in girls while combing, brushing, or blow-drying their hair. Micturition syncope, while more common in the elderly, may occur in all ages of patients. Younger patients tend to be male; predisposing factors may include reduced food intake, fatigue, alcohol ingestion, and recent respiratory infection. The events often occur at night when voiding after awakening from sleep (ie, while standing immediately after being recumbent). Recurrences of micturition syncope are rare in young patients. **Breath-holding spells** in toddlers brought on by anger, pain, fear, or frustration may be

Box 48-1. Causes of Syncope

Neurocardiogenic (Vasovagal Syncope)
Cardiac
- Tachyarrhythmias
  — Supraventricular tachycardia
  — Ventricular tachycardia
- Bradyarrhythmias
  — Second or third degree heart block
  — Sinus node dysfunction
- Left or right ventricular outflow tract obstruction
  — Hypertrophic cardiomyopathy
  — Aortic stenosis
- Idiopathic pulmonary hypertension
- Coronary artery disease
  — Acquired coronary artery disease
    • Kawasaki disease
  — Congenital coronary anomaly
    • Intramural coronary artery
    • Anomalous origin of a coronary artery
- Primary cardiac dysfunction
  — Dilated cardiomyopathy
  — Non-compaction syndrome
Secondary cardiac dysfunction
  — Viral or idiopathic myocarditis
  — Restrictive cardiomyopathy

Noncardiac
- Orthostatic hypotension
- Neurologic (seizures, atypical migraine, dysautonomia)
- Breath-holding spells
- Psychogenic (hysteria, hyperventilation)
- Metabolic abnormality (hypoglycemia, anemia)
- Drug or medication effect

associated with syncope; this is an infantile form of cardioinhibitory neurally mediated syncope. Infants who suffer syncopal breath-holding spells are more likely to grow up and have neurally mediated syncope (see Chapter 38).

Syncope of cardiac etiology will often lack the prodrome of vasovagal syncope. The main cardiac causes of syncope are arrhythmia and left ventricular outflow obstruction. Patients may complain of palpitations, chest pain, or chest tightness. Cardiac syncope commonly occurs during physical activity and may be accompanied by a complete loss of body tone.

Syncope related to **seizures** generally has a longer recovery time associated with the postictal phase; witnesses may describe the patient as being dazed or "having a blank look on their face" prior to fainting. These episodes may occur whether the patient is recumbent or upright.

Pathophysiology

Autonomic

Autonomic causes of syncope are the most common etiology, accounting for up to 80% of cases of syncope that comes to medical attention. They are also referred to as neurally mediated reflexive syncope, vasovagal syncope, neurocardiogenic syncope and, in toddlers, pallid breath-holding spells. They have in common disturbances in autonomic control of heart rate and blood pressure in response to postural changes, bodily functions, pain, fear, or other strong emotional events. Vasovagal syncopal events usually occur when the patient is upright, resulting in decreased venous return, decreased arterial blood pressure, and decreased left ventricular volume. There is a resultant reflex stimulation of vagal fibers leading to bradycardia, vasodilation, and worsening hypotension (Bezold-Jarisch reflex). There are 3 clinical types of neurally mediated syncope: vasodepressor, which starts and is primarily marked by profound hypotension; cardioinhibitory, marked by severe bradycardia or even brief asystole; and mixed response, which is a mixture of both vasodepressor and cardioinhibitory.

Cardiac

Cardiac causes of syncope are more likely to be associated with sudden death, so it is important to identify and treat these abnormalities. Cardiac mechanisms of syncope are mainly related to arrhythmias or to obstructive lesions. Obstructive lesions lead to decreased ventricular outflow, resulting in decreased cerebral perfusion; arrhythmia may lead to decreased ejection volume, also leading to cerebral hypoperfusion and syncope.

Left-sided obstructive lesions, including aortic stenosis and hypertrophic cardiomyopathy, are the most likely cause of obstructive syncope. Rarely, syncope can be caused by pulmonary stenosis or severe primary pulmonary hypertension, mitral stenosis, atrial myxoma, or cardiac tamponade. Cardiac syncope often occurs during exertion, owing to the inability of the heart to increase cardiac output to meet the demands placed on it by increased physical activity. Increased diastolic pressure caused by an obstructive lesion may also decrease myocardial perfusion leading to cardiac ischemia, dyskinesis, or ventricular arrhythmias, which lead to decreased ventricular output.

Anomalous origin of the coronary arteries, though not an obstructive lesion, may also cause syncope with exercise. The left coronary artery may arise from the pulmonary artery, therefore, delivering deoxygenated blood to the left coronary system, or the left coronary artery may arise from the right coronary cusp and course between the aorta and pulmonary arteries. When the patient is in a high cardiac output state, such as during exercise, the left coronary artery may be compressed between the great arteries, leading to ischemia or arrhythmias.

Primary arrhythmias causing syncope are a rare but important cause of syncope. Chest x-ray, echocardiogram, and other imaging modalities will generally be normal, with no evidence of structural heart disease or pulmonary edema. Supraventricular tachycardia may cause syncope or near syncope. In most pediatric patients, the tachycardia is propagated through a concealed pathway, and the resting electrocardiogram (ECG) will be normal if the tachycardia is not occurring while the ECG is being obtained. Supraventricular tachycardia may also be associated with Wolff-Parkinson-White (WPW) syndrome. Wolff-Parkinson-White syndrome is characterized by a short P-R interval followed by an abnormally wide QRS complex with an initial delta wave.

Ventricular tachycardia is rare in children with no underlying structural heart disease, but may be brought on by infection (especially myocarditis or pericarditis), cardiomyopathies, drugs (cocaine, amphetamines), drug interactions (non-sedating antihistamines taken with erythromycin or ketoconazole), and long QT syndrome.

Patients with long QT syndrome have prolonged cardiac repolarization, which will usually manifest on the resting ECG as a prolonged corrected QT interval. The prolongation of the repolarization period of the heart puts patients with long QT syndrome at risk for torsades de pointes, a malignant form of ventricular tachycardia. The genetic forms of long QT syndrome result from mutations in genes that code for ion transport channels or related proteins. Romano-Ward syndrome is an autosomal-recessive form of long QT syndrome that is associated with congenital deafness. Autosomal-dominant long QT syndrome has historically been referred to as Jervell and Lange-Nielsen syndrome. Although the clinical diagnosis of long QT syndrome is based on a QTc that is prolonged for the patient's age, it is estimated that 20% of patients with a gene mutation associated with long QT syndrome will have a normal ECG, therefore, a critical part of the evaluation of the syncopal patient is obtaining a family history of long QT syndrome, sudden death or near sudden death, seizures, or a history of torsade de pointes. Long QT syndrome may also be brought on by electrolyte imbalance, increased intracranial pressure, or medications (see Box 48-1).

Noncardiac

Noncardiac causes of syncope include neurologic etiologies (seizures, migraines), metabolic disturbances (hypoglycemia), hyperventilation (panic attacks or self-induced), and hysteria. Seizures may be difficult to distinguish from vasovagal events because both can have tonic-clonic movements. Unlike vasovagal or cardiac syncope, seizures result in unconsciousness secondary to neurologic dysfunction. Syncope associated with hypoglycemia is due to insufficient substrate being delivered to the brain. Cerebral vasoconstriction secondary to arterial hypocapnia produces syncope with hyperventilation that may be secondary to panic attacks or may be self-induced. Hysterical syncope lacks a true prodrome, and patients usually suffer no injury when they fall. This form of syncope is thought to be related to Munchausen syndrome.

Differential Diagnosis

The differential diagnosis of syncope is presented in Box 48-1. Events that precede and follow the syncopal event are key in determining the etiology of syncope.

Evaluation

History

A thorough history should be obtained from the family and patient, focusing on the patient's symptoms, the situation surrounding the event, and the family history (Questions Box). A primary goal of the history is to identify any underlying cardiac problems because these patients are at the greatest risk for sudden death.

Table 48-1. Drugs Known to Increase the Risk of Ventricular Arrhythmia in Patients With Long QT Syndrome[a]	
Drug	*Class/Clinical Use*
Amiodarone	Antiarrhythmic/abnormal heart rhythm
Arsenic trioxide	Anticancer/leukemia
Bepridil	Antianginal/heart pain
Chloroquine	Antimalarial/malaria infection
Chlorpromazine	Antipsychotic/antiemetic/schizophrenia/nausea
Cisapride	Gastrointestinal (GI) stimulant/heartburn
Clarithromycin	Antibiotic/bacterial infection
Disopyramide	Antiarrhythmic/abnormal heart rhythm
Dofetilide	Antiarrhythmic/abnormal heart rhythm
Droperidol	Sedative; antinausea/anesthesia adjunct, nausea
Erythromycin	Antibiotic; GI stimulant/bacterial infection; increase GI motility
Halofantrine	Antimalarial/malaria infection
Haloperidol	Antipsychotic/schizophrenia, agitation
Ibutilide	Antiarrhythmic/abnormal heart rhythm
Levomethadyl	Opiate agonist/pain control, narcotic dependence
Mesoridazine	Antipsychotic/schizophrenia
Methadone	Opiate agonist/pain control, narcotic dependence
Pentamidine	Antiinfective/pneumocystis pneumonia
Pimozide	Antipsychotic/Tourette tics
Procainamide	Antiarrhythmic/abnormal heart rhythm
Quinidine	Antiarrhythmic/abnormal heart rhythm
Sotalol	Antiarrhythmic/abnormal heart rhythm
Sparfloxacin	Antibiotic/bacterial infection
Thioridazine	Antipsychotic/schizophrenia

[a]For a complete list of drugs to avoid in patients with long QT syndrome, visit www.qtdrugs.org.

Syncope — Questions

- What was the patient doing when the episode occurred?
- What was the position of the patient?
- Did the patient have any symptoms before the syncopal event?
- Did the patient have any chest pain or palpitations during the event?
- How long did it take for the patient to recover from the syncopal event?
- Were any residual symptoms present after the syncopal event?
- Has the patient recently been ill, dehydrated, or fatigued?
- Does the patient have a history of underlying cardiac disease?
- Is the patient taking any type of medication (prescribed, over the counter, or illicit)?
- Does the patient have a history of breath-holding or pallid spells?
- Is there a family history of sudden death, seizures, deafness, or cardiac abnormalities?

Physical Examination

The patient with syncope needs a thorough physical examination. Vital signs should assess the blood pressure to screen for hypotension and hypovolemia. The cardiac examination should include palpation of the chest for the point of maximal intensity, thrills and lifts, and auscultation to assess the intensity of the heart sounds and to detect the presence of murmurs or other adventitial sounds. Upper- and lower-extremity pulses should be palpated for their presence and quality. The remainder of the examination should focus on identifying any abnormal neurologic findings.

Laboratory Tests

The history and physical examination should guide which laboratory tests are necessary. In general, few tests are needed. Serum glucose shortly after the syncopal event may reveal hypoglycemia. Fasting glucose or glucose tolerance tests are usually normal, and such testing is not indicated. In pubertal females, a pregnancy test should be obtained.

Imaging Studies

Every patient who is being evaluated for syncope requires an ECG. The ECG may reveal WPW or a prolonged QT interval, neither of which can be diagnosed by history and physical examination alone. These studies can also be useful in identifying underlying structural abnormalities such as right ventricular hypertrophy secondary to pulmonary hypertension, left ventricular hypertrophy secondary to hypertrophied cardiomyopathy, or Q waves associated with anomalous origin of the coronary arteries. Patients with findings suggestive of cardiac disease (positive history, physical findings, or an abnormal ECG) require referral to a pediatric cardiologist for further evaluation. The cardiac workup of syncope may include a Holter monitor or an event recorder. The Holter monitor is worn for 24 hours and continuously records the heart rhythm. Because this is a limited window of observation, the Holter monitor will capture arrhythmia less than 20% of the time, even in patients with known

arrhythmias. Event recorders are worn for longer periods, often up to several weeks. They can record and retain the cardiac rhythm prior to, during, and following an event. When the patient activates the monitor, the recording is saved for download to the cardiologist. If the monitor is not activated, the event recorder will not save the information but will record over it. Although the event recorder has a higher probability of capturing an arrhythmia if one is present than does a Holter monitor, the tracings are generally lower quality. Exercise stress testing is often used to evaluate the patient's response to exertion and to allow for replication of symptoms in a monitored setting. Electrophysiology studies may be ordered if an arrhythmia is uncovered during the evaluation.

The workup for patients without evidence of cardiac disease (negative family history of cardiac disease or of sudden death and no exertional symptoms such as chest pain) should focus on the noncardiac or autonomic causes of syncope. Patients with prolonged recovery time or persistent neurologic symptoms following an event should be referred to a neurologist and may require an electroencephalogram to rule out seizure disorders.

A tilt test may be used to aid in the diagnosis of vasovagal syncope, although in most cases the history will be sufficient. The patient receiving a tilt test is placed on a table that is then tilted to simulate standing in an upright position, a condition that is commonly associated with vasovagal syncope. Unfortunately, there is great variability in the tilt test with an incidence of up to 20% of false positives. Factors that influence the test results include the time of day, whether the patient has fasted, hydration status, and whether the test was augmented with isoproterenol. There are very few false-negative tilt tests, but due to the high number of false positives, the tilt test should be reserved only for refractory, recurrent, or unexplained syncope.

Management

Management of syncope depends on its cause. Recurrent vasovagal syncope may be treated simply by having the patient increase their fluid intake (including carrying a water bottle in school) and increasing their salt intake. Fludrocortisone, a mineralocorticoid, is the most common medical intervention for vasovagal syncope, although the efficacy is not well established. Other treatments include beta-blockers (propranolol or atenolol), vagolytic drugs (disopyramide), or centrally acting drugs (imipramine, fluoxetine). These medications have varied benefits, and results between small controlled trials are not consistent.

Patients with neurologic syncope secondary to seizures should be treated with anticonvulsants. Patients with hyperventilation, hysteria, or hypoglycemia are most amenable to behavioral interventions. Patients with syncope secondary to a cardiac etiology should be referred to a cardiologist for further evaluation and correction of the underlying problem. These types of syncopal episodes may require more aggressive management, such as surgery or cardiac pacing, because they are more likely to result in sudden death.

Prognosis

The prognosis for autonomic and noncardiac syncope is good. Patients with vasovagal syncope will often suffer only a single event, and those with recurrent events can be treated with increased fluid intake or with medication. One subgroup to be aware of is children with pallid breath-holding spells; while most will have resolution of these spells by 5 years of age, up to 17% may continue to have syncope in adulthood. Patients who have syncope with an underlying cardiac etiology are at the greatest risk for sudden death, and it is only through identification and treatment of these structural or rhythm abnormalities that sudden death may be prevented.

CASE RESOLUTION

The young woman in the opening scenario describes symptoms consistent with vasovagal syncope. Her family history, physical examination, and electrocardiogram do not suggest any underlying cardiac disease. The patient and her family should be informed that certain factors, such as dehydration, fatigue, and hunger, can precipitate syncope. Behavioral changes, such as eating breakfast and drinking plenty of water, should be implemented to prevent or limit recurrence of syncope. The patient should be encouraged to carry a water bottle with her in school, and a note written to the school to allow her to do so, if necessary. Management with medications is not indicated at this time because this is the first syncopal event.

Selected References

Grubb BP. Neurocardiogenic syncope. *N Engl J Med.* 2005;352:1004–1009

Khositseth A, Martinez MW, Driscoll DJ, Ackerman MJ. Syncope in children and adolescents and the congenital long QT syndrome. *Am J Cardiol.* 2003;92:746–749

Klumpf M, Sieverding L, Gass M, Kaulitz R, Ziemer G, Hofbeck M. Anomalous origin of the left coronary artery in young athletes with syncope. *BMJ.* 2006;332:1139–1141

Krongrad E. Syncope and sudden death. In: Emmanouilides GC, ed. *Moss Adams Heart Disease in Infants, Children and Adolescents, Including the Fetus and Young Adult.* 5th ed. Baltimore, MD: Williams & Wilkins; 1995:1604–1619

Piccirillo G, Naso C, Moisè A, et al. Heart rate and blood pressure variability in patients with vasovagal syncope. *Clin Sci.* 2004;107:55–61

Salim MA, DiSessa TG. Effectiveness of fludrocortisone and salt in preventing syncope recurrence in children. *J Am Coll Cardiol.* 2005;45:484–488

Strickberger SA, Benson DW, Biaggioni I, et al. AHA/ACCF Scientific Statement on the evaluation of syncope: from the American Heart Association Councils on Clinical Cardiology, Cardiovascular Nursing, Cardiovascular Disease in the Young, and Stroke, and the Quality of Care and Outcomes Research Interdisciplinary Working Group; and the American College of Cardiology Foundation: in collaboration with the Heart Rhythm Society: endorsed by the American Autonomic Society. *Circulation.* 2006;113:316–327

Sun BC, Emond JA, Camargo CA. Inconsistent electrocardiographic testing for syncope in United States emergency departments. *Am J Cardiol.* 2004;93:1306–1308

Shock

Kelly D. Young, MD

CASE STUDY

A 7-month-old infant boy is brought in by his parents with a history of vomiting and diarrhea for 2 days. He also has had a low-grade fever and, according to his parents, has become progressively more listless. Vital signs show a heart rate of 200/min, respiratory rate of 30/min, and blood pressure of 72/35 mm Hg. The infant is lethargic and mottled. Capillary refill time is 3 seconds. His anterior fontanelle is sunken, and his mucous membranes are dry. The abdomen is flat and non-tender and displays hyperactive bowel sounds.

Questions

1. What is shock, and what clinical signs can help in the recognition and assessment of shock?
2. What are the stages of shock?
3. What different types of shock are there, and what are the possible causes for each type?
4. What are the management priorities in treating shock?

Shock is defined as a state of circulatory dysfunction resulting in insufficient delivery of oxygen and other metabolic substrates to the tissues. Shock is not a disease but rather an abnormal physiological state that may result from many disease processes. Early recognition and prompt therapy of shock are critical to avoid permanent end-organ damage or death.

Epidemiology

The most common type of shock in children is hypovolemic shock, and the most common causes are dehydration from gastrointestinal infections that cause vomiting and diarrhea, and hemorrhage from traumatic injury. Overwhelming sepsis is another common cause of shock. Shock may be seen in any age group, but it is more difficult to recognize the early stages in young children because early clinical signs of shock in children are subjective and may be attributed to other causes. By the time children have developed more typical signs such as thready pulses and hypotension, they are in the late stages of shock.

Clinical Presentation

Early signs of shock include tachycardia; cool, clammy, pale, or mottled skin; and delayed capillary refill time. There may be a history of decreased urine output. In this early stage, perfusion to vital organs such as the brain and heart is maintained by compensatory physiological processes. As the shock state progresses, it becomes uncompensated, resulting in impairment of vital organ perfusion. Signs of uncompensated shock include hypotension; altered mental status (irritability, lethargy, decreased interactiveness); weak, thready, or absent pulses (although pulses may be bounding in "warm" septic shock); and severely mottled or cyanotic skin (Dx Box). Irreversible shock occurs when multiple organs fail and death occurs.

 Shock

Compensated	Uncompensated
• Tachycardia	• Tachycardia or bradycardia
• Normal blood pressure	• Hypotension
• Normal or bounding pulses	• Weak, thready, or absent pulses
• Normal or cool, clammy skin	• Cool, clammy skin
• Pale or mottled skin color	• Severely mottled or cyanotic skin color
• Alert, anxious mental state	• Altered mental state, lethargic
• Mildly delayed capillary refill time	• Delayed capillary refill time
• Decreased urine output	• Decreased or absent urine output

Pathophysiology

Shock occurs when oxygen delivery to tissues is impaired. Adequate oxygen delivery depends on sufficient blood oxygen content and adequate circulatory blood flow (Figure 49-1). The oxygen content in blood depends primarily on the concentration of hemoglobin and the amount of oxygen bound to hemoglobin.

Blood flow, or cardiac output, is determined by heart rate and stroke volume. Stroke volume depends on preload, contractility, and afterload. Preload refers to the amount of blood entering the heart from the systemic vasculature. Increasing preload, for example, via administration of intravenous (IV) fluid boluses, will increase cardiac output until a point of optimal heart muscle fiber length is reached. The Starling curve demonstrates that increased stretching of a muscle fiber results in improved performance of that muscle fiber (ie, improved stroke volume and cardiac output); but after the point of optimal stretching is reached, there is decreased performance (Figure 49-2).

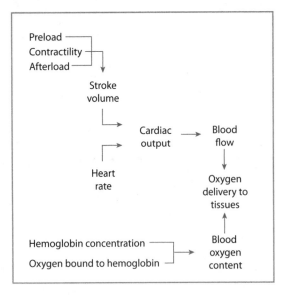

Figure 49-1. Pathophysiology of shock. Factors affecting oxygen delivery to tissue.

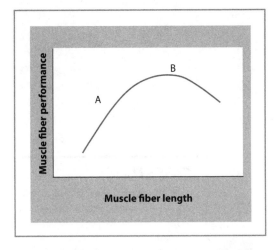

Figure 49-2. Starling curve of cardiac output. A. As muscle fiber length increases, performance increases. B. Muscle fiber reaches its optimal length, after which performance declines.

Contractility, or inotropy, is the heart's intrinsic ability to contract and pump blood to the body. Afterload refers to the systemic vascular resistance impeding ejection of blood from the ventricles. Optimal cardiac output depends on sufficient preload, unimpaired cardiac contractility, and the ability of the heart to overcome any afterload. During states of decreased cardiac output leading to decreased tissue perfusion, adults compensate primarily by increasing cardiac contractility, whereas children compensate primarily by increasing their heart rate. Irreversible shock in adults is most likely to be due to vasomotor collapse, while in children cardiac failure plays a larger role.

Differential Diagnosis

There are several types of shock depending on the underlying pathophysiology (Table 49-1). **Hypovolemic shock** is the most common type seen in children and usually results from dehydration or traumatic hemorrhage. Hypovolemia results in inadequate preload, which leads to impaired cardiac output and impaired perfusion. Other causes of hypovolemic shock include diabetic ketoacidosis (dehydration due to osmotic diuresis) and peritonitis and burns leading to third-spacing of fluids (shifting from intravascular to extravascular sites) with resultant intravascular hypovolemia.

Distributive shock is a relative hypovolemia; vasodilation results in inadequate circulating blood volume relative to the vasodilation (ie, the "tank" has been made larger by vasodilation, and now there is insufficient fluid to fill the tank). Causes include anaphylaxis and sepsis, which result in the release of vasoactive mediators that cause vasodilation. Spinal cord injury (**neurogenic shock**) may result in loss of sympathetic nerve–mediated vascular tone and subsequent vasodilation. Finally, certain intoxications such as iron, barbiturates, and tricyclic antidepressants can cause vasodilation and distributive shock.

Cardiogenic shock is an uncommon but important cause of shock in children. Congestive heart failure from a congenital heart lesion, myocarditis, or cardiomyopathy results in impaired cardiac contractility and decreased cardiac output. Tachydysrhythmias, such as supraventricular tachycardia, do not allow sufficient time for the ventricles to fill with blood, resulting in decreased stroke volume. Closure of the ductus arteriosus in a neonate with a ductal-dependent congenital heart lesion is another cause of insufficient cardiac output and cardiogenic shock.

Table 49-1. Types of Shock		
Type of Shock	**Physiological Mechanism**	**Common Causes**
Hypovolemic	Decreased preload	Dehydration Traumatic hemorrhage Diabetic ketoacidosis Peritonitis Burns
Distributive	Relative hypovolemia due to vasodilation	Sepsis Anaphylaxis Neurogenic Toxin-mediated
Cardiogenic	Decreased contractility	Congestive heart failure from congenital lesions Myocarditis Tachydysrhythmias Ductal-dependent cardiac lesions
Obstructive	Impaired cardiac filling	Pulmonary embolus Pericardial tamponade Tension pneumothorax
Dissociative	Abnormal hemoglobin—inadequate oxygen bound	Carbon monoxide poisoning Methemoglobinemia

Rare causes of shock in pediatric patients include obstructive and dissociative types. In **obstructive shock,** there is obstruction to cardiac filling due to pulmonary embolus, cardiac tamponade, or tension pneumothorax. In **dissociative shock** an abnormal hemoglobin such as methemoglobin or carboxyhemoglobin from carbon monoxide poisoning results in decreased oxygen bound to hemoglobin and decreased oxygen delivered to tissues.

Septic shock combines elements of distributive, hypovolemic, and cardiogenic shock. Vasoactive mediators lead to decreased systemic vascular resistance and a relative hypovolemia. Third-spacing of fluid leads to a true intravascular hypovolemia as well. In addition, mediators of sepsis cause impaired cardiac function.

Evaluation

Early recognition and prompt treatment of shock is the goal. A rapid, focused history and physical examination should be performed to identify patients in shock, and then early therapy should be instituted before returning for a more complete evaluation. Recognition of shock depends on physical examination alone; therapy should never be withheld while awaiting results of diagnostic tests.

History

A history of vomiting with or without diarrhea, decreased oral intake, and decreased urine output, especially in infants, should alert the clinician to possible hypovolemic shock. Children presenting with major trauma should be evaluated for hemorrhagic shock. A history of fever, lethargy, or irritability, and sometimes a rash, may point toward septic shock. Patients with asplenia, sickle cell disease, or indwelling catheters and those who are immunocompromised (eg, young infants or children on chemotherapy) are at increased risk for sepsis. Children in cardiogenic shock may have a history of a murmur, poor feeding, sweating with feeds, cyanosis, tachypnea, and dyspnea and, in the older child, palpitations.

Physical Examination

A brief examination to identify shock focuses on mental status, vital signs, pulses, and skin signs. Impaired level of consciousness, such as lethargy or lack of recognition of parents, occurs later in shock. Earlier, children are anxious or fussy but alert. Tachycardia occurs early in shock but must be interpreted in the context of other signs of shock because tachycardia may also result from fever, pain, or simply the child's fear of the examination process. Bradycardia is a late, ominous sign in shock and often results from hypoxemia. Hypotension is also a late sign in shock. It is important to remember that normal values for heart rate and blood pressure vary by age. The lower limit of acceptable systolic blood pressure in a neonate from birth to 1 month is 60 mm Hg; in an infant from 1 month to 1 year is 70 mm Hg. For a child 1 year or older, the lower limit can be estimated using the formula $70 + (2 \times \text{age in years})$ mm Hg; the lower limit is 90 mm Hg for children 10 years or older. Systolic blood pressures lower than these guidelines represent hypotension and late uncompensated shock.

Presence and quality of pulses should be checked. Weak, thready, or absent peripheral pulses are indicative of shock. However, in warm septic shock, pulses may be bounding. Skin color, moisture, and temperature give valuable clues to diagnosis. Children in shock may have pale, cyanotic, or mottled skin. Early in shock, however, skin color may be normal. Also, some infants may also have mottled skin normally. As with tachycardia, isolated signs must be correlated with the bigger clinical picture to diagnose shock. Decreased perfusion in shock leads to cool and clammy skin. This is often best appreciated in the hands and feet initially.

Capillary refill is tested by compressing the capillary bed of a fingertip, palm, or dorsal foot with gentle pressure until it blanches. On release, color should return in 2 seconds or less; a capillary refill time of 3 seconds or more is abnormal and indicative of shock. Children in warm septic shock may display "flash" (ie, shortened) capillary refill time. Capillary refill should be tested with the extremity elevated above the heart so that arterial, not venous, perfusion is tested. Also, cool ambient temperatures can falsely delay capillary refill times.

In hypovolemic shock due to dehydration, look for signs of dehydration such as dry mucous membranes, lack of tears, sunken eyes, sunken anterior fontanelle in infants, and tenting of the skin. The degree of dehydration can often be estimated clinically (see Chapter 54).

Children with congestive heart failure and cardiogenic shock may demonstrate dyspnea on exertion, tachypnea, orthopnea, rales, hepatomegaly, gallop rhythm, and a heart murmur. Jugular venous distention and peripheral edema are appreciated less often in children compared with adults. Ductal-dependent cardiogenic shock should be suspected in the infant in the first few weeks of life presenting with severe cyanosis unresponsive to oxygen therapy and shock. Other signs may include a cardiac murmur, hepatomegaly, cardiomegaly on chest radiograph, and a differential in pulses or blood pressure between upper and lower extremities.

Approximately 20% of children present with the classic adult form of warm septic shock—including increased cardiac output, hypotension, decreased systemic vascular resistance, warm non-mottled skin, bounding pulses, and flash capillary refill. Children are more likely (60%) to present with cold septic shock—including decreased cardiac output, increased systemic vascular resistance, normal blood pressure to hypotension, cool clammy or mottled skin, thready pulses, and delayed capillary refill. The remaining 20% of children with septic shock present with both decreased cardiac output and decreased systemic vascular resistance.

Laboratory Tests

The suspected cause of the shock will determine which laboratory tests are performed. In hypovolemic shock secondary to dehydration, a chemistry panel should be obtained for electrolyte abnormalities and acidosis. Serial hematocrit determinations and a type and crossmatch are important studies in traumatic hemorrhage. In septic shock, a complete blood count and blood cultures should be obtained, as well as cultures of other potential sources of infection (urine, cerebrospinal fluid, wound, etc). Coagulation studies including panels to rule out disseminated intravascular coagulopathy, and electrolyte studies including calcium and magnesium levels, are frequently abnormal in sepsis. Hypoglycemia is a common finding in any type of shock, and a rapid bedside glucose determination should be performed. Arterial blood gases can demonstrate adequacy of oxygenation and degree of acidosis.

Imaging Studies

Invasive monitoring with arterial lines for systemic arterial blood pressure and central venous lines for central venous pressure or pulmonary artery wedge pressure may be helpful in the ongoing management of shock, particularly fluid-resistant shock. Chest radiography, electrocardiogram, and echocardiogram may be obtained in cardiogenic shock to further elucidate the etiology. Workup of stabilized trauma patients may include radiographs or computed tomography scans.

Management

The first management priority in the treatment of any critically ill child is attention to airway patency and ventilation. If there is significant respiratory compromise, bag-mask ventilation followed by endotracheal intubation is performed. Usually, however, patients in compensated shock do not require immediate attention to airway management. Instead, the immediate priorities are administration of **oxygen** and initiation of **cardiorespiratory monitoring.** Elective, rather than emergent, endotracheal intubation should be considered to reduce metabolic demands caused by increased work of breathing. When intubating patients in shock, induction agents without hemodynamic effects are preferred (ketamine instead of opiates or benzodiazepines), and etomidate may not be ideal due to its effects of cortisol suppression.

Almost concurrently with the above, the next priority is achieving **intravascular access** and, in most cases, administering fluids. Peripheral IV access should be attempted. If this is unsuccessful after 3 attempts or 90 seconds, an intraosseous line may be placed, or IV access may be obtained by placement of a central venous catheter or by cutdown technique. Umbilical venous lines can sometimes be placed in neonates within the first 1 to 2 weeks of life. More than one intravascular line is usually needed for managing patients in shock.

Decreased preload and hypovolemia (actual or relative) are present in the most common causes of shock. Only cardiogenic shock may not benefit from increasing preload via a fluid bolus. Generally, an **initial fluid bolus of 20 mL/kg isotonic crystalloid fluid,** such as normal saline or lactated Ringer's, should be rapidly infused (this may require manually pushing the fluid using a large syringe). The patient should be assessed for improvement in mentation, vital signs, peripheral pulses, and skin signs after each fluid bolus. **Repeat fluid boluses** of 20 mL/kg to a total of 80 mL/kg or more may be necessary to restore intravascular volume. Colloid fluid (eg, albumin)

theoretically has the advantage of staying intravascular longer, but this has not been proved to result in a measurable benefit. Crystalloid fluid is recommended for initial boluses because it is less expensive and more readily available. If a patient with traumatic hemorrhage is still hemodynamically unstable after 2 crystalloid fluid boluses, packed red blood cells at 10 mL/kg may be required.

Further management in addition to fluids depends on the specific etiology. Patients in septic shock should receive empiric broad-spectrum antibiotic coverage. A surgeon must assist in identifying the source of hemorrhage and controlling the bleeding in patients with traumatic hemorrhage. Spinal cord injury is treated with supportive care and high-dose methylprednisolone in consultation with a neurosurgeon. Anaphylactic shock is treated with IV epinephrine, IV diphenhydramine, anti-histamine H_2 receptor blockers, glucocorticoids, and nebulized albuterol. Pericardial tamponade is relieved by pericardiocentesis, tension pneumothorax by needle thoracotomy or tube thoracostomy, and pulmonary embolus with supportive care and thrombolytics. Carbon monoxide poisoning is treated with 100% oxygen and, if severe, hyperbaric oxygen therapy. Patients with methemoglobinemia appear cyanotic even while receiving 100% oxygen and may be treated with methylene blue. Supraventricular tachycardia should be treated with adenosine if the patient is stable and with synchronized cardioversion if the patient is hemodynamically unstable. Ductal-dependent cardiogenic shock should be treated with prostaglandin E_1 (PGE_1) infusion.

Patients with cardiogenic shock require **inotropic agents** to increase cardiac contractility and improve tissue perfusion. Patients in the later stages of other forms of shock (hypovolemic, distributive, septic) may suffer cardiac dysfunction. In such patients, only after adequate fluid resuscitation has been performed and there are still signs of shock or hypotension should inotropic agents be started. Central venous pressure monitoring may be needed to determine whether fluid resuscitation is adequate. Patients with septic shock may require **vasoactive agents** to reduce or increase systemic vascular resistance.

Dopamine or epinephrine is often the first-line inotropic agent. At low doses (2–5 µg/kg/min), dopamine improves renal blood flow and enhances urine output. At mid-range doses (5–10 µg/kg/min), dopamine exerts primarily a β-adrenergic effect, improving contractility and increasing heart rate. At higher doses (10–20 µg/kg/min), dopamine's α-adrenergic effects cause peripheral vasoconstriction to improve hypotension. **Epinephrine** has predominantly β-adrenergic effects at lower doses (0.05–0.1 µg/kg/min) and α-adrenergic effects at higher doses (up to 1.0 µg/kg/min). Because epinephrine is a strong inotrope, it is recommended for dopamine-resistant cold septic shock. **Norepinephrine** (0.01–1.0 µg/kg/min) has predominantly α-adrenergic vasoconstricting effects, and is therefore preferred for warm septic shock with low systemic vascular resistance and for distributive shock states (anaphylaxis, neurogenic shock, certain toxin-induced shock states). **Dobutamine** (1–20 µg/kg/min) may be the most useful drug for cardiogenic shock because it is selective for β-adrenergic effects, increasing cardiac contractility. However, if hypotension is present, dobutamine-mediated peripheral vasodilation may be detrimental. Dobutamine is typically used in a range of 10 to 20 µg/kg/min. Combinations of inotropic agents may be beneficial to maximize improvements in cardiac contractility and cardiac output without compromising renal perfusion or worsening hypotension. Both dopamine and dobutamine may be less effective in children younger than 6 to 12 months. For this reason, some centers recommend epinephrine as the first-line inotropic agent.

Patients in cardiogenic shock or cold septic shock may also benefit from afterload reduction using systemic vasodilators such as **nitroprusside** (0.5–5 µg/kg/min). If these are used, blood pressure should be continuously monitored, typically in the setting of the intensive care unit. Cold septic shock refractory to epinephrine may also be treated with type III phosphodiesterase inhibitors (**amrinone** 1–20 µg/kg/min, **milrinone** 0.25–1.0 µg/kg/min), which exert inotropic and vasodilator actions. Typically, a pediatric intensive care specialist should be involved in the care of the patient, and central venous pressure monitoring should be begun before vasodilator agents are started.

Neonates with duct-dependent lesions present with a sudden onset of shock and cyanosis in the second half of the first week of life. Common lesions include hypoplastic left heart syndrome, aortic coarctation, and tricuspid atresia. **Prostaglandin E$_1$** (0.1 µg/kg/min, titrated to effect), which acts to keep the ductus arteriosus open, should be immediately infused if a duct-dependent lesion is suspected as the cause of shock. Apnea may result from PGE$_1$ therapy, and attention to airway management is key.

It used to be common to mix vasoactive infusions using the **rule of 6 and 0.6.** For dopamine, dobutamine, and nitroprusside, mix 6 mg/kg of drug with enough dextrose 5% in water to produce a final volume of 100 mL. Infusion at 1 mL/h provides a dose of 1 µg/kg/min. For epinephrine, norepinephrine, and PGE$_1$, mix 0.6 mg/kg of drug with enough D5W to produce a final volume of 100 mL. Infusion of 1 mL/h provides a dose of 0.1 µg/kg/min. However, calculations such as these are error prone, and computerized order forms with automatic error alerts, or "smart" pumps that automatically calculate doses based on the patient's inputted weight, may be better choices.

Treatment of patients in shock must include attention to conditions that increase metabolic demand. Acidosis should be assessed and, if severe, treatment with bicarbonate considered. Temperature should be kept neutral with use of antipyretics and cooling measures for fever as needed. Electrolyte abnormalities, particularly hypocalcemia, and hypoglycemia must be assessed and corrected. If a hypothyroid state is suspected, thyroid hormone replacement therapy is important. Blood products may be required for patients with septic shock and disseminated intravascular coagulation. Packed red blood cells, 10 cc/kg at a time, should be given to maintain a hemoglobin of at least 10 g/dL. Fresh frozen plasma may be given to correct abnormalities in prothrombin and partial thromboplastin times, but

should not be pushed due to its propensity to cause further hypotension. Cryoprecipitate should be reserved for documented hypofibrinogenic states.

An expert panel from the American College of Critical Care Medicine created **clinical practice parameters for the treatment of pediatric septic shock.** Recommended therapy is divided between therapies for the first hour (the "golden hour") and therapies beyond the first hour (often with critical care specialists involved). In the first 15 minutes after recognition of septic shock, practitioners should attend to the airway and establish intravascular access, begin fluid boluses in 20 cc/kg increments, and diagnose and correct any hypoglycemia and hypocalcemia. The goal of therapy is normalization of blood pressure, capillary refill, cardiac index more than 3.3 and less than 6.0 L/min/m^2, and superior vena cava (SVC) oxygen saturation (O$_2$ sat) 70% or higher. Patients who are responsive to fluid may be observed in the pediatric intensive care unit. Dopamine therapy should be started for those who are still hypotensive after fluid resuscitation. Once dopamine therapy is titrated up to 20 µg/kg/min, epinephrine should be added for dopamine-resistant cold septic shock, while norepinephrine should be added for dopamine-resistant warm septic shock. A study of patients transferred into a tertiary children's hospital showed significantly improved survival for patients cared for by community practitioners who followed the above guidelines for the first hour of care.

Corticosteroids are controversial in the treatment of sepsis. Guidelines suggest administering "stress doses" of hydrocortisone 2 mg/kg or 50 mg/m^2 body surface area beyond the first hour of therapy for catecholamine-resistant septic shock when adrenal insufficiency is suspected. Adrenal insufficiency may be suspected in patients with a history of a central nervous system abnormality or pituitary abnormality, a known adrenal gland disorder, recent surgery, history of chronic steroid therapy (eg, for asthma, inflammatory bowel disease, or a rheumatologic condition), and in purpura fulminans. "Shock doses" of hydrocortisone (50 mg/kg) may be given in catecholamine-resistant fulminant septic shock and dopamine-resistant purpura fulminans. It is suggested that a baseline cortisol level be drawn prior to giving corticosteroids.

Following the first hour of therapy, a vasodilator (nitroprusside) or type III phosphodiesterase inhibitor (amrinone or milrinone) along with further volume loading may be helpful in catecholamine-resistant cold septic shock with normal blood pressure and SVC O$_2$ sat less than 70%. In cases of "cold" septic shock with low blood pressure and SVC O$_2$ sat less than 70%, continued titration of epinephrine and volume is recommended. For "warm" septic shock, continued titration of norepinephrine and volume is recommended, with the possible addition of vasopressin (0.0003–0.0008 U/kg/min). Vasopressin has not been studied well in children, but shows promise in adults. Finally, for persistent catecholamine-resistant septic shock, consideration may be given to extracorporeal membrane oxygenation. Recombinant activated protein C (drotrecogin alfa) is recommended for some septic adult patients, but not for pediatric patients.

Prognosis

Children in shock are critically ill and at risk for progression to multiorgan failure and death. Prognosis depends on how early shock is recognized and treated, and on the underlying etiology. Pediatric septic shock carries a 9% mortality rate, which is significantly improved from 60% in the 1980s and 97% in the 1960s, and is also lower than the adult septic shock mortality rate. Prompt, appropriate therapy has a significant impact on morbidity and mortality.

CASE RESOLUTION

The boy in the case history is in barely compensated (he is not hypotensive) hypovolemic shock due to diarrhea, vomiting, and dehydration. He should receive oxygen and cardiorespiratory monitoring, and intravenous access should be rapidly established. Isotonic fluid boluses of 20 mL/kg should be given with reassessment between each bolus. As much as 80 mL/kg may be needed before improvements in mentation, vital signs, pulses, and skin signs are seen.

Selected References

American Heart Association. Part 12: pediatric advanced life support. *Circulation.* 2005;112:IV-167–IV-187

Carcillo JA, Fields AI, American College of Critical Care Medicine Task Force Committee. Clinical practice parameters for hemodynamic support of pediatric and neonatal patients in septic shock. *Crit Care Med.* 2002;30:1365–1378

Han YY, Carcillo JA, Dragotta MA, et al. Early reversal of pediatric-neonatal septic shock by community physicians is associated with improved outcome. *Pediatrics.* 2003;112:793–799

Maar SP. Emergency care in pediatric septic shock. *Ped Emerg Care.* 2004; 20:617–624

McKiernan CA, Lieberman SA. Circulatory shock in children: an overview. *Pediatr Rev.* 2005;26:451–460

Saladino RA. Management of septic shock in the pediatric emergency department in 2004. *Clin Pediatr Emerg Med.* 2004;5:20–27

Approach to the Traumatized Child

David B. Burbulys, MD

CASE STUDY

A 6-year-old boy is brought to the emergency department after being struck by an automobile while crossing the street. He was found unconscious at the scene. Initial evaluation shows that he has an altered level of consciousness; shallow respirations; ecchymosis across the upper abdomen; and a deformed, swollen left thigh. The pediatric emergency physician is called in to discuss an initial assessment and management plan for the injured child with the trauma surgeon.

Questions

1. What are the most common mechanisms of injury responsible for trauma in children?
2. What are some of the physiological differences between adults and children that make children more susceptible to certain types of injuries?
3. Which areas of the body are most likely to be injured in a typical automobile versus pedestrian collision?
4. What are the components of a primary survey in pediatric trauma patients?
5. What radiographic and laboratory studies should be performed in children with multiple injuries?

Trauma is often referred to as the neglected disease of modern society. Childhood trauma, in particular, is poorly understood and studied. Death from trauma is higher in pediatric patients than in adult patients. Mechanisms of injury may be similar in adults and children, but children have particular anatomical differences and physiological responses to injury. Health care professionals should realize that children have unique anatomical and physiological features; they are not just small adults (Box 50-1). Evaluation and management of traumatized children may require specialized knowledge, training, and equipment. Recognition of such facts, coupled with expertise in the performance of emergency procedures, should improve the outcome of children who sustain major injuries.

Epidemiology

More than 64% of the deaths of children, who are 1 to 14 years, are caused by traumatic injuries. This number peaks at 8 years of age. Approximately 1.5 million pediatric injuries result in a quarter million to half million hospitalizations, and 15,000 to 25,000 deaths (1.5%) each year. Adolescents are most likely to die in motor vehicle crashes and school-aged children are most likely to die after being struck by automobiles. This figure, unfortunately, may be an underestimation, as most childhood injury fatalities occur in the field prior to arrival at a health care facility. The magnitude of the problem becomes even more evident when morbidity is considered.

Box 50-1. Characteristics of Children That Lead to Increased Susceptibility to Injury

Anatomical Characteristics

- Smaller body size allows for the greater distribution of force with trauma, so multiple system injury is common.
- A prominent occiput, exaggerated head-to-body ratio, weak neck muscles, and higher center of gravity predispose younger children to head injury.
- Cranial bones are thinner and the brain is less myelinated, resulting in more serious head injury.
- Skeletal and ligamentous structures have increased flexibility, which results in greater transmission of force to internal organs.
- Less protective muscle and subcutaneous tissue over internal organs expose them to injury.
- Growth plates are not yet fused, which leads to Salter-type fractures and possible bone growth abnormalities with healing.

Physiological Characteristics

- High body surface area-to-weight ratio predisposes children to hypothermia, which may complicate shock and worsen acidosis if it is not corrected.
- Hypoxia and respiratory failure are increasingly likely in children.
- Hemorrhagic shock is initially well tolerated by increasing heart rate and peripheral vascular resistance without significant changes in systolic blood pressure.

Between 50,000 and 100,000 children per year become permanently disabled as a result of their injuries. Such disabilities have an enormous impact on society; they result in financial and emotional losses for families and many years of lost productivity for individuals.

Blunt trauma, which is more common than penetrating injury in children, represents about 87% of all childhood injuries. Head injuries, followed by thoracoabdominal injuries, are the leading causes of death in this group. In adolescents, however, penetrating injury (suicide and homicide) accounts for a higher percentage of the total, especially among minority populations in urban areas. Causes of non-penetrating trauma are motor vehicle crashes (>40%), falls (25%–30%), drowning (10%–15%), and burns (5%–10%). Included in the remainder are bicycle-related and automobile versus pedestrian injuries. Male children are injured twice as often as female children. Different mechanisms of injury predominate in different age groups; the figures given above refer to overall causes of trauma. Perhaps as much as 25% to 35% of trauma deaths are related to child abuse in some centers.

Clinical Presentation

Children who sustain severe trauma present with multiple organ system injury manifested by shock, respiratory failure, or altered mental status (singly or in combination). Those with mild to moderate injury may present in this way or simply with localized signs and symptoms in the injured area.

Pathophysiology

Patterns of injury are important to identify to develop strategies for injury prevention as well as anticipate injuries during patient management. One common pattern in the United States is the triad of injuries that result from an automobile versus pedestrian collision (Waddell triad) (Figure 50-1).

Multisystem injury is the rule rather than the exception in children. Internal injury should always be suspected, even if no evidence suggestive of external trauma is apparent when the mechanism of injury warrants. Because children are anatomically and physiologically different from adults, they are more susceptible to different types of injuries (Box 50-1). The most striking physiological differences between adults and children concern responses to acute blood loss. Children have a tremendous capacity to maintain systolic blood pressure despite 25% to 30% acute blood loss.

Hypovolemic shock secondary to acute blood loss is the most common cause of shock in pediatric trauma patients. In general, hemorrhagic shock is a clinical state where the cardiac output is unable to meet the metabolic demands of the tissues for oxygen and nutrients; it is not defined by any absolute blood pressure value.

Acute blood loss stimulates peripheral and central receptors and results in an increased production of catecholamines and adrenocorticoids. The body responds by increasing peripheral vascular resistance, stroke volume, and heart rate. Children are able to tolerate increases in heart rate and peripheral vascular resistance very well at first, and they exhibit normal blood pressure in the presence of

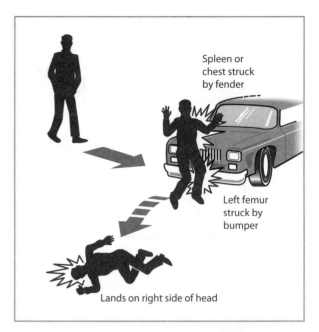

Figure 50-1. Illustration of Waddell triad. Femur, abdominal, and contralateral head injuries (Waddell triad) should be expected to result from automobile versus pedestrian collisions in the United States. A child crossing the street is struck on the left side of the body by an automobile traveling on the right side of the road. The left femur is likely to be injured by the bumper, and the abdomen or chest strikes the grille as the child is lifted into the air and lands on the opposite side of the head, sustaining blunt head trauma. The Waddell triad illustrates the necessity of having a high degree of suspicion for a complex of injuries based on a well-known mechanism.

hypovolemic shock. By the time their blood pressure falls, they commonly have lost 20% to 25% of their circulating blood volume. In adults, blood pressure tends to decline after a less significant blood loss and therefore may be recognized sooner (Figure 50-2). Subtle changes in heart rate, blood pressure, and capillary refill may indicate impending cardiovascular collapse in traumatically injured children and should not be overlooked.

Another obstacle to the recognition of shock in children is the lack of knowledge on the part of many health professionals of age-appropriate vital signs, particularly blood pressure. Table 50-1 gives the normal blood pressure ranges for children of different ages.

Three stages of shock correspond to the progression of volume loss. In the first stage, **compensated shock,** mechanisms for preserving blood pressure are still effective. Decreased capillary refill, diminished pulses, cool extremities, and tachypnea may be apparent, but blood pressure is normal and accompanied by tachycardia. Unrecognized, untreated compensated shock rapidly progresses to **uncompensated shock.** Examination reveals decreased level of consciousness, pallor, reduced urine output, and lower blood pressure with weak, thready pulses and marked tachycardia. With inadequate therapy, or at times despite therapy, uncompensated shock becomes **irreversible shock,** resulting in irreparable organ damage and often unpreventable death. (See Chapter 49 for a more extensive discussion.)

Figure 50-2. Graph showing cardiovascular response to hypovolemia in children. Blood pressure does not begin to decline until the volume deficit is more than 25% because of the compensatory increase in vascular resistance. Cardiac output drops earlier and is manifested clinically as delayed capillary refill; cool, clammy skin; and tachycardia.

Shock has several causes, and it is important to emphasize that, in trauma patients, it should always be initially attributed to hemorrhage. Shock due to obstructive cardiac output causes such as tension pneumothorax or cardiac tamponade are much less common. Shock due to spinal cord injury is exceedingly rare. Shock should never be attributed solely to head trauma. The pathways resulting in decreased blood pressure in patients with head trauma are present only at the terminal stages. Therefore, the possibility of blood loss from internal organs should be pursued promptly.

Evaluation and Management

Because of the high potential for serious morbidity and mortality in trauma patients, evaluation and management are performed simultaneously. This care is best handled using an organized, multidisciplinary team approach, with preestablished criteria for activation of the trauma team. History of the event provides important information when implementing these criteria. For example, the entire team responds for all pedestrians struck by an automobile. The types of subspecialists that make up a trauma team are decided by individual institutions.*

Several approaches to the assessment of trauma patients have been developed by professional organizations. The Advanced Trauma Life Support (ATLS) course of the American College of Surgeons and the Basic Trauma Life Support (BTLS) course of the American College of Emergency Physicians are 2 such approaches. Both the ATLS and the BTLS methods stress the importance of a primary evaluation, or primary survey, to identify and treat life-threatening injuries and a more detailed regional examination, or secondary survey, after stabilization, to identify and treat all other injuries. In addition, they both adhere to the principles of serial examination and

---

*Most institutions have trauma teams composed of pediatric emergency and critical care specialists, anesthesiologists, trauma surgeons, surgical subspecialists, emergency nurses, respiratory therapists, social workers, and x-ray technicians.

Age	Respiration (breaths/min)	Pulse (beats/min)	Blood Pressure (Systolic)
Newborn	30–60	100–160	50–70
1–6 wk	30–60	100–160	70–95
6 mo	25–40	90–120	80–100
1 y	20–40	90–120	80–100
3 y	20–30	80–120	80–110
6 y	12–25	70–110	80–110
10 y	12–20	60–90	90–120

Table 50-1. Normal Vital Signs for Children of Different Ages

reassessment after each intervention. The primary survey and initial resuscitation efforts must occur simultaneously and within the first 5 to 10 minutes of the evaluation. The secondary survey is meant to enhance the primary survey. Vital signs should be repeated every 5 minutes during the primary survey and every 15 minutes during the secondary survey until the trauma team feels the patient has been adequately stabilized. The reader should understand the rationale for the trauma examination and its parts. (See Selected References for articles that explain the rationale for trauma examination and provide detailed descriptions of evaluation and management techniques.)

Physical Examination

The **primary survey** begins with an assessment of **level of consciousness,** patency of the **airway** (Box 50-2), and quality of **breathing** (Box 50-3). When evaluating injured patients, physicians should always assume that the cervical spine has been injured and should use in-line immobilization to secure it. Basic airway maneuvers for positioning should be performed. The safest method is the jaw thrust to avoid moving the cervical spine (Figure 50-3). The oral cavity should be examined for foreign bodies, blood, or secretions. The most common form of airway obstruction in children is a posteriorly displaced tongue, which is relieved by good airway positioning. Advanced airway maneuvers (bag-valve-mask ventilation or endotracheal tube intubation) are performed during the primary survey if children have apnea, significant respiratory distress, severe head

Box 50-2. Airway Assessment and Treatment

Assessment
- Airway patency and ability to protect it
- Level of consciousness
- Stridor

Treatment
- Spinal immobilization
- Jaw thrust and suctioning
- 100% oxygen by non-rebreathing mask
- Intubate for Glasgow Coma Scale score <9, no gag reflex

Box 50-3. Breathing Assessment and Treatment

Assessment
- Respiratory rate and depth
- Chest wall compliance, symmetry, and movement
- Tracheal deviation

Treatment
- 100% oxygen by non-rebreathing mask
- Intubate for respiratory failure, severe flail chest
- Compress obvious bleeding sites
- Seal open pneumothorax with occlusive dressing
- Needle decompress tension pneumothorax
- Place chest tube for pneumothorax or hemothorax

Box 50-4. Circulation Assessment and Treatment

Assessment
- Identify obvious bleeding sites
- Peripheral pulses and capillary refill
- Heart rate
- Level of consciousness

Treatment
- Compress obvious bleeding sites
- 100 % oxygen by non-rebreathing mask
- 2 large-bore intravenous lines
- Fluid resuscitation; 20 mL/kg normal saline
- Packed red blood cells; 10 mL/kg after 60 mL/kg normal saline and still in shock

Figure 50-3. Correct method for positioning the head with chin lift or jaw thrust.

trauma, or an airway that cannot be maintained with basic techniques. All trauma patients are initially given supplemental oxygen by non-rebreathing mask at a concentration of 100%.

After a patent airway and adequate ventilation have been established, **circulatory status** is assessed. All pediatric trauma patients require placement of the largest bore intravenous catheter obtainable for that patient; 2 of these should be placed, if possible. In life-threatening situations, peripheral vascular access is attempted either 3 times or for 90 seconds, whichever comes first. If peripheral attempts fail, then intraosseous infusion or central venous access should be used. A bolus of 20 mL/kg of an isotonic fluid (normal saline or Ringer's lactate) should be given. This may be repeated, if necessary, to treat hypovolemic shock. After 60 mL/kg, administration of blood should be considered, and the likelihood of surgical exploration is high. Acutely exsanguinating wounds are treated using direct pressure bandages (Box 50-4).

A brief neurologic assessment to assess patient **disability** is also performed during the primary survey. One rapid assessment technique is the AVPU system (A, alert; V, responds to verbal stimuli; P, responds to painful stimuli; and U, unresponsive). Subsequently, a Glasgow Coma Scale score or Children's Coma Scale score may be calculated (Table 50-5).

Once life-threatening conditions are stabilized, more information can be collected. The **secondary survey** involves a complete and thorough head-to-toe examination of the child, fully exposed, to identify additional injuries, while taking great care to maintain normothermia. It also includes a **SAMPLE** history (symptoms, allergies, medications, past history/ hospitalizations/surgeries, last meal, events preceding trauma). A detailed history of events preceding trauma should ensure that injuries are consistent with the causal mechanism. Health care professionals should be prepared to consider abuse when specific diagnoses do not correlate with either the history given by the caregiver or the developmental ability of the child. Measurement of vital signs should occur as previously described and other devices such as Foley catheters, nasogastric tubes, and pulse oximetry should be used at this time. Every time an intervention is performed, repeat assessments that incorporate the elements of the primary survey are made.

Laboratory Tests

Most institutions have a standardized trauma panel (complete blood count with differential, electrolytes, blood urea nitrogen, creatinine, glucose, amylase, prothrombin time, partial thromboplastin time, urine analysis, and blood typing and crossmatching). In addition, drug and alcohol screens may provide important information, particularly in the child with altered mental status.

Imaging Studies

When major trauma is suspected, radiographs of at least the chest, pelvis/abdomen, and cervical spine should be obtained. This prevents missing injuries in children who may be unconscious or who need lifesaving procedures during resuscitation, which obscure an area of injury from examination. Additional radiographs, for example, of the

Box 50-5. Glasgow Coma Scale Modified for Pediatric Patients

Eye Opening Response
4   Spontaneous
3   To verbal command/shout[a]
2   To pain
1   None

Motor Response
6   Obeys commands/spontaneous[a]
5   Localizes pain
4   Withdraws to pain
3   Decerebrate posturing to pain (flexion)
2   Decorticate posturing to pain (extension)
1   None

Verbal Response
5   Oriented and conversant/appropriate words[a]
4   Confused/inappropriate words[a]
3   Inappropriate words/persistent crying or screaming[a]
2   Incomprehensible sounds/grunts or moans[a]
1   None

Scoring
14–15 Mild
9–13 Moderate
<9 Severe

[a]Younger than 1 year.

extremities, may be indicated when other areas of injury are detected on secondary survey. Children are often initially distracted from one injury because of the presence of a more painful one.

More sophisticated imaging techniques such as computed tomography scans and ultrasound are a usual part of the evaluation of the seriously injured pediatric trauma patient. The choice of test depends on the experience of the trauma team and the individual characteristics of the patient.

Prognosis

The highest survival rates for seriously injured children have been found among those who are brought to the operating room for treatment within 1 hour of the injury. Definitive care for trauma takes place in the operating room, and initial stabilization takes place in the emergency department. Absolute indications for surgery include hemodynamic instability despite aggressive resuscitation, transfusion of more than 50% of the total blood volume, pneumoperitoneum, intraperitoneal bladder rupture, severe renovascular injury, gunshot wounds to the abdomen, evisceration, and peritonitis. Other injuries are often treated more conservatively in the intensive care unit after complete consultation with all involved providers.

An organized, preestablished, multidisciplinary approach to care is essential. Studies have shown that the single most important

element for any hospital treating injured children is the commitment on the part of the institution and its surgeons. Regional pediatric trauma centers have increased resources for dealing with severely injured patients that include long-term care and rehabilitation. Other non-designated hospitals may do an excellent job in the initial stabilization phase of care. Indications for transfer to a specialty center include inability to provide definitive surgical intervention, inability to provide an appropriate intensive care environment, the presence of multisystem injuries or injuries requiring extensive orthopedic or plastic surgery procedures, or major burns. Health care professionals who treat children should not only become adept at the recognition and initial stabilization of injuries, but should also serve as advocates for injury prevention and coordinated prehospital care services in the community.

CASE RESOLUTION

The 6-year-old boy in the case history sustained multiple trauma from an automobile versus pedestrian collision. He presents with altered level of consciousness; respiratory failure (shallow respirations); potential internal organ injury, which may lead to shock; and probable fracture of the left femur, which may also contribute to the development of shock. These injuries are identified by performance of a primary and secondary survey. Proper management includes stabilization of the cervical spine, airway management, aggressive early shock treatment with fluid replacement, and a vigilant search for additional injuries. Continued reassessment is also an integral part of emergency department stabilization. Due to the presence of multisystem injuries, after initial stabilization, the patient should be transferred to a regional pediatric trauma center for extended care.

Selected References

American Heart Association. 2005 American Heart Association (AHA) guidelines for cardiopulmonary resuscitation (CPR) and emergency cardiovascular care (ECC) of pediatric and neonatal patients: pediatric advanced life support. *Pediatrics.* 2006;117:e1005–e1028

American College of Surgeons. *Advanced Trauma Life Support (ATLS) Student Manual.* 7th ed. Chicago, IL: American College of Surgeons; 2005

Carley S, Driscoll P. Trauma education. *Resuscitation.* 2001;48:47–56

Cantor RM, Leaming JM. Evaluation and management of pediatric major trauma. *Emerg Med Clin North Am.* 1998;16:229–256

Fitzmaurice LS. Approach to multiple trauma. In: Barkin RM, ed. *Pediatric Emergency Medicine Concepts and Clinical Practice.* St Louis, MO: Mosby-Year Book; 1997:223–235

Roaten JB, Partrick DA, Nydam TL, et al. Nonaccidental trauma is a major cause of morbidity and mortality among patients at a regional level 1 pediatric trauma center. *J Pediatr Surg.* 2006;41:2013–2015

Ruddy RM, Fleisher GR. An approach to the injured child. In: Fleisher GR, Ludwig S, eds. *Textbook of Pediatric Emergency Medicine.* 5th ed. Baltimore, MD: Williams & Wilkins; 2005

Swischuk LE. Emergency pediatric imaging: changes over the years (Part I). *Emerg Radiol.* 2005;11:193–198

Ziegler MM, Templeton JM. Major trauma. In: Fleisher GR, Ludwig S, eds. *Textbook of Pediatric Emergency Medicine.* 5th ed. Baltimore, MD: Williams & Wilkins; 2005

Abdominal Trauma

David B. Burbulys, MD

CASE STUDY

An 8-year-old boy who rode a bicycle quickly and unintentionally crashed into a tree presents. On arrival at the trauma center, the paramedics report that the bike handlebars struck the child's stomach, "knocking the wind out of him." The boy complains of dizziness and vomits several times. Initial vital signs show a heart rate of 135/min and a respiratory rate of 24/min. The abdomen is flat but tender to palpation in the mid-epigastric region and left upper quadrant.

Questions

1. What are the most frequent types of intra-abdominal trauma in children?
2. What are the diagnostic studies used to evaluate abdominal trauma?
3. What are the basic components of the treatment of shock that occurs following abdominal trauma?
4. What is a simple rule for establishing the lower limit of normal blood pressure in children?

Abdominal trauma is the leading unrecognized cause of fatal injury, specifically because early shock is not recognized. Death results when the extent and nature of abdominal injuries are neither appreciated nor appropriately managed, fluid replacement is inadequate, and airway maintenance and surgical intervention are not implemented soon enough. Abdominal trauma is the third leading cause of traumatic death, following head and thoracic injury. Clinicians should be knowledgeable about mechanisms of injury that result in abdominal trauma, the early manifestations of shock, and the methods for aggressive treatment of hemorrhagic shock.

Epidemiology

Twenty-five percent of children who sustain multisystem trauma have significant abdominal injury and 9% die from abdominal-associated trauma. When both head and abdominal injury occur simultaneously, the risk of death is higher than when either occurs alone. Blunt-force mechanisms are responsible for almost 85% of abdominal injuries; the remainder are a result of penetrating force. Examples of blunt-force mechanisms, presented in order of frequency, are motor vehicle crashes (also the most lethal), pedestrian versus automobile collisions, falls, bicycle injuries, sports injuries, and direct blows from both abuse and assault. Injuries to the spleen and liver predominate followed by injuries to the kidney, bowel, and pancreas less often. In multiple injuries, the incidence of trauma involving pelvic bones and organs (bladder, ureter, iliac vessels) is also high. A straddle injury (eg, fall that occurs when climbing over a fence) can also result in abdominal and pelvic trauma.

Clinical Presentation

Pain, tenderness, ecchymoses, and peritoneal signs tend to be more reliable signs of pathology, whereas distension or the absence of bowel sounds are less consistent as a marker for injury. (See Dx Box for signs and symptoms suggestive of abdominal trauma.) It is particularly important to note that no sign, however, is completely reliable and that unexplained hypotension or shock mandates further investigations to assess for intra-abdominal hemorrhage.

Dx Abdominal Trauma

- Pain
- Tenderness
- Distention
- Peritoneal signs (absent or diminished bowel sounds, rebound tenderness)
- Ecchymoses
- Tire tracks
- Seat belt marks
- Urine, stool, or nasogastric aspirate positive for blood
- Unexplained hypotension or other signs of hypovolemic shock

Pathophysiology

Blunt trauma largely involves injury to solid, not hollow, intra-abdominal organs (ie, spleen and liver rather than small bowel) for a variety of reasons. First, the rib cage is flexible in children. Therefore, rib fractures are less likely to occur, reducing the potential for penetration of abdominal organs by broken ribs. Second, children have less well-developed abdominal musculature and less adipose tissue than adults and relatively larger organs. Blunt force is therefore transmitted to the solid organs more easily and more diffusely. Third, because the diaphragm is oriented more horizontally in children than in adults, the liver and spleen lie more anteriorly and caudally within the abdomen.

It is important to emphasize that abdominal injury may lead to excessive blood loss. The pathophysiology of hemorrhagic shock is discussed in detail in Chapters 49 and 50. The liver and spleen are highly vascularized organs that bleed profusely when lacerated. Even the accumulation of subcapsular hematomas without rupture may cause a profound drop in hematocrit. Because intra-abdominal organs are not directly visible when a patient is examined, signs and symptoms of injury are not always obvious. Therefore, hemorrhagic shock should always be suspected with abdominal trauma. Likewise, large volumes of blood can accumulate in the pelvis and retroperitoneum, and because of their proximity to the abdomen, they should always be considered as a reservoir for hemorrhage in abdominal as well as pelvic trauma.

Differential Diagnosis

Physicians should be familiar with the most common patterns of abdominal injury, and they should consider the possibility of specific injuries. Any solid abdominal organ can be injured by any mechanism, either blunt or penetrating. The spleen is the most common intra-abdominal organ injured by a blunt force. **Hepatic injuries** are the most common fatal abdominal injuries, although they are less frequent than **splenic injuries.** The right lobe of the liver is injured more frequently than the left lobe.

Injuries to **hollow viscera** such as the stomach and intestines, which represent only about 5% to 15% of injuries from blunt forces, are difficult to diagnose and often present late. Three mechanisms lead to injuries of hollow structures: (1) "crush" between the anterior wall of the abdomen and the vertebral column; (2) deceleration, which causes shearing of the bowel from its mesenteric attachments; and (3) "burst," which occurs when an air-filled or fluid-filled loop of bowel is closed at both ends at the time of impact. Peritonitis may develop in 6 to 48 hours secondary to fecal spillage or devascularization as a consequence of any of these mechanisms. Occasionally, a diagnosis of hollow viscera injury is made incidentally or may be delayed more than 48 hours, highlighting the need for serial examinations. **Duodenal** and **pancreatic** injuries are examples of potentially delayed diagnoses that can have grave consequences. Leakage of bile and enzymes may activate autodigestion of the pancreas and result in sepsis.

Evaluation

Determining which organ or organs may be injured from abdominal trauma is difficult. Children are often uncooperative or unable to assist with the physical examination. Physicians tend to focus on injuries to the extremities, pelvis, face, or chest that are painful and distracting to children and more clinically obvious to the examiner.

Initial clinical impressions may be incorrect, causing delay in diagnosis or unnecessary surgical exploration.

History

The history should focus on the mechanism of injury and the physiological response of the child, especially in the pre-hospital setting (eg, initial hypotension, tachycardia, cyanosis) (Questions Box). A poor history concerning the circumstances of the injury may contribute to a delayed diagnosis.

Questions

Abdominal Trauma

- How was the child injured?
- How long ago did the injury occur?
- What parts of the body were injured?
- Has the child received any treatment prior to coming to the hospital, and what was the response?

Physical Examination

An abnormal physical examination may not always be indicative of pathology. Clinicians should avoid relying on physical examination alone as a predictor of abdominal injury. Studies have demonstrated that patients with and without proven injuries often showed no significant differences with respect to physical findings. In particular, children with abusive abdominal trauma often have no cutaneous evidence of bruising, especially immediately after the injury is inflicted (see Chapter 115). Definitive evaluation of the abdomen often includes rapid computed tomography (CT) scan, ultrasound, diagnostic peritoneal lavage, laparoscopy, or laparotomy.

Vital signs should be monitored. In children, the range for normal heart rate, respiratory rate, and blood pressure is age-dependent. A simple rule for calculating the lower limit of normal systolic blood pressure is 70 + (2 x age in years). Physicians should always remember that a drop in blood pressure is a very late sign in the development of shock in children (see Chapters 49 and 50).

Serial abdominal examinations increase the likelihood of detecting a previously missed condition. Inspection of the abdomen to look for ecchymoses, distention, tire tracks, penetrations, or paradoxical motion should occur first. Auscultation for bowel sounds follows this inspection, and palpation should come last. Palpation should be done in all 4 quadrants to elicit tenderness, rebound, and guarding. If a hepatic or splenic injury is initially suspected, palpation should be minimized to avoid further hemorrhaging.

Laboratory Tests

Laboratory evaluation should be guided by the history and physical examination. A urinalysis to look for hematuria and check for associated genitourinary injuries is helpful. Elevated serum transaminases, amylase, and alkaline phosphatase may be indicative of injury, but normal values do not exclude pathology. A comprehensive trauma panel, which usually includes a complete blood count and differential, serum electrolytes, blood urea nitrogen, creatinine, glucose, prothrombin time, partial thromboplastin time, urinalysis, and blood type and crossmatch, should be carried out for all patients with serious or multiple injuries (see Chapter 50).

Imaging Studies

Multiple imaging modalities are available to assess the pediatric trauma patient with suspected abdominal injuries. The time to perform an imaging study is after the patient is responding appropriately to resuscitation (ie, fluid therapy). Unstable patients will require surgical exploration for definitive treatment of abdominal or pelvic injury.

In the United States, CT scanning is the standard of care for imaging the injured abdomen of a pediatric trauma patient. Computed tomography scans have a greater than 97% accuracy in identifying abdominal injury, are noninvasive, and most notably provide detailed specific information regarding injuries. The images can also be extended to include the pelvis, if necessary. Disadvantages of CT scanning include the lack of proximity to the trauma suite, which may not be ideal for unstable patients; the length of time it takes to perform the procedure; and the need for an intravenous (IV) line and possibly oral contrast, which have inherent risks such as allergic reactions and aspiration.

The use of ultrasonography has become very popular, with encouraging results for the identification of abdominal injury. Ultrasound can rapidly and noninvasively document the presence of intraperitoneal and pelvic fluid (blood). Studies so far show that it is probably at least as effective as CT scanning for documenting the **presence of injury** but does not provide as much specific information about the **nature** of the injury. Ultrasound has a few additional advantages: It is relatively inexpensive; does not require contrast or radiation exposure; can be performed in 5 to 10 minutes in the trauma room, thus minimizing the risk to an unstable patient; and can be used many times for serial assessments.

Over the last several decades, diagnostic peritoneal lavage has been a dependable method of detecting intra-abdominal hemorrhage. However, its use may be limited in the pediatric population because many children with blunt trauma to the abdomen are now managed nonoperatively.

Management

Management of abdominal trauma in children occurs simultaneously with evaluation. The stabilization of children with abdominal trauma, especially in the context of multiple trauma, requires a multidisciplinary team approach that includes surgeons, pediatricians, and emergency physicians. A discussion on the approach to trauma management can be found in Chapter 50.

Hypovolemic shock, if present, is the primary complication of abdominal trauma on which to focus because the leading unrecognized cause of death in affected children is profound blood loss.

Airway problems and **breathing difficulties** should be addressed initially, followed by **vascular access** and **fluid replacement.** No more than 3 attempts at peripheral vascular access should be made (≤90 seconds) before moving on to more invasive procedures.

The intraosseous route should be used for the next vascular access attempt in children who are younger than 6 years. The flat, medial portion of the proximal tibia is most commonly used for the procedure, which is performed with an intraosseous, bone marrow, or spinal needle (Figure 51-1). Fluids and medications, delivered into the marrow cavity, then flow into the venous circulation. Intraosseous cannulation is rapid, simple, and may be lifesaving. It is limited by low flow rates (approximately 30 mL/min), which can be augmented either by using pressure on the IV bag or by pushing fluid by hand through a syringe. Complications associated with intraosseous line placement are rare. All physicians who care for pediatric trauma patients should be familiar with this technique.

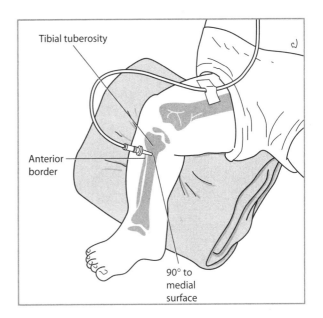

Figure 51-1. Intraosseous cannulation technique. (Adapted with permission from American Heart Association. 2005 American Heart Association [AHA] guidelines for cardiopulmonary resuscitation [CPR] and emergency cardiovascular care [ECC] of pediatric and neonatal patients: pediatric advanced life support. *Pediatrics.* **2006;117:e1005–e1028.)**

A variety of central venous access sites, such as femoral, subclavian, and internal jugular, may be used in older children. Upper and lower saphenous vein cutdowns are also possible access sites. The Seldinger technique, with insertion of a large-bore catheter over a guidewire, is often used. A description of these procedures is beyond the scope of this book but may be found in many other publications, including the 2005 American Heart Association (AHA) Guidelines for Cardiopulmonary Resuscitation (CPR) and Emergency Cardiovascular Care (ECC) of Pediatric and Neonatal Patients: Pediatric Advanced Life Support published by the American Heart Association (see Selected References). Intravenous access above the diaphragm is preferred in patients with blunt or penetrating abdominal trauma who have potential disruption of the vena cava or other large veins.

Fluid replacement begins with a 20- to 40-mL/kg bolus of crystalloid solution, either warmed normal saline or Ringer's lactate. If no improvement in circulation occurs, additional 10- to 20-mL/kg boluses may be given, and type-specific blood should be considered. In most scenarios, type-specific blood is given after 60 mL/kg of crystalloid has failed to improve circulatory parameters. Frequent hematocrits or hemoglobins should be determined to monitor ongoing blood loss. Vital signs should be repeated frequently. Serial examinations, which detect the signs and symptoms of shock (Box 51-1), are the most important gauge of hemodynamic recovery and stability. All children require close hospital observation, preferably in a pediatric trauma center and pediatric intensive care unit.

Box 51-1. Signs and Symptoms of Hemorrhagic Shock in Children

Tachycardia

Delayed capillary refill (>2 s)

Cool and mottled skin, pallor

Respiratory distress

Anxiety, irritability, decreased responsiveness

Thirst

Orthostatic fall in blood pressure and supine hypotension (late sign) must be aggressively managed. If hemodynamic stabilization is not achieved after appropriate vascular access and fluid resuscitation, the trauma surgeon will most likely perform an exploratory laparotomy. If children have been stabilized with initial airway and circulatory support, diagnostic procedures such as CT scans can be performed as part of the emergency department evaluation. Once identified, specific organ injury can be managed.

Other specific management concerns for pediatric patients with abdominal injury are early decompression of the stomach with a nasogastric or orogastric tube to prevent respiratory compromise and urinary catheter insertion to decompress the bladder. Before inserting a urinary catheter, the trauma team should evaluate for possible urethral trauma and check for the presence of blood in the urine, which may indicate other genitourinary trauma.

Prognosis

Morbidity and mortality related to abdominal trauma depend on the specific organ injury and the style of management. More than 40% of patients with major liver injuries die in the prehospital setting. However, a large number of minor liver injuries can be managed nonoperatively. Currently an increasing number of injuries to

the spleen and liver are managed with observation in the pediatric intensive care unit. Surgical exploration and repair are performed only if patients become hemodynamically unstable. Reduction in anesthetic-related mortality, post-splenectomy sepsis, and a decrease in other postoperative complications have resulted from this shift in practice style. Without surgical intervention, however, a severe injury such as complete splenic rupture has a 90% to 100% mortality rate.

CASE RESOLUTION

The boy in the case scenario sustained isolated abdominal trauma. Initial presenting signs and symptoms are consistent with internal organ injury, specifically splenic hematoma, pancreatic injury, internal hemorrhage, and compensated shock (eg, tachycardia, tachypnea). The child should undergo initial resuscitation with attention to the airway, breathing, and circulation, especially fluid repletion. Serial hemodynamic measurement and hematocrits, if stable, permit diagnosis of specific injuries by computed tomography scanning. Surgical consultation with expectant observation is the likely management choice. If the child deteriorates, surgical intervention would ensue. Trauma to the small intestine, particularly a duodenal hematoma, must also be suspected because of the mechanism of injury.

Selected References

American Heart Association. 2005 American Heart Association (AHA) guidelines for cardiopulmonary resuscitation (CPR) and emergency cardiovascular care (ECC) of pediatric and neonatal patients: pediatric advanced life support. *Pediatrics.* 2006;117:e1005–e1028

American College of Surgeons. *Advanced Trauma Life Support (ATLS) Student Manual.* 7th ed. Chicago, IL: American College of Surgeons; 2005

Capraro AJ, Mooney D, Waltzman ML. The use of routine laboratory studies as screening tools in pediatric abdominal trauma. *Pediatr Emerg Care.* 2006;22:480–484

Foltin GL, Cooper A. Abdominal trauma. In: Barkin RM, ed. *Pediatric Emergency Medicine Concepts and Clinical Practice.* St Louis, MO: Mosby-Year Book; 1997:335–354

Haller JA. Blunt trauma to the abdomen. *Pediatr Rev.* 1996;17:29–31

Holmes JF, Brant WE, Bond WF, Sokolove PE, Kuppermann N. Emergency department ultrasonography in the evaluation of hypotensive and normotensive children with blunt abdominal trauma. *J Pediatr Surg.* 2001;36:968–973

Soudack M, Epelman M, Maor R, et al. Experience with focused abdominal sonography for trauma (FAST) in 313 pediatric patients. *J Clin Ultrasound.* 2004;32:53–61

Stylianos S. Outcomes from pediatric solid organ injury: role of standardized care guidelines. *Curr Opin Pediatr.* 2005;17:402–406

Venkatesh KR, McQuay N Jr. Outcomes of management in stable children with intra-abdominal free fluid without solid organ injury after blunt abdominal injury. *J Trauma.* 2007;62:216–220

Wegner S, Colletti JE, Van Wie D. Pediatric blunt abdominal trauma. *Pediatr Clin North Am.* 2006;53:243–256

Head Trauma

Paul Bryan, MD

CASE STUDY

A 2-year-old girl is playing on a window ledge unsupervised. She pushes the screen out and falls onto the concrete sidewalk below, striking her head. A neighbor reports that she is unconscious for 10 minutes. When paramedics arrive, the girl is awake but lethargic. She is transported to the emergency department. Her vital signs are normal. A scalp hematoma is present, and a depressed area of cranial bone is palpated.

Questions

1. What are the priorities in the initial stabilization and management of pediatric head trauma?
2. What is the difference between primary and secondary brain injury?
3. What are the common structural injuries sustained by children with head trauma?
4. What are the various modalities available for treatment of increased intracranial pressure?
5. What are the scoring systems used in the evaluation of mental status in children with head trauma?

Although most childhood head injuries are minor and can be treated on an outpatient basis, it is important for clinicians to become adept at recognizing and managing concussions and more severe forms of head injury. Health care providers can also help lower mortality from head trauma by actively promoting injury prevention to patients and communities.

Epidemiology

Head trauma is one of the most common pediatric injuries and is the leading cause of morbidity and mortality among pediatric trauma patients. Pediatric head trauma accounts for more than 500,000 emergency department (ED) visits, 95,000 hospital admissions, 7,000 deaths, and 29,000 permanent disabilities per year in the United States. The hospital care costs exceed a billion dollars annually. In multiple-injured pediatric patients, 70% of the deaths that occur within 48 hours of hospitalization are the result of trauma to the head. The rates of intracranial injuries in children with only minor head trauma, however, are low with the largest numbers occurring in young children and infants with an incidence of 3% to 6%. Only 0.4% to 1% of children require surgical intervention after minor closed injury.

Falls account for most cases of pediatric head trauma. Other major causes include motor vehicle and vehicle versus pedestrian collisions, bicycle crashes, sports-related injuries, and recreational activities. Non-accidental trauma (ie, child abuse) must be recognized as another important cause of head injury in children, particularly among those younger than 2 years.

Clinical Presentation

Children who have sustained head trauma may present with a history of an antecedent event (eg, fall or collision with another child) or signs and symptoms related to the injury. These include external bruises or lacerations; alterations in the level of consciousness; and neurologic findings, including seizures. Vital signs may be altered; in particular, deep or irregular respirations, hypertension, or bradycardia may be apparent (Dx Box). These changes are indicative of elevated intracranial pressure (ICP).

Pathophysiology

Children have significant anatomical differences from adults that predispose them to head trauma and certain types of intracranial injuries. They have a higher center of gravity, an increased head-to-body ratio, and weaker neck muscles compared with adults. In addition,

Dx **Head Trauma**[a]

- Loss of consciousness
- Somnolence
- Pallor
- Emesis/nausea/anorexia
- Irritability
- Lethargy
- Seizure
- Ataxia
- Weakness
- Pain
- Parasthesias
- Amnesia
- Headache
- Visual changes
- Confusion/altered mental status

[a] All these symptoms may not be present in head trauma.

children have thinner cranial bones and less myelinated brain tissue, predisposing them to intraparenchymal injuries. Whereas adults are more likely to have focal intracranial hematomas, children are more likely to develop diffuse cerebral edema. Cerebral edema can disrupt cerebral blood flow resulting in ischemic injury.

Normally, blood flow to the brain is maintained at a constant rate by a process known as *autoregulation*. With severe brain injury, autoregulation is disrupted and blood flow to the brain is determined by cerebral perfusion pressure (CPP), which is a measure of the mean arterial pressure (MAP) minus ICP [CPP = MAP − ICP]. Cerebral blood flow is therefore compromised when the MAP is too low (ie, hypotension) or the ICP is too high (ie, cerebral edema). Several of the management strategies in severely brain-injured children focus on maintaining MAP and reducing ICP, but control of CPP after head injury can be quite difficult. Children have a greater capacity for recovery than adults, especially infants and very young children, whose open sutures and fontanelles permit expansion of the skull in response to edema and blood.

In head trauma, both primary and secondary brain injury can occur (Figure 52-1). Primary injury is the structural damage that occurs to the cranium and its contents at the time of the injury. Secondary injury is damage to the brain tissue after the initial event. Such damage may result from hypoxia, hypoperfusion, hypercarbia, hyperthermia, and altered glucose or sodium metabolism. The main management strategies for head trauma victims focus on the prevention of secondary brain injury. Primary brain injury can only be prevented through education and safety.

Types of Head Injuries

Even minor head trauma in children can result in fractures to the skull or intracranial injuries. Most skull fractures are simple and linear. Other fracture types are comminuted, diastatic, basilar, and depressed. Comminuted fractures occur when there are multiple skull fragments. Diastatic fractures occur when there is a wide separation at the fracture site. Basilar fractures occur at the base of the skull and often have characteristic findings on physical examination (ie, bilateral periorbital ecchymosis, hemotympanum, postauricular ecchymosis [Battle sign]). Depressed fracture occurs when fragments of the skull are displaced inward, potentially damaging intracranial structures.

Head trauma may result in a **concussion** or concussive syndrome. A concussion is defined as a trauma-induced alteration in mental status. This may occur with or without a loss of consciousness (LOC). Neurologic examination is usually normal, but patients may experience headache, confusion, amnesia, vomiting, and other minor symptoms. Concussions can also have minor and subtle neurologic sequelae, such as dizziness or headache, for months following the injury (post-concussive syndrome). Concussions are normally classified on a 3-point scale. Grade 1 concussions are defined as transient confusion without LOC and mental status abnormalities lasting less than 15 minutes. Grade 2 concussions occur when there is transient confusion without LOC and mental status abnormalities lasting longer than 15 minutes. Grade 3 concussions involve any LOC.

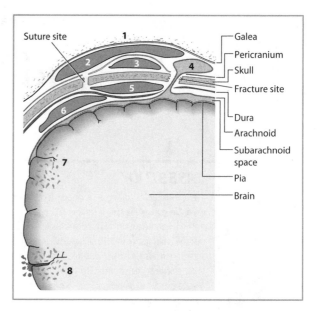

Figure 52-1. Functional anatomy of brain and surrounding structures with sites of pathology. 1. Caput succedaneum. 2. Subgaleal hematoma. 3. Cephalhematoma. 4. Porencephalic cyst or leptomeningeal cyst. 5. Epidural hematoma. 6. Subdural hematoma. 7. Cerebral contusion. 8. Cerebral laceration. (Redrawn with permission from Tecklenburg FW, Wright MS. Minor head trauma in the pediatric patient. *Pediatr Emerg Care.* 1991;7:40–47.)

A **cerebral contusion** is essentially a bruise of the brain tissue and typically occurs with a more severe injury, such as a high-speed motor vehicle crash. A coup-contrecoup type injury may be produced when the brain strikes the skull on direct impact bruising one portion of the brain, and then injury occurs to the opposite portion of the brain when rapid deceleration occurs. Clinical manifestations depend on the location of the contusion but often include altered mental status, excessive sleepiness, confusion, and agitation. Small intraparenchymal hemorrhages and swelling of the surrounding tissues are often seen on computed tomography (CT) scan.

Epidural hematomas are collections of blood that accumulate between the skull bone and the tough outer covering of the brain (dura). They are often the result of tears in the middle meningeal artery caused by skull fractures. Classically, patients have initial LOC followed by a lucid interval and then rapid deterioration secondary to brain compression. On CT scan an epidural hematoma appears as a large collection of blood with convex borders next to the skull (Figure 52-2A). Surgical evacuation is required in most cases.

Subdural hematomas accumulate between the dura and the underlying brain tissue. They are associated with both skull fractures and contusions. On CT scan they appear to have crescent-shaped borders (Figure 52-2B). Large subdural hematomas usually require surgical evacuation. These can be seen in infants and young children as a result of non-accidental trauma.

Diffuse axonal injury occurs when there is extensive damage to the axonal white matter of the brain that results from shearing forces that typically occur with rapid acceleration or deceleration of the brain (Figure 52-2C).

Figure 52-2. A. Epidural hematoma, marked by the asterisk. Note convex borders and midline shift. B. Subdural hematoma. Note crescent shape. C. Diffuse axonal injury. Note ground-glass appearance and tightly compressed ventricles. (Reproduced with permission from Harris JH Jr, Harris WH, Norelline RA. *The Radiology of Emergency Medicine.* 3rd ed. Baltimore, MD: Williams & Wilkins; 1993:15, 16, 17.)

Evaluation

History

Historical data are obtained during the secondary survey or reassessment phase of evaluation. Prehospital health care providers or witnesses to the injury should be asked about details of the event (Questions Box).

Questions

Head Trauma

- What was the mechanism of injury (motor vehicle crash, ejection from motor vehicle, fall, assault)?
- What was the height of the fall?
- What was the type of impact surface?
- What was the shape of the object(s) striking the head?
- What was the child's immediate status after injury?
- What changes in status occurred before arrival at the hospital?
- Did the child lose consciousness? If so, for how long?
- Did the child vomit?
- Did the child have a seizure? If so, when did it occur in relation to the injury and does the child have an underlying seizure disorder?

Physical Examination

Careful attention to the vital signs of children with head injuries is important. The presence of hypertension, bradycardia, and an irregular breathing pattern (**Cushing triad**) all suggest a significant intracranial injury with associated increased ICP.

Secondary survey actions include palpation and inspection of the scalp for soft-tissue swelling, step-offs, lacerations, and fullness of the fontanelle. Facial bones should be tested for stability and deformities. Other clues to possible head trauma include the presence of a septal hematoma, draining blood or fluid from the nose or ears, dental injury, and malocclusion of the mandible. The tympanic membranes should be visualized for the presence of hemotympanum or cerebrospinal fluid (CSF) otorrhea, which along with postauricular ecchymosis (**Battle sign**), periorbital ecchymosis, or cranial nerve

palsies suggest a basilar skull fracture. Funduscopic examination should be performed if possible to look for the presence of papilledema associated with increased ICP or **retinal hemorrhages** that indicate non-accidental trauma.

A comprehensive neurologic examination is the most important part of the secondary survey. This examination should include a mental status assessment, cranial nerve evaluation, presence and quality of deep tendon reflexes, muscle tone, muscle strength, sensation, and cerebellar function. When describing mental status, imprecise terms such as *altered, lethargic,* and *obtunded* should be avoided. Several widely used scoring systems are available for mental status assessment of children who have suffered head trauma that are useful predictors of intracranial injury. A number of scales exist for assessment of the level of consciousness. The most universally accepted and widely used of these scales is the **Glasgow Coma Score** (GCS). It is used routinely in children older than 5 years, but can be modified for younger children. Each scoring system has 3 measured responses (eye opening, verbal, and motor) to a variety of stimuli. Scores should be tabulated when children first present to establish a baseline. They can then be used for reassessment on a regular basis until patients have stabilized or returned to normal mental status. Use of these scores helps promote consistent and accurate communication among health care providers. Tables 52-1 and 52-2 show how to calculate the GCS and modified GCS scores.

The secondary survey should be completed to identify any additional life- or limb-threatening injuries.

Table 52-1. Glasgow Coma Scale	
Elements	**Points**
I. Eye opening	
a. Spontaneous	4
b. To command	3
c. With pain	2
d. No response	1
II. Verbal response[a]	
a. Oriented, converses normally	5
b. Disoriented, confused	4
c. Utters inappropriate words	3
d. Incomprehensible sounds	2
e. No response	1
III. Motor response	
a. Obeys commands	6
b. Localizes pain	5
c. Flexes with pain	4
d. Flexes abnormally with pain	3
e. Extensor response	2
f. None	1
Maximum score	**15**

[a]Assessment of verbal response is modified in children.

Table 52-2. Modified Glasgow Coma Scale for Younger Children	
Elements	**Points**
I. Eye opening	
a. Spontaneous	4
b. To command	3
c. With pain	2
d. No response	1
II. Verbal response[a]	
a. Coos and babbles	5
b. Irritable cry	4
c. Cries to pain	3
d. Moans to pain	2
e. None	1
III. Motor response	
a. Normal spontaneous movement	6
b. Withdraws to touch	5
c. Withdraws to pain	4
d. Abnormal flexion	3
e. Abnormal extension	2
f. None	1
Maximum score	*15*

[a]Assessment of verbal response is modified in children.

Laboratory Testing

All pediatric patients with significant head trauma should have a complete blood cell count and serum electrolytes performed. Bedside glucose should be performed in any child with a head injury with an altered level of consciousness. Toxicological evaluation may be indicated in adolescents who appear to be intoxicated or have an altered level of consciousness. Those infants and children with an intracranial hemorrhage should have screening coagulation studies performed (ie, prothrombin time, activated partial thromboplastin time), as well as a type and screen or crossmatch, should surgery be required.

Imaging Studies

In cases of acute pediatric blunt or penetrating trauma, a non-contrast CT of the head is currently the diagnostic study of choice. It is very sensitive for the detection of acute hemorrhages and skull fractures. It can also provide additional information as to the severity of injury indicating increased ICP, cerebral edema, or pending herniation. Some of the findings on CT that indicate severe brain injury are the shift of midline structures, effacement of the sulci, ventricular enlargement or compression, and loss of the normal gray-white matter differentiation.

A list of suggested criteria for obtaining a CT scan for patients with head injuries can be found in Box 52-1. All children classified

Box 52-1. Indications for Computed Tomography Scans in Children With Head Trauma
• Alteration in level of consciousness, with waxing and waning or deteriorating mental status
• Glasgow Coma Score lower than 14
• Focal neurologic deficit(s) on examination
• Examination findings suggestive of a skull fracture
• Posttraumatic seizures
• Persistent vomiting or headache
• Scalp hematoma in a child younger than 2 years
• Prolonged loss of consciousness
• Possibility of penetration of the skull

with moderate to severe head trauma (GCS <14) should have a head CT performed. There is considerable debate about which children who have suffered minor closed head trauma with a normal examination and a GCS of 14 to 15 warrant imaging. There is no pediatric study thus far that has been able to identify a set of clinical criteria to identify all children with radiographic lesions. Vomiting, LOC, and seizures, which can all be seen in intracranial injuries, are relatively poor predictors of radiographic intracranial abnormality in children. The best predictors in children are altered mental status, focal neurologic deficit, and the presence of a skull fracture. Given the small numbers that require actual surgical intervention, some argue that the goal should not necessarily be to identify all of these clinically insignificant lesions and thereby minimize radiation exposure. Others argue that given the lack of reliable clinical criteria, and the possibility of significant intracranial injury in the face of a normal examination, a more liberal use of CT should be employed. Currently there are large multicenter studies being conducted in the United States, the United Kingdom, and Canada that will hopefully be able to provide management guidance in the future. The decision to perform a CT scan in these children with minor head trauma currently is based on a variety of factors including historical data, physical findings, age of the child, physician experience, and the psychosocial situation of patients and their families.

With the speed and widespread availability of CT scanners, skull x-rays have relatively little role in the acute evaluation of pediatric head trauma patients. Current CT scans can be performed very quickly, often with the need for no or little sedation. Although sensitive for the detection of skull fractures, plain films do not provide any information about associated intracranial injuries. In addition, several studies have demonstrated that intracranial injuries occur in the absence of a skull fracture, particularly among young pediatric patients. The role of plain films is limited to part of the skeletal survey in suspected cases of non-accidental trauma.

Magnetic resonance imaging (MRI) has little role in the management of the acutely injured head trauma victim. Computed tomography scan is often more sensitive at detecting acute intracranial hemorrhages and is sufficient to guide most immediate patient care issues. Magnetic resonance imaging may be superior to CT for identifying diffuse axonal injury and subtle brain injuries. In general, MRI takes longer to complete, often requires sedation, and the scanners are frequently located away from the ED where the child cannot be monitored appropriately.

One important consideration of any trauma victim is the possibility of a cervical spine injury. Although cervical spine injuries are less common in children, the clinician must maintain a high index of suspicion when presented with a child who has suffered significant head trauma. All children with an altered level of consciousness; significant painful/distracting injuries; an inability to communicate; focal neurologic deficits; or localized pain, swelling, or ecchymosis of the cervical spine require careful evaluation and imaging of the cervical spine.

Management

Assessment and management occur simultaneously when an acutely injured child presents. A primary survey is initially performed with attention to airway, breathing, circulation (ABCs), and cervical spine immobilization. Prompt neurosurgical consultation should be obtained for all children with significant head trauma to assess the need for operative management and ICP monitoring. The primary management goal of significant acute head trauma is the prevention of secondary brain injury by (1) maximizing oxygenation and ventilation, (2) supporting circulation to maximize cerebral perfusion, (3) decreasing elevated ICP, and (4) decreasing cerebral metabolic demands.

Individuals with significant intracranial injuries will often require intubation for airway protection. Those individuals with a GCS of 8 or lower should undergo **rapid sequence intubation** to control the airway. These individuals should be premedicated with etomidate and lidocaine prior to the use of paralytics. Etomidate is a sedative that is cardiovascularly neutral with minimal effect on blood pressure. Most other sedatives can result in hypotension thereby lowering MAP and reducing CPP. Lidocaine is recommended to potentially blunt the transient increase in ICP often associated with orotracheal intubation. In the past, moderate hyperventilation was advocated to reduce ICP. Hyperventilation lowers arterial carbon dioxide partial pressure (pCO_2), leading to cerebral vasoconstriction and decreased cerebral blood flow, lowering ICP. This has been shown to have the unwanted effect of disrupting cerebral metabolism and possibly exacerbating ischemic injury. Currently normoventilation is recommended with the goal of maintaining pCO_2 no lower than 34 mm Hg. Moderate hyperventilation may have a role in the transient management of serious or acute life-threatening elevations in ICP (ie, acute herniation).

Circulation and MAP should be aggressively supported with fluids to prevent hypoperfusion to the brain. Hypovolemia or hypotension should never be assumed to result from head trauma alone. Children should be examined carefully for evidence of additional injury. Central venous pressure monitoring is often necessary to accurately assess volume status. Pressors may be necessary to maintain MAP in euvolemic patients. Morbidity has been shown to significantly increase with subsequent episodes of hypotension that occur.

Elevations in ICP may impede cerebral blood flow and exacerbate ischemic injury. Administration of hypertonic solutions (3% saline), osmotic agents (mannitol), diuretics, and elevation of the head of the bed to 30 degrees to promote venous drainage are all examples of methods used to reduce ICP. Use of mannitol and other diuretics is contraindicated in patients with borderline blood pressures because they can cause hypotension, which can in turn lower MAP, worsening cerebral perfusion. Paralytic agents, sedatives, and analgesics may be needed to prevent agitation, which also leads to increased ICP and increases cerebral metabolic demands. Painful procedures (eg, suctioning) should receive adequate pre-medication with sedatives and analgesics. Intraventricular pressure catheters are often necessary to allow for close monitoring of ICP. In addition, they can be used to drain CSF to help lower elevated ICP.

Hyperthermia and seizure activity should be managed aggressively because these all increase cerebral metabolic demands. Hyperthermia should be managed with antipyretics and active cooling measures. There is some evidence that controlled hypothermia may have some benefit in children with severe brain injuries, as does anticonvulsant prophylaxis. It is important to remember that the ability to detect clinical seizure activity is lost if the child is paralyzed.

Serum electrolytes should be followed closely, and any alterations should be minimized. Patients with head injuries should be monitored closely for the development of diabetes insipidus or syndrome of inappropriate secretion of antidiuretic hormone.

Children with large epidural and subdural hematomas will frequently require surgical evacuation. Individuals with depressed skull fractures often require operative management to lift the depressed fragment away from the underlying brain. Children who have suffered significant penetrating head trauma warrant antibiotic and antiepileptic prophylaxis, and may need angiography to assess for vascular injury. They should all have their tetanus status updated if necessary.

Children with minor head injuries (GCS = 14–15) with no LOC or a brief witnessed period of LOC, no focal deficits on neurologic examination, no skull fractures, and no persistent vomiting who demonstrate improvement and normal mental status (GCS = 15) after 4 to 6 hours of observation can be discharged with written instructions if they have adequate transportation back to the hospital, a telephone, and a reliable parent or guardian. Children should be admitted if these criteria cannot be met. Younger children (<2 years of age) are more difficult to assess accurately and consistently and are at higher risk for intracranial injuries. Admission should be strongly considered if their mental status is not completely normal or at baseline. Physicians should be wary of discharging children whose conditions have not improved to baseline following minor injuries or who have persistent emesis, even if their CT scans are normal.

More moderate head injuries (initial GCS = 9–12) necessitate a longer period of evaluation, probably in a monitored setting along with neurosurgical consultation. Severe head injuries (GCS <8) require aggressive stabilization in the ED with the measures described previously and admission to a pediatric intensive care unit.

Children who have suffered a concussion warrant close observation and reevaluation before resuming sporting activities. In general, athletes should not resume competition for a minimum of 1 to 2 weeks following a grade 1 or 2 concussion, and 1 month following a grade 3 concussion. In addition, there should be no signs or symptoms of any kind while at rest or during exertion, they should have a normal neurologic examination, and normal imaging (if performed). Athletes should return to play in a gradual stepwise fashion rather than an abrupt return to full activity and game play.

Prognosis

Age is the most important prognostic factor in outcome. Younger children tend to do better than older children. It is still difficult to predict the outcome of any individual patient. Scalp lacerations, most skull fractures, and concussions are low-risk injuries. Intracranial hemorrhage, specific skull fractures, head injury secondary to nonaccidental trauma, and trauma accompanied by diffuse cerebral edema are high-risk injuries. If untreated, severe head injury may lead to death from herniation.

Other complications from severe head trauma are posttraumatic seizures, requiring lifelong treatment with anticonvulsants; hydrocephalus, necessitating placement of a ventriculoperitoneal shunt catheter; and persistent vegetative or severely impaired mental states. Penetrating head injuries can result in infections (eg, meningitis, abscess) and vascular injuries (eg, aneurysm, arteriovenous malformations). Sequelae such as post-concussive syndrome may result from less severe head trauma. Some of the characteristics of this syndrome include dizziness, headache, irritability, memory deficits, impaired behavior, and impaired cognitive development. These may persist for months after the head injury and can sometimes be permanent. These children may warrant formal neurobehavioral testing.

Prevention

Despite advancing medical knowledge and excellent critical care available to children with head trauma, little can be done to reduce the severity of primary brain injury once it has occurred. Therefore, pediatric health care providers should make every attempt to educate patients and families about prevention strategies. Some of the most successful prevention strategies involve the required use of restraint devices such as seat belts, and of proper safety gear such as bicycle helmets. Anticipatory guidance and home safety recommendations provided to parents are also worthwhile. Finally, communities can contribute to injury prevention by providing playground resurfacing, reducing the height of playground equipment, and changing traffic laws. It is only through a combination of these prevention strategies that morbidity and mortality of pediatric head trauma will be truly reduced.

> ### CASE RESOLUTION
>
> The case scenario involves a young child with a significant mechanism of injury; brief LOC; and a depressed, altered mental status. Initial physical findings prompt suspicion of a depressed skull fracture and overlying soft tissue injury. Appropriate diagnostic tools after evaluation of airway, breathing, and circulation are a cranial computed tomography scan followed by admission for observation, monitoring, and serial neurologic examination. Operative repair of the skull fracture may be necessary.

Selected References

American Academy of Pediatrics Committee on Quality Improvement, American Academy of Family Physicians Commission on Clinical Policies and Research. The management of minor closed head injury in children. *Pediatrics*. 1999;104:1407–1415

Bruce DA. Head trauma. In: Fleisher GR, Ludwig S, eds. *Textbook of Pediatric Emergency Medicine*. 5th ed. Baltimore, MD: Williams & Wilkins; 2005

Dunning J, Daly JP, Lomas JP, Lecky F, Batchelor J, Makaway-Jones K. Derivation of the children's head injury algorithm for the prediction of important clinical events decision rule for head injury in children. *Arch Dis Child*. 2006;91:885–891

Goldstein B, Powers KS. Head trauma in children. *Pediatr Rev*. 1994; 15:213–219

Kirkwood MW, Yeates KO, Wilson PE. Pediatric sport-related concussion: a review of the clinical management of an oft-neglected population. *Pediatrics*. 2006;117:1359–1369

Koestler J, Keshavarz R. Penetrating head injury in children: a case report and review of the literature. *J Emerg Med*. 2001;21:145–150

Michaud LJ, Duhaime A, Batshaw ML. Traumatic brain injury in children. *Pediatr Clin North Am*. 1993;40:553–565

Palchak MJ, Holmes JF, Vance CW, et al. A decision rule for identifying children at low risk for brain injuries after blunt head trauma. *Ann Emerg Med*. 2003;42:492–506

Palchak MJ, Holmes JF, Vance CW, et al. Does an isolated history of loss of consciousness or amnesia predict brain injuries in children after blunt head trauma? *Pediatrics*. 2004;113:e507–e513

Rivara FP. Epidemiology and prevention of pediatric traumatic brain injury. *Pediatr Ann*. 1994;23:12–17

Schutzman SA, Barnes P, Duhaime AC, et al. Evaluation and management of children younger than two years old with apparently minor head trauma: proposed guidelines. *Pediatrics*. 2001;107:983–993

Schutzman SA, Greenes DS. Pediatric minor head trauma. *Ann Emerg Med*. 2001;37:65–74

Sun BC, Hoffman JR, Mower WR. Evaluation of a modified prediction instrument to identify significant pediatric intracranial injury after blunt head trauma. *Ann Emerg Med*. 2007;49:325–332

Tecklenburg FW, Wright MS. Minor head trauma in the pediatric patient. *Pediatr Emerg Care*. 1991;7:40–47

Zuckerman GB, Conway EE. Accidental head injury. *Pediatr Ann*. 1997;26:621–632

Increased Intracranial Pressure

Kenneth R. Huff, MD

CASE STUDY

A 7-year-old boy has a 2-week history of recurrent vomiting. No fever, abdominal pain, or diarrhea has accompanied the vomiting; the vomiting has no particular relationship to meals; and the boy's appetite has decreased only slightly. The vomiting has gradually increased in frequency and is occurring every night. Yesterday there were 4 episodes. The boy's parents have noticed that their son is generally less active; he spends more time playing on the floor of his room and does not want to ride his bicycle or play with neighborhood friends. Some unsteadiness in the boy's gait has developed in the last few days. His parents attribute this to weakness from the vomiting.

The child's vital signs are normal except for a blood pressure of 130/80 mm Hg. Although the boy is somewhat pale and uncomfortable, he does not appear to be in acute distress. His abdominal examination is unremarkable. His speech is grammatically correct but sparse and hesitant, and he seems inattentive. On lateral and upgaze the boy has coarse nystagmus, and upgaze is somewhat limited.

Some diplopia on left gaze is apparent, with slight failure of left eye abduction. The left eye does not blink as much as the right eye. Fundal examination discloses elevated disks with indistinct margins. No upper extremity weakness is evident. The right foot is slightly weaker than the left, ankle tone is bilaterally increased, and 3 to 4 beats of clonus on the right and bilateral positive Babinski reflexes are present. Some tremor occurs in both arms with finger-to-nose testing. The boy walks with shuffling, small steps; his gait has a slight lurching character, and he veers to the right.

Questions

1. What clinical situations are associated with increased intracranial pressure (ICP)?
2. What is the pathophysiological process leading to ICP?
3. What studies are used to evaluate children with ICP?
4. What measures are used to treat children with ICP?

The signs and symptoms of increased intracranial pressure (ICP) are often a signal of a serious intracranial process that may require surgical or intensive care intervention depending on the underlying cause. Because the process is frequently dynamic, it has proven useful to quantitate ICP for management purposes, although values in children are not as well correlated with pathophysiology as in adults. Normal ICP levels are somewhat lower in the neonatal and infantile period at 2 to 5 mm Hg, but in older children, pressures above 13 mm Hg (180 mm H_2O) are abnormal and may become symptomatic above 20 mm Hg. Although it is possible to have normal mental function up to 40 mm Hg, the ICP becomes clinically significant when the perfusion pressure is compromised, which begins when the ICP is 70 mm Hg below the mean arterial pressure, and it becomes more dangerous as the ICP approaches 40 to 50 mm Hg below the mean arterial pressure. Decreased perfusion produces swollen, damaged tissue, which further exacerbates the pressure-volume problem in a snowballing fashion.

Although only a relatively small number of effective treatments for increased ICP are available, greater understanding is accumulating about when to initiate them. It is important to recognize signs and symptoms early and determine the underlying cause; treatment of the cause may resolve the increased ICP, particularly if used early in the course. In other cases, however, increased ICP is a potentially life-threatening critical care issue where management, along with that of the underlying cause, is key for survival.

Epidemiology

Head trauma is a leading cause of increased ICP. Infants may be victims of non-accidental trauma; older children may be stricken pedestrians or bicycle riders, occupants of motor vehicles, or victims of falls; and adolescents may be victims of penetrating trauma such as gunshots. Such trauma is a major source of morbidity in children and requires careful monitoring and management of ICP.

Brain tumors are the most common solid neoplasms in children and frequently lead to increased ICP either by direct mass effect or blockage of cerebrospinal fluid (CSF) flow. Ischemic brain damage resulting from a difficult delivery at birth, a submersion incident, or a major cerebral vessel thrombosis is also a cause of increased ICP. Cytotoxic causes of brain swelling, such as lead intoxication and liver failure in Reye syndrome, are less common etiologies.

Idiopathic intracranial hypertension (also called benign intracranial hypertension or pseudotumor cerebri) may also lead to increased ICP. This condition is seen most frequently in obese adolescent females, but has also been seen with thrombosis of a lateral venous sinus following complicated otitis media, or following the use of high doses of vitamin A or tetracycline or withdrawal of steroid therapy.

Clinical Presentation

Children with increased ICP may present with a history of recurrent vomiting, lethargy, and headaches of increasing frequency or severity or that awaken them from sleep. A prior history of trauma, ischemia, meningitis, or having a CSF shunt, or a concomitant history of intoxication such as with lead or metabolic aberration (ie, Reye syndrome or diabetic ketoacidosis) may also raise suspicions of increased ICP in the child with compatible examination findings. Neonates with intraventricular hemorrhage or meningomyelocele are prone to hydrocephalus. Children with cyanotic congenital heart disease are prone to abscesses, and children with sickle cell disease can present with strokes or hemorrhages causing increased ICP. In endemic areas of the world, cerebral malaria and intraventricular cysticercosis are frequent causes of increased ICP. Physical findings may include elevated optic disk, failure of upward gaze, hypertonicity of the extremities, and depressed alertness or inattention. Localized findings on neurologic examination may point to a lesion indicative of a space-occupying intracranial mass, which could contribute to increased ICP (Dx Box).

Dx Increased Intracranial Pressure

- Loss of appetite, nausea, vomiting, headache, or lethargy
- Inattention, decreased arousability
- Papilledema, upward gaze paresis
- Increased tone, positive Babinski reflex
- Focal signs and history compatible with an intracranial mass
- Mass lesion, cerebral edema, or enlarged ventricles in an imaging study

Pathophysiology

The problem of increased ICP can be understood in terms of the Monro-Kellie doctrine, which applies to the rigid cranial compartment and pressure-volume relationships of the contents. Intracranial volume has 3 main components: brain parenchyma, CSF, and blood. Except in the first 2 years of life before most of the cranial sutures are fused, the skull and dura form a relatively rigid compartment; any increase in 1 of the 3 intracranial volume components must occur at the expense of 1 or both of the other 2. Decreased volume leads to increased pressure in a nonlinear relationship related to compliance of the skull, sutures, and dura. As compliance decreases, pressure rises rapidly. Irreversible damage to brain tissue occurs primarily as a result of pressure of the other components overtaking the arterial blood pressure and not allowing adequate tissue perfusion. In younger children, non-fused sutures allow more compliance if volume increases are relatively slow, but this factor is not true for acute volume increases. In addition, pressure gradients exist across compartments, sites of CSF flow obstruction, or even around lesions within brain parenchyma, which may lead to focal findings that are more difficult to explain by global ICP or perfusion changes.

Changes in any of the 3 components making up the intracranial volume may result in increased ICP in several ways. First, the brain parenchyma component may be directly increased by mass lesions such as neoplasms, abscesses, or hemorrhages. Edema may increase the brain parenchyma volume. Fluid may accumulate because of vascular leakage due to cytokines termed vasogenic edema. Brain edema may also result from cytotoxic damage, cell death, and necrosis. Cytotoxic processes include swelling of intact cells, cell rupture producing increased interstitial oncotic pressure from released proteins and ions, and cellular inflammatory and repair processes. Cytotoxic brain edema may be caused by various cellular insults including hypoxemia; ischemia; toxins, including neuronal excitotoxins; and depletion of energy substrates. These cellular insults may in turn be a consequence of a diversity of local or diffuse brain problems including major vessel thrombosis, trauma (eg, local contusion or diffuse axonal injury), anoxia from cardiac arrest, hypertension, encephalitic infection, or metabolic poisoning. Edema with head trauma may be a combination of vasogenic and cytotoxic edema, but also may be related to neurogenic inflammatory release of substance P and calcitonin gene–related peptide.

Second, the pressure of the CSF volume component (ventricles or subarachnoid spaces) may increase in hydrocephalus. Hydrocephalus can result in 2 ways: (1) from a discrepancy in the rate of formation of CSF relative to absorption, and (2) from an obstruction between the point of formation in the lateral ventricles and the sites of absorption at the arachnoid granulations in the post-neonatal brain or brain parenchyma in the neonatal brain. An obstruction can occur with a congenital malformation; parenchymal or CSF mass such as a cyst or neoplasm; CSF inflammatory cells from meningitis, ventriculitis, or hemorrhage; displaced brain parenchyma; subarachnoid protein or debris; or even overgrowth of dural tissue. The small passageways connecting the ventricular system, the foramen of Monro and the aqueduct of Sylvius; the exits of the ventricular system, the foramen of Magendie and foramen of Luschka; and the cisterns surrounding the brain stem are particularly vulnerable points of obstruction. A third type of brain edema, interstitial edema, is characterized by transependymal transudation of CSF into the adjacent white matter and is generally seen in patients with hydrocephalus.

Third, ICP may rise because the intravascular volume component may increase. One process that leads to this increase is venous outflow obstruction such as occurs with a dural sinus thrombosis. Other processes that raise jugular venous pressure may also increase ICP. In addition, the intracranial arterial vascular volume is affected by carbon dioxide partial pressure. It not only increases with hypercarbia but also decreases with hypocarbia, which allows for central neurogenic or iatrogenic lowering of ICP by hyperventilation.

As ICP increases, brain perfusion pressure may be maintained up to a point by a spontaneous increase in mean arterial pressure, a response referred to as Cushing phenomenon. Although the relationship may not be direct and universally reliable, the rise in systemic pressure can be a useful clinical sign of increased ICP. Normally changes in arterial cerebrovascular resistance meet changes in perfusion pressure to maintain constant cerebral blood flow, a process called *autoregulation*. This process is frequently compromised after head trauma or asphyxia.

Acute or subacute changes in pressure in an intracranial compartment may produce a pressure gradient that may precipitate a brain herniation syndrome (Figure 53-1). An ominous heralding sign of transtentorial herniation of the uncus of the temporal lobe is loss of the pupillary light reflex caused by entrapment of the third cranial nerve. This herniation often leads to irreversible brain stem damage as well as infarcts and additional secondary edema. Focally increased posterior fossa pressure may result in a pressure cone downward through the foramen magnum–compressing medullary centers leading to apnea and death. A marginally compensated system could be decompensated by an ill-advised lumbar puncture when the spinal compartment pressure is acutely lowered, increasing the pressure gradient across the foramen magnum.

Differential Diagnosis

Seizures, metabolic derangements, and complicated migraine sometimes have a clinical presentation similar to increased ICP. In children who are only partially responsive, distinguishing an ictal or postictal state from a condition that may be producing increased ICP is sometimes difficult. Findings that suggest a seizure include rhythmic, clonic movements or sudden myoclonic jerks; rapid or variable changes of tone or posturing that are different from decerebrate posturing; abrupt, fluctuating changes of autonomic function (eg, heart rate, blood pressure, pupillary size); saliva production without swallowing; and history of prior seizures. Sometimes, however, only direct electroencephalogram (EEG) monitoring and ICP monitoring are able to distinguish ongoing seizure activity from increased ICP as the cause of the change in level of responsiveness.

In some cases, diffuse brain dysfunction from a toxic or metabolic etiology mimics increased ICP. Such toxic/metabolic causes include medication toxicity, electrolyte or blood chemistry imbalances, and systemic infections. With toxic/metabolic disorders, inattention is often accompanied by a confusional state with disorientation, incoherence, and sometimes agitation. In contrast, with increased ICP, inattention is frequently accompanied by slowness of thought, perseveration, decreased mental activity, and impaired gait, although these differences are not universal.

The symptoms and signs of complicated migraine sometimes also mimic those of increased ICP. At the initial headache presentation or when only a short headache history is present, the complicated migraine diagnosis may be one of exclusion. If children display focal neurologic signs along with some symptoms of increased ICP, imaging studies to rule out space-occupying lesions and then laboratory

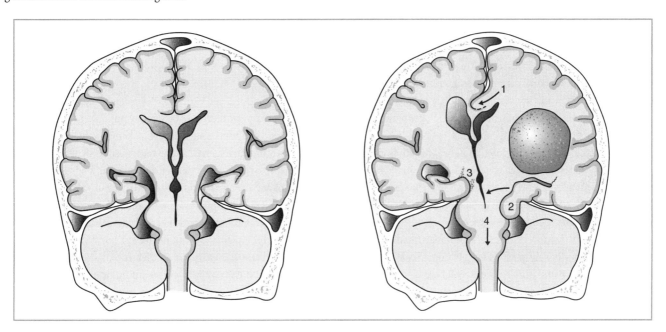

Figure 53-1. Depiction of the anatomy of several potential herniation syndromes caused by intracranial compartment pressure gradients related to a mass (hematoma, neoplasm, or acutely necrotic brain tissue) in a cerebral hemisphere. 1. Transfalcine herniation. 2. Uncal herniation. 3. Contralateral tentorial-midbrain damage. 4. Central herniation and foramen magnum pressure cone. These syndromes often lead to further brain ischemia and additional increases in intracranial pressure. The drawing on the left depicts a normal brain.

confirmation of normal pressure by lumbar puncture manometry may need to be performed.

Evaluation

History

A thorough neurologic history should be taken (Questions Box). Headache, nausea and vomiting, drowsiness, personality change, and changes in visual acuity are important historical factors. The headache history may be "crescendo" in frequency or intensity and of only a few days' or weeks' duration. The headache may be worsened by cough, micturition, or defecation.

Questions

Increased Intracranial Pressure

- How long has the child been vomiting?
- When does the vomiting occur?
- Is the vomiting related to meals?
- Do the headaches awaken the child?
- Has there been a progressive decline in activity level or loss of developmental skills?
- Does the child display weakness or change in gait?
- Does the child have a recent history of trauma or potential ischemic event?

Physical Examination

Vital signs and head circumference should be noted. A careful neurologic examination is warranted whenever increased ICP is suspected. Particular attention should be paid to the mental status and level of responsiveness of patients. The presence of papilledema and cranial nerve function should be assessed. Retinal hemorrhages may raise the suspicion of non-accidental trauma. Cranial nerve VI is particularly susceptible to displacement by increased ICP. Impaired upward gaze and lid retraction may be present. Specific muscle tone and strength as well as gait should be evaluated in cooperative children who are able. Posturing responses and the breathing pattern should be noted in comatose children to help ascertain brain stem localization of the lesion. In such children, findings should be reassessed at frequent intervals to follow a potentially rapid process such as impending tentorial or brain stem herniation, which would necessitate immediate intervention measures.

Useful quick-assessment instruments for initial, rapid evaluation and subsequent monitoring are the Glasgow Coma Scale (GCS) and Children's (ages ≤4 years) Coma Scale (see Tables 52-1 and 52-2 in Chapter 52). However, these scales do not contain adequate information for all clinical decisions related to patients with increased ICP.

In infants, a unique collection of signs—enlarged head circumference; bulging, raised fontanelle; frontal bone bossing with prominent venous distention; "sunset sign" (inability to elevate the eyes and lid retraction from midbrain tectal pressure); hypertonicity; and

hyperreflexia—may be secondary to increased ICP from hydrocephalus. Papilledema is not present, perhaps related to greater compliance of the infant skull.

Chronic hydrocephalus may result in optic atrophy, depressed hypothalamic functions, spastic lower limbs, and learning problems.

Laboratory Tests

If mental status changes are suggestive of a toxic or metabolic aberration, appropriate laboratory screens should be performed. These may include electrolytes, toxicological screen, liver function tests, and kidney function tests. A CSF examination should be done if signs of meningeal irritation or infection are present without lateralized signs of altered tone or strength. Imaging study evidence of an intercompartmental pressure gradient that could lead to herniation after lumbar puncture would also lead one away from that procedure, but CSF analysis and pressure measurements can also be made from ventricular taps after ventriculostomy. If there are clinical signs of increased ICP and no focal clinical or imaging signs of a mass, then a lumbar puncture can be both diagnostic and therapeutic for idiopathic intracranial hypertension.

Imaging Studies

A computed tomography (CT) or magnetic resonance imaging scan should be performed whenever children's signs or symptoms indicate the possibility of increased ICP. Severe head trauma patients frequently have a dynamic pathophysiology and may benefit from serial CT scanning along with their ICP monitoring. Intravenous (IV) contrast should be given if disruption in the blood-brain barrier (eg, infection, inflammation, neoplasia) is suspected and children are not hypersensitive and have adequate kidney function. A magnetic resonance venogram can be obtained if there is a possibility of a venous sinus thrombosis.

Management

If idiopathic intracranial hypertension is diagnosed, pressure should be monitored periodically with lumbar punctures. Increased ICP may respond to diuretics such as acetazolamide at high dose (20 mg/kg/d) or furosemide as well as the removal of CSF during the lumbar puncture. The primary danger in this condition is an expanding blind spot and eventual blindness due to pressure at the optic nerve head. Visual fields should also be monitored, and if medical therapy is not successful, then optic nerve sheath fenestration or lumbar peritoneal shunt placement can be done surgically.

When diagnostic imaging studies reveal an etiology for the increased ICP, if it is a rapidly enlarging surgically accessible lesion such as an epidural hematoma, then management is emergently directed at the cause. In such cases, immediate **neurosurgical craniotomy** may be necessary. Other focal space-occupying lesions seen on scans may not require immediate craniotomy, depending on size, position, and accompanying edema of the lesion as well as the compliance of the surrounding structures and the distortion of normal brain tissue and potential for loss of perfusion; neoplastic lesions may require diagnostic biopsy or excisional biopsy within a few days if surgically accessible. **Mineralocorticoids (dexamethasone 0.25–0.5 mg/kg every 6 hours)** are useful in situations in which the pressure is produced by a component of vasogenic edema, such as that surrounding neoplasms. A histamine H_2 blocker should also be used to help prevent gastric ulcer. Hypotonic IV fluids should be avoided, and the patient should be monitored for the syndrome of inappropriate secretion of antidiuretic hormone with serum and urine osmolalities. Hypoglycemia and hyperglycemia should also be avoided. If acute danger of herniation due to a pressure gradient produced by CSF flow blockage is present, then a temporary ventriculostomy may be indicated to relieve the CSF pressure. If an infectious process is present, including focal lesions, abscess, cerebritis, or encephalitis, **antibiotics** and/or **antiviral** agents are indicated after appropriate cultures, serology, and molecular diagnostic tests have been done. Following directed specific treatment of the underlying lesion, increased ICP may eventually resolve spontaneously. If hydrocephalus due to CSF flow obstruction is still present after initial therapy, **ventriculoperitoneal shunting of CSF** may be necessary. Endoscopic third ventriculotomy avoids long-term hardware complications of obstruction and infection, but is much less successful in the younger children.

Encephalopathic children whose ICP is markedly elevated or likely to rise rapidly require treatment in an intensive care unit. If there is no mass or other space-occupying lesion or necrotic, traumatized tissue able to be surgically removed, then interventional measures are directed toward preventing eventual loss of perfusion of normal brain tissue. In patients with head injury, a GCS score of 8 or less can be used as a guideline for ICP monitoring. Intracranial pressure can be monitored on an ongoing basis with commonly used neurosurgically placed devices including the fiberoptic microtransducer and intraventricular catheter or ventriculostomy. The former device can measure pressure in brain parenchyma as well as in fluid-filled spaces. An advantage of the latter device is that it also allows for therapeutic CSF drainage to relieve pressure. It carries a slight risk of infection (increasing to a plateau at day 4 of 1%–2% per day) or hemorrhage and may be difficult to place if ventricles are small or shifted. Intracranial pressure monitoring with neurosurgically placed devices and therapy based on the measurements, however, have not been helpful in many cases of ischemic damage, infection, or poisoning because of the totality of brain involvement without normal remaining tissue to which perfusion could be maintained.

Children with a decreased or fluctuating level of responsiveness may require EEG monitoring of cerebral electrical activity. The EEG helps diagnose the abnormal responsiveness as seizure threshold may fluctuate and seizures may occur even in the presence of increased ICP. Anticonvulsant therapy is indicated if evidence of clinical or electrographic seizures is present. In addition, the EEG may be used to monitor barbiturate-induced coma, which may be used for severely increased ICP.

Airway patency and ventilation are important in children with increased ICP because hypoxia and hypercarbia can contribute to vasodilation and increased pressure. Rapid sequence intubation should be performed to minimize elevations of ICP. Ketamine and succinylcholine can increase ICP also. Transmission of elevated intrathoracic pressure to intracranial vessels can be avoided by sedation and decreasing the inspiratory phase of the ventilator. If acute lowering of pressure is necessary, hyperventilation to reduce the intracranial arterial blood volume is most effective, but care must be taken to avoid decreasing brain cell perfusion to the point of producing ischemic damage and exacerbating the problem. It is recommended that carbon dioxide partial pressure be kept at 30 to 35 mm Hg. Elevating the head to about 30 degrees and avoiding flexion or excessive turning of the neck to prevent jugular kinking are also effective in reducing ICP. Because the goal is to ensure perfusion while lowering ICP, maintaining and even elevating systemic mean arterial pressure by appropriate use of fluid therapy and pressor agents are key. Central venous pressure monitoring may also be helpful.

Diuretic agents such as mannitol (osmotherapy) (0.25–1 g/kg bolus) may also be useful in reducing brain volume by removing water, changing the rheologic characteristics of blood, and producing reflex vasoconstriction, but caution is advised. Mannitol, as a chronic infusion, can eventually cross the blood-brain barrier and draw more fluid into the brain. It is most effective where the blood-brain barrier is intact. Hypertonic saline (3%) as a continuous infusion may be an effective alternative. Serum osmolarity greater than 320 mOsm/kg can lead to renal failure. By giving diuretic agents at intervals as a bolus and titrating up to the ICP-lowering dose, such effects can generally be avoided. Sometimes these agents are used to counter ICP plateau waves or increased pressure with endotracheal suctioning or other procedures.

In children with severe refractory increased ICP, especially if secondary to an acute focal process, barbiturates such as pentobarbital or the benzodiazepine midazolam can be given as a continuous IV infusion with appropriate monitoring of brain electrical activity, serum levels, and systemic and brain perfusion pressures (Box 53-1). These agents may serve to reduce brain metabolism without impairing vascular autoregulation significantly. Their risk is in reducing cardiac output and with associated infections, particularly pneumonia. Xenon CT measures multiple areas of local blood flow and may be a useful bedside technique to help specify targeted therapies. Decompressive craniotomy or craniectomy in early severe trauma in small series of patients has been associated with up to 50% good outcomes. Hypothermia to 93.2°F (34°C) for head injury and numerous "neuroprotective" agents have been and continue to be studied as means to slow metabolism and reduce the rate of cytotoxic edema increase in the penumbra surrounding the irreversibly damaged brain tissue.

Box 53-1. Management Interventions in Increased ICP

- Maintain serum osmols at 300–320 mOsm
- Keep head elevated to 30 degrees
- Maintain normal or elevated systemic blood pressure
- Controlled hyperventilation to $PaCO_2$ at 30–35 mm Hg
- Supplemental O_2 and PEEP as needed to keep PaO_2 >90 mm Hg and FiO_2 <50%
- If ICP progressively rises, pressure waves higher than 20 mm Hg last longer than 5 minutes, or any pressure in first 24 hours is higher than 30 mm Hg, then give mannitol, 250–1,000 mg/kg IV
- If mannitol needs repeating in <4 hours or osmolality is >320 mOsm:
  — Give pentobarbital, 5 mg/kg IV, then 2 mg/kg/h IV monitoring to blood level of 25–35 µg/mL, burst-suppression pattern with 10 s between bursts on EEG, and cardiac index >2.7 L/min/m²

  or

  — Give midazolam by titrating the dose starting at 0.1 mg/kg/hr IV to the same EEG criteria and limited by the same cardiac index criteria

Abbreviations: ICP, intracranial pressure; $PaCO_2$, carbon dioxide partial pressure; PEEP, positive end-expiratory pressure; PaO_2, oxygen partial pressure; FiO_2, fraction of inspired oxygen; IV, intravenous; EEG, electroencephalogram.

Prognosis

Children may recover fully from increased ICP if brain perfusion pressure is adequately maintained and the underlying brain lesion generating the increased pressure can be resolved. Ultimately the prognosis depends on the nature of the lesion; its propensity to generate ICP that may be refractory to treatment, leading to brain tissue damage or death; and its permanence or potential for recurrence.

CASE RESOLUTION

The boy in the case history has focal signs and symptoms referable to the posterior fossa brain as well as symptoms of increased intracranial pressure (ICP). An emergent computed tomography scan shows subacute hydrocephalus due to obstruction of cerebrospinal fluid flow produced by a large mass in the cerebellum and brain stem on the left side. He begins taking dexamethasone with some relief of the increased ICP symptoms. Two days later the mass is surgically excised and is found to be a medulloblastoma. Because the ICP remains high, a ventriculoperitoneal shunt is subsequently required for the hydrocephalus. The boy's recovery is otherwise uneventful, and he begins evaluation for further brain tumor therapy.

Selected References

American Academy of Pediatrics Committee on Child Abuse and Neglect. Shaken baby syndrome: inflicted cerebral trauma. *Pediatrics.* 1993;92:872–875

Ball A, Clarke C. Idiopathic intracranial hypertension. *Lancet Neurol.* 2006; 5:433–442

Del Bigio M. Cellular damage and prevention in childhood hydrocephalus. *Brain Pathol.* 2004;14:317–24

Fishman RA. *Cerebrospinal Fluid in Diseases of the Nervous System.* 2nd ed. Philadelphia, PA: W. B. Saunders; 1992

Garton H, Piatt J. Hydrocephalus. *Pediatr Clin North Am.* 2004;51:305–325

Huff K. Central nervous system failure. In: Osborn L, DeWitt T, First L, Zenel J, eds. *Pediatrics.* Philadelphia, PA: Elsevier; 2005

Kotagal S. Increased intracranial pressure. In: Swaiman K, Ashwal S, Ferriero D, eds. *Pediatric Neurology Principles and Practice.* 4th ed. Philadelphia, PA: Mosby; 2006

Marcoux K. Management of increased intracranial pressure in the critically ill child with an acute neurological injury. *AACN Clin Issues.* 2005;16:212–231

Fluid and Electrolyte Disturbances

Charlotte W. Lewis, MD, MPH, and Sudhir K. Anand, MD

CASE STUDY

A 2-year-old boy presents to your office after 2 days of vomiting and diarrhea. His siblings were both ill a few days ago with similar symptoms. Two weeks ago his weight was 12 kg at a well-child visit. Today his weight is 10.8 kg. He has a pulse of 130/min, respiratory rate of 28/min, blood pressure of 85/55. He is alert and responsive but appears tired. He has dry mucous membranes, no tears with crying, and slightly sunken-appearing eyeballs. His capillary refill is 2 seconds. He urinated a small amount about 6 hours ago. Despite his mother's best efforts in your office, the patient has vomited all of the oral rehydration therapy given to him. You draw serum electrolytes, blood urea nitrogen, and creatinine and initiate intravenous rehydration.

Questions

1. How does one assess the magnitude of dehydration in children?
2. What are the different types of dehydration?
3. How does one determine the type and amount of fluid that a dehydrated child requires?
4. How does one assess renal status in a dehydrated child?
5. What is the role of electrolyte and acid-base laboratory studies in the evaluation of the dehydrated child?

Pediatrics is unique among fields in medicine in its focus on the growing and developing individual. Within the scope of pediatric practice, patients may range in size and weight from the less than 1 kg preterm infant to the greater than 100 kg adolescent. Young children, like adults, maintain fluid and electrolyte balance under a variety of physiological conditions; however, during illness their homeostatic adjustments may be less efficient than those of adult patients. Clinicians caring for children must feel comfortable in determining fluid and electrolyte needs for healthy children as they grow from infants into adults and understand how fluid and electrolyte needs are altered in dehydration and other illnesses.

Epidemiology

Dehydration is one of the most common medical problems encountered in pediatrics. In the United States, dehydration, as the result of common childhood illnesses, is responsible for 2 million to 3 million clinic visits and approximately 10% of all pediatric hospital admissions. Worldwide, 8,000 children younger than 5 years die *every day* from diarrhea and dehydration.

Maintenance Fluid and Electrolyte Requirements

The body has a **maintenance fluid requirement** to replace daily normal losses that occur through the kidney, intestines, skin, and respiratory tract. Of the various methods available for the determination of fluid needs, the most common is the **caloric method,** which is based on the linear relationship between metabolic rate and fluid needs. For every 100 calories expended in metabolism, a child requires about 100 mL of water. Metabolic rate in children is a function of body surface area. Infants, with higher relative surface areas per unit of body weight, have higher metabolic rates and, therefore, higher fluid requirements per unit weight. As children grow, their relative surface area decreases as does their metabolic rate and fluid requirement per unit weight. Using this relationship, maintenance fluid needs can be calculated for the healthy child using the method outlined in Table 54-1. These calculations of fluid needs are often used to determine the amount of intravenous (IV) fluids provided to a hospitalized child or to calculate the approximate amount of fluid a healthy child requires orally to maintain hydration. However, these calculations may not be appropriate for critically ill children,

Table 54-1. Caloric Method of Determining Maintenance Fluid Requirements in Healthy Children	
Weight	*Maintenance Fluid Requirement for 24 Hours*
3ᵃ–10 kg	100 mL/kg/dᵇ
11–20 kg	50 mL/kg/d for each kg above 10 kg + 1,000 mL (fluid requirement for first 10 kg)
>20 kg	20 mL/kg/d for each kg above 20 kg + 1,500 mL (fluid requirement for first 20 kg)

ᵃChildren weighing less than 3 kg may have altered fluid requirements owing to prematurity or other conditions.

ᵇDuring the first 2 to 3 days of life, normal term infants require less fluid (approximately 80 mL/kg) because they mobilize excess extracellular fluid.

some of whom require fluid restriction and others of whom may have increased fluid needs. Moreover, the caloric method makes no allowance for extra fluid needed for weight gain, growth, activity, or pathophysiological states that increase fluid needs (such as fever). The fluid requirement derived from this method is valid to determine the daily fluid need for an essentially healthy child. Thriving infants normally drink more fluid than this method suggests. On average, growing infants may take 150 to 200 mL/kg/d of milk (breast or infant formula) as desired to support the average weight gain of 30 g/d usually observed in the first few months of life.

Replacement of normal daily losses of electrolytes is considered when a child is not able to take an adequate nutritional intake orally (as in the example in Box 54-1, where the child receives nothing orally in preparation for surgery). Electrolyte quantities are usually expressed as milliequivalent (mEq) or millimole (mmol) amount per 100 mL of fluid required. Traditionally, the recommended **sodium** (Na^+) requirement for a healthy child is 3 mEq/100 mL fluid required, and the **potassium** (K^+) requirement is 2 to 2.5 mEq/100 mL of fluid (see Box 54-1, part B for sample calculation and IV order). As discussed in more detail below, K^+ should only be given to a patient after ensuring adequate renal function. These estimations of Na^+ and K^+ requirements are meant to replace normal daily losses and would not be adequate in the face of increased electrolyte losses that can occur in a number of pathologic conditions (such as diarrhea). Moreover, there has recently been increasing focus on the risk of hyponatremia and related complications developing in hospitalized ill children.

Relatively healthy, well-nourished children receiving IV fluids for a brief period (ie, 1–2 days) while hospitalized do not routinely require supplementation with other electrolytes such as calcium and magnesium. However, it is important to realize that standard IV fluids containing 5% dextrose, sodium chloride (NaCl), and potassium chloride (KCl) provide only minimal caloric needs and do not adequately support weight gain or provide other necessary nutrients. Children who require prolonged IV therapy because of inadequate gastrointestinal (GI) tract function should receive total parenteral nutrition to better meet their caloric and nutritional needs.

Box 54-1. Example of Fluid Calculations

Part A

Case: A 22-kg boy is given nothing orally in preparation for an elective abdominal surgery. How much intravenous (IV) fluid per hour should he receive as he awaits the surgery?

- For first 10 kg: 100 mL/kg/d × 10 kg = 1,000 mL
- For next 10 kg (to get to 20 kg): 50 mL/kg/d × 10 kg = 500 mL
- For next 2 kg (to get to 22 kg): 20 mL/kg/d × 2 kg = 40 mL

1,000 mL + 500 mL + 40 mL = 1,540 mL/24 h

IV rate per hour = 64.2 mL/h (with a healthy child, round off to 65 mL/h for ease of administration)

Part B

Question: How much sodium (Na^+) and potassium (K^+) should this patient receive in his IV fluids?

Answer: 3 mEq Na^+/100 mL (1 dL) of fluid = 3 mEq × 15.4 dL = 46.2 mEq Na^+/d in 1,540 mL of water or 30 mEq NaCl/L

2.5 mEq K^+/100 mL (1 dL) of fluid = 2.5 × 15.4 = 38.5 mEq K^+/d in 1,540 mL of water or 25 mEq KCl/L

One possible way to write an IV order for this patient

D5 0.2 NS with 20 mEq KCl/L to run at 65 mL/h.

Note: D5 = 5% dextrose water; normal saline (NS) contains 154 mEq NaCl/L and 0.2 NS contains 34 mEq NaCl. This solution is a widely available, premade IV solution that provides the approximate daily Na^+ requirement of the patient.

Alterations in Fluid Needs in Illness

A number of conditions alter fluid requirements. Conditions that increase a patient's metabolic rate (eg, fever) will also increase their fluid requirement. A child's metabolic rate is increased 12% for every 1°C temperature elevation above normal. Most otherwise healthy children with free access to fluids will increase their own intake to account for increased needs when febrile. Other less common hypermetabolic states, such as thyrotoxicoses or salicylate poisoning, may have an even more dramatic effect, perhaps increasing metabolic rate by 25% to 50% over maintenance. In these cases and for children who are dependent on others to provide their fluids, clinicians must be aware of the magnitude of increased need and provide supplemental fluids to avoid dehydration.

Other conditions may decrease a child's fluid requirement. In hypometabolic states such as hypothyroidism, metabolic rate and fluid needs are decreased by 10% to 25%. Fluid requirements are decreased by 10% to 25% in high environmental humidity unless the ambient temperature is also high and results in visible sweating. In these situations, a healthy child with normal renal function given extra fluid beyond what is needed can, within limits, effectively excrete any excessive intake. Children with renal failure, however, pose a special challenge for the clinician in the management of fluid and electrolytes. When a child is unable to adequately excrete excessive fluid intake, this fluid can accumulate and lead to complications such as congestive heart failure and pulmonary edema. Without functioning kidneys, only **insensible fluid losses** need to be replaced. Insensible losses occur primarily through the skin and respiratory tract; they account for approximately 40% of maintenance fluid needs. However, fluid needs for patients with renal failure are usually estimated at 30% of the maintenance requirement, with additional fluids provided if needed. This is to avoid giving excessive fluids that may require dialysis for removal.

Fluid requirements may also be decreased under circumstances where **arginine vasopressin** (AVP, also called antidiuretic hormone) is increased. In addition to hypovolemia or hypertonicity (hyperosmolality), AVP release is also stimulated by pain, nausea, surgery (postoperatively), central nervous system (CNS) infections such as meningitis and encephalitis, severe pneumonia or respirator use, and certain medications (including thiazide diuretics, chemotherapeutic agents, and selective serotonin reuptake inhibitors). Arginine vasopressin release in the absence of hypovolemia or hypertonicity results in hyponatremia, and is referred to as **SIADH** (syndrome of inappropriate antidiuretic hormone release). In patients with SIADH, both fluid restriction as well as administration of fluids with a higher Na^+ concentration may be indicated.

What exactly is the most appropriate Na^+ concentration of IV fluids for hospitalized children admitted to a pediatric intensive care unit or in postoperative patients is an area of current controversy. Over the past 25 years most such children have been maintained on a solution containing 5% dextrose water in half normal saline (D5 0.5 NS) or lower Na^+ concentration. There are concerns that such children, due to the kidney retaining free water in response to excessive AVP found in some of these patients, are at risk for developing hyponatremia and resulting hyponatremic encephalopathy, which can lead to brain stem herniation and death or permanent brain damage. Some pediatric nephrologists and intensivists have recently recommended that we should forgo Na^+ calculations in hospitalized very sick children and instead rely solely on isotonic fluids for their management. Other pediatric nephrologists have cautioned that before abandoning previous practices, we must make certain that the new recommendations using isotonic fluids only do not result in excessive congestive heart failure or hypernatremia. Regardless of the approach that is taken, close attention to the type and quantity of fluids provided, quantity of body fluid output, weight change, and serial electrolyte assessments are important in the management of all sick children and must be individualized to prevent serious complications.

Pathophysiology

Dehydration is one of the most common pathophysiological alterations in fluid balance encountered in pediatrics. Although strictly speaking dehydration means deficit of water only, most children with dehydration have lost both water and electrolytes. Dehydration can result from (1) diminished intake, (2) excessive losses through the GI tract (eg, diarrhea or vomiting), (3) excessive losses from the kidney or skin (eg, polyuria due to osmotic diuresis in uncontrolled diabetes), or (4) a combination of these factors.

Children are at increased risk for episodes of dehydration for a number of reasons. Young children have 3 to 4 times the body surface area per unit body weight compared with adults and so have relatively higher fluid needs. It is therefore much easier for children to become dehydrated in the face of the decreased intake or increased losses that often accompany common childhood illnesses. For example, acute gastroenteritis, which is common in young children, often leads to anorexia, recurrent vomiting, and frequent or large-volume stools, with proportionately more severe fluid loss than in older children and adults. In addition, infants and young children are dependent beings who are unable to increase their own fluid intake in response to thirst and must rely on others to provide their fluid needs. If these fluid needs are not met or are underestimated, children can easily become dehydrated.

Dehydration is classified as **isotonic, hypotonic, or hypertonic.** When considering acute dehydration, these terms are often used interchangeably with **isonatremic, hypernatremic,** and **hyponatremic** dehydration, respectively, because it is the Na^+ content of the extracellular fluid (ECF) that largely determines serum osmolality in otherwise healthy dehydrated children. In acute **isotonic** or isonatremic dehydration (serum Na^+ 135–150 mEq/L), the most common type of dehydration, there is net loss of isotonic fluid containing both Na^+ and K^+ (Figure 54-1, top). Sodium, the primary ECF cation, is lost not only to the environment but some also shifts to the intracellular fluid (ICF) to balance the loss of K^+, because K^+ losses from cells are generally not accompanied by intracellular anionic losses in acute dehydration. The Na^+ that has shifted into the ICF will return to the ECF compartment with rehydration. There is no net loss of fluid from the ICF in this process; the total water deficit in dehydration comes primarily from the ECF, although some suggest that two-thirds of the losses come from ECF and one-third from ICF.

Hypertonic or **hypernatremic dehydration** (serum Na^+ >150 mEq/L) occurs when net loss of water exceeds that of solute loss (Figure 54-1, bottom). It is usually seen in clinical conditions where there is rapid loss of hypotonic fluid in stool, vomit, or urine accompanied by failure of adequate water intake due to anorexia or vomiting. Fever or hyperventilation, if present, may intensify the disproportionate loss of water. Occasionally, hypernatremic dehydration may be due to excessive solute intake. The urinary excretion of the excess solute obligates loss of large volumes of water, resulting in dehydration. The history may reveal that the child was accidentally fed a high Na^+ solution or concentrated formula. In hypernatremic dehydration, there is shift of fluid from the ICF to the ECF to attain osmotic balance. As such, the ECF volume is somewhat spared at the expense of the ICF, and signs of dehydration may be delayed. However, fluid loss from the ICF results in intracellular dehydration, the most serious effect of which can occur in the brain. If hypernatremia occurs rapidly, there is not only a decrease in brain size but also a fall in cerebral spinal fluid (CSF) pressure owing to diffusion of water from CSF to the blood. As the brain shrinks, the bridging veins within the skull may stretch and even tear, resulting in subdural hemorrhage or other complications. If the hypernatremic state

Figure 54-1. **Pathophysiology of various types of dehydration. Abbreviations: ECF, extracellular fluid; ICF, intracellular fluid; Na⁺, sodium; K⁺, potassium; H₂O, water.**

develops more slowly, the brain cell size may initially shrink minimally but will gradually return to normal size even in the face of continued hypernatremia. The preservation of the brain cell volume despite hypernatremia is thought to be due to the generation of idiogenic osmoles (myoinositol, trimethylamines, taurine, and other amino acids) that attract water back into the cell and maintain cell volume. Rehydration of the patient with hypernatremia must occur slowly and cautiously to avoid brain cell swelling (Figure 54-2). The skin, on clinical examination, in hypernatremic dehydration may sometimes feel "doughy" due to intracellular dehydration. This finding, however, is inconsistent even in the hands of experienced pediatricians and should not substitute for serum Na⁺ measurements to diagnose hypernatremia.

There are a variety of mechanisms by which **hyponatremia** (serum Na⁺ <135 mEq/L) occurs in association with dehydration. In **hyponatremic dehydration,** the ECF volume is compromised to a greater degree than in isotonic dehydration because of osmotic shifts of ECF into the cell, resulting in more severe signs of dehydration (Figure 54-l, middle). Hyponatremic dehydration typically

occurs in children with gastroenteritis when there are excessive Na⁺ losses in stool along with a parent giving oral replacement with water or very low Na⁺ beverages such as apple juice or tea. In hyponatremic dehydration, the kidney often excretes a concentrated urine (ie, retains free water) despite hyponatremia because AVP is stimulated by the decreased effective circulating volume. Intravascular volume depletion seems to be a potent stimulus for AVP release, overriding the AVP suppressive effect of hypotonicity/hyponatremia. The result is that serum Na⁺ levels are lowered due to dilution. Hyponatremic dehydration may sometimes also occur due to excessive loss of Na⁺ (relative to body water) in stool (eg, cholera) or in the urine (eg, adrenogenital syndrome, cerebral salt wasting, pseudohypoaldosteronism, and other salt-wasting renal disorders).

Evaluation

History

In addition to signs and symptoms of the current illness, the history should focus on the cause of dehydration. Parents should be questioned on the type and amount of oral intake; the duration, quality, and frequency of vomiting and/or diarrhea; whether blood is present in the stool; the presence or absence of fever; frequency of urination; and whether a recent pre-illness weight is known for the child (Questions Box). When parents report change in mental status, it is of particular concern because this may occur because of significant electrolyte (eg, Na⁺) disturbance, marked dehydration, or other serious infection or illness. The most accurate way to assess the degree of dehydration is to compare current weight with a recent pre-illness weight, although a prior weight is often unavailable. In acute dehydration, the loss of weight is primarily due to fluid loss. The difference between pre-illness and current weight can be used to determine the degree of the fluid deficit.

Physical Examination

An important goal of the physical examination of the dehydrated child is to assess the degree of dehydration. In the process, vital signs including blood pressure and a current weight should be obtained. Specific attention should be focused on the general appearance of the child and in particular whether he or she is ill-appearing, listless, or less reactive. In addition to the usual components of the physical examination, assessing for the following is important: whether the oral mucosal membranes appear tacky or dry; whether tears are present or absent; if tenting of the skin is present (abnormal when tenting remains after the skin is pinched between 2 fingers); and perfusion status of the extremities. In the process, it is important that the clinician recognize whether shock is present because this is a life-threatening condition that requires emergent treatment (see Chapter 49).

Because comparison to an accurate recent pre-illness weight usually is not possible, clinicians must rely on vital signs and clinical signs and symptoms to assess the degree of dehydration (Table 54-2). In infants and young children (<5 years), the estimated fluid loss for

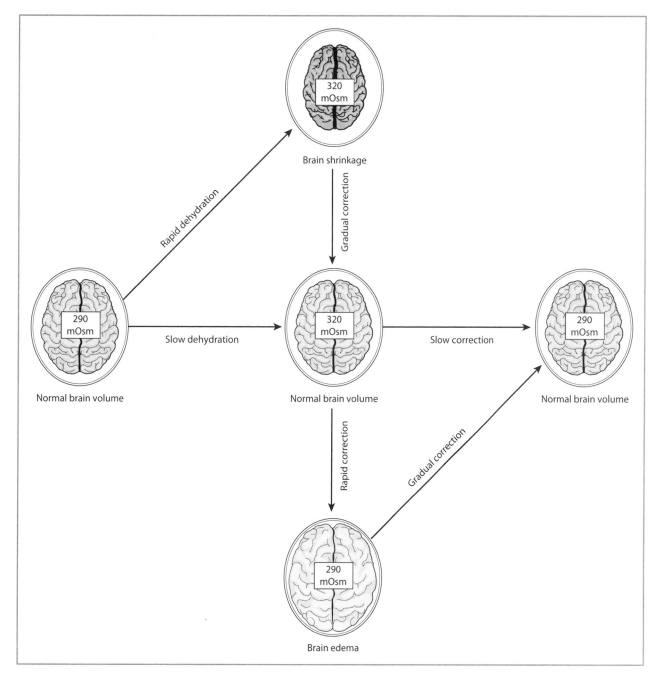

Figure 54-2. Hypernatremic dehydration. Effects on brain volume of rapid versus slow development of hypernatremia and results of rapid versus slow correction of hypernatremia.

Questions

Dehydration

- Has the child had vomiting or diarrhea?
- Has the child had fever?
- What has the child been eating or drinking?
- Has the child been urinating? How many wet diapers did the child have?
- How much did the child weigh at the last visit to the physician?
- Is your child's behavior or level of alertness changed from normal?

mild dehydration is 5% deficit of body water; moderate dehydration, 10%; and severe dehydration, 15%. The corresponding numbers for estimated fluid loss in older children are 3%, 6%, and 9%, respectively. A variety of clinical signs have been proposed to evaluate the degree of dehydration—some more valid and reliable than others. A 2004 systematic review found that assessment of capillary refill was the most useful single sign in detecting 5% or greater dehydration (capillary refill is assessed by placing brief pressure on the distal palmar aspect of a fingertip and assessing the amount of time for the blanched area to refill—normal is considered ≤2 seconds). Two other single signs found to be important in predicting 5% or greater

Table 54-2. Clinical Assessment of Magnitude of Dehydration

Clinical Signs	Mild Dehydration	Moderate Dehydration	Severe Dehydration

Loss of body weight
   Infant/young child
   Older child/adult
	
	5%
	3%
		
		10%
		6%
			
			15%
			9%

Skin turgor	Normal to slightly reduced	Decreased	Markedly decreased (tenting)
Skin color and temperature	Pale or normal	Ashen, cool	Mottled, cool
Dry mucous membranes	±	+	++
Absent tears	±	+	++
Sunken eyeballs	±	+	++
Increased pulse	±	+	++ (may be thready)
Blood pressure	Normal	Normal Postural decrease ±	Reduced (in late shock)
Urine output	Normal or reduced[a]	Oliguria[a]	Oliguria/anuria
Capillary refill time	Slightly prolonged	Prolonged	Prolonged

[a]Usually resumes with restoration of intravascular volume.

dehydration were abnormal skin turgor (ie, tenting) and respiratory disturbance, in particular hyperpnea (deep, rapid breathing without other signs of respiratory distress) suggestive of acidosis. In general, the more signs that are present the greater the severity of dehydration; however, a combination of delayed capillary refill time, absent tears, dry mucosal membranes, and general ill appearance may be equally as good as capillary refill, tenting, and hyperpnea combined in identifying children who have more than mild dehydration.

Laboratory Studies

Laboratory studies typically are not indicated in children who present with mild dehydration. Dehydrated children who are treated with IV fluids after failing oral rehydration should have initial assessment of their serum electrolytes, blood urea nitrogen, and creatinine. Initial and serial measurements of these laboratory studies should also be performed during rehydration in children with (1) shock, (2) severe dehydration, (3) decreased urine output that does not improve after initial restoration of intravascular volume, or (4) a history and clinical findings inconsistent with straightforward isotonic dehydration or found to have dysnatremia (ie, serum Na$^+$ outside of the normal range [135–150], whether too low or too high). Dehydration in association with dysnatremia can have serious complications, and treatment requires special considerations. Hemolytic uremic syndrome, although uncommon, should be considered in any child with gastroenteritis, particularly with a history of grossly bloody stool, who also has decreased urine output.

Very ill children may require an arterial blood gas measurement to more accurately assess their acid-base status; in others, serum electrolytes are sufficient. The usual acid-base derangement in the moderately dehydrated child is a non-anion gap acidosis (with hyperchloremia) due to bicarbonate losses in the stool. Severely dehydrated children may have an anion gap acidosis due to lactic acid and/or ketone accumulation in the peripheral tissues secondary to the decreased perfusion that accompanies hypovolemia. An interesting exception is seen in infants with pyloric stenosis, who typically manifest a hypokalemic, hypochloremic metabolic alkalosis.

Imaging Studies

Imaging studies such as chest x-ray, abdominal series, renal ultrasound, and computed tomography scans are indicated based on the suspected etiology of the dehydration.

Management

The management of the dehydrated child involves consideration of 3 components (1) normal **maintenance** fluid and electrolyte requirement, (2) fluid and electrolyte **deficit** incurred during the present illness, and (3) **ongoing fluid and electrolyte losses.** Most commonly, ongoing losses result from continued vomiting and diarrhea. Losses from diarrhea can be estimated at 10 mL/kg per stool and from vomitus at 5 mL/kg per vomiting episode. Other forms of ongoing losses that occasionally must be considered and replaced include those associated with burns, gastric secretion suctioned via nasogastric tube, hyperventilation, or prolonged fever. The estimation of children's fluid and electrolyte needs and losses are almost always an approximation and require close follow-up, reassessment, and readjustment throughout treatment. At the very least, monitoring during treatment for dehydration requires regular assessment of vital signs, body weight, intake, and output.

Fluid given to dehydrated children may be provided either **enterally** or **parenterally.** Whenever possible, **oral rehydration therapy (ORT)** using oral rehydration solution (ORS) is preferred for children with mild dehydration and most children with moderate dehydration. Parenteral fluid therapy should be used in children with more severe dehydration, when oral therapy has failed despite an adequate trial (eg, due to intractable vomiting or lethargy), in children in shock or impending shock, or when an anatomical defect such as pyloric stenosis or ileus is suspected.

Parenteral Fluid Therapy

The parenteral management of moderate or severe dehydration can be divided into 2 phases: an initial phase (first 1–2 hours) and the main phase of rehydration. The aim of the initial phase is to restore intravascular volume, thus improving perfusion and renal function and reversing tissue hypoxia and acidosis. Regardless of the type of dehydration (isonatremic, hypernatremic, or hyponatremic), NS (0.9% sodium chloride) plain or NS with 5% dextrose at 10 mL/kg/h generally provides the most rapid and effective means to expand the intravascular volume at acute presentation. If shock is present or imminent, the treatment is more aggressive (see Chapter 49). The child should immediately receive a 20 mL/kg bolus of NS given over 20 to 30 minutes. After the first bolus, the child should be reassessed, and if signs and symptoms of intravascular depletion persist, a second IV bolus of 20 mL/kg of NS should be given over 20 to 30 minutes and the child admitted to the hospital for further careful evaluation, including assessment for other causes of shock such as sepsis.

During the second phase of rehydration, the remaining fluid and electrolyte deficits are replaced based on the magnitude of these losses. These replacements are in addition to the daily maintenance requirements as well as any ongoing losses, as discussed previously. Various protocols exist to restore fluid and electrolyte deficits; approaches to treatment of dehydration at different institutions will vary. Many of the differences in rehydration strategies lie in the composition of treatment fluid and the rate at which it is administered. Some clinicians prefer to administer half of the total fluid needs over the first 8 hours and the remainder over the next 16 hours; others replace the fluid at the same rate over the entire rehydration period. The latter method is presented in the case resolution at the end of the chapter. Usually the fluid deficit is replaced within 24 hours. There are noteworthy exceptions. Treating dehydration associated with **dysnatremia** (ie, abnormally low or high serum Na$^+$) should entail slower return (eg, 12–15 mEq serum Na$^+$ change per 24 hours) to a normal range and may require 48 to 72 hours for correction.

Sodium replacement in the dehydrated child depends on the type of dehydration. In isotonic dehydration some clinicians elect to replace the entire fluid deficit with NS, others use a saline solution containing 110 mEq Na$^+$/L and still others 0.5 NS (77 mEq Na$^+$/L). We prefer to use 110 mEq Na$^+$/L to replace the fluid deficit (see Case Resolution for example). This is less than the 154 mEq Na$^+$/L in NS, but we base the use of 110 mEq Na$^+$/L solution on the assumption that some of the Na$^+$ lost from the ECF during isotonic dehydration is shifted intracellularly to balance K$^+$ losses and thus will return to the ECF during rehydration. Although the content of excreted body fluids can be analyzed for electrolyte content for more exact replacement, ongoing losses from, for example, frequent diarrheal stools, are commonly replaced with 0.5 NS. (This should be adequate in Na$^+$ content for most cases given diarrhea in rotavirus contains approximately 30 to 40 mEq Na$^+$/L and enterotoxigenic *Escherichia coli*: 50 to 60 mEq/L; however, Na$^+$ stool losses in cholera are 90–120 mEq/L.)

Management of Dehydration With Dysnatremia

In hypernatremic dehydration, the patient is considered to have a relative free water deficit but usually has lost not only body water, but also some Na$^+$. The amount of free water a patient requires to decrease their serum Na$^+$ to normal (eg, 145 mEq/L is desired serum Na$^+$) is calculated as follows:

$$[\text{patient weight in kilograms}] \times [\text{actual serum Na}^+ - \text{desired serum Na}^+] \times 4 \text{ mL/kg}$$

For serum Na$^+$ greater than 170 mEq/L, 3 mL/kg of free water is estimated to lower the Na$^+$ to the desired level (and thus the 4 mL/kg in the above equation is changed to 3 mL/kg). The quantity of free water provided by this equation is only part of the patient's total needs. The remainder of their fluid needs include isotonic losses that occurred during the dehydration process, ongoing losses, and maintenance fluids as well. Hypernatremic dehydration is corrected slowly to avoid cerebral edema, which can lead to brain stem herniation and death. Many clinicians will provide a higher content Na$^+$ fluid than calculated by various equations to ensure a slow rate of serum Na$^+$ decline. Serial monitoring of electrolytes is important to ensure that the serum Na$^+$ is decreasing at the expected slow rate and not so quickly as to lead to life-threatening brain complications.

Management of **hyponatremic dehydration** also poses challenges. In addition to isotonic losses, additional Na$^+$ loss may have occurred. The amount of additional Na$^+$ (in milliequivalents) to correct the serum Na$^+$ into a normal range (desired Na$^+$ level, eg, 135 mEq/L) has traditionally been calculated by the following equation (where 0.6 represents the body space where Na$^+$ is present):

$$[\text{patient weight in kilograms}] \times [\text{desired serum Na}^+ - \text{actual Na}^+ \text{ level}] \times 0.6$$

This amount of Na$^+$ represents an additional need beyond a patient's isotonic losses, ongoing losses, and maintenance requirements. The use of hypertonic saline (3% containing 513 mEq Na$^+$/L) is generally reserved for children with symptomatic hyponatremia (eg, a child who is seizing). Hypertonic saline is administered as 6.0 mL/kg of 3% saline given by IV over 30 to 60 minutes. This volume of 3% saline will raise the serum Na$^+$ approximately 5 mEq/L, which is usually sufficient to correct the serum Na$^+$ to a level where serious signs and symptoms improve. Some intensivists prefer to give only 3.0 mL/kg of 3% saline and consider raising serum sodium by 2.5 mEq/L sufficient to improve the CNS-related symptoms. The remaining hyponatremia is corrected more slowly so as not to exceed 12 mEq/L per 24 hours because too rapid correction of serum Na$^+$, particularly when hyponatremia has been long-standing, can potentially cause pontine demyelination.

Hyponatremia in hospitalized children, as stated earlier (see Maintenance), can result from other factors besides or in addition to Na$^+$ loss. Arginine vasopressin release in response to hypovolemia, hypertonicity, or other stimuli followed by free water retention can lead to dilutional hyponatremia (water intoxication). Hyponatremia in infants given excessively diluted baby formula (WIC [Special

Supplemental Nutrition Program for Women, Infants, and Children] syndrome) results from inadequate Na$^+$ intake and free water retention. There have been a number of recent reports of encephalopathy, brain stem herniation, and death occurring in hospitalized children with hyponatremia whose low Na$^+$ level was not appreciated or who received inappropriately low Na$^+$ content IV fluids or excessive volumes of IV fluids. The adverse effects of hyponatremia on the CNS seem to be accentuated in the setting of hypoxemia, thus further pointing to the importance of close monitoring of children with electrolyte disturbances. Moreover, with rehydration and provision of Na$^+$, the kidneys excrete relatively more dilute urine that can sometimes lead to rapid and unpredictable increases in serum Na$^+$ levels. As is the case with treatment of hypernatremia, close attention to type and quantity of fluids provided, quantity of body fluid output, weight change, and serial electrolyte assessment is important to prevent serious complications during therapy for low Na$^+$. When faced with such issues, consultation with a pediatric nephrologist or pediatric intensivist experienced in managing alterations in fluid and electrolyte balance is very important.

Potassium Replacement

Potassium deficits are more difficult to determine, and there is no specific method to calculate the exact amount of K$^+$ that a dehydrated child requires. Additionally, as the acidosis that commonly accompanies moderate and severe dehydration corrects, K$^+$ shifts intracellularly. What initially seems to be a normal serum K$^+$ may fall into the hypokalemic zone, potentially resulting in adverse effects on neuromuscular and cardiac function. Frequent reassessment of serum K$^+$ and adjustment of K$^+$ content of the IV fluids may be necessary. In general, once adequate urine output has been established, K$^+$ may be added to the IV fluids to provide 3 to 4 mEq/kg/24 h. Children who have decreased urine output or other indicators of renal impairment should not receive K$^+$ until normal urine output has been restored. Hyperkalemia, a serious and life-threatening condition, may occur if a child is unable to excrete excess K$^+$ via the kidney because of renal impairment.

Oral Rehydration

Oral rehydration therapy refers to specially prepared, balanced preparations of carbohydrates and electrolytes meant for oral consumption. Clinical trials have repeatedly shown that ORT is as efficacious as IV therapy in the treatment of the child with mild or moderate dehydration. Additional advantages of ORT over IV therapy are that it is less expensive and noninvasive, and requires little technology. Oral rehydration therapy has been credited with the dramatic reduction in death associated with diarrhea in the developing world. In 2002 the World Health Organization and UNICEF announced a new ORS with reduced osmolarity (proportionally lower Na$^+$ and glucose concentration) based on a number of clinical studies demonstrating less vomiting, lower stool output, and reduced need for IV fluids relative to the prior formulation.

In the United States, Pedialyte (Ross Laboratories, Abbott) and generic equivalents are the most widely commercially available

products. Flavored solutions and ice-pop versions of these solutions are available and often preferred by older children over the unflavored variety. Enfalyte (Mead Johnson) contains rice syrup solids as its carbohydrate source and is only available in unflavored, 6 oz ready-to-use bottles. It is not necessary to change to ORT in a breastfed child who is tolerating breast milk; these children can continue to receive breast milk for rehydration, though they may require shorter, more frequent feedings.

The composition of various ORS is presented in Table 54-3. The cost of commercially available ORS may be prohibitive for some families. Given the simplicity of the ORS packet in the developing world and commercially available ORS in the developed world, these remain the first choice. However, homemade ORT, using the recipes in Box 54-2, can be effective as long as families have and know how to use measuring spoons and cups and have a clean source of water. Some solutions such as fruit juices or chicken broth do not contain the proper balance of Na$^+$ and carbohydrate to effectively rehydrate a dehydrated patient and should not be used (Table 54-4).

The amount of ORT fluid needed for rehydration can be calculated much the same way as was done when determining the parenteral fluid requirement for a dehydrated child. However, most children with mild dehydration can be rehydrated relatively quickly and then are likely to request, in response to thirst, the amount of fluid they need. Therefore, a simplified method of determining ORT

Table 54-3. Composition of Various ORS					
Solution	Carbohy-drate (gm/L)	Sodium (mEq/L)	Potassium (mEq/L)	Base (mmol/L)	Osmolarity (mOsm/L)
Pedialyte	25	45	20	30	250
Enfalyte	30[a]	50	25	34	170
World Health Organization-UNICEF Oral Rehydration Solution	13.5	70	20	30	245

[a]As rice syrup solids.

Box 54-2. Recipes for 2 Homemade Oral Rehydration Solutions[a]
Starch-Based Solution
• 1 quart *clean* water (4 cups, or 32 ounces)
• ½ teaspoon salt
• 1 cup dry baby rice cereal (about 2 ounces in weight)
Sugar-Based Solution
• 1 quart *clean* water (4 cups, or 32 ounces)
• ½ teaspoon salt
• 6 teaspoons sugar
• One teaspoon of flavored gelatin powder may be added to either recipe to improve palatability.

[a]The proportion of ingredients in these recipes is important. These recipes should only be given to families who have and know how to use measuring spoons and cups. (Courtesy of Kathi Kemper, MD.)

Table 54-4. Composition of Some Clear Liquids Not Appropriate for Rehydration					
Liquid	Carbohydrate (g/L)	Sodium (mEq/L)	Potassium (mEq/L)	Base (mmol/L)	Osmolality
Cola	110	2	0	13	750
Apple juice	120	3	32	0	730
Chicken broth	0	250	8	0	500
Sport beverage	40	20	3	3	330

fluid requirements has been developed (Table 54-5). This quantity of fluid is given over a period of 3 to 4 hours. Children with ongoing losses should have these replaced. For the most part, it is not necessary to calculate the quantity of electrolytes that should be provided because these solutions are designed to adequately replace electrolytes in otherwise healthy children who are dehydrated.

Parents should receive guidance about the volume (converted into common household measures, eg, 5mL = 1 teaspoon and 15 mL = 1 tablespoon of water or ORS) and the frequency and duration of ORT to be given at home. Small volumes of 5 to 15 mL administered with a syringe or teaspoon every 2 to 5 minutes are much more likely to be retained by children who vomit larger volumes. Although this technique is labor intensive, it can be done by the parent and can deliver 150 to 300 mL/h. As dehydration is corrected, vomiting often decreases and the child is then able to tolerate larger volumes. With ORT the frequency and amount of stooling often increases during the initial period of treatment. Parents should be made aware that the primary purpose of ORT is to rehydrate and not to stop diarrhea, which will gradually decrease spontaneously. "Gut rest" is not appropriate in most cases, and early refeeding with a return to the usual formula or milk and solids, if appropriate, should be prioritized.

Prognosis

Children with mild or moderate dehydration as a consequence of a self-limited childhood illness are likely to recover completely when given timely and appropriate rehydration therapy. It is more difficult to predict the prognosis of children with severe dehydration or significant aberrations in electrolyte balance. If managed appropriately, most of these children also completely recover; however, some, despite closely monitored care, may have permanent sequelae or poor outcomes.

CASE RESOLUTION

The opening vignette describes a child who is moderately dehydrated. Based on clinical assessment and weight change since his last clinic visit, he is approximately 10% dehydrated. He does not show evidence of shock. His laboratory studies show a serum sodium (Na^+) of 138 mEq/L, potassium (K^+) of 3.7 mEq/L, chloride of 108 mEq/L, bicarbonate of 14 mEq/L, blood urea nitrogen (BUN) of 13 mg/dL, and creatinine 0.4 of mg/dL. His renal status is likely to be adequate because he is urinating and BUN as well as creatinine are normal for patient age. The child's serum Na^+ is 138 mEq/L, which is in the isonatremic range. The serum K^+ is 3.7 mEq/L, which is within normal range; however, this may not accurately reflect this patient's total body K^+ status. This level may decrease substantially as he is rehydrated and acidosis is corrected, indicating total body K^+ depletion. His serum bicarbonate is 14 mEq/L, and his anion gap is 16 [138 − (108 + 14)], which is mildly increased and probably related to ketosis or mild lactic acidosis.

A calculation of this child's fluid and electrolyte needs follows:
His pre-illness weight was 12 kg.

Maintenance
Fluid needs: 1,000 mL for first 10 kg + 100 mL for next 2 kg = 1,100 mL.
Sodium needs: 33 mEq Na^+ (3 mEq/100 mL of maintenance fluid requirement)

Deficit
Fluid: 10% of child's weight has been lost during this episode of dehydration = 1,200 mL deficit
Sodium: 132 mEq Na^+ (110 mEq/1,000 mL of isotonic losses): 110/1,000 × 1,200 = 132 mEq.

Ongoing Losses
Fluid: Estimate this child's ongoing losses at 10 mL/kg for each stool. He had one loose stool while in the office, so add 120 mL of additional fluid.
Sodium: The Na^+ content of diarrhea is variable; however, it is usually replaced with 0.5 normal saline (NS) or about 75 mEq/1,000/mL. We estimate about 9 mEq of Na^+ in his one loose stool.
Total fluid needs: 1,100 mL (maintenance) + 1,200 mL (deficit) + 120 mL (ongoing losses) = 2420 mL/24 h.

Electrolyte Needs
Sodium: 33 mEq (maintenance) + 132 mEq (deficit) + 9 mEq (ongoing losses) = 174 mEq Na+/24 h.
Potassium: Estimate his maintenance and replacement needs to be 20 mEq K^+/1,000 mL fluid provided.

Treatment
In the initial phase of therapy, provide 10 mL/kg/h NS with 5% dextrose (D5NS) for about 2 hours. During this period, his heart rate normalizes and he urinates. The initial parenteral phase provides 240 mL fluid and 37 mEq Na^+. This amount of fluid and Na^+ is subtracted from the patient's total fluid needs. The remaining amount to be provided is 2,180 mL fluid and 137 mEq Na^+, or about 65 mEq Na+/1,000 mL fluid. It is not necessary to prepare a special intravenous (IV) solution; 0.5 NS (77 mEq NaCl/L) with 5% dextrose ordered as **D5 0.5 NS with 20 mEq KCl/L to run at 90 mL/h** is appropriate. As his gastrointestinal symptoms improve, IV therapy is discontinued and oral rehydration therapy (ORT) instituted. The patient tolerates the ORT well and is discharged home.

Table 54-5. Treatment With Oral Rehydration Therapy (ORT)			
Degree	Dehydration ORT (Given Over 3–4 h)	Replacement of Losses	Dietary Therapy
Mild (5%) (older children = 3%)	50 mL/kg of oral rehydration solution (ORT)	10 mL/kg for each diarrheal stool 5 mL/kg for each vomitus	Return to formula or milk as soon as vomiting resolves. Children who eat solid food can continue their regular diet.
Moderate (10%) (older children = 6%)	100 mL/kg of ORT	10 mL/kg for each diarrheal stool 5 mL/kg for each vomitus	Return to formula or milk as soon as vomiting resolves. Children who eat solid food can continue their regular diet.

Selected References

Holliday MA, Friedman AL, Segar WE, Chesney R, Finbert L. Acute hospital-induced hyponatremia in children: a physiologic approach. *J Pediatr.* 2004;145:584–587

King CK, Glass R, Bresee JS, Duggan C, Centers for Disease Control and Prevention. Managing acute gastroenteritis among children: oral rehydration, maintenance, and nutritional therapy. *MMWR Recomm Rep.* 2003;52:1–16

Moritz ML, Ayus JC. Preventing neurological complications from dysnatremias in children. *Pediatr Nephrol.* 2005;20:1687–1700

Rose BD, Post TW. *Clinical Physiology of Acid-Base and Electrolyte Disorders.* New York, NY: McGraw Hill; 2001

Steiner MJ, DeWalt DA, Byerley JS. Is this child dehydrated? *JAMA.* 2004;291:2746–2754

Winters RW, ed. *The Body Fluids in Pediatrics.* Boston, MA: Little Brown; 1973

Acute Renal Failure/ Acute Kidney Injury

Hali Sherman, MD, and Sudhir K. Anand, MD

CASE STUDY

A 10-month-old girl has a 2-day history of fever, vomiting, and watery diarrhea. The child has previously been healthy. Her diet has consisted of Similac with iron, baby food, and some table food. Since the onset of her illness, she has not been drinking or eating well, and she has thrown up most of what she has eaten. Her mother has tried to give her Pedialyte and apple juice on several occasions but has had limited success. The child has had 8 to 10 watery stools without blood or mucus each day. Her temperature has varied between 98.6°F and 101.8°F (37.0°C and 38.8°C); the mother has given her daughter acetaminophen, which she has vomited. The girl's 4-year-old brother and her parents are doing well and have no vomiting or diarrhea.

The physical examination reveals a severely dehydrated (15%), listless infant. Her weight is 9.4 kg, her height is 74 cm, her temperature is 101.1°F (38.4°C), her heart rate is 168/min, her respiratory rate is 30/min, and her blood pressure is 72/40 with an appropriately sized cuff. Capillary refill is 2 to 3 seconds. The skin appears dry, but no rash is present. Head and neck, chest, heart, and abdominal examinations are normal. Pending the results of her blood studies, an intravenous fluid bolus of 180 mL normal saline (20 mL/kg) over 20 to 30 minutes is administered. This is followed by a second bolus of 180 mL normal saline over 20 to 30 minutes. The girl is catheterized to obtain urine and determine the urine flow rate over the next several hours. A urinalysis is performed.

Questions

1. What are the 3 categories of acute renal failure (ARF)/ acute kidney injury (AKI)?
2. What is the etiology of ARF/AKI?
3. What tests distinguish the 3 causes of ARF/AKI?
4. What is the appropriate management for children with ARF/AKI? What are the indications for dialysis?

For the past 50 to 60 years, a sudden decrease in kidney function, signified by the accumulation of nitrogenous waste products (eg, blood urea nitrogen [BUN], creatinine) and often accompanied by a decrease in urine output, has been called acute renal failure. With better understanding of the pathophysiology of acute deterioration in renal function, many nephrologists and intensivists have suggested that the term **acute kidney injury (AKI)** be used instead of acute renal failure (ARF). Acute kidney injury is a more descriptive term that encompasses the full spectrum of renal dysfunction, from early and mild renal injury with only a small elevation in creatinine, to severe kidney injury requiring renal replacement therapy (dialysis). In this chapter, the terms ARF and AKI are used together as ARF/AKI to reflect both continuity and an evolving concept.

There are more than 30 different definitions of ARF/AKI in the literature. These definitions are undergoing evaluation and standardization to better compare studies. In general, a doubling of the serum creatinine constitutes AKI and a tripling is considered ARF. Most children with AKI/ARF will have oliguria, but urine output may remain normal (or even increase) in some children.

Epidemiology

ARF/AKI occurs in children with a wide variety of medical or surgical conditions and especially in children who are critically ill. The exact incidence of ARF/AKI in children is not known, but a late 1990s study from the United Kingdom estimated an incidence of 0.8 per 100,000 children. ARF/AKI is often observed in patients in pediatric intensive care units (ICUs) who are septic or in the postoperative period. Primary renal disease leading to ARF/AKI seems to be decreasing in incidence when compared with ARF/AKI caused by other systemic illnesses and/or their treatments. The incidence of ARF/AKI is about 5% to 10% in neonatal ICUs.

Clinical Presentation

Most children with ARF/AKI initially present with the clinical findings of the primary condition that ultimately led to the renal problem. In critically ill children, a small increase in the creatinine may be the first indication of incipient ARF/AKI. Other findings, such as decreased urine output, edema, and heart failure (following administration of excessive fluids), are specifically related to declining renal function (Dx Box). Additionally, hyperkalemia with cardiac arrhythmia, hyperventilation due to acidosis, and nausea and vomiting due to uremia may occur as renal failure progresses.

Dx Acute Renal Failure/Kidney Injury

- Decreased urine output
- Hematuria
- Edema
- Elevated serum creatinine
- Elevated blood urea nitrogen
- Elevated fractional excretion of sodium

Etiology and Pathophysiology

The causes of ARF/AKI are usually grouped into 3 categories: prerenal, intrinsic renal, and postrenal disorders (Box 55-1). Although prerenal failure and acute tubular necrosis (intrinsic renal failure) may actually be on opposite ends of a continuum, rather than separate entities, this classification system still aids in the conceptualization of the underlying problem and formulation of the initial treatment plan.

Prerenal Disorders

Prerenal disorders are the most common cause of ARF/AKI in pediatrics and lead to a decrease in total or "effective" circulating blood volume. An absolute decrease in circulating volume can be caused by blood loss from acute hemorrhage secondary to trauma or fluid loss and dehydration secondary to gastroenteritis. Heart failure or postoperative third spacing can lead to a decrease in effective circulating volume. In each of these situations, the resulting decrease in the glomerular filtration rate (GFR) can be readily reversed by improving renal perfusion in its early stages. If hypoperfusion is prolonged, however, ischemic damage to the kidney occurs and intrinsic renal failure develops (see below).

Postrenal Disorders

Urinary obstruction due to posterior urethral valves or other lesions occasionally leads to ARF/AKI, especially during infancy.

Intrinsic Disorders

Intrinsic renal failure occurs because of injury to the vascular, glomerular, interstitial, or tubular components of the kidney (see Box 55-1). Intrinsic ARF/AKI can result from ischemia, sepsis, or toxins. ARF/AKI resulting from renal tubular lesions is also called acute tubular necrosis (ATN), although in many patients with ATN, necrosis of tubular cells visible by light microscopy is minimal. Certain histologic changes that characterize ATN include loss of brush border microvilli in tubular cells, detachment of epithelial cells from basement membrane, and cast formation from cellular debris and protein.

Box 55-1. Etiology of Acute Renal Failure/Kidney Injury in Children

Prerenal Causes
- Decreased plasma volume
- Dehydration, hemorrhage, third spacing of plasma volume in burns, sepsis, bowel obstruction
- Other causes of renal hypoperfusion
- Shock, hypoxia, congestive heart failure, hepatorenal syndrome, bilateral renal artery stenosis, cardiac surgery

Postrenal Causes
- Bilateral obstruction
- Posterior urethral valves, trauma to urethra, neurogenic bladder, bilateral ureteropelvic obstruction
- Obstruction of only functioning kidney
- Ureteropelvic obstruction, stone

Intrinsic Renal Causes
- Vascular: renal artery or vein thrombosis, disseminated intravascular coagulation
- Glomerular: hemolytic-uremic syndrome, severe (rapidly progressive) glomerulonephritis from any etiology
- Interstitial: interstitial nephritis due to allergic reaction to drugs (eg, nonsteroidal anti-inflammatory drugs, methicillin), sepsis
- Tubular (acute tubular necrosis [ATN]): sepsis, post-cardiac surgery, ischemia due to prolonged hypoperfusion: all causes listed in prerenal category, if sufficiently prolonged may lead to ATN
- Nephrotoxins: aminoglycoside antibiotics, indomethacin, radiocontrast agents, ethylene glycol, methanol, heavy metals
- Pigments: myoglobinuria, hemoglobinuria
- Uric acid: hyperuricemia, tumor lysis syndrome
- Congenital renal anomalies (especially in newborns and young infants)
- Bilateral cystic dysplastic kidneys, reflux nephropathy, polycystic kidneys, oligomeganephronia

---

Children with prolonged shock due to sepsis, post-cardiac surgery, trauma (hemorrhage), or dehydration often develop ATN if the effective circulating volume is not expanded. This is the most frequent type of intrinsic ARF/AKI observed in children. Hemolytic-uremic syndrome (HUS) had been the most common cause of ARF/AKI in young children, but its incidence has declined in recent years. Nonsteroidal anti-inflammatory drugs are increasingly being recognized as a cause of ARF/AKI in children, especially when used in volume-depleted patients. In newborns and young infants, ARF/AKI may result from, or be superimposed on, a preexisting congenital renal disorder.

The pathogenesis of ATN in humans is controversial, and no single mechanism completely explains the sequence of events that lead to ATN. Ischemic and toxic ATN result from a complex interplay of hemodynamic, nephronal, and cellular changes. These include hypoperfusion in glomerular and tubular capillaries, resulting in reduced GFR; injury to cortical and medullary tubules with their cellular debris, leading to tubular obstruction; and "back leak" of solute and water from the lumen to the interstitium with further decrease in GFR. Increased production of endothelin and reduced production of nitrous oxide in the capillaries lead to increased vasoconstriction and reduced perfusion, perpetuating the renal injury. Renal tubular cells respond to the injury in many different ways including no or minimal damage, sublethal injury, apoptosis, or necrosis. At the renal cellular level, when the damage is severe, there is decreased production of adenosine triphosphate (ATP), damage to cell membranes and cell cytoskeletons, alterations in cell polarity, and entry of increased amounts of calcium and intracellular free radicals. These changes lead to altered function and cellular swelling and eventually result in cell necrosis. It is hoped that with better understanding of the pathophysiology of ARF/AKI, innovative, improved ways to prevent, diagnose, and treat the disease will be developed.

Differential Diagnosis

The diagnosis of ARF/AKI is established by the demonstration of a sudden increase in serum creatinine and/or BUN. Decreased urine output is also helpful. Identification of the clinical disorder that led to ARF/AKI is sometimes obvious, but at other times extensive evaluation to discover the etiology of the primary disorder may be necessary. It should also be determined whether children have chronic kidney disease or superimposition of ARF/AKI on a preexisting renal condition.

Evaluation

This is one of the few settings in which laboratory and radiologic tests are often more helpful diagnostically than history and physical examination.

History

The possibility of developing ARF/AKI should be anticipated in all critically ill children. A history of decreasing urine output, hematuria, dysuria, and nausea and vomiting should be sought in all patients. The presence of previous genitourinary disorders, delayed growth, and anemia may point to preexisting kidney conditions (Questions Box).

Questions

Acute Renal Failure/Kidney Injury

- How frequently is the child passing urine?
- Is the amount of daily urine decreased, increased, or unchanged?
- Does the child have hematuria or dysuria?
- Does the child have nausea or vomiting?
- Has the child had any previous urinary problems?
- (Older children) Does the child have a history of enuresis or nocturia?
- Is the child's physical development normal or delayed?
- Does the child have a history consistent with a primary condition that may have led to the acute renal failure/acute kidney injury?

Physical Examination

An evaluation of physical growth, hypotension or hypertension, arrhythmia, dehydration, or edema should be made. Examination of the flank area for renal enlargement or tenderness and of the bladder for distention is necessary to help determine the etiology of ARF/AKI.

Laboratory Tests

The following laboratory tests are recommended in all children with ARF/AKI: complete blood count, with red blood cell (RBC) morphology and platelet count; serum sodium, potassium, and bicarbonate; BUN; creatinine, uric acid, calcium, and phosphorus; glucose; total protein and albumin serum concentration; urinalysis and urine culture (if indicated); and spot urinary sodium and creatinine concentration and osmolality. If children are not voiding frequently, catheterization of the bladder is advisable temporarily (4–6 hours) to obtain urine for analysis. Residual volume should also be assessed, and the urinary flow rate (especially the response to initial fluid therapy) and presence of an outflow obstruction should be determined. All children with ARF/AKI and evidence of hyperkalemia should have an electrocardiogram (ECG).

The diagnosis of ARF/AKI can easily be established by laboratory tests and determination of urinary output over a specific time. Oliguria is defined as urine output less than 400 mL/m²/d or less than 1 mL/kg/h in infants younger than 1 year, less than 0.75 mL/kg/h in children 2 to 6 years of age, and less than 0.5 mL/kg/h in children older than 6 years. Urinalysis, urine-specific gravity or osmolality, urine-plasma creatinine ratio, urinary sodium concentration, and fractional excretion of sodium help differentiate prerenal from intrinsic ARF/AKI (Table 55-1). While a BUN-creatinine

Table 55-1. Diagnostic Indices in Acute Renal Failure/Kidney Injury[a]		
Test	*Prerenal*	*Intrinsic Renal*
Urinalysis	Normal, occasional granular casts	Renal epithelial cells; pigment casts
Urine osmolality (mOsm/kg H₂0)	>600	<400
Urine specific gravity	>1.020	<1.015
Urine sodium (mEq/ L)	<15	>40
U-P creatinine	>40	<20
Fractional excretion of sodium[b]	<1%	>2%

Abbreviation: U/P creatinine, urine-plasma creatinine ratio (mg/mg).

[a]Values in patients with nonoliguric ARF/AKI often overlap and fall between prerenal and renal values. In addition, values in newborn infants differ from those in children beyond 1 year of age.

[b]$FE_{Na} = UNa / UCr) \times PCr / PNa) \times 100$; UNa = urine sodium (mEq / L)

FE_{Na}, fractional excretion of sodium; UCr, urine creatinine (mg/dL); PCr, plasma creatinine (mg/dL); PNa, plasma sodium (mEq / L) ratio of greater than 20:1 suggests prerenal azotemia in adults, this is not necessarily true in small children.

Tubular epithelial cells and brown-pigmented casts are often seen in patients with ATN. Evidence of hematuria or proteinuria signifies glomerular disease, especially glomerulonephritis or HUS. Presence of blood on dipstick but absence of RBCs on sediment examination suggests hemoglobinuria or myoglobinuria as the basis of ATN.

Although urinary indices are helpful in differentiating prerenal from intrinsic ARF/AKI, a simple clinical method to distinguish between the two can be used. A therapeutic trial of volume expansion with 20 mL/kg of normal saline is administered intravenously over 1 hour (after the possibilities of congestive heart failure and urinary obstruction are excluded). If oliguria persists at the end of 1 hour, furosemide (2 mg/kg) is given. If urinary output does not increase following furosemide administration, intrinsic ARF/AKI should be suspected and fluid administration reduced. Once intrinsic ARF/AKI has developed, repeated administration of high-dose furosemide has few benefits and can cause toxicity, especially hearing loss.

Many biomarkers have been investigated for the early diagnosis of ARF/AKI in adults and children. The hope is that one day biomarkers found in either the serum or urine will allow us to better detect early kidney injury, differentiate among the multiple etiologies, and predict its severity. While there are many promising biomarker candidates, including KIM-1 and NGAL, none have been validated in large trials.

Imaging Studies

Renal ultrasonography is the most useful test for differentiating postrenal from other forms of ARF/AKI. Renal ultrasound can detect the presence or absence of kidneys, enlarged kidneys, dilated pelvocalyceal system, a distended bladder, and other congenital anomalies. Other investigative tests such as voiding cystourethrography, renal scans, angiography, computed tomography, magnetic resonance imaging, or renal biopsy may occasionally be necessary but are generally not indicated in children with ARF/AKI. A chest x-ray may also be helpful in detecting cardiac enlargement or pulmonary edema due to fluid overload.

Management

Prerenal azotemia is corrected by reestablishing adequate circulating volume, but unfortunately no current treatment leads to rapid recovery of renal function in humans with established intrinsic ARF/AKI. Although low-dose dopamine and furosemide are often used in the initial management of ARF/AKI, many studies have shown that these medications do not enhance recovery of renal function. Certain drugs, such as ATP-magnesium chloride, thyroxine, atrial natriuretic hormone, and insulin-like growth factors (IGF-1) have been used experimentally in animal and some human trials without much success. The goal of therapeutic management of intrinsic ARF/AKI is maintenance of normal body homeostasis while awaiting spontaneous improvement because proximal tubules can undergo repair and regeneration after damage.

After dehydration is corrected, **daily fluid intake** is limited to replacement of insensible water loss (about 30% of daily recommended fluid intake for age), urinary losses, and fluid losses from non-renal sources (eg, nasogastric drainage). Overhydration should be avoided in patients with ARF/AKI because it can cause edema, congestive heart failure, hypertension, hyponatremia, encephalopathy, and seizures.

Patients with complete anuria require no sodium intake. **Sodium** losses should be replaced daily in patients with urinary output, however. Preferably, the amount of sodium required should be determined by measuring daily urinary sodium losses.

Once ARF/AKI is suspected, **potassium** intake from all sources should be restricted. Severe hyperkalemia can often be avoided early in the course of the disease with strict adherence to potassium restriction. The level of serum potassium as well as ECG changes should be closely monitored. Patients with mild hyperkalemia may be treated with ion exchange resins; sodium polystyrene sulfonate (Kayexalate) may be given orally every 4 to 6 hours or by retention enema every 1 to 2 hours. Moderate hyperkalemia can be treated with insulin and glucose infusions or beta-agonists, which will drive the potassium intracellularly. Calcium gluconate should be given to stabilize the myocardium. Dialysis is the most effective treatment for hyperkalemia and may be warranted if serum potassium has been rising slowly over several days or there is evidence of cardiac instability despite conservative treatment. Dialysis is also indicated for other reasons (see below).

Hypocalcemia and hyperphosphatemia are common in ARF/AKI, and small alterations in levels of **calcium** and **phosphorus** require no treatment. For serum phosphate greater than 8 mg/dL, phosphate binders such as calcium carbonate or calcium acetate may be used. If serum calcium is less than 8 mg/dL, intravenous or oral calcium should be given to prevent tetany.

Mild metabolic acidosis is common in ARF/AKI and requires no treatment. If blood pH is less than 7.2 or serum bicarbonate is less than 12 mEq/L, sodium **bicarbonate** may be administered.

Adequate nutrition is important in ARF/AKI because it prevents excessive tissue breakdown. If renal failure is expected to be short in duration (3–4 days), most calories may be provided as carbohydrates. If ARF/AKI is expected to last longer, adequate calories in the form of carbohydrates along with daily protein intake of 1 g/kg should be provided.

Many children with ARF/AKI can be managed by the conservative measures described previously. If renal failure lasts more than a few days or if complications develop, however, **dialysis** should be planned. The usual indications for dialysis include uncontrollable hyperkalemia or acidosis, volume overload with pulmonary edema and/or congestive heart failure, progressive uremia with BUN greater than 120 mg/dL, or creatinine greater than 6 mg/dL. In very small children, peritoneal dialysis is usually preferred over hemodialysis. In critically ill children with multisystem organ dysfunction, early continuous venovenous hemodiafiltration may be indicated for better overall management of the patient.

Acute renal failure/AKI can often be prevented by anticipating its possible occurrence in children with high-risk conditions such as dehydration, trauma, sepsis, and shock, or after cardiac surgery. Prompt recognition of prerenal failure and its aggressive management with volume expansion may prevent the development of intrinsic ARF/AKI. Nephrotoxic agents such as gentamicin should be avoided in high-risk patients if possible. When these drugs are used, they should be monitored meticulously, with frequent measurement of blood levels.

Prognosis

The duration of oliguria in ARF/AKI may be short (1–2 days) or long (a few weeks). Recovery is usually first indicated by an increase in urinary output. Blood urea nitrogen and creatinine may rise during the first few days of diuresis before beginning to return to normal. During diuresis, large quantities of sodium and potassium may be lost in the urine. Serum electrolytes should be closely monitored, and adequate replacements should be made to prevent hyponatremia or hypokalemia.

In children with ARF/AKI, outcome largely depends on the primary condition, the severity of damage to other organs, and physician expertise in managing ARF/AKI. Nonoliguric ARF/AKI is consistently associated with a shorter clinical course and better prognosis than oliguric ARF/AKI. Most children with ATN recover completely. However, children with more severe kidney involvement (cortical necrosis) may have residual renal impairment or chronic renal failure, and critically ill children have a 60% mortality rate.

CASE RESOLUTION

In the case scenario, a series of diagnostic studies are performed. The laboratory results are: hemoglobin, 13.8 g/dL; hematocrit, 41%; white blood cell (WBC) count, 12,400/μL; neutrophils, 58%; band forms, 6%; lymphocytes, 32%; monocytes, 3%; and eosinophils, 1%. The platelet count is 277,500/μL. Serum sodium is 136 mEq/L; potassium, 5.1 mEq/L; chloride, 110 mEq/L; bicarbonate, 10 mEq/L; blood urea nitrogen, 84 mg/dL; creatinine, 2.8 mg/dL; and glucose, 68 mg/dL. The specific gravity is 1.015, the specimen shows protein trace, blood, WBC and nitrite negative, and the sediment has many epithelial cells, 1 to 2 red blood cells, and many granular and pigmented casts. Spot urinary sodium is 65 mEq/L, creatinine is 39 mg/dL, and the fractional excretion of sodium is 3.4%.

These results are most consistent with the diagnosis of intrinsic renal failure/acute kidney injury because the fractional excretion of sodium is increased. Recovery may take a few days to a few weeks. The patient is admitted to the pediatric step-down unit where fluids are adjusted according to her urine output and electrolytes are monitored frequently.

Selected References

Akcan-Arikan A, Zappitelli M, Loftis LL, Washburn KK, Jefferson LS, Goldstein SL. Modified RIFLE criteria in critically ill children with acute kidney injury. *Kidney Int.* 2007;71:1028–1035

Devarajan P. Cellular and molecular derangements in acute tubular necrosis. *Curr Opin Pediatr.* 2005;17:193–199

Himmelfarb J, Ikizler TA. Acute kidney injury: changing lexicography, definitions, and epidemiology. *Kidney Int.* 2007;71:971–976

Lameire N, Biesen WV, Vanholder R. Acute renal failure. *Lancet.* 2005; 365:417–430

Radhakrishnan J, Kiryluk K. Acute renal failure outcomes in children and adults. *Kidney Int.* 2006;69:17–19

Sehic A, Chesney RW. Acute renal failure: diagnosis and therapy. *Pediatr Rev.* 1995;16:101–106, 137–141

Zhou H, Hewittsun SM, Yuen PST, Star RA. Acute kidney injury biomarkers—needs, present status, and future promise. *NephSAP.* 2006;5:63–71

Ingestions: Diagnosis and Management

Kelly D. Young, MD

CASE STUDY

A 2-year-old girl is found by her mother with an open bottle of pills and pill fragments in her hands and mouth. She is rushed into the emergency department. She is sleepy but arousable. The vital signs are temperature of 98.8°F (37.1°C), heart rate of 120/min, respiratory rate of 12/min, and blood pressure of 85/42 mm Hg. Pupils are 2 mm and reactive. Skin color, temperature, and moisture are normal. She has no other medical problems.

Questions

1. What history questions should be asked to help identify the substance ingested?
2. What physical examination findings can give clues to the substance ingested and the seriousness of the ingestion?
3. What other diagnostic tests might be helpful in managing ingestion patients?
4. What are the management priorities?

Ingestions are a common problem faced by pediatric practitioners. Two scenarios frequently encountered are accidental ingestions by preschool-aged children and intentional suicide attempts by adolescents. This chapter discusses the general approach to the child who has ingested a potentially poisonous substance; ingestions of specific substances are beyond the scope of this chapter, as is toxicity occurring by dermal, ophthalmologic, or inhalational routes. However, the general approach to history, physical examination, laboratory tests and diagnostic studies, and management, especially decontamination, is useful for all ingestions.

Epidemiology

Most calls made to poison control centers involve children younger than 18 years. Accidental ingestions by curious preschoolers and intentional ingestions by adolescents predominate. The most common substances ingested overall are analgesics (including acetaminophen, nonsteroidal anti-inflammatory drugs, and narcotics). The most common fatal ingestion in young children is narcotic analgesics (often not their own prescription). Another common fatal poisoning for children is carbon monoxide poisoning. Fatalities are uncommon overall and are more likely to be seen in intentional ingestions by older children. Young children tend to ingest either nontoxic substances or small quantities of toxic substances. There has been a decline in pediatric fatalities due to poisoning over the last few decades, possibly owing to improved child-resistant packaging of medications, increased education of parents and caretakers, and better supportive care.

Clinical Presentation

The clinical presentation varies considerably depending on the substance ingested. Some patients may not present with a clear history of an ingestion. The clinician must maintain a high index of suspicion for poisoning as the cause of symptoms such as altered behavior, depressed level of consciousness, cardiac dysrhythmias, vomiting, seizures, and autonomic changes.

Pathophysiology

The pathophysiological picture depends on the substance. Some toxins act on a particular organ system (eg, acetaminophen on the liver, ethanol on the central nervous system), while others act diffusely at the cellular level (eg, cyanide). Generally, drugs are absorbed, distributed within the body, metabolized, then excreted. Drug levels obtained prior to completion of absorption and distribution may not reflect the peak level. Interventions focus on preventing absorption, sometimes on preventing metabolism into a more toxic by-product, and on enhancing excretion. Toxic effects may be delayed or prolonged when an extended-release form of a drug has been ingested, with drugs likely to form concretions (iron, aspirin, theophylline), or when toxicity is a result of an active metabolite (toxic alcohols, acetaminophen, acetonitrile, dapsone).

Differential Diagnosis

The differential diagnosis of toxic ingestions is broad. If there is a history of ingestion, the differential is narrowed to substances available to the child. If no history of ingestion is given, practitioners should include ingestion in the differential when evaluating symptoms and signs such as altered mental status, altered behavior, metabolic derangements, cardiac dysrhythmias, hypotension and shock states, seizures, respiratory distress or apnea, cyanosis, vomiting, and diarrhea. In fact, almost any symptom complex may result from a toxic ingestion.

Evaluation

A detailed history of what and how much the patient ingested is key to the evaluation. Physical examination should focus on identifying symptoms and serious complications. Patients should be monitored and reassessed frequently. Laboratory and other diagnostic studies can be tailored to the specific ingestion.

History

The most important questions address the ingestion (Questions Box): What did the patient ingest, what is the maximum possible amount that was ingested, when did the ingestion occur, and what symptoms are occurring? History regarding previous medical conditions is also important to identify increased susceptibility to a particular toxin (eg, seizure disorder with ingestion of a substance that causes seizures); assess for factors that may have precipitated the ingestion, such as depression; and assess for medications that may interact with or exacerbate the toxic effects of the ingested substance (eg, acetaminophen ingestion in a patient taking a cytochrome P-450 inhibiting medication).

Questions

Poisonings

- What did the child take? (If unknown, what is available to the child?)
- How much did the child take? (If unknown, what is the maximum amount possible?)
- When did the child take it?
- What symptoms have occurred, and when did the symptoms start relative to the time of ingestion?
- What other medical conditions does the child have? What medications does the child take regularly?

Parents should be encouraged to bring in the container and any remains of the substance ingested. The practitioner should try to obtain the exact formulation because generic and brand name drugs may differ. One must be aware also of possible combination products. Sleuthing methods such as calling or sending a family member to the home to identify the product, calling the pharmacy on a prescription label, or identifying a pill by comparing its picture and imprint to those in a pharmaceuticals reference may be necessary. Internet search engines may be used to search the imprint on a pill, or to identify foreign medications. Parents should be questioned regarding all available drugs or other toxic substances in the household. The practitioner must ask about medications used by recent visitors (eg, grandparents). It is important not to overlook the possibility

of herbal preparations, vitamins, alternative medications, household products (including cleaning and personal care products), gardening products, chemicals used in hobbies or work, and alcohol or drugs of abuse belonging to an adult. It may be helpful to interview siblings or friends of an adolescent suspected of recreational drug use. One must maintain a high index of suspicion for unreported co-ingestants, especially in adolescent suicide attempts.

Although often difficult, it is important to attempt to determine the quantity of drug that was available to the patient and how much is currently missing. One may need to count pills or measure liquid to determine this. For estimating liquids, the approximate volume of a swallow is 0.3 mL/kg. The practitioner should always assume the "worst case" (ie, the patient took all of the drug that is missing). History concerning the amount ingested may be inaccurate, especially when taken from adolescents with intentional ingestion.

The practitioner should try to determine approximately what time the ingestion occurred. Symptoms are usually expected within a defined time range. Recommended observation periods before discharge usually take into account expected symptoms based on the length of time since the ingestion. Timing may also be important in determining expected toxicity. For example, ingestion of mushrooms that cause a self-limited illness usually causes gastrointestinal (GI) upset within 4 to 6 hours, whereas *Amanita* mushrooms that may ultimately result in hepatic failure typically present with GI upset in 6 to 12 hours.

The practitioner should ask about current symptoms and when they started relative to the time of the ingestion. In a patient without a definite history of ingestion, certain combinations of symptoms may point toward a specific substance. Whether the patient is symptomatic and what symptoms are present may guide the workup for an unknown ingestion, determine whether the patient needs to be hospitalized, or dictate therapy.

Physical Examination

If the substance ingested is known, the physical examination should be directed toward identifying expected symptoms of toxicity. A general physical examination should always be performed, however, because co-ingestion of another undisclosed substance must be considered. Particular attention should be paid to vital signs including temperature; pupillary size and reaction; breathing (eg, Kussmaul respiration seen in acidosis); mental status; distinctive breath odors; and skin color, temperature, and moisture. The patient's weight should be measured because toxicity is often estimated based on milligrams of drug ingested per kilogram of body weight. Because symptoms may develop or worsen if peak levels of the toxic substance have not been reached at the time of initial evaluation, continual reassessment and cardiorespiratory monitoring are imperative. A recognizable set of symptoms suggestive of a certain class of medications or toxins is called a toxidrome. If a symptomatic patient is noted to have a typical toxidrome, therapy may be initiated based on the toxidrome without confirmation of the exact substance ingested. Some common toxidromes and their treatments are listed in Table 56-1.

Table 56-1. Toxidromes

Toxin	Symptoms	Treatment
Narcotic	Nausea/vomiting, respiratory depression, miosis, altered mental status, or coma	Naloxone
Organophosphate, cholinergic	SLUDGE mnemonic: salivation, lacrimation, urination, diarrhea, gastrointestinal cramping, emesis; also bronchorrhea, bronchospasm	Atropine 2-PAM (pralidoxime)
Tricyclic antidepressant	Seizures, prolonged QRS complex, altered level of consciousness, dysrhythmias	Sodium bicarbonate
Anticholinergic	Flushing ("red as a beet"), dry skin and mucous membranes ("dry as a bone"), hyperthermia ("hot as a hare"), delirium ("mad as a hatter"); also, mydriasis, tachycardia, urinary retention	Supportive care
Sympathomimetic	Mydriasis, anxiety, tachycardia, hypertension, hyperthermia, diaphoresis	Quiet environment and benzodiazepines
Salicylate	Hyperventilation, nausea/vomiting, tinnitus, hyperthermia, metabolic acidosis	Alkalinization with $NaHCO_3$ (confirm salicylate level)

Laboratory Tests (Box 56-1)

Qualitative drug screens (reporting only presence or absence of the drug) of urine or blood are often used when poisoning is part of a broader differential for symptoms such as altered mental status or acute behavioral changes. Such drug screens are rarely helpful acutely in the poisoned patient because results are typically not rapidly reported, testing can only be done for a limited number of substances, and false-positives and false-negatives may occur. Given the frequency of narcotic ingestions, it is important to note that synthetic opioids (eg, fentanyl, methadone, oxycodone, and hydrocodone) are not detected by typical hospital immunoassay "tox screens."

Box 56-1. Laboratory Tests and Diagnostic Studies to Consider

- Specific drug levels as indicated
- Qualitative urine or blood "tox screen"
- Acetaminophen level, consider ethanol level and salicylate level
- Serum chemistries, calculated anion gap
- Serum osmolarity, calculated osmolar gap
- Liver function panel, renal function tests
- Rapid bedside glucose test
- Urine pregnancy test
- Pulse oximetry
- Electrocardiogram
- Arterial blood gas
- Urinalysis
- Creatinine phosphokinase level
- Chest radiograph
- Abdominal film for radiopaque tablets

However, quantitative drug levels for specific drugs can be helpful to estimate severity of expected symptoms or to rule out ingestion of that drug.

Examples are acetaminophen, salicylate, ethanol, methanol, ethylene glycol, iron, theophylline, lithium, anticonvulsants, and levels of carboxyhemoglobin or methemoglobin by blood gas analysis. Such levels should only be measured when suggested by history or physical examination, with the exception of acetaminophen and ethanol. Many experts in toxicology feel that because acetaminophen overdose produces few acute symptoms, may lead to fulminant hepatic failure, and is readily treatable with an antidote, all patients with a history of ingestion should have an acetaminophen level determined. In adolescents and adults, ethanol is a common coingestant, and ethanol levels are often routinely measured. Routine salicylate levels are likely to be low yield in the absence of suspicion by history or physical examination, although some practitioners also obtain them.

Serum chemistries and osmolarity may offer clues in ingestion of an unknown substance. The **anion gap** is calculated as $[Na] - ([Cl] + [HCO_3])$ and is normally 8 to 12 mEq/L. An elevated anion gap indicates presence of metabolic acidosis and is seen in ingestions and conditions identified by the **MUDPILES** mnemonic: methanol, uremia, diabetic ketoacidosis, paraldehyde and phenformin, iron and isoniazid, lactic acidosis, ethylene glycol and ethanol, salicylates and solvents (eg, toluene). The **osmolar gap** is the difference between the measured serum osmolarity and the calculated osmolarity (given by the formula $2[Na] + [glucose]/18 + [BUN]/2.8$). The normal osmolar gap is less than 10 mOsm. An elevated osmolar gap is seen with ingestion of alcohols such as ethanol, methanol, ethylene glycol, and isopropanol.

Depending on one's suspicion for acidosis, hypoxemia, or abnormal hemoglobins (carboxyhemoglobin and methemoglobin), arterial blood gas analysis may be indicated. Because hypoglycemia may be seen with some ingestions and is easily treated, a rapid bedside glucose test should be done on all patients. Urinalysis and creatinine phosphokinase level tests may be performed to look for signs of rhabdomyolysis if the patient is deemed at risk. All females of childbearing age should have a urine pregnancy test. Assessment of liver and renal function is often important because many substances are metabolized by these routes.

Diagnostic Studies

Pulse oximetry and cardiorespiratory monitoring should be instituted for all serious ingestions. An electrocardiogram may be indicated if cardiac toxicity is expected. Other studies are tailored to the specific ingestion, such as endoscopy after ingestion of caustic acids or alkalis.

Imaging Studies

Specific imaging studies may be indicated for certain ingestions, such as chest radiography in hydrocarbon ingestion, to look for signs of aspiration. An abdominal film may be helpful in identifying ingestion of radiopaque substances and monitoring the effectiveness of GI decontamination procedures for removing such substances. The mnemonic **CHIPS** can be used for radiopaque medications: chloral hydrate, heavy metals, iron, phenothiazines, and slow-release (enteric-coated) medications. In practice, abdominal radiography is primarily used in iron ingestion.

Management

Management strategies are specific for the substance ingested. The regional poison control center should be consulted for advice regarding management and length of time to observe asymptomatic patients. A single number, 1-800-222-1222, automatically routes the caller to one of the appropriate 62 regional poison control centers in the nation. In general, the approach to management includes attention to the basic ABCs (airway, breathing, circulation) of resuscitation, decontamination methods, specific antidotes when available and indicated, and meticulous supportive care, often in an intensive care unit.

Decontamination

Decontamination techniques are strategies used to prevent or minimize absorption of the toxic substance and to enhance its elimination. They are a critical part of the management of acutely poisoned patients and should be used whenever a significant ingestion is suspected (Table 56-2).

Syrup of ipecac was commonly recommended in the past for home use to induce vomiting in the event of an accidental ingestion. **Gastric lavage,** in which a large nasogastric tube is placed and the stomach is washed with normal saline, is the hospital counterpart to syrup of ipecac. Both techniques theoretically remove toxic substance from the stomach, thus preventing absorption. However, at best (immediate performance after ingestion), less than a third of gastric contents are removed by these methods. In addition, these techniques may interfere with the use of activated charcoal, usually a more effective therapy. Gastric lavage is technically difficult to perform in young children owing to the need to pass a large-bore tube. Gastric lavage also has a high rate of complications such as aspiration and esophageal trauma. Neither syrup of ipecac nor gastric lavage is recommended for routine use. The American Academy of Pediatrics released a policy statement in 2003 stating that syrup of ipecac should no longer be kept in homes. The American Academy of Clinical Toxicology (AACT) reserves gastric lavage only for life-threatening ingestions presenting at less than 60 minutes since ingestion, with the caveat that there is no confirmed clinical benefit.

Table 56-2. Summary of Gastric Decontamination Techniques		
Technique	*Dose*	*Contraindications*
Syrup of ipecac	6 months–1 year: 10 mL (use with caution) 1–12 years: 15 mL >12 years: 30 mL Follow with 8 oz water	**Not recommended for routine use** Altered level of consciousness (ALOC) Caustics: acids and alkalis Hydrocarbons Expected ALOC (eg, tricyclic antidepressants)
Gastric lavage	15 mL/kg aliquots normal saline to maximum of 400 mL until lavage fluid is clear (may be several liters)	ALOC with unprotected airway Caustics: acids and alkalis Hydrocarbons Expected ALOC >1 hour since ingestion
Activated charcoal	1–2 g/kg or <6 years: 25–50 g >6 years: 50–100 g	ALOC with unprotected airway Absent bowel sounds or bowel obstruction Substance not bound by charcoal
Cathartics	Magnesium citrate 4 mL/kg 70% sorbitol 1 g/kg	**Not recommended for routine use** Repeated doses can cause dehydration or electrolyte imbalances.
Whole-bowel irrigation	Toddler and preschool age: 500 mL/h 6–12 y: 1,000 mL/h Adolescent and adult: 1.5–2 L/h Continue until rectal effluent is clear	Bowel obstruction, ileus, perforation, or hemorrhage ALOC with unprotected airway

Activated charcoal is the mainstay in treatment of ingestion. Charcoal binds toxins, and because it is not absorbed in the GI tract, the charcoal-toxin complex passes through and is eliminated. Its efficacy decreases with increasing time since the ingestion, and ideally it should be started within an hour of the ingestion. The optimal dose of charcoal is 10 times the amount of substance ingested. Because the exact amount of toxin ingested is often unknown, activated charcoal is usually dosed at 1 to 2 g/kg. The amount of charcoal given is limited only by what the child is able to tolerate. Only a few substances are not absorbed by activated charcoal. The mnemonic **PHAILS** can be used to remember them: pesticides, hydrocarbons and heavy metals, acids, alkalis and alcohols, iron, lithium, and solvents. The main complication of charcoal administration is aspiration pneumonitis, primarily seen in patients with altered level of consciousness and an unprotected airway. If charcoal is not voluntarily taken by the child, it may be administered via nasogastric tube. Endotracheal intubation to protect the airway may be necessary in the patient with altered mental status. It is imperative that nasogastric tube placement in the GI tract (as opposed to the respiratory tract) be confirmed prior to charcoal administration.

Cathartics (most commonly sorbitol) have been used to decrease transit time and improve elimination of the toxin through the GI tract and to counteract activated charcoal-induced constipation. The cathartic is often mixed with the activated charcoal and may serve to improve the palatability of the charcoal. A significant benefit from cathartic use has never been demonstrated, however, and there is a risk of dehydration and electrolyte disturbances, particularly in young children. The AACT recommends *against* use of cathartics. Under no circumstances should repeated doses of cathartics be given.

Multiple-dose charcoal may remove drugs from the bloodstream by promoting diffusion back into the GI tract and subsequent binding to charcoal. It has been called the "GI dialysis." Activated charcoal at the same dose previously used is repeated approximately every 4 hours. Cathartics should *not* be mixed with the charcoal for repeat doses. Multiple-dose charcoal is useful for a small number of drugs, such as phenobarbital, theophylline, carbamazepine, dapsone, and quinine. It should only be used if a potentially life-threatening amount has been ingested. It should not be used for drugs that can cause an ileus (eg, tricyclic antidepressants).

Whole-bowel irrigation involves infusion of a solution usually used for cleansing of the bowel prior to GI surgery (eg, polyethylene glycol). It is especially useful for slow-release medications, for tablets that dissolve slowly and may cause concretions (eg, iron), and in ingestions where charcoal is not likely to be effective (eg, heavy metals). A nasogastric tube is used to infuse the solution at a rate of 500 mL/h in young children, and 1 to 2 L/h in older children and adolescents. Clear rectal effluent is the endpoint; a bedpan may be necessary. Whole-bowel irrigation should not be used when there is bowel obstruction, ileus, perforation, or hemorrhage or altered mental status with an unprotected airway.

Hemodialysis may be used for serious ingestions of ethylene glycol, methanol, phenobarbital, lithium, salicylate, or theophylline. **Charcoal hemoperfusion,** in which blood goes through a charcoal cartridge instead of a dialysis machine, is used rarely for severe theophylline poisoning. **Urinary alkalinization** (by administration of sodium bicarbonate) can increase elimination of weak acids by keeping the drug in its ionic state, thus preventing reabsorption in the renal tubule. It is primarily used for significant salicylate, phenobarbital, and isoniazid poisonings.

Supportive Care

Attention to the basic ABCs (airway, breathing, circulation) of resuscitation is always the first step in management. **Hypoglycemia** must be assessed and managed as soon as possible. Dextrose 0.5 to 1 g/kg intravenously is given; glucagon may be used if dextrose cannot be given. **Seizures** are generally treatable with benzodiazepines. Glucose and electrolyte levels should be normalized. With isoniazid ingestions, pyridoxine may be helpful. **Shock** requires aggressive fluid resuscitation. Fluid-resistant shock may require vasopressors, most commonly dopamine, epinephrine, or norepinephrine. Resistant shock in a beta-blocker ingestion may respond to glucagon, and in a calcium channel blocker ingestion to insulin plus glucose. **Dysrhythmias** should generally be treated by following Pediatric Advanced Life Support (PALS) protocols, although specific ingestions may respond to specific therapies. Sodium bicarbonate is the first-line treatment for dysrhythmias associated with ingestions of antihistamines, class I antiarrhythmics (lidocaine, quinidine, procainamide), cocaine, and tricyclic antidepressants. Beta-blocker ingestions may respond to atropine and glucagon, while ingestions of calcium channel blockers are managed with calcium. Procainamide, found on PALS algorithms, should be avoided for dysrhythmias due to overdoses of antihistamines, quinidine and other class I antiarrhythmics, digoxin, quinine, and tricyclic antidepressants. Amiodarone, also found on PALS algorithms, should also be avoided in the treatment of antihistamine ingestions. Electrolyte imbalances should be assessed and corrected. **Suicidality** should be assessed, often in conjunction with a mental health professional.

Antidotes

Antidotes or medications that counteract the pathophysiological mechanisms of the toxin are available for only a few ingestions (Table 56-3). Important antidotes are N-acetylcysteine for acetaminophen, naloxone for narcotics, oxygen for carbon monoxide poisoning, bicarbonate for tricyclic antidepressant cardiotoxicity, Digibind for digoxin, and deferoxamine for iron. Antidotes are not without adverse effects themselves, and should only be given in cases of symptomatic or potentially symptomatic (acetaminophen) ingestions of significant amounts. The poison control center staff can be very helpful in guiding practitioners in the use of antidotes.

Table 56-3. Antidotes	
Toxin	*Antidote*
Acetaminophen	N-acetylcysteine
Anticoagulants (coumadin-like)	Vitamin K
Anticholinergic	Physostigmine
Benzodiazepine	Flumazenil
Beta-blocker	Glucagon
Calcium channel blocker	Calcium, insulin + glucose
Carbamate pesticide	Atropine
Carbon monoxide	Oxygen
Cyanide	Cyanide antidote kit
Digoxin	Digibind
Ethylene glycol	Fomepizole, ethanol
Iron	Deferoxamine
Isoniazid	Pyridoxine
Lead	Dimercaprol (BAL), ethylene diamine tetraacetic acid, dimercaptosuccinic acid (DMSA)
Mercury	BAL, DMSA
Methanol	Fomepizole, ethanol
Methemoglobinemia	Methylene blue
Narcotics	Naloxone
Organophosphate pesticide	Atropine, 2-PAM (pralidoxime)
Rattlesnake bite	Crofab (crotalidae polyvalent immune fab [ovine])
Sulfonylurea oral hypoglycemic	Dextrose, octreotide
Tricyclic antidepressant	Sodium bicarbonate

Anticipatory Guidance and Prevention

Most ingestions are nontoxic and require only observation for a few hours. They do, however, provide an excellent opportunity to discuss poisoning prevention with parents and caretakers. Possible toxins, including prescription and over-the-counter medications, cleaning and household products, cosmetics and nail care products, toxic plants, gardening and hobby chemicals, and kitchen items such as alcohol should be kept out of reach of children. Visitors to the household should also be cautioned to keep medications out of reach of children. Substances should never be stored in unmarked containers, particularly in containers that typically hold beverages such as old soda bottles or cups. Medications should not be referred to as "candy" to entice youngsters to take them. Parents should have the universal telephone number for the poison control center and telephone numbers for local emergency departments readily available. Carbon monoxide detectors should be placed near children's bedrooms. Activated charcoal for home use is controversial and not currently recommended, although it is available without prescription from many pharmacies. Parents should not give activated charcoal without speaking to poison control center staff or medical personnel first.

Prognosis

Prognosis depends on the toxicity of the substance ingested. For a few substances, a small amount can be fatal (Box 56-2), whereas for others, even large ingestions are generally benign. Prognosis is generally excellent; fatalities in children are rare. Prognosis is worse for intentional ingestions, often because patients delay or fail to reveal that they attempted overdose.

Box 56-2. Substances Potentially Fatal in 1 to 2 Pills or Teaspoons
• Camphor (found in Vicks VapoRub, Campho-Phenique, Tiger Balm)
• Imidazoline decongestants (found in over-the-counter nasal and eye drops)
• Acetonitrile nail glue remover
• Clonidine (available in transdermal patches also)
• Opiates (available in transdermal patches also)
• Methyl salicylate (oil of wintergreen, Ben-gay)
• Calcium channel blockers
• Toxic alcohols (methanol, ethylene glycol, ethanol, isopropanol)
• Tricyclic antidepressants
• Lomotil (opiate diphenoxylate + atropine)
• Sulfonylurea oral hypoglycemics
• Chloroquine and hydrochloroquine antimalarial agents
• Hydrofluoric acid
• Selenious acid (gun bluing solution)
• Buffered saline solution
• Benzocaine-induced methemoglobinemia

> ### CASE RESOLUTION
> Because the respiratory rate of this 2-year-old is slow and there are symptoms of miosis and altered level of consciousness, narcotic ingestion is suspected and naloxone is administered. The child becomes more alert and respiratory rate increases to 24 breaths per minute. The father is instructed to retrieve the bottle, and it turns out to be a prescription narcotic analgesic left in the house by a recent visitor. The child is given activated charcoal, observed overnight in the hospital, and discharged on the following day without sequelae.

Selected References

American Academy of Pediatrics Committee on Injury, Violence, and Poison Prevention. Poison treatment in the home. *Pediatrics.* 2003;112:1182–1185

Barry JD. Diagnosis and management of the poisoned child. *Pediatr Ann.* 2005; 34:937–946

Henry K, Harris CR. Deadly ingestions. *Pediatr Clin North Am.* 2006; 53:293–315

Lai MW, Klein-Schwartz W, Rodgers GC, et al. 2005 annual report of the American Association of Poison Control Centers' national poisoning and exposure database. *Clin Toxicol (Phila).* 2006;44:803–932

Riordan M, Rylance G, Berry K. Poisoning in children 1: general management. *Arch Dis Child.* 2002;87:392–396

White ML, Liebelt EL. Update on antidotes for pediatric poisoning. *Pediatr Emerg Care.* 2006;22:740–746

SECTION IV

Head, Neck, and Respiratory System

57. Approach to the Dysmorphic Child 317

58. Craniofacial Anomalies 323

59. Common Oral Lesions 331

60. Otitis Media 335

61. Hearing Impairments 341

62. Sore Throat 347

63. Nosebleeds 355

64. Strabismus 361

65. Infections of the Eye 367

66. Excessive Tearing 373

67. Neck Masses 377

68. Allergic Disease 387

69. Wheezing and Asthma 393

70. Cough 403

Approach to the Dysmorphic Child

Julie E. Noble, MD

CASE STUDY

A 12-year-old male presents to the office for the first time for an evaluation after moving to the area. Parents note that he has unexplained mental retardation and has had problems with hyperactivity in school. The pregnancy was uncomplicated and the mother, who was a 32-year-old gravida I para I at the time of the child's birth, denies alcohol or drug use or exposure to any teratogens during pregnancy. Delivery was by cesarean section secondary to cephalopelvic disproportion, but Apgar scores were 8 at 1 minute and 9 at 5 minutes. The infant was noted to have macrocephaly and to be large for gestational age. He did well in the newborn period and had no feeding problems. Subsequently, he had no significant medical illnesses including no seizures, but at 1 year of age was noted to be developmentally delayed. This delay continued, and he has been in special education classes throughout his school career. Family history is negative for any family members with retardation.

On physical examination, the boy is greater than 90th percentile for height and weight. He is mildly prognathic with large ears. He has hyperextensible fingers. A complete examination reveals that his testicles appear large (6 cm) and his sexual maturity rating (Tanner stage) is 2. The rest of the examination is normal.

Questions

1. What history is important to elicit in evaluating a child with dysmorphic features?
2. What are the possible causes of errors in morphogenesis?
3. What clues on physical examination can aid in establishing a specific diagnosis?
4. What laboratory tests can confirm a diagnosis?
5. When is it appropriate to obtain a genetics consultation or refer a patient for genetic counseling?
6. What are the benefits of establishing a specific diagnosis?

Evaluation for structural anomalies is an essential part of all pediatric examinations. Visible errors in morphogenesis give the physician valuable information in evaluating a patient with abnormal symptoms, such as seizures. Additionally, major malformations frequently require treatment, and the presence of one anomaly suggests that others may also exist.

The study of these congenital defects was termed dysmorphology by David Smith in 1966. The anomalies fall into 2 categories: minor and major. Minor malformations are those of "no medical or cosmetic consequence to the patient." An example would be a supernumerary nipple that appears as a hyperpigmented papule along the nipple line. Identification of minor malformations is important because they may indicate the presence of a more generalized pattern of malformation. Major malformations are those that have "an adverse effect on either the function or social acceptability of the individual." A cleft lip and palate are major malformations that have functional as well as cosmetic relevance to the patient's health.

Epidemiology

Structural anomalies are common in the general population. Most are minor. In the first comprehensive analysis of minor structural anomalies, Marden in 1964 identified 7% to 14% of newborn infants with at least one minor anomaly on surface examination. Other studies identify up to 40% of newborns with one anomaly. Three or more minor malformations have predictive value in identifying a major malformation. In newborns, 0.8% have 2 minor malformations, and 11% of these patients will have a major malformation. Three or more minor malformations occur in 0.5% of newborns, and 90% of these will have a major malformation. Data from the National Collaborative Perinatal Program revealed that 44.78% of these anomalies were craniofacial and 45.3% were skin. Males are affected with minor malformations more often than females. Autopsies of dead fetuses reveal an increased incidence of both minor and major malformations. Frequencies of both minor and major malformations vary along racial lines, depending on the specific malformations. For example, postaxial polydactyly is seen in 16 of 10,000 births in the white population and 140 of 10,000 births in the African American population. Hemangiomas are seen in 350 of 10,000 births in whites and only 100 of 10,000 births in African Americans.

Three percent of all pregnancies produce a child with a significant genetic disease or a birth defect. These malformations account for a great proportion of morbidity and mortality in the pediatric population. Of all pediatric hospital admissions, one-third to one-half involve a child with a disease with a genetic component.

Clinical Presentation

With the advent of more prenatal tests and diagnostic modalities (see Chapter 11), the detection of anomalies may first occur in the prenatal period. Routine prenatal screening tests that are abnormal raise the possibility that the infant will have an anomaly. For instance, an elevated maternal alpha fetoprotein indicates the possibility of a spinal cord defect. Amniocentesis or chorionic villus biopsy may reveal abnormal chromosomes with associated structural defects. Prenatal ultrasound now demonstrates structural defects that can be diagnosed in utero.

Most structural anomalies develop during the first trimester of gestation and, if not detected prenatally, are noted at birth in the delivery room or the newborn nursery. Many major congenital defects are obvious on a thorough physical examination. Some major defects such as a tracheoesophageal fistula will not be manifest on surface examination but will be readily apparent as the infant adapts to extra-uterine life and experiences symptoms when feeding begins. Minor anomalies may be overlooked on an infant's initial examination. However, if that infant manifests developmental delay at 6 months of age, the physician may be more inclined to evaluate for minor anomalies that may aid in identifying the cause of the developmental delay.

Sometimes dysmorphic features are not present at birth but become apparent later in life as the child grows and develops. These types of features are associated with dysplasias, defects in cellular metabolism that become manifest after birth. An example is a skeletal dysplasia that becomes more apparent as the bones grow.

Pathophysiology

The pathophysiology of structural defects can be separated into 4 different types of errors in morphogenesis: malformations, deformations, disruptions, and dysplasias (Box 57-1).

Previously, the term **malformation** was used descriptively to denote an anomaly; but it is also used to denote a specific pathogenic mechanism. Malformations are permanent defects in a structure caused by an intrinsic abnormality in the development of that structure. An example of a malformation is an endocardial cushion defect in a patient with Down syndrome. Malformations frequently are caused by chromosomal abnormalities and single-gene disorders that program for abnormal structure.

Deformations occur in an infant when external forces exert a mechanical pressure on the developing fetus. There is no intrinsic defect of the fetus. These deformations can be caused by uterine

Box 57-1. Pathophysiology of Structural Defects
Malformation
Chromosomal abnormality
Single gene disorder
Deformation
Disruption
Vascular compromise
Viral infection
Mechanical—amniotic bands
Teratogens—alcohol, drugs, irradiation
Dysplasia
Metabolic disorder

constraint, an abnormally shaped uterus, or multiparous pregnancy. A flexible clubfoot is a deformation caused by uterine constraint. **Disruptions** occur when an agent outside a fetus causes cell death and a permanent defect in development. These disruptive events result in tissue destruction. Disruptions can occur during development when there is tissue ischemia secondary to vascular compromise, when a viral infection disrupts development at a critical gestational age, or when a mechanical disruption interferes with normal development. An amniotic band is an example of a mechanical disruptive agent that can cause an amputation of a limb by constricting the extremity during development. Teratogens can also function as disruptive agents by interfering during a critical period in embryogenesis, causing dysgenesis of fetal organs. Alcohol, drugs, and irradiation are all teratogens. Fewer than 30 drugs have been proved to be teratogenic.

Dysplasias, often caused by a single-gene defect, are structural abnormalities that develop from abnormal cellular metabolism and organization. Mucopolysaccharidosis is a dysplasia that develops secondary to the absence of the lysosomal hydrolase of α-L-iduronidase. As a result, mucopolysaccharides accumulate in parenchymal and mesenchymal tissues. As affected children grow, they develop coarse facies, enlarged tongue, misshapen bones, and hepatosplenomegaly among other features.

Differential Diagnosis

In generating an appropriate differential diagnosis for a dysmorphic child, it is essential to identify all minor and major malformations. The differential will vary depending on the specific findings. A thorough history and physical examination will help greatly to establish the list of conditions to consider. If there are multiple anomalies, identifying the most specific and rarest anomaly can direct the practitioner to a narrower list of possible diagnoses. For example, nail hypoplasia, which is seen in fetal hydantoin syndrome, is much rarer than congenital cardiac disease, which is seen in multiple syndromes. A practitioner should be familiar with the prominent features of the more common syndromes but also should have readily available reference texts, such as *Smith's Recognizable Patterns of Human Malformation,* to aid in establishing differential lists as well as finalizing diagnoses. In addition, the Internet has developed into a valuable tool through Web sites such as PubMed or Google or those specifically developed for the delineation of syndromes and genetic disorders.

In evaluating an infant with congenital anomalies, the practitioner should attempt to separate the findings into 1 of 5 categories: an isolated defect, a developmental field defect, a birth defect association, a sequence pattern, or a dysmorphic syndrome (Box 57-2). The first step is to determine whether the anomaly is **isolated.** If so, does it represent a failure in development in one location, such as a cleft lip? Most isolated anomalies are believed to have a multifactorial inheritance, representing the interaction between multiple genes and unknown external influences. They usually have a recurrence risk of 2% to 5%.

Box 57-2. Categories of Anomalies
Isolated defect
Developmental field defect
Birth defect association
Sequence pattern
Dysmorphic syndrome

A **developmental field defect** is a pattern of anomalies that develops in structures that are together during embryologic development. These defects involve one limited region and are secondary to a disruptive event such as vascular compromise. They therefore have a low recurrence risk. An example would be hemifacial microsomia, where the defects are secondary to disruption in vascular flow to the first and second branchial arches. This disruption results in hypoplasia of the malar, maxillary, and mandibular region on one side with associated microtia and vertebral defects.

Birth defect associations are diagnosed when the combination of anomalies occurs together commonly but the pattern does not fit a known field defect or syndrome. The etiology of association defects is unknown at this time, and the recurrence risk is low. One of the more common associations is the VACTERRL association (vertebral anomalies, anal atresia, cardiac defects, tracheoesophageal fistula, radial defects, and renal and limb defects).

A **sequence pattern** of anomalies occurs when one malformation leads to multiple dysmorphic features. Potter oligohydramnios sequence results from renal agenesis. The renal malformation causes oligohydramnios with resultant fetal contractures, pulmonary hypoplasia, and a flattened face.

A **syndrome** is a pattern of anomalies that are pathologically related. Chromosomal abnormalities such as Down syndrome (trisomy 21), single-gene disorders, and teratogens fall into this category. Alcohol is the most common teratogen to which fetuses are exposed. Alcohol causes growth failure, developmental delay, microcephaly, a short nose, and small distal phalanges. Children with developmental delay and anomalies have a higher likelihood of having a syndrome and should undergo a chromosome analysis.

Evaluation

History

A complete history is essential (Questions Box). The history begins prenatally with information from the mother on duration of pregnancy, possible teratogen exposure, fetal activity, diagnostic test results, and any complications of pregnancy. The delivery history should include type of delivery, infant presentation, and size at birth, including growth percentiles. Neonatal adaptation and feeding patterns are important parameters to assess. The subsequent medical history should be obtained.

A thorough family history is equally important, and a pedigree should be outlined. Specifically, the family should be questioned for parental age, possible consanguinity, and history of fetal loss or early infant deaths. Family history of birth defects or retardation should be documented.

Questions

The Dysmorphic Child

- How long was the pregnancy?
- Did the mother take any medications, smoke cigarettes, or use alcohol or any illicit drug?
- What was the fetal activity?
- Were there any complications of pregnancy?
- What was the type of delivery and presentation of the baby?
- What was the infant's size at birth?
- How did the infant feed?
- What is the subsequent medical and developmental history?
- Are the parents related?
- What are the parents' ages?
- Is there a history of fetal or infant deaths?
- Is there a history of birth defects in the family?
- Are any family members retarded?

Physical Examination

The physical examination should be extremely thorough with all morphological findings noted. As previously mentioned, the craniofacial area and skin are common sites for anomalies. But all organ systems should be extensively evaluated. Even minor anomalies such as a supernumerary nipple or clinodactyly may have significance. Objective measurements should be obtained when possible. Normal grids are available for evaluating inner canthus distance, palpebral fissure length, ear length, etc. Hair whorl patterns and dermatoglyphics should be evaluated. Physical data, including height, weight, and head circumference, should be plotted and the growth percentiles noted. A complete ophthalmologic evaluation may be indicated to detect abnormalities such as cataracts or cherry-red spots.

Laboratory Tests

In assessments of dysmorphic-appearing children, the physical examination is the most important part. Findings on physical examination direct which further studies will be of benefit. Additional studies may give added or confirmatory information regarding a suspected diagnosis. Prenatal screening tests may be used to detect a fetal abnormality, and specific prenatal tests are available to assess a fetus at risk for a given disease. Cytogenetic evaluation is essential in evaluating a child with a suspected syndrome and also in evaluating a child with malformations and developmental delay. Standard chromosomal analysis is the first-line laboratory test, but may not detect many small chromosomal or gene defects. More sophisticated testing may be indicated. Small chromosomal aberrations can be detected by FISH (fluorescent in situ hybridization) analysis, in which labeled probes are applied to chromosomal preparations. These probes are specific for given disorders and should be used to confirm a suspected clinical syndrome. Prader-Willi and DiGeorge syndromes may be diagnosed by FISH analysis. FISH probes can now be applied to subtelomeric regions of the chromosome, which are very gene rich. Whole chromosome painting is another technique in which FISH probes are used to paint the entire chromosome, thus identifying the origin of additional chromosomal material or cryptic translocations. Molecular testing is available for many single-gene disorders.

Many dysplasias and some syndromes can be detected by metabolic testing. Serum amino acids and urine organic acids should be ordered if a diagnosis is suspected. Many states are now including an analysis for metabolic disorders in their expanded newborn screening protocols.

Imaging Studies

Imaging studies are extremely useful in deriving information on internal malformations. X-rays including a skeletal survey may detect skeletal anomalies. Echocardiogram, ultrasound, computed tomography scan, and magnetic resonance imaging (MRI) studies can all be used when appropriate. With the findings of anomalies and global developmental delay in a patient, the American Academy of Neurology recommends routine neuroimaging with an MRI.

Management

When children present with dysmorphic features, they should be evaluated to determine a specific diagnosis. Obtaining a diagnosis is of vital importance to the care of the patient and parental counseling. Knowing the diagnosis can direct subsequent testing for associated abnormalities. Treatment options may also be available for the condition, and a prognosis can be established. Defining the developmental prognosis for children is essential to establish appropriate school planning. If developmental delay is not associated with the diagnosis, such as with cleft lip and palate, the parents should be reassured. Parents also need to know the recurrence risk for themselves and for their children. Occasionally, further testing of the parents may be necessary to determine the accurate recurrence risk. If one of the parents is a translocation carrier, the risk of subsequent children having the abnormality is increased.

Consultation with a geneticist can help the practitioner in establishing the correct diagnosis and provide the practitioner with the latest information regarding evaluation and possible treatment. New information in the field of genetic disease appears daily, and it is difficult for a primary care practitioner to stay abreast. A genetic consultation should also be obtained in most patients with major malformations to confirm the diagnosis and to help counsel parents.

Health supervision strategies have been established for specific disorders. For instance, published guidelines recommend hearing, ophthalmologic, and thyroid screening, among other tests, for patients with Down syndrome. A geneticist can give guidance regarding revised recommendations.

If support groups are available for specific conditions, parents should be referred to these groups. Such groups can be invaluable in helping parents understand as well as adjust to the disorder. They can also advise parents about community and educational resources available for their child's care and help parents advocate for their child's unique needs.

A referral to a genetics counselor can provide parents with education about prenatal testing, recurrence risk, and alternatives for dealing with this recurrence risk. Counseling is extremely useful to help parents understand the inheritance pattern.

Prognosis

As with management, defining an accurate prognosis for each patient depends on recognition of the specific condition. Some conditions such as trisomy 13 are lethal, while other conditions allow for a normal life span.

Malformations are permanent defects that generally have a recurrence risk. They may be correctable with surgery or treatment but frequently leave a residual disability.

Deformations usually resolve with treatment and have no recurrence risk unless the deformation is secondary to a uterine abnormality such as a bicornuate uterus.

A disruption may be treated with surgery or therapy to improve function but, as in malformations, a residual disability frequently remains. When the disruption is due to tissue ischemia or a mechanical agent, there is no recurrence risk. If it is due to a teratogen, the disruption will recur with the same teratogenic exposure.

Dysplasias tend to persist or worsen with time unless a specific treatment is available. Only a limited number of diseases have specific treatments available. Generally, there is a recurrence risk.

CASE RESOLUTION

The child in the case scenario has features that suggest a dysmorphic syndrome. The most specific finding on examination is macro-orchidism. This finding is associated with fragile X syndrome. Specific DNA-based molecular analysis is performed and is positive for a fragile site on the X chromosome at Xq27.3.

Parents are counseled that this condition has an X-linked inheritance pattern. The child will have a normal life span but may need early intervention services and later a special education program, and may not be capable of independent living as an adult. Parents are encouraged to attend a parents' support group and consult with experts to learn how their child's full potential may be realized.

Selected References

Aase JM. Dysmorphologic diagnosis for the pediatric practitioner. *Pediatr Clin North Am.* 1992;39:135–156

Friedman JM. A practical approach to dysmorphology. *Pediatr Ann.* 1990; 19:95–101

Hunter A. Medical genetics: 2. The diagnostic approach to the child with dysmorphic signs. *Can Med Assoc J.* 2002;167:367–372

Jones KL. *Smith's Recognizable Patterns of Human Malformation.* 6th ed. Philadelphia, PA: W. B. Saunders; 2006

Koren G, Pastuszak A, Ito S. Drugs in pregnancy. *N Engl J Med.* 1998; 338:1128–1136

Moeschler J, Shevell M, Committee on Genetics. Clinical genetic evaluation of the child with mental retardation or developmental delays. *Pediatrics.* 2006;117:2304–2316

Shevell M, Ashwal S, Donley D, et al. Practice parameter: evaluation of the child with global developmental delay: report of the Quality Standards Subcommittee of the American Academy of Neurology and The Practice Committee of the Child Neurology Society. *Neurology.* 2003;60:367–380

Toomay KE. Medical genetics for the practitioner. *Pediatr Rev.* 1996;17: 163–174

Walker W, Johnson C. Mental retardation: overview and diagnosis. *Pediatr Rev.* 2006;27:204–212

Craniofacial Anomalies

Carol D. Berkowitz, MD

CASE STUDY

A 3,500-g boy is born by normal spontaneous vaginal delivery to a 28-year-old gravida III para III mother after an uncomplicated full-term gestation. The Apgar scores are 9 and 10. On physical examination, the infant is well but has an incomplete, left-sided unilateral cleft of the lip and palate.

No other family members have such a deformity, but the mother and father are distantly related. The mother had prenatal care. During the pregnancy she had no illnesses; took vitamins but no other medications; and did not smoke, drink alcohol, or use illicit drugs.

The mother is planning to feed the infant with formula and wonders if she should do anything special. She is also wondering if her son's lip deformity can be repaired before she takes him home from the hospital. Except for the cleft, the physical examination is normal.

Questions

1. What craniofacial anomalies are common in children?
2. What are feeding considerations in infants with cleft lip or palate?
3. What is the appropriate timing of surgery for the more common craniofacial anomalies?
4. What are the major medical problems that children with craniofacial anomalies, particularly clefts of the lip or palate, experience?
5. What is positional plagiocephaly? How is its prevalence related to the Back to Sleep campaign?

Infants may be born with readily apparent craniofacial anomalies such as cleft lip, cleft palate, or microtia, or anomalies may emerge as an infant grows older. The latter includes conditions that may be genetically based but do not manifest until later, such as facial asymmetry (hemifacial microsomia) and premature closure of one or more sutures. Alternatively, these anomalies may be environmentally influenced, such as positional or deformational plagiocephaly. Deformational plagiocephaly is defined as a condition in which the infant's head and sometimes face are misshapen as a result of prenatal and, in recent years, postnatal external molding, which occur on the infant's malleable cranium.

Epidemiology

The overall incidence of cleft lip with or without cleft palate is 1 in 1,000, and that of isolated cleft palate is 1 in 2,500. Cleft lip with or without cleft palate is the fourth most common birth defect. There is racial, ethnic, and geographic variation in the incidence of clefts. For example, the incidence of clefts in parts of the Philippines is 1 in 200. The gender distribution varies with the type of cleft. Isolated clefts of the palate occur twice as frequently in girls, but clefts of the lip with or without clefts of the palate appear twice as often in boys.

The type of cleft, the gender of the child, and whether parents or other siblings are similarly affected influence the risk for recurrence of clefts in subsequent offspring. In general, the risk for recurrence of clefts is 4% to 7% for cleft lip with or without cleft palate and 3% for isolated cleft palate.

Clefts may occur either as isolated findings or as part of syndromes such as Pierre Robin syndrome, where they are associated with micrognathia and glossoptosis. In Van der Woude syndrome, clefts of the lip or palate are associated with lip pits. This condition is inherited in an autosomal-dominant manner. There are now approximately 300 disorders associated with clefts, although only 10% to 15% of children with clefts fit a syndrome.

True craniosynostosis occurs in about 1 in 2,000 to 3,000 births, and this incidence is the same in all ethnic groups. There is gender variation among the different types of craniosynostosis. Mild deformational plagiocephaly is reported to be present in up to 13% of newborns, 16% of 6-week-olds, and nearly 20% of 4-month-olds. First born and male gender increase the risk of deformational plagiocephaly at birth. Most cases of deformational plagiocephaly resolve over time without specific medical intervention. When infants slept in the prone position, plagiocephaly occurred in 1 in 300. The prevalence of plagiocephaly increased to 1 in 60 following the recommendation for supine sleep position.

Microtia is less common and occurs in 1 in 6,000 to 8,000 births. Other ear malformations such as auricular dystopia (ear located on the check) or total atresia of the external area are less common and can be associated with other syndromes.

Clinical Presentation

Most craniofacial anomalies are readily apparent (see Dx Box). Some anomalies, such as cleft lips or microtia, are noted immediately in the delivery room. Other anomalies, such as craniosynostosis, develop over time. Because the onset of craniosynostosis may be gradual, parents may fail to recognize the condition, which usually appears as asymmetry of the face or skull. Deformational plagiocephaly also evolves over time and is more often noted by the clinician rather than the parents.

Dx Craniofacial Anomalies

- Cleft of the lip or palate
- Small, atretic, or malformed ear
- Asymmetry of the face
- Misshapen skull
- Recurrent otitis media
- Speech impairment

Children with craniofacial anomalies may also have medical problems that occur secondary to the deformity. Infants with cleft palate may present with failure to thrive because of difficulty feeding. Older infants and children may experience recurrent otitis media, speech impairments, or psychosocial stress. Nasal regurgitation of liquids may occur in children with obvious palatal clefts or more subtle deformities, such as submucous clefts of the soft palate.

Pathophysiology

Clefts of the lip and palate (Figure 58-1) are believed to develop as a result of an interruption in the merging of the middle and lateral portions of the face during the sixth to seventh week of gestation. The palate normally closes with an anterior to posterior progression. Any interference with this progression (eg, tumor or encephalocele in the roof of the mouth) leads to a cleft. A vascular disruption may also result in ischemia in the involved areas. Although the etiology of clefts is not fully determined, it is felt to be multifactorial. Studies establish a link between clefting and transforming growth factor–α (TGF-α). The locus for TGF-α is on the short arm of 2p13. As with other clinical conditions, genetic predisposition interacts with environmental factors to increase the risk of the emergence of a disorder. Infants with the A2 form of the TGF-α gene are 8 times more likely to have facial clefts if their mothers smoke.

The presence of a cleft palate affects normal oropharyngeal functioning, including sucking and speech. Children may exhibit hypernasal speech due to the escape of air through the nose, and have articulation problems. Recurrent otitis media seems to be related to dysfunction of the eustachian tube.

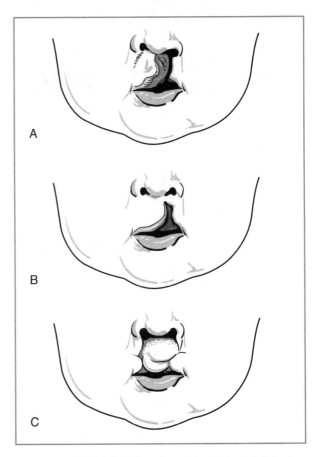

Figure 58-1. Cleft lips. A. Unilateral, complete cleft lip. B. Unilateral, incomplete cleft lip. C. Bilateral, complete cleft lip.

Microtia, a small atretic pinna of the ear, results from failure of development of the pinna and portions of the external auditory canal. It is most likely caused by a vascular accident during the 12th week of gestation. Similar anomalies have been created in laboratory animals by ligature of the stapedius artery. Microtia is considered in the spectrum of branchial arch defects.

Craniosynostosis refers to the premature closure of the sutures, which should remain open until 2 to 3 years of age. What initiates this pathologic ossification is unclear. There is some evidence to suggest that skull compression, such as occurs in utero with breech presentation or twins, contributes to the process. When there are other associated anomalies, such as syndactyly, embryologic disturbances in fibrocartilaginous development are suspected. Abnormalities in one region of chromosome 10 are implicated in syndrome synostosis. Any or all of the sutures can be affected, and the closure may result in asymmetry of the skull or microcephaly. Single suture synostosis is classified as simple; multiple synostosis is classified as compound. When closure is related to pathology at the suture, the condition is primary. When there is underlying brain pathology, the disorder is secondary. Premature closure of all sutures is often associated with diseases of the central nervous system, with failure of the brain to grow.

Microcephaly may result from premature closure of some or all of the sutures as a primary event or from impairment of the brain and its growth related to some other problem, such as hypoxic encephalopathy or congenital infection.

Fusion of individual sutures prevents growth of the skull perpendicular to the suture, and skull expansion proceeds in an axis parallel to that of the suture (Figure 58-2). If the sagittal suture fuses prematurely, the head is long and narrow, a condition referred to as **scaphocephaly** (boat head). This is the most common type of craniosynostosis, occurring in about 54% to 58%. If the coronal sutures fuse too soon, the head is flattened; this condition is called **brachycephaly** and occurs in 18% to 29% of cases of craniosynostosis. The incidence is 1 in 10,000 live births. Premature closure of the metopic suture results in the triangular-shaped head characteristic of **trigonocephaly,** reported in 4% to 10%. Familial cases have been reported, as well as abnormalities of chromosomes 3, 9, and 11.

Premature closure of the lambdoidal sutures leads to **plagiocephaly** (oblique head) (Figure 58-3). Plagiocephaly may also result from malpositioning in utero or after birth, a condition referred to as non-synostotic, deformational, or positional plagiocephaly. The skull has been likened to a parallelogram in appearance when there is also involvement of the facial structures. Torticollis, often related to injury to the sternocleidomastoid muscle at birth (see Chapter 94) and abnormal positioning after birth, may contribute to plagiocephaly. Plagiocephaly-torticollis sequence occurs in 1 in 300 live births. Malar and contralateral occipital flattening related to preferential positioning by infants are characteristically seen in affected infants. Some affected babies also have hip dislocation or positional clubfoot from in utero constraint (see Chapter 88). Positional plagiocephaly may be seen without torticollis and has been attributed to supine sleeping.

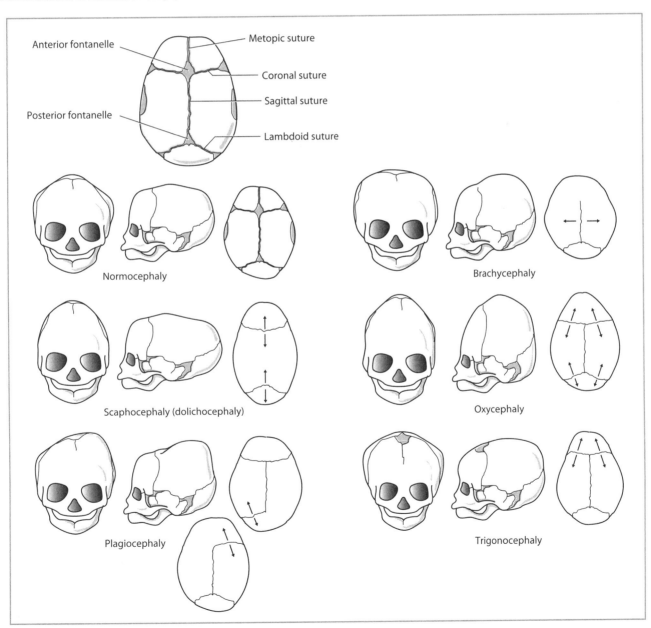

Figure 58-2. Changes in the shape of the skull when sutures fuse prematurely. Growth occurs parallel to the fused suture.

Differential Diagnosis

In general, the differential diagnosis of clefts of the lip and palate presents few problems. However, submucous clefts may be more difficult to diagnose. Children with such clefts may present with recurrent otitis media or hypernasal speech. Physical examination may reveal a bifid uvula and occasionally a notch at the junction of the hard and soft palates.

Determining whether any physical finding represents an isolated anomaly or is part of a genetic syndrome may be challenging. Any associated anomalies (eg, syndactyly or atrial septal defect) suggest the possibility of a genetic problem (Boxes 58-1 and 58-2).

Microtia does not present a diagnostic dilemma. The anomaly usually appears sporadically as an isolated condition although, like a cleft, it may be part of some other syndrome. Microtia is associated with midfacial hypoplasia and antimongoloid slant to the eyes in Treacher Collins syndrome. Microtia may also occur in Goldenhar syndrome, which is characterized by several associated findings, including hemifacial microsomia (one side of the face smaller than the other), epibulbar dermoids, hemivertebrae, microphthalmia, and renal and cardiac anomalies.

Box 58-1. Genetic Syndromes Associated With Clefts	
Ankyloblepharon filiforme adnatum	Optiz
Apert	Oral-facial-digital
Ectrodactyly-ectodermal dysplasia-clefting	Popliteal pterygium
Goldenhar	Stickler
Meckel	Treacher Collins
	Van der Woude

Craniosynostosis may also be an isolated finding or associated with a condition such as Apert syndrome, in which clefts of the palate are also seen (Box 58-3). A careful neurodevelopmental assessment helps determine whether microcephaly is related to an underlying neurodevelopmental disorder. Plagiocephaly may present a diagnostic dilemma: Is the condition related to unilateral craniosynostosis, torticollis, or supine sleeping? A careful assessment of the neck for masses or mobility helps determine the role of the neck musculature in the cranial flattening and defines the management approach (eg, neck exercises).

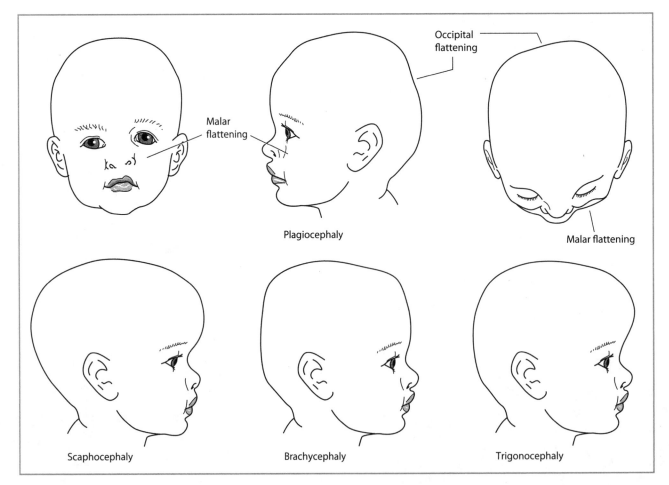

Figure 58-3. Top row. Classic appearance of an infant with facial asymmetry secondary to plagiocephaly. Bottom row. Classic appearance of infants with craniosynostosis.

Box 58-2. Anomalies Associated With Cleft Lips and Palates	
Nasal glioma or meningoencephalocele	Sacral agenesis
Persistent buccopharyngeal membrane	Aniridia
	Cleft larynx
Congenital neuroblastoma	Polydactyly
Congenital heart disease	Anencephaly
Thoracopagus twins	Foot deformities
Congenital oral teratoma	Oral duplication
Forearm bone aplasia	Spina bifida
Lateral proboscis	Aplasia of trochlea
	Laryngeal web

Box 58-3. Genetic Disorders With Craniosynostosis
Apert syndrome
Crouzon disease
Jackson-Weiss syndrome
Pfeiffer syndrome

Evaluation

Care must be taken to assess children and determine if the anomalies are isolated findings or components of a syndrome. This information is important both in terms of patient care and genetic counseling for parents regarding the likelihood of having future offspring with similar anomalies.

History

A medical, family, and psychosocial history should be obtained (Questions Box). Whether the condition appeared at birth or some time later is particularly significant in lesions affecting the skull, such as craniosynostosis. Maternal use of certain medications, such as diazepam, phenytoin, and isotretinoin (Accutane), and alcohol is associated with an increased incidence of clefts of the lip and palate. Maternal smoking also increases the risk of clefting, especially in a genetically vulnerable population. Maternal smoking and high altitude are associated with an increased occurrence of craniosynostosis.

Physical Examination

Height, weight, and head circumference should be measured and plotted at each visit. Head circumference is especially important in children with craniosynostosis or facial asymmetry. The skull should be palpated to detect perisutural ridging. Inner canthal distance may reveal hypotelorism, a finding seen in trigonocephaly. The neck should be palpated for masses and the range of neck motion assessed. The growth of children with craniofacial anomalies must be carefully monitored. Problems with adequate weight gain are frequently experienced by infants with clefts.

The physical examination should focus on defining the extent of the anomaly and determining if associated abnormalities are present. Such abnormalities may involve the face or other parts of the body, including the skeleton. The pharynx should be carefully examined for mobility of the palate. While some children with nasal regurgitation have a structural deformity such as a submucosal cleft, others, including infants with DiGeorge syndrome (22q11), have

Questions

Craniofacial Anomalies

- Did the child suffer any injuries at birth?
- Was the child born in an abnormal position?
- What is the child's usual sleeping position?
- Have the findings been present since birth, or did they appear later?
- Has the anomaly led to any changes in the child's health, such as recurrent ear infections or speech difficulties?
- Does the child have any family history of craniofacial anomalies?
- Does the mother have a history of illness during pregnancy?
- Was the mother exposed to any medications, particularly teratogenic agents, during pregnancy?
- Did the mother use alcohol during pregnancy?
- Did the mother smoke during pregnancy?
- Is the child experiencing difficulties in school (eg, teasing)?
- How is the child performing in school?
- Is development progressing normally? What are the child's milestones?
- Is the child's speech understandable?
- Does the child have any trouble with eating or drinking? Are fluids expelled through the child's nose with swallowing?

functional impairment with decreased palatal mobility. In children with microtia, the position of the ear should be noted. When the ear is displaced to the cheek, the condition is called *auricular dystopia*. Cardiac murmurs may be noted in children with clefts, and these murmurs should be carefully evaluated.

Children with clefts should be carefully assessed for the presence of otitis media at each visit. Periodic hearing assessments should be carried out in children with clefts or microtia. Speech and development should also be evaluated.

Laboratory Tests

Routine laboratory tests are not indicated in most children with craniofacial anomalies. Chromosomal studies are indicated if a genetic disorder is suspected. Refined studies including FISH (fluorescent in situ hybridization) may be needed to detect certain chromosomal abnormalities (see Chapter 57).

Imaging Studies

X-rays and imaging studies may be indicated in children with facial asymmetry, microcephaly and macrocephaly, and craniosynostosis.

A 3-dimensional computed tomography scan of the skull is particularly helpful in defining which if any sutures are fused. Such studies are helpful in differentiating craniosynostosis and deformational disorders. Renal ultrasound may be indicated in children with microtia or other ear anomalies because of the association between ear and renal anomalies.

Management

The management of children with craniofacial anomalies usually requires the expertise of a multidisciplinary team, including a pediatrician; plastic surgeon; ear, nose, and throat specialist; speech pathologist; social worker; psychologist; orthodontist; and prosthodontist. Primary care physicians who are not part of the team can receive information regarding appropriate patient care and follow-up. It is important for primary care physicians to be familiar with the appropriate nomenclature to be able to communicate with consultants. In brief, clefts of the lip are unilateral or bilateral and complete or incomplete. A complete cleft extends into the nares (see Figure 58-1). Clefts of the palate may involve the entire palate or be confined to the secondary or soft palate.

Routine **well-child care,** including monitoring of growth and administration of immunizations, is most important in the management of children with craniofacial anomalies. Some infants with clefts are slow feeders. Mothers should be told that although breastfeeding can be carried out, it may present unique challenges; however, the compliancy of the breast tissue creates a natural seal for the lip and palate. If difficulties are encountered, consultation with a lactation specialist may be especially helpful. Some formula-fed infants require the use of special adaptive nipples or feeders. A specific cleft palate feeder, which consists of a plastic bottle that allows for compression of the unit during feeding, is available. A soft, premature-type nipple can also be obtained. Long nipples, such as lamb's nipples, which are used to feed infant lambs, are not routinely recommended because they cause infants to gag. Infants who gain weight slowly may need to be given concentrated formulas (see Chapter 117).

Hearing and speech should be monitored. Chronic prophylactic **antibiotics** or the insertion of **pressure equalization tubes** may be needed to manage recurrent otitis media (see Chapter 60). Speech problems require the expertise of a speech pathologist and placement of children in **speech therapy** in either the community or school.

Surgical correction is indicated for many anomalies. Clefts are usually repaired as staged procedures during the first 2 years of life. Repair of the cleft lip, the first procedure, is traditionally scheduled when infants weigh 10 pounds, are 10 weeks of age, and when their hemoglobin is 10 (rule of tens). Appropriate weight gain is therefore critical to ensure timely surgery. If skilled anesthesiologists and nurses are available, cleft lip repair can be carried out within the first 2 weeks of life. Early repair is recommended at some centers. Repair of the cleft palate, the second procedure, is usually undertaken when infants are between 12 and 18 months of age. Better speech develops with earlier palatal repair. Surgical correction of clefts does not alter children's propensity to otitis media. This condition improves as children get older, however. Refinement of the

cosmetic results, including rhinoplasty, occurs throughout childhood. Orthodontia is frequently a key component to achieve a cosmetically acceptable result and appropriate occlusion of the dentition for speech and chewing.

Children with isolated unilateral microtia often hear, and surgery is recommended for cosmetic purposes. Surgical correction of microtia is usually initiated when children are 5 years of age, before they start school. At this time the ear has achieved 90% of its growth, and children are spared the potential embarrassment of their deformity in the school setting. Surgical reconstruction can involve the implantation of the child's costal cartilage or a prosthetic device shaped like the pinnae. In either case, several surgical procedures are usually needed. If there are other facial anomalies, more extensive reconstructive surgery is indicated.

Craniosynostosis can be corrected surgically, although the procedure is major and has significant risks. The age of the infant and the site of the synostosis influence the complexity of the procedure. A controversy about whether neurodevelopmental problems are related to craniosynostosis or whether they represent a preexisting condition has arisen. In developmentally normal children with evidence of closure of all the sutures, surgical repair is believed to be warranted. In other cases, the procedure is thought to be reconstructive because it normalizes the appearance of children with a deformation.

In children with plagiocephaly, where the deformation is believed to be related to torticollis, **passive stretching of the neck** 5 to 6 times a day (with each diaper change) is used to manage the condition. In addition, it is recommended that bright objects such as mobiles be placed over children's cribs to encourage head turning. Studies have shown that 90% of infants with congenital torticollis improve with manual stretching. Children who do not improve with stretching, have a deformity related to supine sleeping, or have a deformity that is still present at 6 months of age may be fitted with a specially designed helmet referred to as a *dynamic orthotic cranioplasty device* that reshapes the skull. The device is not used prior to 6 months of age and is generally worn for a minimum of 4 months. In an effort to reverse the trend of increasing positional plagiocephaly related to supine sleeping, the American Academy of Pediatrics has recommended that parents rotate their infant's position when they are awake and allow for "tummy time." Tummy time is time when infants are placed prone, sometimes with a rolled receiving blanket under their upper chest. This promotes the development of the neck musculature and head control. Positional plagiocephaly secondary to supine sleeping usually resolves with either repositioning or the use of a helmet and does not require surgical intervention.

Psychological counseling should be available to affected children and their families to help them adjust to the anomalies and the reactions of society. Parents may be referred to community agencies such as the Cleft Palate Foundation (www.cleftline.org) to help them cope with the potential stress related to giving birth to children with this anomaly and to advise them about the medical and surgical interventions that are available. FACES, the National Craniofacial Association (www.faces-cranio.org), is a referral source for parents.

Prognosis

Some anomalies, such as deformational plagiocephaly, resolve spontaneously or with exercise and positioning. Most other anomalies can be surgically corrected, leaving little residual evidence of the deformity. School success and psychological well-being may be more resistant to remediation and are highly dependent on the supportiveness of the family and their emotional resources. Children who grow up in settings where the deformity is thought to be embarrassing have long-term problems with low self-esteem.

CASE RESOLUTION

The infant in the case history has a cleft of the lip and palate. The mother is advised that the infant can be given formula, and she is given a supply of special feeders. She is given the contact information for a parent's support group and meets other parents of children with similar anomalies. During her visit to the local craniofacial team, she views pictures of children who have undergone a repair and feels relieved.

The mother is advised about the timing of surgery and told that the surgery will be scheduled when the infant is approximately 10 weeks old. A follow-up appointment in about 2 weeks is arranged. Weight gain is monitored, and the adjustment between the mother and the infant is assessed.

Selected References

Balasubrahmanyam G, Schere NJ, Martin JA, Michal ML. Cleft lip and palate: keys to successful management. *Contemp Pediatr.* 1998;15:133–153

Connolly JP, Seto ML, Whelan MF, et al. Progressive postnatal craniosynostosis and increased intracranial pressure. *Plast Reconstr Surg.* 2004;113:1313–1323

DaCosta AC, Walters I, Savarirayan R, Anderson VA, Wrennall JA, Meara JG. Intellectual outcomes in children and adolescents with syndromic and nonsyndromic craniosynostosis. *Plast Reconstr Surg.* 2006;118:175–181

Damiano PC, Tyler MC, Romitti PA, et al. Health-related quality of life among pre-adolescent children with oral clefts: the mother's perspective. *Pediatrics.* 2007;120:e283–e290

Denk MJ. Topics in pediatric plastic surgery. *Pediatr Clin North Am.* 1998;45: 1479–1506

Graham JM, Gomez M, Halberg A, et al. Management of deformational plagiocephaly: repositioning versus orthotic therapy. *J Pediatr.* 2005;146:258–262

Graham JM, Kreutzman J, Earl D, Halberg A, Samayoa C, Guo X. Deformational brachycephaly in supine-sleeping infants. *J Pediatr.* 2005;146:253–257

Harville EW, Wilcox AJ, Lie RT, Vindenes H, Abyholm F. Cleft lip and palate versus cleft lip: are they distinct defects? *Am J Epidemiol.* 2005;162:448–453

Hunt O, Burden D, Hepper P, Stevenson M, Johnston C. Self-reports of psychosocial functioning among children and young adults with cleft lip and palate. *Cleft Palate Craniofac J.* 2006;43:598–605

Ishimoto S, Karino S, Takegoshi H, Kaga K, Yamasoba T. Hearing levels in patients with microtia: correlation with temporal bone malformation. *Laryngoscope.* 2007;117:416–465

Kane AA, Mitchell LE, Craven KP, Marsh JL. Observations on a recent increase in plagiocephaly without synostosis. *Pediatrics.* 1996;97:877–885

Keating RF. Craniosynostosis: diagnosis and management in the new millennium. *Pediatr Ann.* 1997;26:600–612

Liptak GS, Serletti JM. Pediatric approach to craniosynostosis. *Pediatr Rev.* 1998;19:352–358

Meng T, Shi B, Zheng Q, Wang y, Li S. Clinical and epidemiologic studies of nonsyndromic cleft lip and palate in China: analysis of 4268 cases. *Ann Plast Surg.* 2006;57:264–269

Rohan AJ, Golombek SG, Rosenthal AD. Infants with misshapen skulls: when to worry. *Contemp Pediatr.* 1999;16:47–70

Schuster M, Maier A, Haderlein T, et al. Evalaution of speech intelligibility for children with cleft lip and palate by means of automatic speech recognition. *Int J Pediatr Otorhinolaryngol.* 2006;70:1741–1747

Shaw GM, Carmichael SL, Kaidarova Z, Harris JA. Epidemiologic characteristics of anotia and microtia in California, 1989–1997. *Birth Defects Res A Clin Mol Teratol.* 2004;70:472–475

van Vlimmeren LA, van der Graaf Y, Boere-Boonekamp MM, L'Hoir MP, Helders PJM, Engelbert RHH. Risk factors for deformational plagiocephaly at birth and at 7 weeks of age: a prospective cohort study. *Pediatrics.* 2007;119:e408–e418

Common Oral Lesions

Charlotte W. Lewis, MD, MPH

CASE STUDY

A 7-year-old girl is brought to the office for evaluation of a swelling on the inside of her lower lip of 4 to 6 weeks' duration. Her mother reports that it increases and decreases in size. The girl says that the swelling is not painful, and she cannot remember hurting her lower lip. On examination, a raised, bluish, non-tender, 1 x 1 cm swelling is apparent along the mucosa of the lower lip.

Questions

1. What is the differential diagnosis of lip masses?
2. What laboratory or radiographic tests are useful in the evaluation of oral lesions?
3. What management strategies are used to treat cyst-like oral lesions?
4. When should children with oral lesions be referred to subspecialists?

Primary care physicians are often required to evaluate lesions in the oral cavity. Knowledge of common congenital, developmental, infectious, traumatic, and neoplastic conditions that affect the mouth and its structures can help physicians to recognize and manage these lesions appropriately. Although many oral lesions are benign or represent normal variants, others may require specific medical or surgical treatment. Some oral lesions offer clues to underlying syndromic diagnoses, indicate more serious systemic disease, or occur as side effects of certain medications.

Epidemiology

Oral pathology is common and covers a broad range of lesions. Benign oral lesions such as gingival cysts occur in about 75% of newborns. Approximately 20% of the population has at least a small **torus palatinus,** a benign boney overgrowth of the palate that usually begins in childhood. **Ankyloglossia,** commonly referred to as tongue-tie, affects approximately 5% of newborns. **Fissured tongue** affects approximately 2% of the population. Fissured tongue may be associated with **benign migratory glossitis** (geographic tongue), which occurs in approximately 1% to 2% of children. **Tobacco-associated keratosis** occurs at the site of habitual placement of snuff or chewing tobacco and is estimated to affect more than 300,000 US children. **Leukoplakia,** a premalignant condition associated with smokeless tobacco, occurs in approximately half of users.

Aphthous ulcers (commonly known as canker sores) are one of the most common oral lesions seen in developed countries, with typical onset early in childhood. Approximately 20% to 25% of the US population experiences recurrent aphthous ulcers (RAU). Oral lesions resulting from infections are also common. Approximately 35% of newborns and young infants will develop **oral candidiasis,** commonly known as thrush. Oral **herpes** lesions are also common and are due to herpes simplex virus (HSV) group, usually type 1

(HSV-1). By young adulthood, more than half of US individuals will be seropositive for HSV-1. Approximately 20% to 40% of the population has experienced oral herpes at least one time.

Chronic ("ordinary") gingivitis usually has its onset in older children and will ultimately affect as many as 90% of adults.

Clinical Presentation

Oral lesions may come to the clinician's attention in any number of ways. Some may be obvious at birth, most notably a **congenital epulis,** which while benign in histology typically presents as a mass protruding from an infant's oral cavity and potentially interfering with breathing or eating. Oral lesions may be an incidental finding on physical examination. For example, in examining a newborn, the pediatrician may notice small (approximately 2–3 mm) yellow-white papules along the palatal midline and can then reassure the family that these are Epstein pearls, common lesions of no clinical significance. Clinicians may be the first to note swollen, friable, erythematous gingiva along with plaque buildup on and between the teeth representing the initial presentation of chronic gingivitis. Chronic gingivitis is the first stage of periodontal disease. Onset is typically in peripubertal children. Although young children experience gingivostomatitis from other causes, they do not usually harbor *Actinobacillus actinomycetemcomitans* or *Porphyromonas gingivalis,* and thus do not commonly experience chronic gingivitis or periodontal disease. Thickening of the mucosa, usually in the labial vestibule, offers clues to smokeless tobacco use. The severity of tobacco-related oral lesions demonstrates a dose-response relationship with the amount, frequency, and duration of smokeless tobacco exposure. Tobacco-associated keratosis is a predictable lesion that manifests as an area of thickening at the site of habitual placement of snuff or chewing tobacco. Chronic exposure to smokeless tobacco can lead to the development of opaque-white to yellow-brown lesions with a wrinkled appearance, known as leukoplakia and considered to be a premalignant condition.

Either the clinician or parent may be the first to notice thrush. The incidence of oral candidiasis peaks around the fourth week of life; thrush is uncommon in infants older than 6 to 9 months. Thrush can occur, however, at any age in predisposed patients (ie, immunosuppressed or deficient). *Candida albicans* in combination with contact irritation has been implicated in **angular cheilitis,** which appear as crusty or scaling erythematous fissures at the corners of the mouth.

Other benign oral lesions, such as benign migratory glossitis, are brought to the clinician's attention because parents are concerned that they represent pathology; however, reassurance is appropriate. Concerns for ankyloglossia may arise when newborns have difficulty breastfeeding or as a cause of speech problems in older children. Whether treatment for ankyloglossia improves an infant's ability to breastfeed is controversial. Ankyloglossia is a less common cause of speech difficulties than was once assumed. Nevertheless, it can be difficult for children to use their tongue to clean food debris from around their teeth when the lingual frenulum is short. The maxillary labial frenulum can appear quite prominent in young children. It is common for parents to inquire whether this is contributing to what appears to be abnormal spacing between the upper central incisors (midline **diastema**). However, the prominent frenulum may be more a result of a diastema than a cause of it.

Other oral lesions may present in conjunction with systemic symptoms. **Primary herpetic gingivostomatitis** typically occurs in infants and young children with the initial HSV-1 infection and is characterized by multiple oral and labial vesicular or ulcerative lesions, fever, malaise, cervical lymphadenopathy, and decreased oral intake. Oral lesions may indicate underlying serious systemic illness such as Crohn disease, systemic lupus erythematosus, or acute myelogenous leukemia. Some genetic syndromes are first detected because of oral lesions. For example, lip pits or mounds in conjunction with cleft palate are virtually pathognomonic of van der Woude syndrome, an autosomal-dominant cause of orofacial clefting. Hyperpigmented lesions (brown or dark blue, similar to freckles) on the lips or buccal mucosa may provide a clue toward the diagnosis of Peutz-Jeghers syndrome, an autosomal-dominant condition of multiple intestinal hamartomas. Patients with Peutz-Jeghers syndrome may experience recurrent abdominal pain, intestinal obstruction, or bleeding, and have a 15-fold increased risk of intestinal cancer.

Pathophysiology

Neonatal and Other Developmental Lesions

Gingival cysts in the neonate include Epstein pearls, Bohn nodules, and dental lamina cysts and are due to entrapment of tissues during embryologic development. Congenital epulis of the newborn is a rare, gingival tumor of unclear etiology that occurs more commonly in the maxilla than the mandible, with a marked female predilection

(8:1), and may occur as a single or multiple tumors. The etiology of fissured tongue and geographic tongue are unknown. Fissured tongue tends to cluster in families, suggesting a genetic etiology, and can also be seen in Down syndrome. Benign migratory glossitis results from the loss of the tiny finger-like projections, called papillae, on the tongue's surface, giving the tongue a map-like appearance.

Traumatic

Some of the most common oral lesions noted on physical examination result from minor accidental self-bites to the lip or buccal mucosa. Most of these resolve quickly, but recurrent trauma may lead to **pyogenic granuloma** or **fibroma** formation. A **mucocele** results from traumatic rupture of a minor salivary gland with subsequent cyst formation.

Infectious

Although an infectious etiology to aphthous ulcers has been proposed, their true etiology remains unclear. Oral herpes lesions are usually due to infection with HSV-1. **Herpangina** results from Coxsackievirus A infection. *C albicans* causes oral candidiasis. Thrush occurs when normal host immunity is immature (as in neonates) or suppressed (eg, during steroid treatment) or when normal flora is disrupted (eg, while on antibiotics). Infants may be colonized with *C albicans* during birth. Other sources of transmission to neonates include colonized skin (particularly around the breasts for breastfed infants) and/or improperly cleaned bottle nipples.

Chronic gingivitis occurs after build-up of bacterial plaque on the teeth, adjacent gingiva, and pockets between teeth and gums. Bacteria within plaque (most common species involved are Gram-negative anaerobic bacteria *[A actinomycetemcomitans* and *P gingivalis]*) release toxins that cause an inflammatory response.

Other

Drug-induced gingival hyperplasia can occur in patients taking corticosteroids, phenytoin (most common cause in children), cyclosporine, and nifedipine. It results from fibrous tissue overgrowth but is exacerbated by poor oral hygiene and presence of plaque in much the same way as ordinary gingivitis is.

Differential Diagnosis

Age at onset, location and characteristics of the lesion, and accompanying signs and symptoms often help to narrow the differential diagnosis. The appearance of 1- to 3-mm cysts in the mouth of a neonate brings to mind (1) **Epstein pearls,** which are the most common and are usually present along the palatal midline; (2) **dental lamina cysts,** which are usually located bilaterally along the crest of the dental ridge about where the first molars usually will erupt; or (3) **Bohn nodules,** which are found on the buccal and lingual aspects of the ridge, away from the midline. A protuberant mass from the anterior maxillary ridge of a newborn should suggest a congenital epulis; however, examination by a pathologist after resection is important to confirm the diagnosis. A mucocele is a painless, clear or bluish, fluid-filled cyst that results from damage to the salivary duct leading to extravasation of mucus from the gland into the surrounding soft tissue.

White plaques involving the buccal, lingual, and palatal mucosa bring to mind oral candidiasis. Thrush can sometimes be confused with milk remaining in the child's mouth after feeding. Scraping the lesion to determine if the white substance is readily removed (as milk is) helps to differentiate this from oral candidiasis, where the white plaques do not easily scrape off, and after scraping, the base of the thrush lesion may be erythematous or bleed. Thrush involving the tongue may also be confused with the erythematous denuded areas of the tongue seen in benign migratory glossitis. In fissured tongue, grooves that vary in depth are noted along the dorsal and lateral aspects of the tongue.

Common oral ulcers include aphthous ulcers, herpes gingivostomatitis, or herpangina. Oral herpes may be characerized by multiple vesicular lesions, which after rupture appear as ulcers, involving the lips, skin around the mouth, tongue, and mucosal membranes, typically in the anterior portion of the mouth. The initial infection may occur between 1 to 3 years of age. Aphthous ulcers also involve the anterior mouth, typically along the wet vermillion but they usually first appear at a somewhat older age (ie, in the preschool years or later) and with fewer lesions than oral herpes. Herpangina may present similarly to herpes but it more typically involves the posterior pharynx and the palate. Similar lesions on the hands and/or foot, as in hand-foot-and-mouth disease, may lend support to coxsaxievirus A as the etiology.

Trauma to the salivary duct may result in a mucocele. In contrast, a pyogenic granuloma is an erythematous, non-painful, smooth or lobulated mass that often bleeds easily when touched, while a fibroma is a moderately firm, smooth-surfaced, pink, sessile or pedunculated nodule, usually noted on the buccal mucosa in the occlusal plane.

Erythematous and friable gums often indicate the presence of chronic gingivitis. Typically plaque is seen on and between the teeth. In contrast to plaque-associated chronic gingivitis, which is usually painless, **acute necrotizing ulcerative gingivitis** is characterized by painful, edematous, bleeding gums with ulcers, necrosis, and pseudomembrane formation in affected areas. When this spreads to the oropharynx, it is referred to as **Vincent angina** (trench mouth), which can progress rapidly and interfere with speech and swallowing, and obstruct the airway.

Evaluation

History

The history is very important in evaluating oral lesions and determining the need for further treatment or referral. Key factors to include in the history are age at onset, duration, inciting factors, other medical problems, medications, use of tobacco, family history, ill contacts, and associated or systemic symptoms such as fever (Questions Box).

Questions

Common Oral Lesions

- How long has the child had the lesion?
- Is the lesion painful?
- Did the child recently injure the affected area?
- Has the child had any fever?
- Is the child eating as usual?
- Does the child have any other lesions?
- Is the child currently taking any medications? Has the child recently taken any medications?

Physical Examination

Physical examination of the oral structures should start with the lip (both the dry and wet vermillion) and surrounding skin (the "white lip"). The examination should then turn to the mucosa, gingiva, teeth, palate; superior, lateral, and posterior aspect of the tongue; sublingual structures; frena; and posterior pharynx. The clinician should note the number, size, location, and characteristics of the lesions because this information can be helpful in narrowing the differential diagnosis. Whether fever is present should be determined. The rest of the body should be examined with specific attention to the presence of other lesions, rashes, or arthritis.

Laboratory Tests

In otherwise healthy children who present with oral ulcerative lesions, supportive care is typically implemented without pursuing a definitive etiology. When there is need for specific diagnosis, HSV can be diagnosed via polymerase chain reaction techniques, immunofluorescence, or culture. Tzanck smears are no longer commonly performed to diagnose HSV because they require special skills, are not specific to HSV, and more specific tests are available. Likewise, oral candidiasis in an otherwise healthy infant is usually treated without diagnostic tests. However, a potassium hydroxide 10% microscopic slide preparation of scrapings from the lesion should demonstrate the characteristic spherical budding yeasts and pseudohyphae.

An excisional biopsy or resection may be needed to determine histology and diagnosis of an oral lesion.

Laboratory tests including a complete blood count, C-reactive protein, or erythrocyte sedimentation rate may be helpful in the initial evaluation of the ill-appearing child with oral lesions or when serious infection, systemic illness, or inflammatory conditions are suspected.

Imaging Studies

Imaging studies are not indicated in the evaluation of most oral lesions unless the lesions are related to problems of dentition such as dental abscesses, in which case the x-rays are obtained by the dentist rather than the pediatrician.

Management

Many of the common oral lesions are developmental or normal variants and/or are self-limited, and their management entails observation to ensure the lesions follow their expected course. For example, gingival cysts in newborns typically regress spontaneously. Oral lesions such as torus palatinus or benign migratory glossitis do not require treatment. Other oral lesions respond well to supportive care. For example, a child with herpetic gingivostomatitis or other forms of oral ulcers may benefit from regular ibuprofen or Tylenol, topical application of a 1:1 mixture of attapulgite (Kaopectate) and diphenhydramine elixir (Benadryl) to form a protective coating over the lesion, avoidance of acidic beverages such as orange juice that may burn on contact with the ulcers, and close attention to fluid intake and signs/symptoms of dehydration. Because of the risk of systemic absorption and subsequent dysrhythmia or seizure, viscous lidocaine should not be applied to oral lesions. Likewise, over-the-counter topical anesthetic agents contain a high content of alcohol and should not be used in children. Children who have severe presentations of primary herpetic gingivostomatitis or who develop HSV when immunocompromised may benefit from early initiation of therapy with acyclovir. Amlexanox 5% oral paste or high-dose steroid gel reduces pain, duration, and size of aphthous ulcers and is used in adults with RAU; however, safety of these treatments in children has not been established.

Other oral lesions require specific therapy. Thrush is typically treated with nystatin suspension (100,000 units/mL) as 1 mL swabbed to lesions 4 times per day until lesions are resolved. It is important to consider the possibility of an underlying immunodeficiency when thrush occurs outside of infancy or without a reasonable explanation. Angular cheilitis can be treated with nystatin cream or ointment and a low-potency hydrocortisone cream. Some oral lesions are best treated by resection. These would include congenital epulis, mucocele, pyogenic granuloma, and fibroma.

Treatment of gingivitis includes regular rinsing with alcohol-containing phenolic mouth rinse (eg, Listerine) or chlorhexidine gluconate oral preparation, improving oral hygiene (flossing, toothbrushing), and referral for professional dental care. The goals of therapy for gingivitis are to reduce clinical signs of inflammation and gingival bleeding and arrest or reduce the risk of progression of the periodontal disease and maintain dentition. Drug-induced gingival hyperplasia requires similar therapy to ordinary gingivitis. In addition, if the causative medication cannot be discontinued or changed, patients can be referred for surgical removal of excess gingival tissue and fitting of a positive-pressure mouth guard to inhibit further tissue growth. Acute necrotizing ulcerative gingivitis should be treated with penicillin V (or erythromycin for patients allergic to penicillin). Clindamycin can be used in refractory cases.

Management of oral lesions may require consultation and collaboration with dental, oral surgery, head and neck surgery, or other subspecialty colleagues. If the etiology of a lesion is unclear or if an oral lesion does not follow its expected course, referral is essential to ensure appropriate diagnosis and treatment.

Prognosis

Most oral lesions in children respond to appropriate intervention without residual problems. However, oral lesions can signal the onset of or occur in association with serious systemic conditions. In addition, chronic gingivitis represents the first and only reversible stage of periodontal disease, the leading case of tooth loss in adulthood. Because chronic gingivitis has its onset during childhood, physicians can play an important role in prevention of periodontal disease by promoting oral hygiene early in life. Once periodontal disease extends beyond the gums, it is no longer reversible and gradually destroys the bone and tissue that support the teeth, resulting in halitosis and tooth loss.

CASE RESOLUTION

The child described in the case history at the beginning of this chapter seems to have a mucocele. She should be referred to either an oral or head and neck surgeon for surgical excision of the lesion.

Selected References

American Academy of Pediatric Dentistry Council on Clinical Affairs. Guideline on pediatric oral surgery. *Pediatr Dent.* 2005–2006;27:158–164

Ebbert JO, Carr AB, Dale LC. Smokeless tobacco: an emerging addiction. *Med Clin North Am.* 2004;88:1593–1605

Gonsalves WC, Chi AC, Neville BW. Common oral lesions: part I. Superficial mucosal lesions. *Am Fam Physician.* 2007;75:501–507

Gonsalves WC, Chi AC, Neville BW. Common oral lesions: part II. Masses and neoplasia. *Am Fam Physician.* 2007;75:509–512

Scully C. Clinical practice. Aphthous ulceration. *N Engl J Med.* 2006; 355:165–172

CHAPTER 60

Otitis Media

Nasser Redjal, MD

CASE STUDY

An 18-month-old male infant is brought to your office with a 2-day history of fever and decreased food intake. He has had symptoms of an upper respiratory infection for the past 4 days but no vomiting or diarrhea. Otherwise he is healthy.

The infant appears tired but not toxic. On physical examination the vital signs are normal except for a temperature of 101°F (38.3°C). The left tympanic membrane (TM) is erythematous and injected, with yellow pus behind the membrane. The light reflex is splayed, and mobility is decreased. The right TM is gray and mobile, with a sharp light reflex. The neck is supple with shotty anterior cervical adenopathy, and the lungs are clear.

He has a 10- to 15-word vocabulary, and no one smokes in the household.

Questions

1. What are the differences between acute, persistent, and recurrent otitis media (OM)?
2. What factors predispose to the development of ear infections?
3. What are the most common presenting signs and symptoms of an ear infection in infants, older children, and adolescents?
4. How do the treatment considerations differ between acute, persistent, and recurrent ear infections?
5. What are some of the complications of OM?

Otitis media (OM) is the second most common reason after well-child care for a visit to the pediatrician and is the most common reason for which antibiotics are prescribed for children. It is estimated that approximately 30 million office visits per year are for the evaluation and treatment of OM and that billions of dollars are spent annually for OM care. Moreover, more than a quarter of all prescriptions written each year for oral antibiotics are for the treatment of middle-ear infections. In addition, many surgical procedures such as **myringotomy** with **tympanostomy tube** placement or adenoidectomy are performed on children for treatment of recurrent disease. Therefore, the primary care physician must have a good understanding of this very common pediatric condition.

Otitis media can be classified into the following 5 categories: **acute OM (AOM), OM with effusion (OME), recurrent AOM, chronic OME,** and **chronic suppurative OME.** It is important to distinguish between each of these entities because their presentation and management differ.

Acute OM (acute suppurative or purulent OM) is the sudden onset of inflammation of the middle ear, which is often accompanied by fever and ear pain (otalgia) (Box 60-1). Otitis media with effusion is the presence of middle-ear fluid after antimicrobial treatment. Resolution of acute inflammatory signs has occurred, with persistence of a more serous, non-purulent effusion. Although the fluid may persist for 2 to 3 months, it resolves within 3 to 4 weeks in 60% of cases. Recurrent OM is defined as frequent episodes of AOM with complete clearing between each episode. A more specific definition

is 3 new episodes of AOM requiring antibiotic treatment within a 6-month period, or 4 documented infections in 1 year. This condition affects approximately 20% of children who are "otitis prone"; such children are usually infants who have their first infection at

---

Box 60-1. Components of Acute Otitis Media (AOM)[a]

Definition of AOM

A diagnosis of AOM requires

1. A history of acute onset of signs and symptoms
2. The presence of middle-ear effusion (MEE)
3. Signs and symptoms of middle-ear inflammation

Elements of the definition of AOM are all of the following:

1. Recent, usually abrupt, onset of signs and symptoms of middle-ear inflammation and MEE
2. The presence of MEE that is indicated by any of the following:
   a. Bulging of the tympanic membrane
   b. Limited or absent mobility of the tympanic membrane
   c. Air-fluid level behind the tympanic membrane
   d. Otorrhea
3. Signs or symptoms of middle-ear inflammation as indicated by either
   a. Distinct erythema of the tympanic membrane

   or

   b. Distinct otalgia (discomfort clearly referable to the ear[s] that results in interference with or precludes normal activity)

[a]Adapted with permission from American Academy of Pediatrics Subcommittee on Management of Acute Otitis Media. Diagnosis and management of acute otitis media. *Pediatrics.* 2004;113:1451–1465.

younger than 1 year. Chronic OME (serous OM, secretory OM, non-suppurative OM, mucoid OM, glue ear OM) is a chronic condition characterized by persistence of fluid in the middle ear for 3 months or longer. The tympanic membrane (TM) is retracted or concave with impaired mobility and without signs of acute inflammation. Affected children may be asymptomatic. These children are at greater risk for developing hearing deficits and speech delay. Chronic suppurative OM implies a non-intact TM (perforation or tympanostomy tube present) with 6 or more weeks of middle-ear drainage.

Epidemiology

The overall prevalence of OM is 15% to 20%, with the highest peak in children 6 to 36 months of age. An additional smaller peak occurs at about 4 to 6 years. Otitis media is relatively uncommon in older children and adolescents. The condition is more common in boys than girls, and the prevalence is greater in Alaska Natives, Canadian Inuits, and Native Americans than in whites.

Several epidemiological risk factors for OM have been identified, including familial predisposition; siblings in the household; low socioeconomic status; non-breastfed infant; altered host defenses (acquired or congenital immunodeficiencies); environmental factors, such as child care attendance and passive smoke exposure; and the presence of an underlying condition, such as allergic disease of the upper airway, a cleft palate, or other craniofacial anomalies. Children with Down, Goldenhar, and Treacher Collins syndromes also have an increased risk of OM. As one might expect, the highest rate of OM occurs during the winter months and in early spring, coinciding with peaks in the incidence of upper respiratory infections (URIs).

Etiology

Up until the widespread immunization of children with heptavalent pneumococcal vaccine, the causative microorganisms for AOM were *Streptococcus pneumoniae* (25%–50%), *Haemophilus influenzae* (15%–30% most non-typeable strains), and *Moraxella catarrhalis* (3%–20%). Since vaccine licensure, there has been an overall decrease in the incidence of AOM, especially noted in children who are completely immunized. Group A streptococcus, *Staphylococcus aureus,* α-hemolytic *Streptococcus, Pseudomonas aeruginosa,* and anaerobic bacteria are other less common causative organisms. Other uncommon organisms such as *Mycoplasma pneumoniae*, chlamydia, and *Mycobacterium tuberculosis* have also been isolated. Respiratory viruses such as respiratory syncytial virus, adenovirus, rhinovirus, parainfluenza, coronavirus, and influenza A also play a role. Gram-negative enteric bacteria are common etiologic agents in the neonate, occurring in approximately 20% of cases, but are rare in older patients.

No bacterial or viral pathogen is recovered in middle-ear effusions in approximately 16% to 25% of cases of AOM. Currently approximately 50% of *H influenzae* and 100% of *M catarrhalis* isolated from the upper respiratory tract are β-lactamase positive and 15% to 50% (average 30%) of *S pneumoniae* are not susceptible to penicillin. The mechanism of penicillin resistance among isolates of *S pneumoniae* is not associated with β-lactamase production but related to an alteration of penicillin-binding proteins. This effect varies widely by geographic location and results in resistance to both penicillins and cephalosporins.

Clinical Presentation

Children with AOM often have a history of fever and ear pain. Associated symptoms include URI, cough, vomiting, diarrhea, and nonspecific complaints such as decreased appetite, waking at night, generalized malaise, lethargy, or irritability. Purulent otorrhea with minimal ear pain and hearing loss may also occur. Fever occurs in approximately 30% to 50% of patients. Temperatures exceeding 40°C are uncommon and suggest bacteremia or another complication. Older children may complain of tinnitus, vertigo, and hearing loss. Younger children are not able to express such complaints but may appear ataxic.

Pathophysiology

The most important factor in the pathogenesis of OM is abnormal function of the eustachian tube (Figure 60-1). Eustachian tube dysfunction occurs for 2 main reasons: abnormal patency and obstruction of the tube. Obstruction is either functional (secondary to collapse of the tube), mechanical (from intrinsic or extrinsic causes), or both. Functional obstruction or collapse of the eustachian tube occurs commonly in infants and young children because the tube is less cartilaginous and therefore less stiff than in adults, as well as more horizontal and shorter. In addition, the tensor veli palatini muscle is less efficient in this age group. Extrinsically, the presence of lymphoid follicles (adenoidal enlargement) or tumors (rare) surrounding the opening of the tube contributes to reflux, aspiration, or insufflation of nasopharyngeal bacteria into the middle ear. Intrinsic mechanical obstruction of the eustachian tube occurs as the result of inflammation secondary to a URI or allergy in patients older than 5 years. In addition, viral infection that can occur up to 6 to 12 times per year in children younger than 3 years also affects anatomical function, contributing to the risk of AOM (see Figure 60-1).

Hematogenous spread of microorganisms also can lead to infection. Less often, primary mucosal disease of the middle ear from allergies or abnormal cilia contributes to OM.

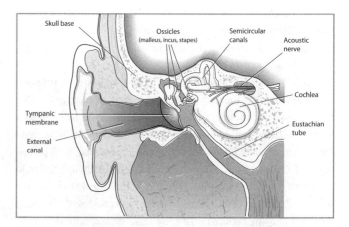

Figure 60-1. Relationship of middle ear to external and inner ears.

Differential Diagnosis

The most common cause of otalgia, or ear pain, is AOM. Other causes include mastoiditis, which is almost always accompanied by OM; otitis externa; and referred pain from the oropharynx, teeth, adenoids, or posterior auricular lymph nodes. A foreign body in the canal can produce similar symptoms. In children with ear pain, a search for any of these other conditions must be undertaken if the TM appears completely normal.

Evaluation

History

The history should carefully delineate the symptoms of OM and differentiate from those indicating a more serious condition such as meningitis (Questions Box).

For infants or children with a history of persistent or recurrent OM, it is important to find out when they had their last documented infection and what treatment they received. It is also critical to monitor development, particularly speech.

Otitis Media **Questions**

- Does the infant or child have fever, ear pain, hearing loss, or otorrhea?
- Is the infant or child inconsolable or lethargic?
- Has the infant or child had a previous ear infection? If so, when?
- Did the child complete the course of prescribed antibiotics?
- How many ear infections has the child had in the past year?
- Is the child taking any medication to prevent recurrent otitis media?
- Does the child attend child care?
- Is the child exposed to passive smoke?
- Is the infant breastfed?
- Does the child seem to hear?
- Is the child's speech development normal?

Physical Examination

To diagnose OM, the TM must be completely visualized and its mobility assessed. Occasionally this may be difficult because of the presence of cerumen or otorrhea. The diagnosis is then made on the basis of the history, and treatment may be initiated without confirmation by physical assessment. In all other cases, the position, color, degree of translucency, and mobility of the TM are evaluated. Classically, in AOM the TM is full, bulging, hyperemic, opaque, and/or has an air fluid level, with limited or no mobility. In addition, the light reflex is usually distorted or absent. In the case of persistent or chronic OM, signs of inflammation are usually absent, and the TM may be retracted, with limited or no mobility.

Associated physical findings with an uncomplicated middle-ear infection may include posterior auricular and cervical adenopathy. Other significant findings on physical examination are pain on movement of the pinna, anterior ear displacement, posterior auricular pain

and, rarely, evidence of peripheral facial nerve (cranial nerve VII) paralysis. The presence of these findings suggests other diagnoses such as an associated otitis externa or mastoiditis.

Positioning of infants or young children for examination of the ear is critical for an adequate examination. Several methods have been described, including allowing parents to hold the child in their arms or on their laps or restraining the child on the examination table with or without a papoose board (Figure 60-2). In addition, it may be difficult to visualize the TM in infants because the external auditory canal is slightly angulated. Lateral retraction of the pinna may help correct this problem.

Figure 60-2. **Three ways to position the infant or child for examination of the ear.**

Laboratory Tests

Although the diagnosis of OM is suspected on the basis of the history and then verified on physical examination, tympanometry may be helpful in distinguishing the normal ear from one with an effusion. In acute cases, audiometry is of limited diagnostic value, but it is helpful in evaluating the effects of a persistent, recurrent, or chronic middle-ear effusion on hearing.

Tympanocentesis is the most definitive method of verifying the presence of middle-ear fluid and of recovering the organism responsible for the infection. Indications for tympanocentesis or myringotomy are listed in Box 60-2. Nasopharyngeal cultures are not helpful because they do not seem to correlate highly with middle-ear fluid cultures.

Box 60-2. Indications for Tympanocentesis or Myringotomy in Children With Otitis Media (OM)

- OM in patients with severe ear pain, serious illness, or appearance of toxicity
- Onset of OM in children receiving appropriate and adequate antimicrobial therapy
- OM associated with confirmed or potential suppurative complications, such as facial paralysis, mastoiditis, or meningitis
- OM in newborns, sick neonates, or immunodeficient patients, in each of whom an unusual organism may be present

Prevention

During infancy and early childhood, the incidence of respiratory tract infections and recurrent OM can be reduced by altering child care center attendance patterns and exposure to passive tobacco smoke.

Immunoprophylaxis with influenza vaccine and pneumococcal conjugate vaccine has proven effective in preventing OM. Avoiding supine bottle-feeding (bottle propping) and reducing or eliminating pacifier use in the second 6 months of life can also decrease the incidence of AOM.

Breastfeeding, which provides infants with immunologic protection against URIs, other viral and bacterial infections, and allergies, also has a protective effect. Facial musculature may mature differently in breastfed infants, thus influencing eustachian tube function and reducing the risk of aspiration of fluid into the middle ear. Positioning during breastfeeding also has some protective effect, although immune factors in breast milk may serve as the most important mechanism for the reduced prevalence of OM.

Increased antibiotic resistance has eliminated the utility of routine antibiotic prophylaxis for recurrent AOM as a means of disease prevention.

Management

Current guidelines regarding the treatment of AOM confine the use of antibiotics to young children (<2 years old) or older ones with severe symptoms (Box 60-3). Otherwise, observation without the use of antibacterial agents in a child with uncomplicated AOM is recommended. Antibacterial treatment is deferred in these other children for 48 to 72 hours and management is limited to symptomatic relief. In an era of conjugated pneumococcal vaccine, the likelihood of bacteremia accompanying AOM is remote. Parents may be provided with a prescription to fill without recontacting the physician if the child remains symptomatic. This option is also recommended to otherwise healthy children 6 months to 2 years of age

Box 60-3. Indications for Antibiotics in the Treatment of Otitis Media[a]
Criteria for antibacterial treatment or observation in children with non-severe illness
1. Younger than 6 months: antibacterial treatment
2. 6 months to 2 years: antibacterial treatment with certain diagnosis or severe illness or observation with uncertain diagnosis or non-severe illness
3. 2 years and older: antibacterial treatment with severe or observe with non-severe illness with certain diagnosis; observation for uncertain diagnosis
• Caregiver is informed and agrees.
• Caregiver is able to monitor the child and return should condition worsen.
• Systems are in place for ready communication with the clinician, reevaluation, and obtaining medication if necessary.

[a]Adapted with permission from American Academy of Pediatrics Subcommittee on Management of Acute Otitis Media. Diagnosis and management of acute otitis media. *Pediatrics*. 2004;113:1451–1465.

with non-severe illness at presentation *and* an uncertain diagnosis. Age younger than 2 years is associated with increased risk of failure of a watchful waiting strategy. Concern for serious infection among children younger than 6 months influences the decision for immediate antibacterial therapy in this age group. The recommended antibiotic therapy is noted in Table 60-1.

Tympanocentesis is rarely performed nowadays prior to the initiation of antibiotics. Indications for tympanocentesis include severe ear pain (provides relief through decompression) or toxic appearance. Tympanocentesis is occasionally carried out in a child who has been receiving appropriate and adequate antimicrobial therapy but fails to improve; or in the face of confirmed or potential suppurative complications, such as facial paralysis, mastoiditis, or meningitis; or in newborns, sick neonates, or immunodeficient patients, in whom an unusual organism may be present (see Box 60-2).

Table 60-1. Recommended Antibacterial Agents for Patients Who Have Failed 48 to 72 Hours of Observation or Initial Management With Antibacterial Agents[a]				
	Clinically Defined Treatment Failure at 48–72 Hours After Initial Management With Observation Option		*Clinically Defined Treatment Failure 48–72 Hours After Initial Management With Antibacterial Agents*	
Temperature ≥39°C (102.2°F) and/or Severe Otalgia	*Recommended*	*Alternative for Penicillin Allergy*	*Recommended*	*Alternative for Penicillin Allergy*
No	Amoxicillin, 80–90 mg/kg/d	Non–type I: cefdinir, cefuroxime, cefpodoxime; type I: azithromycin, clarithromycin	Amoxicillin-clavulanate, 90 mg/kg/d of amoxicillin component, with 6.4 mg/kg/d of clavulanate	Non–type I: ceftriaxone, 3 days; type I: clindamycin
Yes	Amoxicillin, clavulanate, 90 mg/kg/d of amoxicillin, with 6.4 mg/kg/d of clavulanate	Ceftriaxone, 1 or 3 days	Ceftriaxone, 3 days	Tympanocentesis, clindamycin

[a]Adapted with permission from American Academy of Pediatrics Subcommittee on Management of Acute Otitis Media. Diagnosis and management of acute otitis media. *Pediatrics*. 2004;113:1451–1465.

Adjunctive medications such as topical analgesics and antipyretics are important therapeutic options and should be prescribed for children with significant pain or fever. Antihistamines, decongestants, or steroids play no documented role in the treatment of OME. Most resolving middle-ear effusions seen after AOM in otherwise healthy children do not need to be treated and the "wait-and-watch" approach is recommended.

Failure of antibiotic treatment and chronic effusions warrant a referral to an otolaryngologist for further evaluation for pressure equalization tubes or, if the patient is older than 4 years, a possible adenoidectomy. Other reasons for consultation include evidence of hearing loss; the presence of any anatomical abnormality, such as a defect of the TM (perforations, cholesteatomas) or intranasal problems (deviated septum, polyp); signs and symptoms of an OM but normal physical examination; and a predisposition to chronic recurrent OM (eg, children with a cleft palate or Down syndrome).

Prognosis

Complications associated with OM are much less common with appropriate antibiotic therapy and follow-up, but occasionally occur. They can be divided into 2 categories: extracranial and intracranial. Extracranial complications include perforation of the TM, conductive and sensorineural hearing loss, cholesteatoma, mastoiditis, facial nerve (cranial nerve VII) paralysis, osteomyelitis of the temporal bone, and Bezold abscess. Intracranial complications are meningitis, extradural as well as subdural abscesses, lateral venous sinus thrombosis, brain abscess, and hydrocephalus.

CASE RESOLUTION

In the case presented at the beginning of the chapter, the child displays the classic signs and symptoms of acute otitis media: fever, upper respiratory infection, decreased appetite, and an abnormal tympanic membrane on physical examination. Because of his age, fever, and the certainty of diagnosis, he should be treated for 10 days with oral antibiotics. The prognosis is good given his normal speech development.

Selected References

American Academy of Pediatrics. Appropriate use of antimicrobial agents. In: Pickering LK, Baker CJ, Long SS, McMillan JA, eds. *Red Book: 2006 Report of the Committee on Infectious Diseases.* 27th ed. Elk Grove Village, IL: American Academy of Pediatrics; 2006:737–741

American Academy of Pediatrics Subcommittee on Management of Acute Otitis Media. Diagnosis and management of acute otitis media. *Pediatrics.* 2004;113:1451–1465

Apiro DM, Khoon YT, Donald HA, Dziura JD, Baker MD, Shapiro ED. Wait and see prescription for the treatment of AOM. *JAMA.* 2006;296:1235–1241

Arguedas A, Emparanza P, Schwartz RH, et al. A randomized, multicenter, double blind, double dummy trial of single dose azithromycin versus high dose amoxicillin for treatment of uncomplicated acute otitis media. *Pediatr Infect Dis J.* 2005;24:153–161

Brunton S, Pichichero ME. Acute otitis media: influence of the PCV-7 vaccine on changes in the disease and its management. *J Fam Pract.* 2005;54:961–968

Casey JR, Pichichero ME. Changes in frequency and pathogens causing acute otitis media in 1995–2003. *Pediatr Infect Dis J.* 2004;23:824–828

Centers for Disease Control and Prevention. National, state, and urban area vaccination coverage among children aged 19–35 months—United States, 2005. *MMWR Morb Mortal Wkly Rep.* 2006;55:988–993

Damoiseaux RA, van Balen FA, Hoes AW, Vaerheij TJ, de Melker RA. Primary care based randomised, double blind trial of amoxicillin versus placebo for acute otitis media in children aged under 2 years. *BMJ.* 2000;320:350–354

Piglansky L, Leibovitz E, Raiz S, et al. Bacteriologic and clinical efficacy of high dose amoxicillin for therapy of acute otitis media in children. *Pediatr Infect Dis J.* 2003;22:405–413

Rosenfeld RM. Diagnostic certainty for acute otitis media. *Int J Pediatr Otorhinolaryngol.* 2002;64:89–95

Siegel RM, Kiely M, Bien JP, et al. Treatment of otitis media with observation and a safety-net antibiotic prescription. *Pediatrics.* 2003;112:527–531

Wald ER. Acute otitis media: more trouble with the evidence. *Pediatr Infect Dis J.* 2003;22:103–104

Whitney CG, Farley MM, Hadler J, et al. Decline in invasive pneumococcal disease after the introduction of protein-polysaccharide conjugate vaccine. *N Engl J Med.* 2003;348:1737–1746

Hearing Impairments

Julie E. Noble, MD, and Monica Sifuentes, MD

CASE STUDY

A 15-month-old girl is brought to the office because the parents are concerned that she has not yet begun to speak. The child was the full-term product of an uncomplicated pregnancy. Her 25-year-old mother, who began to receive regular prenatal care during the second month of gestation, had no documented infections during the pregnancy, took no medications, and has denied using illicit drugs or alcohol. The 27-year-old father is reportedly healthy. There is no family history of deafness, mental retardation, or consanguinity.

The girl, who is otherwise healthy, has never been hospitalized, but she has had 3 documented ear infections. She rolled over at 4 to 5 months of age, sat at 7 months, and walked at 13 months. She is able to scribble. The parents report that their daughter smiles appropriately, laughs occasionally, and plays well with other children. As an infant, the girl cooed and babbled, but she now points and grunts to indicate her needs. She does not respond to loud noises by turning her head.

The child's growth parameters, including head circumference, are normal for age. The rest of the physical examination is unremarkable.

Questions

1. When should deafness be suspected in infants or children?
2. What is the relationship between hearing loss and language development?
3. What are the major causes of deafness in children?
4. What neonates are at risk for the development of hearing deficits?
5. What methods are currently available to evaluate hearing in infants and children?
6. What are the important issues to address with families who have infants or children with suspected hearing impairment?

Hearing loss, even in a mild degree, is a significant childhood disability that can compromise speech and language development, academic performance, and psychosocial behavior. Its identification as early as possible is essential to implement intervention, which has been shown to prevent many adverse consequences. Children may either be born with a hearing deficit, termed *congenital deafness,* or may acquire the condition during childhood, termed *progressive* or *late-onset.* A mild hearing deficit occurs with a 26 to 40 decibel (dB) loss. Severe hearing loss, on the other hand, is defined as 71 to 90 dB, and profound loss is 90 dB or greater. The most important period for speech and language development is from birth to 3 years of age. Reduced hearing acuity in both or even one ear during this time can greatly interfere with this important process (see Chapter 19). Therefore, primary care physicians must have a clear understanding of when to suspect deafness in infancy and early childhood and must be familiar with its identification, evaluation methods, and treatment.

Epidemiology

The prevalence of congenital deafness in children is approximately 0.1%. In other words, 1 in 1,000 children is born severely to profoundly deaf. It has been estimated, however, that 3 to 5 in 1,000 children have mild to moderate hearing loss. The average age at diagnosis

of most children who were born deaf was 2 to 3 years prior to the initiation of newborn hearing screening. Since its advent, the average age of diagnosis has dropped to 2 to 3 months. At this time in the United States, all 50 states have a policy on newborn hearing screening with mandates in 38 states. But the policies are not followed at every hospital, follow-up of positive tests may not occur, and some forms of early-onset hearing loss are not apparent at birth. Therefore, careful assessment of hearing and language development by the pediatrician is essential at each patient encounter.

An estimated 20% to 30% of children who are hearing impaired developed the condition during childhood. Of these, 70% of children with acquired hearing loss are initially identified by the parents rather than physicians. Any concern by the parent that their child might have a hearing problem should be taken seriously by the physician and objective testing performed.

Graduates of the neonatal intensive care unit have a significant increased risk of bilateral sensorineural hearing loss (1%–3%). Associated factors such as prematurity (birth weight <1,500 g), hyperbilirubinemia, prolonged mechanical ventilation, and neonatal sepsis increase this risk. Other factors associated with deafness in infancy include meningitis, parental consanguinity, craniofacial malformations, congenital viral infections, perinatal asphyxia, and a family history of deafness.

Clinical Presentation

Children with hearing impairments frequently present to physicians with delayed speech. Parents may be concerned that the toddler is indicating his needs by grunting and pointing rather than by using words. Children also may display behavioral problems, such as inattention, temper tantrums, or aggressive play with other children (Dx Box).

> ### Hearing Impairment
>
> - Parental concern or suspicion of hearing loss
> - Delayed speech and language development
> - Associated risk factors including prematurity, exposure to ototoxic drugs, congenital or acquired central nervous system infections, and craniofacial abnormalities
> - History of behavioral problems and/or poor school performance
> - Abnormal hearing test

Hearing impairment can be more difficult to recognize in infants younger than 6 months because they may have no obvious symptoms of hearing loss. They may startle to moderately loud noises and begin to vocalize just as other infants (Figure 61-1). All health care providers should review the newborn hearing screening results and follow up on any abnormal findings (see Newborn Hearing Screening). If the history is suggestive of a hearing loss, repeat testing should be performed.

Pathophysiology

Mechanism of Hearing

Sounds in the form of pressure waves are carried from the external environment through the external auditory canal to the tympanic membrane (TM). These waves are then converted to mechanical vibrations by the ossicles, and the mechanical vibrations are then transmitted from the TM to the inner ear, where they are transformed to fluid vibrations. Finally, these fluid vibrations are converted into nerve impulses by nerve endings located in the cochlea in the inner ear. These impulses are conducted via the auditory nerve to the auditory cortex (Figure 61-2).

Hearing impairments can be classified either according to the part of the auditory system affected or by the cause of the hearing loss.

Types of Hearing Loss

A **conductive hearing loss denotes an abnormality in the outer ear, the TM, or middle-ear ossicles.** Cerumen impaction, otitis externa, serous otitis, recurrent otitis media, TM perforation, and ossicular discontinuity are examples of this type of hearing loss. Middle-ear effusions rarely cause more than a 20- to 30-dB loss.

The cochlea or inner ear or auditory nerve is affected in **sensorineural hearing loss.** Congenital infections, anomalies, and

Figure 61-1. Loudness of everyday sounds. (Reproduced with permission from Northern J, Downs M. *Hearing in Children.* 4th ed. Baltimore, MD: Williams & Wilkins; 1991.)

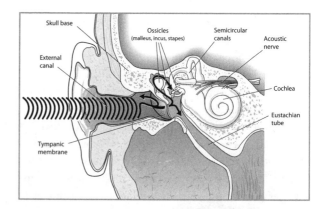

Figure 61-2. Sound waves passing through the external ear into the middle ear.

genetic disorders lead to this type of loss. A **mixed disorder** has characteristics of both conductive and sensorineural losses. In a **retrocochlear hearing loss,** the auditory nerve, brain stem, or cortex is affected.

Etiology of Hearing Impairment (Box 61-1)

Severe to profound hearing loss has 2 main causes: genetic and acquired environmental. Genetic causes account for approximately 68% of cases. There are more than 300 forms of syndromic hearing loss with associated clinical features. An autosomal-recessive syndrome, Pendred syndrome with thyromegaly is a more common example. Down syndrome and Goldenhar syndrome both have frequently associated hearing impairment. But most cases of genetic hearing loss are non-syndromic and are a single gene defect. Mutations in the GJB2 gene account for 30% to 50% of all cases in many populations. Genetic malformations of the ear pinnae or ossicles do occur but are the least common cause of hearing loss. Genetic mutations may result in different types of deafness with various presentations and outcomes (ie, hearing loss may be conductive, sensorineural, or mixed, and may be static or progressive with the initial presentation either in infancy or later childhood).

Acquired environmental causes include prenatal, perinatal, or postnatal events and exposures such as congenital infections, bacterial meningitis, hyperbilirubinemia, complications of prematurity, and exposure to ototoxic medications. Cytomegalovirus (CMV) is probably the most frequently unrecognized congenital infection causing deafness. Ten percent of infants with congenital hearing loss are infected with CMV. However, toxoplasmosis, rubella, herpes simplex virus, human immunodeficiency virus (HIV), and syphilis can also be implicated. Hearing loss associated with bacterial meningitis was as high as 20%, with *Streptococcus pneumoniae* as the prevalent responsible organism. The incidence of both *S pneumoniae* and *Haemophilus influenzae* meningitis have decreased tremendously in young children following the advent of conjugate vaccine, and the prevalence of post-meningitic hearing loss has similarly declined. The role of steroids in the treatment of bacterial meningitis has also contributed to the decrease in sensorineural hearing loss in survivors.

With the recognition and treatment of hyperbilirubinemia in term newborns, this as a cause of hearing loss is now rare in the United States and other developed countries. Prematurity as a cause of hearing loss is, however, not uncommon. Because of associated complications, premature infants have higher rates of severe hearing loss than do full-term infants. Some antibiotics, such as the aminoglycosides, and other medications like furosemide can be irreversibly ototoxic; other drugs may cause only transient effects.

Any head injury causing significant middle-ear trauma may also cause deafness in children. Repeated acoustic trauma from continuous or significant exposure to loud noise can also cause irreversible hearing loss. With children's use of personal listening devices, this cause of hearing loss is increasing.

Differential Diagnosis

In addition to hearing loss, communication disorders should be considered in infants or children with delayed speech and language development. These include problems with speech perception, language comprehension, formulation of language output, and speech

---

Box 61-1. Major Causes of Childhood Deafness[a]

- Genetic (familial or sporadic)
- GJB2 gene defect
- Pendred syndrome
- Ear malformations
- Acquired
  Infections
  — Congenital—cytomegalovirus, rubella, toxoplasmosis, herpes simplex virus, human immunodeficiency virus, syphilis
  — Acquired—bacterial meningitis, mastoiditis, recurrent and chronic otitis media, mumps
  Complications associated with prematurity
  Ototoxic medications and chemicals
  Hyperbilirubinemia
  Head trauma
  Acoustic trauma
- Unknown

[a]Modified with permission from Rapin I. Hearing disorders. *Pediatr Rev.* 1993;14:44.

---

production. Unrecognized conditions such as mental retardation or autism can be responsible for some of these disorders. Other etiologies include specific central nervous system deficits as well as impairments of fine motor control of the oropharynx.

Evaluation

Newborn Hearing Screening

In 1994 the Joint Committee on Infant Hearing, composed of representatives from several professional organizations, endorsed universal newborn hearing screening. Their goal was the early identification of hearing loss in infants before age 3 months and the implementation of intervention services by 6 months of age. As a result of these recommendations, states have implemented legislation mandating newborn hearing screening and intervention programs. A subsequent position statement was issued in 2000 titled Principles and Guidelines for Early Detection and Intervention Programs. The American Academy of Pediatrics endorsed this statement and promotes newborn hearing screening as well as periodic hearing assessment for every child. The clinician should maintain a high index of suspicion for hearing loss and be familiar with the high risk factors associated with sensorineural and/or conductive hearing loss.

History

Because the primary symptom of deafness is failure to learn to speak at the appropriate age, the most important aspect of the history in children with possible hearing loss is determining whether speech is developing normally. Even deaf infants may begin cooing and babbling in infancy, and these early attempts at verbalization are not useful milestones for assessment of hearing deficits. It helps to ask parents whether they are at all suspicious or concerned about their children's speech or hearing. Guidelines to assess language development are found in Box 61-2. (See Chapter 19.) An assessment of risk

Box 61-2. Expected Speech-Language-Auditory Milestones[a]

Birth to 3 months

- Startles to loud noise
- Awakens to sounds
- Blink reflex or eye widening to noises

3 to 4 months

- Quiets to mother's voice
- Stops playing, listens to new sounds
- Looks for source of new sounds not in sight

6 to 9 months

- Enjoys musical toys
- Coos and gurgles with inflection
- Says "mama"

12 to 15 months

- Responds to his/her name and "no"
- Follows simple requests
- Expressive vocabulary of 3 to 5 words
- Imitates some sounds

18 to 24 months

- Knows body parts
- Expressive vocabulary minimum of 20 to 50 words (uses 2-word phrases)
- 50% of speech intelligible to strangers

By 36 months

- Expressive vocabulary of 500 words (uses 4-5–word sentences)
- Speech is 80% intelligible to strangers
- Understands some verbs

[a]Adapted with permission from Northern J, Downs M. *Hearing in Children.* 4th ed. Baltimore, MD: Williams & Wilkins; 1991.

Questions

Hearing Impairment

- Does the infant seem to respond to sounds?
- Does the infant attempt to repeat sounds?
- How does the young child indicate his or her desires or needs?
- How are the parents currently communicating with the child?
- Is there any evidence of a congenital infection, structural anomaly of the head and neck, or syndrome?
- Is there a history of prematurity or other prenatal or perinatal problem?
- Have there been any serious bacterial infections such as meningitis?
- Has the child had a history of repeated ear infections or exposure to ototoxic drugs?
- Aside from the hearing problem, is the child developmentally normal?
- Is there a family history of deafness, consanguinity, or multiple miscarriages or stillbirths?

factors for deafness, such as a positive family history, infection during gestation, history of prematurity, hyperbilirubinemia, neonatal sepsis, and asphyxia, is also important (Questions Box).

Physical Examination

A complete physical examination should be performed on all children. In particular, any dysmorphic facial features that may suggest the presence of a syndrome with an associated hearing deficit should be noted. Other anomalies of the head and neck should be noted as well. Abnormal pigmentary conditions may be important clues. The eyes should be evaluated for heterochromia and hypertelorism. The size and shape of the pinnae and external ear canals should be carefully inspected for abnormalities and patency, respectively. Preauricular pits or tags may be apparent. In addition, the TMs should also be visualized and assessed for the presence of a middle-ear effusion that may influence subsequent audiological tests. Insufflation may be helpful. The oropharynx should be examined for a cleft palate or a bifid uvula, which may be associated with a submucous cleft. The manner in which children communicate with parents should be noted, if possible, and the child assessed for response to sound.

Laboratory Tests

Tympanometry does not measure hearing, but is useful in assessing the presence of middle-ear fluid and the mobility of the TM. Tympanometry can be particularly helpful with uncooperative, crying children in whom assessing the appearance of the TM and insufflation is difficult. Different types of hearing tests for evaluating infants and children for possible hearing deficits are available to general pediatricians (Box 61-3). **Automated auditory brain stem response (ABR)** and **brain stem auditory evoked response (BAER)** are electrophysiological measurements of activity in the auditory nerve and brain stem pathways. Electrodes are placed on the infant or child's head to record brain wave activity while a specific auditory stimulus is presented through earphones to one ear at a time. Auditory thresholds can be estimated. The ABR is used for newborn hearing screening and only takes approximately 10 minutes, whereas the BAER is more comprehensive, requiring up to 90 minutes to perform. **Behavioral observation audiometry** measures a child's response to speech and frequency-specific stimuli presented through speakers in a soundproof room. This method of testing can only assess hearing in the better ear and cannot detect unilateral hearing loss. It is used with children at younger than 6 months' developmental age. **Evoked otoacoustic emissions** can be performed on children of all ages. It measures cochlear function in response to a specific stimulus via a small probe that contains a microphone that is placed in the ear canal. This test can be used for newborn hearing screening and also can be performed in approximately 10 minutes. **Conditioned play audiometry** like **conventional audiometric testing** measures auditory thresholds in response to frequency-specific stimuli presented through earphones to one ear at a time. The patient is instructed to perform a particular task, such as put a block in a container versus raise his or her hand, when the stimulus is heard. Children as young as 3 years can be tested by conditioned play audiometry and 4 or 5 years of age via conventional

Box 61-3. Tests to Evaluate Hearing

- Automated auditory brain stem response (ABR): used for newborn hearing screening
- Behavioral observation audiometry
- Brain stem auditory evoked response (BAER)
- Evoked otoacoustic emissions (EOAE): newer type of newborn hearing screening
- Conditioned play audiometry
- Conventional audiometric testing

audiometric testing. These tests should be used in conjunction with evaluations from audiological and otolaryngologic consultations. In the case of high-risk infants, testing should be repeated at least every 6 months until 3 years of age, and at appropriate intervals thereafter depending on the etiology of the suspected hearing loss and the hearing test results.

Other diagnostic tests to consider in infants whose cause of deafness is unknown include titers for congenital infections such as CMV, toxoplasmosis, HIV, and rubella and fluorescent treponemal antibody absorption tests for syphilis. In the newborn period, a CMV culture may be helpful. Testing for the GJB2 gene, the mitochondrial A1555G mutation that predisposes one to ototoxicity from drugs, and the SLC26A4 gene for Pendred syndrome along with CMV testing would reveal an etiology for 40% of congenital hearing loss and for 60% of late-onset hearing loss. Thyroid function tests are necessary if Pendred syndrome is suspected, especially in school-aged children with goiters. Proteinuria and hematuria should also be ruled out by urine dipstick, especially in boys with a positive family history of deafness and renal failure, findings suggestive of Alport syndrome. An electrocardiogram is recommended to detect conduction defects such as QT prolongation in Jervell and Lange-Nielsen syndrome.

Imaging Studies

Occasionally, a computed tomography or magnetic resonance imaging scan of the temporal bone may be used to view the anatomy of the middle and inner ear, particularly in cases of a suspected cochlear/vestibular malformation or fistula. Necessity should be determined by the audiologist.

Management

Studies have shown that the earlier the hearing deficit is detected and remediation begun in the otherwise normal infant, the greater the likelihood the child will have language development close to that of a hearing infant. Initiation of intervention prior to 6 months of age produces infants who are able to develop language, social, and emotional skills appropriate for their age. School performance and communication skills also have been shown to be better in those identified at a younger age. All infants and children identified with a hearing deficit should be referred to an otolaryngologist and audiologist for immediate assessment and recommendation for assistive devices.

Once infants or children are found to have a hearing impairment, careful follow-up is necessary so that no further reduction in hearing occurs. The role of primary care providers thus becomes even more crucial. Both parents and other family members may initially be devastated by the diagnosis of a hearing impairment, especially if the deficit is severe to profound. They often have multiple questions about children's medical prognosis and educational future. The possibility of further speech and language development may also be a foremost concern in their minds. In addition to providing patients with comprehensive care, all of the parents' questions and concerns must be addressed and anticipated.

Future Audiological Evaluations

In newly diagnosed patients with sensorineural hearing loss, **audiograms** should be repeated every 3 months in the first year and then every 6 months when children are in preschool. The test should be repeated at least annually after children have begun school. Continued monitoring is essential to detect any progression of the hearing deficit, especially in the less affected ear.

Assistive Devices

Although **hearing aids** may not restore normal hearing, all children with conductive as well as sensorineural hearing loss benefit from amplification. Several different types of hearing aids are available for children; these devices should be fitted appropriately and adjusted regularly. In addition, it is also recommended that all patients receive bilateral hearing aids to improve auditory localization and training, particularly in the context of different learning situations. In reality, unfortunately, many children do not use bilateral hearing aids, either because their families do not have the necessary financial resources or because one is lost, damaged, or malfunctioning.

An **FM system** is an additional assistive listening device that can be used in a classroom. A speaker uses a microphone to transmit to a receiver the child wears to improve reception. **Closed-caption television** (signed or subtitled) is another method of auditory training. In addition, **teletype telephone systems** are available for children who can read.

A **cochlear implant** may be surgically placed in the cochlea to improve hearing. It is an electrode array that responds to an external microphone and speech processor and produces an electrical discharge within the cochlea. It is used in children at 12 months of age or older with profound sensorineural hearing loss. There are ongoing improvements in technology with improving results. Speech, language, and special education resources should also be provided. Most patients with implants show significant improvement in communication skills.

Education and Communication

Much controversy exists regarding the optimal method of communication for deaf children. **Oral communication (lip reading)** and **sign language** each have their advantages as well as disadvantages depending on children's age, the type of deafness, and whether the deficit is congenital or acquired. Whether the children already know a language is also important to consider. The preferred methods seem to vary from region to region; therefore, schools, other institutions, and resource groups often use the most popular communication method in a particular area. In general, some authors recommend that children with minimal hearing loss may do better with lip reading than those with greater hearing loss, who will most likely benefit more from sign language.

Whether to "mainstream" children with severe hearing loss in a regular classroom with an interpreter or place them in a school for deaf children is another controversial issue. Parents should be encouraged to explore the possibilities of each option and to make a decision based on the individual needs of their children and not current trends. The expertise of an educator who is knowledgeable in this field can also be helpful when making this decision.

Outside Resources and Referrals

Newly diagnosed children should be evaluated by **otolaryngologists** with pediatric expertise, **audiologists,** pediatric **ophthalmologists,** and medical **geneticists.** Any refractory error should be treated and followed closely because children with severe hearing difficulties are more dependent on vision. A genetics evaluation is important for diagnostic reasons as well as for providing families with information and counseling about the risk of recurrence.

Speech assessment and therapy are an essential part of long-term management as are special education resources. Support groups and referrals to national organizations for hearing impaired individuals can be valuable for parents and families. Resources for financial support should also be explored. Agencies with multidisciplinary teams are particularly important for infants or children with other associated handicaps.

Prognosis

The goal of early recognition and treatment of infants and children with hearing deficits is to minimize the possible long-term sequelae of persistent speech and language problems. An additional goal is to prevent the development of learning disabilities with subsequent educational failure. The earlier the intervention, the more likely children succeed and maximize their potential. With appropriate treatment the child should be able to lead a normal life.

CASE RESOLUTION

In the opening case, the child has a history classic for a hearing deficit. She does not turn to loud noises, she has not developed any specific words, and she indicates her needs nonverbally. Although there are no obvious historical risk factors for hearing loss, a behavioral audiogram or **brain stem auditory evoked response** should be performed. The physician's suspicion should be discussed with the family, and a follow-up visit should be arranged to review the hearing test results as soon as possible.

Selected References

American Academy of Pediatrics Task Force on Newborn and Infant Screening. Newborn and infant hearing loss: detection and intervention. *Pediatrics.* 1999;103:527–530

Cunningham M, Cox E. Hearing assessment in infants and children: recommendations beyond neonatal screening. *Pediatrics.* 2003;111:436–440

Francis C, Niparko J. Cochlear implantation update. *Pediatr Clin North Am.* 2003;50:341–361

Gregg R, Wiorck L, Arvedson J. Pediatric audiology: a review. *Pediatr Rev.* 2004;25:224–233

Joint Committee on Infant Hearing, American Academy of Audiology, American Academy of Pediatrics, American Speech-Language-Hearing Association, and Directors of Speech and Hearing Programs in State Health and Welfare Agencies. Year 2000 position statement: principle and guidelines for early hearing detection and intervention programs. *Pediatrics.* 2000;106:798–817

Kennedy C, McCann DC, Campbell MJ, et al. Language ability after early detection of permanent childhood hearing impairment. *N Engl J Med.* 2006;354:2131–2141

Kerschner J. Neonatal hearing screening: to do or not to do. *Pediatr Clin North Am.* 2004;51:725–736

Lieu JE. Speech-language and educational consequences of unilateral hearing loss in children. *Arch Otolaryngol Head Neck Surg.* 2004;130:524–530

Morton C, Nance W. Newborn hearing screening—a silent revolution. *N Engl J Med.* 2006;354:2151–2164

Smith R, Bale J, White K. Sensorineural hearing loss in children. *Lancet.* 2005;365:879–890

Weichbold V, Nekahm-Heis D, Welzl-Mueller K. Universal newborn hearing screening and postnatal hearing loss. *Pediatrics.* 2006;117:e631–e636

Sore Throat

Stanley H. Inkelis, MD

CASE STUDY

An 8-year-old girl has had a sore throat and fever for 2 days. She also has pain on swallowing, a headache, and a feeling of general malaise but no stridor, drooling, breathing difficulty, or rash. Other than the current illness, the girl is in good health. Although she has had sore throats in the past, she has never had one this severe. One week ago both her mother and father had a sore throat and fever that resolved after 5 days with no medication.

The child has a temperature of 102.2°F (39.0°C). The physical examination is normal except for red tonsils with exudate bilaterally, palatal petechiae, and tender cervical lymphadenopathy.

Questions

1. What are the causes of sore throat in children?
2. What is the appropriate evaluation of children with sore throat? What laboratory tests are necessary?
3. What is the appropriate management for children with sore throat?
4. When should otolaryngologic consultation be obtained?

Sore throat, one of the most common illnesses seen by the primary care physician, is a painful inflammation of the pharynx, tonsils, or surrounding areas. In most cases, children with sore throat have mild symptoms that require little or no treatment. However, sore throat may be the presenting complaint of a severe illness such as epiglottitis or retropharyngeal abscess. Small children are not able to define their complaints very well, which makes a careful history from parents or other caregivers and a good physical examination essential for correct diagnosis. Optimal management of sore throat, especially if group A beta-hemolytic streptococcus (GABHS) is suspected, is still very controversial.

Epidemiology

Five percent of all pediatric visits are for pharyngitis. Sore throats are most common in children 5 to 8 years of age, and they continue to occur during later childhood. They are uncommon in children younger than 1 year. Like other respiratory infections, sore throats occur most often in the late fall and winter months. Approximately 11% of all school-aged children receive medical care for pharyngitis. Fifteen percent to 30% or more of cases of pharyngitis in these children are caused by GABHS.

The organisms that cause bacterial and viral pharyngitis are present in saliva and nasal secretions and are almost always transmitted by close contact. Spread from child to child in school is the common mode of transmission.

Clinical Presentation

The clinical presentation of sore throat is variable and often depends on etiology (Dx Box and see Differential Diagnosis). Most children with sore throat present with sudden onset of pain and fever. The height of the fever is variable and is typically higher in younger children. In older children, especially if the sore throat is associated with a common cold, fever is minimal or absent. The throat or tonsils are red, and the breath may be malodorous. Headache, nausea, vomiting, and abdominal pain

Dx — Sore Throat

Viral	Bacterial
• Pain in throat	• Pain in throat, usually sudden onset
• Fever (variable)[a]	• Fever
• Rhinorrhea (common)	• Marked erythema of pharynx, tonsils, or uvula
• Cough (common)	
• Erythema of pharynx or tonsils	• Headache, nausea, vomiting, abdominal pain
• Follicular, ulcerative, exudative lesions of pharynx or tonsils[a]	• Tonsillar and posterior pharyngeal wall exudate
• Conjunctivitis	• Tender, swollen cervical lymphadenopathy
	• Scarlatiniform rash
	• Absence of rhinorrhea or cough
	• Positive rapid antigen test or throat culture

[a]Dependent on etiology (see Differential Diagnosis).

may occur, especially if children are febrile. The appetite may be decreased. Children may be less active than usual.

In children with the common cold, rhinorrhea and postnasal discharge are present. A pharyngeal and tonsillar exudate is not typical. Although the cervical lymph nodes may be enlarged, they are usually not very tender. In contrast, children with streptococcal pharyngitis typically have high fever, pharyngeal and tonsillar exudate, and tender cervical lymph nodes.

Pathophysiology

Various bacteria and viruses produce sore throat symptoms by causing inflammation in the ring of posterior pharyngeal lymphoid tissue that consists of the tonsils, adenoids, and surrounding lymphoid tissue. This ring of tissue, called *Waldeyer ring,* drains the oral and pharyngeal cavity and defends against infection of the mouth and throat. Other host defenses that protect against infection include the sneeze, gag, and cough reflexes; secretory immunoglobulin A; and a rich blood supply.

Viral sore throats may be acquired by inhalation or self-inoculation from the nasal mucosa or conjunctiva. The local respiratory epithelium becomes infected with the virus, and inflammation occurs. In some instances, inflammatory mediators may be responsible for the pain of sore throat. Group A streptococcus and other bacterial organisms directly invade the mucous membranes. Enzymes produced by this organism, streptolysin O and hyaluronidase, aid in the spread of infection.

Differential Diagnosis

Although most children who present with sore throat have common viral or bacterial pharyngitis, other less common disorders such as infectious mononucleosis, epiglottitis, retropharyngeal abscess, or peritonsillar abscess should be considered.

Viral Infection

Viral infection, the most common cause of sore throat in children, is most often associated with an upper respiratory infection caused by a rhinovirus. Cough and rhinorrhea associated with a sore throat suggest this etiology.

Adenovirus often leads to exudative pharyngitis, frequently in children younger than 3 years. Pharyngoconjunctival fever, caused by adenovirus 3, is characterized by a high fever (temperature: >102.2°F [39.0°C]) for several days, conjunctivitis, and exudative tonsillitis.

Coxsackievirus and **echovirus** (enteroviruses) are the usual cause of herpangina. Vesicles and ulcers are generally apparent on the anterior tonsillar pillars and soft palate. They may also be found on the tonsils, pharynx, or posterior buccal mucosa. Children may have a high fever (temperature: >102.2°F [39.0°C]), be irritable, and refuse to eat or drink; dehydration may result. Coxsackievirus A16 and enterovirus 71 cause hand-foot-and-mouth disease, which is characterized by ulcerative oral lesions on the tongue and buccal mucosa and, less frequently, on the palate and anterior tonsillar pillars. Vesicular and papulovesicular lesions are evident on the hands and feet and occasionally on other parts of the body, most commonly the knees and buttocks. Enteroviral infections typically occur in the late spring, summer, and early fall.

Herpes simplex virus (HSV) may lead to pharyngotonsillitis but can be distinguished from most of the enteroviral infections because HSV almost always involves the anterior portion of the mouth and lips and is associated with gingivitis (herpes gingivostomatitis). The lesions often appear as whitish-yellow plaques with an erythematous base and are sometimes ulcerative. This illness is characterized by a high fever (temperature: 102.2°F [39.0°C]) for up to 7 to 10 days and frequent refusal to eat or drink because of the painful lesions. Dehydration may occur.

Epstein-Barr virus (EBV) may cause exudative pharyngotonsillitis either alone or as part of the infectious mononucleosis syndrome that includes fever, malaise, lymphadenopathy, palatal petechiae, and hepatosplenomegaly. Fatigue, malaise, eyelid or periorbital edema, organomegaly, and a maculopapular rash without the other characteristics of a scarlet fever rash help distinguish between infectious mononucleosis and GABHS infection.

Cytomegalovirus may cause an infectious mononucleosis syndrome similar to EBV but is not as commonly associated with pharyngitis and splenomegaly.

Bacterial Infection

Group A beta-hemolytic streptococcus is the most common cause of bacterial sore throat in children older than 3 years. The pharynx is typically very red and sometimes edematous, and the tonsils are red, enlarged, and covered with exudate. Occasionally, the uvula is very inflamed as well. Children may also have dysphagia, fever, vomiting, headache, malaise, and abdominal pain. Swollen anterior cervical lymphadenopathy and petechiae on the soft palate and uvula are usually apparent. In addition, the occurrence of a scarlatiniform rash, "strawberry tongue," and Pastia lines (petechiae in the flexor skin creases of joints) indicates scarlet fever, which is diagnostic of group A streptococcal infection (see Chapter 110). Sore throat from GABHS typically occurs in the winter and spring. Rheumatic fever and glomerulonephritis are non-suppurative complications of group A streptococcal infection.

Peritonsillar abscess or cellulitis and cervical lymphadenitis are suppurative complications of GABHS. Children with peritonsillar abscess often experience trismus and drooling and speak with a "hot potato" voice. The abscess in the affected tonsil causes a bulge in the posterior soft palate and pushes the uvula away from the midline to the unaffected side of the pharynx. On palpation, the abscess may feel fluctuant. Peritonsillar cellulitis typically produces a bulge in the soft palate but does not cause deviation of the uvula.

Group B, C, and G beta-hemolytic streptococci (non-GABHS) have all been isolated from children with pharyngitis. *Streptococcus pneumoniae* and *Arcanobacterium haemolyticum* infrequently cause pharyngitis in children. The latter organism is associated with a scarlatiniform rash in some patients and is most common in adolescents and young adults. In contrast to scarlet fever, palatal petechiae and strawberry tongue are not present with the pharyngitis caused by this bacterium. Although *Corynebacterium diphtheriae* (diphtheria) rarely causes sore throat in immunized children, this organism should be considered in non-immunized children who have exudative pharyngotonsillitis and a grayish pseudomembrane that bleeds when removal is attempted.

Chlamydia trachomatis may lead to pharyngitis and tonsillitis in adolescents and young adults through sexual transmission. The role of *Chlamydia pneumoniae* as a cause of sore throat in children remains unclear. *Mycoplasma pneumoniae* does not usually produce sore throat in children unless they have lower respiratory tract disease. *Neisseria gonorrhoeae* may lead to sore throat in sexually active adolescents. Its occurrence in prepubertal children is often secondary to sexual abuse. The appearance of the throat is not characteristic, and diagnosis is made by cultures when the degree of suspicion is high. **Tularemia** is a rare cause of exudative pharyngitis in children but should be suspected if contact with wild animals has occurred.

Other Causes

Candida albicans may be responsible for sore throat in infants and in children who are immunocompromised or taking antibiotics. Children with oral candidiasis usually present with whitish plaques on the labial or buccal mucosa that do not wipe off easily. When the pharynx and tonsils are involved, some discomfort or dysphagia, but usually not significant pain, may occur.

Retropharyngeal abscess typically occurs in children younger than 6 years. Sore throat is associated with this condition, but it is usually more evident when the child swallows. Fever, refusal to swallow, drooling, stridor, and meningismus in toxic-appearing children suggest this diagnosis.

Epiglottitis (supraglottitis) may present as sore throat. Prior to the *Haemophilus influenzae* type B (Hib) conjugate vaccine, epiglottitis typically affected children 2 to 7 years of age who would present with signs of toxicity, stridor, difficulty swallowing, and drooling. In relatively well-appearing children with sore throat but no stridor, neither epiglottitis nor retropharyngeal abscess is a likely cause of sore throat. In the past, epiglottitis was almost always caused by Hib. With the widespread use of the Hib conjugate vaccine, this organism is now rarely the etiology, thus diminishing the prevalence of epiglottitis and making this entity an uncommon cause of sore throat in children. Although rare in adolescents, epiglottitis may present with severe sore throat out of proportion to clinical findings. Other signs and symptoms include dysphagia, odynophagia, a muffled voice, and pain on palpation of the anterior neck around the hyoid bone. *S pneumoniae; Staphylococcus aureus;* and group A, B, and C beta-hemolytic streptococci are unusual but reported causative agents of epiglottitis.

Children with croup may have sore throat and stridor, but they do not usually appear toxic and do not have difficulty swallowing. Affected children are usually between 6 months and 3 years of age (see Chapter 46).

Trauma from penetrating objects, burns, or exposure to caustic materials may cause sore throat in children. Household smoking may also lead to pharyngeal irritation. In addition, allergic rhinitis with postnasal drip may result in sore throat. Tumor rarely causes sore throat in children but should be considered if a mass is present or pharyngeal inflammation persists. Persistent sore throat may also be a symptom of Kawasaki disease.

Evaluation

History

A thorough history often reveals the etiology of the sore throat (Questions Box). Questions regarding duration, fever, headache, vomiting, pain on swallowing, rash, oral lesions, abdominal pain, and history of contact with other family members or classmates with similar symptoms suggest the most common causes of sore throat (infections with viruses and GABHS). A history of rapid onset of fever, toxicity, difficulty swallowing, drooling, and respiratory distress suggest epiglottitis and retropharyngeal abscess. Voice changes suggest peritonsillar abscess or tonsillar hypertrophy associated with infectious mononucleosis (EBV). Immunization history or history of immigration from a developing country helps assess the risk of diphtheria. Oral sexual activity suggests the possibility of a sexually transmitted infection. A history of allergies, trauma, and environmental smoke may help diagnose other causes of sore throat. Red eye or pinkeye with a rash, persistent fever (>5 days), and sore throat suggest Kawasaki disease.

Questions

Sore Throat

- How long has the child had a sore throat?
- Does the child have fever, headache, or vomiting?
- How rapid was the onset of fever?
- Does the child have pain on swallowing?
- Are there any voice changes?
- Does the child have a rash or oral lesions?
- Does the child have abdominal pain?
- Does the child have any ill contacts?
- Are the child's immunizations up to date?
- Is the child having any difficulty breathing?
- Does the child have a history of allergies?
- Has the child suffered any trauma to the throat or neck?
- Has the child been exposed to environmental smoke?
- For sexually active adolescents or children with a history of sexual abuse with non-responding sore throats: Has there been any oral sexual activity?

Physical Examination

A general physical examination should be performed. It is important to note whether children appear toxic. The skin should be examined for a scarlatiniform, sandpaper-like rash; a vesicular rash involving the hands and feet; or a generalized maculopapular rash. The eyes should be evaluated for conjunctivitis and the nose for rhinorrhea (serous or purulent). The mouth, pharynx, and tonsils should be examined for vesicular lesions, ulcers, and gingivitis. The pharynx should be checked for redness, exudate, vesicles, edema, and foreign bodies. The tonsils and uvula should be examined for these same findings as well as asymmetry, and the neck should be checked for nuchal rigidity. The lymph nodes should be evaluated for enlargement (adenopathy) and inflammation (adenitis). The abdomen should be examined for hepatosplenomegaly.

Laboratory Tests

Although many signs and symptoms may suggest streptococcal pharyngitis, diagnosis can be confirmed only with laboratory tests. The **throat culture** is the gold standard for diagnosis. When done correctly, throat culture has a sensitivity of 90% to 95% in detecting pharyngeal GABHS. Specimens should be obtained from the surfaces of both tonsils and posterior pharynx without touching other parts of the pharynx or the mouth. The main disadvantage of throat culture is that the results are not available for a day or more after the specimen is obtained. Nevertheless, throat culture is the most reliable way to confirm streptococcal infection.

Rapid antigen detection tests (RADTs) are available for on-the-spot diagnosis. False-positive results are uncommon (specificity: ≥95%), but false-negative results for most RADTs occur commonly (sensitivity: 80%–90%). Because a negative test may not exclude a streptococcal infection, it is currently recommended that this result should be confirmed by throat culture. However, newer RADTs using optical immunoassay (OIA) and chemiluminescent DNA probes may be as sensitive as throat cultures. Recent data suggest that a negative OIA RADT may not always need routine confirmation with a throat culture, especially if physicians confirm in their practice setting that the newer RADT has a sensitivity comparable to the sensitivity of throat culture. In one study of more than 30,000 patients comparing those managed with throat cultures alone to those managed with a high sensitivity RADT without throat culture confirmation, it was determined that throat culture confirmation of a high sensitivity RADT is not necessary to prevent suppurative or nonsuppurative complications of group A streptococcal pharyngitis. In addition, it has been suggested in several studies that the recommendation to obtain a backup throat culture in all patients with a negative RADT is not a cost-effective approach. An antistreptolysin-O titer and an anti-DNase-B titer may help confirm a prior streptococcal infection if the throat culture is negative, particularly in children in whom there is a high suspicion of acute rheumatic fever or acute post-streptococcal glomerulonephritis.

Differentiating between viral and bacterial pharyngitis is often difficult, and the rapid streptococcal antigen tests and throat cultures should be reserved for patients who have signs and symptoms common for both illnesses. There are some children whose clinical findings are not consistent with bacterial pharyngitis. For example, afebrile children with a sore throat, runny nose, and cough who have slight pharyngeal erythema almost certainly have viral pharyngitis and do not need further workup. However, children with a constellation of signs and symptoms suggesting bacterial pharyngitis, such as sudden onset of sore throat, fever, headache, swollen and erythematous tonsils, tonsillar or posterior pharyngeal wall exudate, uvulitis, tender and enlarged cervical lymphadenopathy, absence of runny nose or cough, or exposure to an individual with streptococcal pharyngitis may need further testing with RADT or throat culture to confirm group A streptococcal pharyngitis because an accurate diagnosis cannot be made on clinical grounds alone. Guidelines for clinical prediction have been evaluated and have suggested different approaches to the need for RADT or throat culture and antibiotic management. Some recommend empirical antibiotic treatment for children but may result in unnecessary antibiotic use. Guidelines that recommend identifying patients who are likely to have group A streptococcal pharyngitis based on clinical or epidemiological findings and providing antibiotics for only those confirmed by RADT or throat culture decrease the unnecessary overuse of antibiotics.

Viral throat cultures and acute and convalescent titers to determine viral pharyngitis are rarely indicated unless systemic infection occurs (eg, herpes encephalitis). Epstein-Barr virus infection can be determined by specific serologic antibody assays, but non-specific tests for heterophil antibody (eg, monospot test) are most available and are usually the tests of choice for diagnosing infectious mononucleosis. However, it may be negative in children younger than 4 years or early in the course of the infection. Only 75% of infected children between 2 and 4 years of age, and less than 30% of children younger than 2 years, are identified by this test. The monospot test, a rapid slide test for heterophil antibodies, may remain positive for months after the infection and may suggest the diagnosis of infectious mononucleosis in children who do not have this disorder. A complete blood cell count with more than 50% to 60% lymphocytes or more than 10% atypical lymphocytes is suggestive of mononucleosis. When these tests are inconclusive, the specific serologic antibody tests for EBV infection are helpful in establishing the diagnosis. Cytomegalovirus-specific antibody tests should be considered in the patient with a mononucleosis syndrome and negative laboratory tests for EBV. Culture or fluorescent antibody evaluation of the pseudomembrane may be used to diagnose diphtheria. Culture or presence of serum agglutinins confirms tularemia. Thayer-Martin culture plates should be used to diagnose suspected gonorrheal sore throat.

Imaging Studies

If epiglottitis or retropharyngeal abscess is suspected but is not clinically apparent, a lateral neck x-ray may be obtained. The x-ray should be performed with a physician in attendance who is capable of performing endotracheal intubation in case the child has respiratory difficulties (see Chapter 46).

Management

The management of children with sore throat is based on the etiology of the condition. The early recognition of potentially serious conditions based on history and physical examination is essential to providing optimal care. **Otolaryngological consultation** should be obtained in children with peritonsillar abscess, retropharyngeal abscess, epiglottitis, significant pharyngeal trauma, or pharyngeal tumor. Recurrent tonsillitis, especially in children who miss school, may be a reason for referral to an otolaryngologist.

Outpatient Treatment

For most children with sore throat, the physician must differentiate between viral and streptococcal pharyngitis. Viral sore throat can be managed symptomatically. Treatment of pain and discomfort with **analgesics such as acetaminophen or ibuprofen to relieve pain and maintain hydration** are the mainstays of therapy for young children with viral or bacterial sore throat. Gargling with warm water and sucking on hard candy may provide additional symptomatic relief for older children. The use of steroids for reducing pain for pharyngitis is controversial. There is evidence, particularly in moderate or severe pharyngitis, that the use of dexamethasone (0.6 mg/kg, maximum 10 mg) in children 5 years of age or older results in earlier onset of pain relief and decreases the duration of sore throat pain.

The pain from lesions of herpes stomatitis sometimes responds to acetaminophen or ibuprofen. For those children with persistent pain, acetaminophen with codeine or hydrocodone may be helpful. **Anesthetics** such as lidocaine may also decrease the pain. A convenient way of delivering lidocaine is in a mixture (1 part each) of lidocaine, diphenhydramine (Benadryl), and a liquid antacid. This mixture (called "magical mouth wash" by some) may be inserted into each side of the mouth, gargled, or placed on a gloved finger and applied directly on the oral lesions of the tongue and labial and buccal mucosa. It is best used about 15 to 30 minutes before feeding or drinking, especially in children who refuse to drink. Lidocaine should be used cautiously because it can suppress the gag reflex. The dose should never exceed 3 mg/kg/dose. Too much lidocaine may result in seizures. Parents should also be given instruction on how to monitor fluid intake and of the signs of dehydration.

In children without clear-cut evidence of streptococcal pharyngitis, a positive rapid streptococcal antigen test helps direct antibiotic treatment. A negative test in the presence of positive symptoms should be accompanied by a throat culture. However, the OIA rapid test may preclude the need for culture confirmation. Patients can await the results of culture before beginning antibiotic therapy. **Antibiotics** without confirmation from rapid streptococcal tests or cultures are indicated in children who appear toxic, who have scarlet fever or peritonsillar cellulitis/abscess, or who have a history of rheumatic fever. Most evidence suggests that early treatment results in more rapid clinical improvement, although this is controversial. Rheumatic fever can be prevented if treatment is started within 9 days of sore throat symptom development. Glomerulonephritis probably is not affected by antibiotic therapy.

Evidence suggests that children with streptococcal pharyngitis should be treated with antibiotics to relieve symptoms; shorten the course of their illness; and prevent disease dissemination, suppurative complications, and rheumatic fever. Penicillin is the antibiotic of choice. It may be administered orally as penicillin V (phenoxymethyl penicillin) in a dose of 250 mg 2 to 3 times a day for 10 days for children and 500 mg 2 to 3 times a day for adolescents and adults. Most patients will feel better after 2 to 3 days, but it is important to

stress to parents that their children need to complete the full 10-day course. Amoxicillin, which tastes better, is frequently used to treat streptococcal pharyngitis, but offers no bacteriologic advantage over penicillin. However, there are data to suggest that amoxicillin given once a day for 10 days is as effective as penicillin V given 3 times a day for 10 days, which makes compliance more likely. (See Table 62-1 for dosages.)

If the risk of noncompliance is high or if the risk of complication is great (eg, children have a history of rheumatic fever), the penicillin should be administered intramuscularly. Intramuscular penicillin has 2 disadvantages: (1) pain associated with the injection and (2) increased incidence of a potentially more severe allergic reaction. The dose of benzathine penicillin for children weighing less than 27 kg (60 lb) is 600,000 U. The dose for larger children and adults is 1.2 million U. Bicillin CR, which contains 900,000 U of benzathine penicillin and 300,000 U of procaine penicillin, is a satisfactory alternative form of delivering penicillin intramuscularly in children and may be preferable because it causes less pain and less severe local reaction. This preparation has not been determined to be effective in heavier patients (adolescents and adults) and therefore the benzathine preparation noted previously is recommended. The injection of benzathine penicillin is less painful if it is given after it reaches room temperature. (See Table 62-1 for dosage information.) Macrolides such as erythromycin may be substituted in children who are allergic to penicillin. Some of the newer macrolides, clarithromycin and azithromycin, offer the benefit of fewer gastrointestinal side effects than erythromycin. Azithromycin has the added advantage of once-a-day dosing and a shortened course of therapy of only 5 days. A first-generation oral cephalosporin is also an acceptable alternative, but should not be used in children with an immediate or Type I hypersensitivity to penicillin. Tetracyclines and sulfonamides are not recommended for the treatment of streptococcal pharyngitis.

Studies have shown that a 5-day course of some oral cephalosporins may be used in place of penicillin with equal efficacy. These agents are more costly, have a broader microbiological spectrum, and are therefore not recommended as first-line therapy. These antibiotics, however, may be beneficial in children with recurrent streptococcal tonsillopharyngitis, especially those in whom compliance is an issue. Other options for children having a recurrence soon after completing an oral course of antibiotics are to re-treat with the same antibiotic, give another oral antibiotic (as noted previously and in Table 62-1), or give an intramuscular dose of penicillin.

Many children are asymptomatic carriers of group A streptococci. In general, these children do well, and eradication of the bacteria is not necessary. Cultures after treatment are generally not recommended, except for children with recurring or persistent symptoms or those with a previous history of rheumatic fever. In selected cases of children whose throat cultures remain positive, eradication of the pharyngeal carriage should be strongly considered. These indications are as follows: if there is an outbreak of acute rheumatic fever or poststreptococcal glomerulonephritis, if there is an outbreak of group A streptococcal pharyngitis in a closed or semiclosed community, if there is a family history of rheumatic fever, if repeated episodes of documented symptomatic group A streptococcal pharyngitis recur within a family over several weeks despite appropriate therapy, if there is a high level of anxiety in the family about group A streptococcal infections, or if tonsillectomy is considered only because of persistent group A streptococcal carriage. If cultures remain positive, these children may be treated with benzathine penicillin and oral rifampin for 4 days in an attempt to eradicate the organism. (See Table 62-1 for dosages.) Clindamycin is reportedly more effective in eradication of the organism from symptom-free carriers. (See Table 62-1 for dosages.)

M pneumoniae pharyngitis is usually associated with a generalized infection. Because it is often a self-limited illness, it does not require antibiotic therapy unless symptoms persist. Treatment with any of the macrolide antibiotics may be helpful. However, clarithromycin and azithromycin have fewer side effects and are likely to produce better compliance. Macrolides are also the drugs of choice for children with *A haemolyticum* pharyngitis.

Diphtheria, seen almost exclusively in less advantaged countries, is a life-threatening infection that requires prompt diagnosis and treatment. Penicillin G or erythromycin must be given to kill *C diphtheriae* and, in addition, equine antitoxin must be administered to neutralize the exotoxin. Tularemia pharyngitis is unusual, but if suspected is treated with gentamicin.

For gonococcal pharyngitis caused by *N gonorrhoeae,* intramuscular ceftriaxone is the drug of choice. (See Table 62-1 for dosages.) Additional antibiotic coverage for associated *C trachomatis* infection should be administered. Oral azithromycin or doxycycline should also be given to children 9 years of age or older. (See Table 62-1 for dosages.) Azithromycin or erythromycin may be used for younger children. Children should be examined and cultured for sexually transmitted infections in other sites and should have a serological test for syphilis at the first visit and have a repeat test 6 to 8 weeks later. They should also be evaluated for concurrent hepatitis B and human immunodeficiency virus infection. Sexual abuse should be considered in all cases of gonococcal pharyngitis, particularly in prepubertal children (see Chapters 85 and 116).

Children with croup usually respond to steroids. Oral nystatin can be used in children with oral candidiasis. Adolescents with uncomplicated peritonsillar abscess may be managed as outpatients in selected cases with needle aspiration and oral antibiotics.

Inpatient Treatment

Children with sore throat should be admitted to the hospital if they have airway obstruction or need intravenous (IV) hydration or antibiotics. Children with retropharyngeal abscess and epiglottitis require IV antibiotics and should be managed in consultation

Table 62-1. Antibiotics Used in the Management of Sore Throat in Children	
Drug (for Streptococcal Pharyngitis)	**Dosage**
Penicillin V	250 mg x 2–3/d for children and 500 mg x 2–3/d for adolescents orally for 10 days
Benzathine penicillin	600,000 U (<27 kg or 60 lb); 1.2 million U (>27 kg or 60 lb) as single intramuscular injection
Bicillin CR	900,000 U benzathine penicillin and 300,000 U procaine penicillin for children as single intramuscular injection
Erythromycin estolate	20–40 mg/kg/d in 2–4 divided doses orally for 10 days (maximum 1 g/d)
Erythromycin ethyl succinate	40 mg/kg/d in 2–4 divided doses orally for 10 days (maximum 1 g/d)
Clarithromycin	15 mg/kg/d every 12 hours orally for 10 days
Azithromycin	12 mg/kg/d, once a day orally for 5 days (maximum 500 mg)
Cephalexin	25–50 mg/kg/d every 12 hours orally for 10 days (maximum 500 mg every 12 hours)
Amoxicillin	750 mg once a day <40 kg, 1,000 mg once a day >40 kg for 10 days
Cefpodoxime proxetil	10 mg/kg/d, every 12 hours orally for 5 days (maximum 400 mg/d)
Rifampin	10 mg/kg/dose orally every 12 hours for 4 days (given last 4 days of treatment with penicillin V or benzathine penicillin for chronic streptococcal carriers)
Clindamycin	20 mg/kg/d in 3 divided doses (maximum 1.8 g/d) orally for 10 days (for chronic streptococcal carriers)
Drug (for Gonococcal Pharyngitis)	**Dosage**
Ceftriaxone **Plus**	125 mg intramuscularly in a single dose
Azithromycin **or**	20 mg/kg (maximum 1 g) orally in a single dose
Erythromycin **or (if ≥9 y)**	50 mg/kg/d (maximum 2 g/d) orally every 6 hours for 14 days
Doxycycline	100 mg orally 2 times a day for 7 days

with an otolaryngologist. Preadolescent children or adolescents with complicated peritonsillar abscess also require IV antibiotics. Surgical intervention is indicated if the abscess is fluctuant, the child is toxic or has severe trismus or airway compromise, or if there is no resolution within 24 hours. Needle aspiration may be acceptable in selected cases. Intravenous hydration is occasionally needed for patients with severe herpes stomatitis who will not drink because of pain and who become dehydrated.

The role of tonsillectomy or adenotonsillectomy for children with recurrent sore throat is still controversial. Because the indications for surgery are not clearly defined and many children improve spontaneously, decisions for surgery should be individualized.

Education

Both patients and families should receive general education about sore throats. Medication for pain with drugs such as acetaminophen or ibuprofen is useful, especially if children are having difficulty swallowing. Gargling with warm salt water or sucking on hard candy may soothe the pain of sore throat. Children with bacterial pharyngitis may return to school after 24 hours of antibiotic therapy and the disappearance of fever. The practitioner should recommend that symptomatic family members see a physician. Parents should call or return to the physician if their children have respiratory or swallowing difficulties, drooling, severe pain, or fever (temperature: >101.0°F [38.3°C]) for more than 48 hours after the initiation of appropriate antibiotics.

Prognosis

The prognosis for children with viral sore throat is excellent because of its self-limited nature. The outlook for children with streptococcal sore throat is also excellent. If the infection is not diagnosed and treated appropriately, however, suppurative (eg, peritonsillar abscess) and non-suppurative complications (eg, rheumatic fever, acute glomerulonephritis) may occur. With early diagnosis and prompt treatment, the prognosis for unusual, life-threatening causes of sore throat is also very good.

CASE RESOLUTION

In the case presented, the child has palatal petechiae and tonsillar exudate, which are signs and symptoms consistent with streptococcal pharyngitis. A streptococcal rapid antigen detection test is performed, and is positive. The child is treated with oral penicillin. Neither of her parents have sore throat symptoms.

Selected References

American Academy of Pediatrics. Group A streptococcal infections. In: Pickering LK, Baker CJ, Long SS, McMillan JA, eds. *Red Book: 2006 Report of the Committee on Infectious Diseases.* 27th ed. Elk Grove Village, IL: American Academy of Pediatrics; 2006:610–620

Bisno AL. Acute pharyngitis: etiology and diagnosis. *Pediatrics.* 1996; 97(suppl):949–954

Bisno AL, Gerber MA, Gwaltney JM Jr, Kaplan EL, Schwartz RH, Infectious Diseases Society of America. Practice guidelines for the diagnosis and management of group A streptococcal pharyngitis. *Clin Infect Dis.* 2002;35:113–125

Bulloch B, Kabani A, Tenenbein M. Oral dexamethasone for the treatment of pain in children with acute pharyngitis: a randomized, double-blind, placebo-controlled trial. *Ann Emerg Med.* 2003;41:601–608

Cherry JD. Pharyngitis (pharyngitis, tonsillitis, tonsillopharyngitis, and nasopharyngitis). In: Feigen RD, Cherry JD, eds. *Textbook of Pediatric Infectious Diseases.* 5th ed. Philadelphia, PA: Saunders; 2004:161–170

Clegg HW, Ryan AG, Dallas SD, et al. Treatment of streptococcal pharyngitis with once-daily compared with twice-daily amoxicillin. *Pediatr Infect Dis J.* 2006;25:761–767

Dajani A, Taubert K, Ferrieri P, Peter G, Shulman S. Treatment of acute streptococcal pharyngitis and prevention of rheumatic fever: a statement for health professionals. *Pediatrics.* 1995;96:758–764

Diaz MC, Symons N, Ramundo ML, et al. Effect of a standardized pharyngitis treatment protocol on use of antibiotics in a pediatric emergency department. *Arch Pediatr Adolesc Med.* 2004;158:977–981

Ebell MH, Smith MA, Barry HC, et al. Does this patient have strep throat? *JAMA.* 2000;284:2912–2918

Edmonson MB, Farwell KR. Relationship between the clinical likelihood of group A streptococcal pharyngitis and the sensitivity of a rapid antigen-detection test in a pediatric practice. *Pediatrics.* 2005;115:280–285

Fleisher GR. Sore throat. In: Fleisher GR, Ludwig S, Henretig FM, eds. *Textbook of Pediatric Emergency Medicine.* 5th ed. Philadelphia, PA: Lippincott; 2006:637–641

Gerber MA. Diagnosis and treatment of pharyngitis in children. *Pediatr Clin North Am.* 2005;52:729–747

Gieseker KE, Roe MH, MacKenzie T, et al. Evaluating the American Academy of Pediatrics diagnostic standard for *Streptococcus pyogenes* pharyngitis: backup culture versus repeat rapid antigen testing. *Pediatrics.* 2003;111:666–670

Jaggi P, Shulman ST. Group A streptococcal infections. *Pediatr Rev.* 2006; 27:99–105

Linder JA, Bates DW, Lee GM, et al. Antibiotic treatment of children with sore throat. *JAMA.* 2005;294:2315–2322

Linder JA, Chan JC, Bates DW. Evaluation and treatment of pharyngitis in primary care practice. The difference between guidelines is largely academic. *Arch Intern Med.* 2006;166:1374–1379

Martin JM, Green M, Barbadora KA, et al. Group A streptococci among school-aged children: clinical characteristics and the carrier state. *Pediatrics.* 2004;114:1212–1219

McIsaac WJ, Kellner JD, Aufricht P, et al. Empirical validation of guidelines for the management of pharyngitis in children and adults. *JAMA.* 2004;291:1587–1595

Olympia RP, Khine H, Avner JR. Effectiveness of oral dexamethasone in the treatment of moderate to severe pharyngitis in children. *Arch Pediatr Adolesc Med.* 2005;159:278–282

Paradise JL. Tonsillectomy and adenoidectomy. In: Bluestone CD, Stool SE, Alper CM, et al, eds. *Pediatric Otolaryngology.* 4th ed. Philadelphia, PA: Saunders; 2003:1210–1222

Paradise JL, Bluestone CD, Colborn K, et al. Tonsillectomy and adenotonsillectomy for recurrent throat infection in moderately affected children. *Pediatrics.* 2002;110:7–15

Park SY, Gerber MA, Tanz RR, et al. Clinicians' management of children and adolescents with acute pharyngitis. *Pediatrics.* 2006;117:1871–1878

Rafei K, Lichenstein R. Airway infectious disease emergencies. *Pediatr Clin North Am.* 2006;53:215–242

Van Howe RS, Kusnier LP II. Diagnosis and management of pharyngitis in a pediatric population based on cost-effectiveness and projected health outcomes. *Pediatrics.* 2006;117:609–619

Webb KH. Does culture confirmation of high-sensitivity rapid streptococcal tests make sense? A medical decision analysis. *Pediatrics.* 1998;101:e2

Webb KH, Needham CA, Kurtz SB. Use of a high-sensitivity rapid strep test without culture confirmation of negative results. *J Fam Pract.* 2000;49:34–38

Weber JT. Appropriate use of antimicrobial drugs. A better prescription is needed. *JAMA.* 2005;294:2354–2356

Nosebleeds

Stanley H. Inkelis, MD

CASE STUDY

A 3-year-old boy is brought to the office one winter day. He has had 4 nosebleeds in the past week as well as a cold with a runny nose and cough, which began the day before the first nosebleed. The nosebleeds occurred either at night or during sleep and stopped spontaneously or with gentle pressure. Other than the cold and nosebleeds, the boy is in good health. He is active, with bruises over both tibias but none elsewhere. The many cuts and scrapes he has had in the past resulted in minimal bleeding. His family has no history of a bleeding disorder or easy bruisability.

The child's physical examination is entirely normal except for a small amount of blood in the left anterior naris.

Questions

1. What are the common causes of nosebleeds in children?
2. What systemic diseases are associated with nosebleeds?
3. How should nosebleeds be evaluated in children?
4. How should minor and severe nosebleeds be managed in children?

Nosebleed, or epistaxis, occurs commonly in children, especially in those between the ages of 2 and 10 years. In most cases, nosebleeds are secondary to local trauma and can be cared for by primary care physicians. In rare instances, however, a nosebleed may be difficult to control or may be a manifestation of a serious systemic illness. Referral to an otolaryngologist or a hematologist/oncologist is usually not required except in these situations, and hospitalization is generally unnecessary. Parents and children, who are often frightened by nosebleeds, frequently overestimate the amount of blood lost. Understanding and reassurance are important in allaying anxiety.

Epidemiology

Thirty percent of children have one nosebleed by the time they are 5 years of age. In children between the ages of 6 and 10, the frequency increases to 56%. Nosebleeds are rare in infancy and infrequent after puberty. They occur much more frequently in the late fall and winter months, when upper respiratory infections (URIs) are common, environmental humidity is relatively low, and the use of heating systems results in dryness. Nosebleeds are also more common in children who live in dry climates, especially if they have a URI or allergic rhinitis.

Clinical Presentation

Most children with nosebleeds have a history of bleeding at home and have minimal or no bleeding at the time of presentation (Dx Box). With anterior nosebleeds, blood exits almost entirely from the anterior portion of the nose. With posterior nosebleeds, most of the bleeding occurs into the nasopharynx and mouth, although some blood exits through the nose as well. Posterior nosebleeds are heavier and more difficult to control, and children may present in a hemodynamically unstable condition.

 Nosebleeds

- Blood in anterior nares, nasopharynx, or mouth
- History of any of the following:
  — Frequent digital manipulation (nose picking)
  — Upper respiratory infection (recent)
  — Allergic rhinitis
  — Dry climate
  — Foreign body in nose
  — Trauma to nose
  — Prolonged or difficult-to-stop bleeding or easy bruisability
- Physical examination consistent with any of the following:
  — Rhinorrhea
  — Dry, cracked nasal mucosa
  — Foreign body in nose
  — Trauma to nose
  — Multiple bruises

Children with bleeding disorders may have recurrent nosebleeds and a history of prolonged bleeding, easy bruisability, or multiple bruises in unlikely locations. In unusual situations, children with gastrointestinal or respiratory tract bleeding may present with blood exiting through the nose. Alternatively, some children who present with hematemesis have vomited swallowed nasal blood.

Pathophysiology

Nosebleeds may be either anterior or posterior in origin. Most nosebleeds in children (90%) are anterior and are more easily controlled than posterior nosebleeds. The anteroinferior portion of the nasal septum, about 0.5 cm from the tip of the nose, known as Kiesselbach plexus or Little area, is the most common part of the nose involved in anterior nosebleeds. This area is supplied by the anterior and posterior ethmoidal arteries, the sphenopalatine artery, and the septal branches of the superior labial artery (Figure 63-1). The mucosa covering the area is thin and friable, and the small vessels supplying the nasal mucous membrane have little structural support. Congestion of the vessels caused by conditions such as a URI or drying of the mucosa from low environmental humidity makes this area susceptible to bleeding.

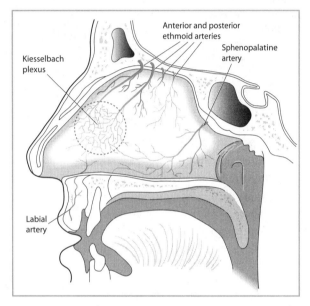

Figure 63-1. Vascular supply of nasal septum. Note the confluence of vessels that forms the Kiesselbach plexus.

Posterior nosebleeds generally arise from the turbinate or nasal wall. Significant bleeding, usually from a branch of the sphenopalatine artery, may occur.

Differential Diagnosis

Trauma from nose picking and **inflammation** of the nasal mucosa from a URI are by far the most common causes of nosebleeds in children. Repetitive, habitual nose picking results in the formation of friable granulation tissue that bleeds when traumatized (epistaxis digitorum). Mucosal inflammation predisposes children to bleeding because of erosion of congested blood vessels. As the nasal mucosa dries, it may lead to crust formation and cracking. Bleeding may occur spontaneously, but more often it results from forceful nose blowing and sneezing that increases venous pressure in the more vascularized nasal septum.

Other viral respiratory infections, such as infectious mononucleosis and influenza, may also predispose children to nosebleeds because of their local inflammatory effect. Nosebleeds in children with these infections are more common in areas of low environmental humidity. Many children with no URI-like symptoms also suffer from nosebleeds in such environments, usually in winter, when inhaling dry, hot air from heating systems causes desiccation of the nasal mucosa (rhinitis sicca). **Allergic rhinitis** with inflammation and subsequent drying may also lead to nosebleeds. Children with allergic rhinitis who take decongestants may be more likely to suffer from nosebleeds.

Foreign bodies may cause direct trauma or pressure necrosis to the vessels of the nasal mucosa. **External trauma** can cause either tears to the nasal mucosa or nasal fractures. If bleeding from mucosal vessels occurs but the mucosa remains intact, a septal hematoma may develop. Abscess formation or septal perforation may occur if the septal hematoma is not drained.

Although nosebleeds are usually benign conditions, they may be the first sign of serious illness. Persistent or recurrent nosebleeds with no obvious cause should raise the suspicion of **bleeding disorders.** Thrombocytopenia is the most common coagulation defect causing nosebleeds. Idiopathic thrombocytopenic purpura is the most frequent thrombocytopenic disorder associated with nosebleeds. Leukemia, aplastic anemia, and human immunodeficiency virus (HIV) infection must be strongly considered and ruled out in children with nosebleeds and thrombocytopenia. Platelet aggregation disorders may also be a cause of recurrent nosebleeds.

The most commonly inherited bleeding disorder associated with nosebleeds is von Willebrand disease, an autosomal-dominant bleeding disorder characterized by varying degrees of factor VIII deficiency and platelet dysfunction (decreased platelet adhesiveness). Hemophilia (factor VIII, IX, or XI) deficiency, factor VII deficiency, Glanzmann thrombasthenia, and Bernard-Soulier syndrome are other inherited bleeding disorders that may lead to nosebleeds. Hepatic disease, severe vitamin K deficiency, or malabsorption syndrome is associated with an acquired coagulopathy, which may present with nosebleed. Valproic acid administration has been associated with acquired von Willebrand disease and nosebleeds.

Nosebleeds may be a manifestation of **blood vessel disorders,** either hereditary or acquired. Osler-Weber-Rendu syndrome (hereditary hemorrhagic telangiectasia) is an inherited autosomal-dominant disease with multiple mucosal telangiectasias, especially in the nose. Because telangiectasias are deficient in muscular and connective tissue, these telangiectasias may rupture spontaneously and bleed profusely. An acquired blood vessel disorder from vitamin C deficiency is a rare cause of nosebleeds. An association between migraine headaches and recurrent nosebleeds has also been reported.

Neoplasms, particularly malignancies, are uncommon causes of nosebleeds in children. Polyps are usually present in association with cystic fibrosis or allergies. Capillary, cavernous, and mixed hemangiomas may occur in the nose. Juvenile nasopharyngeal angiofibroma occurs almost exclusively in adolescent males who present with nasal obstruction and bleeding. Rhabdomyosarcomas, lymphomas, and squamous cell carcinomas of the nose, sinuses, or nasopharynx are rare causes of nosebleeds.

Drugs such as aspirin and nonsteroidal anti-inflammatory drugs, which interfere with platelet function, and warfarin and heparin, which inhibit clotting factors, increase the risk of nasal hemorrhage with minor trauma, infection, or inflammation. Accidental ingestion of these medications should be suspected if they are available. Cocaine or heroin snorting may cause nasal septal perforation and nosebleeds.

Hypertension is rarely associated with nosebleeds in children. Wegener granulomatosis and lethal midline granuloma are rare idiopathic inflammatory diseases in children that lead to nasal tissue destruction and bleeding. Nosebleeds during menstruation may be secondary to endometriosis with ectopic endometrial tissue implants in the nasal cavity.

Evaluation

History

A thorough history often reveals the etiology of the nosebleed (Questions Box). Information concerning the side of the nose from which the bleeding occurred, the amount of bleeding, the measures used to stop the bleeding, and the time required to stop the bleeding may be helpful to quickly assess the severity of the nosebleed.

Questions

Nosebleeds

- Does the child pick his or her nose?
- Has the child suffered any trauma recently?
- Has the child recently had an upper respiratory infection?
- Has the child recently had any systemic viral or bacterial illness?
- Does the child have any allergies?
- Is the child exposed to dry conditions (eg, dry climate, dry heat, dehumidified air)?
- Has the child put or tried to put foreign objects in his or her nose?
- Is there a history of easy bruisability or prolonged, difficult-to-stop bleeding in the child or family?
- Does the child or anyone in the family use any aspirin, aspirin-containing medications, nonsteroidal anti-inflammatory drugs, or warfarin?
- Which side of the nose was bleeding?
- How extensive was the bleeding?
- Did the child spit out or swallow blood? Was there blood in the mouth?
- What measures were used to stop the bleeding? How long did it take to stop the bleeding?
- Was this the first nosebleed? If the nosebleeds are recurrent, how often do they occur and how long do they last?

Physical Examination

A general physical examination should be performed. In children with significant blood loss, particular attention should be directed toward the mental status and vital signs to determine hemodynamic stability. If vital signs are normal, these children should also be evaluated for orthostatic changes. If the blood pressure is elevated, it should be reassessed at a time when the anxiety related to the nosebleed has dissipated.

In addition, the skin and mucous membranes should be checked carefully for petechiae, purpura, and ecchymosis, which are signs of easy bruisability. The abdomen should be examined for hepatosplenomegaly, and the child should be evaluated for lymphadenopathy. Telangiectasias in the oropharynx or mucous membranes suggest Osler-Weber-Rendu syndrome. The oropharynx and nasopharynx should be examined for masses and blood dripping downward from a posterior bleed. The nose should then be inspected for the site of bleeding, with special attention directed toward Kiesselbach plexus in the anterior septum.

Diagnostic Studies

Laboratory tests are rarely indicated in most children with nosebleeds. A hematocrit/hemoglobin should be obtained if the nosebleeds are severe or recur frequently. Blood for type and crossmatch should be sent in children who have signs or symptoms of hypovolemia (increased pulse; cool, clammy skin; increased capillary refill; decreased blood pressure; etc) or a marked drop in hematocrit. If the history or physical examination suggests that a coagulopathy may be present, a complete blood count with platelet count, prothrombin time, and partial thromboplastin time should be obtained and a bleeding time considered if the other laboratory tests are negative.

X-rays and other imaging studies are rarely necessary in children with nosebleeds.

Management

Children who present to primary care physicians with a history of a nosebleed or nosebleeds that have resolved spontaneously or with application of pressure to the nose need no further treatment in the office setting, provided that the history and physical examination are consistent with a benign cause of the nosebleed. These children or their parents should be instructed to apply **petroleum jelly** (Vaseline) or an antibiotic ointment inside the septal portion of the involved naris twice a day for 3 to 5 days with a cotton-tipped swab (Q-tip) or with the little finger. Often the child's little finger is used because it is nonthreatening and it "knows where to go." Further nose picking should be discouraged, and fingernails should be trimmed to minimize trauma. In addition, a bedside **humidifier** helps to moisturize the air, especially in dry climates or during the winter when forced hot-air heat is used. Children whose nares moisten from rhinorrhea and then dry and crack also benefit from humidified air. Buffered saline nasal spray may also be helpful in humidifying the nose. Those children who are prone to recurrent nosebleeds in whom serious causes have been ruled out may benefit from regular use of some of the mentioned measures when they have URIs, allergic manifestations, or are in a dry season or environment. In addition, for those children with allergic rhinitis and recurrent nosebleeds, topical corticosteroid nasal spray may reduce vascular inflammation and decrease the number of recurrences.

Children or parents should be given advice about how to care for nosebleeds at home. These instructions can also be given to parents who seek advice over the telephone about how to stop children's nosebleeds. Practitioners should reassure parents and children that most nosebleeds are easily controlled. Children should sit upright and lean forward slightly while **direct pressure** is applied to the nose. External compression of the nares between 2 fingers for 5 to 10 minutes should be sufficient. Pressure applied to the anterior and mid-portion of the nose rather than at the base is more effective in stopping the bleeding because most nosebleeds occur in these parts of the nose.

Children who are actively bleeding through the nose when seen by primary care physicians should be positioned sitting upright and leaning forward slightly, and they should be given a basin and facial tissue. Direct pressure should be applied by a nurse or physician to the anterior and mid-portion of the nose while following universal precautions. A cotton dental roll may be placed under the upper lip to compress the labial artery in older children in whom concern about displacement and possible aspiration of the cotton is minimal. If the bleeding continues after external compression, children should be instructed to blow their noses to remove as much clot as possible. Fresh blood should be removed with suction. Cotton pledgets moistened with a few drops of a topical **vasoconstrictor,** such as 0.05% oxymetazoline (Afrin), 0.25% phenylephrine (Neo-Synephrine) or epinephrine (1:1,000) mixed with lidocaine if local anesthesia is needed, or topical thrombin, should be inserted into the side of the nose involved. Pressure should then be applied for an additional 10 minutes.

If the bleeding persists, **cauterization** of the bleeding site with a silver nitrate stick is indicated. Continued bleeding is slowed by first cauterizing a small ring around the bleeding point to interrupt flow from surrounding vessels and then rolling the tip of the applicator onto the bleeding site. Cauterization is often difficult in children, and consultation with an otolaryngologist is advisable. Cauterization should not be performed in children with a bleeding diathesis.

If the bleeding continues, or as a modality to attempt prior to cauterization, an absorbable **nasal sponge** made from oxidized cellulose (Oxicel, Surgicel) or gelatin (Gelfoam) may be directly applied to the bleeding site to form an artificial clot. Alternatively, a **nasal tampon** (Merocel), made from a dehydrated material that expands when it becomes moist, may be inserted to tamponade the area of bleeding. Applying antibiotic ointment, preferably mupirocin, to the tampon allows for easier insertion and removal as well as potentially preventing *Staphylococcus aureus* infection, leading to toxic shock

syndrome. Avitene, a microfibrillar collagen material, provides for platelet aggregation and clot formation when applied to the bleeding site. Continued uncontrolled bleeding requires anterior **nasal packing** with antibiotic-impregnated, preferably mupirocin, 1-inch petrolatum gauze strips, which should remain in place for approximately 2 to 3 days. Prophylactic **antibiotics** should be started because sinusitis is a complication of anterior nasal packing. Antibiotics providing coverage for staphylococcal organisms, in particular methicillin-resistant *S aureus*, and sinusitis should be strongly considered.

Posterior nosebleeds, which are more difficult to control, should be suspected if (1) the measures described previously are ineffective, (2) bleeding is vigorous and the cause cannot be identified, or (3) most of the bleeding is into the nasopharynx and mouth. A posterior nasal pack using a Foley catheter or an Epistat inflatable nasal balloon catheter is indicated to control posterior nosebleeds. This pack is left in place for 2 to 5 days, and children should be started on antibiotics to prevent sinusitis.

The need for **otolaryngological consultation** depends on the experience of the individual physician and the availability of consultation. Prompt consultation, if available, should be obtained for children with severe nosebleeds who need volume replacement; with nosebleeds that do not stop or recur after the mentioned measures have been taken; who may need anterior or posterior nasal packing; and with recurrent, difficult-to-stop nosebleeds. In some cases, obtaining consultation before cauterization with silver nitrate is advisable. Children with septal hematomas, tumors, polyps, and telangiectasias should be referred to an otolaryngologist for further care. Children with a documented or suspected bleeding disorder should be referred to a hematologist. Selective angiographic embolization by an interventional radiologist may be necessary for patients with persistent, intractable nosebleeds. Endonasal laser surgery may be indicated in patients with recurrent nosebleeds from abnormal vascular malformations.

Children with severe nosebleeds should have an intravenous line started early; blood sent for type and crossmatch; and fluids replaced, depending on the amount of blood loss and physical evidence of hypovolemia. In children who are frightened or in whom certain procedures (eg, cauterization of bleeding site, drainage of septal hematoma) are performed, procedural sedation should be strongly considered. Intravenous pain medication should be used in children who need anterior or posterior packing. If procedures that cause undue pain or discomfort are necessary, general anesthesia in an operating room setting may be indicated.

Hospitalization is not often necessary for children with nosebleeds. However, children who are hemodynamically unstable on presentation usually require inpatient treatment. Children who need placement of a posterior nasal pack should be admitted to the hospital for close airway observation. Hospitalization may be necessary for children with difficult-to-stop bleeds who need an anterior nasal pack or who have a bleeding disorder or underlying chronic illness such as leukemia, aplastic anemia, or HIV infection.

Prognosis

The prognosis for nosebleeds in children is excellent. Almost all nosebleeds are easily controlled with a minimal amount of home care or medical management. Surgery is rarely indicated. Complications associated with significant nosebleeds include hypovolemia from blood loss, and sinusitis and toxic shock syndrome from anterior or posterior nasal packs. Even for rare causes of nosebleeds, the prognosis is very good with prompt diagnosis and treatment.

CASE RESOLUTION

In the case presented, the boy has experienced several nosebleeds of short duration associated with an upper respiratory infection and winter dryness. His history and physical examination are unremarkable for a bleeding disorder or chronic illness. The small amount of blood in his nose is consistent with an anterior nosebleed originating from Kiesselbach plexus with inflammation and drying of the nasal mucosa. Laboratory tests are not indicated. The parents should be instructed to apply petroleum jelly to the septal portion of the left side of the child's nose twice a day for 3 to 5 days and to humidify the child's bedroom. They should also be reassured that their child has a common condition that he will outgrow.

Selected References

Bernius M, Perlin D. Pediatric ear, nose and throat emergencies. *Pediatr Clin North Am.* 2006;53:195–214

Elden LM, Potsic WP. Otolaryngologic emergencies (epistaxis). In: Fleisher GR, Ludwig S, Henretig FM, eds. *Textbook of Pediatric Emergency Medicine.* 5th ed. Philadelphia, PA: Lippincott Williams & Wilkins; 2006:1669–1671

Jarjour IT, Jarjour LK. Migraine and recurrent epistaxis in children. *Pediatr Neurol.* 2005;33:94–97

Katsanis E, Luke KH, Hsu E, Li M, Lillicrap D. Prevalence and significance of mild bleeding disorders in children with recurrent epistaxis. *J Pediatr.* 1988;113:73–76

Kost SI, Post JC. Management of epistaxis. In: Henretig FM, King C, eds. *Textbook of Pediatric Emergency Procedures.* Baltimore, MD: Williams & Wilkins; 1997:663–673

Manning SC, Culbertson MC Jr. Epistaxis. In: Bluestone CD, Stool SE, Alper CM, et al, eds. *Pediatric Otolaryngology.* 4th ed. Philadelphia, PA: Saunders; 2003:925–931

Nadel F, Henretig FM. Epistaxis. In: Fleischer GR, Ludwig S, Henretig FM, eds. *Textbook of Pediatric Emergency Medicine.* 5th ed. Philadelphia, PA: Lippincott Williams and Wilkins; 2006:263–266

Riviello RJ. Otolaryngologic procedures. In: Roberts JR, Hedges JR, eds. *Clinical Procedures in Emergency Medicine.* 4th ed. Philadelphia, PA: Saunders; 2004:1280–1316

Sandoval C, Dong S, Visintainer P, et al. Clinical and laboratory features of 178 children with recurrent epistaxis. *J Pediatr Hematol Oncol.* 2002;24:47–49

Santamaria JP, Abrunzo TJ. Ear, nose, and throat (epistaxis). In: Barkin RM, ed. *Pediatric Emergency Medicine.* 2nd ed. St Louis, MO: C.V. Mosby; 1997:713–716

Viehweg TL, Roberson JB, Hudson JW. Epistaxis: diagnosis and treatment. *J Oral Maxillofac Surg.* 2006;64:511–518

Werner EJ, Broxson EH, Tucker EL, Giroux DS, Shults J, Abshire TC. Prevalence of von Willebrand disease in children: a multiethnic study. *J Pediatr.* 1993;123:893–898

Strabismus

Teresa Rosales, MD

CASE STUDY

The mother of an 8-month-old infant complains that every time her son looks to either side his eyes seem crossed. Otherwise, he is growing and developing normally. A symmetric pupillary light reflex, bilateral red reflex, and normal extraocular eye movements in all directions are noted on physical examination of the eyes.

Questions

1. What is strabismus?
2. What conditions make infants' eyes appear crossed? What is the differential diagnosis?
3. What tests are used in the office evaluation of children suspected of having strabismus?
4. Which infants with crossed eyes require referral for further evaluation and treatment?

Strabismus refers to any abnormality in ocular alignment, whether the eyes go in or out or one eye is higher than the other. It is one of the most common eye problems observed in infants and children. The pediatrician plays an important role in the early detection and prompt referral of children with suspected ocular alignment abnormalities.

Epidemiology

Strabismus affects approximately 3% of the population, and the condition is seen most commonly in children younger than 6 years. About 50% of all affected children have a positive family history of strabismus, although the exact genetic mode of inheritance is unclear. Up to 75% of normal infants have transient intermittent strabismus during the first 3 months of life.

Clinical Presentation

Children with ocular misalignment have an asymmetrical corneal light reflex test. Eye movement is noted with cover testing. Children with paralytic strabismus may present with torticollis or head tilting in an effort to avoid diplopia (Dx Box).

Dx Strabismus

- Head tilt
- Double vision (diplopia)
- Squint
- Asymmetrical corneal light reflex
- Eye movement with cover testing

Pathophysiology

Normal binocular vision is the result of the fusion of images from both eyes working synchronously across the visual field. Six extraocular muscles control all eye movements. Orthophoria is proper alignment of the eyes, and strabismus results from an imbalance in muscle movements.

Strabismus

The classification of strabismus is complex. Based on etiology, it may be considered non-paralytic (comitant) or paralytic (non-comitant). Strabismus may also be classified as congenital or acquired, intermittent or constant, and alternating or unilateral. In **non-paralytic strabismus,** the extraocular muscles and the nerves that control them are normal. The degree of deviation is constant or nearly constant in all directions of gaze. Non-paralytic strabismus is the most common type of strabismus seen in children, and congenital or infantile esotropia is usually of this kind. Ocular or visual defects such as cataracts or high refractive errors occasionally cause non-paralytic strabismus.

In **paralytic strabismus,** paralysis or paresis of one or more of the extraocular muscles produces a muscle imbalance. The deviation is asymmetrical, and characteristically the degree of deviation is worse when gazing in the direction of the affected muscle. Paralytic strabismus may be congenital or acquired. **Congenital paralytic strabismus** may result from birth trauma, muscle anomalies, abnormal development of the cranial nerve nuclei, or congenital infections affecting the eyes. Congenital strabismus may be seen in association with neurodevelopmental disorders such as cerebral palsy. **Acquired paralytic strabismus** due to extraocular muscle palsies usually indicates the presence of a serious underlying condition, such as an intracranial tumor, a demyelinating or neurodegenerative disease, myasthenia gravis, a progressive myopathy, or a central nervous system (CNS) infection. Children may present with a complaint of double vision or a compensatory torticollis (head tilt) to avoid double vision (diplopia).

Intermittent (latent) misalignment of the eyes is referred to as a **phoria.** Under normal conditions, the fusional mechanisms of the CNS maintain eye alignment. Eye deviation is appreciated only under certain conditions, such as illness, fatigue, stress, or when fusion is interrupted by occluding one eye (eg, during cover testing). Some degree of phoria may be found in almost all individuals and it is usually asymptomatic. Larger degrees of phoria may give rise to troublesome symptoms such as headaches, transient diplopia, or asthenopia (eye strain).

Constant misalignment of the eyes is referred to as **heterotropia.** This condition occurs because normal fusional mechanisms are unable to control eye deviation; children are unable to use both eyes together to fixate on an object. In alternating heterotropias, both eyes appear to deviate equally, and vision generally develops normally in each eye because children have no preference for fixation. If strabismus affects only one eye, the other eye is always used for fixation, and there is a danger of developing amblyopia or loss of vision in the deviating eye.

Convergent deviation, a turning in or crossing of the eyes, is called an esodeviation (eg, esotropia or esophoria). Divergent deviation, a turning out of the eyes, is an exodeviation. Hypertropia is used for upward vertical deviations. Esodeviations are the most common type of ocular misalignment, accounting for 50% to 75% of all cases of strabismus. Vertical deviations represent less than 5% of all cases of strabismus.

Amblyopia

Amblyopia, a potential complication if strabismus is not corrected in a timely manner, refers to poor vision in one eye or, rarely, both despite correction of any refractive errors. If children have no significant refractive error and the visual acuity of one eye is worse than the other, they have amblyopia. To be considered amblyopia, visual acuity, as measured by reading an eye chart, should differ by at least 2 lines (eg, 20/20 in one eye and 20/40 in the other). It is the leading cause of preventable visual loss in children.

Amblyopia may be classified into 3 major categories. **Deprivational amblyopia** generally results when a unilateral lesion or developmental defect in one of the structures of the eye or its visual pathways obstructs vision. Causes of deprivational amblyopia include congenital cataract, ptosis, corneal opacity, retinal detachment, retinoblastoma, colobomas, optic nerve defects (eg, optic nerve hypoplasia), or orbital tumors. These conditions cause a lack of formation of a retinal image or a blurred retinal image, usually in one eye. **Refractive amblyopia** refers to a blurring of the retinal image due to large or asymmetrical refractive errors. Amblyopia is usually considered a unilateral abnormality, but may be bilateral in cases of large refractive errors (usually astigmatism or hyperopia). In

strabismic amblyopia, the immature or developing brain suppresses images from the deviating eye to prevent diplopia. Strabismic amblyopia is most commonly associated with strabismus that develops in children who are younger than 4 years. If the condition leading to the amblyopia is not corrected while the brain's visual pathways are still malleable (eg, before approximately 6–7 years of age), children may have some degree of permanent visual loss.

Differential Diagnosis

The differential diagnosis of strabismus may be divided into 3 categories: transient neonatal strabismus, congenital or infantile strabismus, and acquired strabismus. True strabismus must be differentiated from the illusion of deviation created by facial asymmetry or anatomical variations (ie, pseudostrabismus).

Transient Neonatal Strabismus

Eye alignment in normal infants during the first 2 to 3 months of life may vary from normal to intermittent esotropia or exotropia. These deviations are believed to result from CNS immaturity and resolve spontaneously in most children by 4 months of age. If such deviations are constant or persist beyond this age, children should be referred to an ophthalmologist for further evaluation.

Congenital or Infantile Strabismus

This type of strabismus is defined as a deviation that occurs during the first 6 months of life. Because the deviation may not always be present at birth, the term *infantile* may be more accurate. The differential diagnosis of infantile strabismus is presented in Box 64-1. **Pseudoesotropia** is an illusion or apparent deviation and not a true deviation. In many infants, the broad, flat nasal bridge and prominent epicanthal folds may obscure a portion of the sclera near the nose and create the appearance of esotropia (Figure 64-1). This illusion resolves as children mature. Symmetrical corneal light reflexes or normal cover tests differentiate pseudoesotropia from true esotropia.

Esotropia is one of the more common types of childhood strabismus. The constant deviation of infantile esotropia is usually readily apparent because of the large angle of deviation. Affected children usually have good bilateral vision because of the alternation of fixation from one eye to the other. Cross-fixation, in which children look to the left with the adducted right eye and to the right with the adducted left eye, may be evident because of the large angle of deviation. Rarely, esotropia may be due to palsy of the sixth cranial nerve either in isolation or in association with other cranial nerve palsies (Möbius syndrome).

Infantile exotropia is less common than esotropia. Like esotropia, exotropia develops within the first 6 months of life and is characterized by a large angle of deviation. Other causes of infantile exotropia include congenital third nerve palsy (paralytic strabismus) and abnormalities of the bones of the orbit (eg, Crouzon disease).

Box 64-1. Differential Diagnosis of Strabismus

Congenital or Infantile Strabismus

Esodeviations

Infantile esotropia

Pseudoesotropia

Möbius syndrome

Congenital sixth nerve palsy

Duane syndrome

Exodeviations

Congenital exotropia

Congenital third nerve palsy

Abnormalities of the bony orbit (Crouzon disease)

Both Esodeviations and Exodeviations

Duane syndrome (esotropia more common than exotropia)

Acquired Strabismus

Esodeviations

Accommodative esotropia

Benign sixth cranial nerve palsy

Exodeviations

Intermittent exotropia

Overcorrection after surgery for esotropia

Both Esodeviations and Exodeviations

Poor vision

Orbital trauma causing entrapment of extraocular muscles

Intracranial tumors or tumors involving the orbit (eg, retinoblastoma)

Myasthenia gravis

Central nervous system (CNS) infection (eg, meningitis)

CNS tumor

Orbital cellulitis

Figure 64-1. Child with pseudoesotropia. Note the wide nasal bridge and prominent epicanthal folds.

Acquired Strabismus

Acquired strabismus may result from a variety of causes (Box 64-1). Accommodative esotropia and intermittent exotropia are the 2 most common types of acquired strabismus. **Accommodative esotropia** typically develops in children between 2 to 4 years of age but may appear as early as 6 months or as late as 8 years. Children with hyperopia use accommodation (attempts to focus) to see clearly. The accommodative reflex is closely linked to convergence; when accommodation occurs, so does convergence. If children have severe hyperopia (farsightedness), the amount of convergence that occurs with accommodation may be severe and lead to the development of esotropia. Such esotropia is usually intermittent initially and only gradually becomes constant. The deviating eye frequently becomes amblyopic.

Intermittent exotropia, the most common form of exodeviation seen in children, develops between birth and 4 years of age. Although it begins as an intermittent condition in which children's eyes appear to deviate outward, especially when they are tired, ill, or fixating at a distance, the exotropia can become constant with time. Children may also close one eye in bright sunlight, presumably in an effort to prevent diplopia.

Evaluation

History

The evaluation of infants or children suspected of having strabismus should begin with a thorough family history; strabismus often runs in families (Questions Box). Parental description of the ocular deviation is useful because misalignments, especially intermittent deviations that may only become manifest when children are tired, may not always be evident during the office visit. A history of head or orbital trauma may help in the evaluation of acquired strabismus.

Questions

Strabismus

- Does the child have a family history of strabismus?
- Does the child constantly tilt the head toward one side?
- Does the child squint?
- Has the child complained of blurred or double vision?
- Does the child close one eye in bright sunlight?
- Has the child had any recent trauma to the eyes or head?

Physical Examination

On physical examination, the presence of any dysmorphic features and structural abnormalities of the face or neck (eg, torticollis) should be noted. Children with paralytic strabismus (eg, fourth nerve palsy or superior oblique palsy) may compensate for their paretic lesion by tilting their head to avoid diplopia. It is important that visual screening of children begin during the neonatal period. Newborn screening should emphasize the presence of a bilateral red reflex. An abnormal red reflex or a white reflex may indicate the presence of a cataract or retinoblastoma. These require immediate referral to an ophthalmologist. Evaluation for ocular alignment should begin at the 4-month health maintenance visit. Intermittent misalignment of the eyes is often seen in normal infants who are younger than 4 months. However, constant misalignment requires immediate attention at any age.

Vision Testing

Testing visual acuity is essential in the evaluation of children with suspected strabismus. Such testing may be performed as early as 3 years of age if children are cooperative. Charts with symbols, figures, or letters can be used. The traditional Snellen eye chart with letters can generally be used in children who are 4 years of age. Decreased vision in one eye may be indicative of ocular abnormalities, including ocular deviations.

The 2 basic tests for strabismus that can be easily performed in the office are the corneal light reflex test, or Hirschberg test, and the cover test. The pediatrician should be comfortable performing both tests.

The **corneal light reflex test** is the simplest and quickest test for the evaluation of strabismus. In this test, a penlight is projected simultaneously onto the corneas of both eyes as the child looks straight ahead. The examiner compares the placement of the corneal light reflex in each eye with respect to the center of the pupil. If the eyes are straight, the reflection appears symmetrically in the center of both pupils or on the same point on each cornea. If the light reflex appears off center in one eye compared with the other, an ocular deviation or heterotropia is present. Nasal deviation of the light reflex on the cornea indicates exotropia on that side, temporal deviation signifies esotropia, and inferior deviation indicates hypertropia.

Unlike the corneal light reflex test, which may be performed even in uncooperative children, the **cover tests** require a child's cooperation and ability to fixate on a specified object. These tests are used to detect heterophorias. Two types of cover tests, alternate cover and cover-uncover, are used. Only the alternate cover test detects both heterophorias and heterotropias. This test may be preferred by the primary care physician as a screening tool; the cover-uncover test detects only manifest deviations or heterotropias. In the alternate cover test, one eye and then the other is covered as the child fixates on an object at a distance. If neither eye moves as the cover is moved rapidly between the eyes, the eyes are in alignment or orthophoric. With heterotropia, the deviating eye moves when the fixating eye is occluded; in heterophoria, the deviating eye moves when it is uncovered (Figure 64-2).

The alternate cover test may be illustrated with the following example. A child presents with constant esotropia of the left eye. When the right or fixating eye is occluded, the left eye is forced to fixate so that the child can see, and the left eye moves outward as the right eye is occluded. In the case of a child with an esophoria or latent deviation of the left eye, the eye deviates inward when it is occluded because it is not being forced to fixate. As the occluder is moved from the left eye to the right, the left eye moves outward and returns to a position of fixation.

The alternate cover test may be more difficult to interpret in children with bilateral or alternating strabismus who use both eyes in turn for fixation. It is not necessary for the pediatrician to identify exactly what type of strabismus is present; abnormal movement should be noted and children should be referred for further evaluation. An ophthalmologist is able to perform a more detailed examination.

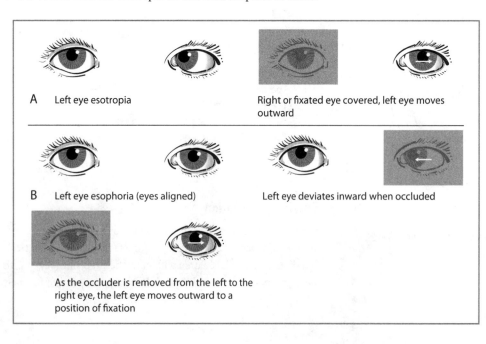

A   Left eye esotropia

Right or fixated eye covered, left eye moves outward

B   Left eye esophoria (eyes aligned)

Left eye deviates inward when occluded

As the occluder is removed from the left to the right eye, the left eye moves outward to a position of fixation

Figure 64-2. Alternate cover test in the detection of strabismus. Normally, both eyes appear to be aligned and centrally fixed. A. Detection of esotropia. The right eye is fixating and a left esotropia is present. When the right or fixating eye is covered, the left eye moves outward (away from the nose). B. Detection of esophoria. The eyes are aligned with a left esophoria. When the left eye is covered, it deviates inward. As the occluder is moved from the left eye to the right eye, the left eye moves outward to a position of fixation.

Management

The goals of management are the attainment of the best possible vision in each eye, straight eyes cosmetically, and fusion. The sooner deviations are corrected, the better the child's chances for equal bilateral vision. Treatment includes correction of any underlying refractive error with **corrective lenses.** Such lenses, which remedy the refractive error and minimize the need for accommodation, are used to treat accommodative esotropia. Glasses are also used in anisometropic amblyopia in which one eye has a significantly different refractive error than the other.

Children who do not see equally well from both eyes may be at risk for amblyopia if they preferentially fixate with only one eye. If detected, amblyopia should be corrected with occlusion therapy of the fixating "good" eye. **Occlusion therapy** forces children to use the amblyopic eye. This treatment is best accomplished by constantly patching the eye with better vision during waking hours, or penalization with dilating drops in the better seeing eye. Children require repeat evaluations and close monitoring during this therapy.

If nonsurgical methods fail to align the eyes, surgical correction may be necessary. **Surgery** may be used to achieve the best possible ocular alignment and is usually required for treatment of infantile esotropia. It is generally performed in children between 6 months and 1 year of age, while the visual system is still pliable enough to allow for development of postsurgical binocular vision. Surgery also may be needed in children with intermittent exotropia if the frequency of the deviation is increasing.

Prognosis

Certain conditions, such as pseudoesotropia or infrequent intermittent exotropia, may resolve as children mature. Others, such as infantile esotropia, require early detection and treatment to achieve the best binocular vision. Amblyopia and permanent vision loss may result if correction of strabismus is delayed.

CASE RESOLUTION

The infant in the case history has pseudoesotropia. Although the boy's eyes appear to deviate, the corneal light reflex and cover tests are normal. Physical examination reveals prominent epicanthal folds and a broad, flat nasal bridge.

Selected References

Bacal DA. Don't be lazy about looking for amblyopia. *Contemp Pediatr.* 1998;15:99–107

Catalano JD. Strabismus. *Pediatr Ann.* 1990;19:289–297

Cheng KP, Biglan AW, Hiles DA. Pediatric ophthalmology. In: Zitelli BJ, Davis HW. *Pediatric Physical Diagnosis.* 3rd ed. St Louis, MO: Mosby-Wolfe; 1997:563–601

Crouch ER Jr, Crouch ER. Pediatric vision screening: why? when? what? how? *Contemp Pediatr.* 1991;8(special issue):9–30

Greenwald M, Parks M. Treatment of amblyopia. In: *Duane's Clinical Ophthalmology.* Philadelphia, PA: Lippincott Williams & Wilkins; 2002: 1–10

Keech R. Practical management of amblyopia. In: Wright K, ed. *Focal Points: Clinical Modules for Ophthalmologists.* Vol. XVIII, No. 2. San Francisco, CA: American Academy of Ophthalmology; 2000:1–3

Lavrich JB, Nelson LB. Diagnosis and treatment of strabismus disorders. *Pediatr Clin North Am.* 1993;40:737–752

Mitchell P, Parks M. Concomitant exodeviations. In: *Duane's Clinical Ophthalmology.* Philadelphia, PA: Lippincott Williams & Wilkins; 2002: 1–17

Parks M. Alignment. In: *Duane's Clinical Ophthalmology.* Philadelphia, PA: Lippincott Williams & Wilkins; 2002: 1–12

Parks M, Mitchell P, Wheeler M. Concomitant esodeviations. In: *Duane's Clinical Ophthalmology.* Philadelphia, PA: Lippincott Williams & Wilkins; 2002: 1–21

Simon J, ed. *Pediatric Ophthalmology and Strabismus.* San Francisco, CA: American Academy of Ophthalmology; 2006–2007: 9–12, 67–118

Spencer RF, Tucker MG, Choi RY, McNeer KW. Botulinum toxin management of childhood intermittent exotropia. *Ophthalmology.* 1997;104:1762–1767

Wallace DK, Chandler DL, Beck RW, et al. Treatment of bilateral refractive amblyopia in children three to less than 10 years of age. *Am J Ophthalmol.* 2007;144:487–496

Infections of the Eye

Teresa Rosales, MD

CASE STUDY

A 10-day-old neonate has a 1-day history of red, watery eyes and nonproductive cough with no fever. The girl is breastfed and continues to eat well. She was the 7-lb, 2-oz (3,238-g) product of a term gestation, born via normal spontaneous vaginal delivery without complications to a 26-year-old woman. The pregnancy was also uncomplicated. No one at home is ill.

On examination, the infant is afebrile with normal vital signs. Examination of the eyes reveals bilateral conjunctival injection with only a mild amount of purulent discharge. Bilateral red reflexes are present. The rest of the physical examination is within normal limits.

Questions

1. What is the differential diagnosis of conjunctivitis both during and following the neonatal period?
2. What laboratory tests, if any, should be performed?
3. When is a chest x-ray indicated in the evaluation of neonates with conjunctivitis?
4. What are management strategies for eye infections?

Infections of the eye and surrounding structures are commonly seen by pediatricians. Such infections range in severity from common problems such as blepharitis and conjunctivitis, which lack serious sequelae, to severe and less common infections such as periorbital and orbital cellulitis. The presenting complaint in many children with eye infections is a red-appearing eye. Familiarity with the common causes of a red eye makes prompt diagnosis and treatment possible.

Epidemiology

Conjunctivitis, which affects children of all ages, is perhaps the most common eye infection of childhood. The incidence of conjunctivitis in the newborn period is estimated to range from 1.6% to 12%. The incidence of chlamydial conjunctivitis is about 8 in 1,000 live births. About two-thirds of acute childhood conjunctivitis has a bacterial etiology, and one-third is viral. *Haemophilus influenzae* and *Streptococcus pneumoniae* are the most common bacterial agents and account for about 40% and 10% of culture-proven cases, respectively. The incidence of *H influenzae* is decreasing with the advent of the *H influenzae* type b vaccine. *Staphylococcus aureus* is isolated from the conjunctivae of children with acute conjunctivitis, but it is found with about the same frequency in the eyes of children without conjunctivitis. Adenovirus is the most common viral isolate. Most cases of acute conjunctivitis in young adults have a viral etiology. Serious eye infections such as periorbital and orbital cellulitis occur far less often.

Clinical Presentation

Red eyes and discharge are the common presenting signs of infections of the eyelids and conjunctivae. Eyelid edema and erythema surrounding the eye characterize periorbital and orbital cellulitis. Proptosis, abnormal extraocular movement, or loss of visual acuity may signal spread of the infection beyond the orbital septum (orbital cellulitis) (Dx Box).

Pathophysiology

Eye infections may be divided into 2 types: those affecting the structures surrounding the orbit and those involving the orbital contents themselves (Figure 65-1). Although all structures surrounding the eye may potentially become inflamed or infected, the eyelids, nasolacrimal drainage system (dacryocystitis; see Chapter 66), conjunctiva, and cornea are most commonly involved. Orbital cellulitis is defined as an infection of the orbital structures posterior to the orbital septum. The orbital septum, an extension of the periosteum of the bones of the orbit, extends to the margins of both the upper and lower eyelids and provides an anatomical barrier to the spread of most infectious and inflammatory processes. Preseptal, or periorbital, cellulitis is localized to structures superficial to the orbital septum, whereas post-septal, or orbital, cellulitis implies that the disease process involves orbital structures extending beyond the septum.

Differential Diagnosis

Infections of the eye are included in the differential diagnosis of conditions presenting with red eye (Box 65-1). Also included in the differential diagnosis are congenital, inflammatory, traumatic, and systemic processes. Although infection and irritation are by far the most common causes of an acute onset of red eye, other possibilities, especially trauma, glaucoma, or underlying systemic disease, must be considered.

Dx Eye Infections

Eyelid Infections
- Redness
- Itching (blepharitis)
- Burning (blepharitis)
- Scales at the base of the lashes (seborrheic blepharitis)
- Swelling (hordeolum or chalazion)
- Pain (hordeolum)

Conjunctivitis
- Conjunctival injection and edema
- Excessive tearing
- Discharge or crusting
- Itching (allergic conjunctivitis)

Uveitis
- Conjunctival injection
- Pain
- Blurred vision
- Photophobia
- Headache

Periorbital Cellulitis
- Unilateral eyelid edema
- Erythema surrounding the eye
- Pain
- Fever

Orbital Cellulitis
- Eyelid edema
- Proptosis
- Decreased extraocular movements
- Loss of visual acuity
- Fever
- Ill appearance
- Associated sinusitis

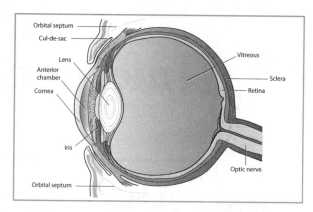

Figure 65-1. **The eye and surrounding structures.**

that may manifest as clusters of vesicles on the eyelids. Acne rosacea may rarely occur in childhood and can present very similarly to chronic blepharitis.

The glands of the eyelid can also be infected. *S aureus* is the most common organism. A **hordeolum,** or common stye, results from an infection of the meibomian glands located along the lid margins. The glands become obstructed and an abscess can form. Affected children present with a well-circumscribed, painful swelling that may

Box 65-1. Differential Diagnosis of Red Eye
Congenital Anomalies
• Nasolacrimal duct obstruction
• Congenital glaucoma
Infection
• Keratitis
• Conjunctivitis
• Dacryocystitis
• Corneal ulcer
• Periorbital and orbital cellulitis
Inflammation
• Blepharitis
• Hordeolum
• Chalazion
Trauma
• Corneal abrasion
• Foreign body
• Blunt trauma: hyphema
• Perforating injuries
• Exposure to chemicals or other noxious substances
Systemic Illnesses
• Kawasaki disease
• Varicella
• Measles
• Lyme disease
• Stevens-Johnson syndrome
• Ataxia-telangiectasia
• Juvenile rheumatoid arthritis

Eyelid Infections

Common conditions affecting the eyelid and its related structures are blepharitis, hordeolum, and chalazion.

Blepharitis is an inflammation of the lid margins. This condition, which is often bilateral, may be chronic or recurrent. The 2 most common causes of blepharitis are staphylococcal infection and seborrheic dermatitis. Children with staphylococcal blepharitis often present with scales at the base of the lashes, ulceration of the lid margin, and loss of lashes. The infection may spread to the conjunctiva or cornea, producing conjunctivitis or keratitis. In contrast, seborrheic blepharitis is characterized by greasy, yellow scales attached to the base of the lashes. In addition, associated seborrhea of the scalp or eyebrows may be present. Mixed staphylococcal-seborrheic infections, which occur as staphylococcal superinfection, may complicate seborrheic blepharitis. Less commonly seen forms of blepharitis are parasitic blepharitis, which results from infestation of the lids by the head louse, *Pediculus capitis,* or crab louse, *Pediculus pubis,* and primary or recurrent herpes simplex virus type 1 infections be at the lid margin or may be deeper in the lid tissue. These generally rupture or resolve without complications when treated aggressively with hot compresses.

A chalazion is a hordeolum that has not resolved over weeks to months. It is no longer an infectious process but has become a chronic granulomatous inflammation of the meibomian glands. The resulting firm, non-tender, slow-growing mass within the upper or lower eyelid may be painful if secondary infection is present.

Infections of the Conjunctiva

Conjunctivitis refers to any inflammation of the conjunctiva. The condition may be allergic, chemical, viral, or bacterial in etiology. In addition, it may be a sign of systemic disease such as Kawasaki disease or Stevens-Johnson syndrome.

Acute conjunctivitis, or pinkeye, is common during childhood and can be extremely contagious. The usual signs are conjunctival injection, tearing, discharge, crusting of the lashes, and conjunctival edema (chemosis). Pain and decreased vision are uncommon symptoms and may signal corneal involvement.

In general, it is difficult to distinguish bacterial conjunctivitis from viral conjunctivitis on clinical features alone. Certain clinical characteristics may guide the diagnosis. The average age of children affected with **bacterial conjunctivitis** tends to be younger than the age of those with viral conjunctivitis, which occurs more frequent in adolescents; however, considerable overlap occurs. Children with bacterial conjunctivitis typically present with an acute onset of unilateral or bilateral injection and edema of both the palpebral and bulbar conjunctiva, minimal to copious purulent discharge, and crusting of the eyelashes. Children may have difficulty opening their eyes on awakening in the morning because of the exudate. An association between conjunctivitis and concomitant otitis media has been well described. *H influenzae,* which is often resistant to ampicillin, is the pathogen most commonly isolated from affected children.

The diagnosis of **viral conjunctivitis** is considered if signs of viral upper respiratory infection (eg, low-grade fever, cough, rhinorrhea) are evident. Viral infection is associated with conjunctival injection, watery or thin mucoid discharge, and only mild lid edema and erythema. Adenoviral infection is usually bilateral, with significant conjunctival injection and chemosis of the lids, and is often accompanied by a tender preauricular lymph node. Epidemic keratoconjunctivitis is a highly contagious form of adenoviral conjunctivitis. Affected children often complain of foreign body sensation beneath the lids or photophobia due to corneal involvement. Pharyngeal conjunctival fever, another presentation of adenoviral conjunctivitis, usually manifests as conjunctivitis in association with pharyngitis and fever.

Infants who suffer from **chronic or recurrent conjunctival discharge** may have an obstruction of the nasolacrimal duct, whereas older children with chronic conjunctivitis may have allergic diseases, recurrent blepharitis, or chlamydial infections. Blepharitis is the most common cause of chronic conjunctivitis in older children. *S aureus* is frequently implicated in these infections.

Itching, tearing, and conjunctival edema are the hallmarks of **allergic conjunctivitis,** a noninfectious form of conjunctival inflammation often seen in children with other allergic disorders such as asthma or hay fever. Conjunctival injection tends to be mild, bilateral, and seasonal. The etiology is most often a hypersensitivity to pollens, dust, or animal dander. Vernal conjunctivitis is a bilateral, severe form of allergic conjunctivitis seen primarily during childhood. Most cases occur during the spring and summer. Severe itching and tearing are the most frequent complaints. The conjunctiva of the upper eyelid may have a cobblestone appearance due to the accumulation of inflammatory cells, or there may be small, elevated lesions of the bulbar conjunctiva at the corneal limbus. The pathogenesis is unclear, but atopy seems to play a role.

Chlamydial conjunctivitis frequently affects both neonates and adolescents. Inclusion conjunctivitis is an acute infection of the eyes caused by sexually transmitted *Chlamydia trachomatis* (usually serotypes D through K). This condition may be seen in neonates or sexually active adolescents. Trachoma, the most common cause of impaired vision and preventable blindness worldwide, is a chronic conjunctivitis usually caused by *C trachomatis* serotypes A, B, and C. Although this disease is rarely seen in North America, it is endemic among certain populations, especially Native Americans. Inclusion conjunctivitis and endemic trachoma are both characterized initially by conjunctivitis with small lymphoid follicles in the conjunctiva.

Neonatal conjunctivitis, or ophthalmia neonatorum, occurs during the first month of life. The major causes of neonatal conjunctivitis are chemical, chlamydial, and bacterial (in decreasing order of frequency). Ophthalmia neonatorum may be produced by the same bacteria that cause childhood conjunctivitis but also results from organisms such as *C trachomatis or Neisseria gonorrhoeae.* Newborns may acquire these latter pathogens following premature rupture of membranes or passage through an infected or colonized birth canal. *C trachomatis* is the organism most commonly identified. It has been isolated from 17% to 40% of neonates with conjunctivitis. Infants born to mothers with active cervical chlamydial infection have a 20% to 50% chance of developing chlamydial conjunctivitis. Viruses are uncommon causes of neonatal ocular infections. Herpes simplex virus (HSV) is the primary viral agent involved in neonatal conjunctivitis. The presence of characteristic vesicular skin lesions or corneal dendritic lesions helps in the diagnosis.

The time of onset of symptoms is related to the etiologic agent. Inflammation secondary to the **silver nitrate** drops instilled at birth to prevent gonococcal infection presents as mild conjunctivitis 12 to 24 hours after birth in 10% to 100% of treated newborns. This condition usually resolves spontaneously in 24 to 48 hours. This is more of historic interest because erythromycin ointment 0.5% has replaced silver nitrate in most hospitals. (Silver nitrate was ineffective against *C trachomatis.*) Conjunctivitis due to *N gonorrhoeae* appears 2 to 5 days after birth and is associated with copious purulent discharge. Conjunctivitis due to *C trachomatis* occurs at 5 to 14 days, a result of a longer incubation period. The time of onset and the severity of symptoms of these 2 conditions may overlap, however. The presentation of gonococcal infection may be delayed for 5 days or more because of the partial suppression of the infection by the prophylactic drops instilled at birth. Chlamydial infection can vary in severity from mild erythema of the eyelids to severe inflammation and copious purulent discharge. Chlamydial infection is primarily localized to the palpebral conjunctiva and only rarely affects the cornea. Gonococcal conjunctivitis is considered a medical emergency because the gonococcus can penetrate the cornea, resulting in corneal ulceration and perforation of the globe within 24 hours if untreated.

Concomitant nasopharyngeal chlamydial infection is commonly seen. Spread of the organism from the nasopharynx to the lungs is a sequela of colonization. Ten percent to 20% of infants with conjunctivitis have chlamydial pneumonia. It may occur either simultaneously with the conjunctivitis or up to 4 to 6 weeks later. Affected infants are usually afebrile and present with symptoms of increasing tachypnea and cough.

Anterior uveitis may be confused with conjunctivitis. The uvea consists of the iris, the ciliary body, the retina, and the choroid. Inflammation of the iris or ciliary body may produce conjunctival injection, which may be associated with decreased visual acuity, pain, headache, and photophobia. Systemic conditions associated with uveitis include Kawasaki disease, juvenile rheumatoid arthritis, Lyme disease, tuberculosis, sarcoidosis, toxocara infection, toxoplasmosis, and spondyloarthropathies.

Infections of the Eye and Surrounding Tissues

Preseptal cellulitis and **orbital cellulitis** are 2 serious infections of the eyelids and surrounding structures. Although these infections are not as frequent as those that are limited to the eye, they have serious sequelae. The preseptal space is defined by the skin of the eyelid on one side and the orbital septum on the other. Children with preseptal cellulitis, or **periorbital cellulitis,** usually present with acute onset, unilateral upper and lower eyelid edema, erythema, and pain. The condition is often associated with systemic signs and symptoms such as ill appearance, fever, and leukocytosis. The eye itself usually appears normal. Infection may follow hematogenous seeding of the preseptal space, most often with *H influenzae* type b or *S pneumoniae*, or after traumatic breaks in the skin that usually lead to *S aureus* infection.

Orbital cellulitis is an infection of the contents of the orbit posterior to the orbital septum. Usually an insidious onset of eyelid edema, proptosis, decreased extraocular movements, and loss of visual acuity occur. As with periorbital cellulitis, children are often febrile and ill-appearing. Contiguous spread of infection from adjacent sinusitis (most often ethmoid) is the most common cause. The organisms most often involved are the same as those in acute sinusitis (*S aureus*, *S pneumoniae*, non-typeable *H influenzae*, and *Staphylococcus pyogenes*). Untreated, the infection may progress to orbital abscess formation or progress posteriorly in the orbit to the cavernous sinus and the brain.

Primary herpes simplex infection can affect the skin surrounding the eyes as well as the eye itself. Most of these infections are caused by HSV type 1, although type 2 infections may be seen in newborns. Children with **herpetic infections of the eye** usually present with unilateral skin vesicles and a mild conjunctivitis or keratitis. Herpetic keratoconjunctivitis can recur following fever, exposure to sunlight, or mild trauma. The characteristic corneal lesion of herpes keratitis is the dendritic corneal ulcer, which appears as a tree branch pattern on fluorescein staining of the cornea. Although this lesion may be seen with primary infection, it is more common in recurrent infections. Skin vesicles may not appear with a recurrence, which makes it difficult to distinguish herpetic infection from other causes of conjunctivitis. Empiric topical steroid treatment for presumed viral conjunctivitis should be avoided for this reason; steroids may lead to progression of the herpetic infection and permanent corneal scarring as well as cataracts and glaucoma. Neonatal herpetic infections of the eye primarily result from HSV 2. Infections may be isolated to the eye or the eye may be infected secondarily due to central nervous system (CNS) or disseminated disease. Proper diagnosis is important because disseminated herpetic disease has a mortality of about 85%, and CNS disease has a mortality of 50%. Isolated herpetic eye disease is actually quite rare in neonates.

Evaluation

History

A careful history taken from the parent or primary caregiver as well as the child can guide the diagnosis (Questions Box). It is important to exclude the possibility of ocular trauma or exposure to noxious chemicals when evaluating children with red, irritated eyes.

Questions

Eye Infections

- How long has the child had symptoms?
- Is the child having any difficulty seeing clearly?
- Is he or she complaining of light sensitivity?
- Has the child had fever, cold symptoms, or purulent nasal discharge (eg, green or yellow)?
- Are the eyes pruritic (itchy) or painful?
- Does the child have difficulty opening the affected eye on awakening in the morning or after naps?
- Have the parents noticed any discharge from the eyes or crusting around the eyelids?
- Is the child complaining of earache or sore throat?
- Does the child have allergies, asthma, or hay fever?
- Has there been any trauma or bug bites?

Physical Examination

A thorough examination of the eyes should be performed. The eyelids, conjunctiva, and cornea should be inspected for evidence of inflammation or foreign bodies. The presence of any discharge or crusting of the eyelids as well as light sensitivity or pain should be noted. Extraocular movements should be checked, and their symmetry should be noted. Visual acuity should be determined, and an ophthalmoscopic examination of the retina should be performed whenever possible. A slit-lamp examination of the eye is indicated if uveitis is suspected. In addition, it is important to perform a thorough head and neck examination, noting the presence of associated sinusitis, otitis media, pharyngitis, or preauricular nodes.

Laboratory Tests

Laboratory assessment is guided by the history and physical examination. Although clinical differentiation between a bacterial and viral etiology is difficult, cultures are usually not required because acute conjunctivitis in children is a self-limited disease. In neonatal conjunctivitis, however, the time of onset of illness and the clinical findings overlap, and Gram stain and cultures are essential. Gonococcal infection is assessed by both Gram stain and culture. Treatment may be initiated on the basis of Gram stain alone because of the serious potential for corneal involvement and subsequent loss of visual acuity.

If HSV is suspected, viral cultures should be obtained. If chlamydial infection is suspected, a nasopharyngeal culture should be sent in addition to conjunctival scraping. Purulent material may be examined for gonococci, but conjunctival scrapings are required for chlamydia because chlamydia is an obligate intracellular organism. Laboratory assessment of periorbital cellulitis includes a complete blood count (CBC), blood culture, and a lumbar puncture in young infants or in children with signs of meningeal irritation. The reported prevalence of meningitis is 1% in children with periorbital cellulitis and 10% in children with bacteremia and periorbital cellulitis. As with periorbital cellulitis, laboratory assessment of orbital cellulitis includes a CBC and blood culture.

Imaging Studies

Imaging studies are required infrequently in the assessment of eye infections. A chest x-ray to detect pneumonia should be taken if infants with neonatal conjunctivitis have respiratory symptoms. Characteristic features on chest x-ray include hyperinflation and diffuse or patchy interstitial infiltrates. In orbital cellulitis, a computed tomography scan of the orbit and sinuses may be useful for assessing the degree of involvement.

Management

Most common eye infections either resolve spontaneously or respond readily to **hygiene** and **topical antibiotics.** Treatment of both staphylococcal and seborrheic blepharitis consists of daily lid hygiene (usually at bedtime), including application of a warm compress and removal of the scales and crusts with a moistened, warm washcloth. The eyelashes and lid margins may also be scrubbed with a washcloth soaked in a 50:50 mixture of baby shampoo and water. When staphylococcal blepharitis is present, an ointment containing an antistaphylococcal antibiotic agent such as erythromycin may be applied to the eyelids after cleansing. Treatment of parasitic blepharitis consists of application of petrolatum ophthalmic ointment (to smother the nits) several times a day for 1 week, followed by removal of the remaining parasites and their ova with tweezers or forceps.

Treatment for hordeola consists of application of hot compresses several times a day. This usually causes the abscess to come to a point and drain. Occasionally, surgical excision and drainage may be required if the abscess does not resolve. Unlike the hordeolum, a chalazion generally requires surgical excision, because spontaneous resolution is uncommon.

Most cases of acute childhood conjunctivitis can be managed successfully by primary care physicians. Acute conjunctivitis in childhood is generally a self-limited disease. However, antibiotic treatment of bacterial conjunctivitis hastens recovery and may help prevent secondary cases by eradicating the bacterial pathogen. It is helpful to determine clinically whether the infection is bacterial and initiate empiric treatment with topical antibiotic preparations. Trimethoprim and polymyxin B sulfate (Polytrim), sodium sulfacetamide (Bleph-10), gentamicin (Garamycin), and tobramycin (Tobrex) are some of the commonly prescribed antibiotics. The newest antibiotic of choice is Vigamox (moxifloxacin). Avoid neomycin-containing products because sensitivity to neomycin occurs frequently. Antibiotic ointments may be easier to instill in infants and young children. Antibiotic drops should be used in older children during the day because the ointments can blur the vision. Ointments may be used at bedtime. Systemic therapy can be considered for concomitant conjunctivitis and otitis media. Good hygiene with special attention to hand washing is important to prevent the spread of the infection to the other eye and to family and friends. Children should not go to school until the discharge and drainage have resolved (even if on antibiotic drops). If symptoms persist for more than 7 to 10 days or if the diagnosis is in question, appropriate cultures should be taken. Complicated cases such as suspected herpetic or gonococcal infection, foreign bodies that cannot be removed easily, loss of visual acuity, presence of significant pain, those involving children with a history of recent penetrating ocular trauma or surgery, and those involving children who use contact lenses should be referred to an ophthalmologist immediately. Contact lens wearers with red eyes are at high risk for corneal ulcers.

Allergic conjunctivitis can be managed with cool compresses. Topical decongestant drops may provide symptomatic relief if treatment is indicated. Vernal conjunctivitis may be treated with topical cromolyn sodium drops or medications designed to relieve redness and itching and stabilize mast cells, such as Patanol (olopatadine) or Acular (ketorolac). Caution should be used when prescribing corticosteroid preparations for the eye because they may lead to progression of an undiagnosed herpetic eye infection. Chronic use of topical steroids can cause cataracts and glaucoma.

Treatment of neonatal conjunctivitis depends on the diagnosis. If **gonococcal infection** is suspected and Gram stain is positive for gram-negative diplococci, immediate parenteral therapy with ceftriaxone should be initiated. **Chlamydial** conjunctivitis should be managed with systemic rather than topical treatment to prevent systemic disease. Oral erythromycin is the drug of choice. Although oral treatment provides adequate local antibiotic levels, topical erythromycin ointment may be used in conjunction with systemic therapy to provide more prompt relief of ophthalmic symptoms. The parents should also be treated.

Empiric parenteral antibiotic therapy (eg, cefuroxime) should be initiated for **periorbital cellulitis.** Repeat evaluations for signs of progression should be performed frequently during the initial 24 to 48 hours. If **orbital cellulitis** is suspected, an ophthalmologist should be consulted, and hospitalization and systemic antibiotics should be instituted. Surgical drainage of the sinuses or of an orbital abscess is sometimes necessary.

Children with suspected **herpetic infection** should be referred to an ophthalmologist. Intravenous acyclovir is often recommended for the treatment of isolated herpetic eye infections in neonates.

Prognosis

Most common eye infections such as blepharitis, hordeolum, and acute childhood conjunctivitis resolve without sequelae. Recurrence is common for hordeola, and periorbital cellulitis may be a potential complication in rare or untreated cases. Unlike acute conjunctivitis, chronic conjunctivitis may not be self-limited. Appropriate diagnosis and management are extremely important to prevent serious sequelae in some children. For example, endemic trachoma may progress to produce conjunctival scarring, pannus formation, and even blindness if not appropriately treated with systemic erythromycin or tetracycline. (In general, systemic tetracycline should not be used in children <8 years to avoid discoloration of the teeth.)

Periorbital cellulitis generally resolves without sequelae if treated promptly with systemic antibiotics. Orbital cellulitis should be considered a true ophthalmologic emergency because the potential for complications is high. The optic nerve may become involved, resulting in loss of vision or spread of the infection into the cranial cavity. This spreading may lead to meningitis, cavernous sinus thrombosis, or brain abscess.

CASE RESOLUTION

The infant presented in the case history has neonatal conjunctivitis. A Gram stain of the purulent discharge should be examined, and cultures should be taken from the eye and nasopharynx. If the Gram stain is negative for gonococci, empiric treatment may begin with oral erythromycin.

Selected References

Gigliotti F. Acute conjunctivitis. *Pediatr Rev.* 1995;16:203–207

King RA. Common ocular signs and symptoms in childhood. *Pediatr Clin North Am.* 1993;40:753–766

Liesegang T, Skuta G, Cantor L. Infectious and allergic ocular diseases. *J Pediatr Ophthalmol Strabismus.* 2006;17:215–238

Mets M, Noffke A. Ocular infections of the external eye and cornea in children. *Focal Points.* 2002;2:1–14

McKinley S, Yen M, Miller A, et al. Microbiology of pediatric orbital cellulitis. *Am J Ophthalmol.* 2007;144:497–501

O'Hara MA. Ophthalmia neonatorum. *Pediatr Clin North Am.* 1993;40:715–725

Powell KR. Orbital and periorbital cellulitis. *Pediatr Rev.* 1995;16:163–167

Silver LH, Woodside AM, Montgomery DB. Clinical safety of moxifloxacin ophthalmic solution 0.5% (Vigamox) in pediatric and non-pediatric patients with bacterial conjunctivitis. *Surv Ophthalmol.* 2005;50(suppl 1):S55–S63

Wagner RS. Eye infections and abnormalities: issues for the pediatrician. *Contemp Pediatr.* 1997;14:137–153

Wagner RS. The differential diagnosis of the red eye. *Contemp Pediatr.* 1991;8:26–48

Weiss AH. Chronic conjunctivitis in infants and children. *Pediatr Ann.* 1993;22:366–374

Excessive Tearing

Teresa Rosales, MD

CASE STUDY

A 4-week-old infant girl has had a persistent watery discharge from both eyes since birth. Her mother has noticed white, crusty material on her daughter's eyelids for the past few days. The infant's birth and medical history are unremarkable. Examination of the eyes, including bilateral red reflexes and symmetrical extraocular movements, is normal, except that the left eye appears "wetter" than the right.

Questions

1. What is the differential diagnosis of excessive tearing in infancy?
2. How do physical findings such as corneal enlargement and haziness influence the differential diagnosis?
3. How should infants with excessive tearing be managed?
4. When should a child with excessive tearing be referred to an ophthalmologist?

Infants or young children with excessive tearing or epiphora in one or both eyes are a common pediatric ophthalmologic concern. The pediatrician must be capable of differentiating benign causes of this common childhood condition from other more serious illnesses, such as glaucoma, that potentially threaten vision.

NASOLACRIMAL DUCT OBSTRUCTION

Epidemiology

Congenital obstruction of the nasolacrimal duct or dacryostenosis, which occurs in 1% to 6% of newborn infants, is the most common cause of excessive tearing in infancy. Eighty percent will resolve spontaneously by 6 months of age.

Clinical Presentation

Infants with dacryostenosis usually present with a history of a mucoid discharge and crusting along the eyelid margins. The affected eye appears "wetter" than the normal eye, and a small pool of tears may be noted along the lower eyelid. Frequent tearing is reported. Commonly, the patient has repeated episodes of infection with purulent discharge (Dx Box).

Pathophysiology

The lacrimal system (Figure 66-1) produces and drains tears away from the eyes and into the nose. Reflex tearing is usually present shortly after birth but may be delayed for several weeks to months until the lacrimal gland begins to function. Tears drain away from the eyes through the superior and inferior puncta into the superior and inferior canaliculi and finally into the nasolacrimal duct, which drains beneath the inferior turbinate into the nose.

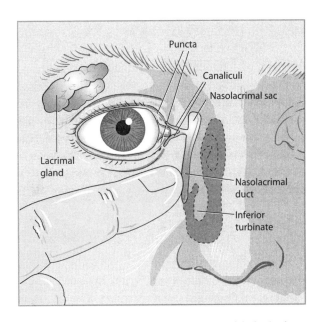

Figure 66-1. The lacrimal system, showing massage of the lacrimal sac.

Outflow obstruction, most often due to obstruction of the nasolacrimal duct or dacryostenosis, is the most common cause of excessive tearing in infancy. The obstruction is usually bilateral and occurs during fetal development. Most commonly a persistent, thin membrane (Hasner membrane) obstructs the opening of the sac in the nose. The membrane is usually located in the distal or nasal segment of the duct rather than in the proximal portion. The term *dacryocystitis* is used if acute infection or inflammation is associated with the obstruction. If both the canaliculi and the nasolacrimal duct are obstructed, a mucocele over the nasolacrimal sac may be noted at birth. This sac appears as a bluish, firm mass located over the lacrimal sac. Atresia of some portion of the drainage system may also occur, but this is extremely rare.

Differential Diagnosis

Box 66-1 outlines the differential diagnosis of excessive tearing in infancy. Although obstruction of the nasolacrimal duct is the most common cause of excessive tearing in infants, it is important to consider and rule out glaucoma when evaluating infants with this complaint. Unlike dacryostenosis, which is usually unilateral, infantile glaucoma may be unilateral or bilateral.

Box 66-1. Differential Diagnosis of Excessive Tearing in Infants

Increased Production
- Infantile glaucoma
- Allergy
- Conjunctivitis
- Corneal abrasion
- Foreign body under the eyelid

Outflow Obstruction
- Nasolacrimal duct obstruction (dacryostenosis)
- Anomalies of the lacrimal drainage system
- Mucocele of the lacrimal sac
- Atresia of the lacrimal punctum or canaliculus
- Nasal congestion
- Craniofacial anomalies involving the midface

Acute onset of excessive tearing in older children is usually due to ocular irritation. Any irritation of the conjunctiva, cornea, or eyelids may produce tearing. Conjunctivitis and corneal abrasion, usually secondary to a retained foreign body or herpes simplex keratoconjunctivitis, are the 2 most common causes. Eye infections are discussed in Chapter 65.

Evaluation

History

Evaluation of excessive tearing should begin with a thorough history. The nature of any discharge (eg, watery, mucoid, or purulent) should be noted. Parents or other caregivers should be questioned about the appearance of the child's eyes (Questions Box). The excessive mucoid discharge in the medial canthal region and on the eyelashes is noticeable to the family as is the increased tearing. Crusting along the eyelashes caused by drying of the mucoid material is usually noted when children awaken in the morning or after a nap. Mucopurulent discharge may be noted if an associated acute infection is present (dacryocystitis).

Physical Examination

A careful examination of the eyes in infants includes inspection, evaluation of extraocular movements, and funduscopic examination. Funduscopic examination may be difficult in this age group, but bilateral red reflexes should at least be elicited. Signs of **dacryostenosis,**

Questions

Excessive Tearing

- How old was the child when the excessive tearing appeared?
- Are one or both eyes affected?
- How does the eye appear? How has its appearance changed?
- Is there a family history of infantile glaucoma?
- Is the child photophobic or light sensitive (eg, closes the eyes in bright sunlight)?
- Has the child had any persistent, watery discharge?
- Does the child have difficulty opening the affected eye on awakening in the morning or after a nap?

which usually appear days to weeks after birth, include tearing, mucoid discharge, and crusting of the eyelids. Tearing may be as mild as an increased wetness of the affected eye; this is best evaluated prior to disturbing the child. Visible overflow of tears from the affected eye is not unusual, and is typically seen when the eye is irritated (eg, due to cold or wind). If dacryostenosis is present, there may be associated erythema and edema of the eyelids. Dacryocystitis may also spread to the surrounding tissues, producing a periorbital cellulitis; systemic signs of infection such as fever may be noted. Gentle pressure along the medial canthal region over the lacrimal sac may produce a reflux of tears or mucoid discharge onto the surface of the eye, thus confirming the diagnosis of obstruction.

Laboratory Tests

Routine laboratory assessment is generally not necessary.

Management

Spontaneous resolution of dacryostenosis is common by 6 to 8 months of age. The primary medical treatment of uncomplicated nasolacrimal duct obstruction consists of **local massage** and **cleansing** beginning when the symptoms are noted. Parents are instructed to massage the nasolacrimal duct several times a day by applying firm, downward pressure over the medial canthal region with their finger and then sliding the finger down toward the mouth (Crigler maneuver) (see Figure 66-1). This maneuver attempts to move fluid trapped within the nasolacrimal sac down through the duct in an attempt to break the obstruction with hydrostatic pressure. Parents may be asked to cleanse the eyes with warm water before performing this maneuver. Antibiotic ointments and drops should be prescribed only if the discharge is purulent or associated conjunctivitis is evident.

Controversy exists regarding when probing of the nasolacrimal duct should be performed. Some ophthalmologists prefer probing the duct before children are 6 months of age because prior to this time the procedure may be performed in the office without general anesthesia. Others state that more than 80% of obstructions resolve with conservative medical management by 6 months of age and prefer to delay probing until the age of 9 to 12 months. At this age the procedure needs to be performed under general anesthesia. Deciding when to proceed with the probing depends on the standard of practice within the community, the severity of symptoms, the response to medical management, and the level of parental concern.

Ophthalmologic referral is necessary for affected infants by 6 months of age if the obstruction has not resolved. Referral should be made sooner if symptoms are severe or infections recur.

Prognosis

Most cases of dacryostenosis resolve spontaneously during the first year of life without further sequelae. If tear duct probing is necessary, it is 90% to 95% successful if performed before 13 months of age. The success rate drops to 70% between 13 to 15 months and 50% over 18 months.

CONGENITAL GLAUCOMA

Epidemiology

Congenital or infantile glaucoma, a serious cause of excessive tearing, is quite rare; the incidence is about 1 in 10,000 live births. Although glaucoma may be present at birth, onset during the first few weeks to months of life is more common. Approximately 25% of cases are diagnosed at birth and 80% by 1 year of age. The severity of the disease is worse with earlier onset. Most affected infants are male; the male-female ratio in older infants is 2:1. Infantile glaucoma seems to have a multifactorial inheritance pattern, but most cases are sporadic. In families with one affected child or a parental history of infantile glaucoma, the chance of having a child with glaucoma is about 5%. Although glaucoma may be unilateral or bilateral, most children (75%–90%) who present before 3 months of age have bilateral glaucoma.

Clinical Presentation

In addition to excessive tearing, other clinical signs of infantile glaucoma include blepharospasm (spasmodic blinking of the eyelids), photophobia, corneal enlargement and corneal haziness due to corneal edema, progressive enlargement of the eye (buphthalmos), and cupping and atrophy of the optic nerve (Dx Box).

 Dx Excessive Tearing

- Conjunctival edema or injection
- Crusting of the eyelids
- Rhinorrhea
- Photophobia
- Corneal haziness
- Reflux of tears with gentle pressure on medial canthus
- Wetness of eye

Pathophysiology

Glaucoma is the most serious and potentially sight-threatening etiology for excessive production of tears. Glaucoma refers to an increase in intraocular pressure that is severe enough to damage the eye and alter vision. In infants and children, glaucoma is usually a result of a developmental abnormality of the iridocorneal angle, interfering with drainage of aqueous humor from the anterior chamber. Young infants differ from adults in that the globe in infants' eyes is distensible; the increased intraocular pressure not only produces corneal enlargement and edema but also expands the globe itself. Breakdown of the corneal epithelium and resultant irritation of the eyes produce reflex tearing and photophobia. Untreated glaucoma may lead to optic nerve damage with resultant loss of visual acuity, decreased visual field, and even blindness. Glaucoma in children younger than 3 years is referred to broadly as infantile glaucoma, and glaucoma that occurs in children between 3 and 20 years of age is called juvenile glaucoma. Infantile glaucoma is further classified as being primary or secondary. Primary glaucoma refers to isolated abnormalities of the iridocorneal angle, whereas secondary glaucoma may be associated with other ocular or systemic diseases. Juvenile glaucoma is a form of open-angle glaucoma.

Differential Diagnosis

Excessive tearing may be due to increased production or to obstruction to outflow (see Box 66-1). Infants with increased production of tears will demonstrate rhinorrhea in association with epiphora, a finding that distinguishes glaucoma from dacryostenosis. Rhinorrhea is not associated with dacryostenosis because the nasolacrimal duct is obstructed and no tears drain out of the nose. Unlike dacryostenosis, which is usually unilateral, infantile glaucoma is most commonly bilateral, though may be unilateral. Ocular irritation as occurs with conjunctivitis, corneal abrasion, or a foreign body under the eyelid can also produce excessive tearing, especially in older children. Allergies are also associated with excessive tearing due to overproduction.

Disorders associated with outflow obstruction include dacryostenosis, anomalies of the lacrimal drainage system (mucoceles of the lacrimal sac and atresia of the lacrimal punctum or caniculus), nasal congestion, and craniofacial anomalies involving the midface.

Evaluation

A corneal diameter greater than 12 mm in infants is suggestive of infantile glaucoma. Corneal edema is more common in younger infants (<3 months of age) and may cause the red reflex to appear dull in the affected eye. The optic cup may be enlarged. A cup-to-disk ratio greater than 0.3 or an asymmetry of the ratio between the eyes may indicate glaucoma.

As in adults, loss of visual fields occurs in children with glaucoma. Visual fields are difficult to evaluate in young children because of their inability to cooperate with the examination.

Management

Suspected cases of glaucoma should be referred to an ophthalmologist immediately for further evaluation, including measurement of intraocular pressure. Pressures greater than 20 mm Hg are suggestive of glaucoma (normal pressures are 10–20 mm Hg in infants and young children as well as in adults).

Surgery is the primary treatment. The goal is to normalize intraocular pressure and minimize irreversible corneal and optic nerve damage.

Prognosis

Infantile glaucoma, if left untreated, may progress to blindness. The visual prognosis depends on several factors, including the age at onset of glaucoma (the earlier the onset, the worse the prognosis), the amount of optic nerve damage, and the degree of myopia caused by the enlargement of the eye. In addition, amblyopia, secondary to either deprivation due to corneal opacities or unequal refractive errors, is often seen (see Chapter 64).

CASE RESOLUTION

The infant presented in the case history at the beginning of the chapter has dacryostenosis. She can be managed with medical treatment such as local massage and cleansing at this stage. If her symptoms persist beyond the age of 6 months, consultation with an ophthalmologist is recommended.

Selected References

Beck AD, Lynch MG. Pediatric glaucoma. *Focal Points: Clinical Modules for Ophthalmologists*. Module 5. San Francisco, CA: American Academy of Ophthalmology; 1997;XV:1–14

Becker BB. The treatment of congenital dacryocystocele. *Am J Ophthalmol.* 2006;142:835–838

Howard CW. The baby with too many tears: what to do and how to do it. *Int Pediatr.* 1990;5:239–242

Isenberg SJ, Apt L, McCarty J, Cooper LL, Lim L, Del Signore M. Development of tearing in preterm and term neonates. *Arch Ophthalmol.* 1998;116:773–776

Kushner BJ. The management of nasolacrimal duct obstruction in children between 18 months and 4 years old. *J AAPOS.* 1998;2:57–60

Lavrich JB, Nelson LB. Disorders of the lacrimal system apparatus. *Pediatr Clin North Am.* 1993;40:767–776

Olitsky S, Medow N, Rogers G. Diagnosis and treatment of congenital nasolacrimal duct obstruction. *J Pediatr Ophthalmol Strabismus.* 2007;44:80–83

Paysse EA, Coats DK, Bernstein JM, et al. Management and complications of congenital dacryocele with concurrent intranasal mucocele. *J AAPOS.* 2000;4:46–53

Robb R. Nasolacrimal duct obstruction in children. *Focal Points: Clinical Modules for Ophthalmologists*. Module 8. San Francisco, CA: American Academy of Ophthalmology; 2004;XXII;1–10

Schnall BM, Christion CJ. Conservative treatment of congenital dacryocele. *J Pediatr Ophthalmol Strabismus.* 1996;33:219–222

Schwartz BA, Manley DR. Disorders of the lacrimal apparatus in infancy and childhood. In: Nelson LB, ed. *Pediatric Ophthalmology.* 4th ed. Philadelphia, PA: W. B. Saunders; 1998:345–352

Stamper RL, Lieberman MF, Drake MV. *Becker-Shaffer's Diagnosis and Therapy of the Glaucomas.* 7th ed. St Louis, MO: Mosby; 1999

Wagner RS. Glaucoma in children. *Pediatr Clin North Am.* 1993;40:855–867

Neck Masses

Stanley H. Inkelis, MD

CASE STUDY

A 2-year-old boy is brought to the office with a 1-day history of an enlarging red, tender "bump" beneath his right mandible. He has a fever (temperature: 101.6°F [38.5°C]) and sores around his nose, upper lip, and cheek. These sores have been present for 3 days and have not responded to an over-the-counter antibiotic ointment. He had an upper respiratory tract infection 1 week ago, which has almost entirely resolved. He is otherwise in good health. The family has no history of tuberculosis or recent travel, and the child has not been playing with cats or other animals.

The physical examination is completely normal except for fever, mild rhinorrhea, honey-crusted lesions on the nares and upper lip, and a 4 × 5-cm, right submandibular neck mass that is erythematous, warm, and tender to palpation.

Questions

1. What are the common causes of neck masses in children?
2. What steps are involved in the evaluation of children with neck masses?
3. What clinical findings suggest that neck masses are neoplasms? When should neck masses be biopsied or removed?
4. What is involved in the treatment of the different types of neck masses in children?
5. When should children with neck masses be referred for further consultation?

Neck masses are any swellings or enlargements of the structures in the area between the inferior mandible and the clavicle. Normal variants, such as the angle of the mandible or tip of the mastoid, may occasionally appear as swellings, and parents sometimes confuse these with neck masses. If the swelling is not a normal structure, a well-directed history and physical examination usually determine the etiology.

Lymphadenopathy from viral or bacterial throat infections is the most common cause of neck **masses** in children. Therefore, neck masses are common because children frequently have sore throats. Most parents know about swollen lymph glands, and they usually do not seek medical advice unless the glands become very large or do not recede in a few days. Neck masses in children may have many other causes besides lymphadenopathy. Most of these masses may be categorized as inflammatory, neoplastic, traumatic, or congenital in origin.

Epidemiology

Most neck masses are benign. Almost 50% of all 2-year-old children and up to 90% of children between 4 and 8 years of age have palpable cervical lymph nodes. Although more than 25% of malignant tumors in children are found in the head and neck region (this is the primary site in only 5%), less than 2% of suspicious head and neck masses are malignant.

The epidemiology of neck masses of infectious origin depends on the infectious agent itself, geographic location of the child, and the child's socioeconomic status. Neck masses of viral origin may be related to focal infection of the oropharynx or respiratory tract but are often associated with generalized adenopathy. Neck masses of bacterial origin typically occur from normal bacterial flora of the nose, mouth, pharynx, and skin that secondarily spreads to lymph nodes. These organisms are not usually transmitted from person to person. Pathologic flora such as group A streptococcus and *Mycobacterium tuberculosis* that result in neck masses can spread by human-to-human contact, however.

Clinical Presentation

Children with neck masses present in a variety of different ways depending on the etiology of the mass. Typically a swelling or enlargement in the neck, which parents often notice more than children, is evident. Associated signs and symptoms include fever, upper respiratory tract infection, sore throat, ear pain, pain or tenderness over the mass, changes in skin color over the mass, skin lesions of the head or neck, and dental caries or infections (Dx Box). Malignant tumors are usually slow-growing, firm, fixed, non-tender masses. Congenital neck masses and benign tumors, which have frequently been present since birth or early infancy, are soft, smooth, and cyst-like and may be recurrent. Neck masses associated with trauma are often rapidly evolving and may lead to airway obstruction.

Dx Neck Masses

Inflammatory/Infectious
- Swelling or enlargement in the neck
- Fever
- Sore throat, dental infection, skin infection of head or neck
- Pain or tenderness over the mass (usually)

Neoplastic
- Slowly enlarging mass
- Unilateral, discrete
- Firm or rubbery
- Fixed to tissue
- Deep within the fascia
- Non-tender (usually)

Congenital
- Enlargement in neck (usually present since birth or soon after)
- Soft, smooth, cyst-like
- Non-tender (unless infected)
- Recurrent

Pathophysiology

The pathophysiology of neck masses in children is dependent on etiology. Most neck masses are related to inflammation or infection of lymph nodes. Enlargement of lymph nodes usually results from proliferation of intrinsic lymphocytes or histiocytes already present in the lymph node (eg, lymphadenopathy caused by a viral infection) or from infiltration of extrinsic cells (eg, lymphadenitis, metastatic tumor). Neck masses from trauma occur from leakage of fluid into the neck, and congenital anatomical abnormalities become apparent because of fluid collection or infection of the defect. The parotid gland may be enlarged from inflammation (eg, blocked salivary gland duct), infection (eg, mumps), or tumor (eg, pleomorphic adenoma), but the swelling primarily involves the face rather than the neck and obscures the angle of the jaw. Other salivary glands may be infected or obstructed and may cause submandibular swelling, erythema, and tenderness.

Differential Diagnosis

Neck masses in children are usually the result of inflammation or infection of lymph nodes, tumors of lymph nodes and other neck structures, trauma, and congenital lesions. The location of the mass is often a clue to its etiology (Figure 67-1).

Lymphadenopathy/Lymphadenitis

Lymphadenopathy is lymph node enlargement or hyperplasia secondary to localized infection or antigenic stimulation proximal to the involved node or nodes. Because lymphoid tissue steadily increases until puberty, palpable lymph nodes, including those in the cervical area, are a common, normal finding in children. Any lymph node in the neck larger than 10 mm qualifies as cervical lymphadenopathy.

Figure 67-1. Differential diagnosis of neck mass by location. 1. Parotid—cystic hygroma, hemangioma, lymphadenitis, parotitis, Sjögren and Caffey-Silverman syndromes, lymphoma. **2. Postauricular**—lymphadenitis, branchial cleft cyst (1st), squamous epithelial cyst. **3. Submental**—lymphadenitis, cystic hygroma, thyroglossal duct cyst, dermoid, sialoadenitis. **4. Submandibular**—lymphadenitis, cystic hygroma, sialoadenitis, tumor, cystic fibrosis. **5. Jugulodiagastic**—lymphadenitis, squamous epithelial cyst, branchial cleft cyst (1st), parotid tumor, normal-transverse process C2, styloid process. **6. Midline neck**—lymphadenitis, thyroglossal duct cyst, dermoid, laryngocele, normal hyoid, thyroid. **7. Sternomastoid (anterior)**—lymphadenitis, branchial cleft cyst (2nd, 3rd) pilomatrixoma, rare tumors. **8. Spinal accessory**—lymphadenitis, lymphoma, metastasis from nasopharynx. **9. Paratracheal**—thyroid, parathyroid, esophageal diverticulum. **10. Supraclavicular**—cystic hygroma, lipoma, lymphoma, metastasis, normal fat pad, pneumatocele of upper lobe. **11. Suprasternal**—thyroid, lipoma, dermoid, thymus, mediastinal mass. (Reproduced with permission from Fleisher GR, Ludwig S, eds. *Textbook of Pediatric Emergency Medicine.* 5th ed. Philadelphia, PA: Lippincott Williams & Wilkins; 2006:433.)

The most common cause of cervical lymphadenopathy is a viral infection of the upper respiratory tract. Lymphadenopathy usually begins and resolves with the acute infection. Occasionally the swelling remains for several days or months, however, and children present because of parental concern. Bacterial pharyngitis, usually from infection with group A beta-hemolytic streptococcus (GABHS), is often associated with cervical lymphadenopathy. Cervical as well as generalized lymphadenopathy may be seen in children with systemic illness (eg, Kawasaki disease, sarcoid, human immunodeficiency virus). Cat-scratch disease, toxoplasmosis, fungal infection, and mycobacterial and atypical mycobacterial infections may be associated with lymphadenopathy that may later progress to lymphadenitis. Viral illnesses, including Epstein-Barr virus (EBV) (mononucleosis), adenovirus, enterovirus, herpes simplex virus, human herpesvirus 6 (HHV-6), and cytomegalovirus (CMV), commonly cause lymphadenopathy and lymphadenitis.

Lymphadenitis is infection or inflammation of the lymph node that occurs when microorganisms and neutrophils infiltrate the node, leading to necrosis and abscess formation. This condition is usually associated with proximal bacterial infection that drains to the affected nodes by connecting afferent lymphatic channels. Lymphadenitis is often a progression of disease, resulting in enlarged nodes that measure 2 to 6 cm. These nodes, which are typical of bacterial disease, are often termed *hot nodes,* and they are erythematous, warm, tender, and sometimes fluctuant. *Cold nodes* or *cold lymphadenitis* usually represents subacute or chronic inflammation of lymph nodes typical in illnesses such as cat-scratch disease, mycobacterial infection, or toxoplasmosis. Unlike hot nodes, cold nodes are not warm to the touch and are usually not as tender. They are usually not suppurative and may be difficult to distinguish from nodes that are simply enlarged (Figure 67-2).

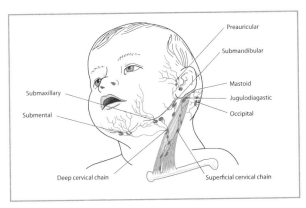

Figure 67-2. **The lymphatic drainage and lymph nodes involved in infants and children with cervical lymphadenitis. (Reproduced with permission from Feigin RD, Cherry JD, eds.** *Textbook of Pediatric Infectious Diseases.* **5th ed. Philadelphia, PA: Saunders; 2004:186.)**

Staphylococcus aureus and group A streptococcus are responsible for 50% to 90% of cases of acute unilateral cervical lymphadenitis. These organisms spread from a primary site to the lymph nodes draining those sites. Common primary sites of infection are the throat; teeth and gums; and skin (lesions), particularly on the scalp or ears. Infections at these sites may result from trauma, such as scratches or scabs, or from primary infection, such as impetigo. *S aureus* or group B streptococcus usually causes cervical lymphadenitis in neonates or very young infants. Such staphylococcal infections, which are often nosocomially spread from contact in the newborn nursery, present as discrete masses. Group B streptococcus causes the "cellulitis-adenitis" syndrome, which presents as cervical adenitis associated with a facial cellulitis. *Pseudomonas aeruginosa* is an unusual cause of cervical adenitis in newborns.

Mycobacterial disease must always be considered in children of all ages who present with cervical adenitis. The child with *M tuberculosis* cervical adenitis often has multiple nodes, sometimes bilateral, usually non-tender, and usually not erythematous or warm. These children are typically older, commonly reside in an urban setting, have a history of tuberculosis exposure, and often have an abnormal chest x-ray. Intradermal placement of a purified protein derivative (PPD) often produces more than 15 mm of induration in most children with typical mycobacterial infection. A reaction of 5 to 14 mm may be caused by tuberculous or non-tuberculous mycobacterial infection. Atypical mycobacterial infection usually occurs in children between 1 and 6 years of age with unilateral rather than bilateral lymph node enlargement and a normal chest x-ray.

Cat-scratch disease should be considered in children who have cats or kittens or who play with them. The infection may result from a cat scratch or from a cat licking a child's broken skin. If the inoculum is near the head and neck area, cervical adenitis develops. Occasionally generalized lymphadenopathy is present. An associated papule or papules where the cat scratch or lick occurred may be apparent. *Bartonella henselae* has been identified as the organism causing cat-scratch disease.

Toxoplasmosis may be accompanied by adenitis, usually in the posterior cervical area. Nodes are painless and may fluctuate in size, and children are often asymptomatic. Multiple lymph nodes are involved in about one-third to one-half of cases.

Children presenting with recurrent cervical adenitis and recurrent fevers may have PFAPA syndrome (periodic fever, aphthous ulcers, pharyngitis, and adenopathy) characterized by periodic fever, aphthous stomatitis, pharyngitis, and cervical adenitis. This entity usually occurs in children younger than 5 years and can be aborted with steroids.

Kikuchi disease, or histiocytic necrotizing lymphadenitis, has an Asian and female predilection and is characterized by fever, leukopenia, and cervical lymphadenopathy. The illness is self-limited, and follow-up is recommended because of a possible association with systemic lupus erythematosus.

Less common bacterial, viral, and fungal causes of cervical adenitis are listed in Box 67-1.

Tumors

Compared with other neck masses, **malignant neck tumors** occur rarely; nevertheless, they should be considered in any children with rapidly enlarging or persistent neck masses. Hodgkin disease and non-Hodgkin lymphoma are the most frequent cause of head and neck malignancies in children, accounting for almost 60% of the cases. Rhabdomyosarcomas are the next most frequent head and neck malignancy followed by thyroid tumors, neuroblastoma, and nasopharyngeal carcinomas. Age is an important factor in determining the likelihood of specific tumors. Neuroblastoma and rhabdomyosarcoma are the most common tumor types in children younger than 6 years. Non-Hodgkin lymphoma typically occurs in preadolescence, and Hodgkin disease and thyroid carcinoma are the most common malignancies in adolescents.

Benign neck tumors, with the exception of those mentioned later in the discussion of congenital lesions, are uncommon. They include epidermoid inclusion cysts, lipomas, fibromas, neurofibromas, pilomatrixomas (benign skin neoplasms of hair follicle origin), keloids, goiters, and ranulas (intraoral mucocysts).

Box 67-1. Differential Diagnosis of Neck Masses

Cervical Lymphadenopathy/Lymphadenitis

Bacterial origin

Staphylococcus aureus (methicillin sensitive; MSSA)

Staphylococcus aureus (methicillin resistant; MRSA)

Group A beta-hemolytic streptococcus

Mycobacterium tuberculosis

Atypical mycobacteria

Cat-scratch disease *(Bartonella henselae)*

Anaerobes

Gram-negative enteric bacteria

Haemophilus influenzae

Plague

Actinomycosis

Diphtheria

Tularemia

Brucellosis

Syphilis

Group B streptococcus (neonates)

Viral origin

Epstein-Barr virus (infectious mononucleosis)

Adenovirus

Cytomegalovirus

Herpes simplex virus, types 1 and 2

Enterovirus

Human immunodeficiency virus

Measles

Rubella

Human herpes virus 6

Influenza virus

Fungal origin

Histoplasmosis

Coccidioidomycosis

Aspergillosis

Candidiasis

Sporotrichosis

Cryptococcosis

Parasitic origin

Toxoplasmosis

Leishmaniasis

Tumor

Malignant

Hodgkin disease

Non-Hodgkin lymphoma

Lymphosarcoma

Rhabdomyosarcoma

Neuroblastoma

Leukemia

Langerhans cell histiocytosis

Thyroid tumors

Nasopharyngeal squamous cell carcinoma

Salivary gland carcinoma

Benign

Epidermoid cyst

Lipoma

Fibroma

Neurofibroma

Pilomatrixoma

Keloid

Goiter

Osteochondroma

Teratoma (may be malignant)

Ranula

Congenital Disorders

Hemangioma

Cystic hygroma (lymphangioma)

Branchial cleft cyst

Thyroglossal duct cyst

Laryngocele

Dermoid cyst

Cervical rib

Sternocleidomastoid tumor

Trauma

Hematoma (acute or organized)

Subcutaneous emphysema

Foreign body

Arteriovenous malformation

Immunologic Disorders

Local hypersensitivity reaction (sting or bite)

Pseudolymphoma (from phenytoin)

Serum sickness

Sarcoidosis

Caffey-Silverman syndrome

Kawasaki disease

Systemic lupus erythematosus

Juvenile rheumatoid arthritis

Kikuchi disease (necrotizing lymphadenitis)

Miscellaneous

Sialadenitis

Parotitis

Storage disorders

   Niemann-Pick disease

   Gaucher disease

Obstructive airway disease (asthma, cystic fibrosis)

Trauma

Trauma to the neck may be associated with bleeding and edema. Large hematomas that affect vital structures are potentially life-threatening. Significant trauma and structural injury usually accompany neck hematomas. In children with mild injuries and neck hematomas, bleeding disorders are a possible cause of the hematoma. Twisting injuries to the neck may lead to muscle spasm of the sternocleidomastoid muscle (torticollis) and an apparent mass that is the contracted muscle. Child abuse should also be considered in children who have neck injuries that are not consistent with their histories.

A foreign body in the neck may present as a mass because of the foreign body itself (eg, piece of glass or metal, bullet) or surrounding inflammation. A crepitant neck mass following trauma to the neck or chest suggests subcutaneous emphysema from tracheal injury or a pneumomediastinum. Crepitant neck masses may also be seen secondary to pneumomediastinum in children with obstructive lung diseases such as asthma or cystic fibrosis.

Congenital Lesions

Children with congenital neck lesions can present with a neck mass in early infancy or later in childhood. Some congenital lesions are not discovered until adulthood. The most common of these benign lesions are thyroglossal duct cysts, branchial cleft cysts, lymphatic malformations (cystic hygromas/lymphangiomas), and hemangiomas (Figure 67-3).

Figure 67-3. Head and neck congenital lesions seen in children in frontal and lateral views. The shaded areas denote the distribution in which a given lesion may be found. A. Dermoid cyst. B. Thyroglossal duct cyst. C. Second branchial cleft appendage. D. Second branchial cleft sinus. E. Second branchial cleft cyst. F. First branchial pouch defect. G. Preauricular sinus or appendage. (Reproduced with permission from Fleisher GR, Ludwig S, eds. *Textbook of Pediatric Emergency Medicine.* 5th ed. Philadelphia, PA: Lippincott Williams & Wilkins; 2006:1594.)

Thyroglossal duct cysts are almost always midline in the neck and inferior to the hyoid bone. They usually move upward with tongue protrusion or swallowing. Most branchial cleft cysts occur anterior to the middle one-third of the sternocleidomastoid muscle. Branchial cleft sinus tracts appear as slit-like openings anterior to the lower third of the sternocleidomastoid muscle and may present as neck masses if they become infected. Thyroglossal duct cysts and branchial cleft cysts may also present for the first time as infected neck masses.

Cystic hygromas are usually large, soft, easily compressible masses found in the posterior triangle behind the sternocleidomastoid muscle in the supraclavicular fossa. They transilluminate well. Two-thirds of cystic hygromas are present at birth, and 80% to 90% are identified before 3 years of age. They are more common on the left side of the neck. Cystic hygromas occasionally become secondarily infected, with findings of erythema, warmth, and tenderness.

Hemangiomas are usually not present at birth but appear in early infancy and may enlarge rapidly. In most cases, they recede spontaneously by 9 years of age. They are usually much smaller than cystic hygromas, do not transilluminate, and may be recognized by their reddish color (capillary or strawberry hemangioma) or by a bluish hue of the overlying skin (cavernous hemangioma).

Small infants who present with torticollis should be examined for a sternocleidomastoid mass ("tumor"), which represents fibrosis and contracture of that sternocleidomastoid muscle so that the head tilts toward the affected side with the chin rotating to the opposite side. Contusion of the sternocleidomastoid muscle from traumatic extraction of the head during delivery with subsequent hemorrhage and healing has been implicated as the cause of the fibrotic mass. However, it is more likely that this mass occurs prior to birth because it contains mature fibrous tissue. In addition, the mass may be present following cesarean section and is associated with hip dysplasia and other congenital lesions, suggesting that the condition is related to abnormal positioning in utero. Venous occlusion of the sternocleidomastoid muscle either in utero or at the time of delivery has also been proposed as a cause.

Evaluation

History

A thorough history is important in establishing the etiology of the neck mass (Questions Box).

> **Questions**
>
> ### Neck Masses
>
> - How old is the child?
> - How long has the neck mass been present?
> - What signs and symptoms are associated with the neck mass?
> - Has the child been exposed to tuberculosis?
> - Has the child ever drunk any unpasteurized cow's milk?
> - Has the child been in contact with any cats or kittens? Rabbits? Other animals?
> - Has the child traveled to areas where endemic diseases such as histoplasmosis or coccidioidomycosis are prevalent?
> - Has the child suffered any trauma recently?
> - Does the child have any allergies?
> - Does the child have any risk factors for human immunodeficiency virus?

Physical Examination

A general physical examination should be performed. The neck mass should be examined for anatomical location, color, size, shape, consistency, tenderness, fluctuance, and mobility. The mass should also be measured. The head, neck, and face should be examined for lesions, most often infections, that drain into neck lymph nodes. Lesions can frequently be found on the scalp, neck, face, ears, mouth, teeth, tongue, gums, and throat. Hairstyles such as tight braids can sometimes provide ports of entry for bacteria. Occasionally, sinus tracts or fistulas may be the entry point of infection. In addition, other lymph node groups should be examined to determine if the lymphadenopathy is local or generalized. Particular attention should be paid to the supraclavicular area because enlarged supraclavicular nodes are more frequently associated with malignant pathology such as Hodgkin disease. The chest should be examined for use of accessory muscles, equality of breath sounds, and wheezing. The abdomen should be examined for hepatosplenomegaly.

Laboratory Tests

Laboratory tests are rarely indicated in children with cervical lymphadenopathy or lymphadenitis of acute onset. Although a rapid streptococcal antigen detection test or throat culture is helpful in children with suspected streptococcal sore throat, it may be unnecessary if antibiotic therapy is empirically prescribed for the lymphadenitis. If the adenitis is fluctuant, aspiration and culture may be helpful in determining the specific bacteriologic diagnosis. Fine-needle aspiration cytology and polymerase chain reaction assays may help differentiate between tuberculous and nontuberculous mycobacterial disease. In addition, a PPD test should be applied to all children who present with lymphadenitis.

If the adenitis does not resolve or improve after 2 to 3 days of observation or therapy, laboratory tests directed by the history and physical examination should be considered. A complete blood count (CBC) with differential and a monospot or serologic antibody tests for EBV may be helpful in the diagnosis of infectious mononucleosis. If the mass in the neck is a hematoma and a bleeding disorder is suspected, a CBC with platelet count, prothrombin time, and partial thromboplastin time should be obtained. Possible additional tests include an erythrocyte sedimentation rate, C-reactive protein and, if indicated, serologic tests for toxoplasmosis, CMV, HHV-6, coccidioidomycosis, histoplasmosis, tularemia, *B henselae,* and syphilis should be performed. Skin tests for fungi should be considered in those patients coming from endemic areas. These tests should be placed after serologic tests are performed so that false-positive serologic test results are not obtained.

Similar laboratory tests should be considered for children who present for the first time with enlarged or enlarging lymph nodes of long duration or those who do not respond after 2 weeks of antibiotic therapy. The physician may choose to do more of these laboratory tests at the initial evaluation or after a therapeutic trial because the likelihood of viral lymphadenopathy decreases and the possibility of a more unusual etiology increases. Human immunodeficiency virus testing should also be considered.

Thyroid function tests and thyroid scans should be considered in children with a thyroid mass or suspected thyroglossal duct cyst.

Unless cat-scratch disease is very likely, immediate lymph node biopsy is indicated for enlarged supraclavicular nodes or lymph nodes in the lower half of the neck, rapidly progressive and enlarging nodes, fixed nodes, nodes deep within the fascia, or firm or hard nodes. Children who have a persistent fever or weight loss should

have a biopsy at 1 week if a diagnosis has not been established. Asymptomatic children without an established diagnosis should have a biopsy at 2 weeks if the node increases in size, at 4 to 6 weeks if the node is not increased in size but is persistent, and at 8 to 12 weeks if the node has not regressed to a normal size. In some cases, the initial biopsy is non-diagnostic but on subsequent biopsy a specific diagnosis may be made. Consequently, children with persistent adenopathy should be followed closely and be biopsied again if indicated. Fine-needle aspiration biopsy in children is controversial, but has some demonstrated benefits. It is being used more often to differentiate between benign and malignant disease and to potentially decrease the need for open biopsy. However, if malignancy is a consideration, consultation with an oncologist is advisable to determine the biopsy method of choice.

Imaging Studies

A chest x-ray should be obtained in all children with suspected tuberculosis or tumor (eg, enlarged supraclavicular nodes) as well as in children with crepitant neck masses or in those children in whom the diagnosis of the adenitis remains uncertain. If a foreign body in the neck is suspected, both anteroposterior and lateral neck x-rays should be obtained.

Almost all neck masses can be evaluated by ultrasonography, computed tomography (CT), or magnetic resonance imaging (MRI). Because there is no ionizing radiation associated with ultrasonography, it is quickly available, is noninvasive, and does not need sedation. It is considered by many to be the initial imaging study of choice, particularly for thyroid masses, thyroglossal duct cysts, branchial cleft cysts, and parotid masses. Ultrasonography with color Doppler is helpful in differentiating cystic from solid masses and determining if the mass is vascular. In addition, demonstration of a normal thyroid gland by ultrasound in patients with thyroglossal duct cysts confirms a source of thyroid hormone. Consequently, a thyroid scan is not necessary.

Computed tomography and MRI scans provide better definition and extent of the mass. Computed tomography scan with contrast is the preferred method of imaging for deep neck abscesses that present with a neck mass and for enlarged salivary glands. Magnetic resonance imaging provides the best anatomical detail, and it is the preferred imaging study for children with vascular and lymphatic malformations and neoplasms; however, it is not as available as CT and often requires a greater degree of sedation.

Management

Neck masses are rarely acutely life-threatening. If neck masses impinge on the airway, children may experience stridor, hoarseness, drooling, increased effort of breathing, unequal breath sounds, or evidence of shock. Resuscitation and stabilization should be initiated immediately. The algorithm in Figure 67-4 outlines the management of cervical lymphadenitis.

Children with lymphadenitis who do not appear toxic and have no evidence of sepsis may be treated empirically with **oral antibiotics**

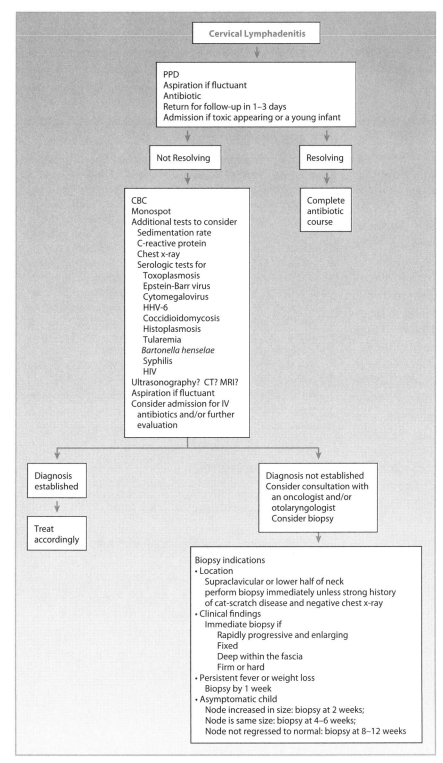

Figure 67-4. Management of cervical lymphadenitis. Abbreviations: PPD, purified protein derivative; CBC, complete blood count; HHV-b, human herpesvirus 6; HIV, human immunodeficiency virus; CT, computed tomography; MRI, magnetic resonance imaging; IV, intravenous.

S aureus (MSSA) is cultured and sensitivities are determined, a first-generation cephalosporin such as cephalexin (50 mg/kg/d), dicloxacillin (50 mg/kg/d), or amoxicillin/clavulanic acid (40 mg/kg/d [amoxicillin]) may provide satisfactory coverage. Treatment should be continued for a minimum of 10 days but for no less than 5 days after resolution of acute signs and symptoms. Lack of clinical improvement after 36 to 48 hours suggests that the diagnosis and proposed therapy need to be reevaluated.

Infants and small children, as well as those older children who do not respond to oral antibiotic therapy, may require admission for **intravenous antibiotics** such as clindamycin or vancomycin (especially for a potentially life-threatening infection) until culture results are available. If MSSA is cultured and sensitivities are determined, oxacillin or a cephalosporin may be satisfactory alternatives. Incision and drainage of large, fluctuant nodes that are clearly from bacterial disease should be done in consultation with an otolaryngologist or surgeon to promote resolution of the lymphadenitis. Alternatively, treatment by needle aspiration instead of incision and drainage has been advocated by some physicians. If *M tuberculosis* or atypical mycobacterial infection is suspected, incision and drainage should not be done because persistent sinus tracts may result.

Atypical mycobacterial infection is generally unresponsive to treatment with antituberculous medications. **Surgical excision** of all visibly affected nodes, deep as well as superficial, is recommended. However, in cases where surgery is problematic or is refused, macrolide monotherapy or a macrolide in combination with ethambutol or rifampin has been helpful in treating non-tuberculous adenitis. Tuberculous mycobacterial adenitis usually responds to short-course medical therapy. Antituberculous medication for 6 to 9 months is recommended.

Lymphadenitis from cat-scratch disease usually resolves on its own. Antibiotic therapy is usually not indicated, but if children are severely ill or appear toxic with systemic cat-scratch disease, have hepatic or splenic involvement, are immunocompromised, or are admitted for a suppurative adenitis, treatment with oral antibiotics such as rifampin, trimethoprim-sulfamethoxazole, azithromycin, or ciprofloxacin may be beneficial. If there is no improvement, the addition of parenteral gentamicin to the regimen may be considered.

that cover *S aureus,* particularly methicillin-resistant *S aureus*, and GABHS. Clindamycin or a combination of cephalexin (administered until the culture from the lymph node, if available, for group A streptococcus is negative) and trimethoprim-sulfamethoxazole may be used to provide coverage for these organisms. If methicillin-susceptible

Aspiration is indicated to relieve symptoms in patients with fluctuant or painful suppurative nodes. Incision and drainage should not be done. Total removal of the node is sometimes necessary to effect a cure.

There is no specific therapy for lymphadenitis caused by *Toxoplasma gondii*. Excision of the affected node may be indicated if the diagnosis is questionable.

If a tumor is suspected, consultation with a pediatric oncologist is recommended. The mass should be biopsied for a definitive diagnosis. If it is malignant, a treatment plan should be generated with the appropriate consultants.

Congenital torticollis from fibrosis of the sternocleidomastoid muscle is best treated with nonoperative intervention. Repetitive passive range-of-motion exercises over several weeks usually result in loosening the tight muscle and increasing the range of motion.

Hemangiomas usually resolve by the time children are 9 years of age, and surgical intervention is rarely indicated. For life-threatening hemangiomas, or those that may cause complications such as vision loss, corticosteroids and interferon alfa-2a are effective medications. Interferon alfa-2a has been associated with transient or permanent neurologic disabilities, so it is important to balance the benefits and risks of this medication. Surgical excision is usually indicated for cystic hygromas (lymphangiomas), branchial cleft cysts, and thyroglossal duct cysts. A thyroid ultrasound should be performed before removal of a thyroglossal duct cyst to confirm that other thyroid tissue is not present. Endocrinologic consultation is recommended in these cases. Thyroid nodules in children may be cancerous, especially in children who have had irradiation to the head and neck region. Consultation with an endocrinologist and surgeon should be obtained. Goiters in children should be evaluated by an endocrinologist.

Prognosis

The prognosis for children with neck masses is generally excellent but differs depending on the cause. Children with an infectious etiology do very well if diagnosed and treated with appropriate antimicrobials. Mycobacterial lymphadenitis may result in sinus tract formation or disseminated disease. Surgical excision usually cures atypical mycobacterial infection. Cat-scratch disease is usually benign and self-limited. Encephalopathy is a rare complication of this disorder.

The prognosis for benign tumors of the neck is excellent. The outlook for children with malignant neck tumors depends on etiology of the tumor and the spread of the malignancy to other organs. Early diagnosis and treatment are clearly important in improving outcome.

Children with neck masses from trauma usually have had significant injury. The outcome often depends on establishment of an airway, provision of ventilatory support, and management of hemodynamic instability. Availability of surgical support is often essential to a good outcome.

Children with congenital lesions of the neck usually have an excellent prognosis. Some lesions resolve spontaneously, while others require simple surgical excision. Cystic hygromas may require multiple operations for complete removal because of their diffuse nature.

CASE RESOLUTION

In the case presented, the boy has signs and symptoms consistent with submandibular bacterial cervical lymphadenitis. The location of the neck mass in relation to the honey-crusted lesions (non-bullous impetigo) implicates spread of bacteria from the primary site of infection to the lymph nodes. Laboratory tests are unnecessary because the child does not appear septic. Culture of the impetigo may be helpful in determining if the organism causing the infection is methicillin-resistant *Staphylococcus aureus* (MRSA). If the affected lymph node is fluctuant, aspiration of fluid for culture is indicated and incision and drainage should be considered. The child should be treated as an outpatient with an oral antibiotic directed against MRSA and group A beta-hemolytic streptococcus, such as clindamycin or a combination of cephalexin and trimethoprim-sulfamethoxazole, as well as an analgesic for pain as needed. If methicillin-susceptible *S aureus* is cultured and sensitivities are determined, cephalexin, amoxicillin-clavulinic acid, or dicloxacillin may be administered. If the child appears toxic, or if there is marked lymph node enlargement, the child should be admitted for intravenous antibiotics. A purified protein derivative skin test should be placed. The child should be followed up in 1 to 3 days for clinical improvement depending on the severity of the infection.

Selected References

Acierno SP, Waldhausen JHT. Congenital cervical cysts, sinuses and fistulae. *Otolaryngol Clin North Am.* 2007;40:161–176

Agarwal RP, Handler SD, Matthews MR, et al. Pilomatrixoma of the head and neck in children. *Otolaryngol Head Neck Surg.* 2001;125:510–515

Bauer PW, Lusk RP. Neck masses. In: Bluestone CD, Stool SE, Alper CM, et al, eds. *Pediatric Otolaryngology.* 4th ed. Philadelphia, PA: Saunders; 2003:1629–1647

Bentz BG, Hughes CA, Ludemann JP, et al. Masses of the salivary gland region in children. *Arch Otolaryngol Head Neck Surg.* 2000;126:1435–1439

Bergman KS, Harris BH. Scalp and neck masses. *Pediatr Clin North Am.* 1993;40:1151–1161

Brown RL, Azizkhan RG. Pediatric head and neck lesions. *Pediatr Clin North Am.* 1998;45:889–905

Chao SS, Loh KS, Tan KK, Chong SM. Tuberculous and nontuberculous cervical lymphadenitis: a clinical review. *Otolaryngol Head Neck Surg.* 2002;126:176–179

Healy CM, Baker CJ. Cervical lymphadenitis. In: Feigin RD, Cherry JD, eds. *Textbook of Pediatric Infectious Diseases.* 5th ed. Philadelphia, PA: Saunders; 2004:185–197

Jha BC, Dass A, Nagarkar NM, Gupta R, Singhal S. Cervical tuberculous lymphadenopathy: changing clinical pattern and concepts in management. *Postgrad Med J.* 2001;77:185–187

Karmody CS. Developmental anomalies of the neck. In: Bluestone CD, Stool SE, Alper CM, et al, eds. *Pediatric Otolaryngology.* 4th ed. Philadelphia, PA: Saunders; 2003:1648–1663

Knight PJ, Mulne AF, Vassy LE. When is lymph node biopsy indicated in children with enlarged peripheral nodes? *Pediatrics.* 1982;69:391–396

Lin HC, Su CY, Huang SC. Kikuchi's disease in Asian children. *Pediatrics.* 2005;115:92–96

Malley R. Lymphadenopathy. In: Fleisher GR, Ludwig S, eds. *Textbook of Pediatric Emergency Medicine.* 5th ed. Philadelphia, PA: Lippincott; 2006:421–428

McAnney CM, Ruddy RM. Neck mass. In: Fleisher GR, Ludwig S, eds. *Textbook of Pediatric Emergency Medicine.* 5th ed. Philadelphia, PA: Lippincott; 2006:429–435

Moran GJ, Krishnadasan A, Gorwitz RJ, et al. Methicillin-resistant *S. aureus* infections among patients in the emergency department. *N Engl J Med.* 2006;355:666–674

Peters TR, Edwards KM. Cervical lymphadenopathy and adenitis. *Pediatr Rev.* 2000;21:399–405

Rosenfeld RM. Cervical adenopathy. In: Bluestone CD, Stool SE, Alper CM, et al, eds. *Pediatric Otolaryngology.* 4th ed. Philadelphia, PA: Saunders; 2003:1665–1680

Turkington JRA, Paterson A, Sweeney LE, et al. Neck masses in children. *Br J Radiol.* 2005;78:75–85

Allergic Disease

Nasser Redjal, MD

CASE STUDY

A 3-year-old girl is rushed to the office by her mother after her daughter developed a pruritic rash, facial swelling, and hoarseness shortly after eating a peanut butter sandwich. Previously she has been well except for recurrent nasal congestion every spring that has responded to antihistamines. She has also had an intermittent skin rash that has been treated with topical steroid creams. She has never had an acute reaction before and has no history of asthma. Her father had asthma as a child.

Physical examination reveals a well-developed, 3-year-old girl with marked facial swelling and a **generalized rash** who is in mild respiratory distress. Vital signs, including blood pressure, are normal. Growth parameters are at the 50th percentile. The girl has a diffuse, blotchy, erythematous rash with central wheals; a hoarse voice; and a mild expiratory wheeze on auscultation of her chest. The remainder of the examination is normal.

Questions

1. What are the various symptoms of allergic disease?
2. What is the appropriate evaluation of children with manifestations of allergic disease?
3. What allergens are common triggers for allergic symptoms?
4. What management is helpful in the treatment of children with manifestations of allergic disease?
5. Can allergic disease be prevented?

Allergic disease, which occurs frequently in the general population, is manifested in many ways. Asthma; atopic dermatitis; allergic rhinitis; allergic conjunctivitis; urticaria; angioedema; anaphylaxis; and food, insect, and drug allergies are all types of allergic diseases. Allergic symptoms result from the production of specific immunoglobulin E (IgE) antibody following exposure to a foreign antigen. The process has 2 steps. The first step is the sensitization or antibody induction stage. The individual develops IgE antibody against an inhaled, ingested, or injected substance. This newly formed IgE antibody adheres to circulating blood basophils or to tissue mast cells. The second step involves reexposure of a sensitized person to the allergen, which then binds to several specific IgE antibodies on the surface of immune cells. The release of inflammatory mediators causes the appearance of the characteristic features of allergic disease, which can range from rhinorrhea to sudden death. Similar non–IgE-mediated symptoms may occur, but these are not true allergic reactions. The reader should refer to Chapter 69 for details concerning asthma and Chapter 109 for a review of atopic dermatitis. This chapter focuses on the remaining manifestations of allergies, including food allergies.

Epidemiology

Allergic disease or some form of allergic symptoms is found in 12% to 20% of the general population. The prevalence of symptoms varies depending on the population being investigated. Factors such as age, genetic background, and place of residence are significant. Allergic rhinitis occurs in 10% of children, as does asthma. Up to 6% of children younger than 3 years develop food allergies. Urticaria occurs at some time in about 10% to 20% of the population.

It is generally accepted that if neither parent is atopic (has the allergic tendency to manufacture IgE on antigen exposure), then the chance that children will develop allergic symptoms is less than 1 in 5. If one parent is atopic, the risk doubles. If both parents are atopic, the chance is greater than 3 in 5.

Clinical Presentation

Children with allergic disease frequently present with persistent, clear rhinorrhea; sneezing; postnasal drip; or injected pruritic conjunctiva. Skin manifestations include dry, scaling, erythematous rashes; wheals; or subcutaneous swelling (Dx Box). A recurrent cough or wheezing on chest examination is further evidence of allergic disease.

Pathophysiology

Allergic rhinitis, like all allergic manifestations, is caused primarily by an antigen-antibody reaction involving IgE. Antigen-specific IgE is produced by the B lymphocytes of allergic patients on exposure to a particular antigen, which attaches to immune cell receptors located on basophils in the circulation and mast cells in the tissue. On reexposure, the antigen reacts with this specific IgE on the mast cells, releasing vasoactive mediators including histamine, leukotrienes, kinins, and prostaglandins. These mediators produce vasodilation and edema, and they also stimulate neural reflexes to produce mucous hypersecretion and sneezing. Eosinophils, and

Dx **Allergic Disease**

- Chronic, clear rhinorrhea
- Nasal congestion
- Conjunctival tearing and pruritus
- Skin findings of atopic dermatitis or urticaria
- Seasonal variability
- Occurrence of symptoms after exposure to an antigen
- Family history of allergic disease
- Conjunctival injection
- Wheezing
- Chronic cough
- Postnasal drip
- Repetitive sneezing
- Acute onset of symptoms following exposure to possible allergen

other inflammatory cells induced by chemotactic factors, enter the affected organ, releasing mediators, thereby worsening the inflammation and damaging tissues. Secretions and released tissue proteins worsen existing edema. Other immunologic mechanisms can also be involved.

Urticaria, the clinical rash produced by vasodilation and edema of the skin, is the allergic condition that occurs when histamine and other mediators such as prostaglandins and leukotrienes are released from the dermal mast cells. The antigen-specific IgE is located on these mast cells. Otherwise, the pathophysiology is similar to that of allergic rhinitis. Exposure to that antigen causes release of chemical mediators from the mast cells. Other mechanisms, including physical stimuli, can produce urticaria.

Angioedema is the extension of the urticarial process deeper into the dermis of the skin, producing circumscribed swelling. The mucous membranes may be affected. The pathophysiology is the same as for urticaria. A hereditary type of angioedema, which is not allergy related, is caused by the inherited deficiency of the C1 esterase inhibitor.

Anaphylaxis is an acute, systemic allergic reaction resulting from antigen-specific IgE on mast cells and basophils. The pathophysiology is similar to allergic rhinitis, but the reaction occurs in mast cells in many locations simultaneously, and prior sensitization to an allergen is essential. Anaphylactic reactions may be life-threatening. Vasodilation may be so severe that decreased venous return can lead to acute myocardial infarctions and arrhythmias. Reactions can occur in seconds or as late as 1 hour after exposure. Common antigens that precipitate anaphylactic reactions include injections of foreign serum, drugs, foods, and insect venom. Anaphylactoid reactions are clinically indistinguishable from anaphylaxis but are non—IgE-mediated, and include reactions to substances such as intravenous (IV) contrast media, opiates, and deferoxamine. The drug most frequently implicated in anaphylaxis is penicillin. Patients initially experience tightness and intense itching of the skin. Nausea, vomiting, and abdominal pain may ensue. Subsequently, the full spectrum of anaphylaxis appears.

A **food allergy** may produce any of the previously described allergic manifestations, including atopic dermatitis and asthma, as well as vomiting, diarrhea, and failure to thrive. Food intolerance, which has a non-immunologic pathogenesis, should be differentiated from food allergy, which is an IgE-mediated allergic reaction. The localization of the IgE-sensitized mast cells to that specific antigen determines the symptoms produced by the allergy. The antigen enters through the gastrointestinal (GI) mucosal barrier. Intact food proteins may enter the circulation, stimulating the production of antigen-specific IgE.

Major food allergens are usually glycoproteins (Box 68-1), but any food can be sensitizing. Sensitized GI mast cells release mediators, causing vomiting and diarrhea. As a result of the edema and vasodilation of the intestinal wall, the mucosa becomes more permeable to enteric antigens, resulting in more hypersensitivity and inflammation.

Box 68-1. Highly Allergenic Foods		
Egg white	Fish and shellfish	Soy
Cow's milk	Wheat	Corn
Nuts		

Differential Diagnosis

In evaluating children with possible allergic disease, other etiologies for the symptoms should be considered and explored. Allergic rhinitis is most often confused with an upper respiratory infection but may also resemble vasomotor rhinitis, nonallergic rhinitis with eosinophilia syndrome, cerebrospinal fluid rhinorrhea (usually associated with a basilar skull fracture), sinusitis, or a nasal foreign body. Unlike allergic rhinitis, infectious etiologies of rhinitis result in inflammatory nasal mucosa and possible fever. Foreign bodies elicit a unilateral, purulent, often foul-smelling discharge. Vasomotor rhinitis is usually transient.

Urticaria can resemble insect bites, erythema multiforme, papular urticaria, mastocytosis, or contact dermatitis. Distinct features of urticaria include pruritus and a transient nature, without any epidermal break. It may result from an allergic reaction or may occur secondary to an infectious etiology. Parasitic, bacterial, fungal, and viral infections can all cause urticaria. Physical stimuli (eg, sun, cold), exercise, or anxiety can also produce the reaction. In addition, a deficiency in factor I in the complement system may cause a genetic form of urticaria.

Anaphylaxis is usually associated with edema, wheezing, and occasionally fever, although it can present like other forms of shock. A history of an acute exposure is more likely to be seen with anaphylaxis.

Food allergies may resemble food intolerances, which are non-allergenic, with regard to clinical presentation. Food intolerances include toxic contamination, metabolic disorders (eg, lactose intolerance), and reactions to pharmacologic properties of the ingested food. Associated allergic findings (eg, asthma, atopic dermatitis) may be seen with true allergies. Specific testing of the food, stool, or patient may be necessary to differentiate allergic reactions from food intolerance.

Evaluation: History and Physical Examination

Allergic Rhinitis and Conjunctivitis

Practitioners should determine if children with possible allergic rhinitis have a history of symptoms of sneezing, itching, and nasal discharge. The eyes, ears, palate, and throat may itch. Children may also have a history of mouth breathing and snoring at night from nasal obstruction, or signs of complications such as sinusitis, postnasal drip, halitosis, cough, and morning sore throat. Symptoms may be seasonal or associated with a specific stimulus. In addition, systemic symptoms of fatigue, headache, anorexia, and irritability may be present.

The history should also include a search for other manifestations of allergies (eg, wheezing, atopic dermatitis) as well as a family history of atopy. An environmental history of allergen exposure, including pets, is also important to obtain.

The physical examination should be thorough. The skin should be inspected for atopic dermatitis and the lungs for evidence of asthma. The nasal mucosa should be examined with an otoscope. In children with allergic rhinitis, the nasal mucosa is swollen, pale, and sometimes cyanotic with copious clear discharge. Nasal polyps, if present, should be noted. Although polyps are most often present on an allergic basis, they may occur with cystic fibrosis. A transverse crease across the nose ("allergic salute") can occur from repeatedly using the palm of the hand in an upward thrust on the nares to relieve itching and open the nasal airway. Dark circles under the eyes ("allergic shiners") may be present from venous stasis. Dennie sign (also called Morgan line), a wrinkle just beneath the lower eyelids,

is present from early infancy and is associated with atopic dermatitis and allergic rhinitis. Allergic gape or adenoid facies is secondary to chronic mouth breathing during the first several years of life and results in a characteristic pattern of maldevelopment of facial bones, causing a high-arched palate, flat maxilla, and angulated mandible with a recessed chin and dental malocclusion. If affected, the conjunctivae are erythematous with a clear discharge and may have a follicular appearance. The mouth may reveal a high-arched palate from chronic mouth breathing, and hypertrophic lymphoid follicles in the oropharynx often can be seen (Figure 68-1).

Complications of chronic allergic rhinitis may be evident on examination. If children have one of these conditions, such as chronic serous otitis, recurrent otitis media, hearing loss secondary to otitis, sinusitis, **nasal polyps,** sleep apnea, or dental malocclusion, the possibility of allergic disease as a cause should be explored.

Urticaria and Angioedema

When children present with an acute rash, questions should focus on recent exposures to drugs, dietary changes, new soaps or detergents, and environmental agents. An urticarial rash is acute in onset, extremely pruritic, and typically evanescent. Evidence of infection and a history of chronic disease or any other allergic disease should be explored. The rash should be evaluated carefully. An urticarial rash appears as erythematous lesions of various sizes with pale, papular centers. Lesions may coalesce, the rash blanches on pressure, and the skin is intact.

The physical examination should also assess whether other contributing problems, such as infection, are present.

Anaphylaxis

An acute exposure to a foreign antigen (eg, medication, food, venom) should be elicited in the history of any patient who presents with anaphylaxis.

Figure 68-1. Characteristic facial features in children with allergic diseases. A. Allergic shiner. B. Nasal crease. C. Adenoid facies.

On physical examination, vital signs indicate hypotension and tachycardia. The skin is erythematous with diffuse edema. Airway edema may produce hoarseness with stridor and wheezing noted on auscultation of the chest. Patients may have severe difficulty breathing. Cardiac examination may reveal arrhythmias.

Food Allergies

An accurate diet diary is essential in diagnosing a food allergy. The timing of symptoms associated with a specific food must be obtained. Personal as well as family history of atopy is important. An elimination diet followed by a challenge helps the diagnostic evaluation. The double-blind, placebo-controlled food challenge is the most accurate assessment for diagnosis.

Evaluation

Laboratory Tests

With allergic rhinitis, as with any allergic disease, the diagnosis can usually be made with a thorough history and physical examination. Frequently, therapy can be initiated with no laboratory data.

Screening tests may include a nasal smear for eosinophils. A result of greater than 10% eosinophils is considered confirmatory data for allergic rhinitis. Although serum IgE levels are elevated in 60% of patients with allergic rhinitis and asthma, they are not sensitive or specific and have limited value. A multi-allergen screening test, which gives reliable results when checking for the presence of allergic disease, is currently available.

Skin testing for specific antigens should be performed if desensitization shots or environmental changes are being considered in the management plan. Skin tests are sensitive and accurate. Positive tests indicate the presence of an antigen-specific IgE. Prick tests are used initially. They may be followed by intradermal tests for allergens that are negative on prick testing. Although skin testing may be less reliable in infants because their skin is less reactive, the tests have been performed in children as young as 4 months.

Radioallergosorbent testing (RAST) of sera, which is also available for the laboratory assessment of allergies, provides a semiquantitative measure of the amount of IgE specific for individual allergens. RAST is much more expensive than skin testing and has no advantage unless skin testing cannot be performed, such as in patients with a history of anaphylaxis, poor skin reactivity, current antihistamine use, or dermatographia.

Objective testing with skin tests by the prick method may be helpful in diagnosing food allergies. Negative tests are accurate for excluding food allergies, but positive tests may occur in patients without symptoms related to a particular food. Intradermal skin tests are not indicated. They do not give additional information, and they increase the risk of a serious reaction. RAST of sera may be used for specific foods.

Management

The first line of therapy for all allergic diseases is **avoidance of any precipitants.** For allergic rhinitis, this begins with environmental control, because the most frequent precipitants are inhalant allergens. Reducing exposure to the dust mite, a common allergen, can help control allergic rhinitis. Environmental humidity, which increases the dust mite population, should be decreased. Specifically, parents should be instructed to remove carpets, drapes, and upholstered furniture, which can harbor dust mites, from the house. They should cover mattresses with plastic covers and remove furry pets. Decreasing humidity also helps reduce mold counts, another important allergen, and air-conditioning units can lower pollen and mold counts as well. Nonspecific irritants such as smoke should be avoided because they can also precipitate any allergic symptom.

Anaphylaxis is considered a **medical emergency.** The first step in management is to establish an airway. Oxygen therapy should be instituted, and IV access established. Epinephrine is the drug of choice because of its potent vasoconstrictive and myocardial stimulating effects. The dose is 0.01 mL/kg of 1:1,000 aqueous solution, up to 0.5 mL, given subcutaneously. If the blood pressure is decreased, epinephrine may be given intravenously, with normal saline fluid boluses to expand intravascular volume. Intravenous administration of an antihistamine, such as diphenhydramine (5 mg/kg/24 hours) is used as well as a steroid, such as methylprednisolone (2 mg/kg).

The management of urticaria should begin with the **identification of the causal agent** and its elimination. Children who have experienced anaphylaxis should be instructed to avoid future exposure to the precipitating allergen. In addition, they should be instructed to wear a medical alert tag that notifies others of the potential for a severe allergic reaction and carry an epinephrine kit for immediate treatment.

A maintenance diet that does not contain the allergen is the basis for management of food allergies. It is essential that the prescribed diet be nutritionally sound. Families should be instructed by a nutritionist and taught to read food labels appropriately to avoid all exposure to the antigen. They should also be advised about what foods children can consume.

Medications should be used in allergic disease when additional management is indicated by persistent symptoms. H_1 receptor antagonists or **antihistamines** are frequently indicated in the treatment of allergic rhinitis. Diphenhydramine, chlorpheniramine, and brompheniramine have all been useful in relieving symptoms but may be very sedating. The newer antagonists, desloratadine, fexofenadine, cetirizine, and loratadine, do not readily cross the blood-brain barrier and are less sedating. Oral decongestants have been effective in decreasing nasal congestion. Pseudoephedrine has been used in children. Topical nasal decongestants, which can cause dependence and rebound swelling, should not be used on a long-term basis.

Antihistamines are also used in the symptomatic treatment of urticaria and angioedema. These agents can relieve the rash as well as the itching of the rash. Diphenhydramine (5–7 mg/kg/d in 4 doses) and hydroxyzine (2–4 mg/kg/d in 4 doses) are both used. If the urticaria is extensive or severe, epinephrine or Sus-Phrine (epinephrine in oil) may be used subcutaneously. This often provides immediate relief of symptoms and is diagnostic as well as therapeutic.

Cromolyn sodium nasal spray is the next line of treatment for allergic rhinitis in children older than 6 years. A very effective mast cell stabilizer, it suppresses mediator release. Cromolyn spray should be used prophylactically on a regular basis 2 to 4 times per day, one spray per nostril, to prevent symptoms.

Steroids have an anti-inflammatory effect and work well topically for allergic rhinitis. Mometasone, triamcinolone, and flunisolide are available as nasal sprays, and all 3 agents may cause stinging and nasal irritation. Systemic steroids may also be used for treatment of urticaria, angioedema, and anaphylaxis.

Immunotherapy should be considered for children with allergic rhinitis when avoidance techniques and medications are not controlling symptoms or when there is a history of anaphylaxis, depending on the allergen. This treatment has been effective in relieving symptoms due to dust mites, pollens, animal dander, molds, insect stings, and drug reactions. Immunotherapy involves a series of injections with extracts of allergens specific for individual patients, producing tolerance to particular antigens. The mechanism of action of immunotherapy is related to the development of allergen-specific blocking antibody (IgG), increased allergen-specific suppressor T cells, decreased lymphocyte cytokine response to an allergen, and decreased basophil histamine release in response to an allergen. The results of skin testing dictate which allergens to use. Initially, injections are given weekly. Then they are tapered and given on a maintenance schedule. Although immunotherapy can be performed at any age, the injections are painful and expensive. They necessitate frequent visits. Patients risk an allergic reaction with each injection.

Prevention

The cost of medical care, lost school days and workdays, disability from complications, and actual lives lost from allergic disease take a great toll on the population. Evidence currently suggests that sensitization to foods is more likely to occur in the first 6 to 12 months of life. Avoidance of these allergens at this age may decrease the subsequent development of allergic disease. For children at high risk for the development of allergic disease, which is usually determined by family history, the following steps are recommended:

- Keep the home free of dust.
- Keep humidity below 50% in the home.
- Prevent smoking in the environment.
- Limit infectious exposures.

To reduce the incidence of food allergies, it is recommended that mothers breastfeed infants exclusively for at least the first 6 months of life. When infants are 6 months old, foods can gradually be introduced. Cow's milk, wheat, corn, and citrus should be avoided until after the age of 1 year. Peanuts, eggs, fish, and shellfish should be delayed until 24 months. Postponing the introduction of food allergens may reduce the rate of sensitization in high-risk infants, but this is a controversial issue. Recent studies demonstrate that such postponement may only delay the sensitization.

Prognosis

The prognosis for children with allergic disease is good when the diagnosis is made correctly. Some patients lose their allergy naturally or following immunotherapy. For others, allergic rhinitis, urticaria, and anaphylactic reactions persist throughout life on exposure to antigens. However, with appropriate management with medication and avoidance of allergens, children with allergic disease can thrive and live a normal life without restrictions on activity. Immunotherapy can be effective in alleviating the allergic response to inhalants in allergic rhinitis and to insect venoms. The chance for resolution of food allergies is very good. Many foods that initially elicit an allergenic reaction can be tolerated after the age of 3 to 4 years; 85% of children with cow's milk, egg, wheat, or soy allergy will experience remission by 5 years, presumably as a result of maturation of the GI mucosa. However, only 20% of young children outgrow peanut allergy.

CASE RESOLUTION

In the case presented at the beginning of the chapter, the girl's symptoms of rash, swelling, and wheezing after exposure to an antigen suggest a systemic allergic reaction with angioedema and asthma. Treatment with epinephrine and antihistamines is clearly indicated. Because of the presence of pulmonary symptoms, admission for observation is warranted. The child and family should be counseled to avoid any foods that contain peanuts in the future. The parents should read all food labels, and carry an epinephrine autoinjector (Epi-pen) at all times for emergency use. The patient should wear a medical alert bracelet indicating peanut allergy.

The patient should be referred to an allergist for further evaluation.

Selected References

American College of Allergy, Asthma and Immunology; Joint Council of Allergy, Asthma and Immunology. Joint task force on practice parameters: the diagnosis and management of anaphylaxis. *J Allergy Clin Immunol.* 1998;101:S465–S528

Barnes ML, Menzies D, Fardon TC, et al. Combined mediator blockade or topical steroid for treating the unified allergic airway. *Allergy.* 2007;62:73–80

Berkowitz RB, McCafferty F, Lutz C, et al. Onset of action of fexofenadine hydrochloride 60 mg/pseudoephedrine hydrochloride 120 mg in subjects aged 12 years with moderate to severe seasonal allergic rhinitis: a pooled analysis of two single-dose, randomized, double-blind, placebo-controlled allergen exposure unit studies. *Clin Ther.* 2006;28:1658–1669

Berger W, Hampel F Jr, Bernstein J, Shah S, Sacks H, Meltzer EO. Impact of azelastine nasal spray on symptoms and quality of life compared with cetirizine oral tablets in patients with seasonal allergic rhinitis. *Ann Allergy Asthma Immunol.* 2006;97:375–381

Bodtger U, Linneberg A. Remission of allergic rhinitis: an 8-year observational study. *J Allergy Clin Immunol.* 2004;114:1384–1388

Burks AW, Sampson H. Food allergies in children. *Curr Probl Pediatr.* 1993;23:230–252

Cutler DL, Banfield C, Affrime MB. Safety of mometasone furoate nasal spray in children with allergic rhinitis as young as 2 years of age: a randomized controlled trial. *Pediatr Asthma Allergy Immunol.* 2006;19:146

Drugs for asthma. *Med Lett Drugs Ther.* 1999;41:5–10

Ellis AK, Day JH. Incidence and characteristics of biphasic anaphylaxis: a prospective evaluation of 103 patients. *Ann Allergy Asthma Immunol.* 2007;98:64–69

Ferguson A. Definitions and diagnosis of food intolerance and food allergy: consensus and controversy. *J Pediatr.* 1992;121:S1–S11

Fireman P. Diagnosis of allergic disorders. *Pediatr Rev.* 1995;16:178–183

Kemp SF, Deshazo RD, Moffitt JE, et al. Expanding habitat of the imported fire ant: a public health concern. *J Allergy Clin Immunol.* 2005;105:683–691

Kim KT, Rabinovitch N, Uryniak T, et al. Effect of budesonide aqueous nasal spray on hypothalamic-pituitary-adrenal axis function in children with allergic rhinitis. *Ann Allergy Asthma Immunol.* 2004;93:61–67

Murphy SJ, Kelly HW. Advances in the management of acute asthma in children. *Pediatr Rev.* 1996;17:227–234

Nash DR. Allergic rhinitis. *Pediatr Ann.* 1998;27:799–808

Norman PS. Immunotherapy: 1999–2004. *J Allergy Clin Immunol.* 2004;113:1013–1023

Patel P, Philip G, Yang W, et al. Randomized, double-blind, placebo-controlled study of montelukast for treating perennial allergic rhinitis. *Ann Allergy Asthma Immunol.* 2005;95:551–557

Pitsios, C, Papadopoulos, D, Kompoti, E, et al. Efficacy and safety of mometasone furoate vs nedocromil sodium as prophylactic treatment for moderate/severe seasonal allergic rhinitis. *Ann Allergy Asthma Immunol.* 2006;96:673–678

Platts-Mills TA. Allergen avoidance. *J Allergy Clin Immunol.* 2004;113:388–391

Rooklin AR, Gaqchik SM. Allergic rhinitis—it's that time again. *Contemp Pediatr.* 1994;11:19–41

Rosen FS. Urticaria, angioedema, and anaphylaxis. *Pediatr Rev.* 1992;13:387–390

Solomon WR. Prevention of allergic disorders. *Pediatr Rev.* 1994;15:301–309

Virant FS. Allergic rhinitis. *Pediatr Rev.* 1992;13:323–333

Wander AA, Bernstein IL, Goodman DL, et al. The diagnosis and management of urticaria: a practice parameter. *Ann Allergy Immunol.* 2005;85:525–544

Weston WL, Badgett JT. Urticaria. *Pediatr Rev.* 1988;19:240–244

Wood RA. Diagnosing allergies: when to test, when to refer. *Contemp Pediatr.* 1994;11:13–28

Zacharisen MC. Pediatrics urticaria and angioedema. *Immunol Allergy Clin North Am.* 1999;19:363–382

Wheezing and Asthma

Nasser Redjal, MD

CASE STUDY

A 7-year-old boy is referred to the office after being seen in the emergency department (ED) for wheezing. He has been treated in the ED for wheezing 4 times in the past month and was once hospitalized for 3 days. The boy's father and paternal grandmother both have asthma.

The child's physical examination is remarkable for end-expiratory wheezing on forced expiration.

Questions

1. What are the most common causes of wheezing in infants and children?
2. What are the causes of reversible bronchospasm?
3. What is the pathophysiology of reversible bronchospasm?
4. How should children with asthma be managed?

Recurrent wheezing is a frequent symptom of obstructive airway disease in children that may be caused by intrinsic or extrinsic compression of the airway, bronchospasm, inflammation, or defective clearance of secretions. Ten percent to 15% of infants wheeze during their first year of life, and as many as 25% of children younger than 5 years present to their clinicians with wheezing during a respiratory illness. Most infants and young children with recurrent wheezing have asthma; however, a wide variety of congenital and acquired conditions can cause narrowing of the extrathoracic or intrathoracic airways, and may present with wheezing. Reactive airway disease (asthma) is the most common cause of wheezing in childhood. Asthma is a chronic illness and requires longitudinal care by a primary care provider to ensure optimal treatment and reduction in costly emergency department (ED) visits and hospital admissions.

Wheezes can originate from airways of any size, from the large extrathoracic upper airway to the intrathoracic small airways. In addition to narrowing or compression of the airway, wheezing requires sufficient airflow to generate airway oscillation and produce sound. Thus the absence of wheezing in a patient who presents with acute asthma may be an ominous finding, suggesting impending respiratory failure. The audible "musical or squeaking sounds" noted with obstruction are caused by the turbulence of the air as it is forced through a narrowed airway. Infants and young children are more prone to wheezing when they have airway obstruction because air forced through smaller airways is more turbulent than air forced through the larger airways of older children and adults. Infection-induced wheezing in children younger than 2 years is associated with respiratory syncytial virus (RSV), especially in infants with passive exposure to smoke and with rhinovirus in children older than 2 years. The most common causes of wheezing in infants and children are asthma, bronchiolitis, and pneumonia. Less common causes include congenital structural anomalies, gastroesophageal reflux and aspiration, cardiac failure, cystic fibrosis, and foreign bodies (Box 69-1).

Infants with RSV infection may present with apnea, inspiratory and expiratory wheezing, fever, and respiratory distress. Treatment is symptomatic and includes hospitalization for apnea and severe respiratory distress. Infants with recurrent bronchiolitis may have underlying reactive airway disease.

Asthma is a common chronic disorder of the airways characterized by variable and recurring symptoms, airflow obstruction, bronchial hyperresponsiveness, and underlying inflammation. Bronchospasm is reversible either spontaneously or with treatment. Development of chronic inflammation in some patients can cause permanent alterations in the airway structure, referred to as *airway remodeling,* that is not prevented by or fully responsive to currently available treatment. Clinically asthma is characterized by recurrent episodes of cough, chest tightness, dyspnea, prolonged expiration, wheezing, hyperinflation of the chest (air trappings), use of accessory chest muscles (retractions) and, in severe cases, cyanosis.

Epidemiology

Asthma is the most common chronic childhood illness. The disease affects 5% to 15% of all children in the United States, an estimated 6.5 million, and is a leading cause of ED visits, hospital admission, and school absenteeism. Over the last several decades, the prevalence of asthma has increased worldwide, an increase that varies from 40% in some areas of the United Kingdom and Australia to 3% in Indonesia, China, and India. Asthma prevalence, mortality, and hospitalization rates are higher in blacks than in whites. One-third of patients initially experience symptoms in the first year of life, and 80% are diagnosed by the time they reach school age. In the United States, asthma is the most frequent admitting diagnosis to children's hospitals. Hospitalization rates have remained relatively stable, with lower rates in some age groups but higher rates in children 0 to 4 years of age. In addition, asthma is a major cause of school absence; 23% of school days missed can be attributed to asthma. The male-

Box 69-1. Causes of Wheezing

Infection
- Bronchiolitis
- Pneumonia
- Bronchitis
- Laryngotracheobronchitis
- Bacterial tracheitis
- Toxocariasis
- Ascariasis

Reactive Airway Disease
- Asthma
- Exercise-induced asthma
- Anaphylaxis
- Nighttime cough asthma
- Toxic exposure (smoke, organophosphate poisoning)
- Allergic aspergillosis

Laryngeal Dysfunction

Congenital Structural Anomalies
- Vascular rings
- Bronchiectasis
- Lung cysts
- Laryngotracheoesophageal cleft
- Tracheobronchomalacia

Defective Secretion Clearance
- Cystic fibrosis
- Immotile cilia syndrome

Tumor
- Mediastinal tumors (lymphoma, teratoma, neuroblastoma, thymoma)

Chronic Aspiration
- Gastroesophageal reflux
- Bulbar palsy
- Tracheoesophageal fistula

Other Causes
- Bronchopulmonary dysplasia
- α_1-Antitrypsin deficiency
- Pulmonary hemosiderosis
- Sarcoidosis

Foreign Body

Cardiac Disease

Immunodeficiency

female ratio is 2:1 until age 10 and is equal from ages 10 to 14; after puberty, asthma incidence is greater in girls and women.

In recent years more serious disease in younger children and adolescents has increased. Low socioeconomic status is associated with an increase in asthma prevalence and morbidity and mortality. Inner-city African Americans are most at risk.

Clinical Presentation

Children with asthma may present with acute symptoms of cough, shortness of breath, prolonged expiration, use of accessory muscles of respiration, wheezing, complaints of chest tightness or congestion, hyperinflation of the chest, cyanosis, exercise intolerance, tachycardia, and abdominal pain.

Wheezing may be audible and detected by the parent or may not be appreciated until the child is examined by a physician. There may be no wheezing in children with severe bronchoconstriction because the flow of air is impeded, but wheezing may appear after broncho-dilator treatment, owing to partial opening of the airway.

Some children have cough, which may be nocturnal or recurrent as a predominant symptom. Some pediatric patients have symptoms such as cough or wheezing that are precipitated or exacerbated by exercise (Dx Box).

Dx **Asthma**

- Recurrent wheezing
- Shortness of breath
- Exercise intolerance
- History of allergies
- History of atopic dermatitis
- Nasal polyps
- History of nighttime cough

Abdominal pain and vomiting also are common in younger children and may be followed by temporary relief of symptoms. During an acute asthma attack, a low-grade fever, profuse sweating, and fatigue from the hard work of breathing may be apparent.

Pathophysiology

Asthma is a chronic inflammatory disorder of the airways. The immunohistopathologic features of asthma include denudation of the airway epithelium, collagen deposition beneath the basement membrane, smooth muscle hypertrophy, edema, mast cell activation, and inflammatory cell infiltration (neutrophils, lymphocytes, eosinophils), which release mediators such as histamine, prostaglandin, major basic protein, etc. These changes lead to airway hyperresponsiveness, airflow limitation, respiratory symptoms, and disease chronicity. The limitation to the flow of air includes acute bronchoconstriction, airway edema, mucus plug formation, and airway wall remodeling. The unique anatomy and physiology of the lung in infants compared with adults predispose infants to obstructive airway disease. These anatomical differences include reduced number and size of the pores of Cohn and Lambert canals, causing deficient collateral ventilation and a predisposition to atelectasis distal to obstructed airway. Mucous gland hyperplasia favors increased intraluminal mucus production. Decreased smooth muscle in the peripheral airway results in less support and narrower airways. Decreased number of fatigue-resistant skeletal muscle fibers in the diaphragm, its horizontal insertion to the rib cage (versus oblique in adult), and a highly compliant rib cage increase the work of breathing in children. Decreased static elastic recoil predisposes to early airway closure during tidal breathing, resulting in mismatching of ventilation and perfusion and resultant hypoxemia.

Atopy, the genetic predisposition to the development of immunoglobulin (Ig) E–mediated response to common aeroallergens, is the strongest predisposing factor for developing asthma. There are at least 50 genes that influence susceptibility to asthma and its clinical expression. Sites located on chromosomes 6p and 12q, 5q, 11q, and 16p are known to be associated with allergic diseases and encoding for major histocompatibility complex, IgE, interferon, and cytokine.

Environmental changes such as wind; temperature fluctuations; and increased exposure to allergens or air pollutants, such as tobacco smoke, ozone, sulfur dioxide, and nitrogen dioxide, and particulate matter, such as diesel exhaust and biological residues (eg, endotoxin), may precipitate clinical attacks. Inhalant allergens, particularly indoors, play an important role. The most important allergens are house dust mite feces (Der p1 and Der p2), cat dander (Feld l), and cockroach saliva (Bla g2, Bla g4, and Bla g5). House dust mite antigen (Der p1) stimulates the response causing an increase in IgE synthesis by impairing T-cell proliferation and interferon-γ secretion. Other inhalant allergens, such as dog dander, and outdoor fungus (ie, *Alternaria),* and some pollens, also play a role in asthma. Infection, particularly respiratory infections, can play a variety of roles in asthma, influencing not only its exacerbation, but also its inception and persistence. Viral infections, such as RSV, influenza, and rhinovirus, are the most frequent precipitants of asthma exacerbations in infancy. *Mycoplasma* and *Chlamydia* infections can cause wheezing and persistence of asthma. Emotional stress may also play a role in the exacerbation of asthma.

The physiological changes involved in asthma occur in 2 phases. An immediate response to the offending agent causes edema and bronchial smooth muscle constriction that lead to narrowing of the airway and plugging with secretions. Air is trapped behind the narrowed airways, resulting in altered gas exchange, increased respiratory rate, decreased tidal volume, and increased work of breathing. The late response, which occurs 4 to 8 hours after the initial symptoms, primarily involves infiltration of the airways with inflammatory cells. The end pathway in the disease process is obstruction to airflow. The pathophysiology of asthma is reviewed in Figure 69-1.

Differential Diagnosis

An extensive differential diagnosis is listed in Box 69-1. Most conditions are differentiated from asthma by the presence of associated symptoms or the child's response to bronchodilators.

The National Heart, Lung, and Blood Institute (NHLBI) expert panel classifies asthma, based on severity, as determined by careful assessment of symptom frequency during the day and at night and pulmonary function testing, into 4 steps (Table 69-1): (1) mild

intermittent, (2) mild persistent, (3) moderate persistent, and (4) severe persistent. The mildest form of the disease is not associated with school absence, sleep disturbance, or loss of pulmonary function. The moderate and severe cases are associated with daily symptoms, limited physical activity, school absence, and sleep disturbances. Pulmonary function is always affected.

Evaluation

An acute asthmatic attack is always considered a medical emergency because it has the potential to deteriorate into respiratory failure. Initially only a brief history should be obtained. If children have recurrent asthma, critical interventions should be started during the evaluation. The initial assessment should include an estimation of the severity of the attack. This can be accomplished by a rapid assessment of the ventilation, oxygenation, and perfusion of the patient.

Signs of respiratory distress include rapid respiratory rate, decreased breath sounds, shortness of breath, use of accessory muscles of respiration, retractions (intercostal, sternal, and supraclavicular), nasal flaring, altered mental status, increased expiratory-inspiratory ratio, changes in skin color, and oxygen saturation. Pulsus paradoxus, the difference between systolic arterial blood pressure during inspiration and expiration, is normally less than 10 mm Hg. During an acute asthmatic attack this difference may be increased; however, this measurement may be difficult to obtain in young children. Children who are older than 6 years and are not in extreme respiratory distress should have their pulmonary function measured; this may include an estimation of peak expiratory flow rate or forced expiratory volume in 1 second (FEV_1).

If signs of a moderate or severe attack are present, children need to be monitored continuously. A severe attack may be heralded by the signs of respiratory distress listed above. In addition, patients may be unable to speak in sentences or may have altered mental status. Therapy includes placing patients in a position of comfort and giving oxygen by mask or nasal prongs, or having oxygen blown in front of the face. Initiation of drug therapy also is indicated.

History

If children are not in respiratory distress, a history should be taken (Questions Box). Practitioners should also find out how children and their families perceive the illness.

Physical Examination

Vital signs should be obtained and breath sounds, work of breathing, the inspiratory-expiratory ratio, use of accessory muscles, presence of retractions, quality of breath sounds (whether decreased), presence of prolonged expiration, and quality of wheezing should be carefully assessed (Table 69-2). Polyphonic wheezing (many different pitches, starting and stopping at varying points in the respiratory cycle) and cough are highly suggestive of asthma. Monophonic wheezing (a single, distinct noise of one pitch and starting and stopping at one discrete time) and cough should always raise suspicion of large airway obstruction caused by foreign body aspiration, vascular ring, or tracheomalacia. The nose and associated nasal passages should

Figure 69-1. **Proposed pathways in the pathogenesis of bronchial inflammation and airway hyperresponsiveness.** (Reproduced from the National Heart, Lung, and Blood Institute. *National Asthma Education Program Expert Panel Report: Guidelines for Diagnosis and Management of Asthma.* Bethesda, MD: National Institutes of Health; National Heart, Lung, and Blood Institute; 1991. NIH Publication No. 91-3042.)

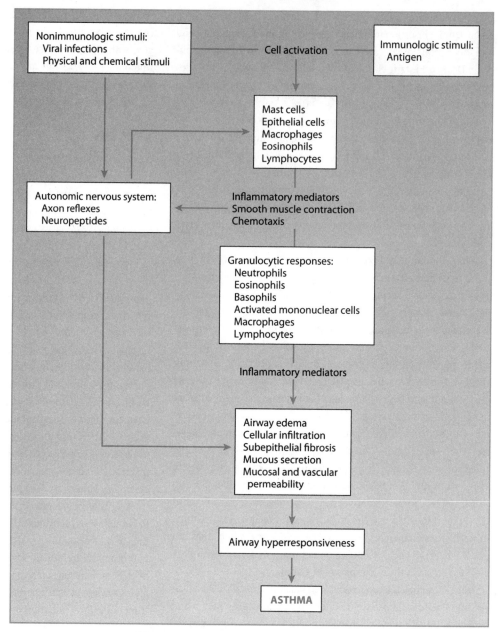

Laboratory Tests

The laboratory assessment of children is indicated if diagnosis is unclear or to rule out disorders that mimic asthma. Pulmonary function tests are noninvasive, objective, and cost-effective in the diagnosis and follow-up of patients with asthma. These tests can be performed in children older than 5 years with appropriate coaching. After the administration of an aerosolized bronchodilator, dynamic tests of airflow increase or return to normal. An improvement in FEV_1 greater than 15% is virtually diagnostic, but lack of improvement in FEV_1 does not preclude asthma. Exercise tolerance tests using a treadmill or free running followed by pulmonary function tests can be performed; a decrease greater than 15% in FEV_1 or 30% in forced expiratory flow (FEF_{25-75}) is diagnostic of exercise-induced asthma. Peak flow meters, which measure forced peak expiratory flow (PEF), are useful in the office and at home to monitor expiratory flow rate. A decrease in PEF predicts the onset of an exacerbation and suggests the need for early intervention, using additional drug therapy. A complete blood count with a differential count may suggest infection or allergies. Peripheral eosinophil counts usually are greater than 250 to 400 mm^3 in asthma. Pulse oximetry assesses the degree of oxygen saturation.

Sputum smear, stained with eosin-methylene blue, may show numerous eosinophils and granules from disrupted white blood cells, eosinophils, and epithelial cells. The presence of more than 5% to 10% eosinophils suggests allergic inflammatory disease. Other findings in the sputum include Curschmann spirals, which are threads of glycoprotein; Creola bodies, which are clusters of epithelial cells; and Charcot-Leyden crystals, which are derived from eosinophils.

The skin should be examined for secretions, edema, pallor, and polyps. The skin should be assessed for eczema and other rashes. The chest should be carefully checked for increased anteroposterior diameter of the chest wall, a sign of air trapping.

Table 69-1. Classification of Asthma Severity[a]

Clinical Features Before Treatment[b]

	Symptoms[c]	Nighttime Symptoms	Lung Function
Step 4: Severe Persistent	• Continual symptoms • Limited physical activity • Frequent exacerbations	Frequent	FEV_1 or PEF <60% predicted PEF variability >30%
Step 3: Moderate Persistent	• Daily symptoms • Daily use of inhaled short-acting β_2-agonist • Exacerbations affect activity • Exacerbations ≥2 times a week; may last days	>1 time a week	FEV_1 or PEF >60%–<80% predicted PEF variability
Step 2: Mild Persistent	• Symptoms >2 times a week but <1 time a day • Exacerbations may affect activity	>2 times a month	FEV_1 or PEF ≥80% predicted PEF variability 20%–30%
Step 1: Mild Intermittent	• Symptoms ≤2 times a week • Asymptomatic and normal PEF between exacerbations • Exacerbations brief (from a few hours to a few days); intensity may vary	≤2 times a month	FEV_1 or PEF ≥80% predicted PEF variability <20%

Abbreviations: FEV_1, forced expiratory volume in one second; PEF, peak expiratory flow.

[a]Reproduced from *National Heart, Lung, and Blood Institute. National Asthma Education and Prevention Program Expert Panel Executive Summary Report: Guidelines for the Diagnosis and Management of Asthma*—Update on Selected Topics 2002. Bethesda, MD: National Institutes of Health; National Heart, Lung, and Blood Institute; 2002. NIH Publication No. 02-5075. The characteristics noted in this table are general and may overlap because asthma is highly variable. Furthermore, an individual's classification may change over time.

[b]The presence of one of the features of severity is sufficient to place a patient in that category. An individual should be assigned to the most severe grade in which any feature occurs.

[c]Patients at any level of severity can have mild, moderate, or severe exacerbations. Some patients with intermittent asthma experience severe and life-threatening exacerbations separated by long periods of normal lung function and no symptoms.

Table 69-2. Parameters Used to Estimate the Severity of Acute Asthma

Sign/Symptom	Mild	Moderate	Severe
Respiratory rate	Normal	Increased	Increased >2 SD
Breath sounds	Normal (some end-expiratory wheezes)	Wheezing in inspiration and expiration	Decreased ± wheezing
Shortness of breath	None (can speak in sentences)	Can speak in phrases	Speaks only single words
Skin color	Normal (pink)	Pale	Pale to cyanotic
Work of breathing	Normal	Moderate retractions; some use of accessory muscles	Severe retractions, nasal flaring, use of accessory muscles
Pulse	Normal	Normal or increased	Increased
Level of consciousness	Normal	Normal	Diminished; may be lethargic or combative
Pulsus paradoxus	<10 mm Hg	10–20 mm Hg	20–40 mm Hg
Oxygen saturation	>95%	90%–95%	<92%
Pulmonary function	80% of predicted	50%–70% of predicted	<50% of predicted

Abbreviation: SD, standard deviation.

Total serum IgE is not as helpful as antigen-specific IgE, and is elevated in 80% of children with allergen-induced asthma. Allergy skin testing or serologic testing, such as radioallergosorbent testing, is indicated to identify potentially important environmental allergens. Allergens may play a significant role in asthma, and 85% of asthma patients have a positive skin test reaction to common aeroallergens. Extensive laboratory testing should be reserved for children with severe disease who may benefit from consultation with an allergy specialist.

Asthma

Questions

- What symptoms (eg, wheezing, exercise intolerance) does the child experience?
- Does the child experience any nocturnal awakening or cough?
- What time of day and year do the symptoms occur?
- When did the symptoms begin? How old was the child?
- Are the symptoms associated with any particular activity? Does anything seem to trigger the symptoms?
- Are the child's activities limited in any way?
- How often do the asthma attacks occur?
- What is the child's living situation? Are there pets in the home?
- Does anyone smoke in the home?
- Do the asthma attacks cause the child to be absent from school?
- Does the child manage the condition at home with any particular treatments or medications?
- Has the child visited any urgent care and emergency departments for treatment for asthma or related episodes in the past? Has the child had any hospitalizations?
- Does the child have a history of allergies?

Imaging Studies

Children suspected of having asthma rarely require a chest radiograph unless there is concern about other pathology. X-ray findings may range from normal to hyperinflation, increased bronchial marking, and atelectasis, especially during acute exacerbation. Infiltration, pneumothorax, pneumomediastinum, and pneumonia are less common findings.

Management

The goals of asthma therapy are as follows:

- Prevent chronic and disabling symptoms (eg, coughing, sleep disturbances, exercise intolerance, shortness of breath).
- Maintain normal or near-normal pulmonary function.
- Maintain normal activity levels.
- Prevent recurrent exacerbations and minimize the need for ED visits and admission to the hospital.
- Provide drug therapy that is effective with minimal side effects.
- Meet the expectations of the child and the family for the care of asthma.
- Encourage self-management of asthma.

Assessment measures for asthma should include monitoring of the following: signs and symptoms, pulmonary function through peak flow or spirometry, quality of life/functional status, acute disease exacerbations, pharmacologic therapy, and satisfaction of the child and family with their asthma care.

Selecting the appropriate therapy for an asthma patient depends on the age and developmental level of the child, the tolerance for a specific pharmacologic agent, and the routes of administration. The pharmacologic treatment for symptom control and reduction of inflammation is predicated on the severity of the asthma, as categorized, according to NHLBI guidelines. Non-pharmacologic

Box 69-2. Pharmacologic Therapy: An Overview of Medications Used to Treat Asthma

Long-Term Control Medications (Controller Class)

Corticosteroids
Most potent and effective anti-inflammatory medication currently available. Inhaled form is used in the long-term control of asthma. Systemic corticosteroids are often used to gain prompt control of the disease when initiating long-term therapy.

Cromolyn Sodium and Nedocromil
Mild-to-moderate anti-inflammatory medication. May be used as initial choice for long-term control therapy for children. Can also be used as preventive treatment prior to exercise or unavoidable exposure to known allergens.

Long-Acting β_2-Agonists
Long-acting bronchodilator used concomitantly with anti-inflammatory medications for long-term control of symptoms, especially nocturnal symptoms. Also prevents exercise-induced bronchospasm (EIB). **Includes salmeterol, fenoterol, procaterol.**

Methylxanthines
Sustained-release theophylline is a mild-to-moderate bronchodilator used principally as adjuvant to inhaled corticosteroids for prevention of nocturnal asthma symptoms. May have mild anti-inflammatory effect.

Leukotriene Modifiers
Montelukast, a leukotriene receptor antagonist, or zileuton, a 5-lipoxygenase inhibitor, may be considered an alternative therapy to low doses of inhaled corticosteroids or cromolyn or nedocromil.

Systemic Corticosteroids
- Used for moderate-to-severe exacerbations to speed recovery and prevent recurrence of exacerbations.
- **Immunomodulators** have been tested for their ability to provide long-term control and/or steroid-sparing effects. Includes omalizumab (anti-immunoglobulin [Ig] E), Ig (Ig intravenous), methotrexate, cyclosporine A, anti-interleukin (IL)-5, soluble IL-4, receptor.
- Omalizimab (anti-IgE) a recombinant DNA-derived humanized monoclonal antibody of the Fc portion of the IgE antibody, binds to that portion thereby preventing IgE binding to its high-affinity receptor (fcER1) on mast cells and basophils, leads to a decrease in the release of mediators in response to allergen exposure.

Quick-Relief Medications (Reliever Class)

Short-Acting β_2-Agonists
Albuterol, levalbuterol, and terbutaline are therapy of choice for relief of acute symptoms and prevention of EIB.

Anticholinergics
Ipratropium bromide may provide some additive benefit to inhaled β_2-agonists in severe exacerbations. May be an alternative bronchodilator for patients who do not tolerate inhaled β_2-agonists.

measures aim at prevention and serve as an adjunct to drug therapy. Box 69-2 contains an overview of these medications. Quick-relief medications are used for acute exacerbations and the long-term control medications for chronic therapy.

Short-Term Management

Acute attacks can be managed in the office if the staff is prepared to deal with children in respiratory distress. Otherwise children can be referred to the ED. Equipment and supplies for resuscitation of infants and children must be available in offices that care for children with asthma.

The goal of therapy is to relieve airflow obstruction and prevent respiratory failure. All children with moderate or severe asthma should be placed in a position of comfort and given oxygen by nasal prongs or mask as tolerated. Assessment of work of breathing and the use of pulse oximetry help guide oxygen therapy. Nebulized β_2-agonists such as albuterol are used until symptoms subside. Children may require drug therapy every 20 to 30 minutes. β_2-agonists may also be given as a continuous nebulized treatment for severe acute attacks. Not only are nebulized β-adrenergic agonists more effective than oral medications, they are associated with fewer side effects. Ipratropium bromide is also used in the initial acute management of asthma. Methylprednisolone, which helps reduce the inflammation associated with clinical attacks, is indicated in most moderate and severe cases. Response to therapy is determined by clinical assessment of work of breathing, respiratory rate, objective changes in pulmonary function, and pulse oximetry. Children with incomplete responses to initial therapy may require several hours of treatment or hospitalization.

Long-Term Management

Asthma is a chronic condition with a varying number of acute exacerbations. The goals of long-term management are shown in Box 69-3.

Box 69-3. Therapeutic Goals for Children With Chronic Asthma

- Maintain a normal, age-appropriate activity level.
- Maintain near-normal pulmonary function.
- Prevent symptoms such as exercise intolerance, chronic cough, and shortness of breath.
- Prevent acute exacerbations of the disease that require acute therapy.
- Minimize adverse effects of the drugs used to treat the disease.
- Promote self-esteem and a sense of well-being.

Continuous and longitudinal primary care of children with asthma can profoundly affect the course of their disease. Primary care practitioners, children, and their families must work together to achieve good control of symptoms. Prevention of exacerbations may be accomplished by removal of offending allergens. Minimization of exposure to known allergens and irritants has been shown to decrease symptoms and exacerbation. The most commonly implicated irritants are tobacco smoke; fumes from gas, oil, and kerosene stoves and wood-burning appliances; and sprays and strong odors. House dust mites are microscopic insects that feed on human scales, require humidity greater than 50%, and are found in stuffed furniture, carpets, and mattresses. House dust mite infestation can be reduced by removing carpeting and decreasing humidity to less than 50%.

Allergen immunotherapy may be considered for asthma patients when there is evidence of a clear relationship between symptom and exposure to an allergen, and symptoms are poorly controlled with pharmacologic management (medication ineffective, multiple medications are required, or patient does not accept or tolerate medication). Adherence with appropriate medications and participation in home pulmonary function testing play a major role for prevention and control of asthma. Periodic assessment ensures appropriate therapy and compliance with treatment. Practitioners should make sure that families can afford the necessary medications. During routine visits, home monitoring and therapy as well as any diaries and records should be reviewed, children's and families' expectations about the course of the disease should be discussed, and all parties should be allowed to express their concerns regarding the development of a treatment plan. Other factors, such as rhinitis, sinusitis, and gastroesophageal reflux, which may influence the severity of asthma or a child's quality of life, should be assessed and treated appropriately.

Family members and children should be given a written action plan based on patients' personal best peak flow (Figure 69-2) and instructed in the use of peak flow meters to indicate when medical treatment is necessary. Some meters have 3 color zones: a green zone, which indicates good airflow; a yellow zone, which signals the need for treatment; and a red zone, which suggests that a visit to the ED may be indicated.

See Figure 69-2 for an example of an asthma action/medicine plan.

Pharmacologic Therapy

The NHLBI expert panel recommends that patients be started at a higher level of medications at the onset, to establish prompt control, and then step-down reduction should be implemented to reach the minimum medication necessary to maintain control (see Table 69-1).

For **Step 1, mild intermittent asthma,** use short-acting β_2-agonists as needed to treat symptoms. In patients who have exercise-induced bronchospasm, prophylactic use of β_2-agonists, cromolyn, or nedocromil shortly before exercise blocks exercise-induced bronchospasm.

For **Step 2, mild persistent asthma,** use daily anti-inflammatory medication; either inhaled corticosteroids at a low dose or cromolyn, or nedocromil. Leukotriene modifier agents, such as montelukast have a good safety profile in children. Use short-acting β_2-agonists for acute exacerbations.

For **Step 3, moderate persistent asthma,** use low- to medium-dose inhaled corticosteroids and long-acting inhaled β_2-agonists. Adding nedocromil, leukotriene modifier, or theophylline decreases the daily dose of corticosteroid that is required to maintain optimal control of asthma. Use β_2-agonists for acute exacerbations.

	Wheeze	Cough	Activity	Sleep	Quick Relief: β_2-Agonist	Cromolyn/Nedocromil	Inhaled Steroids	Other—Inhaled	Oral Steroids	Theophylline	Peak Flow			Comments
Date											AM	PM	Other Times	

Patient Self–Assessment: Example of Patient Diary

Wheeze	None = 0	Some = 1	Medium = 2	Severe = 3
Cough	None = 0	Occasional = 1	Frequent = 2	Continuous = 3
Activity	Normal = 0	Can run short distance or climb 3 flights of stairs = 1	Can walk only = 2	Missed school or work or stayed indoors = 3
Sleep	Fine = 0	Slept well, slight wheeze or cough = 1	Awake 2–3 times, wheeze or cough = 2	Bad night, awake most of the time = 3

Figure 69-2. Asthma management plan based on Peal expiratory flow.

For **Step 4, severe persistent asthma,** use high-dose inhaled corticosteroids and a long-acting bronchodilator. Systemic corticosteroids may also be necessary. A weaning schedule to reduce systemic corticosteroids should be employed once optimal control is achieved so as to use the lowest possible dose (single dose daily or on alternate days). Use short-acting β_2-agonists for acute exacerbations. Specific immediate and long-term management of asthma is indicated.

Prognosis

Asthma can result in significant morbidity and mortality if children are not managed appropriately. Children without longitudinal primary care generally require expensive therapy in EDs or inpatient settings. A significant number of individuals with asthma have fatal outcomes because of lack of timely and appropriate care. Practically all of these deaths are preventable.

CASE RESOLUTION

The 7-year-old boy in the case history who visits the office for asthma requires not only medication but also education and longitudinal primary care. It is particularly important to assess possible environmental factors (eg, pets), exposure to smoke, and poor compliance with previous recommendations, which have contributed to his recurrent symptoms.

Selected References

Abadolgu O, Mungan D, Pasaoglu G, Celik G, Misirligil Z. Influenza vaccination in patients with asthma: effect on the frequency of upper respiratory tract infections and exacerbations. *J Asthma.* 2004;41:279–283

Apter AJ, Szefler SJ. Advances in adult and pediatrics asthma. *J Allergy Clin Immunol.* 2004;113:407–414

Bacharier LB, Strunk RC, Mauger D, White D, Lemanske RF Jr, Sorkness CA. Asthma severity in children: mismatch between symptoms, medication use, and lung function. *Am J Respir Crit Care Med.* 2004;170:426–432

Bisgaard H, Hermansen MN, Loland L, et al. Intermittent inhaled corticosteroids in infants with episodic wheezing. *N Engl J Med.* 2006;354:1998–2005

Boushey HA, Sorkness CA, King TS, et al. Daily versus as-needed corticosteroids for mild persistent asthma. *N Engl J Med.* 2005;352:1519–1528

Bousquet J, Wenzel S, Holgate S, Lumry W, Freeman P, Fox H. Predicting response to omalizumab, an anti-IgE antibody, in patients with allergic asthma. *Chest.* 2004;125:1378–1386

Brussee JE, Smit HA, van Strien RT, et al. Allergen exposure in infancy and the development of sensitization, wheeze, and asthma at 4 years. *J Allergy Clin Immunol.* 2005;115:946–952

Bueving HJ, Bernsen RM, de Jongste JC, et al. Influenza vaccination in children with asthma: randomized double-blind placebo-controlled trial. *Am J Respir Crit Care Med.* 2004;169:488–493

Covar RA, Spahn JD, Murphy JR, Szefler SJ, Childhood Asthma Management Program Research Group. Progression of asthma measured by lung function in the childhood asthma management program. *Am J Respir Crit Care Med.* 2004;170:234–241

Eder W, Ege MJ, von Mutius E. The asthma epidemic. *N Engl J Med.* 2006;355:2226–2235

Greenstone IR, Ni Chroinin MN, Masse V, et al. Combination of inhaled long-acting beta2-agonists and inhaled steroids versus higher dose of inhaled steroids in children and adults with persistent asthma. *Cochrane Database Syst Rev.* 2005;(4):CD005533

Jenkins CR, Thien FC, Whealtely JR, Reddel HK. Traditional and patient-centred outcomes with three classes of asthma medication. *Eur Respir J.* 2005;26:36–44

Masoli M, Weatherall M, Holt S, Beasley R. Moderate dose inhaled corticosteroids plus salmeterol versus higher doses of inhaled corticosteroids in symptomatic asthma. *Thorax.* 2005;60:730–734

Morgan WJ, Crain EF, Grunchalla RS, et al. Results of a home-based environmental intervention among urban children with asthma. *N Engl J Med.* 2004;351:1068–1080

National Center for Health Statistics. Reports From the 2005 National Health Interview Survey. Hyattsville, MD: National Center for Health Statistics, Centers for Disease Control and Prevention; 2005. www.cdc.gov/nchs/about/major/nhis/reports_2005.htm

National Heart, Lung, and Blood Institute. *National Asthma Education and Prevention Program Expert Panel Executive Summary Report: Guidelines for the Diagnosis and Management of Asthma—Update on Selected Topics 2002.* Bethesda, MD: National Institutes of Health; National Heart, Lung, and Blood Institute; 2002. NIH Publication No. 02-5075

Ng D, Salvio F, Hicks G. Anti-leukotriene agents compared to inhaled corticosteroids in the management of recurrent and/or chronic asthma in adults and children. *Cochrane Database Syst Rev.* 2004;(2):CD002314

Pual K, Cover R, Jain N, Gelfand EW, Spahn JD. Do NHLBI lung function criteria apply to children? A cross-sectional evaluation of childhood asthma at national Jewish Medical and Research center, 1999–2002. *Pediatr Pulmonol.* 2005;39:311–317

Saltpeter SR, Buckley NS, Ormiston TM, Salpeter EE. Meta-analysis: effect of long-acting beta-agonists on severe asthma exacerbations and asthma-related deaths. *Ann Intern Med.* 2006;144:904–912

Sigurs N, Gustafsson PM, Bjarnason R, et al. Severe respiratory syncytial virus bronchiolitis in infancy and asthma and allergy at age 13. *Am J Respir Crit Care Med.* 2005;171:137–141

CHAPTER 70

Cough

Nasser Redjal, MD

CASE STUDY

A 3-year-old boy presents with a cough that he has had for 4 weeks. In the past he has had coughs with colds, but this cough is persistent and deeper in quality. The cough seemed to develop suddenly when he was playing at a friend's house. It occurs all day and disrupts his sleep at night. The boy has had no nasal congestion, fever, or sore throat. No one at home is coughing, and the boy has not traveled recently. Neither the boy nor his family has a history of allergies or asthma. Over-the-counter cough preparations have not helped relieve his symptoms. On examination, growth parameters are normal. The child has a persistent cough with no respiratory distress. Chest examination reveals a normal respiratory rate,

no retractions, and no use of accessory muscles, but diffuse expiratory wheezing is noted in the right lower lobe. The remainder of the examination is normal.

Questions

1. What are common parental concerns regarding cough?
2. What diagnoses in children with persistent cough should be considered?
3. What historical factors and physical findings are important to determine the etiology of cough?
4. What diagnostic workup is appropriate?
5. How should children with chronic cough be managed?

Cough is an essential protective reflex that allows for clearance of secretions and particulates from the airways. Its persistence can generate much parental anxiety because of concern about its etiology and the frequently associated disruption of sleep. Cough is either acute or chronic. Acute cough, which may persist up to 2 weeks, is often associated with respiratory tract infections in children. When cough lasts more than 4 weeks, it is considered persistent or chronic. Parental sensitivity as well as accessibility to medical care influence when in the course of disease children present with this problem.

Epidemiology

Cough is a very common complaint initiating pediatric office visits. In the National Ambulatory Medical Care Survey, 6.7% of pediatric office visits involved children who presented with cough. Typically, preschool children have up to 8 upper respiratory infections with associated cough in a winter season. Persistent cough is also very common, with an estimated prevalence of 5% to 7% in preschoolers and 12% to 15% in older children. Cough is more common among boys than girls up to 11 years of age, and may be less common in developing countries than in affluent countries. Many serious diseases, including cystic fibrosis, congenital heart disease, asthma, and immunodeficiency disorders, may result in cough.

Clinical Presentation

The presentation varies greatly depending on the etiology of the cough. Children may present in severe respiratory distress or have no evidence of respiratory compromise. They may have conditions such as failure to thrive or appear totally healthy.

Pathophysiology

Coughing is a complicated reflex process that propels excess mucus up the airways at the pressures of up to 300 mm Hg and at flows of up to 5 to 6 L/sec. It is initiated through irritation of one of the multiple cough receptors (Figure 70-1). These receptors are located in the nose, paranasal sinuses, posterior pharynx, larynx, trachea, bronchi, and pleura. They can also be found outside of the respiratory tract in the ear canal, stomach, pericardium, and diaphragm. Stimulation of any of these receptors by an irritant, whether mechanical, chemical, thermal, or inflammatory, can initiate the cough reflex. The proximal airways (larynx and trachea) are more sensitive to mechanical stimulation, and the distal airways more sensitive to chemical stimulation. The lung parenchymal (bronchiolar and alveolar) tissue contains no cough receptors, so pneumonia may not produce a cough. Impulses from stimulated cough receptors traverse afferent nerves (vagus, glossopharyngeal, trigeminal, or phrenic) to a "cough center" in the medulla, which itself is under some control by higher cortical centers. The cough center generates an efferent signal that travels down the vagus, phrenic, and spinal motor nerves to expiratory musculature thereby producing the cough. The cough center can be voluntarily stimulated or suppressed.

The actual cough experienced by patients may be broken down into 4 phases. First, the glottis opens with an inspiratory gasp. Second, the glottis closes with forceful contraction of the chest wall, diaphragm, and abdominal muscles. Third, the glottis again opens with release of airway pressure in an expiratory phase. The fourth phase involves relaxation in which the chest wall and abdominal muscles relax. This process expels mucus or irritants from the

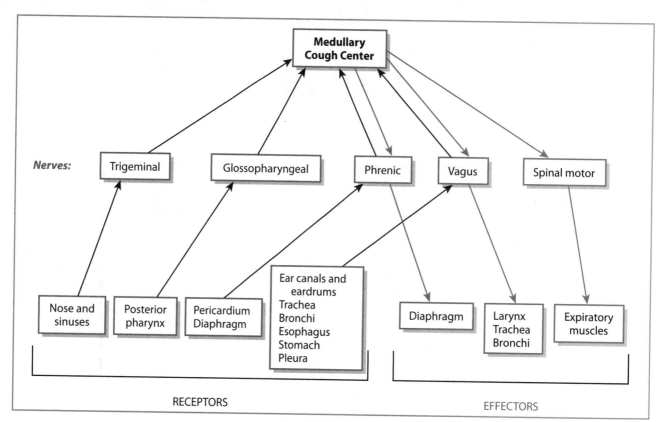

Figure 70-1. The cough reflex.

airways, helping maintain the health of the lungs. Children who do not cough effectively may be at risk for atelectasis, recurrent pneumonia, and chronic airway disease from aspiration and/or retention of secretions.

Differential Diagnosis

The list of differential diagnoses of cough is long (Box 70-1). Narrowing the list of causes can be accomplished by paying attention to several factors (Dx Box).

As with any pediatric symptom, the child's **age** influences the diagnostic possibilities and management of the cough. Congenital anomalies, which are most likely to present in the first few months of life, include tracheoesophageal fistula, laryngeal cleft, vocal cord paralysis, and tracheobronchomalacia. Congenital heart disease can produce a cough from heart failure and pulmonary edema. Congenital mediastinal tumors cause infants to cough if the tumor

Dx **Cough**

- Quality: dry, productive, brassy
- Duration: acute, chronic, recurrent
- Timing: during day, at night, on awakening, with exercise
- Fever or upper respiratory infection associated with infectious origin
- Allergic findings of rhinorrhea, sneezing, wheezing, atopic dermatitis associated with asthma or allergic rhinitis
- Failure to thrive (indicates chronic disease)

presses on the bronchial tree. Many children with asthma experience cough and/or wheezing in infancy, often associated with an episode of bronchiolitis.

The **duration of the cough** also suggests its possible cause. Most acute coughs are infectious in origin. Upper respiratory infections can initiate an acute cough through stimulation of the cough receptors in the nose and posterior pharynx. If nasal congestion and cough persist, a diagnosis of allergic rhinitis or sinusitis should be considered. Serous otitis media can also cause a persistent cough and may occur in children with chronic congestion. Children with pneumonia may present with either acute or chronic cough.

The presence of a nighttime cough can be important. Pathologic coughs, including those caused by sinusitis with postnasal drip, gastroesophageal reflux, and asthma, are more likely to occur at night.

The character of the cough is another factor to consider in the differential diagnosis. Certain etiologies are associated with a very specific type of cough. A barking cough is consistent with laryngeal edema and croup. A stridorous cough may be seen with proximal airway disease, such as laryngomalacia or tracheomalacia, laryngotracheobronchitis, or a foreign body. An inspiratory whoop is characteristic of pertussis or parapertussis. Staccato cough in infants can be the result of infection with *Chlamydia trachomatis*. The psychogenic or habitual cough is a strange, honking sound (Canadian goose-like), disappears at night, and is typically at its worse and most disruptive during school classes. Chronic paroxysmal cough triggered by exercise, cold air, sleep, or allergens is often seen in patients with asthma.

Box 70-1. Causes of Cough

Congenital Anomalies
- Tracheoesophageal fistula
- Laryngeal cleft
- Vocal cord paralysis
- Mediastinal masses
- Pulmonary malformations
- Tracheobronchomalacia
- Congenital heart disease

Infections (eg, upper respiratory infection, sinusitis, pneumonia)

Viral
- Adenovirus
- Influenza
- Parainfluenza
- Respiratory syncytial virus
- Rhinovirus

Bacterial
- Pertussis
- Pneumococcal
- Staphylococcal
- Tuberculosis

Fungal
- Coccidioidomycosis

Parasitic infection
- Paragonimiasis
- Echinococcosis

Other
- Chlamydial
- Mycoplasmosis

Cardiac Disease
- Congestive heart failure
- Pulmonary hypertension

Chronic Disease
- Cystic fibrosis
- Human immunodeficiency virus infection
- Immunodeficiency syndrome
- Dyskinetic cilia

Allergic Conditions
- Allergic rhinitis
- Asthma
- Serous otitis media

Mediastinal Tumors

Foreign Body Aspiration

Gastroesophageal Reflux

Environmental Irritants

Psychogenic Cough

Drug-Induced Conditions

Sarcoidosis

In contrast, a chronic productive (or "wet") cough suggests a suppurative process, and may require further investigation to exclude bronchiectasis, cystic fibrosis, active infection, immune deficiency, or congenital malformation.

Pneumococcus is the most probable causal agent in acute cough with pneumonia, but when the cough becomes chronic, other infectious agents are more likely. Adenovirus and respiratory syncytial virus, which occur more commonly in infants, and influenza and parainfluenza, which affect children of all ages, are common viral agents that produce chronic cough. *Bordetella pertussis,* mycoplasma, and chlamydia also cause chronic cough. Other infections such as tuberculosis and coccidioidomycosis should also be considered in endemic areas or high-risk populations. Chronic infectious coughs, such as those associated with influenza and pertussis, can last up to 6 months. Host factors that may predispose to chronic cough should also be investigated. Children with cystic fibrosis, bronchopulmonary dysplasia, human immunodeficiency virus and other immunodeficiency syndromes, and congenital pulmonary malformations may present with chronic, recurrent cough.

The most common cause of chronic cough is reactive airway disease (asthma) (see Chapter 69). In fact, cough with no notable wheezing may be the only manifestation of asthma. In infants or neurologically impaired children, chronic cough may indicate gastroesophageal reflux **or** recurrent aspiration. An unexplained persistent cough, primarily in toddlers, may be the result of foreign body aspiration if the initial aspiration was not observed. The foreign object acts as a chronic airway irritant that stimulates coughing, and it may be the cause of recurrent infections. Other irritants that initiate cough include dust, allergens, wood- and gas-burning stoves, chemicals, and passive or active exposure to smoke from tobacco, marijuana, cocaine, or other substances. Drugs such as β-adrenergic receptor antagonists and angiotensin-converting enzyme inhibitors

can also induce a chronic cough, probably by increasing the sensitivity of the cough reflex. Patients previously treated with cytotoxic drugs or thoracic radiation are at risk of interstitial lung disease. Cough along with symptoms of pancreatic insufficiency, recurrent bacterial pneumonia, and/or failure to thrive should raise suspicion of cystic fibrosis. Cough with a history of dyspnea or hemoptysis should trigger a search for organic lung disease. Hemoptysis should also raise concerns of bronchiectasis, cavitary lung disease (tuberculosis or bacterial abscesses), congestive heart failure, hemosiderosis, neoplasm, foreign bodies, vascular lesions, endobronchial lesions, catamenial (ectopic endometrial tissue) bleeding, and clotting disorders.

Evaluation

History

A complete history should be obtained when children present with cough (Questions Box). All symptoms should be noted. Vomiting with cough can indicate phlegm production and the accumulation of mucus in the stomach, with resultant delayed gastric emptying. In some children with a chief complaint of vomiting it is actually the cough that precipitates the vomiting. Post-tussive vomiting is characteristic of pertussis.

Physical Examination

A complete physical examination should be performed on all children who present with cough. Growth parameters and vital signs should be assessed. Skin should be examined for evidence of cyanosis or atopy. Facial petechiae or subconjunctival hemorrhage indicates particularly forceful coughing. Extremities should be evaluated for fingernail clubbing, which is a sign of chronic pulmonary disease. The nose should be assessed for evidence of congestion. Allergic disease produces pale,

Cough — Questions

- How old is the child?
- How long has the child had the cough?
- How frequently does the child cough?
- Does the cough occur at night?
- Does exercise make the cough worse?
- Do any factors such as environmental irritants seem to precipitate the cough?
- Does the child have any related infectious symptoms, including fever and nasal congestion?
- Does the child have any other symptoms?
- Has the child had any previous episodes of coughing or associated symptoms?
- Has the child lost weight recently?
- What is the child's birth history?
- Has the child had any pulmonary injuries?
- What is the child's immunization status?
- Does the child have a history of recent travel?
- Has a family member had similar symptoms?
- Does the family have a history of pulmonary disease or allergies?
- Has the child been treated with any medications for the cough? Have they helped?
- Is the child taking any other medications?

edematous mucosa, whereas infection results in more inflammatory mucosa. Tympanic membranes should be examined and mobility tested; halitosis, tonsillar hypertrophy, pharyngeal cobblestoning, and tenderness on the sinus area suggest sinus disease.

The respiratory effort, including the use of accessory muscles, should also be noted. Careful attention should be paid to breath sounds; whether abnormal sounds are in the inspiratory or expiratory phase of respiration should be determined. Stridor is classically an inspiratory sound (see Chapter 46), whereas wheezing is usually an expiratory sound. Chronic cough and wheeze are often noted in combination. Even in the absence of a history of wheeze, clinicians should listen carefully for this finding during the physical examination. Wheezing that is characterized by many different pitches and starting and stopping at varying points in the respiratory cycle is termed *polyphonic* and in association with cough is highly suggestive of asthma. Other causes of polyphonic wheezing include viral bronchiolitis, obliterative bronchiolitis, bronchiectasis, bronchopulmonary dysplasia, congestive heart failure, immunodeficiency, bronchomalacia, and aspiration syndromes.

Monophonic wheezing (a single, distinct, one pitch that starts and stops at one discrete time) and cough should always raise suspicion of large airway obstruction caused by foreign body or by tracheomalacia. Extrinsic airway compression as occurs with vascular rings, lymphadenopathy, and mediastinal tumors is also associated with monophonic wheezing. Tuberculosis should also be considered in a child with a monophonic wheeze, particularly in areas where the disease is prevalent.

Prolongation of the expiratory phase also is associated with wheezing and also indicates airway obstruction. Abnormal breath sounds should be localized if possible. Because the character of the cough can establish the diagnosis, listening to the cough is probably the most important part of the physical examination. A parental description of the cough may be less diagnostic.

Laboratory Tests

After a thorough history and physical examination, laboratory data may not be necessary. Laboratory tests should be ordered when more information is needed to help make a reasonable diagnosis. The laboratory data should be directed at proving or disproving the most likely diagnosis in a specific patient.

If after the history, physical examination, and chest x-ray an infectious etiology for cough is suspected, a complete blood count with differential and a purified protein derivative test should be ordered. Appropriate cultures should be sent, if possible. Most children swallow their phlegm, so sputum cultures may be difficult to obtain. Gastric aspirates can sometimes yield a reasonable sputum specimen for culture. Nasopharyngeal cultures are useful for diagnosing pertussis and viruses.

If a specific diagnosis is suspected, laboratory tests (Table 70-1) should be directed toward that diagnosis (eg, sweat chloride to rule out cystic fibrosis or quantitative immunoglobulins to rule out immunodeficiency). Allergy skin test or radioallergosorbent testing may be indicated to exclude inhalant allergy.

Imaging Studies

The chest x-ray (anteroposterior and lateral views), the mainstay of the diagnostic evaluation of cough, should be the first test ordered in the evaluation of a chronic cough or if definite findings are evident on physical examination. A lateral decubitus film can provide additional information about pleural fluid or air trapping. Inspiratory and expiratory films can be obtained if a foreign body is suspected. An area of inflation that either fails to deflate on exhalation or remains present in the decubitus position is suggestive of a foreign body. Congenital lobar emphysema and unilateral hyperlucent lung (Swyer-James, McLeod) syndrome are rare causes of focal or unilateral hyperinflation. If a nodular pulmonary lesion is found on x-ray, bronchoscopy may be the next step to further define the lesion. Bronchiectasis is a characteristic of cystic fibrosis, immune deficiency, primary ciliary dyskinesia, chronic aspiration, and previous history of severe infection (most commonly adenovirus and pertussis). If sinusitis is suspected, x-rays or a computed tomography scan of the sinuses can be performed. An upper gastrointestinal series of x-rays or a pH probe study would help to define gastroesophageal reflux if the cough occurs after recurrent episodes of vomiting or at night.

In children with asthma, the chest x-ray may be totally normal. Further diagnostic testing with peak flow measurements or pulmonary function tests in children older than 4 years can be done to demonstrate restriction or obstruction of the airway. The most helpful test to diagnose asthma may be a trial of a bronchodilator (see Chapter 69).

Table 70-1. Tests to Consider for Evaluation of Chronic Cough

Allergy	Allergy skin test or blood-specific immunoglobulin E test
Asthma	Pulmonary function test (PFT), bronchial hyperresponsiveness test such as methacholine challenge test, exhaled nitric oxide, trial of asthma treatments
Ciliary dyskinesia	Ciliary function tests
Congenital anomalies	Bronchoscopy, chest x-ray (CXR), computed tomography (CT)/magnetic resonance imaging, angiography
Cystic fibrosis	Sweat chloride test, genetic test
Fibrosing alveolitis, autoimmune disease	PFT and diffusion CT, autoantibodies
Foreign body	CXR, bronchoscopy
Gastroesophageal reflux	Barium swallow, 24-hour pH recording, and bronchoalveolar lavage (BAL)
Pertussis, chlamydia, or other infectious etiologies	Cultures, serology, polymerase chain reaction testing
Purulent infection	Cultures (sputum, BAL), CXR, CT, microbiology immunology, sweat test
Sinusitis	Imaging of sinuses with x-ray or CT scan
Tuberculosis	Mantoux testing

Management

Cough should not be treated until the cause has been identified by a thorough consideration of the differential diagnoses. Therapy should then be directed toward treating that etiology. However, many children do not have any evidence of chronic disease based on a detailed history, physical examination, radiography, and pulmonary function testing. When the initial evaluation outlined previously is unrevealing, cough-variant asthma, post-viral cough, increased cough receptor sensitivity, and functional disorders (including habit cough and tic disorders) should be considered. Empiric courses of therapy for asthma, rhinitis, sinusitis, or gastroesophageal reflux can be considered if suggestive findings exist. The external ear is innervated by the vagus nerve, and removal of irritants from the external auditory canal may reduce the coughing. Airflow obstruction may be apparent at the first visit, and a trial of asthma therapy is warranted, particularly if other signs of allergic disease are present or if the child's cough is precipitated by typical asthma triggers. A cough of an infectious etiology should be treated with the appropriate antibiotics. If the cough is keeping children awake at night, a cough suppressant may be indicated so that children and their families can rest. Cough syrups containing dextromethorphan are efficacious. Cough syrups with codeine can also be used. Such medications can be very helpful in interrupting the cough cycle generated by constant irritation of the cough receptors. Expectorants and mucolytic agents in cough syrups have little effect on relieving coughs.

Prognosis

With thoughtful evaluation, it is usually possible to identify the causes of both acute and chronic cough. Most symptoms resolve with appropriate therapy. If the cough persists with treatment, then alternate diagnoses should be considered.

CASE RESOLUTION

In the case presented at the beginning of this chapter, the child's cough began acutely and developed into a chronic cough. The boy has no history of allergies or symptoms consistent with an infectious process. Physical examination reveals localized wheezing. A chest x-ray is ordered, which reveals hyperinflation of the right lung. His symptoms and presentation are most consistent with foreign body aspiration and he is admitted to the hospital for bronchoscopy.

Selected References

Guilbert TW, Taussig LM. "Doctor, he's been coughing for a month. Is it serious?" *Contemp Pediatr.* 1998;15:155–172

Katcher ML. Cold, cough, and allergy medications: uses and abuses. *Pediatr Rev.* 1996;17:12–17

Stein RT, Holberg CJ, Sherrill D, et al. Influence of parental smoking on respiratory symptoms during the first decade of life: the Tucson Children's Respiratory Study. *Am J Epidemiol.* 1999;149:1030–1037

Chang AB, Powell CV. Non-specific cough in children: diagnosis and treatment. *Hosp Med.* 1998;59:680–684

de Jongste JC, Shields MD. Cough. 2: chronic cough in children. *Thorax.* 2003;58:998–1003

Chang AB. Cough, cough receptors, and asthma in children. *Pediatr Pulmonol.* 1999;28:59–70

Tekdemir I, Aslan A, Elhan A. A clinico-anatomic study of the auricular branch of the vagus nerve and Arnold's ear-cough reflex. *Surg Radiol Anat.* 1998;20:253–257

Morice AH, Geppetti P. Cough. 5: the type 1 vanilloid receptor: a sensory receptor for cough. *Thorax.* 2004;59:257–258

Boat TF. Pulmonary hemorrhage and hemoptysis. In: Chernick V, Boat TF, eds. *Kendig's Disorders of the Respiratory Tract in Children.* 6th ed. Philadelphia, PA: WB Saunders: 1998:623

Eysink PE, Bottema BJ, ter Riet G, Aalberse RC, Stapel SO, Bindels PJ. Coughing in pre-school children in general practice: when are RAST's for inhalation allergy indicated? *Pediatr Allergy Immunol.* 2004;15:394–400

Schwartz J. Air pollution and children's health. *Pediatrics.* 2004;113:1037–1043

Garrett MH, Hooper MA, Hooper BM, Abramson MJ. Respiratory symptoms in children and indoor exposure to nitrogen dioxide and gas stoves. *Am J Respir Crit Care Med.* 1998;158:891–895

Morice AH, Fontana GA, Sovijarvi AR, et al. The diagnosis and management of chronic cough. *Eur Respir J.* 2004;24:481–492

Tan H, Buyukavci M, Arik A. Tourette's syndrome manifests as chronic persistent cough. *Yonsei Med J.* 2004;45:145–149

Chung KF, Chang AB. Therapy for cough: active agents. *Pulm Pharmacol Ther.* 2002;15:335–338

Hematologic Disorders

71. Anemia 411

72. Bleeding Disorders... 419

73. Lymphadenopathy 427

Anemia

Wendy Y. Tcheng, MD

CASE STUDY

An 18-month-old girl is brought to the office with a 3-day history of cough, rhinorrhea, low-grade fever, and increasing scleral icterus and pallor. During her first week of life, the girl had hyperbilirubinemia of unknown etiology that required phototherapy. Her family history is significant for mild anemia in her father; the cause of his condition is unknown. A paternal aunt and grandfather had cholecystectomies while in their 30s.

On physical examination, the girl is tachycardic and tachypneic (no respiratory distress), with scleral icterus and pallor. Her spleen is palpable 3 cm below the midcostal margin. The remainder of her examination is normal.

Questions

1. What hemoglobin/hematocrit values are associated with anemia?
2. What is the appropriate initial evaluation of children with anemia?
3. What emergency situations in children who present with anemia should be recognized by the primary pediatrician?
4. When should a child with anemia be referred to a hematologist?
5. How is the family history relevant in the evaluation of anemia?

Anemia occurs when there is a reduction in hemoglobin concentration or red blood cell (RBC) number, leading to decreased oxygen-carrying capacity of blood. Anemia is defined as a hemoglobin or hematocrit value that is less than 2 SDs below the mean for age and gender. These values vary throughout infancy and childhood as hematopoiesis evolves from fetal to adult type, and it is important to reference normal age-related values when interpreting a hemoglobin or hematocrit result (see Table 71-1 for normal age-related values). In addition, the cardiopulmonary status should be considered as children with cyanotic heart disease or chronic respiratory insufficiency typically have hemoglobin values that are higher than the normal range and may be functionally anemic when the hemoglobin value falls even if it is within the lower range of normal.

Epidemiology

Iron deficiency is the most common cause of anemia in childhood, occurring most frequently during late infancy through the first few years of life and again during adolescence. This prevalence pattern corresponds to periods of rapid growth, and when combined with poor dietary intake can predispose to iron deficiency. Other contributing factors to iron deficiency include prematurity, blood loss (most commonly menstrual or gastrointestinal [GI]), and GI conditions associated with decreased iron absorption.

Other epidemiological factors that contribute to anemia are presented in Box 71-1. Anemias that have a genetic etiology, including hemoglobinopathies (eg, sickle cell disease, thalassemias), RBC enzyme deficiencies (eg, glucose-6-phosphate dehydrogenase [G6PD], pyruvate kinase), and RBC membrane disorders (eg, hereditary spherocytosis), are commonly diagnosed in childhood. The highest incidence of sickle cell disease, thalassemia, and G6PD deficiency is in individuals of African, Mediterranean, and Southeast Asian descent within the "malaria belt" near the equator, likely reflecting an advantage against malaria. Dietary factors can cause impaired hematopoiesis as in iron, folate, or vitamin B_{12} deficiency. Ingestion of oxidants (eg, fava beans, medications) can trigger hemolysis in G6PD deficiency. Ingestion of toxins such as lead can also result in impaired hematopoiesis. Lead poisoning occurs more commonly in children who live in cities and older housing. In an otherwise healthy child, viral infections can cause a pure red cell aplasia (transient erythroblastopenia of childhood), an autoimmune hemolytic anemia, or an aplastic anemia. Children with congenital hemolytic anemias are at risk for hemolytic and aplastic crises associated with infectious illnesses.

Clinical Presentation

The clinical presentation of anemia depends on the age of the child, the severity of the anemia, and the rapidity of onset (Dx Box). Most often anemia is detected on a routine screen or as part of an evaluation for an acute illness and the child is asymptomatic with no significant physical findings. Children who have developed a gradual anemia can be relatively asymptomatic because time has afforded compensatory mechanisms. Easy fatigability and exercise intolerance soon develop and as the anemia worsens, pallor, fatigue, and irritability occur, as well as signs of tachycardia, tachypnea and, in severe cases, outright congestive heart failure (CHF). Children with an abrupt drop in hemoglobin due to blood loss or hemolysis may present more acutely with signs of tachycardia, tachypnea, and

Table 71-1. Values (Mean and Lower Limits of Normal) for Hemoglobin, Hematocrit, and Mean Corpuscular Volume Determinations[a]

Age, y	Hemoglobin (g/dL) Mean	Lower Limit	Hematocrit (%) Mean	Lower Limit	MCV (µ³) Mean	Lower Limit
0.5–1.9	12.5	11.0	37	33	77	70
2–4	12.5	11.0	38	34	79	73
5–7	13.0	11.5	39	35	81	75
8–11	13.5	12.0	40	36	83	76
12–14						
Female	13.5	12.0	41	36	85	78
Male	14.0	12.5	43	37	84	77
15–17						
Female	14.0	12.0	41	36	87	79
Male	15.0	13.0	46	38	86	78
18–49						
Female	14.0	12.0	42	37	90	80
Male	16.0	14.0	47	40	90	80

Abbreviation: MCV, mean corpuscular volume.

[a]Reproduced with permission from Oski FA, Brugnara C, Nathan DG. A diagnostic approach to the anemic patient. In: Nathan DG, Orkin SH, eds. *Nathan and Oski's Hematology of Infancy and Childhood.* 5th ed. Philadelphia, PA: W. B. Saunders; 1998:376.

Box 71-1. Epidemiological Factors Related to Anemia

Genetic
- Autosomal-dominant: hereditary spherocytosis
- Autosomal-recessive: most Embden-Meyerhof pathway enzyme deficiencies (pyruvate kinase deficiency), most hemoglobinopathies (sickle cell disease, β-thalassemia)
- X-linked: glucose-6-phosphate dehydrogenase (G6PD) deficiency

Ethnicity
- Northern European: hereditary spherocytosis, pyruvate kinase deficiency
- Mediterranean (Italian, Greek, North African): β-thalassemia, G6PD deficiency
- African: sickle cell disease, hemoglobin C, hemoglobin D, G6PD deficiency, α-thalassemia trait, hereditary elliptocytosis
- Southeast Asian: α-thalassemia, hemoglobin E, G6PD deficiency

Dietary
Poor dietary intake (iron, folate, or vitamin B$_{12}$ deficiency)
- Iron (excessive cow's milk intake)
- Folate (excessive goat's milk intake)
- Vitamin B$_{12}$ (vegan diet)

Poor gastrointestinal absorption
- Iron, absorbed in duodenum (small bowel disease)
- Folate, absorbed in duodenum and jejunum (small bowel disease)
- Vitamin B$_{12}$, absorbed in terminal ileum (surgical resection, pernicious anemia, small bowel disease)

Ingestion of oxidants (fava beans in G6PD deficiency)
Toxins (lead)

Socioeconomic
- Living near highways: increased incidence of lead poisoning
- Poverty: associated with pica and lead poisoning

Infectious
- Malaria: heterozygous form of sickle cell disease, thalassemia, G6PD deficiency confer protection
- Viral infections: transient erythroblastopenia of childhood, autoimmune hemolytic anemias, hemolytic crisis in patients with congenital hemolytic anemias
- Parvovirus: aplastic crisis in patients with hemolytic anemias
- Viral hepatitis: aplastic anemia

possible hypotension and shock. If the anemia is due to acute hemolysis, accompanying jaundice, icterus, and dark urine may be seen.

Pathophysiology

Erythrocytes develop from pluripotent stem cells within the bone marrow under the influence of various hematopoietic growth factors. The primary function of the erythrocyte is the delivery of oxygen to tissues for aerobic metabolism. To this end, hemoglobin is the main intracellular protein of the erythrocyte. Hemoglobin consists of 4 polypeptide chains, each containing an active heme group that is capable of binding to an oxygen molecule. A normal erythrocyte has a life span of approximately 120 days and is subsequently removed from circulation as it passes through the reticuloendothelial system. Under steady state conditions, the daily loss of aged erythrocytes is compensated by a normal active erythropoiesis.

Anemia occurs when there is an imbalance between erythrocyte production and destruction. It can arise from conditions leading to **decreased production, increased destruction** (ie, hemolysis), or **blood loss.** Deficient production may be due to nutrient deficiency (iron, folate, vitamin B$_{12}$), bone marrow failure (acquired or inherited), or bone marrow infiltration (eg, malignancy). Increased destruction of erythrocytes can occur as a consequence of disorders intrinsic to the erythrocyte (eg, hemoglobinopathies, enzymopathies, membranopathies) or extrinsic factors (immune or nonimmune etiologies).

Dx Anemia

- Pallor, fatigue
- Scleral icterus
- Hepatosplenomegaly
- Lymphadenopathy
- Weight loss
- Congestive heart failure

Differential Diagnosis

The differential diagnosis of anemia can be determined by considering both the underlying mechanism of anemia (decreased production/increased destruction/blood loss) and the size of the erythrocyte (mean corpuscular volume [MCV]). The differential diagnosis of anemia based on pathophysiology and erythrocyte size can be found in Table 71-2 and Box 71-2. In determining the cause of anemia, the reticulocyte count is the most useful test in ascertaining whether the anemia is due to decreased production or increased destruction. A reduced reticulocyte count indicates decreased marrow production, whereas an elevated reticulocyte count is highly suggestive of hemolysis. Anemia based on erythrocyte size can be classified as microcytic (low MCV), normocytic (normal MCV), or macrocytic (high MCV). Microcytic anemias reflect a defect in hemoglobin synthesis and are most commonly due to iron deficiency, thalassemia, lead poisoning, and chronic disease. Macrocytic anemias reflect a relative decrease in DNA synthesis during erythropoiesis and are usually of nutritional origin (vitamin B_{12} or folate deficiency). The many other causes of anemia commonly fall into the normocytic category and can be further divided based on the reticulocyte count. Etiology and erythrocyte size, the 2 systems for classification of anemia, are not mutually exclusive—simultaneous application of these 2 systems will enable the pediatrician to make a primary diagnosis of anemia and determine its probable causes.

Microcytic Anemias

Iron deficiency is the most frequent cause of microcytic anemia in childhood and occurs as a result of (1) inadequate intake, (2) increased requirements due to growth, (3) blood loss, and (4) malabsorption of iron. As iron deficiency evolves, depletion of iron stores occurs first, then iron-deficient erythropoiesis without anemia and, finally, iron deficiency anemia. The combination of rapid growth and inadequate iron intake is responsible for the common occurrence of iron deficiency anemia in toddlers and adolescents. Most young infants are spared because of adequate iron stores acquired in utero and the ingestion of iron-fortified formulas. Premature infants are the exception as they have lower baseline iron stores (much of the iron stores are acquired by the fetus in the third trimester). As iron stores become depleted during late infancy and cow's milk is introduced into the diet, the ever-growing older infant/toddler becomes at risk for iron deficiency. Excessive cow's milk intake during the first few years of life predisposes to iron deficiency because cow's milk has minimal iron (<1 mg/L). Large intake of cow's milk results in early satiety and prevents adequate intake of other iron-containing foods. The iron deficiency is often further compounded by trace amounts of GI blood loss due to lack of cytochrome iron and GI mucosal damage or cow's milk allergy enteropathy. Adolescents, particularly menstruating females, are also prone to iron deficiency because of the pubertal growth spurt and suboptimal dietary habits. In young infants and children older than 3 years, dietary iron deficiency is uncommon, and an evaluation for blood loss or malabsorption is warranted. Blood loss can occur as hematochezia or melena (inflammatory bowel disease, diarrhea, Meckel diverticulum, polyp, ulcer), menorrhagia, epistaxis, hematuria (intravascular hemolysis), or rarely as pulmonary bleeding (pulmonary hemosiderosis). Iron is absorbed primarily in the duodenum, and a number of dietary factors (coffee, tea) as well as primary intestinal disorders can impair absorption.

The **thalassemias** are a heterogeneous group of inherited anemias that are characterized by impaired or absent synthesis of either the α or β chains that make up the normal adult hemoglobin tetramer. The β-**thalassemias** are caused by a decrease in the production of β-globin chains. The anemia observed in the severe forms of β-thalassemia occurs as a result of ineffective erythropoiesis. This is due to the instability of the excess α chains, which precipitate and cause oxidative damage to the cell membrane leading to premature destruction of the erythrocyte within the bone marrow. The erythrocytes that do survive in the circulation have a shortened life span because of increased hemolysis. The severe forms (compound heterozygous or homozygous state) are classified as β-**thalassemia major** or β-**thalassemia intermedia** depending on the clinical presentation and degree of anemia. Individuals with β-thalassemia major develop a severe anemia during the first year of life because decreasing levels of fetal hemoglobin ($\alpha_2\gamma_2$) cannot be replaced by normal adult hemoglobin ($\alpha_2\beta_2$). Hemoglobin values fall in the range of 3 to 4 g/dL and regular transfusions are required. Individuals with β-thalassemia intermedia usually present later in life and do not require early intervention with blood transfusions. Hemoglobin values are in the 7 to 8 g/dL range, and individuals may be intermittently transfusion-dependent. Individuals with β-**thalassemia trait** (β-thalassemia minor), the heterozygous form, have a mild microcytic anemia with a hemoglobin that is approximately 2 g/dL below the normal mean for age. Clinically, it is an asymptomatic anemia, however, it is of diagnostic relevance in that it must be distinguished from iron deficiency anemia.

The α-**thalassemias** are caused by a decrease in the production of α chains and are generally milder than the β-thalassemias. This reflects the fact that the excess of β chains that occurs in α-thalassemia is more stable, resulting in less membrane damage and intramedullary erythrocyte destruction. In humans, there are 4 α-globin genes. Individuals with a deletion of one α-globin gene are **silent carriers** and are asymptomatic with a normal hemoglobin value and MCV. Individuals with 2-gene deletions have α-**thalassemia trait** and have a very mild microcytic anemia that is asymptomatic. Three α-globin gene deletions causes **hemoglobin H disease,** a moderately severe chronic hemolytic anemia that may be intermittently transfusion-dependent. This occurs primarily in individuals of Southeast Asian descent. Four-gene deletion causes **hydrops fetalis,** an almost universally fatal condition.

Although **lead** inhibits heme synthesis and red cell function on many levels, microcytic anemia is a late finding of lead intoxication. Iron deficiency and lead poisoning often occur together and the relationship is complex. In the presence of lead, iron uptake by the erythrocyte is diminished and iron deficiency increases lead retention and toxicity. Intestinal absorption and uptake of lead by red cells is decreased in the presence of iron. In addition, iron deficiency and lead poisoning tend to occur in the same lower socioeconomic population, and both are exacerbated by concomitant nutritional deficiencies.

Table 71-2. Differential Diagnosis of Anemia Based on Pathophysiology[a]

Pathophysiological Mechanism	General Diagnostic Features	Specific Diagnostic Features
Decreased Production of RBCs	Evidence of decreased production: ↓ reticulocytes	**Pancytopenia due to bone marrow infiltration with**
Marrow infiltration		Leukemia, neuroblastoma, etc
Secondary to tumor infiltration		
Secondary to infiltration with nonmalignant cells		
Lipidoses		Lipid-filled macrophages
X-linked lymphoproliferative disorder		Erythrophagocytosis
		Hepatosplenomegaly
Decreased production of hematopoietic elements (bone marrow failure)		
Decreased RBC production only		
Constitutional: Diamond-Blackfan syndrome		Multiple physical deformities
Acquired		
Acquired pure red cell aplasia		Associated with thymoma
Transient erythrocytopenia of childhood		Associated with parvovirus infection
Decreased RBC and WBC production		
Constitutional		
Fanconi anemia		Multiple physical deformities
Shwachman syndrome		Pancreatic insufficiency
Decreased production of RBC, WBC, and platelets		
Constitutional		
Fanconi anemia		Multiple physical deformities
Shwachman syndrome		Pancreatic insufficiency
Acquired: aplastic anemia (idiopathic or secondary to toxins, drugs, or infection [eg, hepatitis B])		History of hepatitis B, toxin exposure
Dietary deficiency		
Iron deficiency		↓ MCV, ↓ MCH, ↑ RDW, ↓ serum iron, ↓ serum ferritin, excessive milk intake
Folic acid deficiency		↑ MCV, ↑ RDW, megaloblastic marrow, low serum and RBC folate
Vitamin B₁₂ deficiency		↑ MCV, ↑ RDW, megaloblastic marrow, low serum B₁₂ levels, Schilling test
Vitamin C deficiency		Clinical scurvy
Protein deficiency		Kwashiorkor
Hypothyroidism		Low T4, elevated TSH
Increased Production (Hemolysis)	Evidence of hemolysis: ↑ reticulocytes	
Intrinsic RBC defects		
RBC membrane defects (spherocytosis, elliptocytosis)	Hyperbilirubinemia	+ Osmotic fragility, spectrin deficiency (HS)
RBC enzyme defects (G6PD deficiency, pyruvate kinase)	↑ LDH (RBC)	+ Enzyme assays
Hemoglobin defects	MCV may be ↑ if reticulocytes high	
1. Qualitative defects (sickle cell anemia, Hb C, Hb E)		Hb electrophoresis
2. Quantitative defects (thalassemia)		↑ Hb A2 (β-thalassemia), targets cells, basophilic stippling
Extrinsic RBC disorders		
Immune		
Isoimmune hemolytic anemia (eg, ABO, Rh incompatibility)		+ Coombs test
Autoimmune hemolytic anemia		
Idiopathic		
Secondary: postviral, autoimmune disorders, Evans syndrome		+ ANA
Nonimmune (eg, DIC, HUS)		Concomitant renal disease (HUS)
Blood Loss	Reticulocytes normal (acute loss)	
Overt (eg, splenic sequestration, gastrointestinal, or nasal bleeding)	↑ Reticulocytes (chronic loss, not iron deficient)	Sickle cell anemia (splenic sequestration)
Occult (eg, bleeding Meckel diverticulum, pulmonary hemosiderosis)	↓ Reticulocytes (chronic loss, iron deficient); may have rapidly falling hematocrit	Pulmonary infiltrates iron deficiency (pulmonary hemosiderosis)

Abbreviations: RBC, red blood cell; WBC, white blood cell; MCV, mean corpuscular volume; MCH, mean corpuscular hemoglobin; RDW, red cell distribution width; TSH, thyroid-stimulating hormone; G6PD, glucose-6-phosphate dehydrogenase; Hb, hemoglobin; LDH, lactate dehydrogenase; HS, hereditary spherocytosis; DIC, disseminated intravascular coagulation; HUS, hemolytic-uremic syndrome; ANA, antinuclear antibodies.

[a]Adapted from Lanzkowsky P. *Manual of Pediatric Hematology-Oncology*. New York, NY: Churchill Livingstone; 1989:2–3.

Anemia of inflammation or chronic disease can be seen in children with chronic infections, generalized inflammatory disorders (rheumatoid arthritis), and some cancers. It is characterized by a decrease in serum iron and iron binding capacity, an increase in ferritin, and the presence of iron in bone marrow macrophages indicating impaired iron mobilization from storage sites. Increased synthesis of hepcidin, an iron regulatory hormone, under the influence of inflammatory cytokines seems to be responsible for the hypoferremia observed in anemia of inflammation. In general, the anemia of inflammation is mild and may be microcytic or normocytic.

Macrocytic Anemias

Both **folate** and **vitamin B_{12} deficiency** cause a macrocytic anemia as a consequence of defective erythroid precursor nuclear maturation and megaloblastic changes in the bone marrow. Folate is absorbed in the duodenum and jejunum and is widely available in meats, green leafy vegetables, and cereals. Because of the ubiquity of folate, dietary deficiency is uncommon; however, infants fed exclusively goat's milk are at risk because of the exceedingly low levels of folate in goat's milk. Individuals with chronic hemolytic anemias may also become folate-deficient because of high bone marrow activity and increased demand.

Vitamin B_{12} is available from animal sources and is actively absorbed in the terminal ileum in association with intrinsic factor. Vitamin B_{12} deficiency can occur in individuals with a strict vegan diet (or in exclusively breastfed infants of women following a strict vegan diet); however, it usually occurs as a consequence of malabsorption. Decreased absorption can occur in the setting of pernicious anemia (decreased intrinsic factor), surgical resection, or GI disease.

Other causes of macrocytic anemias include congenital hypoplastic anemias (eg, Diamond-Blackfan anemia), myelodysplastic syndromes, and chemotherapeutic agents (eg, methotrexate).

Normocytic Anemias

Normocytic anemias can be classified as hemolytic anemias (associated with a reticulocytosis) and hypoplastic anemias (reticulocytopenic). **Hemolytic anemias** can be further divided into disorders that are intrinsic to the RBC or extrinsic to it. Intrinsic RBC disorders include hemoglobinopathies, enzymopathies, and membranopathies.

Sickle cell disease is most common in individuals of African or mixed African and Latino descent. Inheritance of 2 sickle β-globin genes (hemoglobin SS) is the most common form, however, other significant sickle syndromes include hemoglobin SC, Sβ+ thalassemia, and Sβ° thalassemia. Hemolytic anemia and vaso-occlusive episodes are the hallmarks of sickle cell disease. The anemia is generally well tolerated with hemoglobin values in the 6.5 to 8.5 g/dL range with an associated reticulocytosis (5%–15%). The 2 most common hematologic complications in sickle cell disease are aplastic crises and splenic sequestration—both of which can cause an acute drop in hemoglobin. Aplastic crises are generally the result of infection with parvovirus, which temporarily causes the complete cessation of red cell production. Splenic sequestration occurs most commonly in infants and young children with sickle cell disease, often in association with a viral illness. Large amounts of blood can be quickly trapped in the spleen causing hypovolemia, shock, and massive splenomegaly.

Pyruvate kinase deficiency is the most common red cell enzyme defect causing a chronic congenital hemolytic anemia. The degree of hemolysis is variable, ranging from a mild fully compensated hemolytic process without anemia to a transfusion-dependent anemia. Individuals with severe hemolysis may be chronically jaundiced and may develop the clinical complications of chronic hemolytic states (gall stones, transient aplastic crises in association with infections, folate deficiency and, infrequently, skin ulcers.) The enzymatic activity of G6PD is essential in protecting the red cell proteins from oxidative damage. **Glucose-6-phosphate dehydrogenase deficiency** renders the red cell susceptible to oxidant stress and hemolysis. A number of variants have been defined; however, the most common variants are those associated with acute intermittent hemolytic anemias with exposure to oxidant stresses (fava beans, medications). Variants associated with chronic hemolytic anemias are very rare.

Hereditary spherocytosis is the most common red cell membranopathy and is characterized by the presence of spherical-shaped erythrocytes on the peripheral blood smear. Increased membrane fragility due to defects in proteins of the red cell membrane (spectrin, ankyrin, band 3, protein 4.2) leads to membrane vesiculation and membrane loss and the assumption of a spheroidal shape. Hemolysis occurs as these spherocytes are then trapped within the spleen. Clinically, the degree of hemolysis varies from mild anemia to severe transfusion dependence. The complications of a chronic hemolytic state such as gallstones, aplastic crises, and folate deficiency can also be observed.

Hemolytic anemias that are due to factors extrinsic to the red cell can be further classified as immune-mediated or nonimmune. **Immune-mediated anemias** may be due to alloantibodies that occur in the setting of neonatal Rh or ABO incompatibility or transfusion reactions. Autoantibodies may occur in association with infection, autoimmune disorders, malignancy, or drugs. In children, autoantibodies (warm immunoglobulin G) are often seen in association with a viral illness. **Nonimmune hemolytic anemias** include microangiopathic and macroangiopathic hemolytic anemias due to a myriad of etiologies including infections, drugs, toxins, burns, and heart valves.

Reticulocytopenic anemias can be congenital or acquired and can occur in isolation or in the setting of pancytopenia. **Diamond-Blackfan anemia** is a ribosomal disorder that causes a congenital pure red cell aplasia that presents early in infancy. The bone marrow typically shows red cell aplasia with a paucity of red cell precursors, and the red cells may be normocytic or macrocytic. Associated congenital anomalies such as craniofacial anomalies, radial abnormalities, and renal and cardiac defects are seen in approximately 25% of affected individuals. **Transient erythroblastopenia of childhood** is an acquired reticulocytopenic anemia that typically occurs following a viral illness. The usual age of presentation is between 2 to 3 years and complete recovery is the natural course.

Evaluation

History

When evaluating an infant or child with anemia, the age, rapidity of onset of symptoms, MCV, and suspected underlying mechanism of anemia will direct the history (Questions Box). In most instances, it is important to inquire about dietary habits, with particular attention to the type and amount of milk ingested per day (number of bottles/ounces). Ingestion of more than 24 oz of cow's milk should raise the suspicion for iron deficiency anemia. Medication use, potential toxin ingestion (lead), or a history of pica should be determined as well. In addition, inquiries to potential sources of blood loss (hematochezia, melena, menorrhagia, hematuria, epistaxis, pulmonary) should be addressed. Acute onset of jaundice, icterus, or dark urine is suggestive of hemolysis and should elicit questions regarding possible triggers (fava beans, medications, illnesses). A personal history of neonatal hyperbilirubinemia or a family history of anemia, gallstones, cholecystectomy, or splenectomy is highly suggestive of a congenital hemolytic anemia. Acute

> ## Questions
>
> ### Anemia
>
> - Does the child eat meat?
> - Does the child drink too much milk (>24 oz/d)?
> - Has the child lost a lot of blood recently?
> - Have the child's eyes appeared yellow?
> - Does the child have a family history of anemia, jaundice, or gallstones?

onset of hemolysis with a viral illness is consistent with an autoimmune hemolytic anemia. Marrow failure syndromes often present with a prolonged history of increased fatigue and pallor, with occasional history of previous red cell transfusions prior to diagnosis. In acquired marrow failure states such as aplastic anemia, the history is occasionally consistent with antecedent hepatitis, a viral syndrome, or, rarely, exposure to toxins such as benzene and toluene-containing compounds, or oral chloramphenicol use (commonly available over the counter in Latin America).

Physical Examination

Most children who present with anemia will have a normal physical examination. Depending on the degree of anemia, pallor, tachycardia, or tachypnea may be present. In severe cases of anemia (hemoglobin <3 g/dL) with chronic onset and moderate anemia (hemoglobin of 3–7 g/dL) with acute onset (blood loss), CHF can occur. Other physical findings are unique to certain red cell disorders. Infants with sickle cell disease may present with dactylitis, a form of painful crisis that manifests as swelling of 1 to 4 digits associated with pain and sometimes fever. Splenomegaly can be seen in sickle cell disease (in younger children prior to autosplenectomy), β-thalassemia major and intermedia, and red cell membrane disorders, most commonly hereditary spherocytosis. In children with severe chronic hemolysis, regardless of etiology, classic facies (often called thalassemic facies) can develop, with frontal bossing and flattened nasal bridge, due to thinning of the facial bones from brisk intramedullary hematopoiesis. Children with Diamond-Blackfan anemia or Fanconi anemia may have physical anomalies such as thumb or radial abnormalities, short stature, cardiac or renal anomalies, and mental retardation. Aplastic anemia or malignant infiltration of the bone marrow may present with concomitant neutropenia and thrombocytopenia. If neutropenic (absolute neutrophil count <1,000/mL), signs of fever or infection may be present. If thrombocytopenic, bruises; petechiae; and mucosal bleeding from the mouth, nose, and GI tract may also be present. With malignancy, such as leukemia, lymphadenopathy and hepatosplenomegaly may also be observed.

Laboratory Tests

The complete blood count (**CBC**) and peripheral blood smear provide a wealth of information and should be evaluated closely to narrow the differential diagnosis. The first step is to determine if the child is truly anemic by referencing the normal **hemoglobin/hematocrit** values for the child's age and gender. The second step is to evaluate the red cell indices. The **MCV** is a direct measure of red cell size and allows for classification of the anemia as microcytic, normocytic, or macrocytic. The mean corpuscular hemoglobin (**MCH**) is a calculated value that typically parallels the MCV. The MCH concentration is a measure of the red cell hydration status and is useful when elevated as this reflects the presence of spherocytes. The red cell volume distribution width reflects the variation in red cell size (usually normal with thalassemia trait and elevated in iron deficiency). The RBC count can be useful because it is typically elevated (>5 million/μL) in a child with thalassemia trait and decreased in iron deficiency anemia. Review of the **white blood cell and platelet count** will provide information as to whether other cell lines are affected. The **peripheral blood smear** provides information regarding RBC morphology characteristic of different red cell disorders (sickle cells, spherocytes, elliptocytes, schistocytes). The presence of polychromasia is suggestive of a hemolytic process. White blood cell morphology can also suggest the etiology of the anemia (hypersegmented neutrophils in folate or vitamin B_{12} deficiency). The **reticulocyte count** provides clues to the underlying mechanism of anemia. An elevated reticulocyte count is consistent with a hemolytic or blood loss picture whereas a reduced or normal reticulocyte count in the face of anemia suggests a production problem. If hemolysis is evident, a **Coombs test** should be performed to determine if this is an immune-mediated process.

With the CBC, peripheral blood smear, and reticulocyte count, a focused differential diagnosis can be generated and more specific testing can be performed. Further studies specific for individual hemolytic diseases or particular diseases secondary to marrow failure are summarized in Table 71-2.

Imaging Studies

Few children routinely need imaging studies in the evaluation of their anemia. Hemolysis is reflected on x-ray by the "hair-on-end" appearance of bones. Patients who have anemia associated with lead poisoning may have lead deposition, referred to as **lead lines,** in their long bones.

Management

The treatment of anemia varies depending on the etiology. Nutritional anemias require dietary counseling and nutrient supplementation. With **iron deficiency anemia,** oral iron supplementation (6 mg/kg/d divided into 2–3 doses) should generate a brisk reticulocytosis within 7 days, and the hemoglobin should increase by 1.0 g/dL/wk thereafter. Therapy should be continued for an additional 6 to 8 weeks after the hemoglobin has normalized to replete iron stores. Failure to respond to iron therapy is most commonly due to noncompliance; however, alternative diagnoses (thalassemia trait), ongoing blood loss, or malabsorption states should also be considered.

Depending on the degree of hemolysis and compensation, individuals with congenital hemolytic anemias may require no transfusions, intermittent transfusions (due to aplastic crises), or regular transfusions. In general, all individuals should receive folate supplementation and be monitored for potential complications such as gallstones and aplastic crises. The more severely affected individuals may benefit from splenectomy. Individuals with G6PD deficiency should be counseled on the avoidance of potential triggers of hemolysis.

Two anemia-related conditions constitute emergencies. Prompt recognition of these conditions is vital if proper treatment is to be initiated. **Splenic sequestration** occurs in infants and young children with sickle cell disease who sequester large volumes of sickling blood within the spleen over a period of hours. This results in a rapidly dropping hemoglobin, clinically resembling anemia due to massive blood loss. The blood pooled in the spleen is not available to the circulation, and affected children are subject to fatal splenic rupture. Treatment involves transfusion or exchange transfusion. **Severe autoimmune hemolytic anemia** is the second anemia-related emergency. Children with this disorder can occasionally present with severe Coombs-positive anemia and clinical evidence of rapid hemolysis; their hemoglobin may fall as much as 1 g/dL per hour. These patients generally require hospitalization, transfusion, and treatment with high-dose steroids.

Prognosis

The prognosis for a child with anemia depends on the underlying cause. Children with some conditions (thalassemia trait) require no treatment and have an excellent prognosis. Early diagnosis and intervention through newborn screening for children with sickle cell disease has significantly reduced early mortality for this disease. Some children, such as those with β-thalassemia major or severe congenital hemolytic anemias, will be transfusion-dependent and will be subject to the complications of iron overload, which can be addressed with chelation therapy using deferoxamine. Some children with transfusion-dependent congenital hemolytic anemias may be candidates for splenectomy, with normalization of their hemoglobin values post-splenectomy. The prognosis for children with Diamond-Blackfan anemia depends on their responsiveness to steroid therapy and the need for transfusions. These individuals are at risk for certain malignancies.

CASE RESOLUTION

The girl described in the case history at the beginning of the chapter has hereditary spherocytosis. Her history is highly suggestive of a hereditary hemolytic disorder, and the combination of spherocytes in the peripheral smear; a negative Coombs test; and a positive, incubated, osmotic fragility test are diagnostic of the condition. At the age of 6 years, she undergoes a splenectomy and has no more hemolytic episodes that require transfusions.

Selected References

American Academy of Pediatrics Committee on Environmental Health. Screening for elevated blood lead levels. *Pediatrics.* 1998;101:1072–1078

Charache S, Lubin B, Reid CD, eds. *Management and Therapy of Sickle Cell Disease.* Bethesda, MD: National Institutes of Health; 1995. NIH Publication No. 96–2117

Fixler J, Styles L. Sickle cell disease. *Pediatr Clin North Am.* 2002;49:1193–1210

Hermiston ML, Mentzer WC. A practical approach to the evaluation of the anemic child. *Pediatr Clin North Am.* 2002;49:877–892

Lo L, Singer ST. Thalassemia: current approach to an old disease. *Pediatr Clin North Am.* 2002;49:1149–1164

McKie VC. Sickle cell anemia in children: practical issues for the pediatrician. *Pediatr Ann.* 1998;27:521–524

Oski FA, Brugnara C, Nathan DG. A diagnostic approach to the anemic patient. In: Nathan DG, Orkin SH, Ginsburg D, Look AT, eds. *Nathan and Oski's Hematology of Infancy and Childhood.* 6th ed. Philadelphia, PA: W. B. Saunders Company; 2003:409–418

Recommendations to prevent and control iron deficiency in the United States. Centers for Disease Control and Prevention. *MMWR Recomm Rep.* 1998;47:1–29

Bleeding Disorders

Wendy Y. Tcheng, MD

CASE STUDY

A 6-year-old girl presents with a several-month history of recurrent epistaxis. Episodes occur every 2 to 3 weeks and last 15 to 20 minutes at a time. Both nares are affected. Her mother also notes that the girl has always bruised easily. On physical examination, several 2- to 3-cm ecchymoses are noted on her lower extremities. Initial laboratory evaluation includes a complete blood count, which is normal (platelet count 300,000), normal a partial thromboplastin time of 30 seconds and prothrombin time of 12.5, international normalized ratio 1.1.

Questions

1. What conditions should be considered when easy bruisability is the chief complaint?
2. What is the appropriate laboratory evaluation for children with clinical signs of bleeding?
3. What management is appropriate for the most common pediatric bleeding disorders?
4. What are the common medical complications that children with bleeding disorders face?
5. When is consultation with a hematologist appropriate in a child with easy bruisability?

When evaluating a child with bruising or bleeding symptoms, the major challenge facing the pediatrician is to ascertain whether the degree of bleeding is appropriate for the hemostatic stress or whether further evaluation for a potential bleeding disorder is warranted. Bruising and bleeding are common childhood complaints and usually follow minor injury or trauma. However, in the child with an underlying hemostatic disorder, non-accidental trauma, or both, the bruising or bleeding may be more extensive than expected. A thorough medical history and physical examination and an understanding of hemostasis will aid in focusing the laboratory evaluation and elucidating the underlying etiology.

Epidemiology

Bleeding disorders can be inherited or acquired. Of the inherited bleeding disorders, von Willebrand disease is the most common, with a reported incidence ranging between 1 in 100 and 1 in 1,000. Von Willebrand disease is autosomally inherited, affecting males and females equally; however, more females are diagnosed because of the inherent hemostatic challenges that females face (menses, childbirth). Hemophilia is the most common severe bleeding disorder affecting about 1 in 5,000 males. Approximately 80% of cases are hemophilia A (factor VIII [FVIII] deficiency) and 20% are hemophilia B (factor IX [FIX] deficiency). Hemophilia is inherited in an X-linked fashion, but a third of newly diagnosed males have no previous family history and represent new mutations. Other inherited coagulation disorders and platelet disorders are rare and are listed in Table 72-1.

Acquired abnormalities of coagulation or platelets are much more common. These can occur in the setting of liver disease, vitamin K deficiency, renal disease, disseminated intravascular coagulation (DIC), infection, medications, malignancy, massive transfusion, post-surgery, and autoimmunity or alloimmunity. Immune thrombocytopenic purpura (ITP) is a common acquired childhood bleeding disorder with an incidence of 4 to 8 per 100,000 children per year. Neonatal alloimmune thrombocytopenia occurs in approximately 1 in 1,800 live births. Common acquired bleeding disorders are also listed in Table 72-1.

Clinical Presentation

Bleeding disorders can present in various ways depending on the etiology. Inherited bleeding disorders will often present during infancy or early childhood; however, mild disorders may go undiagnosed until later in life. In general, disorders of primary hemostasis (ie, von Willebrand disease, platelet disorders, collagen vascular disorders) will present with superficial, immediate, mucocutaneous-type bleeding. Characteristic bleeding symptoms include easy bruising, epistaxis, gum bleeding, menorrhagia, postpartum bleeding, and bleeding with dental extractions or surgeries. Disorders of secondary hemostasis, such as hemophilia A or B, will often present with deep, delayed bleeding, such as hemarthroses or muscular hematomas.

Acquired bleeding disorders typically present with an acute onset and often involve abnormalities of both primary and secondary hemostasis. Acute onset of bleeding symptoms in a toxic or ill-appearing child suggests a systemic process such as sepsis, DIC, malignancy, or hepatic or renal dysfunction. A well-appearing child with acute bleeding symptoms suggests ITP, an acquired inhibitor, or a medication-related cause.

	Table 72-1. Inherited Versus Acquired Bleeding Disorders	
Disorder	*Inherited*	*Acquired*

Coagulation	• von Willebrand disease
	• Hemophilia A (FVIII)
	• Hemophilia B (FIX)
	• Hemophilia C (FXI)
	• FII, FV, FVII, FX, or FXIII deficiency
	• Disorders of fibrinogen
	   — Dysfibrinogenemia, hypofibrinogenemia,
	     or afibrinogenemia
	• Disorders of fibrinolysis
	   — α_2-antiplasmin
	• PAI-1 deficiency
		• Vitamin K deficiency
		• Liver disease
		• DIC
		• Massive transfusion syndrome
		• Disorders of fibrinogen (dysfibrinogenemia or hypofibrinogenemia)
		   — Liver disease
		   — Renal disease
		   — Medication
		• Disorders associated with malignancy
		• Coagulation inhibitors

Platelet	• Quantitative
	   — Thrombocytopenia absent radii syndrome
	   — Amegakaryocytic thrombocytopenia
	   — Fanconi anemia
	• Qualitative
	   — Glanzmann thrombasthenia
	   — Storage pool disorders
	   — Release defects
	• Quantitative/qualitative
	   — Bernard-Soulier syndrome
	   — Wiskott-Aldrich syndrome
	   — Gray platelet syndrome
		• Quantitative
		   — Increased destruction
		     ~ Nonimmune-mediated
		       ◆ HUS
		       ◆ TTP
		       ◆ DIC
		     ~ Immune-mediated
		       ◆ ITP
		       ◆ Evan syndrome
		       ◆ NAIT
		       ◆ Medications
		   — Decreased production
		     ~ Aplastic anemia
		     ~ Malignancy infiltrating bone marrow
		     ~ Medications
		• Qualitative
		   — Medication
		   — Liver disease
		   — Uremia
		   — Post-cardiopulmonary bypass surgery

Abbreviations: DIC, disseminated intravascular coagulation; F, factor; PAI, plasminogen activator inhibitor; HUS, hemolytic uremic syndrome; TTP, thrombotic thrombocytopenic purpura; ITP, immune thrombocytopenic purpura; NAIT, neonatal alloimmune thrombocytopenic purpura.

Pathophysiology

Following vascular injury, hemostasis is initiated by exposure of flowing blood to subendothelial collagen and tissue factor. The primary phase of hemostasis leads to the production of a platelet plug. Von Willebrand factor (vWF), a multimeric glycoprotein of varying size, attaches to exposed subendothelial collagen and binds platelets via the platelet glycoprotein IB/IX receptor. Von Willebrand factor also serves as a carrier protein for FVIII, thereby localizing FVIII to areas of endothelial disruption. Once platelets adhere to vWF, they become activated and release their granular contents, produce thromboxane A_2, and express the fibrinogen receptor glycoprotein IIb/IIIa (GPIIB/IIIA). The release of thromboxane A_2 and other granular contents leads to local vasoconstriction and activation of additional platelets and their respective GPIIB/IIIA receptors, allowing for platelet aggregation. Fibrinogen binds to all of the exposed activated GPIIB/

IIIA sites, clumping the platelets together to form a platelet plug. The platelet plug stops local bleeding and provides a phospholipid surface for the coagulation reactions of secondary hemostasis to occur to form a definitive fibrin plug.

Secondary hemostasis is also initiated at the time of endothelial disruption with exposure of tissue factor to circulating blood. Tissue factor binds to FVIIa and this complex serves as the key initiator of in vivo hemostasis and by activating other tissue factor FVII (TF:FVII) complexes, as well as FIX, and factor X (FX). Once activated (either by FIXa or TF:FVIIa), FXa along with its cofactor, factor Va (FVa), activates prothrombin (FII) to thrombin (FIIa). Thrombin cleaves circulating fibrinogen to fibrin monomers that self-polymerize. Factor XIII then stabilizes the fibrin clot by forming cross-links within the clump of fibrin polymers. These coagulation reactions occur on the surface of the platelet plug and, with the generation of cross-linked fibrin, the primary platelet plug is converted into a definitive fibrin plug that prevents further bleeding. An overview of hemostasis is depicted in Figures 72-1 and 72-2. Deficiencies or impairments in any of these elements can lead to inadequate hemostasis and excessive hemorrhage.

The delicate balance of hemostasis and thrombosis is maintained by inhibitors (protein C, protein S, antithrombin, tissue factor pathway inhibitor) at each step of the coagulation cascade. These natural anticoagulants serve to prevent excessive thrombus formation. Fibrinolysis is mediated by plasmin, which cleaves both fibrinogen and fibrin within a thrombus, allowing for restoration of vessel patency following hemostasis. Plasmin is activated by tissue plasminogen activator (tPA) and urokinase. Fibrinolysis is

kept in check by plasminogen activator inhibitor (PAI-1), which inactivates tPA, and α_2-antiplasmin, which inactivates plasmin (Figure 72-3). Any defects in the fibrinolytic system that leads to an increase in fibrinolysis can result in excessive bleeding.

Differential Diagnosis

In developing the differential diagnosis for a child with bleeding symptoms, it is important to obtain a thorough bleeding history and physical examination. The age, bleeding pattern, duration of symptoms, family history, and overall clinical status of the child will help to narrow the spectrum of possibilities.

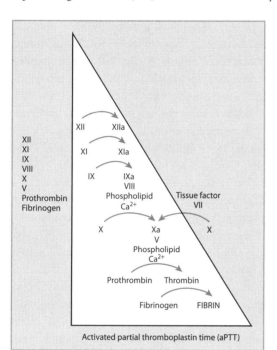

Figure 72-1. Intrinsic pathway reflected by aPTT.

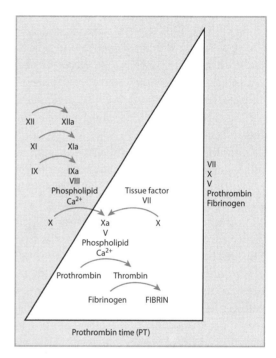

Figure 72-2. Coagulation pathway. Extrinsic pathway reflected by PT.

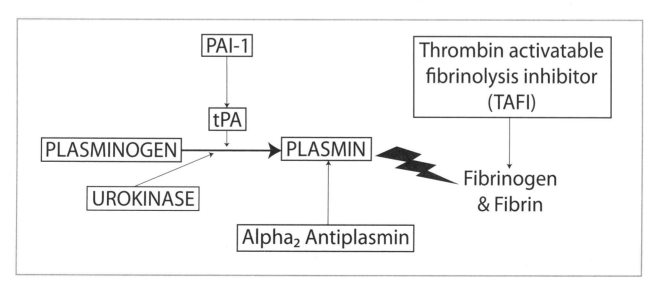

Figure 72-3. Fibrinolysis. Abbreviations: PAI, plasminogen activator inhibitor; tPA, tissue plasminogen activator.

Child With Chronic History of Mucocutaneous Bleeding

In a child who presents with a history of easy bruising, epistaxis, or menorrhagia, the primary differential diagnosis includes von Willebrand disease, platelet disorders, and collagen vascular disorders (disorders of primary hemostasis). **Von Willebrand disease** is caused by a quantitative or qualitative defect of vWF. Von Willebrand factor plays an important role in both primary hemostasis (mediates platelet adhesion at sites of vascular injury) and secondary hemostasis (stabilizes FVIII in plasma). Von Willebrand disease is autosomally inherited and classified into 3 different types. Type 1 refers to a partial quantitative deficiency of vWF. Type 2 refers to qualitative abnormalities of vWF and is further subclassified as type 2A, 2B, 2M, and 2N. Type 3, the most severe form, refers to a complete deficiency of vWF. Type 1 is the most common form, accounting for 70% to 80% of cases. Bleeding symptoms tend to be mild and are characterized by easy bruising, epistaxis, menorrhagia, and prolonged oozing after minor or major surgeries. Only the most severely affected patients (type 3), with very low FVIII levels, will have soft tissue bleeding and hemarthroses similar to an individual with moderate or severe hemophilia.

Qualitative platelet disorders also present with mucocutaneous bleeding, often during infancy. In **Bernard-Soulier syndrome,** the platelets lack a functional glycoprotein IB/IX receptor complex on the platelet surface, resulting in defective platelet adhesion to vWF at sites of vascular injury. It is an autosomal-recessive disorder and is usually seen in consanguineous families. The platelets tend to be large on peripheral smear, and there may be a degree of thrombocytopenia. **Glanzmann thrombasthenia** is characterized by an absence or defect in the platelet membrane GPIIB/IIIA receptor, the main fibrinogen receptor on the platelet surface that allows for platelet aggregation. It is autosomal-recessively inherited and is more common in the presence of consanguinity. Other qualitative platelet disorders such as **storage pool disorders** and **platelet release defects** can also present in a similar manner.

Collagen-vascular disorders, such as Marfan syndrome, Ehlers-Danlos syndrome, and pseudoxanthoma elasticum, can present with bruising and bleeding symptoms. This increased bleeding diathesis is due to an easy disruption of the integrity of the vascular endothelium.

Other rare coagulation disorders to consider in a child with recurrent bleeding symptoms include deficiencies of FXI, FXIII, PAI-1, and α_2-antiplasmin. **Factor XI deficiency,** also known as *hemophilia C,* is a rare bleeding disorder with a high prevalence in the Ashkenazi Jewish population. It differs from the other hemophilias in that it is autosomally inherited and tends to have milder symptoms. Bleeding episodes are typically in response to trauma or surgery, and the deep tissue or intra-articular bleeds characteristic of FVIII or FIX deficiency are not seen. **Factor XIII deficiency** is characterized by delayed or prolonged bleeding because the clots formed are friable owing to the lack of cross-linkage of fibrin monomers by FXIII. It is inherited in an autosomal-dominant pattern, and in the homozygous state usually presents in infancy with umbilical cord bleeding or delayed separation, as well as intracranial hemorrhage. Heterozygotes may present later in life with delayed or prolonged bleeding following trauma or surgery and poor wound healing. **Disorders of fibrinolysis** (deficiency of PAI-1 or α_2-antiplasmin) can also present with prolonged bleeding following trauma.

Child With History of Deep, Delayed Bleeding

Deep tissue and intra-articular bleeding is the hallmark bleeding pattern of **hemophilia.** The differential diagnosis for a child who presents with this type of bleeding is hemophilia A (FVIII deficiency) or B (FIX deficiency), FVII deficiency, and type 3 von Willebrand disease. Clinically, hemophilia is classified according to the factor level with less than 1% factor activity as severe, 1% to 5% as moderate, and greater than 5% as mild. The factor level correlates well with the bleeding tendency and, in general, males with severe hemophilia will have spontaneous bleeds or bleeding with minimal trauma. Males with moderate or mild hemophilia will bleed with trauma. The bleeding complications of hemophilia vary as the child grows. Infants may present with a cephalohematoma or intracranial hemorrhage, particularly if the delivery was complicated with the use of forceps or vacuum extraction. Bleeding with circumcision, heel sticks, or blood draws may also occur. As the infant starts crawling, bruises and soft tissue hematomas on the lower extremities become common. As the toddler becomes upright, the first hemarthroses can occur, typically involving the ankle. The older child has hemarthroses primarily involving the knees and elbows.

Factor VII deficiency is very rare; however, it can present with a bleeding pattern similar to hemophilia A or B. Type 3 von Willebrand disease, which is characterized by an absence of vWF (the carrier protein for FVIII), can have FVIII levels as low as an individual with severe or moderate hemophilia A. In addition to the characteristic mucocutaneous bleeding seen with von Willebrand disease, these individuals can also have deep tissue and intra-articular bleeding.

Well-Appearing Child With Acute Onset of Bleeding Symptoms

An acute onset of bleeding symptoms is consistent with an acquired abnormality of hemostasis. Acute **ITP** is a common acquired bleeding disorder of childhood due to the development of autoantibodies directed against the patient's platelets. These autoantibodies, which cross-react with platelet surface antigens, are thought to develop in response to an infection. Typically, a healthy child (usually between the ages of 2 to 10 years) presents with an abrupt onset of bleeding symptoms, diffuse petechiae and bruising and, occasionally, "wet" bleeding (epistaxis, gum bleeding, gastrointestinal [GI] bleeding). There is often a history of a viral illness or immunization. The complete blood count (CBC) reveals an isolated thrombocytopenia, and large platelets are seen on peripheral smear reflecting an active marrow with the production of young platelets. In approximately 80% of cases, ITP is an acute, self-limited process resolving within 6 months of diagnosis with or without therapy. Chronic ITP exists when the thrombocytopenia persists beyond 6 months. Although it is not possible to predict at diagnosis whether a patient will go on to have chronic ITP, there are certain presenting features that are associated with a higher risk for chronicity. These include older age at presentation (>10 years), female gender, existing autoimmune disease, and insidious onset of symptoms. In most cases of chronic ITP, the platelet count ranges between 40,000 to 80,000, and bleeding symptoms are minimal.

Acquired coagulation inhibitors are rare in children without an underlying coagulation disorder; however, they can occur in the setting of malignancy, infection, or post-surgery. Antiphospholipid antibodies can cause a prolongation of the partial thromboplastin time (PTT) or prothrombin time (PT); however, these antibodies are not associated with bleeding and are typically transient following a viral illness. The exception is if the antiphospholipid antibody is directed against prothrombin, resulting in low levels of prothrombin. In this situation, bleeding may be associated but is usually mild and intervention unnecessary.

Acquired abnormalities of coagulation or platelet function can also occur in association with **medications.** Aspirin and nonsteroidal anti-inflammatory drugs are common medications that affect the function of platelets. Warfarin, a vitamin K antagonist, is commonly used as an anticoagulant. One percent to 3% of patients on therapeutic warfarin can experience bleeding complications. Chronic antibiotic use can result in vitamin K deficiency and a depletion of the vitamin K–dependent factors (II, VII, IX, X).

Ill-Appearing Child With Acute Onset of Bleeding Symptoms

Acute onset of bleeding in an ill-appearing child suggests an acquired systemic process. **Disseminated intravascular coagulation** is a consumptive coagulopathy that can occur secondary to a number of disorders including sepsis, trauma, or malignancy. Disseminated intravascular coagulation occurs as a result of endothelial disruption and initiation of abnormal coagulation; fibrin deposition; and depletion of multiple clotting factors, inhibitor proteins, and platelets.

Because the liver is the primary site of synthesis for most of the coagulation factors, **liver dysfunction** due to any illness can result in an imbalance in the hemostatic system. In addition, thrombocytopenia may be present with chronic liver disease because of portal hypertension and associated splenomegaly with sequestration. Causes of the depletion of vitamin K–dependent factors such as obstructive jaundice, malabsorptive states (cystic fibrosis), parenchymal liver disease, and chronic antibiotic use can also predispose to bleeding.

Renal disease with uremia impairs platelet function and can present with bleeding symptoms as well. A **malignancy** infiltrating the bone marrow, such as leukemia, lymphoma, or neuroblastoma, can cause thrombocytopenia and resultant platelet bleeding. Acquired von Willebrand disease can occur with Wilms tumor and present with mucocutaneous bleeding. **Bone marrow failure syndromes** can also present with thrombocytopenia and associated bleeding.

Infant With Bleeding Symptoms

An infant who presents with bleeding symptoms may have a congenital bleeding disorder or an acquired condition. **Inherited coagulation deficiencies** (VII, VIII, IX, XI, XIII, type 3 von Willebrand disease) and qualitative platelet disorders may present in the newborn period with intracranial hemorrhage or cephalohematoma, bleeding with heel sticks or blood draws, umbilical cord bleeding, and bleeding with circumcision. **Congenital thrombocytopenias** usually present within the first year of life and are associated with other syndromic features. Thrombocytopenia–absent radius (TAR) syndrome is an autosomal-recessive condition, typically recognized in the newborn period, characterized by thrombocytopenia, skeletal anomalies (most commonly radial agenesis), and renal and cardiac abnormalities. Other congenital thrombocytopenias include amegakaryocytic thrombocytopenia, Fanconi anemia, and Wiskott-Aldrich syndrome.

Neonatal alloimmune thrombocytopenia (NAIT) is a rare condition in which an infant inherits platelet antigens from the father that are different from the mother. The mother becomes alloimmunized to the infant's platelet antigens during pregnancy, similar to erythrocyte alloimmunization from Rh incompatibility. The maternal immunoglobulin G alloantibodies cross the placenta and destroy the infant's platelets, resulting in a transient but severe thrombocytopenia in the infant. Thrombocytopenia in the infant lasts a few weeks to several months until the maternal antibody is cleared. Unlike Rh alloimmunization, NAIT can occur in the first pregnancy. The risk of intracranial hemorrhage is significant, with a reported incidence of up to 20% in some series, and can occur in utero. Neonatal thrombocytopenia can also occur as a consequence of **maternal ITP** with maternal transfer of antibody. Bleeding tends to be mild in this setting and intracranial hemorrhage is rare. The thrombocytopenia resolves after several weeks. An acquired thrombocytopenia most often occurs in the setting of an ill infant with sepsis, congenital viral infection, necrotizing enterocolitis, respiratory distress syndrome, asphyxia, or congenital heart disease. Drug-associated thrombocytopenia can also occur in the hospitalized infant.

Vitamin K deficiency in the neonate has 3 different presentations. **Classic hemorrhagic disease of the newborn** presents between days 2 to 7 of life and is due to the immature neonatal liver and impaired clotting factor synthesis, inadequate vitamin K intake, and a sterile neonatal gut. With the advent of vitamin K prophylaxis at birth, this form of vitamin K deficiency is rarely seen. **Early hemorrhagic disease of the newborn** presents in the first 24 hours of life and is due to maternal medications that affect vitamin K metabolism (anticonvulsants). **Late vitamin K deficiency** occurs after the first week of life and is associated with a number of conditions in which vitamin K stores may be low, such as inadequate intake in breastfed infants, impaired absorption in infants with chronic diarrhea, antibiotic use, cystic fibrosis, and other GI disorders. Bleeding symptoms associated with vitamin K deficiency can be quite severe with a significant incidence of GI, deep tissue, and intracranial hemorrhage.

Evaluation

History

A thorough bleeding history and physical examination should enable the pediatrician to determine the likelihood of an underlying bleeding disorder. The pattern of bleeding, the timing of the symptoms (acute vs chronic), the overall health of the child, and the family history are important in helping to determine the underlying etiology. Box 72-1 lists the pertinent questions to ask when obtaining a bleeding history.

Bruises are a common childhood complaint. Normal bruising that occurs in an active child must be differentiated from pathologic bruising owing to a possible bleeding disorder or non-accidental trauma. Bruises over exposed bony prominences such as the anterior tibial region or the knees are common. Bruises of a size inconsistent with the degree of reported trauma, and bruises in nonexposed or unusual areas (back, chest, shoulders, or upper arms) should alert the pediatrician to a possible bleeding disorder or non-accidental trauma. Linear or geometric bruises are concerning for non-accidental trauma. Epistaxis, another common complaint, is most often due to digital trauma or allergic rhinitis. However, epistaxis unrelieved by 15 minutes of appropriately applied pressure or epistaxis requiring packing, cautery, or transfusions is highly suggestive of a bleeding disorder. Menorrhagia, defined as menstrual flow greater than 7 days, frequently stained clothes, and iron deficiency anemia in an adolescent female are concerning. Persistent or recurrent bleeding with dental extractions (beyond the day of the procedure) or with surgeries also merits a closer evaluation. However, if a child has undergone previous dental extractions or surgeries without bleeding complications, an underlying bleeding disorder is unlikely.

Physical Examination

Depending on the underlying bleeding disorder and the timing of presentation, the physical examination may be completely normal at the time of presentation. If there is active bleeding, physical signs may include petechiae, ecchymoses, mucosal bleeding (nasal, oral, vaginal), hematuria, swollen joints (hemarthrosis), or limited range of motion. Children with bleeding associated with an acquired disorder such as infection, malignancy, autoimmunity, or liver or renal dysfunction may have physical signs specific to the underlying illness. Children with bleeding associated with a genetic disorder may have a normal examination or congenital anomalies associated with a particular syndrome.

Laboratory Tests

The extent of the laboratory evaluation is dependent on the bleeding history and clinical presentation. Initial laboratory studies for a potential bleeding disorder should include a CBC with a peripheral smear, a PT, and an activated PTT (aPTT).

The **CBC** is useful in providing a platelet count to identify suspected thrombocytopenia. In addition, abnormalities in the white blood cell count or red cell indices can provide clues to the underlying

---

> **Box 72-1. Pertinent Questions for a Bleeding History**
>
> - Is the bleeding acute or chronic?
>   - For acute onset bleeding
>   - ~ What type of bleeding is the child experiencing?
>   - ~ Is the child well-appearing or toxic?
>   - ~ Is there a history of recent illness?
>   - ~ Is the child taking any medications?
>   - ~ Does the child have any medical problems?
>   - For chronic history of bleeding
>   - ~ What type of bleeding is the child experiencing?
>   - ♦ Bruising (location, size, palpable hematoma)
>   - ♦ Epistaxis (duration of bleeding, history of packing, cauterization, or transfusion)
>   - ♦ Bleeding with vaccinations, injections, minor cuts
>   - ♦ Bleeding with dental extractions/surgeries
>   - ♦ Menses (total number of days of bleeding, leaking, alteration of activities during menses, diagnosis of iron deficiency, use of oral contraceptives, history of transfusion)
>   - ~ Medications
>   - ~ Family history (obstetric and gynecologic history of female relatives)

process. A microcytic anemia consistent with iron deficiency would suggest chronic blood loss and raise the suspicion for an underlying bleeding disorder. Pancytopenia would suggest an underlying bone marrow failure syndrome or a possible malignancy such as leukemia. Review of the **peripheral smear** can confirm the presence of true thrombocytopenia and allow for an assessment of platelet, white blood cell, and red blood cell morphology.

The **PT** reflects the extrinsic and common pathway and the **aPTT** reflects the intrinsic and common pathway. A prolonged PT or PTT should be followed up with a 1:1 mixing study to determine whether the prolongation is due to a factor deficiency or the presence of an inhibitor. The **bleeding time** is a reflection of primary hemostasis (platelets, vWF, vascular integrity), but is rarely performed in pediatrics because of the unreliability and difficulty of performing this test in children. The **PFA-100 screen** is a relatively new laboratory test that is superior to the bleeding time and can identify most defects in primary hemostasis.

A stepwise approach to more specific testing is dictated by the clinical presentation and screening test results and is best performed with the consultation of a pediatric hematologist. When an abnormality of primary hemostasis is suspected, the initial evaluation should focus on von Willebrand disease because it is the most common disorder. A **vWF panel,** which includes vWF antigen, ristocetin cofactor activity (functional measures of vWF), FVIII activity, and a vWF multimer analysis, should be performed. Many factors may transiently increase vWF levels (stress, inflammation, hormones, exercise, oral contraceptives), and normal results are frequently encountered in patients with type 1 von Willebrand disease. Repeat testing is often necessary to make the diagnosis and should be pursued if the suspicion is high. For hemophilia or any other suspected factor deficiency, a specific **coagulation factor assay** must be performed. For patients with suspected qualitative platelet disorder, **platelet aggregation studies** (measuring the degree and pattern of platelet aggregation to various agonists) or **flow cytometry** (measuring the platelet surface GP expression) can be performed. On a case-by-case basis, additional studies such as fibrinogen, d-dimer, fibrin split products, thrombin time, factor inhibitor assay, autoimmune studies, liver function tests, creatinine, or blood urea nitrogen may be indicated. Table 72-2 lists the major screening tests for hemostasis.

Imaging Studies

In general, imaging studies are not indicated. Bone films may be taken of the upper extremities in patients with thrombocytopenia to rule out Fanconi anemia and TAR syndrome.

Management

The management of bleeding disorders is dependent on the underlying abnormality. However, general supportive measures such as local pressure for bleeding, avoidance of blood draws, and avoidance of medications that affect the function of platelets or hemostasis can be applied to most clinical scenarios of bleeding.

Treatment of **von Willebrand disease** is dependent on the subtype and the severity of bleeding symptoms. For mild bleeding symptoms, supportive measures alone may be all that is necessary—applying appropriate pressure for epistaxis, ice pack for bruises, and avoidance of antiplatelet medications. For type 1 von Willebrand disease, DDAVP (synthetic vasopressin) can be used and is available as a concentrated nasal spray or intravenously. DDAVP stimulates endothelial release of vWF and can increase levels 2- to 3-fold. For type 3 and most cases of type 2 von Willebrand disease, replacement therapy with FVIII concentrates that contain vWF is necessary for significant bleeding episodes. Antifibrinolytic agents such as aminocaproic acid are very effective for mucosal bleeding and can be used either alone for mild cases or in conjunction with DDAVP or FVIII concentrates in more severe episodes of bleeding. For females with menorrhagia, a trial of oral contraceptives is reasonable because estrogen can increase vWF levels. This response is variable, however, and if not effective, aminocaproic acid and nasal DDAVP may be necessary

The treatment for most **qualitative platelet disorders** is supportive. Mild bleeding episodes can be treated nonspecifically with antifibrinolytic agents or DDAVP. Platelet transfusions should be reserved for life-threatening bleeds and otherwise avoided because of the risk for developing antibodies.

The management for **acute ITP** consists of family education, supportive measures and, in selected cases, pharmacologic therapies. The natural course of acute ITP is for the platelet count to rise within 1 to 3 weeks of presentation. The impetus to treat is the theoretical prevention of intracranial hemorrhage; however, the incidence of

Table 72-2. Laboratory Evaluation for Hemostasis

Laboratory Test	Measured Hemostatic Function
CBC	Platelet count
Peripheral blood smear	Platelet morphology
aPTT	Factors I, II, V, VIII, IX, XI, XII (intrinsic and common pathway)
PT	Factors I, II, V, VII, X (extrinsic and common pathway)
aPTT and PT mixing studies	Performed when aPTT/PT is prolonged; patient plasma and normal plasma is mixed 1:1, and then aPTT/PT repeated; if the aPTT/PT corrects, there is a factor deficiency, if not, there is an inhibitor
Bleeding time (not recommended)	Primary hemostasis (platelets, vWF, endothelial integrity)
PFA-100 screen	Primary hemostasis (platelets, vWF)
Thrombin time	Fibrinogen
vWF panel	vWF antigen (amount of vWF) Ristocetin cofactor activity (function of vWF) Factor VIII activity vWF multimer analysis (distribution of multimers)
Coagulation factor assays	Specific factor activity
Platelet aggregation studies	Platelet function; patient platelets are exposed to agonists and the degree of aggregation and pattern of the response is unique for various qualitative platelet disorders

Abbreviations: CBC, complete blood count; aPTT, activated partial thromboplastin time; PT, prothrombin time; vWF, von Willebrand factor.

this complication is less than 1%, and there are no data to confirm that any of the currently available therapies actually prevent this complication. Pharmacologic intervention does increase the platelet count more rapidly and may prevent a significant bleeding complication. The decision to treat must be individualized taking into consideration the child's age, bleeding symptoms, child's activity level, and parental anxiety level. Treatment options include observation without medical therapy, steroids, intravenous (IV) gammaglobulin, and anti-D immunoglobulin. Anti-D immunoglobulin can only be used in patients who are Rh positive. In all cases, parents should be instructed to avoid the use of aspirin, ibuprofen, and other antiplatelet medications; to avoid intramuscular injections; and to postpone immunizations and allergic desensitization injections that may exacerbate the degree of thrombocytopenia. Physical activity should be limited with specific instruction to avoid activities that may cause head injury. Parents should also be educated to the signs and symptoms of an intracranial hemorrhage and given instructions as to what to do in the event of an emergency. Therapeutic options for **chronic ITP** include observation without therapy, regular infusions of IV immune globulin (IVIG) or anti-D immunoglobulin (for Rh+ patients), immunosuppressive agents, and laparoscopic splenectomy. Treatment for acute bleeding in **neonatal alloimmune thrombocytopenia** includes transfusion of maternal platelets and IVIG.

Prevention and early treatment of bleeding episodes, family education, and good well-child care are important in providing comprehensive **hemophilia** care. The current standard of care for patients with severe hemophilia is prophylaxis, the IV administration of factor on a regular schedule (every other day, 3 times a week, or twice a week depending on the type of hemophilia) to prevent bleeding episodes. Prophylaxis is usually initiated during the first few years of life. A subcutaneous central venous catheter is inserted for this purpose and, as the child grows, he is eventually taught how to administer factor by peripheral infusion. For acute bleeds, prompt treatment is essential to prevent long-term complications. In 30% of patients with hemophilia A and 2% to 3% of patients with hemophilia B, an inhibitor to the respective factor can develop. In the presence of an inhibitor, acute bleeds must be treated with bypassing agents such as prothrombin concentrates or recombinant FVIIa. In the long term, immune tolerance is attempted by exposing the child to high doses of factor on a daily basis in an attempt to eradicate the inhibitor. A number of immune tolerance regimens have been in use with varying success.

Acquired causes of coagulation or platelet abnormalities can be treated supportively or by replacing the deficiency or removing the offending causative agent. Children with DIC should be given fresh frozen plasma, cryoprecipitate, and platelets as needed while the underlying etiology of the **DIC** is treated. In children in whom **vitamin K deficiency** is suspected as the cause of bleeding, one dose of vitamin K should correct the coagulopathy within 12 to 36 hours.

Prognosis

Most patients with inherited bleeding disorders will have an excellent prognosis if the diagnosis is made in a timely fashion and appropriate intervention is initiated.

Patients with **von Willebrand disease** usually have mild bleeding symptoms and, with appropriate education and intervention, the prognosis is excellent. Patients with **hemophilia** will also have an excellent prognosis assuming early diagnosis, family education, prophylaxis, and early treatment of bleeds. With the advent of prophylaxis, the severe hemophilic arthropathy that plagued older generations of males with hemophilia has been largely averted or minimized. In addition, the use of recombinant factor products and highly purified plasma-derived products in the pediatric population has minimized the risk for viral transmission. **Acute ITP** resolves spontaneously by 6 months in 80% of cases, regardless of pharmacologic intervention, and the risk for significant hemorrhage is exceedingly low. For individuals with **chronic ITP,** most cases will also resolve with time, and individuals do not usually have significant bleeding complications.

CASE RESOLUTION

A von Willebrand factor (vWF) panel was performed and revealed a vWF antigen of 20%, ristocetin cofactor activity of 30%, factor VIII activity of 40%, and a normal multimer analysis. The girl was diagnosed with type 1 von Willebrand disease. A DDAVP challenge was performed in clinic, and she was found to have an excellent response. She was prescribed nasal DDAVP (Stimate) and aminocaproic acid for significant bleeding episodes.

Selected References

Allen GA, Glader B. Approach to the bleeding child. *Pediatr Clin North Am.* 2002;49:1239–1256

Lusher JM. Clinical and laboratory approach to the patient with bleeding. In: Nathan DG, Orkin SH, Ginsburg D, Look AT, eds. *Nathan and Oski's Hematology of Infancy and Childhood.* 6th ed. Philadelphia, PA: W. B. Saunders Company; 2003:1515–1526

Lymphadenopathy

Wendy Y. Tcheng, MD

CASE STUDY

A 12-year-old girl is brought to the office with swelling of the anterior cervical nodes, which she has had for 4 weeks. Intermittent fever with temperatures as high as 101°F (38.3°C) and decreased appetite have been associated with the condition. The girl appears pale. On examination, her temperature is 100.4°F (38.0°C), and her other vital signs are normal. Three to 4 non-tender nodes 1 to 2 cm in diameter are present bilaterally. The remainder of the examination is normal.

Questions

1. When is lymphadenopathy of medical concern?
2. What are the clinical features of childhood diseases that present as cervical lymphadenopathy?
3. What are the diagnostic approaches to the evaluation of children with lymphadenopathy?
4. What is an appropriate therapeutic approach to cervical lymphadenopathy in children?

Lymphadenopathy is a common finding in children and is most often due to a benign, self-limited infectious process. However, in some children lymphadenopathy will signal a serious underlying systemic illness, and it is essential for the pediatrician to make this distinction so that appropriate diagnostic and therapeutic measures can be initiated.

Epidemiology

Lymphadenopathy occurs frequently in childhood, and even healthy children may have palpable lymph nodes in the anterior cervical, inguinal, and axillary regions. Localized lymphadenopathy is largely due to an infectious etiology, whereas generalized lymphadenopathy occurs with systemic illnesses such as systemic infections (viral, bacterial, protozoal, fungal), autoimmune disorders, storage disorders, and malignancies.

Clinical Presentation

Lymphadenopathy may be localized or generalized on presentation. **Localized** or **regional** lymphadenopathy refers to enlargement of lymph nodes within contiguous regions, whereas **generalized** lymphadenopathy involves more than 2 noncontiguous lymph node groups (Dx Box). Infection is the most common cause of localized lymphadenopathy in children, and the anterior cervical lymph node region is the most commonly involved area reflecting the high frequency of upper respiratory infections (URIs). Bilateral cervical lymphadenopathy is often seen with viral and bacterial URIs, and the nodes tend to be soft, mobile, and non-tender. Viruses such as Epstein-Barr virus (EBV) or cytomegalovirus (CMV) can present with prominent posterior cervical lymphadenopathy as well as generalized adenopathy, and occasionally hepatosplenomegaly. Direct bacterial invasion of lymph nodes produces a lymphadenitis, which is often unilateral, tender, erythematous, and fluctuant. Chronic lymphadenopathy may be due to atypical mycobacterial infections, tuberculosis, cat-scratch disease, EBV, CMV, toxoplasmosis, or human immunodeficiency virus (HIV). Generalized lymphadenopathy is concerning for a systemic infection, autoimmune process, storage disease, or malignancy. Lymphadenopathy due to malignancy is typically characterized by fixed, firm, non-tender lymph nodes in the setting of other signs and symptoms such as fever, pallor, night sweats, and weight loss.

Dx Lymphadenopathy

- Enlarged lymph nodes
- Fever
- Tenderness or warmth over the lymph nodes (lymphadenitis)
- Antecedent infection (eg, pharyngitis, upper respiratory infection, otitis media)
- Pallor
- Weight loss
- Bone pain

Pathophysiology

Lymph nodes are an integral part of the immune system where phagocytic cells filter microorganisms and particulate matter, and antigens are presented provoking a cellular or humorally mediated lymphocyte response. Lymph nodes are distributed throughout the body in groups that drain specific regions (Table 73-1). Enlargement of a lymph node may be due to proliferation of lymphocytes intrinsic to the lymph node (as a physiological immune response or a

Table 73-1. Lymph Node Drainage Patterns

Group	Drainage Pattern
Occipital	Posterior scalp
Preauricular	Superficial orbital and periorbital tissue, temporal scalp
Submental/ submandibular	Mouth
Cervical	Mouth, pharynx, ear, parotid gland, deep structures of neck (thyroid, larynx, trachea, upper esophagus)
Supraclavicular	Head, neck, arms, lungs, mediastinum, and abdomen
Mediastinal	Lungs, heart, thymus, esophagus
Axillary	Chest wall, breast, upper extremity
Abdominal	Abdominal organs, pelvis, lower extremities
Iliac and inguinal	Lower extremities, genitalia, buttocks, pelvis

malignant transformation) or may be due to infiltration by extrinsic inflammatory or metastatic malignant cells.

Differential Diagnosis

The duration and extent of lymphadenopathy (localized vs generalized) and the presence of associated symptoms will help to focus the differential diagnosis. A list of the common causes of lymphadenopathy in children is provided in Table 73-2.

Localized lymphadenopathy is most often due to an infectious etiology. Acute bilateral cervical lymphadenopathy is most frequently due to viral URIs (respiratory syncytial virus, adenovirus, influenza virus) or EBV and CMV, which can also cause generalized adenopathy. Bacterial pharyngitis (most commonly *Streptococcus* species) and oral infections/dental abscesses can also present with cervical adenopathy. Unilateral lymphadenitis is most often due to *Staphylococcus aureus,* followed by *Streptococcus pyogenes,* anaerobes, and other species. When the condition appears subacute, cat-scratch disease, tuberculosis (scrofula), atypical mycobacteria, toxoplasmosis, tularemia and, less commonly, histoplasmosis, brucellosis, and syphilis should be considered.

Generalized lymphadenopathy may be due to systemic infections (eg, EBV, CMV, HIV, toxoplasmosis), autoimmune disorders (eg, juvenile rheumatoid arthritis, systemic lupus erythematosus), storage disorders (eg, Niemann-Pick, Gaucher disease), histiocytic disorders (eg, Langerhans cell histiocytosis, hemophagocytic lymphohistiocytosis), drug reactions (eg, phenytoin), or malignancies. Malignancies include leukemia and lymphoma (Hodgkin disease and non-Hodgkin lymphoma) as well as solid tumors that can metastasize to lymph nodes (eg, neuroblastoma, rhabdomyosarcoma, fibrosarcoma, and thyroid carcinoma). With neoplastic infiltration, enlarged nodes are generally non-tender, firm, rubbery, and immobile. In Hodgkin disease, the nodes enlarge sequentially, with involvement spreading from one chain to the next, rather than bilaterally

(in contrast to non-Hodgkin lymphoma). Supraclavicular or epitrochlear adenopathy is suggestive of malignancy.

A number of head and neck lesions that occur in the pediatric population merit comment because they are often confused with cervical lymphadenopathy. These lesions include cystic hygromas, branchial cleft cysts, thyroglossal duct cysts, and epidermoid cysts. These are congenital malformations that often present as a neck mass in the young child and can easily be mistaken for a lymph node, particularly if infected (see Chapter 67).

Evaluation

History

A thorough history and review of symptoms is essential in determining the underlying etiology of lymphadenopathy in children. Inquiries should be made regarding the duration of the lymphadenopathy, the rate of nodal enlargement, and the occurrence of associated fever and other constitutional symptoms such as bone pain, weight loss, fever, and night sweats. Recent illnesses or infections, insect or animal bites, and local trauma should be determined. A history of distant travel; recent emigration from countries with endemic tuberculosis (eg, Mexico, Central America, Southeast Asia), recent travel to areas with endemic histoplasmosis (southeastern United States) or coccidioidomycosis (San Joaquin Valley, CA), a detailed history of pet contact (cats, which transmit toxoplasmosis and cat-scratch disease), and exposure to ill contacts, particularly individuals known to have tuberculosis, are also important (Questions Box).

Questions

Lymphadenopathy

- How long have the nodes been enlarged?
- Was the child sick before the swelling began?
- Does the child have any symptoms now, such as fever, weight loss, pallor, or anorexia?
- Does the child come in contact with any animals, particularly cats?
- Has the child traveled anywhere?
- Is the child taking any medications?
- Has the child been in contact with anyone who is ill?

Physical Examination

When evaluating a child with lymphadenopathy, the enlarged nodes should be measured and examined at their widest diameter and evaluated for evidence of erythema, tenderness, and warmth, all of which are suggestive of infection. The characteristics of the enlarged lymph node should be noted (eg, soft, firm, rubbery, mobile, matted, tender, discrete). The surrounding skin and soft tissue region that is drained by the involved lymph node should be examined for signs of inflammation or skin breakdown. The extent of the lymphadenopathy should be determined, as well as the presence or absence of hepatosplenomegaly.

Table 73-2. Differential Diagnosis of Lymphadenopathy			
Diagnostic Category	*Clinical Features*	*Epidemiological Features*	*Laboratory Features*
Infections			
Viral (EBV, CMV, rubella, HIV)	Usually generalized, not purulent or tender		EBV/CMV with activated lymphocytes on peripheral blood smear
Mycobacterial (TB, atypical mycobacteria)	Usually localized; often tender, red, flocculent		
Bacterial (staphylococcal and streptococcal infections, cat-scratch disease, tularemia, plague, diphtheria)	Usually localized; often tender, red, flocculent		
Protozoal (toxoplasmosis)	Generalized		
Spirochete (syphilis)			
Fungal (histoplasmosis, coccidioidomycosis)	May be generalized	Suspicion should be raised based on regional incidence	
Neoplastic Conditions			
Hodgkin lymphoma	Often associated with "B" symptoms (eg, fever, weight loss, night sweats)	Common among higher socioeconomic groups, only children	↑ ESR (can be >100), ↑ LDH, anergy
Non-Hodgkin lymphoma	See Hodgkin lymphoma		
Leukemia	Generalized lymphadenopathy, hepatosplenomegaly		Blasts on peripheral blood smear
Solid tumors (eg, rhabdomyosarcoma, neuroblastoma)	Depends on underlying malignancy		
Langerhans cell histiocytosis	Eczema, failure to thrive, bony lesions, diabetes insipidus, proptosis, hepatosplenomegaly all possible		
Sinus histiocytosis with massive lymphadenopathy			
Autoimmune Disorders			
JIA	Generalized lymphadenopathy seen in systemic form (Still) (eg, fever, hepatosplenomegaly, evanescent rash, arthritis)	Equal incidence in males and females	↑ ESR, anemia, negative ANA and rheumatoid arthritis in Still JRA
Lupus	Arthritis, butterfly facial rash, effusions (lung, joint, cardiac), CNS, nephrotic syndrome	Increased incidence in girls, Jewish heritage	↑ ESR, positive ANA, anti-ds DNA, ↓ C3, C4, or CH50, anemia, ↑ platelets, proteinuria
Other			
Storage disorders (eg, Niemann-Pick, Gaucher disease)	Generalized lymphadenopathy, hepatosplenomegaly		
Drugs (eg, phenytoin)	Generalized lymphadenopathy		
Sarcoidosis	Bilateral hilar lymphadenopathy, noncaseating granulomas (lung, liver)	↑ in African Americans and those of Irish heritage	↑ serum angiotensin-1 converting enzyme, ↑ serum lysozyme

Abbreviations: EBV, Epstein-Barr virus; CMV, cytomegalovirus; HIV, human immunodeficiency virus; TB, tuberculosis; ESR, erythrocyte sedimentation rate; LDH, lactate dehydrogenase; JIA, juvenile idiopathic arthritis; ANA, antinuclear antibody; CNS, central nervous system.

Laboratory Tests

In most cases, a thorough history and physical examination can establish the likely diagnosis without any laboratory testing. If further testing is deemed necessary, the tests performed should be limited and dictated by the nature of the lymphadenopathy. A complete blood count and peripheral blood smear are useful screening tests that will provide clues to the underlying etiology. A lymphocytosis with activated lymphocytes on peripheral blood smear is consistent with a viral etiology such as EBV or CMV. Leukocytosis with a left shift suggests a bacterial etiology. Cytopenias or blasts on peripheral blood smear are concerning for malignancy. Depending on the clinical scenario, serum antibody studies for various infections may be warranted (ie, EBV, CMV, HIV, *Bartonella henselae* for cat-scratch disease). In addition, a purified protein derivative or skin tests for fungal disease should be considered. In lupus and rheumatoid arthritis, an antinuclear antibody may be positive and complement levels may be reduced.

If infectious lymphadenitis is suspected, a fine-needle aspirate (FNA) for a Gram stain and culture is often helpful, particularly if the infection has been unresponsive to empiric antibiotics. However, if there is a significant concern for malignancy, an FNA is not the preferred method. An excisional biopsy should be performed so that the entire lymph node can be visualized and adequate samples for testing will be available.

Imaging Studies

A chest x-ray should be performed in any child with suspected scrofula or malignancy. In particular, if leukemia or lymphoma is suspected, a chest x-ray should be performed to evaluate for an anterior mediastinal mass. Other imaging studies are not routinely performed; however, if the nature of an enlarged lymph node requires further definition, an ultrasound can be done. In the setting of malignancy, additional radiographic studies are performed for staging purposes.

Management

Management is dictated by the underlying cause of lymphadenopathy. Cervical lymphadenopathy associated with URIs will typically resolve without intervention. Bacterial lymphadenitis can be treated with a trial of **antibiotics** with anti-staphylococcal and streptococcal coverage. Underlying fungal and mycobacterial diseases should be treated with appropriate **antifungal or antibacterial agents,** with the exception of cervical adenopathy due to atypical mycobacteria, which requires **surgical removal.** Malignant disorders require **multimodal therapy** with surgery, chemotherapy, or radiation, depending on the specific disorder and the extent of disease (see Chapter 127).

Prognosis

The outcome of lymphadenopathy depends entirely on the underlying disorder. In most cases, the cause is infectious, and the lymphadenopathy is self-limited or resolves with the use of appropriate antibiotics.

CASE RESOLUTION

In the case history, the bilateral nature of the swelling and the lack of tenderness of the nodes are very worrisome and suggest a noninfectious etiology. The girl had a throat culture, an intermediate purified protein derivative, and a chest x-ray, all of which were negative. A complete blood count reveals leukocytosis with 28,000 white blood cells per deciliter (60% lymphocytes), with a normal hemoglobin and platelet count. A heterophil test for infectious mononucleosis is positive. Bed rest is recommended, and the child makes a complete recovery in 3 weeks.

Selected References

Filston HC. Common lumps and bumps of the head and neck in infants and children. *Pediatr Ann.* 1989;18:180–186

Ginsburg AM. The tuberculosis epidemic: scientific challenges and opportunities. *Public Health Rep.* 1998;113:128–136

Hicks RB, Melish ME. Kawasaki syndrome. *Pediatr Clin North Am.* 1986;33:1151–1176

Huebner RE, Schein MF, Gauthen GM, Geiter LJ, O'Brien RJ. Usefulness of skin testing with mycobacterial antigens in children with cervical lymphadenopathy. *Pediatr Infect Dis J.* 1992;11:450–456

Knight PJ, Mulne AF, Vassy LE. When is lymph node biopsy indicated in children with enlarged peripheral nodes? *Pediatrics.* 1982;69:391–396

Knight PJ, Reiner CB. Superficial lumps in children: what, when and why? *Pediatrics.* 1983;72:147–153

Kurtzberg J, Graham ML. Non-Hodgkin's lymphoma: biologic classification and implications for therapy. *Pediatr Clin North Am.* 1991;38:443–456

Leventhal BG, Kato GJ. Childhood Hodgkin and non-Hodgkin lymphomas. *Pediatr Rev.* 1990;12:171–179

Marcy SM. Infections of lymph nodes of the head and neck. *Pediatr Infect Dis.* 1983;2:397–405

Pollock BH, Krischer JP, Vietti TJ. Interval between symptom onset and diagnosis of pediatric solid tumors. *J Pediatr.* 1991;119:725–732

Zangwill K. Therapeutic options for cat-scratch disease. *Pediatr Infect Dis J.* 1998;17:1059–1061

Zitelli BJ. Evaluating the child with a neck mass. *Contemp Pediatr.* 1990;7:90–112

Cardiovascular System

74. Heart Murmurs 433

75. Cyanosis in the Newborn 437

76. Congestive Heart Failure 443

77. Chest Pain 449

78. Hypertension 455

Heart Murmurs

Robin Winkler Doroshow, MD

CASE STUDY

A 6-year-old girl is brought to the office for a physical examination for school. Her medical history is unremarkable, and her growth and development have been normal. She is asymptomatic. Her physical examination is normal except for a grade II/VI low-pitched vibratory systolic ejection murmur that is loudest at the left lower sternal border, with radiation to the apex and upper sternal border. The murmur increases to III/VI in the supine position.

Questions

1. What is the significance of a heart murmur in asymptomatic children? How reassuring are a negative history and the absence of other physical findings?
2. What workup should be done by primary care physicians?
3. What are the costs of excessive tests and unnecessary consultation? What are the costs of an inadequate workup?
4. When should physicians refer children to specialists for consultation?

Asymptomatic children with heart murmurs are commonly encountered by physicians. Murmurs are a finding rather than a medical sign or symptom because they are detected incidentally at an examination conducted for another purpose.

Correct assessment of the significance of a heart murmur is important to ensure appropriate management of children with heart disease. Complications of undiagnosed cardiac disease in children include progressive hemodynamic impairment, endocarditis, and even sudden death.

The misinterpretation of an innocent murmur as organic in nature can also take its toll, primarily on parental anxiety. Unnecessary restriction of activities may result, which can have a negative impact on children's school and social lives as well as self-image. As adults these children may be denied health insurance, life insurance, and certain types of employment. In addition, misdiagnosis costs money and uses limited resources, with unnecessary tests and doctor visits, as this "non-disease" is evaluated and followed.

Epidemiology

An estimated 50% of healthy children have heart murmurs. The overall incidence of congenital heart disease (CHD), including symptomatic cases, is just under 1%, and some children with CHD have no murmur. Therefore, about 99 out of 100 murmurs noted during childhood are "innocent" (ie, have no organic basis).

Clinical Presentation

Heart murmurs are usually detected on routine examination for well-child care or on evaluation for an unrelated problem. Innocent murmurs are not associated with signs or symptoms because they are normal findings. Most of the symptoms sometimes associated with organic murmurs (ie, murmurs of heart disease) are related to the presence of congestive heart failure (CHF) (see Chapter 76) and usually appear during infancy. Some children with murmurs come to medical attention with complaints of exercise intolerance or chest pain. It is necessary to determine whether these problems are actually referable to the heart.

Pathophysiology

A murmur is a sustained sound that can be detected with a stethoscope placed on the chest. This sound is produced by turbulence of blood flow in the heart or great vessels. This turbulence may be due to structural abnormalities (eg, aortic valve stenosis), benign or normal flow patterns (see below), or exaggeration of normal flow patterns (seen in high output states such as fever, exercise, anxiety, or anemia, and sometimes termed *functional*).

Not all significant heart disease in children is heralded by a murmur. Structural heart disease may be silent and be indicated by other findings. For example, transposition of the great arteries results in cyanosis, anomalous pulmonary venous return in pulmonary edema and hypoxia, and anomalous origin of the left coronary artery in CHF. Acquired heart disease such as Kawasaki disease, myocarditis, or cardiomyopathy often produces no murmur.

The common innocent murmurs are better recognized than understood. Because they occur in normal, healthy individuals, there are few hemodynamic or anatomical data to correlate with the murmur, and pathophysiology is in some cases conjectural. **Still's murmur,** which was once thought to be due to easily appreciated aortic valve flow, is now believed to result from vibration of normal fibrous bands that cross the left ventricle. This murmur may also be heard in children who have undergone spontaneous closure of a membranous ventricular septal defect, with a small residual aneurysm in the septum. The **pulmonary flow murmur** seems to be caused by normal flow across the pulmonary valve, perhaps made more apparent because of high cardiac output, close proximity to the chest wall, and (in adolescent females) mild anemia. The **venous hum** is attributed to turbulence at the confluence of the innominate veins, which is exacerbated in the upright position by gravity.

The **physiological peripheral pulmonic stenosis (PPPS) murmur** in newborns is produced by turbulence at the origins of the left and right pulmonary arteries. Because less than 10% of the combined ventricular output of the fetus goes to these branches, they are small and arise at a sharp angle from the main pulmonary artery. When postnatal circulation abruptly requires the entire cardiac output to enter these vessels, a relative stenosis is encountered (Figure 74-1). This physiological stenosis resolves gradually with remodeling of the pulmonary artery tree by 2 to 3 months of age.

Figure 74-1. Configuration of the central pulmonary arteries in the fetus, the newborn, and the child. Abbreviations: MPA, main pulmonary artery; RPA, right pulmonary artery; LPA, left pulmonary artery; DA, ductus arteriosus; AO, aorta.

Differential Diagnosis

In healthy children, the differential diagnosis of a heart murmur includes innocent murmurs and murmurs resulting from structural lesions, most of which are congenital. The specific features of a particular murmur usually provide most if not all necessary clues to the diagnosis. It is therefore important to develop and maintain auscultatory skills. A good quality stethoscope, with both diaphragm and bell correctly sized for the patient, is essential. Conditions should be optimized: the patient should be kept comfortable and, if necessary, distracted, and extraneous environmental noise should be minimized.

Some features may alert examiners to the organic nature of a murmur. Although very loud murmurs (grades IV–VI; ie, with associated precordial thrill) are usually not innocent, some innocent murmurs may be as loud as grade III, particularly with high cardiac output (eg, fever, anxiety, or anemia). Diastolic murmurs and continuous murmurs, other than the easily recognizable venous hum, are usually pathologic, as are high-pitched and harsh murmurs, which are better heard with the diaphragm of the stethoscope.

The common innocent murmurs of childhood are recognizable on auscultatory examination. **Still's murmur,** or the **innocent vibratory murmur,** is a low-pitched, vibratory, or musical murmur that sounds like a groan. Because of its low frequency, the murmur is better heard with the bell. It is loudest at the left lower sternal border but is often distributed widely over the precordium. This murmur is often quite loud, particularly in the supine position, and is extremely common in school-aged children. The characteristics of the murmur are diagnostic, although the absence of other findings is supportive.

The **pulmonary flow murmur,** usually heard in older children, is a short, blowing systolic ejection (ie, crescendo-decrescendo) murmur localized to the left upper sternal border. It may be louder in the supine position.

The **venous hum** is a soft continuous murmur, similar to the sound heard in a seashell. Because of its constancy, it is often overlooked. This murmur is very commonly heard in preschool and school-aged children. Loudest in the right infraclavicular area, it may also be heard on the left. This murmur is highly variable with head and neck position and compression of the neck veins, which may increase or diminish it. It usually disappears in the supine position.

The **PPPS** murmur is an innocent murmur found in newborns. Best heard at the upper sternal border, this blowing systolic ejection murmur radiates strikingly over the lung fields into the back and both axillae.

Evaluation

History

The history may be helpful in assessment of children with a murmur. If a thorough history shows that children have no symptoms, this suggests the absence of severe heart disease and helps exclude many major or complex defects as well as CHF. The absence of symptoms does not, however, exclude several common defects that may require intervention (Table 74-1).

Table 74-1. Common Organic Murmurs in Asymptomatic Children	
Lesion	**Other Clues**
Atrial septal defect	Fixed split S_2
Ventricular septal defect (small to moderate)	Loud heart sounds
Patent ductus arteriosus (small to moderate)	Full or bounding pulses
Pulmonic stenosis	Systolic ejection click (SEC)
Aortic stenosis	SEC; suprasternal thrill
Coarctation of the aorta	Weak or absent femoral pulses

The most common symptom reported by children or parents is easy fatigability (Questions Box). This is difficult to quantitate. Determining exercise intolerance on the basis of history is very subjective; it may be due, of course, to noncardiac causes and may be unrelated to the murmur. Easy fatigability during infancy may be reported as slow or poor feeding. Chest pain, a common symptom in adults with heart disease, is rarely cardiac in origin in children. A history of rapid breathing, excessive sweating, and other complaints referable to CHF suggests organic heart disease. Central cyanosis (ie, involving the oral mucosa rather than the perioral area or the fingers) may be reported by parents of children with cyanotic CHD but is often not recognized.

Questions

Heart Murmurs

- Is the child easily tired? Is his sleeping/napping pattern normal for age?
- Does the child keep up with others of his or her age?
- If the child is having a good time—for example, at a park or a party—how is the child's endurance?
- Does the child have a family history of congenital heart disease?
- Was the child exposed antenatally to possible teratogens such as maternal diabetes?
- Does the child ever complain of chest pain? At rest or with activity?
- Does the child ever appear blue?
- Does the child perspire excessively?

Physical Examination

The physical examination often gives strong clues to the cardiac diagnosis beyond the murmur itself. Even in children with known CHD, the non-auscultatory portions of the examination are critical in assessing the cardiac status (ie, how the patient is tolerating the defect). **Vital signs,** preferably obtained with the child at rest or sleeping, yield information regarding cardiac status more than specific diagnosis. Tachypnea and tachycardia are present in CHF. A normal resting respiratory rate (ie, <60/min in infants) argues strongly against CHF. Blood pressure is normal in most patients with CHD. It may be useful to measure blood pressure in the legs, especially if coarctation of the aorta is suspected because of diminished pulses in the lower extremities.

The **growth pattern** may reflect the presence of any chronic illness, including hemodynamically significant CHD. Affected patients, particularly infants and children with large left-to-right shunts (with or without CHF) gain weight poorly. Height and head circumference are usually normal, although in more severe or prolonged situations height may also be affected.

A complete **cardiac examination** should be performed. Is the chest asymmetrical, a sign of long-standing cardiomegaly? Is the precordial impulse hyperdynamic? Are extra sounds (eg, clicks, rubs, gallops) heard? Is the second sound normal in intensity and in width and motion of splitting (ie, variation with respiration)?

Additional pertinent findings include lethargy, dysmorphic features suggestive of a genetic syndrome, central cyanosis, and clubbing. Hepatomegaly is found in children with CHF. The peripheral pulses should be normal in volume, neither diminished (eg, pedal pulses in coarctation) nor bounding (eg, in patent ductus arteriosus), and equal in all extremities. The temperature and capillary refill of the extremities in children who are not chilled reflect adequacy of the peripheral circulation.

Imaging Studies

Routine laboratory studies are not warranted in the evaluation of most murmurs. An **electrocardiogram (ECG)** is indicated when heart disease is known or strongly suspected, but a normal ECG may not rule out significant CHD. A chest x-ray may be helpful in this setting, but its potential benefits are usually outweighed by the risks of discomfort and radiation exposure. In the case of some tests, such as echocardiography, the manner in which the examination is actually carried out may vary depending on the suspected diagnosis; direct input from a cardiologist may be necessary to maximize the yield from these studies. Such tests are not suitable for screening purposes and should be obtained only after consultation with a pediatric cardiologist.

Management

If a heart murmur is suspected of being organic in origin because of its features or associated findings, referral to a pediatric cardiologist is indicated. In the case of asymptomatic children there is no urgency, but parental and physician anxiety can best be allayed by proceeding to consultation promptly (ie, within weeks). In some cases, a repeat examination may be useful before deciding whether to consult a specialist, particularly if the murmur is initially heard under non-physiological conditions such as fever. Tests are usually best used if selected and ordered by specialists. Not all cardiologists perform all tests on all patients. Management of organic heart disease in infants or children is also best handled by specialists. Treatment may include **medications, interventional catheterization,** or **cardiac surgery.** Communication with the primary care provider, however, is essential to delivery of optimal patient care.

If the murmur is innocent, physicians must complete the following steps:

1. Children and their families must be informed about the presence of the murmur. Even if the murmur is benign, patients have a right to know that it was heard. In addition, they are likely to be examined by other practitioners who will report it, which may lead to the erroneous suspicion of either a new murmur or negligence on the part of the first examiner.
2. The diagnosis must be clearly explained to parents and children (depending on the age). It is essential that they understand that this is a normal finding rather than a minor abnormality. In some cases, notification of teachers or athletic coaches may be appropriate to prevent misunderstanding. Physicians must stress that no further evaluation is needed and no restrictions are indicated. Printed brochures that

explain innocent murmurs are available from organizations such as the American Heart Association.

3. The description of the murmur and the diagnosis itself must be documented in the medical record. A murmur that is clearly and unequivocally innocent, with no evidence of heart disease, should not affect the child's access to insurance, participation in sports, etc. Medical documentation also helps protect patients from unnecessary reevaluations in the future.

4. Physicians should proceed no further. No laboratory studies or consultations need be performed. If the evaluation has been completed by a specialist because of suspicion of CHD by the referring physician, no follow-up with the specialist is indicated. The child is referred back to the primary practitioner.

Prognosis

The prognosis for children with heart murmurs depends on the cause of the murmur. Children with an innocent murmur, who by definition have normal hearts, have a normal prognosis—with one exception. If children or their parents mistakenly believe children to have heart disease, parents may treat the children inappropriately (eg, unnecessary testing, restriction of activities). As a result, children may develop sedentary habits and inferior self-image.

With appropriate medical attention, the prognosis is normal or near normal in most cases of CHD. Children with minor defects not requiring intervention (eg, small ventricular septal defect, mild pulmonic stenosis) need only endocarditis prophylaxis (eg, for dental procedures) and infrequent cardiology follow-up. With the development of refined cardiac surgery and interventional catheterization, even children with the most complex cardiac anomalies now have a good outlook with respect to both daily living and life expectancy.

CASE RESOLUTION

In the case presented, a healthy girl with no history of cardiovascular symptoms has a heart murmur and an otherwise unremarkable physical examination. The murmur is a typical Still's (innocent vibratory) murmur, which is identifiable by its low-pitched, vibratory quality. No further evaluation is necessary. The diagnosis is explained, the girl and her parents are reassured, and the murmur and diagnosis are noted in the medical record.

Selected References

Bergman AB, Stamm SJ. The morbidity of cardiac nondisease in school children. *N Engl J Med.* 1967;276:1008–1013

Danford DA, Nasir A, Gumbiner C. Cost assessment of the evaluation of heart murmurs in children. *Pediatrics.* 1993;91:365–368

Gaskin PR, Owens SE, Talner NS, Sanders SP, Li JS. Clinical auscultation skills in pediatric residents. *Pediatrics.* 2000;105:1184–1187

Geggel RL, Horowitz LM, Brown EA, Parsons M, Wang PS, Fulton DR. Parental anxiety associated with referral of a child to a pediatric cardiologist for evaluation of a Still's murmur. *J Pediatr.* 2002;140:747–752

Haney I, Ipp M, Feldman W, McCrindle BW. Accuracy of clinical assessment of heart murmurs by office based (general practice) paediatricians. *Arch Dis Child.* 1999;81:409–412

Hohn AR. Congenital heart disease—the first test. *West J Med.* 1992;156:435–436

Mangione S, Nieman LZ. Cardiac auscultatory skills of internal medicine and family practice trainees. *JAMA.* 1997;278:717–722

Moss AJ. Clues in diagnosing congenital heart disease. *West J Med.* 1992;156:392–398

Newburger JW, Rosenthal A, Williams RG. Noninvasive tests in the initial evaluation of heart murmurs in children. *N Engl J Med.* 1983;308:61–64

Smythe JF, Teixeira OH, Vlad P, Demers PP, Feldman W. Initial evaluation of heart murmurs: are laboratory tests necessary? *Pediatrics.* 1990;86:497–500

Vukanovic-Criley JM, Criley S, Warde CM, et al. Competency in cardiac examination skills in medical students, trainees, physicians, and faculty. *Arch Intern Med.* 2006;166:610–616

Cyanosis in the Newborn

Robin Winkler Doroshow, MD

CASE STUDY

A 3,500-g, term male infant born to a 29-year-old, gravida II para II, healthy mother by spontaneous vaginal delivery is well until 24 hours of age, when a nurse notes that he is cyanotic. On examination, he appears blue but in no distress. The vital signs are temperature (axillary), 37°C (98.6°F); pulse, 130/min; respirations, 40/min; and blood pressure, 80/60 in the right arm. His general appearance is normal except for the cyanosis. His heart sounds are normal, and no murmur is heard. His liver is not palpable, and the peripheral pulses are normal and equal in all extremities. Capillary refill is normal. Oxygen saturation is 65% by pulse oximetry.

Questions

1. What are the causes of cyanosis in newborns?
2. What is the appropriate evaluation of cyanosis in newborns?
3. How urgent is the assessment? What are the risks and benefits of further evaluation?
4. Which aspects of management should be initiated by a primary physician at a community hospital?
5. Which types of treatment should be undertaken by the consulting pediatric cardiologist at the referral center?

Cyanosis is a bluish appearance of the skin due to the presence of reduced hemoglobin in the tissues. Central cyanosis, which is detected initially in the oral mucosa and nail beds but is generalized when severe, indicates at least 4 to 5 g of reduced hemoglobin per 100 mL blood. Hypoxemia is usually the cause. This condition is frequently present in neonates with pulmonary pathology but is also one of the most common presentations of severe congenital heart disease (CHD).

Because cyanotic CHD in newborns may be life-threatening, it must not go undiagnosed. Most diagnostic studies have minimal risk. Even the risk of cardiac catheterization in this setting is relatively low. Most of the lesions that cause cyanotic CHD can be palliated or corrected, and the prognosis is good.

Epidemiology

Cyanotic CHD occurs in about 2 to 3 of every 1,000 live-born infants. Approximately 80% to 90% of these cases, usually the most severe ones, are detected in the first 30 days of life. However, failure to diagnose major CHD *before newborn discharge* occurs in at least 10% of cases, leading to increased morbidity and mortality. Infants with low pulmonary blood flow or lesions causing poor mixing most often present with obvious cyanosis, although initially they otherwise appear well and comfortable. Those with high pulmonary flow are less blue and often present first with congestive heart failure (CHF) or a murmur.

Most cyanotic CHD is not diagnosed before birth. The antenatal history, gestational age, birth weight, and delivery room examination are unremarkable. Failure to identify CHD in the setting of a routine obstetric ultrasound study does not rule it out; the sensitivity of such scans in the general population is very low. Congenital heart disease is more likely in some situations that can be anticipated prenatally (Box 75-1). In these settings, increased suspicion may lead to antenatal detection using specialized echocardiography.

Box 75-1. Settings With Increased Risk of Congenital Heart Disease

- Genetic syndromes (eg, trisomies, DiGeorge syndrome)
- Certain extracardiac anomalies (eg, omphalocele, forearm anomalies)
- High incidence of congenital heart disease in the family
- Maternal diabetes if poorly controlled during first trimester
- Fetal exposure to cardiac teratogen (eg, lithium, isotretinoin)
- Fetal or neonatal arrhythmia other than premature atrial beats

Clinical Presentation

Children with cyanotic CHD often present within the first week of life with cyanosis of the oral mucosa. In more severe cases, generalized cyanosis occurs. The abnormal color may be more apparent with effort (eg, feeding, passing stool) or crying. Respiratory distress, heralded by grunting, nasal flaring, and retractions, is minor or absent in many newborn infants with cyanotic CHD. In cases of severe hypoxia, metabolic acidosis leads to poor perfusion and compensatory tachypnea with hyperpnea. Additional findings depend on the nature of the causal lesion (Dx Box). It is important to note that the absence of associated physical findings does not exclude cyanotic CHD.

Cyanosis in the Newborn: Possible Associated Findings

- Low oxygen saturation
- No improvement with oxygen
- Heart murmur
- Tachypnea
- Increased perspiration
- Abnormal cardiac silhouette on x-ray
- Abnormal electrocardiogram
- Abnormal echocardiogram

Pathophysiology

Cardiac cyanosis is due to **right-to-left shunting** so that systemic venous blood bypasses the pulmonary circulation and enters the systemic circulation. Two conditions are necessary to produce this type of shunting: a communication, such as a septal defect, for the blood to shunt across and a cause, such as pulmonic stenosis, for the blood to be shunted away from the lungs. The most notable exception is simple transposition of the great arteries (TGA), where the fundamental connections are abnormal, and all systemic venous blood is directed to the systemic arterial circulation. Lesions associated with cyanosis may be divided into 3 groups.

1. The **low pulmonary blood flow (LPBF) group** consists of tetralogy of Fallot, pulmonary atresia with intact ventricular septum, and virtually any combination of defects that includes pulmonary atresia or severe pulmonic stenosis. Pulmonary flow is diminished and may derive entirely from the ductus arteriosus while it remains patent. Aside from obvious cyanosis, infants often appear well.

2. The **high pulmonary blood flow (HPBF) group** includes truncus arteriosus, single ventricle, and combinations of defects that involve mixing of oxygenated and unoxygenated blood and little or no obstruction to pulmonary flow. Although a right-to-left shunt is present, the left-to-right shunt is even greater. Pulmonary venous return is therefore voluminous and contributes disproportionately to systemic output. Cyanosis is less apparent. Pulmonary flow increases over the first days and weeks of life as the pulmonary vascular resistance falls, and CHF develops, as in patients with isolated shunt lesions (eg, ventricular septal defect). Some children with HPBF lesions also have obstruction to systemic blood flow (eg, coarctation of the aorta, hypoplastic left heart syndrome) and may depend on the ductus arteriosus to carry some or all of this flow.

3. The **poor mixing group** is limited to TGA and its variants. The right and left circuits are in parallel rather than in series, and survival depends on interchange of oxygenated and unoxygenated blood between them. Most newborns with poor mixing present with marked cyanosis, like patients in the LPBF group.

Severe hypoxemia (oxygen partial pressure [pO_2] <35 mm Hg for the average newborn) is not compatible with prolonged survival. Death ensues in a matter of hours. Infants experience tissue hypoxia, anaerobic glycolysis, and metabolic acidosis. Respiratory compensation may occur at first. Even with a normal pH, however, the presence of metabolic acidosis (large base deficit) indicates life-threatening hypoxia, necessitating immediate intervention.

Differential Diagnosis

The major causes of cyanosis are cardiac and respiratory (Box 75-2). Diagnoses in the latter group include problems of the lung, chest, airway, or respiratory drive.

Box 75-2. Noncardiac Causes of Neonatal Cyanosis

- Upper airway obstruction (eg, choanal atresia)
- Pulmonary infection (eg, group B streptococcal infection)
- Aspiration (eg, meconium aspiration syndrome, tracheoesophageal fistula)
- Pulmonary hypoplasia (eg, Potter syndrome, diaphragmatic hernia)
- Respiratory distress syndrome (eg, in prematurity)
- Thoracic hypoplasia (eg, thanatophoric dwarfism)
- Hypoventilation (eg, neurologic depression)
- Persistent fetal circulation

The syndrome of **persistent fetal circulation** is perhaps most often confused with cyanotic CHD. It is also known as **persistent pulmonary hypertension of the newborn.** In this syndrome the heart and great vessels are structurally normal, but high pulmonary vascular resistance, which is often seen in post-term infants with perinatal distress or pulmonary disease, causes blood to shunt away from the lungs at the foramen ovale and ductus arteriosus. Profound cyanosis that is unresponsive to supplemental oxygen may be the only abnormal finding, and echocardiography is required to exclude CHD.

Pulmonary cyanosis may be due to **infection** (eg, group B streptococcal pneumonia); **aspiration** (eg, meconium, tracheoesophageal fistula); **pulmonary hypoplasia** (eg, Potter syndrome, diaphragmatic hernia); **respiratory distress syndrome** (eg, prematurity); or a host of other problems of the lung, chest, or airway. Neurologic depression may produce hypoventilation with resultant hypoxia.

Evaluation

Evaluation of the cyanotic newborn must be expeditious so that management is not delayed. In some cases, therapy may be initiated before the evaluation is complete. All available information, the statistical likelihood of CHD, and the risk-benefit ratio of the treatment must be taken into account.

History

Review of the history may be helpful, particularly in certain situations, such as in children with pulmonary disease (Questions Box). It is important to note that a negative response to any or all of the questions does not render cyanotic CHD unlikely; in fact, negative responses are noted in most cases.

> ### Questions
>
> **Cyanosis in the Newborn**
>
> - Has the infant been in any distress?
> - Has the infant had difficulty feeding?
> - Was the infant suspected of having a heart problem prior to birth (eg, fetal arrhythmia, abnormal heart on ultrasound)?
> - Is the mother diabetic?
> - Did the mother take any drugs (prescribed or not) during the pregnancy?
> - Was the mother ill during the first trimester?
> - Is there a positive family history of congenital heart disease or other birth defects?
> - Did any perinatal problems (eg, passage of meconium in utero) occur?

Physical Examination

Cyanosis may be the only abnormal physical finding in cardiac patients, but a careful, thorough examination often yields information about the underlying cardiac defect and the overall circulatory status. External anomalies or abnormal phenotypic appearance may indicate a genetic disorder with associated cardiac anomalies. Dyspnea (grunting, nasal flaring, intercostal retractions) is more often seen with lung disease, but tachypnea (rapid respiration) is common with both severe heart disease and pulmonary problems. Tachypnea results from CHF in HPBF lesions, and hyperpnea (deep breathing) from metabolic acidosis in severe hypoxia or impaired perfusion. Poor perfusion is also manifested by abnormal color (a gray or ashen appearance if combined with cyanosis), cool extremities, delayed capillary refill, and generally diminished pulses.

The peripheral pulses are palpated in all extremities. Abnormalities or discrepancies between extremities must be confirmed by measuring blood pressure. Weak pulses may be found in cardiogenic shock, and bounding pulses may be noted with diastolic runoff lesions such as patent ductus arteriosus or aortic insufficiency. Pulse quality and blood pressure may differ in different extremities if an aortic arch abnormality such as coarctation is present. The abdominal examination may reveal hepatomegaly (in CHF) or abnormal situs (as in asplenia syndrome, usually associated with complex cyanotic CHD).

The cardiac examination may disclose a loud murmur if an obstruction such as pulmonary stenosis is present. The physician should note, however, that atresia, being a total obstruction, produces no murmur. Heart sounds may be loud and the precordium

hyperdynamic, particularly in children with HPBF. Splitting of the second sound confirms that 2 patent semilunar valves are present, but this finding is often difficult to appreciate even in normal newborns.

Laboratory Tests

A number of laboratory studies are available (see Chapter 76, Table 76-1). As in CHF, it is initially more important to determine whether patients have heart disease than to obtain a precise, complete diagnosis. In cyanotic CHD, sophisticated studies such as echocardiography, magnetic resonance imaging, and catheterization are usually needed to make a detailed diagnosis.

The suspicion of arterial hypoxemia should be confirmed by **pulse oximetry,** an indirect measurement. It is readily available and noninvasive but has shortcomings. Perfusion must be adequate to obtain a reading. Accuracy is diminished at saturations below 75%, although the presence of profound hypoxia can still be confirmed. Cyanotic CHD cannot be ruled out by pulse oximetry, however, because readings of 100% saturation may reflect pO_2 values that range anywhere between 75 and 250 mm Hg (Figure 75-1). **Arterial blood gases** are more accurate and give important additional information about ventilation and acid-base status. Arterialized capillary gases may suffice if perfusion is adequate.

Figure 75-1. Comparison between oxygen partial pressure (pO_2) by arterial blood gas measurement and oxygen saturation by pulse oximetry. (Reproduced with permission from Niehoff J, DelGuercio C, LaMorte W, et al. Efficacy of pulse oximetry and capnometry in postoperative ventilatory weaning. *Crit Care Med.* 1988;16:701.)

Oxygenation may differ between the extremities in infants with certain lesions (eg, coarctation). The site of sampling should be noted. If possible, the saturation should be measured at sites both proximal and distal to the ductus arteriosus (ie, from the right arm and either leg).

A **shunt study,** also known as a hyperoxia challenge, should be performed to determine whether a right-to-left cardiac shunt is present. Pure oxygen (fraction of inspired oxygen in gas [FIO_2] = 1.00) is given for 5 to 10 minutes by hood. In patients with LPBF or TGA, increasing the inspired oxygen does not affect the oxygenation of the blood because the blood is unable to enter the lungs; this is a positive result. In patients with pulmonary disease or hypoventilation, oxygenation increases strikingly, often to a pO_2 exceeding 200 mm Hg; this negative result rules out cyanotic CHD.

A blunted shunt study, characterized by a rise in pO_2 but rarely to levels above 150 mm Hg, is seen in patients with severe pulmonary disease and in those with HPBF lesions. With such lesions the pulmonary venous blood is high in volume, and the rise in its saturation causes a definite rise in arterial oxygenation. This effect is exaggerated by the further increase in pulmonary flow due to the vasodilating effect of oxygen.

A positive shunt study may be identified with pulse oximetry. It is difficult or impossible, however, to distinguish between a blunted study and a negative one with this tool. The oxyhemoglobin dissociation curve is flattened at the upper end, and the saturation changes very little over a wide range of pO_2 (Figure 75-2). Capillary gases may be equally inaccurate in this range, but directly measured arterial blood gases are highly reliable. In addition, they may reveal hypercapnia, with or without respiratory acidosis, suggesting a pulmonary cause for the hypoxia.

Figure 75-2. Oxyhemoglobin dissociation curve. Note that the position of the curve itself may vary with temperature, pH, oxygen partial pressure (pO_2), and 2,3-diphosphoglycerate.

Electrocardiogram (ECG), a fairly inexpensive test, is readily available and noninvasive. However, it does not often help distinguish cyanotic CHD from other causes of cyanosis, particularly for those practitioners who lack experience with neonatal ECGs. The normal range is large in neonates, with much overlap between normal and CHD. Care must also be taken in placing the leads correctly and minimizing artifacts.

Imaging Studies

The **chest x-ray,** a relatively inexpensive and readily available test, is often extremely helpful in differentiating between cardiac and noncardiac disease. Pulmonary disease is often readily apparent on chest x-ray. The x-ray also helps define the cardiac diagnosis broadly but not precisely. Patients with LPBF lesions have small hearts and diminished pulmonary flow. In contrast, patients with HPBF lesions have large hearts and increased flow, such as is seen in infants with simple left-to-right shunts. With many cyanotic lesions, the cardiac silhouette is abnormal in configuration (eg, boot-shaped heart in tetralogy of Fallot) or position (eg, dextrocardia in patients with heterotaxia syndromes). Transposition of the great arteries may be more misleading; pulmonary flow may be increased despite the severe cyanosis, and the heart size may be normal. An apparently normal x-ray does not exclude TGA.

Under optimal conditions, **echocardiography** enables the physician not only to recognize CHD but to identify details of anatomy and physiology. Conversely, a properly performed, complete, negative echocardiogram rules out CHD. The performance of a high-quality study requires the appropriate equipment (with high-resolution imaging), an experienced sonographer, and an experienced cardiologist for interpretation. In the absence of these elements, preliminary echocardiography may be used cautiously as a screening device as part of the initial assessment to confirm heart disease prior to referral to a specialist. Recently, availability of telemedicine for echocardiography has helped to fill this gap in some hospitals and avoid some unnecessary transports. However, referral should not be delayed until echocardiography can be performed.

Management

Initial management prior to cardiac consultation (often with transfer to another institution) includes surveillance, assistance, direct medical management, and supportive care.

Close **surveillance,** including transfer to the highest level of neonatal care available, use of a cardiopulmonary monitor and continuous pulse oximetry, frequent monitoring of vital signs, and repeat physical examinations, is begun as soon as cyanotic CHD is identified. Even if the infant is feeding well, it is best to suspend feedings because of the likelihood of invasive procedures or spontaneous deterioration in the near future. An orogastric tube is placed to decompress the stomach, reducing the work of breathing as well as the risk of aspiration. At least one secure intravenous (IV) line should be placed for administration of fluids, glucose, and medications. If umbilical arterial catheterization can be expeditiously established, it will allow close monitoring of arterial blood gases and blood pressure. The latter may be difficult to measure by cuff in the compromised infant.

While undertaking these measures, the physician should make every effort to seek **assistance** from a pediatric cardiologist. A neonatologist may be consulted if a pediatric cardiologist is not immediately available. Much advice may be obtained over the telephone. In addition, plans for immediate consultation or transfer of patients may be discussed in this way.

The need for **supportive care** depends on the case. In the absence of metabolic acidosis or impaired perfusion, no special measures are indicated in this category. In some cases, IV fluid boluses, inotropic agents, and other treatments may be needed as part of the early management. Mechanical ventilation should be used in patients with metabolic acidosis, whether compensated or uncompensated, because of the increased oxygen requirement produced by hyperventilation and the tendency for tiring, leading to superimposed respiratory acidosis.

The temptation to give supplemental oxygen for more than the few minutes necessary to perform a shunt study is great but must be resisted. Oxygen is rarely helpful and may be harmful in this setting. In infants with TGA or LPBF lesions, oxygenation is not affected. In infants with HPBF lesions, oxygenation is usually adequate in room air (saturation: >80%), and an increase in FIO_2 may exacerbate the CHF. Oxygen may also constrict the ductus arteriosus on which the patient may depend.

The possibility of ductal dependency should prompt consideration of administering the ductus dilator, **prostaglandin E_1 (PGE_1).** The definitive diagnosis of cyanotic CHD need not be made prior to institution of this lifesaving treatment. In infants who remain adequately oxygenated (no acidosis) and perfused, the drug can be prepared but administration deferred pending consultation. The benefits of giving PGE_1 to severely hypoxic infants or infants with compromised perfusion far outweigh the risks, which include apnea and fever. A dramatic improvement is often seen within seconds to minutes, confirming the diagnosis of a ductal-dependent lesion, and enabling the physician to stabilize the patient until more definitive evaluation and intervention can occur.

Prognosis

If untreated, LPBF lesions and TGA are usually fatal during infancy, most often during the neonatal period, because of severe hypoxia. Untreated HPBF lesions may lead to death in infancy from either CHF or complications such as pneumonia. If the systemic blood flow is ductus-dependent (eg, interruption of the aortic arch), death occurs shortly after ductal closure, usually during the first week of life. Delayed diagnosis, even when not fatal, may result in a suboptimal outcome including end-organ injury such as renal dysfunction or neurologic sequelae.

With early recognition and intervention, however, the prognosis for infants with cyanotic CHD is surprisingly good in the absence of a genetic syndrome (eg, trisomy 18) or a major complicating extracardiac malformation (eg, neural tube defect). If diagnosed before the onset of severe circulatory compromise, infants can be stabilized

and evaluated promptly, and palliative or corrective procedures can be performed in the operating suite or catheterization laboratory. Most of these patients can survive for decades with fair-to-good quality of life. Infants with lesions in which all 4 chambers are adequate in size (eg, tetralogy of Fallot) have a better lifetime prognosis than those with a hypoplastic chamber (eg, tricuspid atresia). Even infants with abnormalities such as asplenia syndrome or hypoplastic left heart syndrome now have a reasonable outlook with complex reconstructive surgery or heart transplantation.

CASE RESOLUTION

In the case presented at the beginning of the chapter, marked hypoxia is present in the absence of other cardiac findings such as a heart murmur. The oxygen saturation does not rise after the infant breathes 100% oxygen for 10 minutes. The chest x-ray shows a small, boot-shaped heart and diminished pulmonary blood flow, and the electrocardiogram is normal. Transport is arranged. Because of the marked cyanosis, infusion of prostaglandin E_1 is begun, and saturation increases to 80%, with the oxygen partial pressure rising from 33 to a safer 48 mm Hg. The infant is transferred to a tertiary care center, where consultation is obtained. An echocardiogram is also performed, which demonstrates tetralogy of Fallot with pulmonary atresia. A Blalock-Taussig shunt is placed in the newborn period, and complete repair using a pulmonary artery homograft is performed at 1 year of age.

Selected References

Brown KL, Ridout DA, Hoskote A, Verhulst L, Ricci M, Bull C. Delayed diagnosis of congenital heart disease worsens preoperative condition and outcome of surgery in neonates. *Heart.* 2006;92:1298–1302

Freed MD, Heymann MA, Lewis AB, Roehl SL, Kensey RC. Prostaglandin E1 in infants with ductus arteriosus-dependent congenital heart disease. *Circulation.* 1981;64:899–905

Jones RW, Baumer JH, Joseph MC, Shinebourne EA. Arterial oxygen tension and response to oxygen breathing in differential diagnosis of congenital heart disease in infancy. *Arch Dis Child.* 1976;51:667–673

Liske MR, Greeley CS, Law DJ, et al. Report of the Tennessee Task Force on Screening Newborn Infants for Critical Congenital Heart Disease. *Pediatrics.* 2006;118:e1250–e1256

Niehoff J, DelGuercio C, LaMorte W, et al. Efficacy of pulse oximetry and capnometry in postoperative ventilatory weaning. *Crit Care Med.* 1988;16:701–705

Pfammatter JP, Stocker FP. Delayed recognition of haemodynamically relevant congenital heart disease. *Eur J Pediatr.* 2001;160:231–234

Sasidharan P. An approach to diagnosis and management of cyanosis and tachypnea in term infants. *Pediatr Clin North Am.* 2004;51:999–1021

Sable CA, Cummings SD, Pearson GD, et al. Impact of telemedicine on the practice of pediatric cardiology of community hospitals. *Pediatrics.* 2002;109:e3

Victorica BE. Cyanotic newborns. In: Gessner IH, Victorica BE, eds. *Pediatric Cardiology: A Problem Oriented Approach.* Philadelphia, PA: W. B. Saunders; 1993

Congestive Heart Failure

Robin Winkler Doroshow, MD

CASE STUDY

A 2-month-old infant is brought to the office by his mother, who complains that her son has been eating poorly and breathing oddly for the past few days. The perinatal history is unremarkable. A heart murmur was noted at the 1-month checkup.

The infant is scrawny and irritable. Physical examination shows that the baby's weight, which was at the 50th percentile at birth, is now at the fifth percentile; his height, which was at the 50th percentile, is now at the 25th percentile. He is afebrile, and his heart rate is 165/min, with respirations 60/min and shallow but without respiratory distress. The skin is pale and diaphoretic, and the mucous membranes are pink. Examination of the head and neck is normal; no jugular distention is present. The lungs are clear. The precordium is hyperdynamic, and the heart sounds are loud; a prominent systolic murmur is audible at the left lower sternal border. The liver edge is palpable 4

cm below the right costal margin in the right midclavicular line, and the spleen is not palpable. The extremities are thin, with normal pulses and no edema. Capillary refill is slightly delayed.

Questions

1. What are acute and chronic signs of cardiac disease in children?
2. What are the signs of congestive heart failure (CHF) in children? How do these signs in children differ from those in adults?
3. What underlying disorders can cause CHF in young infants?
4. What is the appropriate emergent management for infants with CHF? What are the risks of treatment if the diagnosis is incorrect?

Congestive heart failure (CHF) is the most common presentation of serious heart disease in infants. Although this condition also occurs in older children, an estimated 90% of cases of CHF in the pediatric population begin in the first year of life. In children CHF is most often caused by structural congenital heart disease (CHD). Compensatory mechanisms are fewer and less successful in small infants. Other causes of CHF are included in Box 76-1.

Epidemiology

The precise incidence of CHF in children is unknown; it is approximately 0.1%. Most cases result from CHD, which occurs in 0.8% of live births. The incidence of CHD varies little with geography, ethnic group, or gender. It is far more common in children with recognizable genetic syndromes (eg, trisomy 21 [Down syndrome], Turner syndrome).

Clinical Presentation

Most commonly, complaints about CHF take the form of concerns about an infant's feeding. Comments are often vague (eg, "my baby is not a good eater") but may be more precise (eg, "he is taking less formula with each feeding," "he is taking longer to nurse"). Parents may also describe rapid breathing, excessive sweating, or decreased activity, but usually only on specific questioning.

Box 76-1. Causes of Congestive Heart Failure in Children

Volume Overload
- Left-to-right shunts (eg, ventricular septal defect)
- Bidirectional shunts (eg, truncus arteriosus)
- Valvular insufficiency (eg, mitral regurgitation)
- Extracardiac conditions (eg, anemia, arteriovenous malformation)

Pressure Overload
- Outflow obstruction (eg, coarctation of the aorta)
- Inflow obstruction (eg, obstructed anomalous pulmonary veins)
- Vascular resistance (eg, hypertension, chronic pulmonary disease)

Myocardial Dysfunction
- Intrinsic conditions (eg, cardiomyopathy, anthracycline toxicity)
- Inflammatory conditions (eg, viral myocarditis, rheumatic fever)
- Coronary insufficiency (eg, anomalous left coronary artery)

Arrhythmias
- Tachyarrhythmia (eg, paroxysmal supraventricular tachycardia)
- Bradyarrhythmia (eg, third-degree atrioventricular block)

Congestive heart failure is also often detected on examination for routine infant checkups or for unrelated complaints. Careful assessment of the physical findings, including vital signs, reveals **tachypnea, tachycardia,** and **hepatomegaly** and frequently signs of underlying structural heart defects, such as a murmur (Dx Box).

Dx Congestive Heart Failure

- Tachycardia
- Tachypnea
- Hepatomegaly
- Sweating
- Decreased feeding
- Irritability
- Easy fatigability
- Murmur

Pathophysiology

High cardiac output may lead to CHF in infants with large left-to-right shunts. Myocardial contractility is relatively normal, and children remain on the "normal" line of the Frank-Starling curve, which relates cardiac output to diastolic volume (also called *preload*) or pressure (Figure 76-1). The shunt requires a very large volume of output, primarily to the pulmonary bed. Although the heart may be able to meet this demand, preload is high, leading to "congestive" signs and symptoms (eg, tachypnea, hepatomegaly). In more severe cases, systemic output may be compromised, resulting in hypotension, renal failure, and metabolic acidosis.

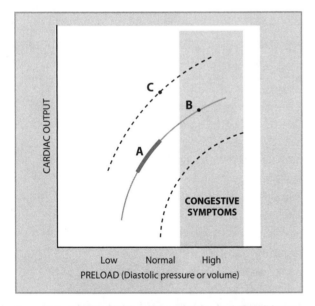

Figure 76-1. **Relationship of cardiac output to preload. The solid curve represents normal myocardial contractility, and the dotted curves represent impaired function (shifted downward) and the positive inotropic state (shifted upward). A. Normal range (no heart disease). B. Left-to-right shunt with congestive heart failure (CHF). Note that overall output is high but most of it is shunted. C. Same situation as B but after treatment for CHF. Cardiac output is the same or better, but preload is now out of the range that results in congestive symptoms.**

Left-sided failure caused by elevated pulmonary venous pressure produces increased lung water. Initially, this fluid is interstitial, and it does not interfere with gas exchange but does trigger reflex tachypnea. Minute volume is kept normal by decreasing tidal (breath-to-breath) volume, leading to shallow as well as rapid breathing (sometimes called "happy tachypnea" because of the absence of dyspnea). Only when the ability of the pulmonary lymphatics to drain this fluid is overcome by large volume does fluid accumulate in the alveoli; rales and respiratory distress, or dyspnea, then result.

Right-sided failure caused by an elevated systemic venous load usually produces more volume than pressure load on this system, possibly as a result of the greater venous compliance in infants compared with adults. The liver becomes very distended and is easily palpated. As long as the liver can absorb the increased venous volume, the portal pressure does not rise, and splenomegaly does not occur. Because the venous pressure rises very little, jugular distention, which is difficult to detect in young infants in any case, is rarely seen, and edema is also rare.

The left and right (systemic and pulmonary) circulations are more interdependent in infants and younger children than they are in older children or adults. As a result, bilateral heart failure is much more common than right-sided or left-sided failure alone. Although this means that recognition of CHF may be easier, determination of the underlying condition may be more difficult because the clues are less specific. For example, in an adult with left-sided failure, the differential diagnosis includes mitral, but not tricuspid, valve disease.

Differential Diagnosis

When tachycardia, tachypnea without dyspnea, and hepatomegaly are present, the diagnosis of CHF is straightforward. Congestive heart failure is most commonly confused with major respiratory infections such as bronchiolitis or pneumonia. Pulmonary infections are frequently associated with dyspnea as well as tachypnea, impaired gas exchange, and other respiratory findings. Rhinorrhea, cough, fever, or wheezing may also be present. Rales may accompany pneumonia but are rare in CHF in infancy or early childhood. Hyperinflation due to lung disease may lead to a false impression of hepatomegaly. In some children, CHD, CHF, and respiratory infections coexist.

Clues to the presence of structural heart disease, such as a murmur or absent femoral pulses, may support the diagnosis of CHF. Severe CHF, with low cardiac output or even shock, has a broader differential diagnosis. In addition to cardiac causes, sepsis, hypovolemia, and disorders associated with inborn errors of metabolism should be considered.

Evaluation

History

The history should include specific questions about feeding and growth (Questions Box). Poor feeding, often a nonspecific complaint in chronically or subacutely ill infants, results from tachypnea and fatigability in infants with heart disease. Growth failure may result from poor feeding and increased cardiopulmonary work. The physician should specifically query parents about possible excessive sweating or rapid breathing in infants, because parents may not volunteer this information (see Chapter 49).

Questions

Congestive Heart Failure

- How has the infant been feeding? Does he or she get out of breath or appear exhausted?
- Has the infant's growth pattern changed recently?
- Does the infant tire easily? With eating? With playing?
- Does the infant perspire excessively, especially with efforts such as feeding?
- Does the infant breathe rapidly, even at rest?

Physical Examination

The diagnosis of CHF is primarily based on clinical findings, and physical examination is essential. The resting respiratory rate must be precisely counted because infants in CHF most often have tachypnea without dyspnea. The liver edge is palpable more than 1 cm below the right costal margin in the midclavicular line, and the degree of enlargement mirrors the severity of the CHF.

In the older child or adolescent, the physical findings are more similar to those of the adult with CHF. Additional findings that may be present include jugular venous distension, basilar rales, and peripheral pitting edema.

Laboratory Tests

Many laboratory tests can be performed to assess infants' hearts (Table 76-1), including electrocardiogram and echocardiogram. However, some procedures are very costly, and some are invasive and therefore carry risk. The value of most of these tests depends on the expertise of the individuals who perform and interpret them. It is important to remember that although test results and consultation with a pediatric cardiologist may be invaluable in the identification of the underlying lesion, *these procedures are not usually required in the diagnosis of CHF.*

Pressure or volume overload of the ventricles causes them to release a neurohumoral peptide, B-type natriuretic peptide, or B-NP, which acts as a natural natriuretic, diuretic, and vasodilator. Studies in adults have demonstrated that blood levels of B-NP are elevated in CHF, and the degree of elevation closely reflects severity of CHF. This new test, which may be performed at the bedside, may be used to distinguish between CHF and other similar disorders such as acute pulmonary disease. Because it closely parallels changes in severity of CHF, it may also be used to track response to treatment. Recent studies in children suggest that it may be similarly useful in the pediatric population; B-NP levels may be very effective in distinguishing between cardiac and noncardiac causes of CHF in children (Figure 76-2).

Table 76-1. Laboratory Tests Used in the Evaluation of Heart Disease in Children

Test	Information
Chest x-ray	Presence and direction of shunt Hints concerning specific diagnosis (possible pulmonary disease ruled out)
Serum B-type natriuretic peptide (B-NP)	Presence and severity of congestive heart failure
Electrocardiogram (ECG)	Cardiac rhythm and conduction Chamber overload Coronary insufficiency
Ambulatory ECG (24-hour ECG)	Subacute rhythm assessment Correlation of symptoms with rhythm
Oximetry	Presence and degree of hypoxemia
Arterial blood gases	Hypoxemia Acid-base status
Hematocrit	Anemia Polycythemia
Exercise test	Quantitation of exercise tolerance Provocation of symptoms or arrhythmia
Echocardiogram	Specific structural diagnosis and hemodynamics Chamber enlargement and function Presence of pericardial effusion
Cardiac catheterization	Specific structural diagnosis and hemodynamics Cardiac electrophysiology
Tilt table test	Autonomic function

Imaging Studies

The most useful supportive study is a **chest x-ray,** preferably in anteroposterior and lateral projections. The chest x-ray may show cardiomegaly, pulmonary venous congestion, and hyperinflation. Cardiomegaly is most commonly due not to myocardial dysfunction, but to volume overload from the shunt. In the absence of cardiac enlargement, the diagnosis of CHF must be seriously questioned. (However, CHF may occur in the absence of cardiomegaly in total anomalous pulmonary venous return with obstruction, which usually presents in the first week of life in association with hypoxia.) Pulmonary venous congestion occurs in left-sided heart failure, but increased pulmonary arterial flow from a left-to-right shunt often obscures the congestion. Hyperinflation resulting from peribronchial edema is also a common finding.

In children with severe CHF, further studies are indicated. **Arterial blood gases** show evidence of metabolic acidosis due to tissue anoxia, with respiratory compensation in early stages and superimposed respiratory acidosis in later stages. A **complete blood count** shows leukocytosis due to stress. It may not differentiate between heart disease and sepsis.

Figure 76-2. Utility of B-type natriuretic peptide (B-NP) in differentiating congestive heart failure (CHF) from lung disease in pediatric patients with respiratory distress. (From Koulouri S, Acherman RJ, Wong PC, Chan LS, Lewis AB. Utility of B-type natriuretic peptide in differentiating congestive heart failure from lung disease in pediatric patients with respiratory distress. *Pediatr Cardiol.* 2004;25:341–346.)

Table 76-2. Therapy for Pediatric Congestive Heart Failure	
Category	**Example**
Chronic (Ambulatory)	
Cardiac glycosides	Digoxin
Diuretics	Furosemide, spironolactone
Angiotensin-converting enzyme inhibitors	Enalapril, captopril
Selective beta-blockers	Carvedilol, metoprolol
Acute (Inpatient)	
Diuretics	Furosemide, bumetanide
Beta agonists	Dobutamine, dopamine
Phosphodiesterase inhibitors	Milrinone, amrinone
Vasodilators	Nitroprusside, oxygen, inhaled nitric oxide
Severe, Refractory	
Mechanical support	Extracorporeal membrane oxygenation, ventricular assist
Cardiac or cardiopulmonary transplantation	
Exogenous B-type natriuretic peptide	Nesiritide

Management

All infants and children with CHF should be under the care of a pediatric cardiologist, often in concert with a pediatrician, intensivist, or neonatologist. Prompt referral to a cardiologist will aid not only in management of the CHF, but also in assessment and management of the underlying disorder.

The numerous pharmacologic treatments for pediatric CHF fall into a small number of categories based on mechanism of action (Table 76-2). Preload can be optimized by the administration of diuretics and venodilators, and afterload by the use of arteriolar dilators, some of which also have inotropic effects. Contractility is enhanced by inotropic agents and antiarrhythmics control tachycardias and bradycardias to optimize heart rate. The most effective control of CHF is attained when more than one mechanism is used.

Inotropes and **diuretics** are used in the initial management of CHF in children. Inotropic support results in a shift to a higher Frank-Starling curve (see Figure 76-1), which allows affected patients to maintain the high volume output necessitated by the underlying CHD at lower diastolic pressures, thus alleviating congestive symptoms. **Digoxin,** a form of digitalis, is the drug of choice in such cases, where cardiac output is not severely impaired, and is therefore often used in outpatients. This agent is readily available, easily absorbed, safe in the therapeutic range, and easy to administer (elixir for oral administration). If digoxin is initially given at the maintenance dose

(10 µg/kg/d), therapeutic levels are not attained for about a week; therefore, loading is preferable (Table 76-3) but may require hospitalization. Digoxin is well tolerated and rarely causes side effects. Because of the safety and reliability of absorption, blood levels need not be checked unless overdose is suspected (eg, history of overadministration, toxic ingestion, unexplained vomiting, or second- or third-degree heart block). In the neonate, blood levels may be difficult to interpret because of the presence of natural digoxin-like immunoreactive substance in the blood.

The elevated diastolic preload of CHF is the result of neurohumorally mediated sodium and water retention. **Diuretics** reverse this phenomenon. **Furosemide,** a potent loop diuretic that is available in an oral suspension and is fairly well absorbed, the most frequent drug of choice for the outpatient. The starting dose is 1 mg/kg once or twice daily. Initially, furosemide may be given intravenously or intramuscularly rather than orally, which reduces the time to onset of action and is more effective. Such treatment also supports the patient while digoxin loading is in progress. **Spironolactone,** a less potent diuretic, may be used in combination with furosemide for its potassium-sparing effects, and may also reduce the deleterious histopathologic and structural changes known as *myocardial remodeling* that can accompany CHF.

Fluid and sodium restriction, often used in adults with CHF, is difficult to achieve with infants because their diet is predominantly or exclusively liquid. High-calorie diets using concentrated formulas, complex carbohydrate additives, or medium-chain triglyceride oils

Table 76-3. Digoxin: Total Oral Loading Dose in Children[a]	
Age	Dose (µg/kg)
Preterm newborns	20–30
Term newborns and infants	25–35
1–5 y	30–40
5–10 y[b]	20–30
10 y to adult[b]	10–15

[a]Intravenous loading dose = 75%–89% of oral dose. Usually given ½, followed 8 hours later by ¼, followed 8 hours later by ¼, followed 12 hours later by initiation of maintenance dose. Assumes normal renal function; the maintenance dose must be adjusted downward for renal failure.

[b]In children older than 5 years, loading dose is more often based on surface area (0.5–1.0 mg/m²).

may reduce the intake of free water and the effort of feeding without compromising caloric intake. Breast milk and most proprietary formulas have a low sodium load. In older infants and children with CHF, salt intake is more easily modified and should be minimized.

Certain pediatric patients with chronic CHF may benefit from the addition of **angiotensin-converting enzyme inhibitors** to their regimen. These arteriolar dilators help control afterload and have been shown to be effective in children with dilated cardiomyopathy and those with large left-to-right shunts such as ventricular septal defects (VSDs). Recent observations suggest that third-generation **beta-blockers** such as carvedilol may be useful to control chronic CHF in children with dilated cardiomyopathy. Randomized, controlled clinical trials in adults with similar pathology have been very encouraging, despite the poor understanding of the mechanism involved; similar trials in children are now underway.

Children with acute, severe, or refractory cases of CHF may require additional medications or interventions, necessitating hospitalization, often in an intensive care unit. These therapies include **beta-agonists** and **phosphodiesterase inhibitors** for inotropic support and **vasodilators** for afterload reduction, **correction of anemia** (eg, transfusion), **treatment of fever** (eg, antipyretics), and **reduction of metabolic demands** (eg, ventilatory support, bed rest, sedation). **Diuretics,** usually given intravenously, provide effective control of congestive symptoms. Because of the importance of fluid balance and nutrition in the child hospitalized with CHF, close and accurate monitoring of fluid intake and output, measurement of daily weight, and measurements of serum electrolytes are essential data in the management of CHF.

In a minority of cases, CHF is refractory to all of the above measures. This may be seen in very severe acute myocarditis, longstanding cardiomyopathy of various causes, and during the postoperative period after complex CHD surgery. Additional options include short-term **mechanical support** such as extracorporeal membrane oxygenation and ventricular assist devices. **Exogenous recombinant B-NP** (nesiritide), which has shown some promise in the setting of adult CHF, may be helpful. In some cases, replacement of the ailing heart or heart-lung unit by **transplantation** may be the only remaining alternative.

Ultimately, the best management for CHF is **treatment of the underlying disorder.** In many cases, failure to treat the underlying disorder will result in limited or no success of other treatment modalities. The degree of urgency depends on the nature of the disorder and the severity of the CHF. For example, in neonates with ductus-dependent lesions such as hypoplastic left heart syndrome, maintenance of ductal patency with prostaglandin E_1 is crucial to initial management. In infants with CHF due to supraventricular tachycardia, prompt conversion to normal sinus rhythm is often the only treatment necessary. Congestive heart failure caused by severe anemia responds dramatically to correction of hemoglobin levels. Cor pulmonale, often seen in children with severe chronic lung disease, is most responsive to measures directed at improving the lung disease and/or decreasing pulmonary vascular resistance, such as supplemental oxygen or inhaled nitric oxide. When CHF is due to structural CHD (the most common situation), surgery or interventional catheterization to palliate the problem (eg, pulmonary artery banding in certain cases with large net left-to-right shunts) or correct the defect (eg, repair of VSD) usually reverses the CHF. Fortunately, it is rarely necessary to "tolerate" prolonged, uncontrolled CHF in children or to treat the condition aggressively at the expense of a major change in lifestyle.

Family counseling, which should begin when CHF is identified, is essential. Several important points should be included, in addition to a general description of both the cardiac defect and CHF. The term *heart failure,* which is commonly thought by laymen to refer to a sudden deterioration of heart function or even cardiac arrest, must be clarified. It is also important to stress that affected infants should be treated as normally as possible, with the exception of administration of medicines and keeping medical appointments. Contrary to popular belief, most infants with cardiac conditions are not fragile. Addressing quality-of-life issues such as parental concern, assuaging guilt, and normalizing existence are key responsibilities of the physician.

Prognosis

In most young infants and children with CHF, the prognosis is excellent. Congestive heart failure responds well to treatment, and the underlying defect can usually be corrected or at least palliated. Without cardiac surgery for CHD, CHF often remits spontaneously over months or years as a result of maturation of compensatory mechanisms, spontaneous improvement in the defect (eg, decrease in the size of a VSD), or increase in pulmonary vascular resistance because of long-standing high pulmonary artery pressure and flow (Eisenmenger syndrome). "Catch-up" growth occurs with remission of CHF, and children have the potential to reach their genetically determined height and weight.

CASE RESOLUTION

The case presented at the beginning of the chapter is typical of an otherwise normal infant with a large ventricular septal defect who becomes symptomatic after the development of congestive heart failure (CHF). The boy's growth failure can be attributed to the chronicity of his illness.

The loud murmur and presentation in infancy strongly suggest the existence of underlying structural congenital heart disease as the cause of CHF. The time of onset of CHF also suggests a specific mechanism. When the onset is slightly delayed after birth, a lesion with changing postnatal hemodynamics, such as left-to-right shunt, which has increased as pulmonary resistance has fallen, is suggested. (Note that a ductus-dependent defect would have presented more acutely and severely in the first week of life.)

Selected References

Bruns LA, Chrisant MK, Lamour JM, et al. Carvedilol as therapy in pediatric heart failure: an initial multicenter experience. *J Pediatr.* 2001;138:505–511

Costello JM, Goodman DM, Green TP. A review of the natriuretic hormone system's diagnostic and therapeutic potential in critically ill children. *Pediatr Crit Care Med.* 2006;7:308–318

Koulouri S, Acherman RJ, Wong PC, Chan LS, Lewis AB. Utility of B-type natriuretic peptide in differentiating congestive heart failure from lung disease in pediatric patients with respiratory distress. *Pediatr Cardiol.* 2004;25:341–346

Mahle WT, Cuadrado AR, Kirshbom PM, Kanter KR, Simsic JM. Nesiritide in infants and children with congestive heart failure. *Pediatr Crit Care Med.* 2005;6:543–546

Maisel AS, Krishnaswamy P, Nowak RM, et al. Rapid measurement of B-type natriuretic peptide in the emergency diagnosis of heart failure. *N Engl J Med.* 2002;347:161–167

O'Laughlin MP. Congestive heart failure in children. *Pediatr Clin North Am.* 1999;46:263–273

Price JF, Thomas AK, Grenier M, et al. B-type natriuretic peptide predicts adverse cardiovascular events in pediatric outpatients with chronic left ventricular systolic dysfunction. *Circulation.* 2006;114:1063–1069

Shaddy RE. Optimizing treatment for chronic congestive heart failure in children. *Crit Care Med.* 2001;29(10 suppl):S237–S240

Chest Pain

Robin Winkler Doroshow, MD

CASE STUDY

A previously healthy 13-year-old boy comes to the office complaining of recurrent chest pain, occurring approximately once a week over the past 2 months. The pain is stabbing in nature, located over the mid-sternum, not associated with any other symptoms, and occurs randomly, both at rest and with exercise. It lasts for 2 to 3 minutes, is ranked as 4 on a severity scale of 10, and subsides spontaneously. He does not appear very concerned about the pain, but his mother is quite anxious to have it checked out. His teacher has sent him home from school twice because of the pain, and the soccer coach will not let him play until he is cleared by a doctor. His physical examination is unremarkable.

Questions

1. What is the significance of chest pain in an otherwise healthy child?
2. How likely is serious heart disease to be heralded by chest pain?
3. How much testing, and what type, is appropriate in working up chest pain?
4. Which chest pain patients should be referred to a cardiologist? To other specialists?

Chest pain in children is one of the most common reasons for referral to a pediatric cardiologist, and is second only to heart murmurs. It is, however, one of the least common presenting complaints of cardiac disease. In fact, from an etiologic standpoint, it would be more suitable for this chapter to be located in the section on gastrointestinal (GI) disorders, respiratory problems, psychological and psychogenic disorders, or hematology, rather than cardiology.

Why, then, approach it in the cardiology section, along with discussions of heart murmurs, cyanosis, and congestive heart failure? Perhaps the strongest reason is that it is the greatest fear of the patient, parent, and physician that chest pain could herald a serious—even lethal—heart problem in an otherwise healthy youngster. This fear is exacerbated by 2 social phenomena in our culture: the widespread press given to cases of sudden unexpected death in young, apparently healthy athletes (who had not, in fact, experienced chest pain in most cases), and the appropriately high level of concern over the underdiagnosis of ischemic heart disease in the adult population. Public information targeting the adult with chest pain may, unfortunately, be misinterpreted as applying also to the child. It is this apprehension, and the associated medicolegal defensive posture, that can so often drive the patient, and his referring primary care physician, to seek cardiology consultation and testing.

Epidemiology

The epidemiology of pediatric chest pain is not well studied. Published series have looked retrospectively at patients seen in an emergency department (ED), with a rate of about 0.25%; an outpatient clinic, at about 0.3%; or, as mentioned previously, a pediatric cardiology clinic, where the rate is disproportionately high. In the primary care office setting, chest pain is the third most frequent pain complaint, after abdominal pain and headache. The most common age range is 8 to 18 years, peaking between 11 and 13 years of age. There is no gender or racial predilection, although the etiologic distribution may vary by gender.

Cardiac causes of chest pain are very uncommon for 2 reasons. Such pain is either a rare symptom in a common cardiac disorder (eg, aortic stenosis) or caused by a very rare condition (eg, anomalous origin of coronary artery [AOCA]).

Clinical Presentation

There is substantial variability in the complaint of chest pain in children (Questions Box). Some youngsters experience a single, protracted, severe episode that brings them to the ED. More frequently, children report repeated episodes occurring sporadically over a period of months or even years. The pain may be induced or exacerbated by exercise, deep breathing, lying down, or eating. It can begin and end abruptly or gradually. It may be accompanied by other symptoms, which can give major clues to the diagnosis. In cases where the pain occurs on exercise, is this a consistent, predictable experience, or is it unpredictable?

Most (up to 97%) of children seen for chest pain have no serious medical history, and most have an unremarkable physical examination.

Chest Pain

Questions

- What is the pain like? Where is it located? Does it radiate? How severe is it?
- How long has the child been having pain? Did it begin after trauma? How often does the pain occur? How long does it last? Does it start and end suddenly?
- What brings the pain on? Is it related to exercise and, if so, is it consistent?
- Does the child have associated symptoms with the pain, such as syncope, shortness of breath, palpitations, fever, nausea, sour taste, wheezing, or cough?
- Does the child at other times have cardiac symptoms, such as easy fatigability, cyanosis, exertional dyspnea, edema, or syncope?
- Does the child's medical history include potentially pertinent disorders such as asthma, gastroesophageal reflux disease, psychiatric problems, heart disease, or sickle cell disease?
- How much impact is the pain having on the child's life? Is he or she missing school or sports?
- Is there a family history of sudden unexpected death, recurrent syncope, or known genetic syndrome?

Pathophysiology

The pathophysiology varies with the underlying cause of the pain, for which there is a broad differential diagnosis (Box 77-1). It is important for the patient, parent, and physician to understand that truncal pain, and particularly visceral pain, is poorly localized, making it difficult to distinguish between, for example, esophagitis and cardiac ischemia; hence, the term "heartburn" for the former. Thus precordial pain may originate from any intrathoracic organ or from the chest wall itself, and the patient cannot identify the source of his discomfort, which in itself is a cause of distress.

Cardiac causes are a heterogeneous category, which can best be viewed as ischemic and non-ischemic in origin (Box 77-2). Ischemic chest pain, or angina, is caused by a drop, often sudden, in the myocardial oxygen supply-demand ratio, causing pain or in rare cases, sudden death. This may occur because of diseased coronary arteries as in adults, due to accelerated coronary atherosclerosis, which is very rare and may be seen in progeria, mucopolysaccharidosis, post-transplantation coronary disease, and severe familial hypercholesterolemia. It may occur as a result of previous inflammation (as in Kawasaki disease with coronary aneurysms) leading to coronary artery stenosis. A congenital AOCA from the opposite sinus of Valsalva (Figure 77-1) or from the pulmonary artery may result in ischemia due to compression of the anomalous vessel between the great arteries, obstruction from a slit-like orifice at the origin or, in the case of the pulmonary artery, low pressure and low saturation in the perfusing blood.

The chest pain seen in patients with left ventricular outflow obstruction (aortic valve stenosis and hypertrophic obstructive cardiomyopathy) is likely also due to ischemia. The already high

Box 77-1. Differential Diagnosis of Chest Pain in Children and Adolescents

Chest Wall
- c Trauma
- c Overuse
- c Inadequate breast support
- c Chronic cough
- u Costochondritis
- u Precordial catch syndrome
- r Slipping rib syndrome

Gastrointestinal
- c Gastroesophageal reflux disease
- u Esophagitis due to repeated vomiting
- r Esophageal stricture
- r Foreign body

Pulmonary
- c Exercise-induced asthma
- c Pneumonia
- u Pleurodynia, pleurisy
- r Pneumothorax/pneumomediastinum
- r Pulmonary embolism

Psychological
- c Anxiety disorder
- u Depression
- u Conversion reaction
- r Munchausen syndrome
- r Bulimia nervosa

Miscellaneous
- c Idiopathic
- u Acute chest syndrome (sickle cell disease)
- r Thoracic tumors
- r Herpes zoster

Cardiac
See Box 77-2

Abbreviations: c, common cause of chest pain; u, uncommon cause of chest pain; r, rare cause of chest pain.

supply-demand ratio due to hypertrophy and hypertension of the left ventricle rises further with strenuous exercise, causing pain and/or arrhythmia.

Although most children with cardiac arrhythmias present with palpitations, dizzy spells, or syncope, and many are entirely asymptomatic, some do complain of chest pain. In the case of the younger child, this may reflect an inability to express the discomfort of palpitations as other than "hurting." In addition, ischemia does occur in some individuals with tachyarrhythmias such as paroxysmal supraventricular tachycardia (SVT), due to high myocardial oxygen consumption and shortened diastole, compromising perfusion. In these patients, ST segment depression may be seen on the electrocardiogram (ECG) during the arrhythmia and persisting for several minutes after the arrhythmia is terminated.

Box 77-2. Cardiac Causes of Chest Pain in Children

Ischemic

u Tachyarrhythmia (supraventricular tachycardia, ventricular tachycardia)

u Cocaine abuse

r Aortic stenosis

r Hypertrophic obstructive cardiomyopathy

r Anomalous origin of a coronary artery

r Accelerated coronary atherosclerosis (eg, progeria, hyperlipidemia, cardiac transplantation)

r Coronary artery stenosis secondary to Kawasaki disease

Non-ischemic

u Pericarditis (viral, bacterial, autoimmune, postoperative)

u Mitral valve prolapse

r Myocarditis

r Aortic root dissection (eg, in Marfan syndrome)

Abbreviations: c, common cause of chest pain; u, uncommon cause of chest pain; r, rare cause of chest pain.

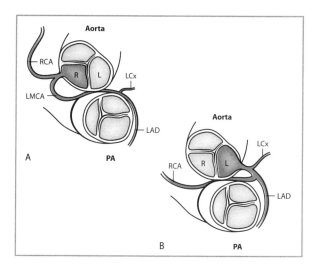

Figure 77-1. Schematic diagram of the 2 forms of anomalous origin of a coronary from the wrong sinus that are associated with myocardial ischemia. A. Anomalous origin of the left main coronary artery (LMA) from the right sinus of Valsalva. B. Anomalous origin of the right coronary artery (RCA) from the left sinus of Valsalva. In each case, the anomalous coronary artery can be seen coursing between the aorta and pulmonary artery (PA). Abbreviations: R, right aortic sinus; L, left aortic sinus; LCx, left circumflex; LAD, left anterior descending.

Non-ischemic cardiac causes of chest pain include pericardial inflammation (eg, acute viral pericarditis, purulent pericarditis, connective tissue disease such as lupus, postpericardiotomy syndrome). Here the pain is due to inflammation of the pericardium and epicardium, directly stimulating the many sensory nerve endings in this area. Aortic dissection also results in direct stimulation of pain fibers, in this case in the aortic wall. Chest pain is also seen in patients with mitral valve prolapse, but it is often difficult to establish a clear causal relationship in this setting. Interestingly, gastroesophageal reflux disease (GERD) can be demonstrated in a high percentage of these patients.

Differential Diagnosis

The differential diagnosis of pediatric chest pain is presented in the Box 77-1, and cardiac causes are listed in greater detail in Box 77-2. The relative frequencies of these causes vary in reported series, but all report higher frequencies of respiratory, idiopathic, traumatic, and psychogenic etiologies and low frequencies of cardiac etiologies, usually in the range of 1% to 5% in patients with no previous cardiac history. These data must be viewed as approximations because the ultimate etiologic classification of cases in these series is not usually based on a definitive result but rather an attribution by the physician involved. Therefore, cultural factors and individual preferences may lead to higher reported rates of "idiopathic" chest pain in some centers, "chest wall pain" in others, and "anxiety disorder" in still others. Some studies report a higher incidence of cardiac etiologies because they so classify any chest pain patient with a cardiac finding (eg, premature beats, abnormal ECG), regardless of whether it may explain the pain.

Evaluation

The keystones to the evaluation of the child with chest pain are a thorough, methodical history and careful physical examination;

indeed, in many cases these will suffice to arrive at a diagnosis and formulate a management plan.

History

The major questions to be addressed are outlined in the Questions Box. Because there are many pertinent details to be included in the **history of present illness,** and they are often provided in a variable sequence, some physicians find it helpful to use a printed format as a guide. Some offer a questionnaire for the patient or parent to complete. Witnesses to the episodes may provide additional helpful information, especially if the patient is not verbally expressive. The witness may estimate a pain score based on observation, which may differ substantially from the score assigned by the patient himself.

Pain that occurs repeatedly over time is less likely due to an organic cause of a serious nature, particularly if it is not reproducible. A severe, protracted episode (eg, lasting hours) is more likely to be organic in origin. The location of the pain has not been a strong predictor of diagnosis in reported series. Its timing and association with other symptoms, however, may provide major clues. Reflux esophagitis may occur after eating, more often when supine or very active, and may be accompanied by a sour taste; it may be relieved by eating. Associated symptoms that may raise a red flag for a cardiac cause include syncope, palpitations, sweating, and nausea; reproducible pain at a given level of exertion is also more likely anginal. Because pain and accompanying anxiety may cause sinus tachycardia, which can be interpreted by the patient as palpitations, it is important to get a sense of the heart rate experienced by patients with that complaint. The child can be asked to tap his chest or clap his hands as fast as his heart was racing during the palpitations; serious tachyarrhythmias such as supraventricular tachycardia and ventricular tachycardia are usually very rapid.

Recent fever and malaise are often present in pneumonia, pleurisy, or pericarditis. Exercise-induced asthma (EIA), in addition to being related to exertion, is sometimes accompanied by cough and/or wheezing. Shortness of breath is very frequently reported by patients in association with their pain; this may reflect anxiety or sensitivity to movement rather than pulmonary pathology.

In youngsters with psychogenic pain, other symptoms of anxiety or depression may be reported, although not necessarily occurring at the same time as the chest pain, and a history of recent stressors may be uncovered. These patients may also report other recurrent somatic complaints.

The nature, severity, and abruptness of the pain may also yield diagnostic clues. Exercise-induced asthma is often described as a chest "tightness," is usually gradual in onset, and lasts beyond the exertion itself. The precordial catch syndrome, a poorly understood disorder also known as *Texidor twinge,* is a sudden, sharp, localized pain that is exacerbated by deep breathing, and lasts only seconds or minutes. In contrast, the slipping rib syndrome, in which the cartilaginous tips of the 8th, 9th, and 10th ribs become transiently subluxated, produces pain at the costal margin, is very sensitive to movement, and is often associated with a "popping" or "slipping" sensation in the affected area. Gastroesophageal reflux disease pain is usually described as "burning," and may awaken the patient from sleep. In contrast, the pain of angina is reported as "crushing," and may radiate to the left arm or the neck. The diffuse pain of pericarditis is often ameliorated by sitting forward. Aortic dissection results in an acute, tearing sensation.

A history of recent chest trauma will naturally suggest chest wall injury as the cause, but the fall or sports mishap may be forgotten if the onset of the pain is not very recent. Chest wall pain may also result from overuse, as seen in weight lifters, or from inadequate breast support, as seen in female runners. Drug abuse, particularly with cocaine, may be disclosed if the patient is questioned in private. In some cases this may have occurred several days before the onset of pain.

The patient's **medical history,** if positive, may lead the diagnostician toward the underlying diagnosis. In children with sickle cell disease, acute chest syndrome must be considered early in the assessment. A history of respiratory disease may point to an acute respiratory infection or to EIA. Children with known heart disease, who are certainly subject to benign chest pain, are more likely to have a cardiac etiology than their peers, but this likelihood will depend on the cardiac diagnosis. Most congenital heart defects, for example, do not cause pain but may raise the level of anxiety in the family and lead to the perception or exaggeration of chest pain. Of greater concern is a history of heart disease that may affect myocardial perfusion, such as Kawasaki disease or cardiac surgery involving the coronary arteries (eg, arterial switch operation for transposition of the great arteries).

The **family history** must not be overlooked. Although most pediatric chest pain is not due to hereditary disorders, some of the more severe causes may be hereditary, such as hypertrophic cardiomyopathy, some arrhythmias, asthma, sickle cell disease, and aortic dissection in Marfan syndrome. It is also noted that in children with nonorganic chest pain, such as psychogenic pain, there is often a history of a close relative having had recent heart surgery or a heart attack, bringing attention to this area during a time of emotional stress.

A complete **review of systems** is essential in the assessment of children with chest pain, due to the wide range of systems potentially involved.

Physical Examination

A careful physical examination is imperative; in children with no history of serious illness, this should be focused on, but not limited to, the chest. General inspection will immediately aid in distinguishing between the acutely ill child and the otherwise well child with chest pain. Abnormal vital signs, such as fever, tachycardia, or tachypnea, are frequently associated with acute etiologies such as infection or inflammation. The child's current pain should be quantified with the aid of a pain scale. If the patient is dyspneic, pulse oximetry should be measured.

The chest wall should be examined for signs of trauma and for tenderness. Care must be taken with the latter because it is easy to obtain a false-positive examination for costochondritis, for example, because the costochondral junctions have some degree of normal tenderness, as do the female breasts. Asymmetry of tenderness, and a report that the pain produced is similar to that complained of, is more suggestive of chest wall injury. In patients with rib injury, the pain can be elicited not only on direct palpation but also indirectly by compression of the thoracic cage from another location. In girls with inadequate breast support, the breast ligaments may be symmetrically tender.

Auscultation of the lungs and heart will, of course, yield useful clues to diagnosis, especially in children with acute inflammatory processes (rales, rub) and in those with left ventricular outflow obstruction such as aortic stenosis (murmur). It must be remembered, however, that many of the organic causes of chest pain, such as GERD, EIA, intermittent arrhythmias, and AOCA, will have a normal examination if the patient is not experiencing the pain at the time of the visit.

The other portions of the physical examination may also aid in the evaluation of the child with chest pain. Jugular distention, hepatomegaly, and peripheral edema suggest congestive heart failure or pericardial effusion with tamponade. The child's behavior pattern and interaction with his parents may suggest a psychological disorder such as anxiety or depression. Poor dentition and halitosis in an adolescent with weight loss may be a sign of bulimia. Excessive signs of trauma such as multiple ecchymoses may indicate a coagulopathy, and also raise the possibility of non-accidental trauma.

Laboratory Studies

A wide variety of diagnostic studies is available to help in arriving at an etiology; it is incumbent on the physician to select those appropriate to the individual patient, guided by the findings of the history and physical examination.

In the patient presenting with **acute chest pain,** often seen in the ED, there is a suitably greater need for tests because the differential diagnosis more often includes serious, even life-threatening, disorders than in the child with chronic recurrent pain. Reported series show the chest x-ray to have a reasonably high yield of positive findings; a negative x-ray is reassuring in ruling out pathology such as pleural effusion, pneumonia, pneumothorax, pneumomediastinum, and thoracic tumor, but cannot be used to exclude most cardiac etiologies. More detailed imaging such as magnetic resonance imaging may be needed when major chest trauma is reported or aortic dissection suspected. Dyspnea or hypoxemia, particularly in the setting of recent immobilization or in an adolescent female taking oral contraceptives, should lead one to suspect pulmonary embolism, for which a nuclear perfusion scan is indicated.

Although ECG is routinely performed as part of the evaluation for acute chest pain in children, it is rarely helpful in establishing a diagnosis other than arrhythmia, which may be suspected from the history or examination. ST segment changes may reflect pericardial irritation or myocardial ischemia if the ECG is done at the time of the pain. If ongoing myocardial ischemia is suspected, myocardial enzymes (creatine phosphokinase-MB fraction, troponin-I) should be measured and a toxicology screen performed. If signs of acute infection such as fever are noted, a complete blood count, sedimentation rate or C-reactive protein, and appropriate cultures are indicated. Echocardiography is highly sensitive and specific for pericardial effusion and should be performed early in the evaluation of the chest pain patient with jugular distention, a friction rub, fever, or ST segment elevation on ECG.

In patients presenting with **chronic recurrent chest pain,** the likelihood of serious pathology is very low. When the examination is normal and the history reassuring, the yield of "screening" tests such as chest x-ray and ECG is extremely poor, and the cost in dollars and anxiety not justifiable. In most cases the history and physical examination are adequate to lead to a focused selection of diagnostic tests, if any are needed. A description of pain suggestive of esophagitis, for example, may lead to endoscopy or upper GI series. When EIA is suspected, pulmonary function testing is appropriate, in some cases with an exercise challenge. Strong suspicion of psychogenic causes should prompt further psychological evaluation at the initial encounter, including querying the patient about suicidality; further testing or consultation may be indicated.

The finding of a murmur of left ventricular outflow tract obstruction is an indication for echocardiography, which will confirm the diagnosis and yield further details that will guide management. A history of palpitations or syncope raises the possibility of arrhythmia; an ECG may give clues such as Wolff-Parkinson-White syndrome as a substrate for SVT, but a normal ECG does not rule out arrhythmia. Here an ambulatory ECG (Holter) monitor or transtelephonic event detector may enable the diagnostician to document the rhythm during an episode of pain. Consistent exertional pain merits evaluation for ischemia, using resting ECG and often exercise stress testing. These studies, unfortunately, can be negative between episodes in patients with AOCA. This diagnosis can, however, be identified by echocardiography, but only if the study is deliberately directed toward that diagnosis; therefore, the study should be done in a pediatric echocardiography laboratory, and the sonographer must be aware of the diagnosis in question.

Management

The management of pediatric chest pain depends on the underlying diagnosis or lack thereof. For management of GERD, acute chest syndrome, pneumonia, pericarditis, connective tissue disorders, thoracic tumors, anxiety disorder, pneumothorax, cocaine abuse, and chest wall trauma, as well as other serious disorders discussed under differential diagnosis, the reader is directed to other sources within and beyond this text.

When there is a strong suspicion of cardiac pathology, either on the basis of history and physical examination or on the basis of subsequent testing as described previously, prompt referral to a pediatric cardiologist is indicated. Management may include surgery (eg, AOCA, aortic stenosis), antibiotics, anti-inflammatories, pericardiocentesis (eg, pericarditis), antiarrhythmics (eg, SVT), interventional catheterization (eg, balloon angioplasty, radiofrequency ablation), or a combination.

Short-term nonsteroidal anti-inflammatory medication is helpful for chest wall pain due to overuse, trauma, costochondritis, or slipping rib syndrome. In a minority of cases, local injection with anesthetic may be necessary.

Therapeutic trials may be considered in some cases to arrive at a diagnosis. A child with suspected esophagitis may be given a liquid antacid at the time of the pain. If the pain is relieved, further workup and treatment can proceed accordingly. Similarly, a youngster with suspected EIA, particularly if there is a previous history of reactive airway disease, may benefit from a trial of an inhaled bronchodilator at the time of the pain.

In the exceedingly common setting of benign chest pain, such as seen in minor chest wall trauma, mild somatization, or occasional reflux esophagitis, the most important step in management is reassurance of the patient and family that this is not an indication of a serious disorder. It is essential to clarify how one has arrived at this conclusion, and why further testing is not appropriate.

A frequent observation in this setting is that most families do not require a definitive diagnosis of the cause of the pain. If a serious disorder is excluded—necessary because 50% of patients believe that chest pain means heart disease—all participants are reassured to their satisfaction. Follow-up studies have demonstrated that at least 80% of patients in this category do not seek further medical attention for their chest pain or return for follow-up.

Prognosis

The outcome is dependent on the underlying diagnosis. In benign chest pain, most cases experience spontaneous resolution, often within a short time of their evaluation. Even in serious and potentially life-threatening causes of chest pain, early diagnosis and intervention will usually lead to an excellent outcome.

CASE RESOLUTION

The patient and his parents are assured that he has no evidence of a serious medical problem. His heart is strong, his lungs clear, and his circulation good. They are told that chest pain in otherwise healthy children may be mysterious but is common, and very rarely a sign of illness. They are told in a gentle but definitive manner that he does not need any more evaluation at this time, but that if the problem does not resolve itself, the child should return for reevaluation.

The boy is delighted to hear that he may return to full sports participation, confirmed in writing to the coach. The parents are very relieved and grateful for the attention and reassurance of the physician.

Selected References

Abdurrahman L, Bockoven JR, Pickoff AS, Ralston MA, Ross JE. Pediatric cardiology update: office-based practice of pediatric cardiology for the primary care provider. *Curr Probl Pediatr Adolesc Health Care.* 2003;33:318–347

Cava JR, Sayger PL. Chest pain in children and adolescents. *Pediatr Clin North Am.* 2004;51:1553–1568

Gumbiner CH. Precordial catch syndrome. *Southern Med J.* 2003;96:38–41

Lipsitz JD, Masia C, Apfel H, et al. Noncardiac chest pain and psychopathology in children and adolescents. *J Psychosom Res.* 2005;59:185–188

Massin MM, Bourguignnont A, Coremans C, Comte L, Lepage P, Gerard P. Chest pain in pediatric patients presenting to an emergency department or to a cardiac clinic. *Clin Pediatr (Phila).* 2004;43:231–238

Rowe BH, Dulberg CS, Peterson RG, Vlad P, Li MM. Characteristics of children presenting with chest pain to a pediatric emergency department. *CMAJ.* 1990;143:388–394

Selbst SM. Chest pain in children. *Pediatrics.* 1985;75:1068–1070

Wiens L, Sabath R, Ewing L, Gowdamarajan R, Portnoy J, Scagliotti D. Chest pain in otherwise healthy children and adolescents is frequently caused by exercise-induced asthma. *Pediatrics.* 1992;90:350–353

Zavaras-Angelidou KA, Weinhouse E, Nelson DB. Review of 180 episodes of chest pain in 134 children. *Pediatr Emerg Care.* 1992;8:189–193

Hypertension

Sudhir K. Anand, MD, and Hali Sherman, MD

CASE STUDY

A 10-year-old girl is seen in the emergency department with a history of severe headache and generalized seizures lasting 2 minutes. Her medical history is remarkable for several episodes of unexplained fever as an infant and an episode of urinary tract infection at age 3 years; no radiologic studies were done. She also has a history of headaches for the past 2 years, which have been treated primarily with acetaminophen. There is no known history of drug ingestion or hypertension in the patient or family members.

The physical examination is remarkable for a pulse of 100/min and a blood pressure of 210/130 mm Hg in the right arm in supine position. Equal pulses are palpable in all 4 extremities. Blood pressure is 216/134 mm Hg in the right lower extremity. The funduscopic examination reveals evidence of petechial hemorrhages and mild papilledema. Chest examination finds normal breath sounds and an active precordium with the apical impulse shifted to the left; no murmurs are heard. The liver is palpable 1 cm below the right costal margin. The neurologic

examination is remarkable for altered sensorium with lethargy; no focal neurologic deficit is present. A routine urinalysis shows 2+ protein and normal urinary sediment. The hemoglobin is 11.2 g/dL and hematocrit is 33%. Sodium is 139 mEq/L, potassium 3.8 mEq/L, chloride 102 mEq/L, and bicarbonate 22 mEq/L. Blood urea nitrogen is 35 mg/dL and serum creatinine is 1.8 mg/dL. An electrocardiogram shows left ventricular enlargement. Computed tomography scan of the head is normal.

Questions

1. What is the definition of hypertension in children?
2. What are the causes of hypertension in children?
3. What is the appropriate evaluation of hypertension in children?
4. What acute and long-term management is used in hypertensive children?
5. What is the appropriate emergency treatment of symptomatic hypertension?

Hypertension is a major public health problem in the adult population. Because of its effects on the heart, central nervous system (CNS), kidneys, and eyes, it is one of the leading causes of increased mortality and morbidity. Hypertension is frequently identified in children also. As with adults, the etiology of elevated blood pressure (BP) in children may be idiopathic (eg, essential or primary hypertension); however, it may also signify the presence of a serious underlying disorder.

Normal Blood Pressure

Both systolic and diastolic BP in children gradually increase, from the newborn period through adolescence; therefore, age-appropriate norms should be used to classify a given BP reading as normal or hypertensive. For example, a BP reading of 120/76 mm Hg would be regarded as normal for a 16-year-old adolescent, but it would signify severe hypertension in a 2-year-old child. Blood pressure measurements should be part of routine physical examinations in all children older than 3 years and in all hospitalized children. Children younger than 3 years who have a history of prematurity, congenital heart disease, recurrent urinary tract infections (UTIs), or chronic systemic illnesses should have their BP measured as a routine part of their well-child care. An appropriately sized BP cuff should be used; the

cuff width should be approximately 40% of the arm circumference midway between the olecranon and the acromion (Dx Box).

 Dx Hypertension

- Blood pressure (BP) elevated >95th percentile for age, gender, and height on at least 3 consecutive occasions with the child in a quiet, non-apprehensive state and with BP cuff of appropriate size
- BP checked in both upper and at least one lower extremity
- Fundus examination: vascular changes, exudates, and papilledema
- Abnormal urinalysis

Epidemiology

Blood pressure values in children are a continuum, with no clear dividing line between normal and high. Despite this limitation, the most recent report on high BP in children and adolescents (2004) defines hypertension as average systolic BP and/or diastolic BP that is greater than the 95th percentile for gender, age, and height on at least 3 occasions (Table 78-1). Patients with BP readings between the 90th and 95th percentile are now considered to be pre-hypertensive and they should receive counseling regarding therapeutic lifestyle

Table 78-1. Definitions of Hypertension[a]

Term	Definition
Normal blood pressure (BP)	Systolic and diastolic BPs <90th percentile for age, gender, and height
Pre-hypertension	Average systolic and/or average diastolic BP between 90th and 95th percentiles for age, gender, and height
	Any BP >120/80 regardless of age
Stage 1 hypertension	Average systolic and/or average diastolic BPs ≥95th percentile to 5 mm above 99th percentile for age, gender, and height with measurements obtained on at least 3 occasions
Stage 2 hypertension	Average systolic and/or diastolic BP >5mm above the 99th percentile for age, gender, and height

[a]National High Blood Pressure Education Program Working Group on High Blood Pressure in Children and Adolescents. The fourth report on the diagnosis, evaluation, and treatment of high blood pressure in children and adolescents. *Pediatrics.* 2004;114:555–576

changes such as increasing physical activity and improving their diet. The report further classifies hypertension into 2 categories: (1) stage 1 hypertension (BP persistently between the 95th percentile to 5 mm above the 99th percentiles) and (2) stage 2 hypertension (BP persistently >5 mm Hg above the 99th percentile). Because this is a statistical definition, 5% of all children (those with BP readings >95th percentile) should be diagnosed with hypertension; however, most providers screening healthy children identify persistent hypertension in fewer than 1% of children rather than the expected 5%. See Tables 78-2 and 78-3 for BP values.

Clinical Presentation

Mild or stage 1 hypertension in most children is usually asymptomatic. Symptoms often associated with high BP such as headache, dizziness, and nosebleeds probably occur no more frequently in these children than in those without elevated BP. Acute presentations of hypertension are divided into 2 categories: hypertensive urgencies and hypertensive emergencies. A hypertensive urgency is defined by the sudden development of elevated BP without evidence of severe end-organ damage but can be associated with headache and vomiting. A hypertensive emergency, in comparison, is defined by obvious signs of significant end-organ damage such as encephalopathy, seizures, papilledema, retinal hemorrhages, or kidney injury and must be dealt with immediately.

Etiology and Pathophysiology

An increase in BP results from an increase in peripheral resistance or cardiac output or a mixture of the two. The exact cause of hypertension in 90% to 95% of adults is still uncertain; hence, the term essential, primary, or idiopathic hypertension. In the past it was often stated that in more than 80% of children, hypertension was secondary to an underlying disorder and that fewer than 20% of cases were idiopathic; however, this is true only in children with very severe hypertension. In most children, especially in adolescents, with mild

increases in BP (ie, slightly beyond the 95th percentile), no etiology of hypertension is found, and they are classified as having idiopathic or essential hypertension.

Many factors play a role in the development of essential hypertension, and this is a very active area of research. Alterations to a variable degree have been found in cardiac output, extracellular fluid volume, peripheral resistance, renin-angiotensin system, aldosterone, electrolyte balance, catecholamines, sympathetic nervous system, natriuretic hormones, prostaglandins, kinins, antidiuretic hormone, insulin response, endothelins, nitric oxide (endothelium-derived relaxation factors), and others. Whether these abnormalities are primary or secondary and their exact role in the pathogenesis of essential hypertension is still uncertain.

Other important factors include heredity, stress response, sleep apnea, and obesity. Recently obesity has been strongly implicated in the increase in incidence of hypertension in the United States. Mirroring the increase in obesity, average BPs rose by 1.4 to 3.3 mm Hg between 1990 and 2000. Studies showing that weight reduction in obese patients lowers BP strengthen the argument that obesity contributes to hypertension. There also seems to be strong associations between sleep disordered breathing, sleep apnea, and hypertension.

Secondary hypertension is more likely in very young children with hypertension, those who meet the criteria for stage 2 hypertension, and those with systemic symptoms of hypertension. The etiology of secondary hypertension varies with the age of the patient and with the nature of the hypertension (ie, whether the condition is acute or chronic) (Boxes 78-1 and 78-2). Renal abnormalities account for 70% to 80% of secondary hypertension in children, the pathogenesis of which may be related to either an increase in extracellular fluid volume (eg, acute glomerulonephritis or chronic renal failure), an increase in renin-angiotensin II activity (eg, renal artery stenosis, renin-producing tumor, or reflux nephropathy), or a combination of both mechanisms (eg, a patient with chronic renal failure caused by reflux nephropathy).

Differential Diagnosis

A reasonable effort should be made to identify the cause of hypertension in all young children who are diagnosed with hypertension because only 30% of them are likely to have essential hypertension (see Boxes 78-1 and 78-2). In older children and adolescents with mildly elevated BPs, essential hypertension is the most likely diagnosis, but must remain a diagnosis of exclusion. The cause of hypertension is often obvious from a detailed history, complete examination, and simple laboratory tests. However, extensive evaluation is sometimes necessary to determine the etiology of hypertension, especially in cases of renovascular hypertension.

Evaluation

When a child is identified as having an elevated BP on any occasion, the finding should be verified with at least 2 additional measurements. The physician should also verify that an appropriately

Table 78-2. Blood Pressure Levels for the 90th and 95th Percentiles of Blood Pressure for Boys Aged 1–17 Years by Percentiles of Height

Age (Year)	BP Percentile ↓	Systolic BP (mm Hg) ← Percentile of Height →							Diastolic BP (mm Hg) ← Percentile of Height →						
		5th	10th	25th	50th	75th	90th	95th	5th	10th	25th	50th	75th	90th	95th
1	50th	80	81	83	85	87	88	89	34	35	36	37	38	39	39
	90th	94	95	97	99	100	102	103	49	50	51	52	53	53	54
	95th	98	99	101	103	104	106	106	54	54	55	56	57	58	58
	99th	105	106	108	110	112	113	114	61	62	63	64	65	66	66
2	50th	84	85	87	88	90	92	92	39	40	41	42	43	44	44
	90th	97	99	100	102	104	105	106	54	55	56	57	58	58	59
	95th	101	102	104	106	108	109	110	59	59	60	61	62	63	63
	99th	109	110	111	113	115	117	117	66	67	68	69	70	71	71
3	50th	86	87	89	91	93	94	95	44	44	45	46	47	48	48
	90th	100	101	103	105	107	108	109	59	59	60	61	62	63	63
	95th	104	105	107	109	110	112	113	63	63	64	65	66	67	67
	99th	111	112	114	116	118	119	120	71	71	72	73	74	75	75
4	50th	88	89	91	93	95	96	97	47	48	49	50	51	51	52
	90th	102	103	105	107	109	110	111	62	63	64	65	66	66	67
	95th	106	107	109	111	112	114	115	66	67	68	69	70	71	71
	99th	113	114	116	118	120	121	122	74	75	76	77	78	78	79
5	50th	90	91	93	95	96	98	98	50	51	52	53	54	55	55
	90th	104	105	106	108	110	111	112	65	66	67	68	69	69	70
	95th	108	109	110	112	114	115	116	69	70	71	72	73	74	74
	99th	115	116	118	120	121	123	123	77	78	79	80	81	81	82
6	50th	91	92	94	96	98	99	100	53	53	54	55	56	57	57
	90th	105	106	108	110	111	113	113	68	68	69	70	71	72	72
	95th	109	110	112	114	115	117	117	72	72	73	74	75	76	76
	99th	116	117	119	121	123	124	125	80	80	81	82	83	84	84
7	50th	92	94	95	97	99	100	101	55	55	56	57	58	59	59
	90th	106	107	109	111	113	114	115	70	70	71	72	73	74	74
	95th	110	111	113	115	117	118	119	74	74	75	76	77	78	78
	99th	117	118	120	122	124	125	126	82	82	83	84	85	86	86
8	50th	94	95	97	99	100	102	102	56	57	58	59	60	60	61
	90th	107	109	110	112	114	115	116	71	72	72	73	74	75	76
	95th	111	112	114	116	118	119	120	75	76	77	78	79	79	80
	99th	119	120	122	123	125	127	127	83	84	85	86	87	87	88
9	50th	95	96	98	100	102	103	104	57	58	59	60	61	61	62
	90th	109	110	112	114	115	117	118	72	73	74	75	76	76	77
	95th	113	114	116	118	119	121	121	76	77	78	79	80	81	81
	99th	120	121	123	125	127	128	129	84	85	86	87	88	88	89
10	50th	97	98	100	102	103	105	106	58	59	60	61	61	62	63
	90th	111	112	114	115	117	119	119	73	73	74	75	76	77	78
	95th	115	116	117	119	121	122	123	77	78	79	80	81	81	82
	99th	122	123	125	127	128	130	130	85	86	86	88	88	89	90

Age (Year)	BP Percentile ↓	Systolic BP (mm Hg)							Diastolic BP (mm Hg)						
		← Percentile of Height →							← Percentile of Height →						
		5th	10th	25th	50th	75th	90th	95th	5th	10th	25th	50th	75th	90th	95th
11	50th	99	100	102	104	105	107	107	59	59	60	61	62	63	63
	90th	113	114	115	117	119	120	121	74	74	75	76	77	78	78
	95th	117	118	119	121	123	124	125	78	78	79	80	81	82	82
	99th	124	125	127	129	130	132	132	86	86	87	88	89	90	90
12	50th	101	102	104	106	108	109	110	59	60	61	62	63	63	64
	90th	115	116	118	120	121	123	123	74	75	75	76	77	78	79
	95th	119	120	122	123	125	127	127	78	79	80	81	82	82	83
	99th	126	127	129	131	133	134	135	86	87	88	89	90	90	91
13	50th	104	105	106	108	110	111	112	60	60	61	62	63	64	64
	90th	117	118	120	122	124	125	126	75	75	76	77	78	79	79
	95th	121	122	124	126	128	129	130	79	79	80	81	82	83	83
	99th	128	130	131	133	135	136	137	87	87	88	89	90	91	91
14	50th	106	107	109	111	113	114	115	60	61	62	63	64	65	65
	90th	120	121	123	125	126	128	128	75	76	77	78	79	79	80
	95th	124	125	127	128	130	132	132	80	80	81	82	83	84	84
	99th	131	132	134	136	138	139	140	87	88	89	90	91	92	92
15	50th	109	110	112	113	115	117	117	61	62	63	64	65	66	66
	90th	122	124	125	127	129	130	131	76	77	78	79	80	80	81
	95th	126	127	129	131	133	134	135	81	81	82	83	84	85	85
	99th	134	135	136	138	140	142	142	88	89	90	91	92	93	93
16	50th	111	112	114	116	118	119	120	63	63	64	65	66	67	67
	90th	125	126	128	130	131	133	134	78	78	79	80	81	82	82
	95th	129	130	132	134	135	137	137	82	83	83	84	85	86	87
	99th	136	137	139	141	143	144	145	90	90	91	92	93	94	94
17	50th	114	115	116	118	120	121	122	65	66	66	67	68	69	70
	90th	127	128	130	132	134	135	136	80	80	81	82	83	84	84
	95th	131	132	134	136	138	139	140	84	85	86	87	87	88	89
	99th	139	140	141	143	145	146	147	92	93	93	94	95	96	97

Abbreviation: BP, blood pressure.

*The 90th percentile is 1.28 SD, 95th percentile is 1.645 SD, and the 99th percentile is 2.326 SD over the mean.

sized cuff is being used to take the measurements and that efforts have been made to put the child at ease. Many children develop mild increases of BP (which can extend into the hypertensive range) when they visit a doctor's office because of anxiety or apprehension (white coat hypertension). Sometimes 24-hour ambulatory BP readings are necessary to confirm whether hypertension is present. An isolated finding of a mild increase in BP with normal subsequent readings does not indicate hypertension. Once hypertension is confirmed, a detailed history, complete physical examination, and appropriate laboratory evaluation should be performed.

History

Information should be obtained about the child's symptoms associated with hypertension, such as headaches and visual difficulties (Questions Box). Inquiry should also be made about the child's history of renal disease, especially previous UTIs, unexplained fevers during infancy and early childhood, edema, hematuria, enuresis or nocturia, and the use of umbilical artery catheterization during the newborn period. Information regarding the child's physical growth; BP recordings during previous physical examinations; eating habits, especially salt intake; use of drugs, especially illicit drugs; and the family's history of hypertension and renal disease should be obtained.

Age (Year)	BP Percentile ↓	Systolic BP (mm Hg)							Diastolic BP (mm Hg)						
		← Percentile of Height →							← Percentile of Height →						
		5th	10th	25th	50th	75th	90th	95th	5th	10th	25th	50th	75th	90th	95th
1	50th	83	84	85	86	88	89	90	38	39	39	40	41	41	42
	90th	97	97	98	100	101	102	103	52	53	53	54	55	55	56
	95th	100	101	102	104	105	106	107	56	57	57	58	59	59	60
	99th	108	108	109	111	112	113	114	64	64	65	65	66	67	67
2	50th	85	85	87	88	89	91	91	43	44	44	45	46	46	47
	90th	98	99	100	101	103	104	105	57	58	58	59	60	61	61
	95th	102	103	104	105	107	108	109	61	62	62	63	64	65	65
	99th	109	110	111	112	114	115	116	69	69	70	70	71	72	72
3	50th	86	87	88	89	91	92	93	47	48	48	49	50	50	51
	90th	100	100	102	103	104	106	106	61	62	62	63	64	64	65
	95th	104	104	105	107	108	109	110	65	66	66	67	68	68	69
	99th	111	111	113	114	115	116	117	73	73	74	74	75	76	76
4	50th	88	88	90	91	92	94	94	50	50	51	52	52	53	54
	90th	101	102	103	104	106	107	108	64	64	65	66	67	67	68
	95th	105	106	107	108	110	111	112	68	68	69	70	71	71	72
	99th	112	113	114	115	117	118	119	76	76	76	77	78	79	79
5	50th	89	90	91	93	94	95	96	52	53	53	54	55	55	56
	90th	103	103	105	106	107	109	109	66	67	67	68	69	69	70
	95th	107	107	108	110	111	112	113	70	71	71	72	73	73	74
	99th	114	114	116	117	118	120	120	78	78	79	79	80	81	81
6	50th	91	92	93	94	96	97	98	54	54	55	56	56	57	58
	90th	104	105	106	108	109	110	111	68	68	69	70	70	71	72
	95th	108	109	110	111	113	114	115	72	72	73	74	74	75	76
	99th	115	116	117	119	120	121	122	80	80	80	81	82	83	83
7	50th	93	93	95	96	97	99	99	55	56	56	57	58	58	59
	90th	106	107	108	109	111	112	113	69	70	70	71	72	72	73
	95th	110	111	112	113	115	116	116	73	74	74	75	76	76	77
	99th	117	118	119	120	122	123	124	81	81	82	82	83	84	84
8	50th	95	95	96	98	99	100	101	57	57	57	58	59	60	60
	90th	108	109	110	111	113	114	114	71	71	71	72	73	74	74
	95th	112	112	114	115	116	118	118	75	75	75	76	77	78	78
	99th	119	120	121	122	123	125	125	82	82	83	83	84	85	86
9	50th	96	97	98	100	101	102	103	58	58	58	59	60	61	61
	90th	110	110	112	113	114	116	116	72	72	72	73	74	75	75
	95th	114	114	115	117	118	119	120	76	76	76	77	78	79	79
	99th	121	121	123	124	125	127	127	83	83	84	84	85	86	87
10	50th	98	99	100	102	103	104	105	59	59	59	60	61	62	62
	90th	112	112	114	115	116	118	118	73	73	73	74	75	76	76
	95th	116	116	117	119	120	121	122	77	77	77	78	79	80	80
	99th	123	123	125	126	127	129	129	84	84	85	86	86	87	88

Table 78-3. Blood Pressure Levels for the 90th and 95th Percentiles of Blood Pressure for Girls Aged 1–17 Years by Percentiles of Height

Table 78-3. Blood Pressure Levels for the 90th and 95th Percentiles of Blood Pressure for Girls Aged 1–17 Years by Percentiles of Height, continued

Age (Year)	BP Percentile ↓	Systolic BP (mm Hg) ← Percentile of Height →							Diastolic BP (mm Hg) ← Percentile of Height →						
		5th	10th	25th	50th	75th	90th	95th	5th	10th	25th	50th	75th	90th	95th
11	50th	100	101	102	103	105	106	107	60	60	60	61	62	63	63
	90th	114	114	116	117	118	119	120	74	74	74	75	76	77	77
	95th	118	118	119	121	122	123	124	78	78	78	79	80	81	81
	99th	125	125	126	128	129	130	131	85	85	86	87	87	88	89
12	50th	102	103	104	105	107	108	109	61	61	61	62	63	64	64
	90th	116	116	117	119	120	121	122	75	75	75	76	77	78	78
	95th	119	120	121	123	124	125	126	79	79	79	80	81	82	82
	99th	127	127	128	130	131	132	133	86	86	87	88	88	89	90
13	50th	104	105	106	107	109	110	110	62	62	62	63	64	65	65
	90th	117	118	119	121	122	123	124	76	76	76	77	78	79	79
	95th	121	122	123	124	126	127	128	80	80	80	81	82	83	83
	99th	128	129	130	132	133	134	135	87	87	88	89	89	90	91
14	50th	106	106	107	109	110	111	112	63	63	63	64	65	66	66
	90th	119	120	121	122	124	125	125	77	77	77	78	79	80	80
	95th	123	123	125	126	127	129	129	81	81	81	82	83	84	84
	99th	130	131	132	133	135	136	136	88	88	89	90	90	91	92
15	50th	107	108	109	110	111	113	113	64	64	64	65	66	67	67
	90th	120	121	122	123	125	126	127	78	78	78	79	80	81	81
	95th	124	125	126	127	129	130	131	82	82	82	83	84	85	85
	99th	131	132	133	134	136	137	138	89	89	90	91	91	92	93
16	50th	108	108	110	111	112	114	114	64	64	65	66	66	67	68
	90th	121	122	123	124	126	127	128	78	78	79	80	81	81	82
	95th	125	126	127	128	130	131	132	82	82	83	84	85	85	86
	99th	132	133	134	135	137	138	139	90	90	90	91	92	93	93
17	50th	108	109	110	111	113	114	115	64	65	65	66	67	67	68
	90th	122	122	123	125	126	127	128	78	79	79	80	81	81	82
	95th	125	126	127	129	130	131	132	82	83	83	84	85	85	86
	99th	133	133	134	136	137	138	139	90	90	91	91	92	93	93

Abbreviation: BP, blood pressure.

*The 90th percentile is 1.28 SD, 95th percentile is 1.645 SD, and the 99th percentile is 2.326 SD over the mean.

Physical Examination

A thorough examination is essential for determining the etiology of hypertension and the extent of target organ damage caused by hypertension. Poor physical growth or short stature may indicate the presence of a chronic disorder, such as Turner syndrome or chronic renal disease with or without renal failure; it may also be the consequence of long-standing severe hypertension alone. Fundus examination is essential to determine if hypertension has been severe and chronic leading to arterial changes, exudate, hemorrhages, and/or papilledema. Tachycardia may signify heart failure or thyrotoxicosis. The child's pulses should be felt in both the upper and lower extremities and the BP should be measured in all 4 extremities to evaluate for coarctation of the aorta and other vascular lesions. A heart murmur may also be present in patients with coarctation of the aorta. Some patients may present in heart failure secondary to chronic severe hypertension or renal disease with fluid retention. The abdomen should be carefully examined for presence of masses caused by cystic kidneys, Wilms tumor, or neuroblastoma and for tenderness especially in the costovertebral angle (CVA). Bruits sometimes may be heard over the CVA in patients with renal artery stenosis. Presence of café-au-lait spots or depigmented spots on the skin may signify hypertension secondary to neurofibromatosis or tuberous sclerosis, respectively.

Box 78-1. Causes of Acute or Intermittent Increases in Blood Pressure in Children

Renal Causes
- Acute glomerulonephritis
- Hemolytic-uremic syndrome
- Henoch-Schönlein purpura nephritis
- Renal trauma
- Renal artery or vein thrombosis
- After renal biopsy
- Acute obstructive uropathy
- Post-genitourinary surgery
- Blood transfusions in patients with renal failure
- After kidney transplant or with transplant rejection

Drug-Induced Causes
- Corticosteroids
- Amphetamine overdose
- Phencyclidine overdose
- Cocaine overdose
- Anabolic steroids
- Oral contraceptives
- Excessive erythropoietin use in patients with end-stage renal disease
- Cyclosporine A and tacrolimus

Central Nervous System Causes
- Increased intracranial pressure (eg, subdural hematoma, meningitis, tumors)
- Encephalitis
- Poliomyelitis
- Guillain-Barré syndrome
- Porphyria
- Familial dysautonomia

Miscellaneous Causes
- Wrong blood pressure cuff size
- Anxiety, apprehension (white coat hypertension)
- Pain
- Fractures
- Orthopedic procedures (especially leg lengthening and those requiring traction)
- Burns
- Leukemia
- Stevens-Johnson syndrome
- Bacterial endocarditis
- Hypernatremia
- Hypercalcemia
- Heavy metal poisoning

Box 78-2. Causes of Chronic Hypertension in Children

Renal
- Scarred kidney: due to pyelonephritis and/or vesicoureteral reflux nephropathy
- Chronic glomerulonephritis
- Connective tissue disease: systemic lupus erythematosus, Henoch-Schönlein purpura
- Hydronephrosis
- Congenital dysplastic kidneys, multicystic kidney
- Polycystic kidney disease
- Solitary renal cyst
- Tumors: Wilms, pericytoma (renin-producing tumor)

Renal Vascular Lesions
- Renal artery stenosis (fibromuscular dysplasia)
- Renal artery thrombosis (especially in the newborn following umbilical artery catheterization)
- Renal vein thrombosis
- Renal artery lesions with neurofibromatosis, tuberous sclerosis

Other Vascular Lesions
- Coarctation of aorta: thoracic, abdominal
- Polyarteritis nodosa and other vasculitides

Endocrine
- Corticosteroid treatment
- Neuroblastoma or other neural crest tumors
- Pheochromocytoma
- Congenital adrenal hyperplasia with 11β- or 17α-hydroxylase deficiency
- 11β-hydroxysteroid dehydrogenase deficiency
- Liddle syndrome
- Primary hyperaldosteronism
- Dexamethasone: suppressible hyperaldosteronism
- Hyperthyroidism
- Hyperparathyroidism
- Cushing syndrome

Central Nervous System
- Intracranial hemorrhage
- Intracranial mass
- Sleep apnea/disordered breathing

Essential (Primary) Hypertension

Laboratory Tests

The extent of laboratory evaluation depends on the clinical findings, the nature of the hypertension (eg, stage 1 or stage 2, acute or chronic), and whether an etiology is apparent or obscure. Box 78-3 outlines suggested laboratory workups for a patient with asymptomatic stage 1 hypertension and for a patient with symptomatic or stage 2 hypertension.

Presence of hematuria, heavy proteinuria, pyuria, and/or elevated blood urea in nitrogen or plasma creatinine would clearly imply a renal disorder as the cause of hypertension and require an appropriate renal evaluation. A kidney biopsy should be performed to diagnose glomerulonephritis, and radiographic investigations, such as ultrasound and nuclear medicine scans, can help identify scarred kidneys, hydronephrosis, cystic kidneys, or tumors.

The presence of electrolyte abnormalities such as hypokalemia, hypochloremia, or metabolic alkalosis would indicate the

Hypertension — **Questions**

- Does the child have any symptoms associated with hypertension (eg, headache, dizziness, nosebleed, visual difficulty, or shortness of breath)?
- Have blood pressure readings been taken during previous routine physical examinations?
- Has the child had any hematuria, generalized swelling of the body (edema), enuresis (nocturia), burning urination, previous urinary tract infection, or other kidney problems?
- How much salt does the child take? Does he or she love to put extra salt on most foods and frequently like to eat salty foods?
- How has the child been growing?
- Is there a history of use of illicit drugs or oral contraceptives?
- Is there a family history of hypertension or renal disease?

Box 78-3. Laboratory Evaluation of Hypertension

A. Stage 1 hypertension
   1. Urinalysis (urine culture if indicated)
   2. Complete blood count, serum electrolytes, blood urea nitrogen, and creatinine, lipid profile for obese patients
   3. Plasma renin activity along with 24-hour urinary sodium excretion may sometimes be indicated
   4. Echocardiography

B. Stage 2 hypertension (in addition to tests for mild hypertension listed above)
   1. Chem-20 panel
   2. 24-hour urine for creatinine, catecholamines, and aldosterone
   3. Renal Doppler ultrasonography
   4. Enalapril- or captopril-enhanced iodine-131 MAG3 renal scan
   5. Renal arteriography (selective if necessary)

---

presence of an increased mineralocorticoid hormone either on a primary basis (primary hyperaldosteronism, adrenogenital syndrome with 11β- or 17α-hydroxylase deficiency, Liddle syndrome, 11β-hydroxysteroid dehydrogenase deficiency, etc) or secondary to increased renin activity in renovascular hypertension, renin-producing tumor, or reflux nephropathy; these values would also indicate a need to measure plasma renin activity and urinary or plasma aldosterone levels. Endocrine-based causes of hypertension in children are uncommon, and tests like plasma or urinary catecholamines, plasma cortisol, thyroid-stimulating hormone, and triiodothyronine are measured on an individual basis depending on the clinical evaluation of the patient.

Imaging Studies

Although electrocardiograms and chest x-rays are often requested to evaluate the effects of hypertension on the heart, they typically yield normal results until the patient enters the late stages of severe hypertension. Echocardiography is now the recommended primary tool for assessing for the presence of target organ damage. In several studies, left ventricular hypertrophy is present even in children with untreated mild hypertension, especially in those who are overweight. Newer recommendations also include obtaining sleep studies in overweight patients to evaluate for sleep apnea.

If the history, physical examination, and initial investigation do not reveal the etiology of severe hypertension in a young child, renovascular disease should be investigated with a renal Doppler ultrasound, enalapril- or captopril-enhanced iodine-131 MAG3 renal scan, renal vein renin measurements, or selective renal arteriography (sometimes magnetic resonance imaging angiography may be used as a substitute).

Management

As previously stated, an effort should be made to identify a remediable cause in all children diagnosed with hypertension so that an appropriate medical or surgical treatment can be offered.

Patients with stage 1 hypertension should be initially managed with non-pharmacologic measures unless the patient is symptomatic or has significant cardiovascular risk factors such as diabetes or hyperlipidemia. These strategies include supportive care, reduction in sodium intake to about 80 to 100 mEq/d, weight reduction if the child is obese, and biofeedback. The 2004 report also recommends treating sleep apnea if present. If after a 3- to 6-month observation period BP remains persistently elevated, drug treatment should be initiated and a decision should be made whether the child needs a more thorough laboratory evaluation. Drug therapy may begin with a beta-blocker (eg, atenolol), an angiotensin converting enzyme (ACE) inhibitor (eg, enalapril), or a diuretic (eg, hydrochlorothiazide).

Patients with stage 2 hypertension may require combination therapy of the above drugs or additional drugs, such as calcium channel blockers, alpha-blockers (eg, prazosin), combined alpha-beta–blockers (eg, labetalol), peripheral vasodilators (eg, hydralazine, minoxidil), or centrally acting drugs (eg, clonidine). The use of one or more of these drugs can control BP in most patients within a satisfactory range and has a limited number of side effects. Patients with renal artery stenosis can be successfully treated with balloon dilatation of the stenosis. If this procedure is unsuccessful or restenosis occurs, surgical correction of the stenosis is usually successful.

Hypertensive emergencies require immediate and rapid intervention with intravenous (IV) medications such as labetalol, nicardipine, or fenoldopam. Hypertensive urgencies may be treated initially with either the above IV medications or oral labetalol or an ACE inhibitor. In both cases, the aim is to lower BP by about 20% to 25% of the presenting values in the first 8 hours. Over the following days to weeks, BP can gradually be controlled to come within normal values for age.

Prognosis

The long-term outcome of hypertension in children depends on the underlying etiology. In children with severe hypertension, BP control improves growth and overall well-being. The very long-term (30–50 years) prognosis of children with persistent, mild essential hypertension is largely unknown; however, one would anticipate that adequate BP control would prolong life and reduce cardiovascular, CNS, renal, and retinal morbidity. In untreated or poorly controlled hypertension the prognosis is probably not good because it is well known that, in combination with obesity and hyperlipidemia, hypertension is linked with severe cardiovascular morbidity and mortality in adults.

Prevention

While there are no specific predictors for the development of hypertension later in life, it is likely that early childhood health plays a role. Children who are small at birth and undergo rapid catch-up growth seem to have a higher incidence of both obesity and hypertension later in life, while breastfed infants have a slower catch-up rate and subsequently have lower rates of hypertension as adults. As a result, it has been postulated that encouraging breastfeeding may have a protective effect. In addition, limiting intake of sodium and caffeine may reduce rates of hypertension in adolescents. Of course, programs aimed at preventing childhood obesity will likely prevent hypertension as well.

CASE RESOLUTION

Because of the elevated blood pressure (BP) and evidence of end-organ dysfunction, the case presented is a clear-cut hypertensive emergency. The history of previous urinary tract infection and the laboratory findings of proteinuria and elevated plasma creatinine suggest chronic pyelonephritis with scarred kidneys secondary to vesicoureteral reflux and chronic renal failure. The elevated creatinine also suggests that both kidneys are affected either by the primary process or as a consequence of severe hypertension. After controlling the initial severe increase in BP, a renal Doppler ultrasound is the appropriate test to determine the kidney size, the extent of kidney damage, and possibly the etiology.

Selected References

Constantine E, Linakis J. The assessment and management of hypertensive emergencies and urgencies in children. *Pediatr Emerg Care.* 2005;21:391–396

Flynn JT. Neonatal hypertension: diagnosis and management. *Pediatr Nephrol.* 2000;14:332–341

Flynn J. Hypertension in childhood and adolescence. In: Kaplan NM, ed. *Clinical Hypertension.* 9th ed. Philadelphia, PA: Lippincott, Williams & Wilkins Company; 2006:465–485

National High Blood Pressure Education Program Working Group on High Blood Pressure in Children and Adolescents. The fourth report on the diagnosis, evaluation, and treatment of high blood pressure in children and adolescents. *Pediatrics.* 2004;114:555–576

Sorof JM, Lai D, Turner J, Poffenbarger T, Portman RJ. Overweight, ethnicity, and the prevalence of hypertension in school-aged children. *Pediatrics.* 2004;113:475–482

Genitourinary Disorders

79. Ambiguous Genitalia 467

80. Inguinal Lumps and Bumps 473

81. Hematuria.. 477

82. Proteinuria... 485

83. Urinary Tract Infection.. 491

84. Vaginitis 497

85. Sexually Transmitted Infections 503

86. Menstrual Disorders 513

87. Disorders of the Breast.. 521

Ambiguous Genitalia

Jennifer K. Yee, MD, and Catherine S. Mao, MD

CASE STUDY

A term infant is being evaluated in the newborn nursery. The mother received prenatal care from the 8th week of gestation, reportedly had no problems during the pregnancy, and took no medications except prenatal vitamins with iron. She specifically denies taking any progesterone-containing drugs. Her previous pregnancy was uneventful, and her 3-year-old son is healthy.

On physical examination, the infant is active and alert, with normal vital signs. Aside from a minimum amount of breast tissue bilaterally, the physical examination is unremarkable, except for the genitalia. The labia are swollen bilaterally and slightly hyperpigmented with what appear to be rugae. No masses are palpable in the labioscrotal folds. The clitoris is 1 cm in length. The introitus is difficult to visualize, but a vaginal opening and urethra are apparent.

Questions

1. What conditions should be considered in newborns with ambiguous genitalia?
2. What should families of such infants be told regarding the gender of the newborns?
3. What key historical information should be obtained from families of such newborns?
4. What laboratory studies must be obtained to aid in the diagnosis?
5. What psychosocial issues should be addressed with families while infants are in the newborn nursery?

Ambiguous genitalia result from disorders of sex development (DSD) in newborns and are classified according to the gonads present. This standard classification, using newer nomenclature with previously used nomenclature in parentheses, includes 46XX DSD (female pseudohermaphroditism) and 46XY DSD (male pseudo-hermaphroditism), ovotesticular DSD (true hermaphroditism), and 46XX testicular DSD or 46XY complete gonadal dysgenesis (mixed gonadal dysgenesis). Individuals with pure gonadal dysgenesis, another DSD, present with primary amenorrhea during adolescence (see Chapter 86).

A multidisciplinary health care team should be involved in the care of infants with ambiguous genitalia. In addition to the general pediatrician, nurses, social workers, neonatologists, pediatric endocrinologists, geneticists, and surgeons are all significant members of the team. The role of primary care physicians, however, cannot be underestimated because they are always involved in the initial evaluations of the newborns and often have already developed relationships with the families.

Epidemiology

The prevalence of ambiguous genitalia in newborns is approximately 1:3,000 to 1:4,000 live births. 46XX DSD is characterized by female chromosomes (46XX), normal ovaries and müllerian structures, and virilized external genitalia. The most common DSD, 46XX DSD, is most often caused by congenital adrenal hyperplasia (CAH). Neonatal screening studies suggest that the incidence of CAH is 1:5,000 to 1:15,000.

46XY DSD occurs in genetic males (46XY) who have testes but abnormal masculinization of the external genitalia. This disorder most commonly results from androgen insensitivity. Ovotesticular DSD is a rare condition in which both ovarian and testicular tissues are present. Seventy percent to 80% of affected individuals have the 46XX karyotype, and the morphology of the external genitalia varies widely.

Mixed gonadal dysgenesis is characterized by one testis and an abnormal streak gonad. Reports indicate that this condition is the second most common form of ambiguous genitalia. Affected newborns often have chromosomal mosaicism (45X/46XY).

Clinical Presentation

Variability in the phenotypic as well as clinical presentation of these disorders is considerable (Dx Box). The newborn with ambiguous genitalia may have an enlarged clitoris or small phallus and varying

---

 Dx Ambiguous Genitalia

- Indeterminate or ambiguous genitalia
- Enlarged clitoris or small phallus
- Hyperpigmented, rugated labia majora that may be fused
- Blind-ending or completely absent vaginal pouch
- Phenotypic male neonate with hypospadias and/or bilateral cryptorchidism
- Phenotypic female neonate with an inguinal hernia or mass

degrees of labioscrotal fusion. Signs of virilization in the female infant might include hyperpigmented labia and the presence of labial rugae. Other findings suggestive of a DSD in a female are perineal hypospadias or an inguinal hernia. More dramatic presentations, such as severe dehydration and shock in a neonate, are associated with CAH of the salt-wasting form.

Pathophysiology

In order to appropriately evaluate and interpret laboratory results of neonates with ambiguous genitalia, it is important to understand the physiology of sexual differentiation and how deviations from this process lead to DSD.

Normal Sexual Differentiation

Normally, before embryos are 6 weeks old, undifferentiated bilateral gonads into which germ cells migrate from the yolk sac have developed. Both wolffian and müllerian duct systems are present at this time, making the embryonic gonads of males and females indistinguishable. The tendency of this bipotential fetus, however, is to develop as a female.

If a Y chromosome is present, a testes-determining factor (known as the sex determining region of the Y chromosome, or SRY) induces differentiation of these gonads into testes, thus blocking female development. This process involves the formation of seminiferous tubules that surround the germ cells. Leydig cells begin to produce testosterone, which in turn acts on the wolffian duct to result in the male internal genitalia: vas deferens, epididymis, and seminal vesicles. Concurrently, regression of the müllerian ducts occurs secondary to testicular production of anti-müllerian hormone (AMH), also called müllerian-inhibiting substance. For normal male external genitalia to form, testosterone must be converted to dihydrotestosterone (DHT) via 5 α-reductase. Dihydrotestosterone then combines with a specific androgen receptor, which allows formation of the phallus and scrotum from the previously undifferentiated external genitalia. The process primarily involves growth and fusion. Later in gestation, the testes migrate into the scrotum.

For the undifferentiated gonads to develop into female organs, the Y chromosome must be absent and 2 intact and normal functioning X chromosomes must be present. Because androgens are not produced and there is no AMH, the wolffian duct degenerates, and the müllerian duct develops into the internal female structures: fallopian tubes, uterus, and upper vagina. Fusion of undifferentiated external genitalia does not occur in the absence of DHT, so folds and swellings become the labia, and the genital tubercle becomes the clitoris.

Development of Ambiguous Genitalia

Congenital adrenal hyperplasia is the most common cause of virilization of the female and is an autosomal recessively inherited defect. Congenital adrenal hyperplasia is the result of an enzymatic deficiency

in the synthesis of cortisol as well as aldosterone from cholesterol. The most common of these enzymatic defects is 21-hydroxylase deficiency. Other less common defects are 11 β-hydroxylase deficiency and 3 β-hydroxysteroid dehydrogenase deficiency. Prenatally, circulating levels of androgens are abnormally high from the overproduction of intermediate steroids. Hence, the external genitalia of the fetus, which are controlled by androgens, are virilized in the female. Internal female organs, however, are normal, because their development is not influenced by androgens.

The salt-wasting form of 21-hydroxylase deficiency is found in approximately two-thirds of patients with classic CAH. As a result of low levels of aldosterone, sodium resorption in the renal tubules is reduced, leading to hyponatremia and hyperkalemia. If this salt-wasting condition goes undiagnosed and untreated, shock and death may result in the first few weeks of life.

46XY DSD is secondary to insufficient testosterone production or insensitivity at the cellular level. Androgen insensitivity, the most common cause of this disorder, is the result of either an abnormality or a reduction in the number of androgen receptors. Not all affected individuals present with ambiguous genitalia at birth because the spectrum of sensitivity is broad. If the androgen receptor is completely nonfunctional or absent, the external genitalia are those of a normal female (complete testicular feminization). This is a recessive condition. In the incomplete forms, which are X-linked recessive, genital ambiguity does occur.

Other causes of male pseudohermaphroditism are (1) inadequate testosterone production secondary to low levels of fetal gonadotropins; (2) defects in testosterone synthesis from enzyme deficiencies; (3) failure to convert testosterone to DHT as a result of 5α-reductase deficiency; (4) deficient müllerian duct–inhibiting substance, which can be autosomal recessive or X-linked recessive; and (5) intrauterine loss of both testes secondary to torsion or another prenatal event.

Although most causes of ambiguous genitalia are related to chromosomal abnormalities and inherited enzymatic defects, exogenous sources of hormones can affect the differentiation of sexual organs. In most cases, the effect is minimal, and no ambiguity develops. Masculinized female external genitalia can occur, however, depending on the timing and duration of prenatal exposure to androgens or other virilizing drugs. Currently the most commonly used androgens are probably anabolic steroids. An adrenal tumor or poorly controlled CAH in the mother will also lead to virilization of the female fetus. Birth control pills do not contain sufficient androgens to cause a problem.

Differential Diagnosis

The differential diagnosis of ambiguous genitalia depends on the classification of the DSD (Table 79-1). Some causes of this condition can be life-threatening and therefore must be recognized immediately (eg, salt-wasting CAH).

Table 79-1. Classification and Causes of Ambiguous Genitalia in the Newborn

Disorder	Causes
46XX DSD	Congenital adrenal hyperplasia
	Maternal androgen ingestion
	Maternal virilizing hormones
	Idiopathic, associated with dysmorphic syndromes
46XY DSD	Biochemical defects in testosterone biosynthesis (enzyme deficiencies)
	Androgen insensitivity (receptor defects)
	5α-reductase deficiency
	Persistent müllerian duct syndrome
	Gonadotropic failure
	Dysgenetic testes
	Bilateral vanishing testes syndrome
Ovotesticular DSD	Chimerism
46XX testicular DSD or 46XY complete gonadal dysgenesis	Chromosomal mosaicism

Abbreviation: DSD, disorders of sex development.

Evaluation

History

The general obstetric history should be reviewed, although it may not be helpful in all cases. Probably the most important source of information on family history can be derived from family pedigrees (Questions Box). Undiagnosed chromosomal disorders, consanguinity, and recurrent medical conditions may be established or inferred from the family background.

Questions

Ambiguous Genitalia

- Did the mother take any medications containing estrogen, progestins, or androgens during the pregnancy? Did she use any other virilizing drugs, such as danazol, during pregnancy?
- Was the mother in contact with anyone using hormonal creams or gels?
- Does the mother have poorly controlled congenital adrenal hyperplasia or an adrenal tumor?
- What is the mother's prior obstetric history?
- Did she have any problems with any previous pregnancies?
- Is there a history of any unexplained neonatal deaths, particularly in male offspring?
- Are her other children growing and developing normally?
- Is there a family history of ambiguous genitalia, including microphallus, hypospadias, and cryptorchidism?
- Is there a family history of sterility, female hirsutism, or amenorrhea?
- Are the parents or other family members consanguineous?

Physical Examination

A complete physical examination of newborns must be performed in the nursery, in addition to a detailed assessment of the genitalia. In particular, the presence of dysmorphic features (eg, microcephaly, low-set ears, micrognathia), which suggests the presence of a chromosomal abnormality, should be appreciated. The areola should be examined for any evidence of hyperpigmentation, and the inguinal area should be palpated for any masses or hernias.

A thorough genital examination should then be performed. The appearance and size of the labioscrotal folds should be noted in terms of pigmentation, presence of rugae, and size. Physicians should keep in mind that normal female labia majora may not completely cover the labia minora. Practitioners should determine whether any masses are palpable in what appear to be the labia and whether the testes are palpable in what appears to be the scrotum. The size of the phallus/clitoris should be measured; a normal stretched phallus is at least 2.5 cm long, whereas a normal clitoris should not exceed 1 cm in term infants. The labioscrotal folds should then be spread apart to look for a vaginal introitus. The presence of posterior labioscrotal fusion, which may preclude this, confirms the suspicion of indeterminate genitalia. Finally, the location of a urethral meatus should be noted, because if hypospadias and cryptorchidism occur together, the chance of a DSD disorder is approximately 50%. A rectal examination may help detect the presence of a uterus or prostate but may be difficult.

Laboratory Tests

The most important study to obtain is a karyotype, which can be performed in 24 to 48 hours by many laboratories. Examination of Barr bodies in a buccal smear is not recommended because this test is unreliable. In addition, serum electrolytes should be ordered in the nursery and monitored closely if CAH is suspected. Certain biochemical studies such as a serum 17α-hydroxyprogesterone and a measurement of 17-ketosteroids and pregnanetriol in the urine are mandatory in newborns with ambiguous genitalia, especially in newborns whose gonads are not palpable. If these initial studies are normal, other intermediate metabolites, such as 11-deoxycortisol, androstenedione, dehydroepiandrosterone sulfate, and sex steroids (eg, testosterone and dihydrotestosterone) can also be measured at a later date.

A human chorionic gonadotropin stimulation test may be performed to measure testosterone if hermaphroditism is suspected or if testes are not palpable.

Imaging Studies

Pelvic ultrasonography is effective in determining if müllerian structures are present, but this technique is not as useful for locating the gonads. If the gonads are not palpable, computed tomography or magnetic resonance imaging of the pelvis may be considered. Genitography can aid in visualizing the duct structures under fluoroscopy.

Management

An interdisciplinary team consisting of a pediatrician, pediatric endocrinologist, medical geneticist, urologist, and psychologist or psychiatrist should be involved in the care of infants with ambiguous genitalia. All aspects of treatment can then be addressed in an efficient and comprehensive manner.

Initial Phase: Delivery Room and Newborn Nursery

If the gender of the newborn is uncertain, it should not be assigned in the delivery room. Parents and nursing staff should be notified immediately of the ambiguity, and a unisex name should be assigned such as "Baby Smith" instead of "Baby Boy Smith" or "Baby Girl Smith." Physicians should then reassure parents that they will soon discuss the issue with them and tell them that until confirmatory tests are done, it is best not to speculate on the gender of the infant.

During the initial hours after birth, parents may have difficulty comprehending the condition. An open line of communication must be maintained with the family, however. Parents should be assured that gender assignment will be made as soon as possible—definitely within 3 to 5 days. Gender can be assigned even earlier in some institutions because most preliminary laboratory results are reported in 24 to 48 hours. Necessary radiographic studies should be ordered as soon as possible.

Intermediate Phase: Psychological Issues

Several psychological issues should be addressed at the time of diagnosis. Alleviation of parental anxiety regarding the cause of the condition should be the priority; general questions can also be answered. For example, parents may be unclear about what to tell others about the gender of the infant and find this process very awkward. In addition, parents should be educated about the normal sexual differentiation. Pediatricians must emphasize that during the first 6 to 8 weeks of gestation, sexual organs are undifferentiated. Ambiguous genitalia should be explained as overdevelopment or underdevelopment rather than as freaky or highly unusual.

Primary care physicians must also assess parents' level of sophistication and their cultural and religious beliefs about gender identity and sexuality. The gender preference for newborn infants should be addressed. Were the parents hoping for a boy or girl? Do they feel strongly about one gender? The medical team can also help families establish a plan for newborns regarding what they want to tell the extended family and in what detail they want to disclose the information. After the initial meeting and while awaiting laboratory data, other questions regarding sexual orientation, puberty, fertility, and self-esteem may arise.

Final Phase: Gender Assignment

After the karyotype is confirmed and the type of DSD has been considered, team members should meet with families to discuss gender assignment before discharge from the hospital. Possible male gender assignment based on factors such as size of the phallus, presence of corporal tissue, and the response to androgen stimulation must be considered. Otherwise, female gender assignment should probably be made regardless of the cause of the DSD. Potential for fertility should also be considered. Parents must be involved in this decision and must agree with the final outcome. Some investigators strongly believe that gender reassignment and genital surgery should be discussed with the patient at a later date rather than assigned during the neonatal period. Such an approach involves consistent counseling for the patient, open discussion among the family, and a primary care physician willing to work diligently with both the patient and the family. Support groups should also be offered regardless of the decision regarding gender reassignment.

Detailed information should be given once again regarding the origin of the condition. The timing and nature of any future hormonal treatment and surgical procedures should be addressed as well. Parents should be urged to move beyond the issue of ambiguous genitalia once a decision regarding gender has been made. They must then deal with activities such as birth announcements and inquiries regarding gender from extended family, siblings, and babysitters. The entire medical team should offer parents encouragement concerning their parenting ability.

Treatment

Hormone replacement therapy is indicated for some newborns with ambiguous genitalia. Cortisol replacement is mandatory in infants with CAH at daily physiological doses of 10 to 20 $mg/m^2/d$. In infants with salt-wasting or classic 21-hydroxylase deficiency, mineralocorticoid replacement is indicated. Oral fludrocortisone should be administered at doses that suppress plasma renin activity to normal levels without causing hypertension.

Testosterone or estrogen replacement is needed at puberty in disorders in which the gonads failed to develop or were surgically removed. For disorders involving microphallus, injections of testosterone enanthate at regular intervals may be used to increase the length and width of the phallus. Recombinant human growth hormone replacement may also be considered for short stature in mixed gonadal dysgenesis.

Surgical procedures may be necessary in many cases, but can be done later in infancy. Although laparoscopy or laparotomy may be indicated for a gonadal biopsy, this is generally not needed in the neonatal period for gender assignment. A gonadectomy is indicated prophylactically in all phenotypic females with all or part of a Y chromosome because of the potential for malignancy. Clitoral recession, vaginoplasty, and labioscrotal reduction are usually performed if infants are to be raised as females. For children to be raised as males, orchiopexy, hypospadias repair, and chordee release are often indicated, but these surgical procedures may be difficult. In some specific cases, however, surgical procedures should be delayed until response to medical treatment is evaluated. For example, in CAH, clitoral size may decrease with glucocorticoid replacement.

Psychological support for the patient and family will be necessary during the child's growth and development into adulthood. Issues revolving around gender identity, gender role, and sexual orientation require ongoing discussion with the patient and the parents. Gender dissatisfaction may occur later in life.

Prognosis

The prognosis for most infants with ambiguous genitalia is excellent. Problems arise with undiagnosed CAH, which may lead to shock and death in the neonatal period if unrecognized and untreated. Otherwise, children should be able to live long healthy lives once their families have come to grips with the diagnosis. Amenorrhea and sterility will need to be addressed with phenotypic females during adolescence, at which time psychological services should be provided.

CASE RESOLUTION

In the case described at the beginning of the chapter, the infant has ambiguous genitalia. The parents should be informed immediately of this finding, and all references related to gender should be avoided. A karyotype and 17α-hydroxyprogesterone analyses should be performed immediately. In addition, serial serum electrolyte should be performed starting at 12 to 24 hours of life. The physician should then meet with the family to further discuss disorders of sex development and explain the diagnostic workup. General psychological services and information regarding support groups should also be provided.

Selected References

American Academy of Pediatrics Committee on Genetics, Section on Endocrinology, and Section on Urology. Evaluation of the newborn with developmental anomalies of the external genitalia. *Pediatrics.* 2000;106:138–142

Blizzard RM. Intersex issues: a series of continuing conundrums. *Pediatrics.* 2002;110:616–621

Hughes IA, Fekete-Nihoul C, Thomas B, Cohen-Kettenis PT. Consequences of the ESPE/LWPES guidelines for diagnosis and treatment of disorders of sex development. *Best Pract Res Clin Endocrinol Metab.* 2007;21:351–365

Krone N, Dhir V, Ivison HE, Arlt W. Congenital adrenal hyperplasia and P450 oxidoreductase deficiency. *Clin Endocrinol (Oxf).* 2007;66:162–172.

Lee PA, Houk CP, Ahmed SF, Hughes IA. Consensus statement on management of intersex disorders. *Pediatrics.* 2006;118:488–500

Ogilvy-Stuart AL, Brain CE. Early assessment of ambiguous genitalia. *Arch Dis Child.* 2004;89:401–407

Rangecroft L. Surgical management of ambiguous genitalia. *Arch Dis Child.* 2003;88:799–801

Verkauskas G, Jaubert F, Lortat-Jacob S, Malan V, Thibaud E, Nihoul-Fekete C. The long-term followup of 33 cases of true hermaphroditism: a 40-year experience with conservative gonadal surgery. *J Urol.* 2007;177:726–731

Inguinal Lumps and Bumps

Julie E. Noble, MD

CASE STUDY

A 2-month-old male infant presents to your office for evaluation of a lump in his right groin for 1-week duration. The lump has been coming and going, and his mother notices that it is larger when he cries. Today, the lump is prominent, and the infant seems fussy. He has been crying more often and vomited once today. His history is remarkable for having been born at 32 weeks' gestation by spontaneous vaginal delivery. Birth weight was 1,500 g, and he did well in the nursery with no respiratory complications. He was sent home at 4 weeks of age and has had no other medical problems. He breastfeeds well and has normal stools.

Physical examination reveals a well-nourished, irritable infant in no acute distress. His vital signs demonstrate mild tachycardia and temperature to 100°F (37.8°C). His abdomen is soft, and the genitourinary examination is significant for a swelling in the right inguinal area that extends into his scrotum. The mass is mildly tender and cannot be reduced. The rest of the examination is normal.

Questions

1. What are the possible causes of inguinal masses?
2. How does age affect the diagnostic possibilities?
3. How do you differentiate between acute and non-acute conditions?
4. What diagnostic modalities can help with the diagnosis?
5. What are the treatment choices for inguinal masses?
6. Are there long-term consequences?

Inguinal masses occur either from disease in normal tissue in the inguinal area or from ectopic tissue, frequently of embryological origin. A child may present with the chief complaint of an inguinal mass, and the mass may vary in position from anywhere along the inguinal canal to the scrotum or labia (Figure 80-1). Along the inguinal canal, a mass might be an enlarged **lymph node,** a **retractile testis,** an **ovary,** or a **synovial cyst.** At the inguinal ring, a mass might also be a testis or an ovary, or an inguinal hernia. In the scrotum, swelling could be due to a **hernia, hydrocele, varicocele, trauma,** or **testicular pathology.** Labial lesions could be secondary to trauma, an **ectopic ovary, mixed gonadal tissue,** an actual testis as in testicular feminization, or a **Bartholin gland cyst.** The differential diagnosis and the subsequent evaluation will vary not only according to the location of the mass and the patient's age but also with the acuity of presentation of the mass.

Epidemiology

Inguinal masses are a fairly frequent complaint in the office setting. The usual cause is an enlarged lymph node, but **hernias and hydroceles** are also common. Surgical repair of hernias and hydroceles are the most common surgical procedures performed in children. The incidence of inguinal hernias has been estimated at 10 to 20 per 1,000 live births. Hernias are present on the right side in 60% of cases, on the left in 30%, and bilateral in 10%. Of affected children, males outnumber females 4:1. Certain conditions are associated with a higher incidence of hernias (Box 80-1). The most significant predisposing factor is prematurity, with hernias reported in 30% of infants weighing less than 1,000 g at birth. Incarcerated hernias are seen in 10% to 20% of patients presenting for hernia surgery. More than 50% of these incarcerated hernias occur in the first 6 months of life.

The other common acute scrotal lesions—**testicular torsion** and **torsion of the appendix testis**—have an incidence of 1:160 in males. The peak incidence of testicular torsion occurs in the perinatal period

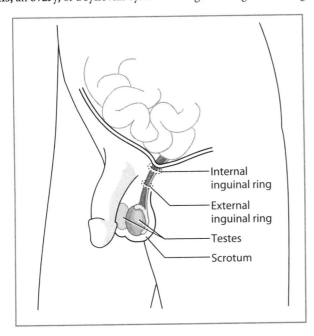

Figure 80-1. The inguinal area.

- Internal inguinal ring
- External inguinal ring
- Testes
- Scrotum

Box 80-1. Conditions Associated With Hernias	
• Abdominal wall defect	• Low birth weight
• Ascites	• Mucopolysaccharidosis
• Connective tissue disease	• Prematurity
• Cystic fibrosis	• Undescended testis
• Family history	• Urologic malformations

and again at puberty. Torsion of the appendix testis is most likely to occur between ages 7 and 10. **Varicoceles** occur in pubertal and postpubertal males, with a fairly high incidence of 2% to 11%. **Testicular tumors** are rare in childhood. They occur at an incidence of 0.5 to 2.0 per 100,000 children and account for only 1% of all pediatric solid tumors.

Clinical Presentation

The child with an inguinal mass presents either acutely or non-acutely. In the acute presentation, the swelling occurs rapidly and is associated with pain. There may be systemic symptoms of nausea and vomiting. The involved area may be extremely tender. Nonacute masses appear more slowly. Some may be present from birth. They may come and go, especially with crying or straining. Nonacute masses usually are not tender and are not associated with systemic symptoms (Dx Box).

Inguinal Masses

Acute
- Rapid onset
- Painful
- Tender
- Nausea and vomiting
- Fever
- Overlying skin red
- Cremasteric reflex absent

Nonacute
- Slower onset
- Not painful
- May fluctuate in size
- Cremasteric reflex present

Pathophysiology

Pathophysiological developmental features of an inguinal mass vary depending on the cause of the mass. An enlarged lymph node may result from proliferation of intrinsic lymphocytes or inflammatory infiltrate from infection (lymphadenitis). The etiology of lymphadenopathy is extensive (see Chapter 73). Any of these processes can appear in the inguinal nodes. An enlarged node can also be secondary to metastatic infiltration from another cell line and represent tumor spread.

A hydrocele develops secondary to failure of obliteration of the patent processus vaginalis during embryologic development. During the 27th to 28th weeks of gestation, the testicle, gubernaculum, and processus vaginalis descend from the peritoneum through the inguinal canal into the scrotum. The processus vaginalis begins closing prior to birth and attaches to the testis, forming the tunica vaginalis

testis. The closure is complete by 1 to 2 years of age. Failure of closure results in a hydrocele (a peritoneal connection with fluid) or a hernia, with intra-abdominal contents. Either may bulge into the inguinal canal and scrotum. If the hernia cannot be reduced and abdominal contents are at risk for vascular compromise, the hernia is termed *incarcerated*.

This condition is a surgical emergency. Sometimes a parent may misinterpret a normal testicle in the process of descent as an abnormal mass. A delay in the normal descent process occurs occasionally, and the testicle may not be in the scrotum at the time of birth. Torsion of the testis after it has reached the scrotum can occur in the newborn if the testis twists on the spermatic cord. Similarly, the testicle can also twist in the pubertal period on its own vasculature within the tunica vaginalis. This is frequently secondary to a high attachment of the tunica vaginalis to the spermatic cord, allowing the testis to hang freely, like a bell clapper. Both types of torsion cause vasculature compromise and an ischemic testis.

Likewise, a vestigial remnant called the *appendix testis* can twist, resulting in vascular compromise of that localized part of the testis.

Pathologically, a traumatic scrotal mass is usually a hematoma, although testicular rupture may occur if the tunica albuginea is torn as a result of trauma. Testicular neoplasms in prepubertal children tend to be germ cell tumors. Yolk sac carcinoma, teratomas, and mixed germ cell tumors with infiltration of their respective cell lines are the usual diseases found.

A varicocele, another scrotal mass, is caused by increased pressure within the venous drainage of the testicle with subsequent dilatation of the veins, producing a mass. Because of the anatomy of the veins, 90% of varicoceles occur on the left side. They are a common finding in adolescent males.

Infections of the epididymis or testis can cause an inflammatory infiltrate and swelling. In the female, infection of Bartholin gland in the labia creates an abscess and leads to an acute, painful mass.

Differential Diagnosis

Location, acuity, and patient age aid in establishing the differential diagnosis.

Non-acute masses, which have a slow onset and are not painful, include lymphadenopathy, a retractile testis, hydrocele, hernia, varicocele, tumor, and ectopic ovary.

Acute masses that have a sudden onset and are associated with pain include epididymitis, orchitis, testicular torsion, traumatic hematoma, torsion of the appendix testis, lymphadenitis, and incarcerated hernia (Box 80-2).

Skin changes can mimic an acute scrotal mass. Henoch-Schönlein purpura, a vasculitis of unclear etiology, can develop in the scrotal area. Scrotal edema can also occur acutely.

Testicular torsion occurs most commonly in the newborn period and again at puberty. Incarcerated hernias are seen most often in the first 6 months of life. Varicoceles are noted almost always at adolescence and beyond.

Box 80-2. Differential Diagnosis of Inguinal Masses

Non-acute	Acute
• Ectopic ovary	• Bartholin abscess
• Hernia	• Epididymitis
• Hydrocele	• Henoch-Schönlein purpura
• Lymphadenopathy	• Idiopathic scrotal swelling
• Retractile testis	• Incarcerated hernia
• Synovial cyst	• Lymphadenitis
• Testicular tumor	• Orchitis
• Varicocele	• Testicular torsion
• Venous aneurysm	• Torsion of appendix testis
	• Trauma

The gender of the patient will also influence the differential diagnosis of the lesion as well as the workup.

Evaluation

History

A thorough, focused history will help define the differential diagnosis (Questions Box). Inquiring about systemic symptoms should always be included and, if positive, may suggest a more generalized process such as a tumor or systemic infection. Symptoms of dysuria would point to epididymitis or orchitis. A history of trauma or possible sexual abuse should always be sought. Hernias and testicular torsion may have a family history positive for the same condition.

Physical Examination

A complete physical examination should always be performed in assessing any pediatric complaint. With an inguinal mass, a concentrated, thorough examination of the inguinal area and lower extremity is needed. If the mass is not apparent on inspection and it comes and goes, ask the parent to point to its location. Observe the skin for evidence of erythema, swelling, or bruising. Gently palpate the

Questions

Inguinal Masses

- How long has the mass been present?
- Is it painful?
- Does it come and go?
- Was there a history of trauma?
- Does the child have dysuria?
- Is there fever or vomiting?
- Are there any other masses?
- Has the child had any lower extremity infections?
- Is there a history of renal disease?
- Is there a history of preterm delivery?
- Is there a positive family history?

inguinal canal to see if you can feel a mass, then assess the scrotal or labial area. If the mass is of acute onset, observe the scrotum and try to localize the tenderness. An incarcerated hernia, testicular torsion, torsion of the appendix testis, epididymitis, and orchitis are extremely tender. If there is torsion of the appendix testis, there may be a classic blue dot at the upper pole of the testis. Try to elicit a cremasteric reflex. If present, it virtually eliminates testicular torsion. The pain of epididymitis and orchitis is relieved partially when the testis is elevated (Prehn sign). Transilluminating the mass may be helpful. A fluid-filled mass such as a hydrocele will definitely transilluminate. But incarcerated bowel may also transilluminate.

Any mass should be accurately measured. Evaluating the borders of an inguinal mass is important. A hydrocele does not extend into the inguinal canal; therefore, the top border can be felt below the pubis. A hernia will extend into the inguinal canal, so an upper border will not be apparent. Reduction of any hernia with gentle pressure should be attempted. To detect a hernia that is not readily apparent, causing the infant to cry increases intra-abdominal pressure and may demonstrate the hernia. An older child can be asked to stand and cough while the inguinal canal is palpated. A varicocele, which feels like a bag of worms, is a non-tender mass over the spermatic cord and is readily palpated.

Laboratory Tests

The laboratory tests should be directed toward the most likely diagnosis as determined by the history and physical examination.

If an infection is suspected, a complete blood count (CBC) should be obtained. If the infection is thought to be epididymitis or orchitis, a urinalysis and urine culture along with gonorrhea and chlamydia cultures should also be obtained. If lymphadenopathy is suspected, a CBC, mononucleosis test, cat-scratch disease test, and possible biopsy may be necessary. If an inguinal mass occurs in a female, chromosomal evaluation is indicated to diagnose testicular feminization syndrome. If a tumor is suspected, the α-fetoprotein level, which is elevated in 90% of yolk sac tumors, and β-human chorionic gonadotropin should be assayed.

Imaging Studies

Ultrasound is the best test to define scrotal contents. It can be useful in differentiating between a hydrocele or hernia and enlarged lymph nodes where a characteristic central echolucent area can be seen. It gives accurate information in evaluating tumors. Ultrasound can provide information in identifying a mass as ovarian or testicular because the ovary is smaller, more echogenic, and may have follicular cysts. Color Doppler ultrasonography is the test of choice in evaluating the acute scrotum to identify a testicular fracture and also assess blood flow in testicular torsion. If incarceration of a hernia is suspected, a flat plate x-ray of the abdomen is helpful to detect signs of intestinal obstruction.

Management

Many inguinal masses require surgical treatment. The acute scrotum is a surgical emergency. There may not be time to perform diagnostic studies. If there is a high probability of a testicular torsion, the scrotum should be surgically explored immediately. There is only a 6- to 8-hour window of time after presentation to save a viable testis. If the testis is nonviable, it is removed. Torsion of the appendix testis does not need to be explored if the diagnosis is certain.

All hernias require surgical repair at some time. Immediate surgery is indicated for an incarcerated hernia that cannot be reduced. If it is reduced, then elective surgical repair can be scheduled. There is controversy regarding the indications for surgery on the contralateral side. An infant younger than 1 year has a 20% chance of developing a hernia on the other side, and most surgeons repair both sides at the same time. As a child gets older, the chance is smaller. Currently some surgeons use laparoscopy at the time of the hernia repair to define a patent processus vaginalis on the opposite side and repair it if patency is found. Hydroceles do not have to be repaired surgically unless they persist beyond 1 year of age. This persistence implies a peritoneal connection and an impending hernia, so repair is indicated. A fracture of the testicle also dictates the need for surgical repair. Varicoceles are removed if the testicle shows growth retardation. All testicular tumors are removed. Additional antitumor therapy is dependent on the stage and cell line of the tumor.

Infectious inguinal masses are treated according to the specific bacteriologic diagnosis.

Prognosis

After surgical treatment for either an inguinal hernia or testicular torsion, the child generally does well. The most significant long-term complication of hernia surgery is subsequent impaired testicular function, and decreased testicular size is noted in up to 27% of cases. Damage to the vas deferens and testicular vessels may impair spermatogenesis and result in a higher incidence of impaired fertility. Surgery for testicular torsion may also be associated with subsequent infertility, particularly if an affected testis is left in place. Two-thirds of affected testicles demonstrate atrophy.

There may be recurrence of a hernia following repair. A hydrocele may develop following varicocele repair.

CASE RESOLUTION

In the case presented at the beginning of the chapter, the infant's history of prematurity associated with a mass that comes and goes most likely indicates an inguinal hernia. With the additional symptoms of pain, fever, and vomiting and the findings of an inflamed, non-reducible mass on examination, there is a high likelihood that the hernia is incarcerated. The infant is taken to the operating room where this diagnosis is confirmed. The hernia is reduced and repaired, and the intestine is noted to be viable. The contralateral side is explored and found to be normal. The infant makes an uneventful recovery.

Selected References

Kapur P, Caty MG, Glick PL. Pediatric hernias and hydroceles. *Pediatr Clin North Am.* 1998;45:773–789

Kass E. Adolescent varicocele. *Pediatr Clin North Am.* 2001;48:1559–1569

Katz DA. Evaluation and management of inguinal and umbilical hernias. *Pediatr Ann.* 2001;30:729–789

Kay R, Ross JH. Testis tumors. In: King LR, ed. *Urologic Surgery in Infants and Children.* Philadelphia, PA: W. B. Saunders; 1998:255–262

Leslie J, Cain M. Pediatric urologic emergencies and urgencies. *Pediatr Clin North Am.* 2006;53:513–527

Maisonet L. Inguinal hernia. *Pediatr Rev.* 2003;24:34–35

Mesrobian H, Balcon A, Durkee C. Urologic problems of the neonate. *Pediatr Clin North Am.* 2004;51:1051–1062

Palmer L. Pediatric urologic imaging. *Urol Clin North Am.* 2006;33:409–423

Sheldon C. The pediatric genitourinary examination: inguinal, urethral and genital diseases. *Pediatr Clin North Am.* 2001;48:1339–1380

Yerkes EB, Brock JW. Diagnosis and management of testicular torsion. In: King LR, ed. *Urologic Surgery in Infants and Children.* Philadelphia, PA: W. B. Saunders; 1998:239–245

Hematuria

Elaine S. Kamil, MD

CASE STUDY

A 5-year-old boy is brought to the office for a school entry examination. He was the full-term product of an uncomplicated pregnancy, labor, and delivery. Although he has had 4 or 5 episodes of otitis media, he has generally been in good health. He has never been hospitalized or experienced any significant trauma. He has no known allergies, has been fully immunized, and is developmentally normal.

In addition, the physical examination is completely normal. The boy's height and weight are at the 75th percentile, and his blood pressure is 100/64. Screening tests for hearing and vision are completely normal. The boy's hematocrit is 42. His urinalysis comes back with a specific gravity of 1.025, pH 6, 2+ blood, and trace protein. Microscopic examination shows 18 to 20 red blood cells per high-power field; 0 to 1 white blood cell per high-power field; and a rare, fine, granular cast.

Questions

1. What disease entities cause hematuria?
2. How should hematuria be evaluated?
3. How does the approach to hematuria differ in children who complain of dark or red urine?
4. What is the appropriate follow-up of children with asymptomatic microscopic hematuria?

Hematuria is a common problem in pediatrics, and primary care physicians should have a clear understanding of its pathophysiology, etiology, evaluation, and therapy. Hematuria can be caused by a serious medical problem, or it may only be an incidental finding with no potential for impairment of patients' health. In general, hematuria is categorized as either gross or microscopic (microhematuria). The etiology and approach to hematuria vary with its severity. Gross hematuria is defined as red or brown urine caused by the presence of red blood cells (RBCs). Microhematuria is defined as 3 or more consecutive urine samples with a positive dipstick and 6 or more RBCs per high-power field in a fresh, spun urine sample.

Epidemiology

The incidence of **gross hematuria** is about 1.3 in 1,000 patient visits (Table 81-1). In one series, the causes in about half of the patients were readily apparent from the intake history or physical examination. The incidence of gross hematuria may increase in the community during an epidemic of a disease, such as acute glomerulonephritis, a condition often associated with gross hematuria. In another series, approximately 30% of children with gross hematuria had glomerular diseases, most commonly immunoglobulin (Ig) A nephropathy.

Microscopic hematuria is a more common pediatric problem. Prevalence rates for persistent, microscopic hematuria range from 0.5% to 2.0%, but 4% to 5% of school-aged children may have microhematuria on a single voided specimen. The incidence is artificially increased in late summer because at that time children tend to visit pediatricians for school physicals that typically include a screening urinalysis.

Table 81-1. Etiology of Gross Hematuria in an Unselected Pediatric Population[a]	
Causes	**Patients (%)**
Readily Apparent Causes	
Documented urinary tract infection (UTI)	26
Perineal irritation	11
Meatal stenosis with ulcer	7
Trauma	7
Coagulopathy	3
Stones	2
Total	56
Other Causes	
Suspected UTI	23
Recurrent gross hematuria	5
Acute nephritis	4
Ureteropelvic junction obstruction	1
Cystitis cystica	<1
Epididymitis	<1
Tumor	<1
Unknown	9
Total	44

[a]Modified with permission from Ingelfinger JR, Davis AE, Grupe WE. Frequency and etiology of gross hematuria in a general pediatric setting. *Pediatrics.* 1977;59:557–561.

Clinical Presentation

Children with gross hematuria present with the sudden appearance of red or brown urine, which may be associated with flank or urethral pain or with a history of trauma.

Children with microscopic hematuria may have urinary complaints (eg, dysuria). In children who appear well, microhematuria is usually detected on screening dipstick examination.

Pathophysiology

Gross Hematuria

Gross hematuria occurs because of the presence of large numbers of RBCs in the urine. Blood may enter the urine because of rupture of blood vessels following trauma or inflammation in the glomeruli or interstitial regions of the kidney. It may also occur as a result of severe inflammation of the bladder wall.

Causes of gross hematuria are listed in Table 81-2. The presence of casts in the urine suggests the diagnosis of glomerulonephritis. The most common causes of glomerulonephritis in children include acute poststreptococcal glomerulonephritis, anaphylactoid purpura, IgA nephropathy, membranoproliferative glomerulonephritis (MPGN), and systemic lupus erythematosus (SLE).

Table 81-2. Common Causes of Gross Hematuria in Pediatric Patients	
Glomerular Causes	**Structural Causes**
• IgA nephropathy	• Renal trauma
• Acute poststreptococcal GN	• Tumor
• Lupus nephritis	• Obstruction
• Membranoproliferative GN	• Renal stones
• Anaphylactoid purpura GN	• Polycystic kidney disease
• Alport syndrome	**Vascular Abnormalities**
• Thin basement membrane disease	• Hemangiomas
• Rapidly progressive GN	• Nutcracker syndrome
• Vasculitis, ANCA positive	• Arteriovenous malformations
• Anti-glomerular basement membrane disease	
• Hemolytic uremic syndrome	
Hematologic Causes	**Infectious Causes**
• Sickle cell disease or trait	• Bacterial urinary tract infection
• Hemophilia	• Viral cystitis
• Thrombocytopenia	• Interstitial diseases
• Thrombosis (renal arterial or venous)	• Acute interstitial nephritis
	• Tubulointerstitial nephritis with uveitis
Other	
• Hypercalciuria	

Abbreviations: IgA, immunoglobulin A; GN, glomerulonephritis; ANCA, antineutrophil cytoplasmic autoantibody.

Common causes of gross hematuria in the absence of RBC casts include urinary tract infection (**UTI**), **renal trauma, bleeding diathesis** (eg, hemophilia or idiopathic thrombocytopenic purpura), **renal tumors, obstruction of the urinary tract, renal stones,** or perhaps **hemolytic uremic syndrome (HUS)**. A hemangioma in the urinary tract is an extremely rare cause of gross hematuria.

Microhematuria

Microhematuria occurs when small numbers of RBCs enter the urine via tiny ruptures in the glomerular capillary walls or in the capillaries of the tubular or bladder lining. One study showed that otherwise healthy children with microscopic hematuria had increased erythrocyte deformability, making it easier for the RBCs to slip through the glomerular capillaries. For purposes of discussion, the following causes of microscopic hematuria are considered: infectious, structural, traumatic, glomerular, and interstitial. Separate consideration of the causes of microscopic and gross hematuria is often helpful, although significant overlap exists. The presence of gross hematuria calls for a more rapid, and usually more extensive, evaluation.

Urinary tract infection is one of the most common **infectious causes** of hematuria. Bacterial infections of the bladder or kidney occur much more frequently than viral cystitis. Adenovirus is the most common viral cause of hemorrhagic cystitis and is usually associated with dysuria. Vaginitis in girls and prostatitis in teenage boys may also result in hematuria.

Any type of congenital obstructive uropathy may lead to massive dilatation of the urinary tract, which makes the urinary tract more susceptible to bleeding, even with trivial trauma. **Chronic urinary tract obstruction** in children (eg, posterior urethral valve or congenital ureteropelvic junction obstruction) is often asymptomatic. In the past these conditions were typically diagnosed when children presented with UTIs or with gross hematuria after relatively trivial trauma. Now they are commonly diagnosed after a prenatal ultrasound reveals hydronephrosis. Nevertheless, urinary tract obstruction may be detected during an evaluation for asymptomatic microhematuria.

Any **tumor** of the genitourinary tract may be associated with both gross and microscopic hematuria. Pelvic tumors rarely cause urinary obstruction in children, although such tumors frequently cause obstruction in adults. Children with Wilms tumor, the most common childhood renal tumor, usually present with an abdominal mass, but it may cause hematuria.

Congenital renal malformations are quite common. Any of these may be associated with hematuria and include polycystic kidney disease, renal dysplasia, medullary sponge kidney, and simple cysts. Patients with polycystic kidney disease may even have severe, painful hematuria.

Vascular problems may also lead to hematuria. Hemangiomas of the kidney, bladder, or ureter are very rare. Arteriovenous malformations also occur infrequently. Hematuria may be a sign of a renal artery or vein thrombosis, particularly in sick neonates.

Young children are more susceptible to **renal injury,** which may result in hematuria, than older children or adults because their kidneys are relatively less protected by the rib cage. In addition, children may insert foreign objects into the urethra and bladder that cause pain and hematuria. Microhematuria has also been described after extremely vigorous exercise such as marathon running. Child abuse should be considered if any suspicions are raised on the basis of the history or physical examination.

Hypercalciuria is another cause of microscopic hematuria. Children with hypercalciuria often have a family history of urinary calculi. Calcium oxalate crystals may be present on the microscopic examination of the urine. A urinary calcium-creatinine ratio is best obtained on a first morning, fasting urine sample. Calcium excretion varies with age. Normal values are listed in Table 81-3.

Table 81-3. Normal Values for Urinary Calcium-Creatinine Ratios[a]		
Age	Urine Calcium-Creatinine	24-Hour Urine Calcium
Preterm	≤ 0.82	≤8.9 mg/kg/d[b]
<7 mo	≤0.86	
7–18 mo	≤0.60	
19 mo–6 y	≤0.42	
6 y–adult	≤0.22	<4 mg/kg/d

[a]Samples for calcium-creatinine ratio should be obtained on a fasting, first voided morning specimen. The calcium and creatinine concentrations must be in the same units (eg, milligrams per deciliter) before the ratio is calculated.

[b]For healthy preterm infants taking no medications. Calcium excretion varies with diet and phosphorus intake and it is higher if patients are treated with furosemide, xanthines, or glucocorticoids.

There are 2 types of hypercalciuria: absorptive and renal leak. Children with absorptive hypercalciuria over-absorb calcium from the gastrointestinal tract, probably because of an exquisite sensitivity to vitamin D, and can be treated with a reduced calcium diet. Children with renal leak hypercalciuria have an inherently higher rate of urinary calcium excretion and may require thiazide diuretics to reduce urinary calcium excretion. **Interstitial nephritis,** usually from drug exposure, may also cause hematuria. Generally patients with interstitial nephritis may exhibit other signs of tubular disease such as glucosuria or proteinuria.

Differential Diagnosis

When children complain of gross hematuria or "red" urine, practitioners must first determine if they have hematuria or pigmenturia by using a urine dipstick. If the dipstick is negative for blood, then the dark urine is due to dyes, drugs, or pigments (Table 81-4). If the dipstick is positive for blood, the red color is caused by intact RBCs, hemolyzed RBCs, or myoglobin; the clarification is based on microscopic examination of fresh, spun urine.

Children whose dipsticks are positive for blood but show no RBCs may have hemoglobinuria or myoglobinuria. Hemoglobinuria may be seen with acute autoimmune hemolytic anemia, drug-induced

Table 81-4. Distinguishing Hematuria From Pigmenturia			
Problem	Urine Color	Hemastix	Microscopic Appearance
Hematuria	Red, brown, or red-brown	Positive	Red blood cells
Hemoglobinuria	Red, brown, or red-brown	Positive	Negative
Myoglobinuria	Red, brown, or red-brown	Positive	Negative
Porphyrins	Red	Negative	Negative
Exogenous pigments[a]	Red or orange	Negative	Negative

[a]Some common exogenous pigments include phenytoin, beets, rifampin, nitrofurantoin, sulfas, amitriptyline, methyldopa, phenothiazine, and chloroquine.

hemolysis, paroxysmal nocturnal hemoglobinuria, a mismatched blood transfusion, cardiopulmonary bypass, freshwater drowning and, in some cases, HUS. Myoglobinuria is seen in individuals with rhabdomyolysis. Acute rhabdomyolysis can occur after a crush injury or a very prolonged seizure and in certain susceptible individuals with an inborn error of muscle metabolism. Both free hemoglobin and myoglobin are toxic to the renal epithelial cells, mandating a generous fluid intake and close monitoring.

Evaluation

Gross Hematuria

History

The history is crucial to an accurate, efficient, and cost-effective evaluation of patients with hematuria (Questions Box). The family should be questioned carefully about trauma (to trunk, abdomen, or perineum), recent skin infection or pharyngitis, dysuria, and abdominal or flank pain. Parents should be asked whether their children appear "puffy." A family history of kidney disease, bleeding diathesis, hemolytic anemia, or inborn error of muscle metabolism may be important.

Questions

Hematuria

- Has the child suffered any recent trauma?
- Has the child had fever or dysuria?
- Does the child have any flank or abdominal pain?
- Does the child have any rashes, joint pains, or edema?
- Does the child have a family history of hematuria, kidney disease, kidney stones, or gross hematuria?
- Is there a family history of bleeding disorders or inborn errors of muscle metabolism?

Physical Examination

A complete physical examination is also essential. Blood pressure should be measured accurately. The skin should be examined thoroughly for rashes or petechiae; the abdomen should be checked carefully for renal masses or tenderness; the genitalia should be examined thoroughly for signs of trauma, masses, or rashes (see Chapter 116); and the joints should be checked carefully for signs of arthritis. Fundi should be examined for any hypertensive changes. Children should be assessed for the presence of edema.

A careful cardiac and chest examination is necessary to detect signs of congestive heart failure (CHF), a finding sometimes seen in acute glomerulonephritis.

Laboratory Tests

Recent studies have shown that careful microscopic examination of a urine sample can help determine whether bleeding originates from the upper urinary tract or the lower urinary tract. Red blood cells originating in the glomerulus have a dysmorphic appearance. The first morning urine sample is the most reliable but is not appropriate in some settings, such as after a motor vehicle crash. Sometimes the gross hematuria is so substantial that spinning the urine results in a large pellet of debris that is difficult to examine. In such instances, it is prudent to examine an unspun sample. The presence of RBC casts indicates glomerulonephritis, but the absence of such casts does not rule out this condition.

If the urine shows RBC casts, then the evaluation should include an antistreptolysin-O (ASO) titer, antinuclear antibody (ANA), C3, complete blood count (CBC) and differential with platelet count, blood urea nitrogen (BUN) and creatinine, serum albumin, and a random urine for a urinary total protein-creatinine ratio.

If the urine shows only large numbers of RBCs, no RBC casts, and no bacteriuria, a CBC with differential and platelet count, a urine

culture, and a prothrombin time (PT) and partial thromboplastin time (PTT) should be obtained. A sickle cell test should be considered as well.

Imaging Studies

If the urine has large numbers of RBCs and no bacteriuria, a renal ultrasound should be obtained. With gross hematuria and a history of serious trauma, an abdominal computed tomography scan should be performed. Children with RBC casts should also have a chest x-ray to evaluate for signs of CHF.

Microhematuria

The evaluation of microscopic hematuria is similar to that of gross hematuria. Figure 81-1 outlines an approach to the evaluation of microscopic hematuria.

History and Physical Examination

Because many conditions may cause either gross or microscopic hematuria, the same historical questions apply to both conditions, and the same careful physical examination is indicated.

Laboratory Tests

Generally, the initial evaluation includes a urine culture and a careful microscopic examination of the urine. If the culture is negative, the hematuria is minimal with no associated proteinuria, and children are otherwise healthy, the urinalysis should be repeated once or twice over the following 2 weeks. Red blood cell casts always signify a glomerular origin. Casts are best preserved in acidic, concentrated urine. Thus the first morning urine is the best sample to examine for casts. Red blood cell morphology should be assessed. Red blood cells originating in the glomerulus are **dysmorphic** and of smaller caliber, whereas those that come from lower downstream appear like normal **biconcave** disks. Although RBC morphology is best appreciated

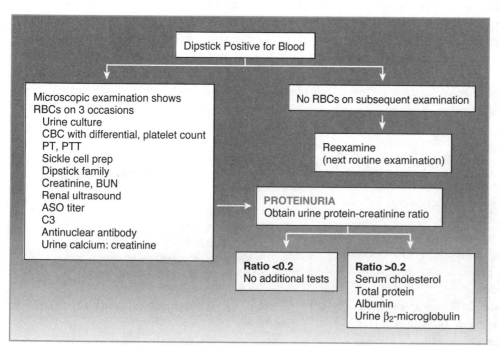

Figure 81-1. **Evaluation of asymptomatic, microscopic hematuria.** Abbreviations: RBCs, red blood cells; CBC, complete blood count; PT, prothrombin time; PTT, partial thromboplastin time; BUN, blood urea nitrogen; ASO, antistreptolysin-O.

with the use of a polarizing microscope, with experience, dysmorphic RBCs can be recognized using an ordinary microscope. Red blood cells of glomerular origin have a mean cell volume of 50 μL or less. In contrast, RBCs of non-glomerular origin have a mean cell volume of 80 to 90 μL. The presence of a newly described, special form of dysmorphic erythrocyte, the G1 cell, is even more specific for glomerular bleeding. These cells are doughnut shaped and contain one or more blebs on their surfaces. Clotting ability should be determined with a platelet count, PT, and PTT. A sickle cell test should be performed. Renal function should be screened with a BUN and creatinine, and a urine calcium-creatinine ratio should be determined. A C3, ANA, and ASO titer should also be checked. If a urine dipstick shows more than a trace of protein, a urinary protein-creatinine ratio should also be determined. If there is a family history of renal disease, a hearing screen should be ordered. All immediate family members should have their urine checked for blood.

If a bloody urine sample is analyzed with a Coulter counter, characteristic distribution curves are seen for glomerular and non-glomerular hematuria. This test is not readily available, however.

Imaging Studies

A renal ultrasound should be performed to rule out structural abnormalities and tumors. Chest x-rays should be obtained if acute glomerulonephritis is suspected.

Renal Biopsy

The definitive diagnosis of the etiology of hematuria may require a kidney biopsy. Generally, pediatric nephrologists perform kidney biopsies only in selected instances after ruling out non-glomerular causes for the hematuria. Indications for renal biopsy in a child with hematuria would include an associated abnormal urinary protein excretion, decreased renal function, recurrent macroscopic hematuria, persistently depressed serum complement levels, serologic evidence for SLE, hypertension, or a family history of renal insufficiency of unknown etiology.

Glomerular Diseases Associated With Hematuria

Glomerulonephritis

Both acute and chronic glomerulonephritis are associated with hematuria. The diagnosis of acute poststreptococcal glomerulonephritis requires a "nephritic" urine sediment (RBCs, RBC casts), a low serum complement, and an elevated streptococcal titer (ASO titer, anti-deoxyribonuclease B, or positive streptozyme). It is important to document that the serum complement returns to normal within 3 months because MPGN may present in a similar way. The serum complement is chronically depressed in MPGN.

The most common form of glomerulonephritis in children is **acute poststreptococcal glomerulonephritis.** Many cases are asymptomatic, however, and do not come to the attention of physicians. The resulting hematuria, which may be gross or microscopic,

is rarely seen before the age of 2 years. The condition is most commonly diagnosed in preschool-aged and school-aged children, who typically present with gross hematuria, often with some edema and hypertension. The hypertension may be severe, and occasionally children even have hypertensive seizures. The edema results from transient, acute renal failure with salt and fluid retention.

Most children with acute poststreptococcal glomerulonephritis recover completely and have an excellent long-term prognosis. Proteinuria is rarely severe enough to cause nephrotic syndrome, and renal failure is rarely serious enough to require dialysis. If hypertension occurs, the chest x-ray often shows some degree of pulmonary edema, even in the absence of overt clinical signs of CHF. Any hypertension requires treatment.

Other infections cause postinfectious glomerulonephritis, but they are less common and less well characterized. The most common form of chronic glomerulonephritis that affects children is **IgA nephropathy.** On kidney biopsy, patients have mesangial proliferation with mesangial deposits of IgA as the dominant Ig. In the later stages, glomerulosclerosis and interstitial fibrosis are apparent. More than one-third of adults with IgA nephropathy develop end-stage renal disease; the percentage of children who progress to this point is less well known. Gross hematuria in IgA nephropathy is occasionally so severe that patients may pass clots and have flank pain. The presence of persistent proteinuria is considered a poor prognostic sign.

Other forms of primary chronic glomerulonephritis include **MPGN, mesangial proliferative glomerulonephritis,** and **membranous nephropathy,** which is technically not a form of glomerulonephritis because it usually lacks a significant proliferative component. Children with these diseases present with hematuria, almost always associated with heavy proteinuria.

Secondary forms of glomerulonephritis include the nephritis of SLE, anaphylactoid purpura, and the nephritis associated with various vasculitides such as Wegener granulomatosis and pauci-immune crescentic glomerulonephritis. Children with lupus tend to present with multisystem disorders but may have only renal manifestations of the disease. Antinuclear antibody is a good screening test for lupus. If the ANA is positive, C3, C4, antidouble-stranded DNA, and a Coombs test should be checked.

Anaphylactoid Purpura

This disease is almost always accompanied by the classical cutaneous vasculitis rash, which is prominent over the lower arms and lower extremities. Abdominal pain may be severe, and affected patients are at risk for the development of intussusception. Children with anaphylactoid purpura have microscopic hematuria, which usually clears, but is occasionally associated with heavy proteinuria and nephrotic syndrome. These children are at risk for developing progressive renal disease. All children with anaphylactoid purpura should have their urine monitored for cessation of hematuria or development of proteinuria. Children with heavy proteinuria and suspected anaphylactoid purpura should have a diagnostic renal biopsy.

Hemolytic Uremic Syndrome

Hemolytic uremic syndrome is a disease characterized by microangiopathic hemolytic anemia, thrombocytopenia, and acute renal failure. It typically follows a prodrome of bloody diarrhea from acute colitis caused by a verotoxin-producing strain of *Escherichia coli* (O157/H7). The verotoxin is believed to be toxic to human endothelial cells. The damaged endothelial cells incite the deposition of fibrin within the glomerular capillaries. These fibrin thrombi lead to the shearing of RBCs and consumption of platelets. Several other organisms, such as pneumococcus and *Shigella*, may precipitate HUS. In atypical cases of HUS, the precipitating event may be an upper respiratory infection. Some cases are familial. Children present with pallor and severe abdominal pain. Urine output may be diminished as a result of renal failure, and in many cases dialysis is required. Hypertension may be severe.

Other Glomerular Diseases

Alport syndrome, thin basement membrane disease (benign familial hematuria), focal segmental glomerulosclerosis (FSGS), and minimal change disease (MCD) are also associated with hematuria. **Alport syndrome** is a disease of the glomerular basement membrane, where thinning and duplication of the basement membrane occur. The renal involvement eventually leads to end-stage renal disease. Patients or their family members often have nerve deafness or keratoconus. The inheritance of Alport syndrome varies by kindred; it may be either autosomal-dominant, autosomal-recessive, or sex-linked. Thin basement membrane disease also is characterized by thinning of the glomerular basement membrane, but the glomeruli are otherwise normal, and the clinical course is benign. Patients with MCD and FSGS present with nephrotic syndrome but may also have microscopic hematuria.

Management

Gross Hematuria

The management of gross hematuria depends on the underlying cause. Children with a history of trauma should be placed on bed rest pending surgical consultation (see Chapter 51). If the evaluation indicates acute glomerulonephritis and if children are not hypertensive, they can be followed carefully as outpatients with monitoring of blood pressure and renal function with consultation with a pediatric nephrologist. Children with coagulopathies require specific treatment of their bleeding disorders (eg, intravenous gamma globulin for idiopathic thrombocytopenic purpura).

If some degree of renal insufficiency is present, then children should be referred to a pediatric nephrologist to rule out more unusual causes of glomerulonephritis, for consideration of renal biopsy, and for treatment.

Microhematuria

Laboratory tests other than urinalysis may be negative in otherwise healthy children with microscopic hematuria. Some of these children may be recovering from subclinical cases of poststreptococcal glomerulonephritis, which can cause microscopic hematuria for up to 1 year. Others may have early IgA nephropathy and not yet have significant proteinuria, and some may have thin basement membrane disease. As long as children have normal renal function, normal blood pressure, a negative renal ultrasound, no significant proteinuria, and all other tests are normal, it is safe to monitor them every 3 to 6 months until the problem resolves. Healthy children with an otherwise negative workup who show no change in their clinical state for a period of 1 year may subsequently be monitored annually. If hypercalciuria is detected, a low-calcium diet or treatment with thiazide diuretics may be tried. Increased urinary microalbuminuria has been shown to be predictive of glomerular lesions in children with isolated microscopic hematuria.

Prognosis

The prognosis for children with hematuria depends on the underlying cause. Gross hematuria is more often associated with serious renal disease such as acute glomerulonephritis, HUS, or renal trauma. Even so, most children with gross hematuria have a good prognosis, provided the diagnosis is rapidly discovered and appropriate specific therapy is given. Children with persistent microscopic hematuria who have no family history of the condition, have a negative evaluation, and do not develop hypertension or proteinuria have an excellent long-term prognosis.

> ### *CASE RESOLUTION*
>
> The boy in the opening scenario shows no worrisome clinical signs such as hypertension or significant proteinuria. His urine should be rechecked twice more, and if the hematuria persists, his evaluation should follow the algorithm in Figure 81-1.

Selected References

Adams ND, Rowe JC. Nephrocalcinosis. In: Bailie MD, ed. *Clinics in Perinatology.* Philadelphia, PA: W. B. Saunders; 1992:179–195

Assadi FK. Value of urinary excretion of microalbumin in predicting glomerular lesions in children with isolated microscopic hematuria. *Pediatr Nephrol.* 2005;20:1131–1135

Ingelfinger JR, Davis AE, Grupe WE. Frequency and etiology of gross hematuria in a general pediatric setting. *Pediatrics.* 1977;59:557–561

Kashtan CE. Alport syndrome and thin glomerular basement membrane disease. *J Am Soc Nephrol.* 1998;9:1736–1750

Lettgen B, Wohlmuth A. Validity of G1-cells in the differentiation between glomerular and non-glomerular haematuria in children. *Pediatr Nephrol.* 1995;9:435–437

Meglic A, Kuzman D, Jazbec J. Erythrocyte deformability and microhematuria in children and adolescents. *Pediatr Nephrol.* 2003;18:127–132

Meyers KEC. Evaluation of hematuria in children. *Urol Clin North Am.* 2004;31:559–573

Pan CG. Evaluation of gross hematuria. *Pediatr Clin North Am.* 2006;53:401–412

Patel HP, Bissler JJ. Hematuria in children. *Pediatr Clin North Am.* 2001;48:1519–1537

Piqueras AI, White RHR, Raafat F, Moghal N, Milford DV. Renal biopsy diagnosis in children presenting with haematuria. *Pediatr Nephrol.* 1998;12:386–391

Sargent JD, Stukel TA, Kresel J, Klein RZ. Normal values for random urinary calcium to creatinine ratios in infancy. *J Pediatr.* 1993;123:393–397

Savige J, Rana K, Tonna S, et al. Thin basement membrane nephropathy. *Kidney Int.* 2003;64:1169–1178

Tsukahara H, Yoshimoto M, Morikawa K, Okada T, Kuroda M, Sudo M. Urinary erythrocyte volume analysis: a simple method for localizing the site of hematuria in pediatric patients. *J Pediatr.* 1989;115:433–436

Youn T, Trachtman H, Gauthier MB. Clinical spectrum of gross hematuria in pediatric patients. *Clin Pediatr.* 2006;45:135–141

Proteinuria

Elaine S. Kamil, MD

CASE STUDY

A 14-year-old boy is brought to the office for a preparticipation sports physical examination. He has been previously healthy but had one hospital admission at the age of 2 years for treatment of a fractured humerus. He has no acute complaints. The family history is positive for diabetes mellitus in the paternal grandfather and lung cancer in the maternal grandfather. It is negative for renal disease or hypertension. The boy's height and weight are at the 75th percentile for age, and his blood pressure is 110/70 mm Hg.

On physical examination he is a well-developed, well-nourished, athletic teenager. No abnormal findings are present. The complete blood count reveals a hemoglobin of 14.8 g/dL, a hematocrit of 48.3%, and a white blood cell (WBC) count of 8,400/mm^3 with a normal differential. The urine has a pH of 5, a specific gravity of 1.025, and a 3+ protein on dipstick. The rest of the dipstick is negative. Microscopic examination shows 0 to 1 WBC count per high-power field and 0 to 2 hyaline casts per low-power field.

Questions

1. What conditions cause proteinuria?
2. When should children with proteinuria undergo further evaluation?
3. What type of evaluation should be carried out to assess proteinuria?
4. When should children with proteinuria be referred to a pediatric nephrologist?

A small amount of **protein** is normally present in the urine. Urine protein levels increase somewhat in certain conditions such as vigorous exercise, febrile illnesses, accidental trauma, and congestive heart failure. Most of the protein in the **glomerular filtrate** is reabsorbed by the tubular cells. Pathologic amounts of protein are present in the urine when the **glomerular leak** of protein is increased, when the **tubules fail to reabsorb** the protein filtered by the glomerulus, or if **inflammation in the renal interstitium** leads to the addition of tubular proteins to the urine.

Urinary protein is initially detected by **urine dipstick,** but this method is unreliable in alkaline urine. Dipstick protein is also affected by urine concentration. A dipstick positive for protein of 1+ in concentrated urine may not correlate with an abnormal 24-hour urinary protein excretion, whereas a dipstick of 1+ in very dilute urine may be associated with an abnormal 24-hour urinary protein excretion. Proteinuria may be more accurately determined by performing a timed urine collection or a random sample for chemical determination of the total protein concentration divided by the urinary creatinine concentration.

Epidemiology

The prevalence of **proteinuria** depends on how the condition is defined. In a Texas study, 10 mg/dL of proteinuria was found consistently in the urine of 2% to 3% of children in 3 consecutive urine samples. When 50 mg/dL was used as the cutoff for proteinuria, however, only 0.4% to 0.7% of boys and 0.4% to 2.5% of girls had proteinuria in 2 of 3 consecutive samples. The prevalence of proteinuria increased with age. In Finland, about 11% of school-aged children had at least one episode of proteinuria of 25 mg/dL by dipstick when the urine was tested 4 times. Approximately 2.5% of the children had proteinuria on 2 of 4 occasions.

Clinical Presentation

Proteinuria is a laboratory finding that may present incidentally on a screening urinalysis or be detected during the evaluation of a complaint, such as edema, that may be caused by renal disease. When proteinuria is detected as an incidental finding in otherwise normal children, the laboratory evaluation of the proteinuria should be delayed until its persistence is confirmed on repeat dipstick (Dx Box). **Edematous children** with proteinuria most likely have renal lesions or more rarely congestive heart failure. Additional findings on examination could include the presence of hypertension, ascites, pleural effusions, or the rash of systemic lupus erythematosus or anaphylactoid purpura.

Dx Proteinuria

- Presence of dipstick proteinuria (>1+ confirmed on 3 occasions)
- Random urine total protein-creatinine ratio greater than 0.2 *or* 24-hour urine protein greater than 4 mg/m^2/h
- Orthostatic proteinuria (assessed through separate measurement of afternoon and first-morning urine for total protein-creatinine ratios)

Pathophysiology

The glomerular capillaries are adapted to permit the filtration of minimal amounts of plasma proteins, particularly those with a small molecular radius. Approximately 320 mg of albumin and 360 mg of lower molecular weight proteins are filtered by the glomerular capillaries each day. Ninety-five percent of this is reabsorbed by the proximal tubular cells. Normally, children may excrete up to 100 mg/m^2/d of protein. Urinary protein excretion is increased in newborns to about 240 mg/m^2/d and in adolescents to about 300 mg/d. Adults may normally excrete up to 150 mg of protein per day. Only 10% to 15% of this is albumin; the rest of the proteins are other plasma proteins and urinary glycoproteins.

When increased proteinuria results from glomerular disease, higher levels of urinary proteins are primarily due to the enhanced filtration of albumin. Protein excretion may be increased transiently by any condition that raises intraglomerular capillary pressure such as congestive heart failure, strenuous exercise, epinephrine use, fever, or surgery.

Orthostatic proteinuria, which affects some children, is a poorly understood, benign condition. Individuals excrete pathologic amounts of protein in their urine while they are upright, but their urinary protein excretion returns to normal when they are recumbent. This condition seems to be more common in athletic individuals. Some investigators believe that orthostatic proteinuria is due to increased pressure in the renal vasculature while patients are upright.

Differential Diagnosis

The proteinuria may be **physiological** (secondary to fever, congestive heart failure), **orthostatic, tubular** (as seen in allergic interstitial nephritis), or **glomerular.** Aminoaciduria as a form of tubular proteinuria may occur, as is seen in certain inborn errors of metabolism.

Evaluation

History

It is important to elicit a complete history (Questions Box) in children with proteinuria. When asking about a history of swelling, the practitioner should note that subtle periorbital edema may be present only in the early morning hours. If the proteinuria is detected at a routine screening examination, the conditions under which the urine was obtained should be determined. Children may have been sick with a high fever or have just participated in an athletic event such as a track meet.

Physical Examination

The physical examination should include a determination of blood pressure and measurement of height and weight. A careful assessment for edema should be made. The skin should be examined for signs of rashes such as that seen in Henoch-Schönlein purpura or healing impetigo. The joints should be inspected for any signs of

swelling or joint inflammation. The abdominal examination should include a careful search for ascites or organomegaly.

Laboratory Tests

The extent of the laboratory evaluation depends on the child's general health (eg, the child is ill with another problem), the amount of proteinuria on dipstick, and whether the child has edema. The suggested evaluation is outlined in Figure 82-1. In non-edematous, otherwise healthy children, it is prudent to examine the urine sediment, and if negative, recheck the dipstick in a few days. If proteinuria of 1+ is consistently present and no hematuria is evident, a first-stage evaluation is indicated. If children are ill with a fever or are hospitalized with a serious illness, it is often appropriate to delay the evaluation of the proteinuria until the acute illness is under control, providing no associated hematuria, hypoproteinemia, hypertension, or azotemia is present.

In healthy ambulatory patients with persistent, isolated dipstick proteinuria on 3 occasions, it is important to quantitate the proteinuria (Box 82-1). This may be done simply by ordering a urinary protein-creatinine ratio. If the ratio is abnormal (>0.2), children need to be evaluated first for orthostatic proteinuria. Orthostatic proteinuria can be ruled out in several ways. The simplest evaluation involves checking a urine dipstick on a first voided morning sample and again on an afternoon specimen. This procedure should be repeated on 2 different days. It is critical to be sure that children empty their bladders before going to bed, because urine produced when they are nonrecumbent may contain protein and give an inaccurate result. If the dipstick from the morning urine is negative on a concentrated, acid urine, and if the afternoon sample is positive on a concentrated, acid urine, children most likely have orthostatic proteinuria.

A more accurate way of checking for orthostatic proteinuria involves the determination of urine protein-creatinine ratios on the first morning and afternoon urine samples. A diagnosis of orthostatic

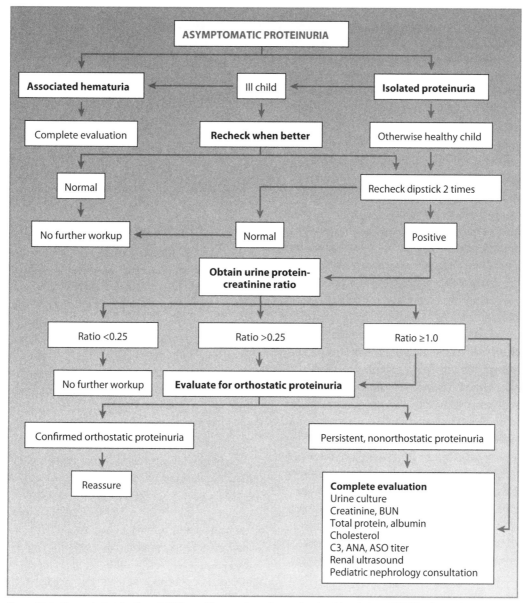

Figure 82-1. Suggested evaluation of children with asymptomatic proteinuria. Abbreviations: BUN, blood urea nitrogen; ANA, antinuclear antibody; ASO, anti-streptelysin O.

proteinuria can be made if the ratio is normal on the recumbent sample and elevated on the daytime sample. The most accurate way of diagnosing orthostatic proteinuria entails collecting 2 timed urine samples, one during the hours that children are up during the day and the other while they are in bed at night. In most instances of orthostatic proteinuria in children, the total urinary protein excretion is less than 1 g. The urine collected in the recumbent period should contain less than 50 mg/m² of protein. If these 2 timed samples meet the criteria for orthostatic proteinuria, they do not need to be repeated. It is important to remember, however, that even in renal disease proteinuria improves somewhat when patients are recumbent.

If children do not have orthostatic proteinuria, a 24-hour urine protein excretion should be determined. If the collection of a 24-hour urine sample is impractical, the urine protein-creatinine ratio is a

reliable alternative. Blood chemistries (eg, blood urea nitrogen [BUN], creatinine) should be obtained to determine renal function. Electrolyte status should be assessed with total carbon dioxide, total protein, albumin, and cholesterol. Serologies should be obtained for antinuclear antibodies, C3, antistreptolysin-O titer, and hepatitis B surface antigen if children come from a population at risk for hepatitis B.

Twenty-four–hour urine protein excretion should be less than 4 mg/m²/h. Neonates may excrete as much as 150 mg/m²/12 h, however. Table 82-1 gives a summary of normal urinary protein excretion. If children have nephrotic range proteinuria or symptoms consistnet with nephrotic syndrome (heavy proteinuria accompanied by hypoalbuminemia and hypercholesterolemia), they require further evaluation for nephrotic syndrome (see Chapter 131). If they do not have nephrotic range proteinuria, abnormal tubular

Table 82-1. Urinary Protein Excretion by Age

Age	24-hour Urine Protein (mg)	Urine Protein-Creatinine
Premature infant	14–60	—
Full-term infant	15–68	—
2–23 mo	17–85	≤0.50
2–4 y	20–121	≤0.2
4–10 y	26–194	≤0.2
10–16 y	29–238	≤0.2

Management

Most children with normal renal function and normal blood pressure whose evaluation reveals physiological or orthostatic proteinuria should have repeat urinalysis on an annual basis. If the proteinuria worsens or if hematuria develops, a repeat evaluation of renal function is indicated. Children whose initial evaluation reveals persistent, significant proteinuria require careful follow-up to detect and monitor signs of serious renal disease. This follow-up should include repeat blood pressure measurement and urinalysis every 3 months and repeat chemistries (BUN, creatinine, serum albumin) and urine protein-creatinine ratios every 6 months. These children should be managed in consultation with the pediatric nephrologist, whose experience is helpful in reassessing the need for kidney biopsy.

Children with physiological or orthostatic proteinuria who have minimal, persistent proteinuria should be able to follow a full school schedule and be allowed to participate in sports, provided there are no other contraindications. The usual immunization schedule should not be interrupted, and children should follow a regular diet. No increase in dietary protein is necessary to compensate for the minimal amounts of protein lost in the urine. Results of recent studies in nephrotic patients have found that a high-protein diet may actually increase urinary protein losses.

Prognosis

The outlook for children with proteinuria depends entirely on the underlying cause of the proteinuria. Children whose proteinuria is associated with edema or hematuria are more likely to have significant renal disease, such as glomerulonephritis, however, and the prognosis may be less favorable. If the proteinuria is due to a form of chronic glomerulonephritis, children may ultimately develop end-stage renal disease. In individuals with glomerular diseases, persistent proteinuria is a strong risk factor for progressive loss of renal function. If the proteinuria is physiological or orthostatic, however, the long-term prognosis is excellent. The likelihood that these children will develop renal functional impairment is no greater than for the rest of the general population.

proteinuria should be ruled out. A normal urinary β_2-microglobulin rules out tubular proteinuria. In general, consultation with a pediatric nephrologist is recommended if children have an abnormal 24-hour urinary protein excretion (see Table 82-1). If the proteinuria exceeds 1 g/d or if any other minor signs of renal dysfunction or hematuria are present, a biopsy is warranted. Sometimes, otherwise healthy children with small amounts of isolated proteinuria of less than 750 to 1,000 mg/d are followed by the pediatric nephrologist without a kidney biopsy. However, if this degree of proteinuria persists for 1 year or more, a renal biopsy is warranted.

Imaging Studies

A renal ultrasound should be obtained to rule out any structural abnormalities but may not be indicated in the child with simple orthostatic proteinuria.

CASE RESOLUTION

In the case presented at the beginning of the chapter, odds are that the evaluation of the healthy teenage boy with isolated proteinuria will reveal that he has orthostatic proteinuria, and his long-term prognosis is good.

Selected References

Abitbol C, Zilleruelo G, Freundlich M, Strauss J. Quantitation of proteinuria with urinary protein/creatinine ratios and random testing with dipsticks in nephrotic children. *J Pediatr.* 1990;116:243–247

Ginsberg JM, Chang BS, Matarese RA, Garella S. Use of single voided urine samples to estimate quantitative proteinuria. *N Engl J Med.* 1983;309:1543–1546

Hogg RJ, Portman RJ, Milliner D, et al. Evaluation and management of proteinuria and nephrotic syndrome in children: recommendations from a pediatric nephrology panel established at the National Kidney Foundation Conference on Proteinuria, Albuminuria, Risk, Assessment, Detection, and Elimination (PARADE). *Pediatrics.* 2000;105:1242–1249

Houser MT, Jahn MF, Kobayashi A. Assessment of urinary protein excretion in the adolescent: effect of body position and exercise. *J Pediatr.* 1986;109:556–561

Koss S, Perl A, Wieder A, et al. Proteinuria and renal disease: prognostic value of urine dipstick testing for leukocytes. *Pediatr Nephrol.* 2006;21:584–587

Pradhan M, Kaplan BS. Proteinuria. In: Kaplan BS, Meyers KEC, eds. *Pediatric Nephrology and Urology: The Requisites in Pediatrics.* Philadelphia, PA: Elsevier; 2005:103–109

Reuben DB, Wachtel TJ, Brown PC, Driscoll JL. Transient proteinuria in emergency medical admissions. *N Engl J Med.* 1982;306:1031–1033

Trachtman H, Bergwerk A, Gauthier B. Isolated proteinuria in children. Natural history and indications for renal biopsy. *Clin Pediatr (Phila).* 1994;33:468–472

Vehaskari VM. Mechanism of orthostatic proteinuria. *Pediatr Nephrol.* 1990;4:328–330

Yoshikawa N, Kitagawa K, Ohta K, Tanaka R, Nakamura H. Asymptomatic constant isolated proteinuria in children. *J Pediatr.* 1991;119:375–379

Urinary Tract Infections

Hali Sherman, MD, and Sudhir K. Anand, MD

CASE STUDY

A 7-month-old girl is brought to the office with a 1-day history of fever (temperature: 103°F [39.4°C]), vomiting, and mild diarrhea. The mother has not noticed any change in urination pattern or any unusual urine odor. The child has been somewhat irritable but fully alert.

Physical examination reveals an active infant. The temperature is 102.6°F (39.2°C), the heart rate is 122/min, the respiratory rate is 30/min, and the blood pressure is 90/60 mm Hg. The neck is supple. The head, eye, ear, nose, throat, chest, heart, abdominal, and genital examination is normal. Urinalysis shows specific gravity 1.025, pH 6.0, leukocyte esterase and nitrite both strongly positive, protein trace, and blood trace; the sediment has 15 to 20 white blood cells per high-power field and 2 to 4 red blood cells per high-power field. The gram stain shows more than 100,000 gram-negative rods, and the urine culture is pending.

Questions

1. What are the possible diagnoses of children with positive leukocyte esterase or nitrite on urinalysis?
2. What are the indications for hospital admission of children with urinary tract infections (UTIs)?
3. What antibiotics are used in the treatment of UTIs?
4. What is the appropriate diagnostic workup for children with suspected UTIs? When are renal ultrasound, technetium 99m-DMSA renal scan, and voiding cystourethrogram included in the evaluation?
5. If workup reveals vesicoureteral reflux, how should children be managed over the long term?

Urinary tract infection (UTI) is now the most common serious bacterial infection that affects infants and children. A UTI may be asymptomatic, associated with urinary symptoms, or occasionally complicated by sepsis. In most children UTIs resolve completely with appropriate antibiotic therapy. However, in children with underlying anatomical abnormalities (eg, vesicoureteral reflux [VUR]) or delayed or inadequate antibiotic treatment, UTIs may result in renal scarring that sometimes leads to hypertension or end-stage renal disease.

Urinary tract infection is a nonspecific, generic term implying significant bacteriuria, irrespective of the site of bacterial growth in the urinary tract. In many young children with bacteriuria, clinical findings overlap and precise classification cannot be easily made. We clarify some of the commonly used terms below.

Asymptomatic, covert, and **screening bacteriuria** are synonymous terms usually used when bacteriuria is detected during surveys of healthy children. The term *screening bacteriuria* is more accurate because some affected children may actually have urinary symptoms on close questioning.

Cystitis implies infection of the bladder only. Its major feature is voiding symptoms (eg, dysuria, frequency, urgency, enuresis, and foul-smelling urine). Fever, if present, is usually low-grade.

Acute pyelonephritis is a symptomatic infection of renal parenchyma characterized by systemic symptoms such as high fever, chills, flank pain, and vomiting in addition to dysuria.

Recurrent UTI generally refers to reinfection with a new organism (often same species but different strain). This condition is a common problem, especially in the first year after initial UTI. Reinfection with the same organism is infrequent and may indicate underlying structural problems of the urinary tract, the presence of stones, or inappropriate antibiotic therapy.

Chronic pyelonephritis is a term that has been used in various ways. Ideally, it should be employed only after renal biopsy specimens reveal renal scarring on histology due to repeated infections. Practically, the term often refers to scarred kidneys as demonstrated by nuclear medicine studies and/or reduced kidney function.

Urethritis implies infection of the urethra and is usually seen in the setting of sexually transmitted infections. The usual symptoms are dysuria and urethral discharge.

Epidemiology

Bacteriuria is detected in approximately 1% of girls and 2% of boys during routine screening of healthy newborns and young infants. Approximately 1% of girls continue to have asymptomatic bacteriuria throughout childhood. Bacteriuria in boys older than 1 year is very uncommon. In most affected infants and children, bacteriuria resolves spontaneously with time and does not lead to renal damage.

Symptomatic UTI occurs in approximately 2.5% of children annually and accounts for more than 1 million office visits per year. In early infancy, UTI is about twice as common in boys than in girls and about 10 times more common in uncircumcised boys than circumcised boys. After the first 6 months of life, the incidence of symptomatic UTI becomes considerably higher in females than males, and the difference between circumcised and uncircumcised males disappears. Among vaccinated febrile infants, UTI is the source of fever in approximately 4% to 8% of patients, even in those who have upper respiratory infection symptoms.

Clinical Presentation

Signs and symptoms of UTI in neonates and young infants are usually nonspecific and include fever, irritability, poor weight gain (or weight loss), diarrhea, vomiting, and jaundice. Occasionally, bacteremia or sepsis with temperature instability, cyanosis, and disseminated intravascular coagulation may occur. Older children often have similar signs and symptoms, and they are often able to describe abdominal or flank pain, dysuria, frequency, urgency, enuresis, foul-smelling or cloudy urine, and occasionally gross hematuria (Dx Box).

Dx **Urinary Tract Infection**

- Abdominal pain
- Burning or pain on urination
- Urgency
- Frequency
- Fever
- Leukocyturia
- Positive urine culture

Pathophysiology

The pathogenesis of UTI involves interaction between various bacterial factors and protective host factors.

Bacterial Factors

Escherichia coli accounts for 80% to 90% of first infections. The remainder are caused by other gram-negative enteric bacilli (*Proteus, Klebsiella, Enterobacter*) and gram-positive cocci (enterococci, *Staphylococcus saprophyticus*). Most organisms that cause UTI originate from the fecal flora. *S saprophyticus* (a coagulase-negative staphylococcus) infections are primarily seen in adolescents with UTI.

Microorganisms that cause UTI usually enter the urinary tract by an ascending route. To initiate colonization and infect the urinary tract, these organisms must first adhere to uroepithelium so they are not swept away during voiding. Bacterial adhesion in *E coli* is mediated by fimbriae, which are fine, hairlike proteins emanating from the bacterial cell wall. One important type of fimbriae, called P-fimbriae, adheres to receptors (Gal-Gal) on the uroepithelium, and some studies have shown that women and children with recurrent UTI have increased numbers of these receptors. In most young children with normal anatomy, acute pyelonephritis is caused by *E*

coli with P-fimbriae. In most patients with VUR and scarred kidneys, however, the infection is caused by *E coli* lacking P-fimbriae. Hence, the role of P-fimbriae in the pathogenesis of renal scarring is uncertain. Additionally, many of these bacteria, which are typically extracellular organisms, are able to survive and flourish intracellularly by taking advantage of the host cell's nutrients and evading immune defenses. Other bacterial virulence factors include K and H antigens, colicin, and hemolysin, but their role in the pathogenesis of UTI is not clearly defined.

Host Factors

There are many unalterable host factors that contribute to the pathogenesis of UTI including age, sex, genetics, anatomy, and immune response to infection. Females seem to be at increased risk because the female urethra is shorter than the male urethra and closer to the anus. As previously stated, the uroepithelium of older girls and adult women who develop recurrent UTI binds *E coli* more avidly than uroepithelium from non-susceptible patients. In addition, individuals with certain P and Lewis blood groups develop more UTIs than others. Urinary obstruction or other anomalies may contribute to the development of UTIs in about 2% of girls and 5% of boys, especially infants.

Vesicoureteral reflux signifies retrograde passage of urine from the bladder to the ureter. After passage through the bladder wall, the normal ureter tunnels under the bladder mucosa before it opens into the bladder lumen. Under normal circumstances the submucosal segment is compressed when the bladder is filled and during voiding, preventing reflux of urine into the ureter. Most VUR is primary and caused by a congenital abnormality of the ureterovesical junction, with the ureter having a short submucosal segment and more laterally placed openings. Reflux may also occur in the presence of normal ureteral anatomy when bladder pressures exceed 40 cm of water, as seen in patients with posterior urethral valves or neurogenic bladders. Vesicoureteral reflux is graded on a scale of I through V, with stage V being the most severe (Figure 83-1).

The incidence of VUR in normal infants is less than 2%. In infants with UTI, the incidence of VUR is about 25% to 50%; in school-aged children, about 25% to 30%; and in adolescents, about 10% to 15%. These figures suggest that, with increasing age and maturation of the bladder wall, VUR often spontaneously resolves. Vesicoureteral reflux may also be a familial disorder and has been reported in 10% to 30% of siblings of index cases. The incidence of UTI is increased in the presence of VUR probably because of incomplete emptying of the bladder; the urine refluxed into the ureters or kidneys returns to the bladder via the abnormally tunneled ureters at the end of voiding. This also provides infected urine direct access to the kidneys, which can lead to pyelonephritis and potential renal scarring.

Intuitively, it would seem that the greater the severity of VUR in children with UTI, the greater the likelihood of renal scarring. Recently, however, it has been clearly recognized that many neonates (especially boys) with antenatal VUR, even in the absence of UTI, have congenital dysplastic renal parenchymal defects, which

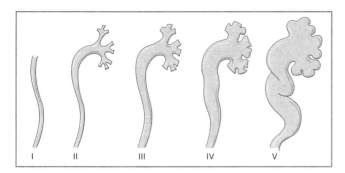

Figure 83-1. Grading of vesicoureteral reflux by vesicoureterogram based on international classification. I. Ureter only. II. Ureter, pelvis, and calyces, but without dilatation. III. Mild or moderate dilatation of ureter and mild or moderate dilatation of renal pelvis, but no or slight blunting of fornices. IV. Moderate dilatation or tortuosity of the ureter with moderate dilatation of renal pelvis and calyces and complete obliteration of the sharp angles of fornices, but maintenance of papillary impressions in most calyces. V. Gross dilatation and tortuosity of ureters, renal pelvis, and calyces; papillary impressions are no longer visible in most calyces.

had been misidentified as infective scars. Therefore, it is unclear whether the progression of renal scarring in this group is simply the natural history of the congenital defect or a result of many superimposed UTIs.

While there are many predisposing host factors that cannot be changed, there are several behavioral issues that are often associated with UTI in older children. School-aged children with frequent complaints of dysuria or recurrent UTIs who do not have a history of UTI as infants should be questioned for symptoms of dysfunctional voiding. The term *dysfunctional voiding* is often applied in the setting of children (especially girls) who have no neurologic or anatomical abnormalities, but who exhibit abnormal voiding behavior. These girls will often hold their urine for so long that they need to rush to the bathroom only to incompletely empty their bladder, leading to urinary stasis and the potential for infection. Additionally, constipation and abnormal stooling patterns are frequently associated with dysfunctional voiding and can also lead to the development of UTI.

Differential Diagnosis

In infants and young children, symptoms of UTI are often nonspecific. Thus a high degree of suspicion for UTI must be maintained. An acute abdomen may rarely be confused with UTI. Some children with dysuria may have chemical irritation from exposure to materials such as bubble baths. Overweight girls may retain urine in their labial folds, which can cause maceration, urethral irritation, or vulvitis. Similarly, some young girls do not sit with their legs spread wide enough on the toilet, which can lead to reflux into the vagina and cause post-void dribbling with subsequent urethral irritation or vulvitis. In these cases, urinalysis and urine culture findings usually help differentiate UTI from vulvitis or urethral irritation.

Evaluation

In all infants and young children with fever without an apparent source, urinalysis, urine gram stain, and urine culture should be obtained to evaluate for UTI.

History

In older children, a history of fever, dysuria, frequency, abdominal pain, and nausea and vomiting is suggestive of UTI (Questions Box). History of previous UTIs, abnormal voiding, and constipation should also be sought.

Questions

Urinary Tract Infection

- Does it hurt when the child urinates? Does the child scream when urinating?
- Does the child void more frequently?
- Does the urine have an unusual odor?
- Has the child had previous urinary infections?
- Does the child have a good urinary stream? Or does the child dribble?

Physical Examination

The abdomen should be examined for masses and tenderness, the genitalia for local lesions, and the lumbosacral area for anomalies such as deep sacral dimples. Blood pressure should be measured to evaluate for hypertension.

Laboratory Tests

The diagnosis of UTI is established by documenting significant bacteria in a urine specimen sent for culture. In young infants the specimen should always be obtained by bladder puncture or catheterization. In infants and children, because of the risk of contamination, a "bag urine" sample is not reliable. In older children with bladder control, a midstream urine collection is satisfactory. The diagnosis of UTI should never be based on the presence or absence of white blood cells alone. Although most older children with symptomatic UTI have pyuria, many neonates and young infants with UTI (25%–50%) may not manifest this finding. Furthermore, leukocyturia may occur in other renal disorders in the absence of UTI. A positive urinary nitrite test is suggestive of UTI, but the false-negative rate is nearly 50%.

Most patients with UTI (>85%) have urine bacterial counts greater than 100,000/mL on a voided specimen (ie, significant bacteriuria), although some adult women and teenage girls with symptomatic recurrent UTI have catheterized or "clean catch" urine colony counts less than 1,000/mL. In general, this has not been observed in young children. Colony counts between 10,000 and 100,000/mL obtained via clean catch are generally unlikely to be significant unless children have symptoms of UTI, associated leukocyturia, and/or cultures that are pure growths of a single organism. Any growth of an organism from a suprapubic tap is considered significant. A colony count of at least 10,000/mL in samples obtained by catheterization is usually necessary to diagnose a UTI. However, in most children with UTIs, urine collected by either of these techniques grows more than 50,000 organisms/mL.

C-reactive protein is usually increased in infants and children with high fever and clinical findings suggestive of acute pyelonephritis. Several other laboratory studies, including erythrocyte sedimentation rate, urinary lactic acid dehydrogenase isoenzymes, urinary concentrating ability, and antibody-coated bacteria, have been used with varying success to differentiate upper (renal) from lower (bladder) UTI in older children and adults. Overall, the reliability of these studies in pediatric patients, especially infants and young children, is not adequate to recommend their routine use. More recently, there has been some focus on serum procalcitonin, and preliminary studies suggest that it might have some predictive value in terms of pyelonephritis and VUR.

Imaging Studies

Although there is controversy regarding the recommendations, the most recent position statement from the American Academy of Pediatrics (AAP) (1999) states that all girls younger than 2 years and all boys (irrespective of age) should have renal ultrasonography and voiding cystoureterogram (VCUG) performed following detection of the first UTI. These 2 studies detect structural renal anomalies and VUR in most patients. In girls, nuclear VCUG instead of contrast VCUG is an acceptable alternative. Renal ultrasound can be performed as soon as feasible after diagnosis. Voiding cystoureterogram may be done once there is clinical evidence that the UTI is resolving, or it may be delayed 4 to 6 weeks depending on the clinical circumstances. Antibiotic prophylaxis, according to the AAP position statement, must be administered until completion of the studies. An excretory urogram (intravenous pyelogram) is no longer recommended.

In recent years, some authorities have recommended a routine 99mTc-DMSA renal scan to differentiate upper from lower tract infection. Although the test is positive in 60% to 90% of children with a clinical diagnosis of acute pyelonephritis, the cost of the nuclear scan, the high dose of radiation, and the fact that therapy is usually not altered, preclude the routine use of this study. The scan is most helpful in a child where the diagnosis of acute pyelonephritis is in doubt or when used in follow-up to detect development of renal scars, especially in patients with VUR.

Management

All infants younger than 2 months with UTIs should be treated with parenteral **antibiotics,** starting with broad-spectrum antibiotic coverage such as ceftriaxone, cefotaxime, or ampicillin and gentamicin, pending results of sensitivity studies. Children older than 2 months who appear well and are able to tolerate liquids may receive oral antibiotics on an outpatient basis. Most physicians recommend cephalexin for the first infection until the results of bacterial

sensitivity tests are available and treatment is continued for 10 days. In older children with clear-cut lower tract infection, shorter courses of trimethoprim-sulfamethoxazole are also effective. One should be aware of the local *E coli* resistance patterns, however, because some communities have a high incidence of *E coli* resistant to trimethoprim-sulfamethoxazole. Children who appear toxic and/or are vomiting should be admitted to the hospital and started on parenteral antibiotics until they show clinical improvement, at which time they can be sent home on oral therapy.

Although recent studies have suggested that antibiotics do not necessarily prevent infections or renal scarring and may cause increased risk of resistant infections, most children with VUR are still placed on low-dose antibiotics (trimethoprim-sulfamethoxazole, cephalexin, or nitrofurantoin) that are continued for 12 to 18 months following treatment for an acute infection. At the end of this period, a radionuclide VCUG is repeated to determine whether reflux has resolved. Development of new renal scars can be best detected by 99mTc-DMSA renal scanning.

Surgery is not necessary in most infants with VUR, including many with severe disease (grades IV and V) because most grade I through III and some grade IV and V reflux in infants disappears with increasing age. In children older than 5 years with grade IV or V reflux, the rate of disappearance with medical treatment is much lower (about 20%–25%). The results of the International Vesicoureteral Reflux Study Group show no difference in the rate of renal scarring between prophylactic medical treatment and surgery. Therefore, surgical reimplantation of the ureter is usually recommended only for those patients who have poor adherence with prophylaxis or breakthrough infections, especially if the upper tract is involved. This latter group seems to have benefited the most from surgery.

An alternate to surgical reimplantation, Deflux is a gel composed of dextranomers and hyaluronic acid that can be injected endoscopically into the ureters. It was approved by the US Food and Drug Administration in September 2001 after having been used extensively throughout Europe with great success. Most pediatric urologists agree that Deflux should be used for persistent grades II through IV, while grade I can be managed expectantly. Severe grade V reflux usually requires surgical intervention.

Prognosis

In most children, UTI is a minor illness with very few long-term or serious consequences. However, UTI commonly reoccurs, especially during the first year following the initial UTI. Repeat urine cultures should be obtained during follow-up assessments in all children with VUR, first at 1- to 2-month intervals and later at 3- to 4-month intervals for at least 1 year or until disappearance of reflux.

The risk factors for the development of renal scars and eventual hypertension and/or renal failure include young age (<1 year), recurrent episodes of acute pyelonephritis, delay in starting effective antibiotic therapy, high-grade reflux, and anatomical or neurogenic obstruction. If repeat infection is prevented in these children, however, development of fresh scars is uncommon, and renal function and growth remain normal. As a group, infants and children younger than 3 years with UTI and high-grade VUR are more likely to develop calyceal clubbing and renal scarring, whereas progressive renal scarring as a result of UTI or reflux after 5 years of age is relatively less common.

CASE RESOLUTION

In the case history, the young girl is hospitalized because of the vomiting. She is started on intravenous ceftriaxone and she improves in 48 hours. Her inpatient renal ultrasound is normal, and she is discharged home with oral antibiotics. Because a radionuclide voiding cystoureterogram (VCUG) is planned in 4 weeks, she is also given a prescription for prophylactic antibiotics to take until the VCUG is completed.

Selected References

American Academy of Pediatrics Committee on Quality Improvement, Subcommittee on Urinary Tract Infection. Practice parameter: the diagnosis, treatment, and evaluation of the initial urinary tract infection in febrile infants and young children. *Pediatrics.* 1999;103:843–852

Conway PH, Cnaan A, Zaoutis T, et al. Recurrent urinary tract infections in children: risk factors and association with prophylactic antimicrobials. *JAMA.* 2007;298:179–186

Wald E. Urinary tract infections in infants and children: a comprehensive overview. *Curr Opin Pediatr.* 2004;16:85–88

Hellerstein S. Acute urinary tract infection–evaluation and treatment. *Curr Opin Pediatrics.* 2006;18:134–138

Chang S, Shortliffe L. Pediatric urinary tract infections. *Pediatr Clin North Am.* 2006;53:379–400

Wald E. Vesicoureteral reflux: the role of antibiotic prophylaxis. *Pediatrics.* 2006;117:919–922

Hoberman A, Charron M, Hickey RW, Baskin M, Kearney DH, Wald ER. Imaging studies after a first febrile urinary tract infection in young children. *N Engl J Med.* 2003;348:195–202

Vaginitis

Monica Sifuentes, MD

CASE STUDY

An 11-year-old girl is brought to your office with vaginal itching for 1 week and a yellow discharge on her panties for the past 4 days. The girl reports no associated abdominal pain, vomiting, or diarrhea. She has no urinary problems and also denies any history of sexual abuse. Although she occasionally bathes with bubble bath, she most often takes showers. Except for the vaginal complaint, she is healthy, and she takes no medications.

The physical examination is notable for a soft, nontender abdomen with no organomegaly. Bowel sounds are audible in all quadrants. The genitalia are sexual maturity rating (Tanner stage) 2. The labia majora and minora and the clitoris all appear normal, and the hymen is annular in shape with a smooth rim. A scant amount of yellow discharge, along with minimal perihymenal injection, is noted at the vaginal introitus. The anal examination is normal, with an intact anal wink.

Questions

1. What are the most common causes for vaginal discharge in prepubescent and adolescent females? How do they differ?
2. What basic historical information must be obtained from all females whose chief complaint is vaginal discharge?
3. What specific methods are used to perform a gynecologic examination in prepubescent and adolescent females?
4. What is the appropriate laboratory evaluation for prepubescent and adolescent females who complain of vaginal discharge? How does this evaluation differ for adolescent females who are sexually active?
5. What are the various treatment options for females with vaginitis?

Vaginal discharge is not an uncommon occurrence in prepubescent and adolescent females. Practitioners are largely responsible for differentiating between a physiological discharge, or leukorrhea, and a pathologic discharge, which occurs, for example, with a bacterial or yeast infection. In cases of an abnormal discharge, the possibility of abuse needs to be considered and investigated appropriately (see Chapter 116). Primary care physicians should become familiar with the various causes of vaginal discharge in both prepubescent and adolescent females. More importantly, they should be comfortable performing gynecologic examinations in these patients so that the appropriate treatment can be initiated.

Vulvovaginitis, which is often used interchangeably with vaginitis or vulvitis, signifies inflammation of the perineal area, often accompanied by vaginal discharge. The discharge may be bloody, malodorous, or purulent, depending on the etiology (Table 84-1).

Epidemiology

Vulvovaginitis is the most common gynecologic complaint in prepubescent girls. Most cases of vulvovaginitis in these girls result from **nonspecific inflammation;** vaginal cultures show normal flora in 33% to 85% of such cases. The incidence of more specific **bacterial causes,** such as group A beta-hemolytic streptococcus (GABHS), has been reported in approximately 14% of patients. However, its occurrence seems to be seasonal, and confirming the diagnosis depends

Table 84-1. Characteristics and Specific Causes of Vaginal Discharge

Color	Consistency	Amount	Cause
Clear/white	Thin	Variable	Physiological
White	Cottage cheese–like	Moderate	*Candida*
White/yellow	Variable	Variable	Chemical irritation, *Chlamydia trachomatis*
Yellow/green	Thick	Moderate–profuse	*Neisseria gonorrhoeae*, foreign body, *Trichomonas vaginalis*
Bloody	Variable	Variable	*Shigella*, group A streptococcus, foreign body

on the use of proper culturing techniques using the appropriate media. Other bacterial causes include respiratory pathogens such as *Haemophilus influenzae, Neisseria meningitidis, Streptococcus pneumoniae,* and enteric organisms such as *Shigella.* A positive culture for *Chlamydia trachomatis* or *Neisseria gonorrhoeae* can be found in approximately 5% of children who are evaluated for sexual abuse. Higher figures have been reported from selected centers and when data from adolescent victims are included. These organisms are not considered part of the normal flora in prepubescent girls. Vaginal and rectal infections with *C trachomatis* can be acquired perinatally, however, but usually are not considered perinatally acquired after 2 to 3 years of age.

Parasitic infections may also lead to vaginal symptoms. Twenty percent of females with a rectal infestation of *Enterobius vermicularis*, the organism known as pinworm, have vulvovaginitis. Affected patients often complain of anal pruritus in addition to the vaginal discharge. **Mycotic infections** with organisms such as *Candida albicans* also can cause symptoms in prepubescent girls, although many of these girls have a previous history of oral antibiotic use.

Clinical Presentation

Prepubescent and adolescent females with vulvovaginitis most commonly present with a vaginal discharge, which may be white, purulent (ie, yellow or green), or serosanguineous. Its consistency can range from smooth and thin to thick and cottage cheese–like. The discharge may also be malodorous. In addition, females may complain of associated pruritus, erythema, urinary problems such as dysuria and increased frequency, and abdominal pain (Dx Box). Sexually active adolescent females with vaginitis from a sexually transmitted infection (STI) (eg, gonorrhea) generally have a more profuse, purulent discharge.

Dx Vaginitis

- Nonphysiological vaginal discharge
- Malodorous vaginal discharge
- Perineal erythema
- Pruritus
- Dysuria

Pathophysiology

Prepubescent girls are at risk for developing vulvovaginitis for both anatomical and physiological reasons. Unlike pubertal adolescents and young women, prepubescent girls have no pubic hair and a smaller labial fat pad to protect the vaginal introitus. The labia minora are small and tend to open when girls are in a squatting position, thereby exposing the vaginal introitus. The relative proximity of the anus to the vagina in young girls also contributes to vaginal contamination with enteric organisms. More importantly, poor hygienic practices (ie, wiping back to front after urination or defecation) can further compound the problem.

In addition, the normal physiology of the vaginal epithelium in prepubescent girls predisposes to vaginitis. The unestrogenized vaginal epithelium is relatively thin, immature, and easily traumatized. In addition, the pH of the vagina is neutral to alkaline, compared with the acidic environment of the vagina in adult females. Local antibody production also may be lacking in the vagina of prepubescent girls.

Differential Diagnosis

A vaginal discharge is normal at 2 distinct times in prepubescent girls: shortly after birth, secondary to the effects of maternal estrogen, and approximately 6 months to 1 year before the onset of menarche, which occurs, in most girls, after sexual maturity rating (SMR) (Tanner Stage) 3. The other causes of other vaginal discharges in prepubescent and pubescent females are presented in Box 84-1.

Box 84-1. Causes of Vaginal Discharge in Prepubescent and Pubescent Females

Prepubescent Females
- Estrogen withdrawal (neonates)
- Chemical irritation secondary to soaps and detergents
- Mechanical irritation from nylon panties or tight-fitting clothes
- Foreign body in vagina
- Poor hygiene
- Pinworms
- Yeast infection (eg, *Candida*)
- Bacterial infection (eg, group A streptococcus, *Shigella*)
- Sexually transmitted infection (eg, gonococcal infection, chlamydial infection, trichomoniasis)
- Congenital abnormality (eg, ectopic ureter [local inflammation])
- Acquired abnormality (eg, labial fusion [pooling of urine in vagina])
- Urethral prolapse
- Systemic illness (eg, scarlet fever, Crohn disease)

Pubescent Females
- Physiological leukorrhea
- Foreign body in vagina (eg, retained tampon)
- Yeast infection (eg, *Candida*)
- Bacterial infection (eg, group A streptococcus, *Staphylococcus aureus*)
- Sexually transmitted infection (eg, gonococcal infection, chlamydial infection, trichomoniasis)
- Chemical irritation (eg, douches, spermicides, latex [condoms])
- Local trauma (eg, penile studs)

Evaluation

Prepubescent Females

History

A complete history should be obtained in all females with a vaginal discharge (Questions Box). Practitioners should inquire about the appearance of the discharge, its duration, and the relative amount. A profuse, purulent discharge is probably more consistent with one specific etiology (eg, *N gonorrhoeae*) than is a scant, thin discharge that suggests a nonspecific etiology. The existence of urinary problems should also be determined. Pooling of urine in the vagina secondary to labial fusion can lead to vulvovaginitis in addition to a urinary tract infection. Changes in bowel or bladder habits and sudden changes in behavior such as nightmares or inappropriate stranger anxiety may also be noted. Such changes in behavior warrant a further inquiry into the possibility of sexual abuse, regardless of the practitioner's index of suspicion. Depending on the information disclosed and the age of the patient, a decision might be made to interview the child and parents independently. Other points to discuss include the type of detergents or soaps used for laundry as well as for bathing, because these may be irritating. Any recent illnesses should also be documented as a possible source of autoinoculation or, if oral antibiotics were required, as a reason for the alteration of the normal vaginal flora. In addition, patients' hygienic practices should be reviewed. Adolescent patients should always be interviewed alone (see Chapter 5). In particular, a reproductive history must be obtained, keeping in mind that puberty and sexual activity both alter vaginal flora.

Questions

Vaginitis

Prepubescent Females
- What is the color of the discharge?
- What is the consistency of the discharge?
- How profuse is the discharge?
- Is the discharge malodorous?
- How long has the discharge been present?
- How often does the discharge occur (ie, is it found on the panties daily)?
- Are there any associated problems (eg, dysuria, abdominal pain)?
- What types of laundry soaps or detergents are used?
- Does the child take bubble baths?
- Has the child had any recent illnesses?
- Does the child clean herself after using the toilet, or does she require help?
- In what direction does she tend to wipe after a bowel movement?

Adolescent Females
(all of the above questions plus the following)
- What is the reproductive history (menstrual and sexual)?
- Is there a history of sexual assault/abuse?
- If appropriate, is the adolescent using any form of barrier or hormonal contraception? When was the last episode of unprotected intercourse?
- How many sexual partners has the patient had?
- Does the patient or partner have any history of a previous sexually transmitted infection, including hepatitis B?

Physical Examination

Although the genital examination is the priority, a complete physical examination should be performed. This not only allows clinicians to identify other abnormal physical findings, but it also alleviates some of the anxiety often associated with a genital examination. Because most vaginal discharges in prepubescent girls result from nonspecific vulvovaginitis, visualization of the cervix with a speculum is not indicated.

The overall demeanor of young girls at the onset of the genital examination should be noted. Overly compliant, apathetic behavior in children may be a cause for concern regarding abuse, especially in the context of a chronic or recurrent purulent discharge.

On physical examination, children's SMR must be noted and recorded. In addition, the external genitalia should be examined closely for the presence of any lesions or any evidence of erythema. Chronic changes in labial skin, such as those associated with constant scratching, also should be documented.

Girls should be placed in the modified lithotomy or "frog leg" position, and the labia majora should be gently spread apart to visualize the hymen. The knee-chest position can also be used, depending on the comfort of the practitioner as well as the patient. If the labia cannot be spread apart, the girl may have labial fusion. Perihymenal and periurethral erythema and injection should be noted, in addition to any evidence of edema, trauma, or abnormal masses such as urethral prolapse. Hymenal size and appearance should be carefully evaluated for any evidence of abuse (see Chapter 116). The appearance, consistency, and amount of the vaginal discharge, including the presence or absence of an odor, also should be documented. These findings may vary depending on the characteristics and cause of the discharge. Finally, the anus should be inspected for tone and any evidence of trauma or abnormal lesions such as genital warts. An anal wink is normally elicited. Although not usually indicated, a rectal examination should be performed in an attempt to palpate a foreign body or mass in those patients with a chronic vaginal discharge.

Laboratory Tests

Laboratory studies are often unnecessary in prepubescent girls with a nonspecific, non-bloody vaginal discharge, diffuse vulvar erythema, and no suspicion or history of sexual abuse. A vaginal culture for isolation of GABHS is indicated in girls with an abrupt onset of a serosanguineous discharge and a history of a systemic illness. The cellophane tape test may be helpful in diagnosing a pinworm infection in girls with associated anal pruritus. A KOH wet mount reveals hyphae if a monilial infection is present.

If the discharge is purulent or malodorous or if abuse is suspected, vaginal cultures must be obtained for *N gonorrhoeae* and *C trachomatis*. For suspected cases of sexual abuse or assault, culture remains the gold standard because of the risk of a false-positive result with non-amplified probe tests (direct immunofluorescent smears, enzyme immunoassays) and nucleic acid amplification tests (NAATs). With genital and anal specimens, false-positive results can occur because of cross-reaction with fecal flora. In certain cases, a normal saline wet mount to check for mobile trichomonads may be indicated.

Pubescent Females

History

In adolescent or pubescent females with vaginal discharge, physicians should inquire about a history of sexual activity or assault in addition to other information that relates to their condition (see

Questions Box). Questions concerning the possible acquisition of an STI also must be asked in a nonjudgmental manner.

Physical Examination

Virginal adolescents with an uncomplicated history should be examined in a similar fashion as the prepubescent female. The external genitalia should be examined to evaluate the SMR of the patient and the presence of any lesions. Perihymenal or periurethral erythema and hymenal size and appearance should be noted. In the absence of a mucopurulent or bloody discharge, a speculum examination is usually not warranted.

In addition to an overall physical examination, a complete genital examination using a speculum is indicated in the sexually active female. The purpose of the speculum examination is to visualize the cervix, properly obtain vaginal and cervical specimens, and examine the vagina for lesions (eg, condylomata acuminata). A bimanual examination must also be performed to check for cervical motion tenderness as well as adnexal masses or tenderness, which are associated with pelvic inflammatory disease (PID).

Laboratory Tests

Adolescent females who are not sexually active should have a laboratory evaluation similar to that described for prepubescent girls. Sexually active teens, however, warrant a more thorough evaluation to establish the etiology of their symptoms. In general, because a speculum examination is being performed in these adolescents, a single-swab endocervical sample should be obtained and sent for gonorrhea and chlamydia via NAATs (eg, ligase chain reaction, polymerase chain reaction). Urine can also be sent for *N gonorrhoeae* and *C trachomatis* in those adolescents who refuse a pelvic examination or for screening purposes. A Pap smear also can be performed at this time, but recommendations have changed for teenagers regarding when cervical cancer screening is indicated (see Chapter 30 for details). A culture for herpes simplex is indicated only if the history of exposure is positive and ulcerative or vesicular lesions are present.

Other causes of vaginal symptoms can be determined by the pH and microscopic analysis of a fresh sample of the vaginal discharge. A normal saline wet mount should be made, especially if a nonspecific discharge is present or bacterial vaginosis (BV) is a concern. A 10% KOH mount is appropriate in cases of suspected candidiasis. Mixing 10% KOH with the discharge may also produce a "fishy" odor (positive "whiff test"), which is consistent with BV. In addition, a vaginal pH greater than 4.5 is commonly seen with BV or trichomoniasis, but it is not specific. A Gram stain of any purulent material may lead to an early diagnosis of gonorrhea. Serologies for syphilis and hepatitis should also be obtained in adolescents with suspected or proven STIs. In addition, these patients should be offered testing for human immunodeficiency virus (HIV), with appropriate pretest and posttest counseling.

Management

Management of a **nonspecific vaginal discharge** is aimed at relieving the uncomfortable symptoms associated with this type of inflammation. Prepubescent females should be instructed to **discontinue use of all chemical irritants,** including bubble baths, in the genital area. Warm water **sitz baths** are also recommended twice daily for approximately 1 week, or until patients feel better. In addition, females should be instructed in **proper hygiene** (eg, wiping front to back after a bowel movement). The use of cotton or cotton-crotch panties and loose-fitting skirts or pants should be recommended.

Antifungal medications such as **clotrimazole** (Lotrimin) or **miconazole** (Monistat) cream may be prescribed if a monilial infection is present. Empiric treatment may be warranted in children or adolescents with a previous history of oral antibiotic usage, diabetes mellitus, or other chronic conditions that may alter the normal vaginal flora.

Pinworms are treated with a single oral dose of **mebendazole** (Vermox), 100 mg, or **pyrantel pamoate** (Antiminth), 11 mg/kg/dose (to a maximum of 1 g). Most authorities recommend repeat treatment after 2 weeks.

If a retained foreign body is suspected in prepubescent girls, then examination under general anesthesia may be necessary. Alternatively, practitioners can attempt vaginal irrigation in cooperative children by placing a small feeding tube at the hymenal opening and injecting warm saline. Toilet paper is the most commonly retrieved material in prepubescent girls.

Adolescent females who are not sexually active should be treated as outlined above. If the discharge is believed to be physiological leukorrhea, practitioners should reassure patients and educate them about other issues related to puberty (eg, menarche, body odor). Sexually active adolescents with positive vaginal cultures, NAATs, or highly suspicious vaginal discharges should receive treatment depending on the causal organism (see Chapter 85 for details concerning treatment). Table 84-2 briefly outlines current recommendations.

Any disclosure of molestation by prepubescent or adolescent females must be reported to the appropriate authorities. In addition, abnormal physical findings and positive cultures of STIs in prepubescent females and adolescent females who have never been sexually active must be reported to law enforcement and investigated.

Prognosis

In most prepubescent females, vaginitis resolves spontaneously or after appropriate treatment with no permanent sequelae. In contrast, adolescent females treated for vulvovaginitis or uncomplicated cervicitis from an STI are at some risk for the development of PID, HIV, and pregnancy given their high-risk behavior.

Table 84-2. Treatment Recommendations for Adolescents With Infectious Vaginitis

Organism	Treatment[a]
Neisseria gonorrhoeae	Ceftriaxone, 125 mg intramuscularly, once, or cefixime, 400 mg orally, once
Chlamydia trachomatis	Azithromycin, 1 g orally, once
Trichomonas vaginalis	Metronidazole, 2 g orally, once, or tinidazole 2 g orally, once
Bacterial vaginosis	Metronidazole, 500 mg, twice a day for 7 days, or clindamycin cream 2%, one applicatorful at bedtime for 7 days, or metronidazole gel 0.75%, one applicatorful at bedtime for 5 days
Candida albicans	1% clotrimazole, cream, one applicatorful vaginally at bedtime for 7 days; 2% miconazole cream, 1 applicatorful vaginally at bedtime for 7 days; 0.8% terconazole cream, 1 applicatorful vaginally at bedtime for 3 days; fluconazole, 150 mg orally once

[a]For a complete list of treatment options, refer to Centers for Disease Control and Prevention, Workowski KA, Berman SM. Sexually transmitted disease treatment guidelines. MMWR Recomm Rep. 2006;55:1–94.

CASE RESOLUTION

In the case presented at the beginning of the chapter, the girl and her parents should be assured that the discharge is consistent with a nonspecific process. She should be instructed to take sitz baths for 1 week, discontinue bubble baths and the use of soap in the genital area, and wear loose-fitting clothes with cotton underwear. The girl should be reexamined in 1 to 2 weeks.

Selected References

Altchek A. Finding the cause of genital bleeding in prepubertal girls. *Contemp Pediatr.* 1996;13:80–92

Baldwin DD, Landa HM. Pediatric gynecology: evaluation and treatment. *Contemp Pediatr.* 1995;12:35–60

Blake DR, Duggan A, Quinn T, Zenilman J, Joffe A. Evaluation of vaginal infections in adolescent women: can it be done without a speculum? *Pediatrics.* 1998;102:939–944

Centers for Disease Control and Prevention, Workowski KA, Berman SM. Sexually transmitted disease treatment guidelines, 2006. *MMWR Recomm Rep.* 2006;55:1–94

Emans SJ, Laufer MR, Goldstein DP, eds. Vulvovaginal problems in the prepubertal child. In: *Pediatric and Adolescent Gynecology.* 5th ed. Philadelphia, PA: Williams & Wilkins; 2005:83–119

Pierce AM, Hart CA. Vulvovaginitis: causes and management. *Arch Dis Child.* 1992;67:509–512

Sobel JD. Vaginitis. *N Engl J Med.* 1997;337:1896–1903

Stricker T, Navratil F, Sennhauser FH. Vulvovaginitis in prepubertal girls. *Arch Dis Child.* 2003;88:324–326

Sugar NF, Graham EA. Common gynecologic problems in prepubertal girls. *Pediatr Rev.* 2006;27:213–223

Syed TS, Braverman PK. Vaginitis in adolescents. *Adolesc Med.* 2004;15:235–251

Sexually Transmitted Infections

Monica Sifuentes, MD

CASE STUDY

A 17-year-old male presents with a small red lesion on the tip of his penis. He noticed an area of erythema a few weeks before, but it resolved spontaneously. He reports no fever, myalgias, headache, dysuria, or urethral discharge. He is sexually active and occasionally uses condoms. He did not use a condom during his last sexual encounter 2 weeks ago, however, because his partner uses oral contraception. The adolescent has never been treated for any sexually transmitted infections (STIs) and is otherwise healthy.

On examination, he is a sexual maturity rating (Tanner stage) 4 circumcised male with a 2- to 3-mm vesicle on the glans penis. Minimal erythema is present at the base of the lesion, and there is no urethral discharge. The testicles are descended bilaterally, and no masses are palpable. Shotty, non-tender, inguinal adenopathy is evident.

Questions

1. What conditions are associated with vesicles in the genital area?
2. What risk factors are associated with the acquisition of an STI during adolescence?
3. What screening tests should be performed in patients with suspected STIs?
4. What recommendations regarding partners of patients with STIs should be given?
5. What issues of confidentiality are important to address with adolescents who desire treatment for STIs?

Most teenagers in the United States have their first sexual experience before they graduate from high school. In a recent survey conducted by the Centers for Disease Control and Prevention (CDC), nearly half of all students in high school reported having had sexual intercourse during their lifetime, with 6% of students nationwide reporting sexual intercourse for the first time before age 13 years. More importantly, nearly 17% of boys and 12% of girls in grades 9 to 12 reported having had 4 or more sexual partners during their life. The consequences of sexual activity in adolescents include increased rates of bacterial and viral sexually transmitted infections (STIs), unintended pregnancy, and the possible acquisition of long-term infections such as human immunodeficiency virus (HIV) in the 15- to 24-year age group. Without adequate antiretroviral therapy, the average time from acquisition of HIV infection to the development of acquired immunodeficiency syndrome (AIDS) is approximately 10 to 11 years. Given the complex nature of these consequences, the physician must be skilled in obtaining a complete sexual history in teenaged patients and in diagnosing and treating STIs.

Increasing levels of sexual activity directly affect STI trends in adolescents. Other influential factors include multiple (sequential or concurrent) sexual partners; inconsistent use of condoms and other barrier methods; experimentation with drugs, including alcohol, which results in poor judgment concerning sexual activity; poor compliance with antibiotic regimens; and biological factors, such as an earlier age of menarche and the presence of cervical ectopy in adolescent females. The feeling of invulnerability and the associated risk-taking behavior that occurs during adolescence make sexual activity spontaneous rather than premeditated. As a result, preventive measures are hindered, ignored, or simply unheard of, allowing adolescents to deny the possible consequences of their actions. Other factors influencing STI trends are related to societal norms. Traditionally, educational materials and STI services have not been readily available to adolescents in some areas of the United States, unlike other industrialized countries. In addition, the depiction of casual sexual relationships in television sitcoms, music videos, and motion pictures may play a major role in glamorizing sex. Advances in technology via Internet access also gives teenagers the opportunity to communicate with peers that were previously unreachable.

Epidemiology

The overall prevalence of STIs in adolescents is difficult to estimate because not all STIs are reportable, and collected data are often influenced by the particular population studied. It has been estimated, however, that more than 25% of STIs diagnosed annually in the United States occur among teenagers. *Chlamydia* remains the most common cause of cervicitis and urethritis in adolescents, with age-specific rates highest among girls and young women 15 to 24 years of age and young men 20 to 24 years of age. Additionally, studies have shown that certain adolescent subpopulations are at greater risk for chlamydial infection, such as homeless and incarcerated youth, teenagers attending family planning clinics, and pregnant adolescents. Complications of untreated chlamydial cervicitis occur in 10% to 30% of cases and include pelvic inflammatory disease (PID), ectopic pregnancy, chronic pelvic pain, and infertility. Epididymitis, a result of urethral infection, occurs in 1% to 3% of infected males. Other conditions that are uncommon but may occur in males as a result of an infection with chlamydia include proctitis, prostatitis, and Reiter syndrome.

Teenagers have the highest incidence of **gonorrhea** of any other age group, although the prevalence rates have decreased since 2001. The highest rates of gonorrhea reportedly occur in adolescent females, young men in their 20s, young adult inner-city minorities, incarcerated youth, men who have sex with men, and prostitutes. A large number of sexual partners, injection drug use, exposure to prostitutes, and casual sexual contacts also contribute to the risk of infection. In 2005 the CDC reported gonorrhea rates to be highest among adolescents and young adults. The incidence of gonorrhea in the 15- to 19-year-old age group was 624.7 per 100,000. Of the more than 1 million cases of PID reported annually in the United States, 20% to 30% are in sexually active adolescents. The risk of developing PID is increased 10-fold in this age group compared with adults for several reasons. Failure to use condoms consistently, new partners within the previous 2 to 3 months, and a history of STIs have been cited as risk factors. Complications of PID such as tubo-ovarian (TOA) abscess formation are more likely in adolescents as a result of late presentation, delayed diagnosis, and noncompliance with prescribed treatment regimens.

Although the rate of primary and secondary **syphilis** declined from 1990 to 2000, the number of cases is now increasing, primarily among men. During 2005 the incidence of syphilis was highest among women in the 20- to 24-year-old age group and among men in their mid-30s. Studies have shown that people with syphilis, as well as other STIs causing genital ulcers, also are at increased risk for HIV acquisition.

Human papillomavirus (HPV) is the most common STI in the United States, with the highest infection rates among adolescents and young adults. Recent studies report the prevalence in sexually active adolescents to range from 30% to 60% and to decline with age. The prevalence of HPV in adolescents varies widely for 2 reasons: (1) infection with HPV is often latent and generally regresses spontaneously and (2) HPV is not a reportable condition. Behavioral and biological risk factors for HPV infection have been identified and include early age of sexual initiation, multiple sexual partners, partner's number of sexual partners, a lack of consistent condom use, and a history of another STI such as genital herpes, which may facilitate HPV acquisition by compromising mucosal integrity. Cigarette use also increases the risk of infection and HPV-related disease, as does an altered immune system.

Infection with **herpes simplex virus type 2 (HSV-2)** is underestimated and is the most common cause of genital ulcerative disease in the United States. Reportedly, HSV-2 occurs in approximately 4% of whites and 17% of African Americans by the end of their teenage years.

By 2005 the number of HIV/**AIDS** cases reported in the United States in adolescents aged 13 to 19 years was 6,324; the number of cases in young adults between 20 and 24 years of age was 34,987. Because the incubation period for AIDS is believed to be from 8 to 10 years for adolescents, estimates of asymptomatic or early HIV infection are often based on reported cases of AIDS in young adults in their 20s. Acquired immunodeficiency syndrome cases in adolescents occur primarily in males and ethnic minorities. Most of these individuals are infected through sexual contact or injection drug use. Teen subpopulations who are at particularly high risk for acquiring HIV are youth who are gay, bisexual, transgendered, homeless, injection drug users, incarcerated, mentally ill, in the foster care system, or sexually or physically abused.

Clinical Presentation

Adolescents with an STI may go to their physicians with specific complaints related to the genitourinary system, such as painful urination or vaginal discharge. They also may report more generalized complaints, like fever and malaise, especially in cases of primary HSV or HIV (Dx Box: Sexually Transmitted Infections). In addition, some teenagers will use a vague complaint to see their primary care practitioner with the hope that the physician inquires about sexual activity. It is only then that they will disclose their true concern.

Dx **Sexually Transmitted Infections (STIs)**

Males
- Dysuria
- Urethral discharge or pain
- Testicular pain
- Presence of any lesions in the genital area such as ulcers, vesicles, or warts
- Sexual partner who has an STI

Females
- Dysuria
- Abnormal vaginal discharge
- Intermenstrual or irregular bleeding
- Dysmenorrhea
- Dyspareunia
- Postcoital bleeding
- Lower abdominal pain
- Systemic symptoms such as fever, nausea, vomiting, malaise
- Presence of any lesions in the genital area such as ulcers, vesicles, or warts
- Sexual partner who has an STI

Pathophysiology

A number of biological factors contribute to the increased prevalence rates of STIs in adolescents, particularly in females. At the onset of puberty, the columnar epithelial cells in the vagina transform to squamous epithelium while columnar cells at the cervix persist (Figure 85-1). With increasing age, the squamocolumnar junction recedes into the endocervix. In adolescent females, however, this junction, referred to as ectopy, is often located at the ectocervix and is relatively exposed, which places these females at particular risk for gonococcal and chlamydial infections. The infectious organisms preferentially attach to cervical columnar cells and infect them. Of note is that the use of oral contraceptives also prolongs this immature histologic state.

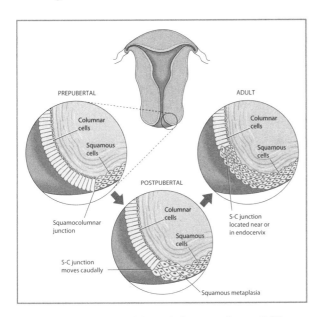

Figure 85-1. Development of the cervical squamocolumnar (S-C) junction, from puberty to adulthood.

The cytologic changes seen in cervical cells of adolescents with HPV infection are also believed to be age-related. The immature cervical metaplastic or columnar cells seem to be more highly vulnerable to infection and neoplastic changes. In addition, exposure to other cofactors (eg, tobacco use, multiple episodes of new HPV infections) is likely to promote the development of squamous intraepithelial neoplasia (SIN) and cervical carcinoma. Not all young women exposed to HPV develop lesions or progress to SIN, and most will not remain positive for HPV throughout their lifetime.

The presence of genital ulcers has been shown to facilitate both the transmission and the acquisition of HIV. Such ulcers provide a point of entry past denuded epithelium. In addition, it is hypothesized that many activated lymphocytes and macrophages are located at the base of the ulcer and are therefore susceptible to infection by HIV.

Pelvic inflammatory disease usually develops from an ascending mixed polymicrobial infection, often related to an untreated STI of the cervix and vagina. The infection spreads contiguously upward to the upper genital tract, resulting in inflammation, scarring, and crypt formation in the fallopian tubes. The most common causal organisms, which account for more than half of the cases of PID in most studies, are *Chlamydia trachomatis* and *Neisseria gonorrhoeae*. Other agents include *Escherichia coli;* other enteric flora; and microbes implicated in bacterial vaginosis, such as *Mycoplasma hominis, Mycoplasma genitalium, Ureaplasma urealyticum, Bacteroides* species, and anaerobic cocci. Viruses such as HIV and herpes simplex can facilitate the process of this ascending infection by disrupting normal immunologic barriers to infection such as altering the vaginal pH and flora and the cervical mucous barrier.

Differential Diagnosis

Most patients with STIs present with 1 of 5 clinical syndromes—urethritis/cervicitis, epididymitis, PID, genital ulcer disease, or genital warts, all of which can be easily diagnosed (Box 85-1). Other conditions that mimic STIs, however, must be considered in certain cases where the adolescent denies sexual activity or where the disorder does not respond to routine treatment. These disorders include **mucocutaneous ulcers** associated with systemic lupus erythematosus and Behçet disease. Often, systemic disorders such as these can be ruled out historically. **Benign oral lesions** such as aphthous ulcers also can be confused with herpetic ulcers. When evaluating an adolescent female with acute lower abdominal pain, surgical conditions such as **appendicitis, ovarian torsion,** and **ectopic pregnancy** must be ruled out. In the sexually active male with testicular pain, **testicular torsion** must be considered and thoroughly evaluated before a diagnosis of acute epididymitis is made.

Evaluation

In all sexually active adolescents, a complete history, including a sexual history, should be obtained (Questions Box). A detailed gynecologic history also should be reviewed with females. The rest of the history should then focus on the particular complaint and any associated symptoms. Sexually active adolescents should have a complete physical examination, including a thorough genital examination. Although diagnostic tests should be determined by the adolescent's risk for a specific STI based on historical and physical findings, one must keep in mind that many adolescent patients are asymptomatic, and screening for common STIs such as chlamydia and gonorrhea should be performed on most sexually active teenagers.

Urethritis and Epididymitis

History

Because urethritis is more common in young men, all sexually active adolescent males should be asked about the presence of dysuria, urethral discharge, and urethral erythema or pruritus. In females, symptoms such as dysuria may appear more gradually, and dysuria is reported more frequently than other symptoms like meatal edema, erythema, or urethral discharge, which are rarely noticed. General urinary symptoms such as acute urinary frequency or urgency are

Box 85-1. Differential Diagnosis of Sexually Transmitted Disease by Clinical Syndrome

Urethritis
- *Neisseria gonorrhoeae*
- Non-gonococcal disease
  - *Chlamydia trachomatis*
  - *Ureaplasma urealyticum*
  - *Trichomonas vaginalis*
  - Herpes simplex virus
  - Yeasts

Cervicitis
- *C trachomatis*
- *N gonorrhoeae*
- *Trichomonas vaginalis*
- Herpes simplex virus (especially primary type 2)

Pelvic Inflammatory Disease
- *N gonorrhoeae*
- *C trachomatis*
- Anaerobes
- Gram-negative rods
- Streptococci
- *Mycoplasma hominis*
- *U urealyticum*

Vaginitis
- *T vaginalis*
- *Candida albicans* and other yeast
- *Gardnerella vaginalis*

Genital Ulcers
- *Treponema pallidum* (syphilis)
- Herpes simplex virus, types 1 and 2
- *Haemophilus ducreyi* (chancroid)
- *C trachomatis* (lymphogranuloma venereum)

Genital Warts
- *T pallidum* (condyloma latum)
- Human papillomavirus (condyloma acuminatum)

Proctitis
- *N gonorrhoeae*
- *C trachomatis*
- *T pallidum*
- Herpes simplex virus
- Particular to homosexual youth (in addition to the above)
  - Hepatitis A and B virus
  - *Shigella*
  - *Campylobacter*
  - *Giardia lamblia*
  - *Entamoeba histolytica*

Pharyngitis
- *N gonorrhoeae*
- Herpes simplex virus, types 1 and 2

Questions

Sexually Transmitted Infections—Questions to Ask the Patient

- Are you currently sexually active?
- At what age did you begin to have sex?
- Do you have sex with men, women, or both?
- How many partners have you had? When was your last contact?
- Have you ever been forced to have sex, or have you ever exchanged sex for food, shelter, money, or drugs?
- Do you or your partner(s) use contraception? What type?
- Do you or your partner(s) use drugs or alcohol?
- Have any of your sexual contacts ever been diagnosed with a sexually transmitted infection?
- Do you have abdominal pain, dysuria, increased urinary frequency, or hesitancy?
- Have you noticed any ulcers, blisters, warts, or other bumps in the genital area?
- For females: Do you have a vaginal discharge or itching? Is sex uncomfortable or painful? Do you have bleeding between periods or after intercourse?
- For males: Do you have a discharge from your penis? Any testicular pain or swelling? Any associated burning or itching?

uncommon, especially in males, but all patients should be asked about these symptoms. More often, urethritis is asymptomatic, and the diagnosis is made by routine screening in sexually active adolescents or through known contact with a partner with a STI (eg, *C trachomatis* or *Trichomonas vaginalis*).

To diagnose acute epididymitis, sexually active males should be asked about testicular pain and swelling. Symptoms associated with urethritis may be present or may have preceded the scrotal symptoms.

Physical Examination

In males, the urethra should be the focus of the genital examination. The presence of a urethral discharge and its consistency (ie, mucoid or purulent) should be noted. Any other urethral or genital lesions should also be assessed. The epididymis, spermatic cord, and testes should be palpated carefully for tenderness and swelling.

In females, a full pelvic examination should be performed after careful examination of the external genitalia for any ulcerative or wart-like lesions. Urethritis is most often caused by *C trachomatis*, but HSV and trichomoniasis can be other causes. The urethra should be inspected for edema, erythema, or any evidence of a discharge prior to speculum insertion. The presence or absence of a vaginal or endocervical discharge also should be noted during the pelvic examination.

Laboratory Tests

A Gram stain of the urethral discharge may confirm the diagnosis of urethritis in both males and females. The specimen should be obtained using a Dacron or cotton swab because calcium alginate inhibits the growth of *Chlamydia*. The presence of gram-negative, intracellular diplococci with the typical "kidney bean" morphology is indicative of an infection with *N gonorrhoeae*. Five or more polymorphonuclear (PMN) leukocytes per high-power field but no organisms indicates the more common type of infection, non-gonococcal urethritis, usually found in males. If no PMN leukocytes are seen on Gram stain or if the patient is asymptomatic, assessment for leukocyte esterase with a urine dipstick should be made using the first 10 to 15 mL of a first-voided urine specimen. The sediment also should be examined under the microscope for PMN leukocytes. A routine urine culture is generally not recommended in males and may be of little help in females.

Newer screening tests using urine samples are now available and considered standard of care for detecting gonorrhea and *C trachomatis,* especially in asymptomatic sexually active adolescents. These non-culture tests rely on amplification of DNA (ie, polymerase chain reaction and ligase chain reaction) and are highly sensitive and convenient for screening teenagers because the test can be performed on a urine specimen. A disadvantage is that these tests are costly and may have a greater potential for false-positive results, making a definitive diagnosis questionable in a judicial setting. In the adolescent population, however, these urine nucleic acid amplification tests (NAATs) are generally more acceptable than tests requiring a direct urethral swab specimen and can be used to initiate treatment for the suspected STI.

Color duplex Doppler ultrasound may be necessary to make an accurate diagnosis of epididymitis, especially if there is any consideration for testicular torsion. If the diagnosis is questionable, a urologic consult should be obtained immediately.

Cervicitis

History

Cervicitis in females is parallel to urethritis in males. Because cervicitis is a local infection, systemic symptoms may not occur. However, a variety of important historical points and associated complaints should be addressed. Is a vaginal discharge present? If so, does it have an odor? Is the patient experiencing any urinary frequency, urgency, or dysuria? Has she had any non-menstrual vaginal bleeding, including postcoital bleeding? A known exposure to an STI also must be ascertained. Is the partner symptomatic or currently receiving treatment? Does the patient or her current partner have a history of an STI?

More generalized symptoms such as moderate lower abdominal pain (either acute or chronic) associated with nausea, vomiting, and fever may indicate a complication of untreated cervicitis such as PID.

Physical Examination

After completing the full physical examination, the physician should focus on the genitourinary examination. The sexual maturity rating should first be noted, then the presence of any lesions on the external genitalia or inflammation of the perineum. Any urethral erythema or discharge also should be noted. The presence of a vaginal discharge can be assessed more completely when performing the speculum examination, which should be performed in all sexually active adolescent females with vaginal or lower urinary tract complaints.

During the speculum examination, the vaginal mucosa should be inspected and the appearance of the cervical os should be noted. The physician should determine whether a mucopurulent exudate is visible in the endocervical canal and should look for any evidence of cervical friability or sustained endocervical bleeding as a cotton swab is gently passed through the cervical os. Cervical inflammation must be differentiated from normal adolescent ectopy. A presumptive diagnosis of mucopurulent cervicitis is made when there is a discharge from the cervical os, cervical erosion, or friability. A bimanual examination also must be performed to evaluate for cervical motion tenderness (CMT) and adnexal masses or fullness.

Laboratory Tests

According to the CDC, NAATs for *N gonorrhoeae* and *C trachomatis* are preferred for the diagnostic evaluation of cervicitis and can be performed on either urine or endocervical specimens. If a pelvic examination is being performed, an endocervical or vaginal swab specimen can be collected by direct visualization for NAATs. A Gram stain of the discharge also can be performed to detect the presence of gram-negative diplococci or PMN leukocytes. The presence of 30 or more PMN leukocytes per oil immersion field is presumptively positive for cervicitis. A wet mount to diagnose associated STIs such as trichomoniasis is recommended, especially if the discharge is foul smelling or frothy. Adolescents who are diagnosed with a new STI or assessed as high risk also should receive testing for other STIs such as HIV, syphilis, and viral hepatitis.

Pelvic Inflammatory Disease

History

When considering a diagnosis of PID, the history should include a discussion of known risk factors such as sexual activity, including the number of sexual partners, especially new partners in the previous 2 months; a previous history of an STI or recent episode of an STI; the type and consistency of contraceptive use; and the timing of the last menstrual cycle because most women present with PID during the first half of their menstrual cycle. The physician also should ask patients about the presence of symptoms that are often associated with PID: the onset, duration, quality, and location of abdominal pain; urinary symptoms that may indicate concomitant urethritis; intermenstrual bleeding; dysmenorrhea or dyspareunia; abnormal vaginal discharge; right upper quadrant pain; and systemic symptoms such as nausea, vomiting, fever, and malaise. The classic symptoms of PID, which include lower abdominal pain, vaginal discharge, fever, and irregular vaginal bleeding, may not be present. More often symptoms are nonspecific, and the practitioner must maintain a high index of suspicion in any sexually active female with abdominal pain.

Physical Examination

Classic signs of acute PID include fever with tenderness of the lower abdomen, cervix, and adnexa. However, the clinical presentation can vary from nearly asymptomatic to severe disease. A thorough physical examination should be completed before performing the pelvic examination, including a review of the vital signs, looking for fever or tachycardia. The blood pressure also must be reviewed carefully because hypotension can be seen with a ruptured ectopic pregnancy, which may present with similar symptoms including abdominal pain and vaginal bleeding. The abdomen should be assessed for tenderness and guarding. The location of the pain is particularly relevant because certain acute surgical conditions such as appendicitis, ovarian torsion, and ectopic pregnancy are important considerations in the differential diagnosis of PID. In addition, right upper quadrant pain is consistent with perihepatitis, or Fitz-Hugh–Curtis syndrome, which can be seen with a gonorrheal or chlamydial infection. The speculum examination should then be performed, looking for a mucopurulent endocervical exudate or any evidence of cervicitis (cervical friability or erosion). The bimanual examination is the most important part of the physical examination. The cervix should be carefully palpated for any evidence of CMT and the adnexa for tenderness or masses.

Laboratory Tests

The diagnosis of PID is based on clinical findings and a high index of suspicion. Previous CDC criteria for the diagnosis of PID included 3 major components: lower abdominal pain, cervical motion tenderness, and adnexal tenderness. Current recommendations now outline 2 minimal clinical criteria and 5 additional criteria to support the diagnosis (Dx Box: Pelvic Inflammatory Disease). Particularly when evaluating an adolescent for PID, early conservative treatment and maximum sensitivity for clinical findings are paramount to avoid a delayed or missed diagnosis. An NAAT for *N gonorrhoeae* and *C trachomatis* should be sent on the endocervical or vaginal swab specimen obtained during the pelvic examination. If readily available, a Gram stain of any cervical discharge should be performed. The specimen should be examined microscopically for PMN leukocytes as well as gram-negative, intracellular diplococci. The presence of numerous PMN leukocytes per oil immersion field is one of the clinical criteria for making a diagnosis of PID. (See Laboratory Tests section for urethritis and epididymitis.)

Other laboratory studies to be obtained include a complete blood count with differential and a sedimentation rate or C-reactive protein, although in many cases the laboratory tests are normal. A urine pregnancy test should be performed to exclude the possibility of a concomitant intrauterine or ectopic pregnancy. Additionally, a

Dx Pelvic Inflammatory Disease

- Uterine/adnexal tenderness
- Cervical motion tenderness

Additional Findings
- Fever >38.3°C (101°F)
- Abnormal vaginal or cervical mucopurulent discharge
- Presence of abundant numbers of white blood cells on saline microscopy of vaginal secretions
- Elevated erythrocyte sedimentation rate or C-reactive protein
- Laboratory documentation of cervical infection with *Neisseria gonorrhoeae* or *Chlamydia trachomatis*
- Inflammatory tubal mass or tubo-ovarian complex seen on magnetic resonance imaging, transvaginal ultrasound, or laparoscopy[a]
- Endometritis on biopsy[a]

[a]Centers for Disease Control and Prevention, Workowski A, Berman SM. Sexually transmitted diseases treatment guidelines, 2006. *MMWR Recomm Rep.* 2006;55:1–94.

urinalysis and urine culture should be obtained, as well as a serologic test for syphilis. Human immunodeficiency virus testing also should be offered after appropriate pretest counseling has occurred. Testing for syphilis and viral hepatitis is recommended.

Laparoscopy can be performed to make a definitive diagnosis of PID or to obtain diagnostic cultures in cases where the diagnosis is equivocal or the patient is not responding to standard antimicrobial therapy. A gynecologist should be consulted for these cases.

Imaging Studies

A pelvic ultrasound may help exclude diagnoses such as ectopic pregnancy or ovarian torsion and also can aid in the detection of associated complications of PID such as TOA. Of note is that although transvaginal ultrasound is more sensitive for detecting a TOA, many adolescent females are uncomfortable with the procedure. Fluid in the cul-de-sac may also be seen on ultrasound in these patients, however, it is not specific for the diagnosis of PID.

Genital Ulcers

History

Probably the most important information to obtain from the adolescent with genital ulcers is whether they are painful. A painless chancre on the penis, around the mouth, in the oropharynx, or on the external genitalia in females is consistent with syphilis. If the lesions are painful or are associated with a grouped vesicular eruption, HSV is the likely cause. The presence of systemic symptoms such as fever, chills, headache, or malaise is also important to discern because these symptoms can be seen with a primary infection with either organism. Generalized complaints, however, are associated with secondary syphilis only 50% of the time. A history of adenopathy, either localized or generalized, also must be noted, along with dysuria, which may be present in females with HSV. In addition, a history of a viral-like illness accompanied by a rash should be explored further. A diffuse maculopapular rash, especially on the palms and soles, is a classic sign of secondary syphilis. A known exposure to other STIs should also be ascertained.

Physical Examination

All adolescents who present with chancres, or ulcers, should receive a complete physical examination. The skin, including the palms and soles, should be examined closely for any dull red to reddish-brown macular or papular lesions. The oropharynx should be carefully checked for chancres or blisters. All lymph nodes should be palpated for pain, enlargement, or induration. Suppurative or fluctuant nodes are often associated with chancroid caused by *Haemophilus ducreyi*. The genital examination should then focus on the appearance of the lesions. The following questions should be asked of the patient: Are the lesions ulcerative, clustered, and painful (HSV or chancroid)? Are they associated with grouped vesicles on an erythematous base (HSV)? Is tender inguinal adenopathy present (HSV or chancroid)? Or is there a single, painless chancre with a clean base and a sharply defined, slightly elevated border (syphilis)? The lymph nodes associated with this syphilitic type chancre are often non-tender but enlarged. Other less common STIs produce genital ulcers that are often painful and deep and may be accompanied by some purulence. Adenopathy can be quite impressive with chancroid and lymphogranuloma venereum *(C trachomatis)*.

Laboratory Tests

The necessary diagnostic tests depend on the patient's clinical picture. However, all adolescents who present with an ulcerative lesion should have dark-field microscopy performed for syphilis. Direct fluorescent antibody testing of the lesions is also available and is very specific. Non-treponemal serologic tests for syphilis, such as the Venereal Disease Research Laboratory (VDRL) or rapid plasma reagin (RPR) tests, should be done if direct examination is not available or the clinical appearance of the ulcer is nonspecific. In cases of early primary syphilis where the VDRL or RPR may not be reactive initially, the test should be repeated in 1 week. Treponemal tests, such as the fluorescent treponemal antibody absorption test, should be used only as confirmatory tests and not for screening purposes.

A viral culture for HSV also should be obtained from the base of an unroofed vesicle. Herpes simplex virus monoclonal antibody can be performed in older lesions that may be culture-negative and can differentiate between types 1 and 2. Herpes simplex virus serology is generally not helpful. Given the well-described correlation between genital ulcers and HIV, it is recommended that all patients with a diagnosis of syphilis be tested for HIV as well. Conversely, annual syphilis screening is recommended for an adolescent with multiple sexual partners; a history of injection drug use; a history of sex with men, women, or both; or a diagnosed STI.

Genital Warts

History

Risk factors for HPV infection should be assessed. These include a history of multiple sexual partners, age younger than 25 years, a previous history of an STI, lack of consistent condom use, pregnancy, altered immune response, and tobacco use. Symptoms may include pruritus, pain, or dyspareunia, but often the condition is asymptomatic. Adolescents may inadvertently palpate a papule on the external genitalia and be concerned or may note bleeding from large, traumatized lesions.

Physical Examination

A complete pelvic examination should be performed on all sexually active female adolescents. Before the speculum is inserted, the external genitalia should be carefully inspected for lesions. Genital warts, or condylomata acuminata, most commonly appear on squamous epithelium as irregular polypoid masses with an irregular, cauliflower-like surface that may coalesce into larger lesions. They are usually located at the posterior introitus, labia minora, and in the vestibule in females, and may be found on the cervix and vagina as well. In males, warts are found more commonly on the penile shaft, glans, or corona. They also may appear as flat, flesh-colored papules on the scrotum and anus. Because this is a common location for lesions, the anus should be inspected carefully in both males and females. Condylomata plana are subclinical lesions that are not grossly visible but are apparent on colposcopy and histology. Condylomata lata are flat, flesh-colored warts that occur in moist areas (anus, scrotum, vulva) and may be associated with other signs of secondary syphilis.

Laboratory Tests

A Pap smear should be performed on all females with any evidence of condylomata acuminata. Cytologic findings associated with HPV include atypia, koilocytosis, and dysplasia. When considering a referral to the gynecologist, the grade of the lesion should be reviewed because most abnormalities in adolescents resolve on their own. A definitive diagnosis of HPV infection is based on detection of viral nucleic acid or capsid protein. Tests that detect specific types of HPV DNA are available but are not routinely recommended in teenagers except if atypical squamous cells of undetermined significance or low-grade squamous intraepithelial lesion are persistent after repeat cytologic testing.

Subclinical HPV infection can be detected using acetic acid, Schiller iodine, and colposcopy. Suspicious areas of white epithelium or a specific vascular pattern consistent with HPV infection should be biopsied. Females may be referred to a gynecologist for this procedure. Subclinical lesions in males should also be evaluated using 3% acetic acid. Biopsy may be difficult to perform. Of note is that subclinical genital HPV infections are generally not treated in the absence of cervical squamous intraepithelial lesions or obvious genital warts.

NAATs for the detection of gonorrhea or chlamydia can be performed on a urine, cervical, or vaginal specimen. Additionally, a nontreponemal antibody test for syphilis (RPR or VDRL) is indicated. An HIV antibody test should be offered to all adolescents who are deemed appropriately at risk after receiving pretest counseling.

A urinalysis for asymptomatic hematuria is indicated in males with visible condyloma. Its presence would indicate a urethral lesion.

Management

Although many states differ with regard to the details of health care delivery for adolescents, a policy allows health care providers to evaluate and treat adolescents for an STI without parental consent in most states. Notification of partners is usually anonymous and carried out by local public health officials. Contacts are informed that a partner has been diagnosed with an STI and are instructed to be evaluated for treatment. The evaluation and treatment of the sexual partners of patients diagnosed with an STI is extremely important to prevent reinfection. However, because partners are often asymptomatic and do not seek treatment, and persistent and recurrent infection rates are reported to be particularly high among adolescents, expedited partner therapy (EPT) is now advocated in a few states. Expedited partner therapy is the practice of treating the sex partners of persons with STIs without an intervening medical evaluation or professional prevention counseling. A permutation of EPT, patient-delivered partner therapy is another practical means for providing patients medications or prescriptions for their partners. Care must be taken when treating the female partners of men with gonorrhea or chlamydia because of the potential for undiagnosed PID. Therefore, as per the CDC guidelines, EPT for female partners should include a review of the symptoms of PID and advice to seek medical attention in addition to accepting the prescribed medications. Antibiotic recommendations and dosing schedules are noted in Box 85-2 as well as in Chapters 84 (Table 84-2) and 116 (Table 116-1). For further details regarding specific conditions and therapies, the reader may consult Selected References at the end of the chapter, particularly the CDC 2006 treatment guidelines.

In addition to antimicrobial therapy, management of an STI in an adolescent should include preventive services. Adolescents with a first-time STI as well as those with recurrent STIs should be educated about disease transmission, consequences of delayed treatment, and methods for prevention. Other associated STIs, such as HIV, should also be addressed. The physician should spend time with adolescents with recurrent STIs and explore the reasons why preventive methods have failed in the past. Several factors are extremely important to consider, including an untreated partner, poor sexual judgment secondary to substance use or abuse, and noncompliance with prescribed treatment regimens because they influence current treatment.

Box 85-2. Parenteral Regimens for the Treatment of Pelvic Inflammatory Disease

Parenteral Regimen A

Cefotetan, 2 g IV every 12 h

or

Cefoxitin, 2 g IV every 6 h

plus

Doxycycline, 100 mg IV

or PO every 12 h

Parenteral Regimen B

Clindamycin 900 mg IV every 8 h

plus

Gentamicin loading dose IV or IM (2 mg/kg body weight), followed by a maintenance dose of 1.5 mg/kg every 8 h (Single daily dosing may be substituted.)

The above regimens are continued for at least 48 hours after the patient improves clinically. On discharge from the hospital, doxycycline is continued orally for a total of 14 days. Clindamycin, 450 mg PO 4 times a day, can be used as an alternative to complete 14 days of treatment. When tubo-ovarian abscess is present, clindamycin is recommended rather than doxycycline.

Abbreviations: IV, intravenously; PO, orally; IM, intramuscularly.

Prognosis

If diagnosed and treated in a timely manner, the prognosis for most STIs is good, especially since the advent of single-dose, oral therapies. Sequelae of PID, however, regardless of treatment, include TOA and Fitz-Hugh–Curtis syndrome (perihepatitis). Long-term consequences of PID are chronic abdominal pain, ectopic pregnancy, and infertility. Currently there is no pharmacologic agent to eradicate HSV or HIV. Although acyclovir, famciclovir, and valacyclovir are useful in treating the signs of primary herpes and reducing the incidence of recurrences, long-term safety of using valacyclovir or famciclovir for longer than 1 year is currently unknown. The prognosis for HIV is variable, depending on the individual's progression at the time of diagnosis and their adherence to antiretroviral therapy.

CASE RESOLUTION

In the case presented at the beginning of the chapter, a diagnosis of herpes simplex virus can be made clinically. The adolescent should be counseled with regard to the mode of transmission, the natural history of primary versus recurrent infection, and the role of antiviral agents. A first-void urine sample should be checked for leukocyte esterase or polymorphonuclear leukocytes and sent for nucleic acid amplification tests for the detection of gonorrhea and chlamydia. A rapid plasma reagin or Venereal Disease Research Laboratory test should be performed as well as a thorough assessment for human immunodeficiency virus risk. Human immunodeficiency virus testing should be offered after appropriate pretest counseling has been performed.

Selected References

American Academy of Pediatrics Committee on Pediatric AIDS, Committee on Adolescence. Adolescents and human immunodeficiency virus infection. *Pediatrics.* 2001;107:188–190

Banikarim C, Chacko MR. Pelvic inflammatory disease in adolescents. *Adolesc Med.* 2006;15:273–285

Burnstein GR, Murray PJ. Diagnosis and management of sexually transmitted disease pathogens among adolescents. *Pediatr Rev.* 2003;24:75–82

Centers for Disease Control and Prevention, Workowski A, Berman SM. Sexually transmitted diseases treatment guidelines, 2006. *MMWR Recomm Rep.* 2006;55:1–94

Centers for Disease Control and Prevention. *Expedited Partner Treatment in the Management of Sexually Transmitted Diseases.* Atlanta, GA: US Department of Health and Human Services; 2006

Decker MR, Silverman JG, Raj A. Dating violence and sexually transmitted disease/HIV testing and diagnosis among adolescent females. *Pediatrics.* 2005;116:e272–e276

Futterman DC. HIV and AIDS in adolescents. *Adolesc Med.* 2006;15:369–391

Hogben M, Burstein GR. Expedited partner therapy for adolescents diagnosed with gonorrhea or chlamydia: a review and commentary. *Adolesc Med.* 2006;17:687–695

Kane ML, Rosen DS. Sexually transmitted infections in adolescents: practical issues in the office setting. *Adolesc Med Clin.* 2004;15:409–421

Lappa S, Moscicki AB. The pediatrician and the sexually active adolescent. A primer for sexually transmitted diseases. *Pediatr Clin North Am.* 1997;44:1405–1445

Niccolai LM, Hochberg AL, Ethier KA, Lewis JB, Ickovics JR. Burden of recurrent *Chlamydia trachomatis* infections in young women: further uncovering the "hidden epidemic." *Arch Pediatr Adolesc Med.* 2007;161:246–251

Saslow D, Runowicz CD, Solomon D, et al. American Cancer Society guideline for the early detection of cervical neoplasia and cancer. *CA Cancer J Clin.* 2002;52:342–362

Scholes D, Stergachis A, Heidrich FE, Andrilla H, Holmes KK, Stamm WE. Prevention of pelvic inflammatory disease by screening for cervical chlamydial infection. *N Engl J Med.* 1996;334:1362–1366

Shafii T, Burnstein GR. An overview of sexually transmitted infections among adolescents. *Adolesc Med Clin.* 2004;15:201–214

Shrier LA. Sexually transmitted disease in adolescents: biologic, cognitive, psychologic, behavioral, and social issues. *Adolesc Med Clin.* 2004;15:215–234

Simpson T, Oh MK. Urethritis and cervicitis in adolescents. *Adolesc Med Clin.* 2004;15:253–271

Menstrual Disorders

Monica Sifuentes, MD

CASE STUDY

A 16-year-old female presents with a 9-day history of vaginal bleeding. She has no history of abdominal pain, nausea, vomiting, fever, dysuria, or anorexia, and she reports no dizziness or syncope. Her menses usually last 4 to 5 days and, in general, occur monthly. Her last menstrual period was 3 weeks ago and was normal in duration and flow. Menarche occurred at 14 years of age. She is sexually active, has had 2 partners, and reportedly uses condoms "most of the time." Neither she nor her current partner has ever been diagnosed with or treated for a sexually transmitted infection. She has no family history of blood dyscrasias or cancer, no history of chronic illness, and takes no medications.

On physical examination, she is an obese adolescent female in no acute distress. Her temperature is 98.4°F (36.9°C). Her heart rate is 100/min, and her blood pressure is 110/60. The physical examination, including a pelvic examination, is unremarkable except for minimal blood noted at the vaginal introitus.

Questions

1. What menstrual disorders commonly affect adolescent females?
2. What factors contribute to the development of menstrual disorders, particularly during adolescence?
3. What relevant history should be obtained in adolescents with menstrual or pelvic complaints?
4. What treatment options are currently available for primary dysmenorrhea?
5. What conditions must be considered in adolescents with abnormal uterine bleeding?
6. How is dysfunctional uterine bleeding managed in adolescent patients?

Gynecologic concerns and complaints are common reasons for adolescent females to visit their primary care physicians. The challenge for practitioners is to differentiate between an organic etiology, functional condition, and psychogenic complaints. When this cannot be readily done or if the physical examination is equivocal, multiple diagnostic procedures may be performed, often with variable results. In addition, many pediatricians are uncomfortable evaluating gynecologic problems in adolescents and performing pelvic examinations, which contributes to this diagnostic dilemma. The purpose of this chapter is to review some of the more common gynecologic conditions affecting the adolescent female and to highlight the significant historical and physical findings associated with each problem. For a discussion of the infectious conditions that cause pelvic pain, see Chapter 85.

Epidemiology

The overall prevalence of menstrual disorders during adolescence is estimated to be 50%, with the most common gynecologic complaint being dysmenorrhea, or painful menstruation. At least 70% to 90% of women have some pain associated with menses regardless of the degree of discomfort. Although most menstruating women report mild to moderate discomfort, severe dysmenorrhea occurs in 10% to 15% of women and has been reported to be responsible for significantly limiting daily activity in these females. Uterine anomalies or pelvic abnormalities such as endometriosis can be found in approximately 10% of adolescents and young women with severe dysmenorrhea.

Prevalence estimates regarding premenstrual syndrome (PMS) are difficult to assess because most studies in adolescents are retrospective and self-reports can be unreliable and misleading. In these studies, between 30% and 75% of older adolescents report significant PMS-type complaints. An estimated 20% to 40% of adult women experience PMS symptoms bothersome enough to impair daily functions, and 5% to 10% have debilitating symptoms. Other menstrual problems in adolescents include abnormal uterine bleeding, vaginal discharge, and amenorrhea.

Several factors contribute to the occurrence of gynecologic problems during adolescence. The average age of menarche in the United States is 12.5 years (range: 9–16 years). Bleeding may be irregular or prolonged initially because 50% to 80% of menstrual cycles are anovulatory and irregular during the first 2 years after menarche. Once ovulatory cycles are established, bleeding problems may resolve, but menstrual symptoms such as pain, headache, and vomiting may predominate. Early sexual activity among adolescents and associated sexually transmitted infections also may contribute to the presence of certain gynecologic conditions in this age group, particularly vaginitis and abnormal uterine bleeding.

Clinical Presentation

Adolescents with menstrual disorders may present in a variety of ways. They may have specific symptoms, such as heavy bleeding, irregular periods, or painful menses, or more general complaints such as fatigue, dizziness, and syncope (Dx Box). In addition, adolescents or their parents may have questions or concerns about delayed pubertal development and amenorrhea.

Dx Menstrual Disorders

Primary Dysmenorrhea

- Painful menstruation
- Lower abdominal pain associated with menstruation, usually worse on the first few days of bleeding
- Associated back pain
- Pain sometimes accompanied by nausea, vomiting, fatigue, headache, bloating, and diarrhea
- Symptoms began 6 to 12 months after menarche

Dysfunctional Uterine Bleeding

- Prolonged bleeding (>8 days) *or*
- Excessive bleeding (>6 tampons/pads per day) or
- Frequent uterine bleeding (≤21 days)
- No demonstrable organic etiology
- Normal laboratory studies, except may have anemia

Primary Amenorrhea

- No spontaneous menstruation in a female of reproductive age
- Absence of menarche by age 16 in a female with normal pubertal development *or*
- Absence of menarche by age 14 in a female with no secondary sexual development *or*
- Absence of menarche within 1 to 2 years of reaching full sexual maturation (sexual maturity rating 5)

Pathophysiology

Puberty and the Normal Menstrual Cycle

Figure 86-1 depicts the menstrual cycle, which typically lasts for 21 to 35 days, with a mean length of approximately 28 days. Normal duration of menses is 4 to 7 days. Blood loss is usually 30 to 40 mL per cycle, and most women do not lose more than 60 mL per cycle. Regular ovulatory cycles usually do not occur until 2 to 3 years after menarche, although 10% to 20% of cycles can remain anovulatory as long as 5 years after menarche.

One quarter of females begin menstruating when they reach sexual maturity rating (SMR) (Tanner stage) 3 of sexual maturation, but approximately two-thirds do not menstruate until they reach SMR 4 breast and genital development. It is important to note that several other processes occur before the onset of menstruation. Thelarche, or the beginning of breast development, takes place approximately 2 to 3 years before menarche, and growth acceleration usually begins about 1 year before thelarche.

Dysmenorrhea

This condition is often accompanied by other symptoms such as nausea, vomiting, diarrhea, and headaches. It can be classified as either primary or secondary. Primary dysmenorrhea occurs in the absence of any pelvic pathology and is most commonly seen in adolescents once ovulatory cycles are established. Secondary dysmenorrhea refers to painful menses associated with some underlying pelvic pathology, such as pelvic inflammatory disease, endometriosis, ovarian cysts or tumors, or cervical stenosis. A complete list of causes of secondary amenorrhea can be found in Box 86-1. In adolescents, endometriosis is the most common cause of secondary dysmenorrhea.

Numerous studies have shown that endometrial prostaglandins and leukotrienes play a role in the pathogenesis of primary dysmenorrhea. During menses, prostaglandin $F_{2\alpha}$ is produced locally by the endometrium from arachidonic acid. Prostaglandin $F_{2\alpha}$ is a potent vasoconstrictor and myometrial stimulant that causes uterine contractions, leading to tissue ischemia and pain. Another prostaglandin, $E_{2\alpha}$, causes hypersensitivity of the pain nerve terminals in the uterine myometrium. The cumulative effect of these prostaglandins may cause the pain of primary dysmenorrhea. Hormonal and endocrine factors also may play a role in the etiology of primary dysmenorrhea because ovulatory cycles with estrogen and progesterone are necessary for development of the condition.

Most cases of primary dysmenorrhea begin 6 to 12 months after menarche, and symptoms gradually increase until patients reach their mid-20s. Parity and advancing age are associated with a decrease in symptomatology.

Dysfunctional Uterine Bleeding

Dysfunctional uterine bleeding (DUB) is defined as abnormal or excessive endometrial bleeding in the absence of any pelvic pathology. Menstruation is considered excessive if the cycles are short (<21 days) and the bleeding is prolonged (≥8 days). Although DUB is the most common cause of abnormal or excessive vaginal bleeding in adolescents, it should be considered a diagnosis of exclusion. Other causes of abnormal bleeding should first be investigated by obtaining a thorough history, performing a complete physical examination, and obtaining laboratory studies as indicated.

Dysfunctional uterine bleeding is usually the result of anovulatory, immature menstrual cycles. In adolescents, 50% of menstrual cycles are anovulatory within the first 2 years of menarche. If menarche occurs later in adolescence (ie, at SMR 5), this period of anovulation reportedly lasts even longer. Most cases of DUB in adolescence are thought to result from the delayed maturation of the hypothalamic-pituitary-ovarian axis. Normally, a positive feedback mechanism develops with rising estrogen levels, resulting in a surge in luteinizing hormone (LH) and follicle-stimulating hormone (FSH), which triggers ovulation. The progesterone-producing corpus luteum

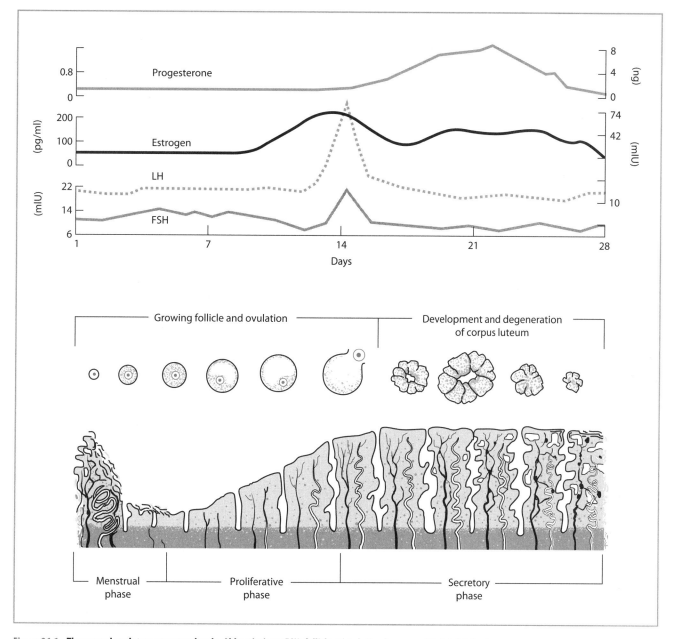

Figure 86-1. **The normal ovulatory menstrual cycle. Abbreviations: FSH, follicle-stimulating hormone; LH, luteinizing hormone.**

then stimulates development of the secretory endometrium, with subsequent shedding after approximately 14 days if no fertilization occurs (menses). With anovulation, there is no progesterone-producing corpus luteum and, therefore, no development of a secretory endometrium. Thus estrogen remains unopposed, and proliferative endometrium continues to accumulate. Finally, when the tissue can no longer maintain its integrity, it sloughs. In addition, without progesterone, the normal vasospasm that helps limit endometrial bleeding does not occur. Hence, bleeding is prolonged, frequent, and heavy.

Premenstrual Syndrome

Premenstrual syndrome refers to a group of physical, cognitive, affective, and behavioral symptoms that occur prior to menses (during the luteal phase of the menstrual cycle) and resolve within a few days following the onset of menstruation. A variety of mechanisms have been proposed, including an increased sensitivity to the normal cyclic fluctuations in steroid hormones and releasing factors and alterations in neurotransmitters such as endorphins, γ-aminobutyric acid, and serotonin. The exact etiology remains unknown, however, despite multiple studies aimed at pinpointing the cause of this complex condition. Various other hormonal factors have been implicated as

Box 86-1. Differential Diagnosis of Common Menstrual Disorders

Dysmenorrhea
- *Primary*
- *Secondary*
- Endometriosis
- PID
- Uterine myomas, polyps, or adhesions
- Adenomyosis
- Ovarian cysts or tumors
- Presence of an intrauterine device
- Cervical stenosis or strictures
- Congenital malformations (ie, septate uterus, imperforate hymen)

Abnormal Vaginal Bleeding
- Dysfunctional uterine bleeding: anovulation
- Complications of pregnancy: threatened/incomplete abortion, ectopic pregnancy, hydatidiform mole
- Infections of the lower and upper genital tract: PID, cervicitis/vaginitis
- Blood dyscrasias: vWD, ITP, leukemia, platelet defects
- Endocrine disorders: hypothyroidism and hyperthyroidism, hyperprolactinemia, late-onset 21-hydroxylase deficiency, Cushing or Addison disease
- Vaginal anomalies: carcinoma
- Cervical/uterine abnormalities: endometriosis, polyps
- Ovarian abnormalities: PCOS, tumors, cysts
- Systemic illness: IBD, malignancy, SLE
- Foreign body: condoms, tampons, IUDs
- Medications: aspirin, anticoagulants, hormonal contraception
- Trauma or sexual assault

Amenorrhea
- Pregnancy
- Systemic abnormalities: endocrinopathies (hypothyroidism, Cushing syndrome), chronic diseases (IBD, sickle cell disease), poor nutrition (anorexia nervosa), obesity, intense exercise, stress, drugs (opiates, valproate)
- Hypothalamic lesions: tumors, infiltrative lesions (TB, CNS leukemia)
- Pituitary lesions: prolactinoma, drugs causing elevated prolactins (marijuana, cocaine), cranial irradiation
- Ovarian failure: gonadal dysgenesis, autoimmune failure, galactosemia
- Congenital abnormalities of the reproductive tract: imperforate hymen, transverse vaginal septum, absence or abnormality of the uterus, complete androgen insensitivity (46, XY-testicular feminization)
- Androgen excess: PCOS, benign ovarian androgen excess

Abbreviations: PID, pelvic inflammatory disease; vWD, von Willebrand disease; ITP, idiopathic thrombocytopenic purpura; PCOS, polycystic ovary syndrome; IBD, inflammatory bowel disease; SLE, systemic lupus erythematosus; IUD, intrauterine device; TB, tuberculosis; CNS, central nervous system.

possibly having a relationship with PMS including prolactin, growth hormone, thyroid hormone, FSH, antidiuretic hormone, insulin, and cortisol. Vitamin deficiencies also have been considered, but have not been documented consistently in the medical literature.

Amenorrhea

Amenorrhea is defined as the lack of spontaneous menstruation in women of reproductive age. Like dysmenorrhea, it can be considered primary or secondary. **Primary amenorrhea** can be further defined by the following criteria: (1) an absence of menarche by age 16 years in females with otherwise normal pubertal development, (2) an absence of menarche by the age of 14 years in females with no secondary sexual development, and (3) an absence of menarche within 1 to 2 years of reaching SMR 5 pubic hair. Causes of primary amenorrhea range from congenital anatomical anomalies to genetic and endocrine conditions. A detailed discussion of each of these etiologies is beyond the scope of this chapter. See Selected References for more information.

Secondary amenorrhea occurs in females who have already established menstruation but have had no periods for 6 months or the equivalent of 3 cycles. The most common cause of secondary amenorrhea is pregnancy, which must be ruled out in all adolescents presenting with this complaint, regardless of their acknowledgment of sexual activity. Other causes include infections, systemic illnesses, significant weight loss, stress, exercise, eating disorders (eg, anorexia nervosa), and certain medications.

Vaginal Discharge

Vaginal discharge can be normal. A thin, white discharge, known as leukorrhea, occurs approximately 1 year prior to the onset of menarche. A purulent, malodorous, or bloody discharge is considered abnormal, however. Etiologies are varied and may be infectious, inflammatory, or traumatic (see Chapters 84 and 85).

Differential Diagnosis

The differential diagnosis of the disorders described above can be found in Box 86-1. Other etiologies of pelvic pain include midcycle menstrual disorders (eg, mittelschmerz), urinary tract infections, and abdominal conditions such as inflammatory bowel disease and irritable bowel syndrome. Psychogenic pain also should be considered as a cause of recurrent pelvic pain and may be secondary to depression, anxiety, previous sexual abuse, or another psychological condition.

Evaluation

History

A thorough history should be obtained in adolescent females with suspected menstrual disorders because many non-gynecologic conditions can affect menses as well. A complete psychosocial assessment also should be performed. The acronym **HEADDSSS** (home environment, employment and education, activities, diet, drugs, sexuality/sexual activity, suicide/depression, safety) serves as a useful tool when interviewing adolescents (see Chapter 5).

Most of the interview should then focus on the gynecologic history (Box 86-2) and any associated problems (Questions Box). With primary dysmenorrhea, pain that radiates to the anterior thighs or the lower back is not uncommon. The color of the blood may be helpful when assessing abnormal uterine bleeding. Brown or dark blood may be associated with a cervical obstruction or endometriosis, whereas red or pink blood is found with most other conditions. More importantly, the timing of the bleeding is extremely significant. Cyclical bleeding beginning at menarche is more consistent with the presence of a blood dyscrasia. In contrast, breakthrough bleeding throughout the cycle may indicate an infection, endometriosis, or perhaps a polyp. The passing of blood clots on rising in the morning is not uncommon secondary to the vaginal pooling of blood while the patient is supine. Clots throughout the day, however, are not normal and require further investigation.

Box 86-2. Gynecologic History

- Age at menarche
- Last menstrual period
- Regularity of menses
- Duration of bleeding
- Amount of flow (number of pads/tampons used per day and amount of saturation)
- Associated symptoms such as bloating, headache, lower abdominal pain, and cramping
- Sexual activity
- Age at debut
- Number of partners and ages
- Consensual versus nonconsensual sex
- Date of last encounter
- Protected versus unprotected vaginal intercourse
- Current method of contraception
- Maternal and sibling gynecologic history
- Symptoms with menses
- Treatment of symptoms

Physical Examination

A complete physical examination, including an evaluation for stigmata of a systemic illness, must be performed in adolescent females with suspected menstrual disorders. Patients' height and weight should be plotted on the growth chart and compared with previous measurements. Depending on the SMR, physicians can then determine if they have experienced their expected growth spurt. Body mass index (body mass index = weight, kg/[height, m]^2) also should be calculated and compared with previous values, especially in females with amenorrhea. Vital signs, including orthostatic measurements, are a screen for significant blood loss with resultant anemia and are especially important in patients with excessive uterine bleeding. The skin should be inspected for any evidence of androgen excess (eg, hirsutism, acne), bruising, or petechiae. The thyroid gland should be palpated for masses or any evidence of hypertrophy, and the abdomen and suprapubic area also should be palpated for masses.

Questions

Menstrual Disorders

Dysmenorrhea
- What is the pain like?
- When did the pain first begin?
- How frequently does the pain occur?
- How long does the pain last?
- Are any symptoms associated with the pain (eg, nausea, vomiting, diarrhea, headache)?
- Does the adolescent miss a lot of school as a result of painful menses?
- Do the painful menses interfere with other activities?
- What does the adolescent do for the pain? Has she tried any medications or home remedies?
- Is there a maternal or sibling history of painful menses?

Abnormal Uterine Bleeding
- Does the adolescent have any symptoms of anemia?
- Is she fatigued, easily tired, dizzy, or short of breath?
- Has she experienced any syncopal episodes?
- Does the adolescent have any history of blood loss in the urine or stool?
- Is there any evidence or a family history of a bleeding disorder (eg, easy bruisability, bleeding from the gums or nares)?
- Does the adolescent have any symptoms of pregnancy (eg, breast tenderness, nausea, fatigue)?
- Is there any known exposure to sexually transmitted infections?
- Is there a marked change in the adolescent's weight? Has the adolescent been on any diets recently?
- Is the adolescent using any medications such as aspirin, oral contraceptives, or anticoagulants?
- Does the adolescent have a history of trauma?
- Is the bleeding cyclic in nature?
- Is there breakthrough bleeding throughout the cycle?
- Does the adolescent have a family history of bleeding disorders, thyroid disease, or exposure to diethylstilbestrol?

Amenorrhea
- Has the adolescent *ever* had a period?
- Has she noticed any other changes associated with puberty (eg, breast development, pubic hair)?
- Does she have any other symptoms such as galactorrhea, weight loss, or hirsutism?
- Has the adolescent experienced significant changes/stressors in her life (eg, parental divorce, new school)?
- How often does the adolescent exercise?
- What is the adolescent's diet or are there any dietary restrictions (eg, vegetarian)?

In addition, the SMR of the breasts should be noted and compared with pubic hair development, particularly in adolescents with primary amenorrhea. The presence or absence of galactorrhea also should be noted. The external genitalia should then be carefully inspected for clitoral size and patency of the hymen. A bimanual or rectoabdominal examination should be performed in adolescents who are not sexually active to ensure the presence of a normal vagina, uterus, and adnexa. A speculum examination is generally not necessary for the virginal adolescent with suspected DUB or primary dysmenorrhea. In adolescents who are sexually active and have an abnormal vaginal discharge, however, complete pelvic and bimanual examinations are indicated.

Laboratory Tests

The performance of laboratory studies depends on the particular menstrual complaint. No laboratory studies are necessary for primary dysmenorrhea because the diagnosis is usually based on history and physical examination. The same is true for PMS. For a discussion of the diagnostic evaluation of amenorrhea, refer to the article by Bravender and Emans listed in Selected References.

In the case of abnormal uterine bleeding, baseline studies must include a hemoglobin or hematocrit. Other initial laboratory studies should include a complete blood count to evaluate the red cell indices and platelets, a reticulocyte count, and a pregnancy test. Further diagnostic studies depend on the severity of the anemia and findings on history and physical examination. These may include coagulation studies (bleeding time, prothrombin time/partial thromboplastin time), erythrocyte sedimentation rate, and thyroid function tests. Other tests for the evaluation of a blood dyscrasia should be performed in the patient presenting with severe anemia, especially at menarche. The studies should be performed in consultation with a pediatric hematologist and obtained prior to the administration of any estrogen-containing medications, which may affect the results of certain assays. If the patient is sexually active and a pelvic examination is performed, an endocervical specimen can be obtained for nucleic acid amplification tests for *Chlamydia trachomatis* and *Neisseria gonorrhoeae*. Nucleic acid amplification tests of the urine to screen for gonorrhea and chlamydia are also available (eg, ligase chain reaction, polymerase chain reaction), however, a speculum examination is still generally indicated for abnormal vaginal bleeding. Follicle-stimulating hormone, LH, prolactin, testosterone, and dehydroepiandrosterone sulfate studies should be performed in patients with a history of chronic anovulation or in whom androgen excess is suspected.

Imaging Studies

A pelvic or intravaginal ultrasound or computed tomography scan of the pelvis can be helpful in patients with abnormal uterine bleeding or amenorrhea if a mass is suspected or palpated on physical examination. Plain radiographs are not indicated.

Management

With each of these adolescent gynecologic conditions, effective treatment is multifaceted and includes patient and parent education, reassurance regarding the ease with which the condition can be treated, and appropriate medications for those conditions requiring therapy. In general, a menstrual calendar or diary initially can be very helpful with most gynecologic conditions to gain a more objective idea of the problem and to assess the pattern of the menstrual cycle.

Dysmenorrhea

General measures in the treatment of dysmenorrhea include education about menstruation, proper diet, application of heat, simple exercise, and psychological support.

For mild symptoms of dysmenorrhea, over-the-counter analgesics, such as ibuprofen, aspirin, or acetaminophen, are appropriate. Physicians most often suggest that patients use ibuprofen because it is probably the most efficacious. The dose is 400 to 600 mg every 4 to 6 hours. Ibuprofen should be taken at the onset of the menstrual cycle and continued for 24 to 72 hours.

For moderate to severe dysmenorrhea in patients who are not sexually active and do not desire birth control, a stronger nonsteroidal anti-inflammatory drug **(NSAID),** such as naproxen, is the treatment of choice (Table 86-1). The major mechanism of action of NSAIDs is the inhibition of prostaglandin synthesis. Side effects of these drugs, which most commonly relate to the gastrointestinal tract, are nausea, vomiting, and dyspepsia. These reactions can be minimized by taking the medication with food or an antacid. Other adverse reactions include renal effects; skin reactions, such as erythema multiforme and urticaria; and central nervous system effects, including headache and dizziness. Contraindications to NSAID use include peptic ulcer disease, clotting disorders, and renal disease. All NSAIDs should be administered with food and taken for 3 to 4 menstrual cycles before their efficacy is judged.

Table 86-1. Nonsteroidal Anti-inflammatory Drugs in the Treatment of Primary Dysmenorrhea

Generic	Trade Name(s)	Dosage
Ibuprofen	Motrin, Advil	400–600 mg every 4–6 h for 24–72 h
Naproxen	Aleve, Naprosyn	500 mg at onset, then 250 mg every 4–6 h
Naproxen sodium	Anaprox	500 mg at onset, then 275 mg every 6–8 h
Mefenamic acid	Ponstel	500 mg at onset, then 250 mg every 6–8 h

Low-dose combination oral contraceptives are indicated in adolescents with severe dysmenorrhea who are sexually active or in patients whose symptoms are not relieved by NSAIDs alone. Oral contraceptives decrease the production of prostaglandins by inhibiting ovulation as well as endometrial growth. Because the symptoms of dysmenorrhea are prevented only after several cycles of oral contraceptive pill (OCP) usage, patients should be told not to expect complete resolution of symptoms during the first month of treatment.

Oral contraceptives should be used for a minimum of 3 to 4 months. If symptoms do not improve, then an NSAID can be added to the treatment regimen. Oral contraceptives are more than 90% effective in cases of severe dysmenorrhea, and physicians should emphasize this benefit to both patients and their parents.

If the patient continues to have dysmenorrhea despite the judicious use of NSAIDs and oral contraceptives, a search for other pelvic pathology is warranted.

Dysfunctional Uterine Bleeding (Table 86-2)

The management of DUB depends on the severity of the bleeding and the degree of anemia. The goal of treatment is 4-fold: (1) to control the bleeding, (2) to correct the anemia, (3) to replenish iron stores, and (4) to prevent further episodes of bleeding. Patients with mild or moderate anemia can be treated as outpatients with weekly to monthly follow-up depending on how quickly the bleeding stops. Although **combination oral contraceptives** are appropriate in the treatment of DUB if the condition is moderate or if birth control is desired, **other hormone regimens** such as estrogen (alone) or synthetic progestin (alone) also can be used.

Most adolescent females with severe bleeding and anemia require a more extensive evaluation, and such patients usually are hospitalized for appropriate parenteral therapy and possible blood transfusion. Intravenous conjugated estrogens may be required every 4 to 6 hours for the first 24 hours to stop the bleeding. This therapy is then followed by a combination oral contraceptive containing 50 μg of estrogen (Ovral); the progesterone component is necessary to stabilize the endometrium. In addition, an antiemetic is often required 1 hour prior to the OCP during the first few days of therapy. Once bleeding is controlled, adolescents can continue a monophasic combined oral contraceptive such as Ovral for a total of 21 days and then switch to a low-dose combination oral contraceptive for at least 3 cycles. Studies have shown that 20% to 25% of adolescents who require hospitalization for severe anemia within the first year following menarche have an underlying coagulopathy. In cases of DUB where oral contraceptives are used but patients do not desire birth control, oral contraceptives should not be stopped until at least 3 months after the anemia has resolved to ensure restoration of iron stores.

Surgical treatment such as dilatation and curettage is rarely indicated in the adolescent patient and is reserved for patients refractory to aggressive medical treatment.

Premenstrual Syndrome

Although various sources have advocated many different treatment regimens for the management of PMS, no definitive studies have been reported, and no single effective treatment has been found. Therapies for mild to moderate symptoms include diet modification for patients who complain predominantly of bloating, promotion of regular aerobic exercise, education regarding menstrual physiology and the relationship of changing hormones to symptoms, stress management, and cognitive-behavior therapy or group therapy. Calcium supplements also can be recommended initially. Although positive outcomes have been reported with vitamin and mineral supplementation as well as with certain herbal preparations, more research is needed to definitively recommend their usage. Of note, some therapies that had been used extensively in the past also have been associated with undesirable outcomes such as the development of peripheral neuropathy with pyridoxine (B₆) at high doses. Combined OCPs, NSAIDs, and spironolactone may be helpful if physical symptoms predominate. Other medications that may be used when mood symptoms predominate and are significantly impairing function are the selective serotonin reuptake inhibitors such as fluoxetine and/or an anxiolytic, specifically alprazolam.

Vaginitis

See Chapters 84 and 85 for a discussion of the management of vaginal discharge in adolescents.

Prognosis

Most adolescents with common menstrual complaints who receive aggressive, appropriate care are symptom-free after 3 to 4 months of continuous therapy. Complications associated with oral contraceptive use and NSAIDs are rare in this otherwise healthy patient population. Symptoms associated with an immature hypothalamic-pituitary-ovarian axis, such as anovulatory bleeding and DUB, often resolve spontaneously. The prognosis for adolescents with amenorrhea depends in part on the underlying etiology.

Table 86-2. General Guidelines for the Management of Dysfunctional Uterine Bleeding in Adolescents			
	Mild Anemia	*Moderate Anemia*	*Severe Anemia*
Hemoglobin (g/dL)	>11	9–11	<9
Management	Menstrual calendar, oral iron twice daily, OBCP (if sexually active)	Initially, 2–3 OBCPs (1/35) every day to control the bleeding, then cycle with OBCP (1/35) for minimum of 3 mo; oral iron supplementation	Hospitalization if signs of hypovolemia; consider intravenous estrogen until bleeding stops; begin 2–4 OBCPs (1/50) every day and taper over 21 d, then cycle with OBCPs (1/35) for 3–6 mo; oral iron supplementation
Follow-up	2–3 mo	2–3 wk, then every 2–3 mo	1–2 wk, then every month

Abbreviations: OBCP, oral birth control pill; (1/35), monophasic pill with 35 μg ethinyl estradiol; (1/50), monophasic pill with 50 μg ethinyl estradiol.

Selected References

Adams Hillard PJ, Deitch HR. Menstrual disorders in the college age female. *Pediatr Clin North Am.* 2005;52:179–197

American Academy of Pediatrics Committee on Adolescence. Menstruation in girls and adolescents: using the menstrual cycle as a vital sign. *Pediatrics.* 2006;118:2245–2250

Bevan JA, Maloney KW, Hillery CA, Gill JC, Montgomery RR, Scott JP. Bleeding disorders: a common cause of menorrhagia in adolescents. *J Pediatr.* 2001;138:856–861

Bravender T, Emans SJ. Menstrual disorders. *Pediatr Clin North Am.* 1999;46:545–553

Braverman PK. Premenstrual syndrome and premenstrual dysphoric disorder. *J Pediatr Adolesc Gynecol.* 2007;20:3–12

Braverman PK, Sondheimer SJ. Menstrual disorders. *Pediatr Rev.* 1997;18:17–25

Chumlea WC, Schubert CM, Roche AF, et al. Age at menarche and racial comparisons in US girls. *Pediatrics.* 2003;111:110–113

Ellis MH, Beyth Y. Abnormal vaginal bleeding in adolescence as the presenting symptom of a bleeding diathesis. *J Pediatr Adolesc Gynecol.* 1999;12:127–131

Gray SH, Emans SJ. Abnormal vaginal bleeding in adolescents. *Pediatr Rev.* 2007;28:175–182

Harel Z. Dysmenorrhea in adolescents and young adults: etiology and management. *J Pediatr Adolesc Gynecol.* 2006;19:363–371

Iglesias EA, Coupey SM. Menstrual cycle abnormalities: diagnosis and management. *Adolesc Med.* 1999;10:255–273

Kadir RA, Lee CA. Menorrhagia in adolescents. *Pediatr Ann.* 2001;30:541–546

Montgomery RR, Kroner PA. von Willebrand disease: a common pediatric disorder. *Pediatr Ann.* 2001;30:534–540

O'Connell BJ. The pediatrician and the sexually active adolescent. Treatment of common menstrual disorders. *Pediatr Clin North Am.* 1997;44:1391–1404

Rimza ME. Dysfunctional uterine bleeding. *Pediatr Rev.* 2002;23:227–235

Smith YR, Quint EH, Hertzberg RB. Menorrhagia in adolescents requiring hospitalization. *J Pediatr Adolesc Gynecol.* 1998;11:13–15

Disorders of the Breast

Monica Sifuentes, MD

CASE STUDY

A 2-year-old girl is brought to the office for bilateral breast swelling first noticed 3 weeks ago by her mother. The swelling is non-tender and does not appear to be increasing in size. There is no history of galactorrhea. The child is otherwise healthy, takes no medications, and is not using any estrogen-containing creams.

On physical examination, the vital signs are normal, and the child is at the 50th percentile for height and weight. A 1.5-cm firm, non-tender mass is palpated below her left nipple. Below the right nipple, a 1-cm non-tender mass of similar consistency is present. There is no discharge from either nipple and no areolar widening. The abdomen is soft with no masses palpated. The genitalia are those of a normal prepubescent female with no pubic hair.

Questions

1. What is premature thelarche, and how can it be differentiated from true precocious puberty?
2. What are the most common causes of breast hypertrophy in the infant?
3. When does pubertal breast development normally occur in females?
4. What are the most common causes of breast masses in adolescent females and how should they be managed?
5. How can transient pubertal gynecomastia be differentiated from pathologic causes of gynecomastia in young males?

Breast disorders can occur in all pediatric age groups. The neonate may present to the pediatrician with bilateral breast hypertrophy and galactorrhea or mastitis. A bewildered parent might bring in a young daughter because of early breast development. An anxious adolescent female may notice for the first time that her breasts are asymmetrical, or she may feel a lump beneath the skin. An adolescent male can present with unilateral or bilateral gynecomastia that causes him severe psychological distress. Whatever the underlying cause, breast problems can be disconcerting at any age. Primary care providers should be equipped to differentiate between normal variants of growth and pathologic conditions in infants, children, and adolescents. Although rare, significant disorders can then be diagnosed and treated appropriately.

Epidemiology

Breast problems range from congenital anomalies and benign disorders related to hormonal stimulation to breast masses and tumors. Serious disorders such as breast cancer are practically unheard of in children and adolescents, although inappropriate breast enlargement or gynecomastia as a sign of another neoplastic process is not uncommon.

Benign breast hypertrophy can occur in 60% to 90% of neonates and is seen in both male and female term infants. It may occur unilaterally or bilaterally. Occasionally there is a nipple discharge.

Congenital anomalies of the breast include polythelia, athelia, polymastia, and amastia. Breast deformities such as a tuberous breast anomaly also can be thought of as a congenital anomaly, although it

is not manifested until puberty when breast growth normally occurs. Polythelia, or extra nipples, can be found anywhere along the embryonic "milk line" from the axilla to the groin and is seen in 2% of the general population (Figure 87-1). Reportedly, abnormalities of the urologic and cardiovascular systems have been associated with polythelia. Polymastia refers to supernumerary breasts along the milk

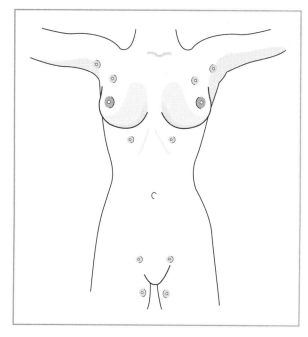

Figure 87-1. Polythelia. Supernumerary nipples along the embryonic mammary ridge (milk line).

line and is seen less frequently than polythelia (Figure 87-2). The usual locations for supernumerary breasts are below the breast on the chest or the upper abdomen. Both polythelia and polymastia may be familial and can occur bilaterally as well as unilaterally.

Amastia (absence of a breast) and athelia (absence of a nipple) are rare occurrences, but their presence often is associated with other anomalies of the chest wall such as pectus excavatum. Amastia also is seen in Poland syndrome (Figure 87-3), which includes

Figure 87-2. **Polymastia. Supernumerary breasts (accessory breast tissue).**

Figure 87-3. **Amastia. Unilateral (left) complete absence of breast tissue.**

absence of the ipsilateral pectoral muscles, various rib deformities and upper limb defects such as syndactyly (webbed fingers), and radial nerve aplasia.

Premature thelarche is isolated unilateral or bilateral breast development in girls between 1 and 4 years of age without other signs of sexual maturation. It has been estimated that 60% of cases occur between 6 months and 2 years of age. In contrast, precocious puberty is the appearance of any sign of secondary sexual maturation before age 7 in white girls or age 9 in boys. In young females, this involves either breast or pubic hair development, and in males, pubic hair or testicular enlargement.

Gynecomastia commonly occurs in males progressing through puberty and is often called transient pubertal gynecomastia (Figure 87-4). An estimated 70% of adolescent males are said to be affected, with a peak prevalence between ages 12 and 15. This generally corresponds to sexual maturity rating (SMR) (Tanner stage) 2 to 3 in the young male but is most prominent at genital SMR 4. Like breast development in the pubertal female, transient pubertal gynecomastia may be asymmetrical, although concurrent or sequential involvement of both breasts can occur.

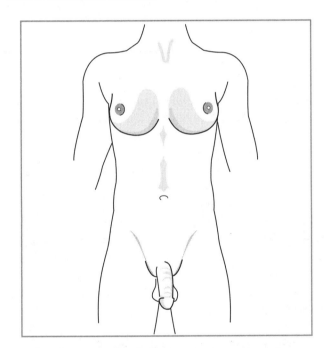

Figure 87-4. **Gynecomastia. Breast tissue development in a male.**

In the adolescent female, breast masses are not uncommon; however, clinically significant lesions are rare. Breast cancer per se has an estimated annual incidence of 0.1:100,000 adolescents. In most patient series through age 20, the most common breast tumor is the fibroadenoma, which has been reported in 60% to 95% of biopsied lesions. Two-thirds of these lesions are located in the lateral quadrants of the breast, with most in the upper outer quadrant. Their peak incidence is in late adolescence (17–21 years of age), and they tend to occur more commonly in African American females. In addition, 25% of cases involve multiple fibroadenomas.

Fibrocystic changes are the second most common histologic diagnosis after fibroadenomas. Other breast masses include solitary cysts; abscesses; lipomas; and cystosarcoma phyllodes, a rare, slow-growing, painless breast tumor that is nearly always benign.

Malignancy is reported in less than 1% of excised lesions. There are fewer than 50 cases of primary breast cancer in children and adolescents reported in the literature to date. Rhabdomyosarcoma and fibrosarcomas are among the other rarely reported primary tumors of the breast in adolescents. Metastatic cancer of the breast has been reported in children with primary hepatocellular carcinoma, Hodgkin and non-Hodgkin lymphoma, neuroblastoma, and rhabdomyosarcoma. Of note is the increased lifetime risk for breast cancer in pubertal girls who receive chest wall irradiation, generally given to treat Hodgkin lymphoma.

Normal Breast Development

In the adolescent female, the first sign of puberty is breast development. This begins with the appearance of a breast bud beneath the areola. Under the influence of estrogen, there is an increase in the adipose tissue along with the beginning of ductal and stromal growth. Progesterone initiates alveolar budding and lobular growth and contributes to the development of secretory lobules and alveoli. The alveoli are later lined by milk-secreting cells under the influence of prolactin when full maturation occurs.

The normal progression of breast growth is divided into 5 stages or SMRs. These descriptions are used to follow normal breast development, which increases in parallel with pubic hair development. It usually takes 2 to 4 years for the completion of breast development although, as in all aspects of puberty, variations do occur. The practitioner should keep in mind that many females will remain in SMR 3 or 4 breast development until pregnancy. Additionally, especially between SMR 2 and 4, significant breast asymmetry can be quite common in the adolescent without indicating a disorder. Once both breasts are fully mature and reach SMR 5, adequate catch-up growth usually has occurred.

Clinical Presentation

Infants with breast disorders usually present in the first few weeks of life with bilateral breast enlargement that may be asymmetrical (Dx Box). There may be an associated clear or cloudy nipple discharge. If an infection is present, the overlying skin may be warm and erythematous. Fever or other nonspecific symptoms such as poor feeding and irritability also may be present because mastitis involves the entire breast bud and, although rare, septicemia can occur.

In prepubertal females, premature thelarche will present as unilateral or bilateral non-tender subareolar swelling without other secondary sexual characteristics. In contrast, girls with precocious puberty may have axillary hair, nipple and areola enlargement and thinning, and pubic hair in addition to early breast development. Adolescent females with a breast problem often will complain of a unilateral breast lump noted incidentally by the teenager. It may be tender, fluctuant, firm, rubbery, or nodular. The adolescent also may

Dx ## Breast Disorder

Infants, Prepubescent Children, and Adolescent Males
- Unilateral or bilateral subareolar mass
- Possible associated nipple discharge
- Skin changes such as erythema in infants

Adolescent Females
- Firm, rubbery, freely movable mass
- Possible tenderness
- Breast asymmetry
- Skin changes such as shininess, venous distention, or dimpling (rare)
- Possible associated nipple discharge

complain of painful breasts (mastalgia) that can be cyclic in nature. For most breast masses, the overlying skin is normal, but occasionally skin changes do occur. Rarely, an associated nipple discharge also may be present.

Because most breast masses occur in females, gynecomastia is particularly anxiety provoking in young adolescent males. It usually appears as a unilateral or bilateral 2- to 3-cm firm mass beneath the areola, which may or may not be tender. There may be irritation of the skin of the nipple from rubbing against the clothing. Galactorrhea rarely accompanies pubertal gynecomastia and may indicate self-stimulation or illicit drug use, especially marijuana.

Pathophysiology

Neonatal breast hypertrophy seems to be a response to maternal estrogen exposure in utero. Constant stimulation can lead to persistent swelling, galactorrhea, and overt infection. In general, preterm infants are less responsive to maternal hormones and, therefore, breast hypertrophy occurs less often in this age group. It also may be delayed for weeks.

Central precocious puberty is due to early activation of the hypothalamic-pituitary-gonadal axis and the secretion of gonadotropin-releasing hormone (GnRH)–dependent pituitary gonadotropins in a pulsatile pattern. Although a search for an underlying central nervous system (CNS) or gonadal abnormality may be undertaken, most cases in females are idiopathic. In contrast, less than 10% of males with precocious puberty do not have an identifiable cause. Central nervous system tumors cause precocious puberty by impinging on the neuronal pathways that inhibit the GnRH pulse generator in childhood. Cranial irradiation, received as a part of tumor therapy, also can lead to sexual precocity. Pseudoprecocious puberty is GnRH-independent and is caused by the extrapituitary secretion of gonadotropins or the secretion of gonadal steroids independent of pulsatile GnRH stimulation.

Premature thelarche is a variation of normal pubertal development with transient elevations in estrogen levels from either functional ovarian cysts or fluctuations in pituitary gonadotropin secretion. Often the breast enlargement occurs without other estrogen effects such as an increase in uterine size or changes in the appearance of the external genitalia. In general, no linear growth or bone age advancement is associated with this condition.

The cause of fibroadenomas in adolescent females is postulated to be an abnormal sensitivity to estrogen. Observations supporting this hypothesis include the presence of estrogen receptors in the tumor and an increased incidence of this type of tumor during late adolescence. Thus prolonged exposure to estrogen may play a role in its development. Enlargement can occur during pregnancy or toward the end of the menstrual cycle.

Transient pubertal galactorrhea is thought to occur from a temporary imbalance of estrogen and androgens. Alterations in the ratio of these hormones leads to an increase in estrogen relative to testosterone. Certain medications can cause elevations in serum prolactin and lead to gynecomastia and/or galactorrhea (Box 87-1). Some illicit drugs, such as marijuana, contain phytoestrogens that can mimic estrogen or stimulate estrogen receptor sites. Others (eg, spironolactone, cimetidine) interfere with androgen receptors or induce inhibition of enzymes needed in steroid synthesis.

Box 87-1. Causes of Galactorrhea[a]

- Mechanical stimulation of the nipple
- Drugs
- Estrogenic drugs
- Digitalis
- Marijuana
- Heroin
- Dopamine receptor blockers
- Phenothiazines
- Haloperidol
- Metoclopramide
- Isoniazid
- Dopamine depleters
- Tricyclic antidepressants
- Reserpine
- Methyldopa
- Cimetidine
- Benzodiazepines
- Hypothalamic-pituitary disorders

[a]Reproduced, with permission from O'Grady LF. Nonmalignant breast disease. In: O'Grady LF, Lindfors KK, Howell LP, Rippon MB, eds. *A Practical Approach to Breast Disease.* Boston, MA: Little, Brown and Company; 1995:9–22.

Differential Diagnosis

The differential diagnosis of breast disorders in children and adolescents depends on gender and age at onset. In addition, the presence or absence of other secondary sexual characteristics is helpful to differentiate between a variation of normal pubertal development and a pathologic process.

Infants and Children Younger Than 9 Years

In prepubertal children, the differential diagnosis of isolated early breast development includes exposure to exogenous sources of estrogen such as skin creams, makeup, and medications (oral contraceptives). For patients with suspected precocious puberty, other etiologies must be considered in addition to exogenous hormones (Box 87-2). Central nervous system tumors, lesions, and insults are among the most common causes. Congenital tumors such as hypothalamic hamartomas are especially important to rule out because they often present before age 3 years. Other CNS tumors to consider are neurofibromas, optic gliomas, astrocytomas, and ependymomas. Specific CNS lesions include cysts in the area of the third ventricle and congenital brain defects. Hydrocephalus, postinfectious encephalitis or meningitis, head trauma, and static cerebral encephalopathy also can lead to sexual precocity. Endocrine disorders include

---

Box 87-2. Differential Diagnosis of Precocious Puberty[a]

- Central (true)—gonadotropin-releasing hormone (GnRH)–dependent
- Idiopathic
- Central nervous system
  - Tumor
    - Optic and hypothalamic gliomas (often associated with neurofibromatosis), hypothalamic hamartoma, astrocytoma, ependymoma, craniopharyngioma
    - Lesion
      - Congenital defects, hydrocephalus, cyst in the third ventricle
    - Insult
      - Postinfectious encephalitis or meningitis, static encephalopathy
    - Infection
      - Abscess, tuberculous granulomas of the hypothalamus
    - Head trauma
    - Sequela of cranial radiation
    - Sarcoid granuloma
- Endocrine
  - Hypothyroidism (mechanism unknown)
  - Secondary to GnRH-independent precocious puberty (21-hydroxylase deficiency, McCune-Albright syndrome)
  - Peripheral (pseudo-)—GnRH-independent
  - Adrenal
    - Tumor
    - 21- or 11-hydroxylase deficiency
- Gonadal
  - Tumor
    - McCune-Albright syndrome
    - Familial testotoxicosis
  - Ectopic human chorionic gonadotropin–secreting tumor
  - Exogenous steroids

[a]Modified and reproduced with permission from Kulin HE, Muller J. The biological aspects of puberty. *Pediatr Rev.* 1996;17:75–86.

hypothyroidism, estrogen-producing tumors of the ovary or adrenal gland, and ovarian cysts.

Adolescents

The differential diagnosis of breast masses in adolescent females is extensive (Box 87-3). Conditions can be distinguished from one another based on the location of the lesion; its texture, mobility, and size; and how rapidly it is enlarging.

Box 87-3. Most Common Causes of Breast Masses in the Adolescent Female

- Fibroadenoma
- Juvenile (giant) fibroadenoma
- Cystosarcoma phyllodes
- Breast abscess
- Breast cyst
- Breast carcinoma
- Fat necrosis (secondary to trauma)
- Lipoma
- Hematoma
- Papilloma

Gynecomastia is classified as type I or II. Type I is benign adolescent male hypertrophy. The differential diagnosis for type II includes physiological gynecomastia (no evidence of an underlying disease process), organic disorders, and side effects of medications (Box 87-4). Types I and II also can be differentiated by the size of the breast tissue: enlargement up to 3 cm is type I; enlargement beyond the areolar perimeter is type II.

Persistent galactorrhea can be caused by several conditions in addition to excessive stimulation from sexual activity or jogging without a support bra. Etiologies include neurologic, hypothalamic, pituitary, and endocrine disorders. Common causes in the adolescent female are prolactin-secreting tumors and hypothyroidism. Drugs that induce galactorrhea in females are the same ones that can cause gynecomastia in males (see Boxes 87-1 and 87-4).

Evaluation

History

In the infant or child, the history should focus on endogenous as well as exogenous sources of estrogen (Questions Box). With teenagers, it is important to rule out drug use and systemic illness. All adolescent patients should be interviewed alone, especially when being asked about illicit substance use (see Chapter 119). The adolescent male may feel particularly embarrassed given the nature of his visit; thus the clinician should be especially sympathetic during the interview.

Physical Examination

The physical examination includes an assessment of the patient's linear growth, especially in cases of suspected precocious puberty. The height and weight should be plotted on the growth curve and

---

Box 87-4. Causes of Type II Gynecomastia in the Adolescent Male[a]

- Idiopathic
- Tumors
  — Seminomas, Leydig cell tumor, teratoma, feminizing adrenal tumor, hepatoma, bronchogenic sarcoma (ectopic human chorionic gonadotropin production)
- Thyroid dysfunction (hyperthyroidism and hypothyroidism)
- Renal failure and dialysis
- Cirrhosis of the liver
- Klinefelter syndrome (XXY)
- Testicular feminization syndrome (partial androgen insensitivity syndrome)
- Drugs
  — Marijuana, amphetamines, heroin, methadone
  — Anabolic steroids
  — Birth control pills
  — Cimetidine
  — Digitalis
  — Spironolactone
  — Tricyclic antidepressants
  — Isoniazid
  — Ketoconazole
- Pseudogynecomastia (adipose tissue in obese male)

[a]Modified and reproduced with permission from Greydanus DE, Parks DS, Farrell EG. Breast disorders in children and adolescents. *Pediatr Clin North Am.* 1989;36:634.

---

compared with previous measurements. Accelerations in height occur in sexual precocity. Excessive weight gain should be noted because obesity can stimulate breast enlargement in young females and gynecomastia in males.

The extent of the breast examination depends on the age of the patient. In infants and young children, the breast tissue should be measured and the size recorded so that growth can be monitored over time. Consistency of the tissue and mobility also should be evaluated. Breast growth as a result of neonatal breast hypertrophy and premature thelarche is non-tender, firm, and freely mobile. The nipple should be examined for a clear or cloudy discharge by gently compressing each one separately.

In the adolescent female, the breast examination should include visual inspection of the breasts as well as palpation of any lesion and axillary nodes. Ideally this would be performed in the sitting and supine positions, as is done in adult women. Most adolescent females, however, would be uncomfortable with so extensive an examination. The physician must take the time to explain the reasons for the examination to help the patient feel less self-conscious.

Visual inspection should assess for SMR, appearance of the skin, breast asymmetry, and evidence of trauma. Shiny skin or superficial venous distention on one breast would indicate the presence of a large mass. A peau d'orange (orange peel) appearance of the skin or erythema and warmth should be noted as a sign of an infiltrative lesion or infection, respectively.

Breast Disorder

Prepubertal Children

- How old is the child?
- When was the breast mass first noted?
- Does it seem to be increasing in size?
- Is it tender or erythematous?
- Is there associated discharge from the nipple?
- Has the child been exposed to any estrogen-containing skin creams or medications?
- In the male patient, is he taking any medications known to cause gynecomastia, such as digoxin?
- Is the child experiencing any neurologic symptoms such a headaches, ataxia, or visual disturbances?
- Is there a history of head trauma, central nervous system infection, or insult?
- Has the parent noted any other signs of early pubertal development (eg, pubic hair, acne, sudden inappropriate increase in height)?

Adolescent

- When was the breast mass first noticed, and where is it located?
- Does it seem to be increasing in size?
- Is the lesion tender?
- Is there a history of trauma to the breast?
- Is there any discharge from either nipple?
- In the female, when was the last menstrual period?
- Is there a history of headache or visual disturbances?
- Are there any signs or symptoms of systemic illness, such as weight loss?
- Is there a family history of breast cancer in a close relative, particularly the mother?
- Is there a history of chest wall radiation or treatment with chemotherapeutic agents?
- In the male, is he taking any medications that can cause gynecomastia, such as cimetidine?
- Is the adolescent male using anabolic steroids?
- Is the adolescent using any other illicit substances such as marijuana or heroin?

Palpation of the breast mass can be accomplished with the patient in the supine position using 1 of 3 methods. Using the second, third, and fourth fingers of one hand, the examiner should gently palpate each breast in a pattern of concentric circles, spokes of a wheel, or vertical and horizontal lines. The location of the mass should be noted; a mass beneath the areola might indicate an intraductal lesion, whereas the upper outer quadrant is the classic location for a fibroadenoma. The consistency of the lesion is important. Is it firm, rubbery, and fluctuant, or irregular and lumpy? Is it freely movable or attached to the chest wall? Fibroadenomas tend to be firm, discrete, freely movable, and rubbery. A tender, poorly defined mass is consistent with a contusion; a hematoma is more sharply defined with associated skin ecchymoses. Fat necrosis can develop after trauma and is painless, firm, well circumscribed, and mobile. The size of the mass should be measured and recorded. One must keep in mind

that tumor size does not correlate with malignant potential. Finally, each nipple should be gently squeezed to check for a discharge. If present, note whether it is clear, milky, or bloody. A serosanguineous or sanguineous discharge would indicate the presence of an intraductal mass. In addition, a retracted nipple indicates involvement of the areolar area.

The examiner should also palpate for axillary lymphadenopathy. Although most clinicians think of its association with breast cancer, it also may be found with infection or necrosis of a benign tumor. In the adolescent male, in addition to palpation of the breast tissue, it is important to determine the SMR of the genitalia to determine whether pubertal development is consistent with the gynecomastia. The testicles should be palpated carefully for masses and evidence of atrophy (decrease in testicular size). In addition, findings suggestive of hypothyroidism or hyperthyroidism or liver disease must be noted.

A detailed neurologic examination should be performed, especially in children with sexual precocity to confirm or detect a CNS disorder.

Laboratory Tests

The laboratory workup for breast disorders is dictated by the findings on history and physical examination. Isolated neonatal breast hyperplasia and premature thelarche require no laboratory studies. Serum gonadotropin concentrations (luteinizing hormone [LH] and follicle-stimulating hormone) and estradiol level should be obtained in girls with precocious puberty. In addition, a morning testosterone level should be ordered in boys. Based on these results, further studies may be indicated such as a serum human chorionic gonadotropin (hCG) level.

For most breast lesions in adolescent females, no laboratory studies are needed. A fine-needle aspiration (FNA) of the lesion may be performed for those cases that seem to be cystic or if the diagnosis is uncertain. The aspirated fluid should be sent for cytologic analysis if the mass does not completely disappear with this procedure. Sometimes it is necessary to perform the procedure to relieve patient and parental anxiety. An excisional biopsy of the mass allows for more accurate histologic information but is rarely indicated for most lesions.

In the healthy adolescent male with no evidence of systemic illness, no history of drug use, and a normal physical examination, no further laboratory studies are necessary. If pubertal gynecomastia and other systemic illnesses are ruled out, an endocrine workup is appropriate to elucidate the cause of non-pubertal gynecomastia. This should begin with levels of hCG, LH, and serum testosterone and estradiol. If these laboratory studies are normal, the diagnosis is idiopathic gynecomastia. If they are abnormal, consultation with a pediatric endocrinologist or adolescent medicine specialist should occur.

A pregnancy test and serum prolactin level should be ordered in the adolescent female with galactorrhea, regardless of the menstrual history.

Imaging Studies

Hand and wrist radiographs to determine the child's bone age should be obtained in children with a diagnosis of precocious puberty. In addition, boys should have magnetic resonance imaging (MRI) of the head to evaluate for a CNS lesion or structural abnormality. Depending on the history, an MRI may be indicated in some girls. Pelvic ultrasound, although rarely necessary, can be performed to rule out the presence of an ovarian tumor in girls.

Mammograms are not helpful in the pediatric age group, especially in adolescents, and are never indicated in the evaluation of a breast mass. They can be very difficult to interpret because of the dense breast tissue of adolescents. In addition, the risk of breast malignancy is very low. An ultrasound may help distinguish between a cystic lesion and a solid tumor. It can also provide more accurate measurement of the size of the lesion and its location prior to the FNA or excisional/diagnostic biopsy.

A testicular ultrasound to search for a tumor is indicated in the adolescent male if the level of hCG or estradiol is elevated.

Management

In neonates, mastitis most often is caused by *Staphylococcus aureus* and group B streptococcus. Gram-negative bacilli also have been reported. Parenteral antibiotics should be initiated when the diagnosis is made. Incision and drainage of a breast abscess should only be undertaken by an experienced physician familiar with the anatomy of the breast to minimize the likelihood of injury to the affected breast bud.

Congenital anomalies such as polythelia and polymastia do not require any treatment. If, however, the patient or parent wants the tissue removed for aesthetic or psychological reasons, it is recommended to do so before puberty. Reconstructive surgery for amastia, as in Poland syndrome, is typically delayed until late adolescence to allow full development of the unaffected breast.

Although no treatment is required for premature thelarche, parents need to be reassured that the condition is self-limited. The patient should be reexamined periodically to check for any further progression of puberty, such as persistent breast growth or the appearance of pubic hair.

The treatment for central precocious puberty is directed at controlling the secondary sexual development with GnRH agonists. When GnRH is administered continuously, gonadotropin secretion decreases. Currently leuprolide acetate is the only GnRH agonist available for use in the United States. Children should be followed every 1 to 3 months in conjunction with a pediatric endocrinologist to monitor their progression and response to therapy.

Unless otherwise indicated by the type of tumor, children with a CNS lesion as a cause of precocious puberty usually do not require neurosurgical intervention. Therapy should focus on minimizing the degree of growth acceleration and the development of secondary sexual characteristics.

Most breast masses in adolescent females are small, well demarcated, firm or rubbery, and non-tender and can be managed with the "wait and watch" approach. The patient can be followed for 2 to 4 months, preferably allowing a few menstrual cycles to pass. If there is no change in the lesion or just a small increase in its size, no studies or procedures are indicated because it is most likely a fibroadenoma. As previously noted, a biopsy may be requested to relieve the anxiety that accompanies the presence of a breast lesion. Total excision of the tumor mass and a careful histologic evaluation may be warranted in some cases. Surgical removal of rapidly enlarging tumors such as a giant fibroadenoma is important. When the lesion becomes very large, an acceptable cosmetic result is more difficult. Accordingly, the lesion should be removed shortly after the time of diagnosis rather than "waiting and watching."

The primary treatment for transient pubertal gynecomastia, or type I, is reassurance for the adolescent male and his family that the condition is self-limited and should resolve in 1 to 2 years. The teenager should be told explicitly that he is not "becoming a girl." In most cases, he should be reexamined periodically until resolution occurs. Type II gynecomastia may need surgical reduction of the mammary gland. Plastic surgery intervention is warranted for cases of persistent breast growth or moderate to severe gynecomastia (SMR 3–4 breasts) with psychological difficulties. Surgical correction involves a combination of liposuction and direct excision of the breast tissue beneath the nipple and areola. The young man may benefit from concurrent psychological counseling as well.

Prognosis

The prognosis of a breast disorder in the child or adolescent depends on the particular lesion. In general, most lesions such as neonatal breast hyperplasia and premature thelarche are self-limited and resolve on their own. Breast development persists for 3 to 5 years in 50% of cases of premature thelarche, but in one retrospective study, most cases regressed within 6 months to 6 years after the diagnosis. Aside from the short stature that may accompany idiopathic central precocious puberty, these females also tend to have a good prognosis. Fibroadenomas in the adolescent female can recur but typically are benign and have no proven link to the development of breast cancer. Most cases of transient pubertal gynecomastia resolve within 1 to 2 years.

CASE RESOLUTION

The child in the case history has a diagnosis of premature thelarche. She has no known exposure to exogenous sources of estrogen and has isolated breast tissue development with no other signs of pubertal maturation. Her parents should be informed of this diagnosis and reassured that the condition is self-limited and does not indicate that the child is starting puberty. The child should be scheduled for a follow-up visit in 3 to 4 months to remeasure the breast buds and reexamine the genitalia for the appearance of pubic hair.

Selected References

Bock K, Duda VF, Hadji P, et al. Pathologic breast conditions in childhood and adolescence: evaluation by sonographic diagnosis. *J Ultrasound Med.* 2005;24:1347–1354

Braunstein GD. Gynecomastia. *N Engl J Med.* 1993;328:490–495

De Silva N, Brandt ML. Disorders of the breast in children and adolescents, Part 1: disorders of growth and infections of the breast. *J Pediatr Adolesc Gynecol.* 2006;19:345–349

De Silva N, Brandt ML. Disorders of the breast in children and adolescents, Part 2: breast masses. *J Pediatr Adolesc Gynecol.* 2006;19:415–418

Dehner LP, Hill DA, Deschryver K. Pathology of the breast in children, adolescents, and young adults. *Semin Diagn Pathol.* 1999;16:235–247

Denk MJ. Topics in plastic surgery. *Pediatr Clin North Am.* 1998;45:1479–1506

Hindle WH, Pan EY. Breast disorders in female adolescents. *Adolesc Med State Art Rev.* 1994;5:123–129

Elger BS, Harding TW. Testing adolescents for a hereditary breast cancer gene (BRCA1). *Arch Pediatr Adolesc Med.* 2000;154:113–119

Greydanus DE, Matytsina L, Gains M. Breast disorders in children and adolescents. *Prim Care.* 2006;33:455–502

Klein KO, Mericq V, Brown-Dawson JM, Larmore KA, Cabezas P, Cortinez A. Estrogen levels in girls with premature thelarche compared with normal pre-pubertal girls as determined by an ultrasensitive recombinant cell bioassay. *J Pediatr.* 1999;134:190–192

Kronemer KA, Rhee K, Siegel MJ, et al. Gray scale sonography of breast masses in adolescent girls. *J Ultrasound Med.* 2001;20:491–496

Neinstein LS. Breast disease in adolescents and young women. *Pediatr Clin North Am.* 1999;46:607–662

Neinstein LS, Joffe A. Gynecomastia. In: Neinstein LS, ed. *Adolescent Health Care: A Practical Guide.* Baltimore, MD: Lippincott Williams & Wilkins; 2002: 264–270

Pacinda SJ, Ramzy I. Fine-needle aspiration of breast masses. A review of its role in diagnosis and management in adolescent patients. *J Adolesc Health.* 1998;23:3–6

Root A. Precocious puberty. *Pediatr Rev.* 2000;21:10–19

Simmons PS. Breast disorders in adolescent females. *Curr Opin Obstet Gynecol.* 2001;13:459–461

Styne DM. New aspects in the diagnosis and treatment of pubertal disorders. *Pediatr Clin North Am.* 1997;44:505–529

Templeman C, Hertweck SP. Breast disorders in the pediatric and adolescent patient. *Obstet Gynecol Clin North Am.* 2000;27:19–34

Weinstein SP, Conant EF, Orel SG, et al. Spectrum of US findings in pediatric and adolescent patients with palpable breast masses. *Radiographics.* 2000;20:1613–1621

SECTION VIII

Orthopedic Disorders

88. Developmental Hip Dysplasia 531

89. Rotational Problems of the Lower Extremity:
    In-toeing and Out-toeing 537

90. Angular Deformities of the Lower Extremity:
    Bow Legs and Knock-Knees 543

91. Orthopedic Injuries and Growing Pains 547

92. Sports-Related Acute Injuries 555

93. Evaluation of Limp 561

94. Musculoskeletal Disorders of the Neck and Back 567

Developmental Hip Dysplasia

Hamid R. Redjal, MD, and David P. Zamorano, MD

CASE STUDY

A 4-month-old girl is seen for her routine health maintenance visit. She is doing well and has no complaints. The results of the entire examination are within normal limits except for limited abduction of the left hip, which is approximately 45 degrees, in comparison to that of the right hip, which is almost 90 degrees.

Questions

1. What factors are responsible for normal growth and development of the hip joint?
2. What specific physical maneuvers help in the evaluation of infants with decreased range of motion of the hip?
3. What are the clinical findings of hip dislocation during and after the neonatal period?
4. What are some of the conditions often seen in conjunction with hip dysplasia that may be noted on physical examination?
5. What is the appropriate diagnostic workup of infants with suspected hip dysplasia?

Developmental dysplasia of the hip (DDH) is a common pediatric orthopedic concern that requires a thorough understanding of normal development, pathoanatomy, natural history, and treatment. Developmental dysplasia of the hip defines a range of hip pathology from congenital dysplasia of the hip, partial dislocation of the femoral head, acetabular dysplasia, and complete dislocation of the femoral head from the true acetabulum. Developmental dysplasia of the hip may either exist at birth or develop during infancy. In a newborn with true congenital dislocation of the hip, the femoral head dislocates into and out of the acetabulum. In an older child, the femoral head remains dislocated, leading to secondary changes in the head and acetabulum. When DDH is recognized and treated appropriately, children potentially develop completely normally. If the diagnosis is missed or delayed, however, children may suffer significant morbidity, including severe degenerative hip disease.

Epidemiology

Historically, the incidence of DDH is 1 in 1,000 live births. The literature has observed that pediatricians diagnose DDH in 8.6 in 1,000 live births, orthopedic surgeons in 1.5 in 1,000 live births, while the use of ultrasound has resulted in 25 in 1,000 diagnoses. Neonatal hip instability is estimated to range from 11.5 to 17 in 1,000 live births. Approximately 50% of these cases resolve by 1 week of age,

and 90% resolve by 2 months of age. Approximately 60% of affected infants are firstborn.

Girls are affected 5 times more frequently than boys. The firstborn child has an increased risk of DDH. Ethnic variations are observed with increased incidence among the Native American Navajo, then whites, followed by African Americans. Approximately 20% of all dislocations occur in infants born in the breech position. A positive family history of DDH increases the risk by 10%. A female born in the breech position has a 1 in 35 chance of having DDH.

The left hip is involved in 60% of children with DDH, the right hip in 20% of cases, and 20% of the time DDH is bilateral. Developmental dysplasia of the hip has an increased association with lesions believed to be secondary to mechanical molding such as congenital torticollis (approximately 8% of affected children may have DDH), metatarsus adductus (approximately 2%–10% of these children may have DDH), and talipes calcaneovalgus.

Clinical Presentation

The clinical presentation and signs of DDH in children vary with age. Diagnosis is made primarily by the physical examination (eg, Ortolani and Barlow maneuvers) during the neonatal period. Asymmetrical skin folds, limitation of hip abduction, and a positive Galeazzi sign are the classic signs of DDH in older infants. Physical signs, which become more obvious once children are walking, include limping and toe-walking (Dx Box).

Dx Developmental Hip Dysplasia

- Breech presentation
- Oligohydramnios
- Female gender
- Positive family history or ethnic background
- Persistent hip asymmetry (asymmetrical skin folds, abduction of one hip and adduction of the other)
- Lower-limb deformity (limp, toe-walking)
- Torticollis

Pathophysiology

Developmental dysplasia of the hip encompasses a wide variety of conditions ranging from hip instability to dislocation. For normal growth and development of the hip joint to occur, there must be a genetically determined balance of growth of the acetabular and tri-radiate cartilages and a well-located and centered femoral head. In a normal hip at birth there is a tight fit between the femoral head and acetabulum; however, in DDH or dislocation this tight fit is lost. Dysplasia refers to a hip with a positive Ortolani sign, meaning that it can be provoked to dislocate or one that is dislocated and can be relocated into the acetabulum. The term *dislocation* refers to any hip with a negative Ortolani sign, meaning that the hip is not reducible and is associated with secondary adaptive changes such as shortening, decreased abduction, and asymmetrical skin folds.

Dysplasia of the acetabulum is also associated with hip instability. The dysplastic acetabular cavity is shallower with a more vertical inclination than normal. An understanding of the pathophysiology that relates primarily to ligamentous laxity and bony abnormalities of the acetabular cavity enables one to see that although most dislocations occur at or near the time of delivery, they can occur later in infancy as well. Late hip dislocations are reported in 3% to 8% of affected infants.

The etiology of DDH is multifactorial, involving genetic and intrauterine environmental factors. The primary **intrauterine environmental factors** are tight maternal abdominal and uterine musculature, breech presentation (causes abnormal hip flexion leading to dislocation of the femoral head), and positioning of the fetal hip against the mother's sacrum. In utero mechanical factors relate to molding and restriction of fetal movement. It is believed that the tight, unstretched maternal abdomen and uterine musculature of primigravidas may prevent fetal movement, thus predisposing firstborn infants to DDH. The increased occurrence of other conditions thought to be secondary to molding (eg, congenital muscular torticollis) with DDH supports this theory of space restriction. **Physiological factors** relate to ligamentous laxity. Female infants may be more sensitive to maternal hormones such as estrogen and

relaxin, which are present around the time of delivery, resulting in generalized ligamentous laxity, including laxity of the hip capsule. **Environmental factors** that may predispose infants to DDH include swaddling with the legs in extension and adduction, which is still practiced in some societies (eg, those who use cradle boards, such as Navajos in North America), and muscle contractures secondary to neuromuscular disease such as cerebral palsy.

Differential Diagnosis

The differential diagnosis of hip dysplasia depends on the age of the child and the presenting complaint. Infants may have a "click" on abduction of the hip that represents the snapping of a ligament rather than the reduction of the dislocated hip into the joint. Infants who have limited abduction may have a neuromuscular disorder such as spastic diplegia. Older children who present with gait disturbances such as limp, waddling gait, or toe-walking may have neuromuscular conditions, fractures, or infection (eg, osteomyelitis, septic arthritis).

Evaluation

History

Family history of DDH should be reviewed. A careful neonatal history detailing the type of presentation (eg, breech versus vertex), type of delivery, history of prenatal problems such as oligohydramnios, and presence of congenital torticollis or metatarsus adductus should also be taken (Questions Box).

Questions

Developmental Hip Dysplasia

- Was the infant a breech presentation?
- Does the child have any muscular problems, such as torticollis?
- When did the gait disturbance begin?
- Does anything make the child's gait better or worse?
- Is the child in any pain?
- Did any member of the family have hip dysplasia?

Physical Examination

It is important to evaluate the hip joint for instability or dislocation throughout the first year of life or until the child begins to walk. The **Ortolani and Barlow maneuvers** may be used in the neonatal period to evaluate for DDH (Figure 88-1). Both tests are performed with infants in a supine position and the hips and knees flexed to 90 degrees. Infants should be quiet and relaxed because both tests require a cooperative child. Adequate results are difficult to obtain with crying or fussy infants.

In the Ortolani sign or click of entry, a palpable "clunk" is caused as the examiner relocates a dislocated hip by gentle abduction and lifting of the femoral head anteriorly. By gently abducting and adducting the flexed hip the examiner may detect reduction or dislocation of the femoral head from the acetabulum. This "clunk" differs from the audible hip click, which is secondary to non-pathologic processes such as ligamentous snapping. Each leg should be examined separately, not simultaneously.

The Barlow maneuver, also referred to as the *click of exit,* is another diagnostic test. It detects any potential subluxation or posterior dislocation of the femoral head by direct pressure on the longitudinal axis of the femur while the hip is in adduction. It is a provocative maneuver that attempts to dislocate the hip by adduction and posterior axial pressure on the thigh. These tests are not useful after approximately 6 to 8 weeks of age because the surrounding soft tissues and muscles adapt to the dislocated hip, making it more difficult to reduce.

If the diagnosis of DDH or dislocation is not made shortly after birth, there is a different set of physical findings. There is asymmetry of hip abduction that is secondary to adductor muscle shortening and contracture on the affected side. Limited hip abduction is the most reliable late diagnostic sign.

As the femoral head dislocates posteriorly, the thigh is shortened on the affected side, producing an asymmetry of the gluteal, thigh, and labial folds and limb shortening. Asymmetrical gluteal folds result from bunching of skin and subcutaneous tissue on the affected side, thus producing extra skin folds. Asymmetrical skin folds have been shown to not be reliable indicators for further evaluation. **Galeazzi sign** is noted when the femoral head displaces laterally and proximally, causing apparent shortening of the femur on the affected side. On examination a positive Galeazzi sign may be observed with discrepancy in knee heights noted when infants are supine with the sacrum flat on the examination table and hips and knees bent.

In children of walking age, the physician may notice a limp secondary to shortening of the leg on the affected side, leading to a leg length discrepancy (Figure 88-2). (Children may try to disguise the limp by toe-walking.) A Trendelenburg test may be positive. Normally, when a child stands on one leg, the hip abductors straighten the pelvis and keep the center of gravity over the femoral head. If the abductors are weak, the weight shifts to the opposite side, causing it to droop. A child with bilateral involvement may display hyperlordosis and a waddling gait.

Figure 88-1.   Ortolani and Barlow tests. A. Ortolani (reduction) test. B. Barlow (dislocation) test.

Figure 88-2.   Late signs in the diagnosis of developmental dysplasia of the hip. A. Asymmetry of thigh folds. B. Asymmetry of hip abduction. C. Discrepancy of knee heights.

Imaging Studies

Radiologic and ultrasound evaluations may aid in the diagnosis. Hip sonography helps to confirm the diagnosis and to identify more subtle forms of the disorder. Ultrasonography is the only diagnostic test that allows real-time evaluation and a 3-dimensional view of the neonate's hip. Reliable x-ray changes begin to become evident at about 4 to 6 months of age, when the ossific nucleus of the femoral head appears in most infants (Figure 88-3). A flat, shallow acetabulum and delayed ossification of the femoral head are the simplest, most easily recognized findings.

Management

The need for repeat examinations of the hips during the first year of life cannot be overemphasized. Children suspected of any hip instability or any children with less than 60 degrees of hip abduction should be evaluated with appropriate imaging studies and referred

Figure 88-3. Radiographic findings associated with developmental dysplasia of the hip. The left hip is dislocated. The femur is lateral and proximal, the acetabulum is shallow and flat, and there is delayed ossification of the femoral head, as evidenced by the absence of the ossific nucleus on the left.

to an orthopedic surgeon for further evaluation and management. An orthopedic surgeon can aid the primary care physician in the management of DDH.

The goal of treatment is to return the femoral head to its normal position within the acetabulum and restore normal hip functioning. The common practice of triple diapering should be discouraged because it is unreliable, often delays definitive therapy, and may produce complications (eg, avascular necrosis of the femoral head).

There are 5 different treatment groups in the management of DDH

1. Newborn to 6 months
2. Infant (6–18 months)
3. Toddler (18–36 months)
4. Child and juvenile (3–8 years)
5. Adolescent to young adult (beyond 8 years)

The **Pavlik harness** is the primary method of treating DDH during infancy. This device has evolved as the clear method of choice for treatment of infants with DDH and has become accepted as the standard of treatment worldwide. The Pavlik harness consists of a chest strap, shoulder straps, and anterior and posterior stirrup straps that maintain the hips in flexion and abduction while restricting extension and adduction. When properly used, the harness holds the hips in a flexed and abducted position while allowing infants to move their legs within safe limits of abduction and adduction until

stability is achieved. In the newborn with DDH the harness should be worn for 23 hours daily until findings of clinical and radiographic examination are normal. The harness must be worn for a minimum of 3 months by children 3 months and younger, whereas children 4 months or older usually must wear the harness for approximately double their age. A newborn with a diagnosis of true dislocation must wear the harness full time until the dislocatable hip has stabilized in the acetabulum.

The harness should be applied and monitored by an orthopedic surgeon because inappropriate application also may produce adverse outcomes such as inferior dislocation and, the most serious, avascular necrosis of the femoral head. Parents play a key role in the successful use of the harness and must be educated on the disease process and the proper use of the harness. Overall, the Pavlik harness has an 85% to 95% success rate, it is a dynamic flexion abduction orthosis that loses efficacy as the child ages due to the soft tissue contractures that develop.

If this treatment method is ineffective or the diagnosis is not made until after 6 months of age, **traction** followed by either open or closed **reduction and spica cast immobilization** may be used. Good results are more difficult to obtain with increasing age, especially after children are walking. Operative treatment is required in children older than 18 months to safely reduce the dislocated hip and to surgically recreate normal anatomy. These procedures include (1) **femoral shortening,** (2) **acetabuloplasty** to correct acetabular dysplasia, and (3) **capsulorrhaphy** (suturing the joint capsule).

Prognosis

The prognosis of DDH depends on age at the time of diagnosis and severity of the deformity. The long-term prognosis for satisfactory hip function is good for children when DDH is recognized early and treated appropriately. Generally children with DDH that is diagnosed after the first year of life have a poorer prognosis for satisfactory hip function than those with DDH that is diagnosed during infancy. Left untreated, DDH may result in significant disability, ranging from limp to pain and stiffness in the hip to degenerative joint disease in adult life.

CASE RESOLUTION

The infant presented in the case history has less than 60 degrees of abduction of the left hip, a sign of developmental dysplasia of the hip. An anteroposterior view of the pelvis may be ordered to confirm the diagnosis. Regardless of the radiographic findings, the infant should be referred to an orthopedic surgeon for further evaluation and management. If hip dislocation is confirmed, the initial treatment will involve bracing with the Pavlik harness.

Selected References

Aronsson DD, Goldberg MJ, Kling TF Jr, Roy DR. Developmental dysplasia of the hip. *Pediatrics.* 1994;94:201–208

Ballock RT, Richards BS. Hip dysplasia: early diagnosis makes a difference. *Contemp Pediatr.* 1997;14:108–117

Bialik V, Bialik GM, Blazer S, Sujov P, Wiener F, Berant M. Developmental dysplasia of the hip: a new approach to incidence. *Pediatrics.* 1999;103:93–99

Bond CD, Hennrikus WL, DellaMaggiore ED. Prospective evaluation of newborn soft-tissue hip "clicks" with ultrasound. *J Pediatr Orthop.* 1997;17:199–201

Hensinger RN. Congenital dislocation of the hip: treatment in infancy to walking age. *Orthop Clin North Am.* 1987;18:597–615

Mooney JF, Emans JB. Developmental dislocation of the hip: a clinical overview. *Pediatr Rev.* 1995;16:299–303

Novacheck TF. Developmental dysplasia of the hip. *Pediatr Clin North Am.* 1996;43:829–848

Theophilopoulos EP, Barrett DJ. Get a grip on the pediatric hip. *Contemp Pediatr.* 1998;15:43–65

Wientroub S, Grill F. Ultrasonography in developmental dysplasia of the hip. *J Bone Joint Surg.* 2000;82:1004–1018

Rotational Problems of the Lower Extremity: In-toeing and Out-toeing

Hamid R. Redjal, MD, and David P. Zamorano, MD

CASE STUDY

A 3-year-old girl is brought to the office. Her mother is concerned because beginning a few months ago her daughter's feet appeared to "turn in" when she walked. The girl has never walked like this before, and she has no history of trauma, fever, pain, or swelling in the joints. The physical examination is within normal limits except for the in-toeing gait.

Questions

1. How can observation of children's gaits help determine the etiology of their in-toeing and out-toeing (rotational problems)?
2. What are the common causes of in-toeing and out-toeing?
3. Does evaluation of in-toeing and out-toeing require any laboratory or radiologic studies?
4. What is the natural history of most rotational problems?

Benign rotational variations of the lower extremities such as in-toeing and out-toeing are seen in many healthy children. Although rotational problems that produce in-toeing and out-toeing may initially be physically alarming, spontaneous resolution occurs in most cases. They are a common cause of parental concern during infancy and childhood; however, they rarely lead to physical limitation. Most of these problems can be managed adequately by primary care physicians and do not necessitate orthopedic referral. A thorough understanding of the normal rotational variations that occur in children younger than 10 years is essential to properly treat and educate and, more importantly, identify more serious underlying structural problems.

Epidemiology

In neonates or young infants, in-toeing is most likely the result of clubfoot (talipes equinovarus), isolated metatarsus adductus, or metatarsus varus. The incidence of clubfoot is 1 in 1,000 live births, with a male-female ratio of 2:1. The condition is bilateral in approximately 50% of cases. The incidence of metatarsus adductus, a much more common problem, is about 1 in 500 live births. It is often bilateral. Internal tibial torsion is the primary cause of in-toeing in the second year of life, and femoral torsion (femoral anteversion) accounts for most cases of this condition during early childhood.

Physiological out-toeing is classically evident in infants who have not yet begun to walk. This condition, which is believed to be secondary to an external rotatory contracture about the hip due to intrauterine positioning, is the most common cause of out-turning in both feet. Lateral tibial torsion may result in out-toeing in older infants and children.

Physical Examination

Normal variability in young children must be differentiated from more serious structural problems. A careful, detailed physical examination, including assessment of gait and neurologic and musculoskeletal function, is essential for making the correct diagnosis. The evaluation should determine whether the rotational problem has caused a functional impairment such as tripping, pain, or shoe wear difficulties. This evaluation should include examination of the hips for signs of hip dysplasia, which may be associated with metatarsus adductus (see Chapter 88).

Evaluation of postural conditions requires both static and dynamic physical examination. Static examination includes an overall evaluation of the patient and a rotational profile. The child's rotational profile as described by Staheli consists of 5 components (Figure 89-1). The 5 components of this profile are internal and external hip rotation, thigh-foot axis, transmalleolar

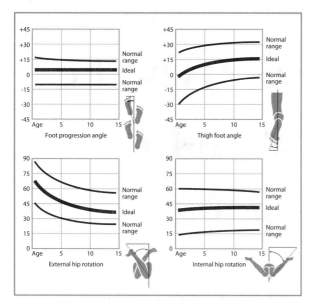

Figure 89-1. Rotational profile. (Reproduced with permission from Wenger DR, Rang M. *The Art and Practice of Children's Orthopedics.* **New York, NY: Raven Press; 1993.)**

Figure 89-2. Evaluation of foot progression angle. (Reproduced with permission from Staheli LT. *Fundamentals of Pediatric Orthopedics.* **New York, NY: Raven Press; 1992.)**

axis, heel-bisector angle, and foot progression angle during gait (Figure 89-2).

Hip rotation in infants averages 40 degrees of internal rotation and 70 degrees of external rotation, and by 10 years of age internal hip rotation averages 50 degrees and external rotation 45 degrees. Internal rotation measuring between 70 and 90 degrees is evidence of femoral torsion.

The **thigh-foot axis** consists of the rotation of the tibia and hindfoot in relation to the longitudinal axis of the thigh and indicates the amount of tibial torsion. In infants the thigh-foot angle averages 5 degrees internal (range: -30 to +20 degrees). Excessive internal tibial torsion spontaneously resolves by 3 to 4 years of age and by 8 years of age averages 10 degrees external.

The **transmalleolar axis** also aids in determining the amount of tibial torsion. It is formed by the angle at the intersection of an imaginary line from the lateral to medial malleolus and a second line from the lateral to medial femoral condyles. At gestational age 5 months, the fetus has 20 degrees of internal tibial torsion and the tibia externally rotates until at adulthood there is an average of 23 degrees of external rotation.

The **heel-bisector** line examines the foot, and is a line drawn through the midline axis of the hindfoot and forefoot. In a neutral foot the heel-bisector line passes through the second web space.

And finally, the **foot progression angle during gait** is the angle of the foot relative to an imaginary straight line in the patient's path (see Figure 89-2). Patients who in-toe are assigned a negative value and patient's who out-toe are assigned a positive value. This value represents the sum total effect of the child's structural alignment and dynamic torsion forces resulting from muscle forces.

The examination of infants with clubfoot should include a careful examination of the back for signs of possible spinal dysraphism (eg, skin dimples and hairy patches) and a thorough neurologic examination.

Internal tibial torsion may be diagnosed by having children sit at the end of the examination table with both knees flexed to 90 degrees and palpating the medial and lateral malleoli with the thumb and index finger. Normally, the medial malleolus lies anterior to the lateral malleolus (approximately one fingerbreadth). If the lateral malleolus is on the same plane or anterior to the medial malleolus, internal tibial torsion is indicated.

The diagnosis of tibial torsion can also be made by measuring the thigh-foot angle (Figure 89-3). Measurement of the thigh-foot angle involves having children lie prone on the examination table and observing the relationship of the long axis of the foot compared with the axis of the thigh as viewed from above. The shape of the foot itself can also be assessed with children in this position. Slight internal rotation is normal as children first learn to walk.

Figure 89-3. Evaluation of the thigh-foot axis. A. Observation with the child in the prone position is best. B. Determination of the thigh-foot axis. C. Assessment of the shape of the foot. (Reproduced with permission from Staheli LT. *Fundamentals of Pediatric Orthopedics.* **New York, NY: Raven Press; 1992.)**

Diagnosis of medial femoral torsion can be made by observing children's gaits and measuring hip rotation. The knees and the feet appear to turn inward when children with medial femoral torsion walk. Internal and external hip rotation are evaluated with the children in a prone position, the pelvis flat, and the knees flexed 90 degrees (Figure 89-4). The degrees of normal rotation vary with age (see Figure 89-1). During childhood, internal hip rotation greater than 70 degrees implies medial femoral torsion.

Figure 89-4.   **Evaluation of hip rotation. A. The child is prone and knees are flexed to 90 degrees. B. Medial rotation is measured. C. Lateral rotation is measured. (Reproduced with permission from Staheli LT. *Fundamentals of Pediatric Orthopedics.* New York, NY: Raven Press; 1992.)**

Imaging Studies

Routine imaging studies are not necessary for rotational deformities. Imaging studies may be considered by the orthopedic surgeon in severe deformities if operative correction is being considered. X-rays are used in clubfoot to assess the relationship and development of the bones of the foot and for monitoring cast correction.

Clinical Presentation

Children with congenital clubfoot, metatarsus adductus, and metatarsus varus present with in-toeing during infancy. Congenital clubfoot is usually readily evident at birth. A severe medial, midline, plantar crease is present, and the foot appears C-shaped, with both the heel and forefront turned inward. The affected foot is small, wide, and stiff, and the lower leg appears small due to hypoplasia of the calf muscles. In contrast to clubfoot, only the forefoot turns inward in metatarsus adductus and varus.

Tibial torsion is apparent during the second year of life. Children's feet turn inward as they walk, but their knees point straight. Medial femoral torsion is evident at 3 to 4 years of age. Affected children are usually girls; they can sit in the "W" position with both legs behind them. As children walk, both the knees and the feet appear to turn inward.

Physiological out-toeing is seen in infancy. Classically, parents note that when they hold their children in a standing position, both feet turn outward. Approximately 5 degrees of out-toeing is normal after age 3. Further degrees of out-toeing may be due to lateral tibial torsion.

Pathophysiology

Several factors are involved in the etiology of rotational conditions. Most of these problems are deformations secondary to intrauterine positioning. Metatarsus adductus and medial tibial torsion result from intrauterine positioning, and certain sleeping and sitting positions may perpetuate these problems in infants and children. For example, sleeping in the prone position with the legs internally rotated may lead to continued internal tibial torsion or metatarsus adductus. Heredity is also believed to play a role in the development of rotational problems. Sometimes parents have the same rotational deformity as their children. In addition, **bony and neuromuscular abnormalities** are part of the etiology of clubfoot.

Specific terminology is used to describe the position of the limb. **Version** is normal variation in limb rotation, whereas **torsion** refers to abnormal conditions (ie, >2 SDs above or below the mean). **Adduction** is movement toward the midline, in contrast to **abduction,** which is movement away from the midline. **Varus angulation** is deviation toward the midline, whereas **valgus angulation** is deviation away from the midline. An **inverted** foot is one turned toward the midline on its long axis. An **everted** foot is one turned away from the midline on its long axis.

Internal rotation of the lower extremity brings the big toe to the midline during the early intrauterine period, whereas external rotation occurs during the later intrauterine period, infancy, and childhood. Alterations in this normal lateral process caused by either genetic or environmental factors such as intrauterine molding and sleep positions may lead to rotational problems. Conditions influenced by intrauterine position, such as metatarsus adductus and developmental hip dysplasia, are sometimes found in the same children.

The primary pathology of congenital clubfoot is related to deformity and hypoplasia of the bones of the foot, especially the talus and tarsal bones, and environmental factors such as intrauterine position and molding. In addition, hypoplasia of the calf muscles and thickening of the ligaments contribute to the deformity.

In-toeing usually is caused by benign conditions such as metatarsus adductus, excessive internal tibial torsion, and excessive femoral torsion. Less frequently, patients have pathologic conditions such as clubfoot, skewfoot, hip disorders, and neuromuscular diseases. Out-toeing typically is caused by external rotation contracture of the hip, external tibial torsion, or external femoral torsion. We will now review the conditions associated with rotational variations in children.

In-toeing

Metatarsus Adductus and Metatarsus Primus Varus

Metatarsus adductus, with or without internal tibial torsion, is the most common cause of in-toeing from birth to 1 year of age. It is a functional deformity in which the forefoot is adducted with respect to the hindfoot with a neutral or slightly valgus heel. It is the most common pediatric foot problem referred to orthopedic surgeons and occurs in 1 in 5,000 live births and in 1 in 20 siblings of patients with metatarsus adductus. The rate is higher in males, twin births, and preterm babies. Numerous theories exist on the cause of metatarsus adductus including in utero positioning, sleeping position of the baby, muscle imbalance, and medial cuneiform abnormality.

Presenting complaints include cosmesis, in-toeing gait, or excessive shoe wear. On physical examination the foot appears C-shaped with a concave medial border and convex lateral border. The forefoot can be brought into the neutral position either by stroking the lateral border of the foot or by gently straightening it. Metatarsus adductus can be classified into flexible or inflexible based on physical examination. Most cases of flexible metatarsus adductus resolve spontaneously and do not require splinting, bracing, or special shoes. However, patients with rigid metatarsus adductus should undergo early casting; uncommonly resistant cases may require surgery.

Congenital **metatarsus primus varus** is a bony abnormality characterized by an isolated adducted first metatarsal. Unlike flexible metatarsus adductus, metatarsus varus is a fixed deformity. The foot cannot be brought into the neutral position. There is a deep vertical skin crease along the medial border of the foot tarsometatarsal joints and a normal lateral border. Because it is a more rigid deformity, early casting is recommended and persistent deformity requires surgery.

Skewfoot or Congenital Metatarsus Varus

Also known as *serpentine metatarsus adductus,* it is characterized by adducted metatarsals combined with a valgus deformity of the heel and plantar flexion of the talus. It is theorized that improper casting of metatarsus adductus or clubfoot may result in a skewfoot; however, most cases are idiopathic. Patients present with pain or callus formation under the head of the talus and base of the fifth metatarsal. Some feet undergo spontaneous correction, while surgery is indicated for a persistently symptomatic foot.

Dynamic Hallucis Abductus/Searching Toe

Dynamic hallucis abductus/searching toe, also known as *wandering* or *atavistic,* can cause in-toeing. Children with a so-called searching toe have a big toe that points medially when they walk. Unlike the other causes of in-toeing, which are structural and present at rest, this condition is a dynamic deformity. Searching toe results from the contraction of the abductors of the big toe during the stance phase of gait, which pulls the toe toward the midline. It usually resolves with age and subsequent development of fine motor coordination.

Clubfoot

Congenital **clubfoot,** a pathologic deformity of the foot, may be identified at birth (Figure 89-5). Clubfoot may be either an isolated deformity or seen in association with other neuromuscular anomalies such as arthrogryposis, myelomeningocele, amniotic band syndrome, cerebral palsy, or poliomyelitis.

Figure 89-5. **Congenital clubfoot.**

The diagnosis of congenital clubfoot is made at birth on the basis of 3 conditions: forefoot varus, heel varus, and ankle equinus. Clubfoot can range in severity from a rigid deformity, in which the forefoot cannot be brought into a neutral position by passive abduction, to nonrigid deformities, in which the forefoot can be gently brought toward the midline. Normal dorsiflexion of the ankle helps distinguish severe forms of metatarsus varus from clubfoot.

Internal Tibial Torsion

This condition is the most common cause of in-toeing from ages 1 to 3 years and is usually first noticed by parents when children begin to walk. Parents often complain that the child is clumsy and trips frequently. In two-thirds of affected children internal tibial torsion is bilateral; when it is unilateral, it more commonly affects the left leg. Most cases are thought to be caused by intrauterine positioning. Observation of children's gaits reveals that the knees point forward but the feet turn inward. Because the knees are straight, the site of the rotational deformity is below this joint. If the feet are normal and no metatarsus adductus or varus is present, the rotational deformity can be isolated to the lower leg. It is important to measure the thigh-foot and transmalleolar axes in the physical examination. Expectant observation is recommended because the natural history of internal tibial torsion strongly favors spontaneous resolution by 4 years of age.

Internal Femoral Torsion

Femoral torsion is the angular difference between the femoral neck axis and the transcondylar axis of the knee. This condition can be conceptualized in the following way: When children lie on their backs, the torsion causes the femoral head to protrude instead of lie flat within the acetabulum. The presence of medial femoral torsion causes the entire distal limb to turn inward when the femoral head articulates normally with the acetabulum. The condition is usually bilateral. Increased femoral anteversion is the most common cause of in-toeing in early childhood.

Children who are 3 to 4 years of age present with this classic story: Their parents report that children, who showed no previous in-toeing have a problem that is becoming severe. Excessive medial femoral torsion, which may have been present at birth, has been masked by the external rotatory forces present during infancy. Children with excessive femoral anteversion characteristically sit with their legs in the "W" position and run with an eggbeater-type motion. No treatment is necessary for most cases of femoral torsion, which usually resolves by 8 years of age.

Out-toeing

Physiological Out-toeing

Out-toeing of infancy, which is most commonly seen in children who are just learning to walk, is caused by an external rotatory contracture of the soft tissues surrounding the hip secondary to intrauterine position. This condition may be perpetuated in children who sleep in the prone, frog-leg position, which does not allow for stretching of the external rotators of the hips. Although both feet turn outward when infants stand, the lateral rotation of both hips is normal on examination (Figure 89-6). More serious conditions, such as slipped capital femoral epiphysis, hip dysplasia, or coxa vara, are less common but should be considered.

External Tibial Torsion

This condition may be suspected in children who are 3 to 5 years of age and present with out-toeing that worsens with time. Increased external tibial torsion is often associated with neuromuscular conditions such as myelodysplasia and polio. Because the tibia normally rotates laterally with development, the condition may become more severe with age. Malalignment between the knee and the direction of gait may produce knee pain.

In-toeing and out-toeing comprise a long list of differential diagnoses and a methodical and meticulous history and physical examination are necessary.

Differential Diagnosis

In-toeing and out-toeing may be classified according to anatomical level and usual age at presentation (Table 89-1). These conditions may be localized to one of 4 areas: toe, foot, tibia, and femur. If in-toeing problems are placed in chronological order by age of presentation, the affected area follows a toe-to-femur sequence.

Figure 89-6. Physiological out-toeing of infancy. (Reproduced with permission from Staheli LT. Torsional deformity. *Pediatr Clin North Am.* 1977;24:799–811.)

Table 89-1. Site and Age of Onset of Rotational Problems of the Lower Extremity in Children		
Problem	**Site of Problem**	**Age of Onset**
In-toeing		
Searching toe	Toe	Infancy
Clubfoot	Foot	Birth
Metatarsus adductus/varus	Foot	Birth/infancy
Medial tibial torsion	Tibia	Toddler stage (12–24 mo)
Medial femoral torsion	Femur	Early childhood (3–5 y)
Out-toeing		
Physiological out-toeing	Hips	Infancy
Lateral tibial torsion	Tibia	Childhood

Evaluation

History

The clinical history must delineate the onset, duration, and progression of any structural problems. The typical natural history of benign rotational conditions shows improvement over time, whereas a more serious condition would have a more progressive deformity. Relevant family and birth history, including gestational age, length of labor, complications, Apgar scores, birth weight, and length of hospital stay, should be noted. These details may heighten suspicion for cerebral palsy or the presence of hereditary disorders such as vitamin D–resistant rickets, mucopolysaccharidoses, achondroplasia, epiphyseal dysplasia, or metaphyseal dysplasia that may affect rotational profiles. A thorough developmental history is important because developmental delays may be a sign of underlying neuromuscular or neurologic disorders (Questions Box).

Questions

In-toeing and Out-toeing

- Is there any family history of in-toeing or out-toeing?
- What is the birth history? Was the child a breech presentation?
- At what age did the child begin walking?
- When did the rotational deformity appear? Is it getting better or worse?
- Does the rotational problem produce any disability (eg, tripping or falling a great deal when walking or running)?
- Has any previous treatment been tried?
- In what position does the child sleep? In what position does the child sit?

Management

In-toeing

Metatarsus adductus generally resolves spontaneously, but stretching exercises for the foot can be advised, particularly if parents are anxious to "do something." Parents are instructed to manipulate the foot with each diaper change. Referral to an orthopedic surgeon for evaluation should be made if the deformity is still present at 3 to 4 months of age (most cases resolve within the first 3 months of life). Cast correction may be required for rigid deformities or those that persist beyond 3 to 4 months. Shoe modifications (eg, putting shoes on the wrong foot) should be avoided because they have not been shown to have any long-term benefits.

Because metatarsus varus may progress when children begin walking, referral to an orthopedic surgeon should be made as soon as the condition is detected. Serial casting followed by corrective shoes or inserts is the first line of treatment. Surgery is only rarely required. Treatment for medial tibial torsion is rarely required because this problem generally corrects with time when children learn to walk. Night splinting, although still occasionally instituted, has not been shown to affect the natural history of this condition. If the deformity is severe or persists without improvement beyond the age of 18 months or after children have been walking for 1 year, referral to an orthopedic surgeon for evaluation should be made. Surgical correction (eg, tibial rotational osteotomy) may be required if the deformity is severe or persists beyond 8 to 10 years of age.

Like the other conditions that produce in-toeing, medial femoral torsion generally does not require treatment. Even if it persists into adulthood, it usually produces no disability nor does it increase the risk for degenerative arthritis in the involved joint. Nonoperative treatment is ineffective. Surgical correction may be required if there is a history of repeated falls or severe gait problems. A derotational femoral osteotomy is the only effective method of treatment. It should not be performed until children are at least 8 to 10 years of age.

Clubfoot, unlike other problems, is a pathologic lesion that requires treatment. Treatment, which should begin during the first week of life, consists of serial manipulations of the foot and casting. Several months of casting may be required to attain full correction. Surgery is often required for resistant or recurrent cases. As many as 50% to 75% of patients with clubfoot may eventually require surgery. Surgery is usually delayed until infants are 6 to 12 months of age.

Out-toeing

Physiological out-toeing of infancy is a rotational problem that spontaneously resolves when children learn to walk. Most cases resolve by about 18 months of age. Severe lateral tibial torsion may require surgical correction with a tibial rotational osteotomy.

Prognosis

Because the lower extremity rotates laterally with growth, the natural history of internal rotational problems, such as internal tibial torsion and medial femoral torsion, is resolution over time. In contrast, lateral tibial torsion may become worse with time.

The prognosis for most rotational problems is excellent. Parental reassurance and education regarding the natural history of these deformities may decrease anxiety and prevent needless visits to specialists in search of treatments that may not be necessary. Functional disability or degenerative arthritis is not associated with these conditions.

Left untreated, clubfoot often leads to considerable pain and disability. The affected foot can be difficult to fit with shoes. And finally, clubfoot can be unsightly and cause children significant emotional distress.

> ### CASE RESOLUTION
>
> The girl described in the case history seems to have medial femoral torsion because she has no history of rotational problems. Her entire leg turns in when she walks. Internal hip rotation greater than 70 degrees confirms the diagnosis. The mother can be reassured that this is a normal, age-related phenomenon that will most likely resolve over time. The child can be reevaluated in 4 to 6 months. Orthopedic referral is not required at this time.

Selected References

Craig CL, Goldberg MJ. Foot and leg problems. *Pediatr Rev*. 1993;14:395–400

Fuchs R, Staheli LT. Splinting and intoeing. *J Pediatr Orthop*. 1996;16:489–491

Hoekelman RA. Foot and leg problems. In: Hoekelman RA, ed. *Primary Pediatric Care*. 3rd ed. St Louis, MO: Mosby-Year Book; 1997:971–979

Hoffinger SA. Evaluation and management of pediatric foot deformities. *Pediatr Clin North Am*. 1996;43:1091–1111

Staheli LT. Lower positional deformity in infants and children: a review. *J Pediatr Orthop*. 1990;10:559–563

Wenger DR, Rang M. *The Art and Practice of Children's Orthopedics*. New York, NY: Raven Press; 1993

Angular Deformities of the Lower Extremity: Bowlegs and Knock-Knees

Carol D. Berkowitz, MD

CASE STUDY

During the routine health maintenance examination of a 2-year-old child, you observe moderate to severe bilateral bowing of both legs. The child's mother reports that her son began walking at 10 months. She has noticed no problems with his gait and says he does not trip or fall excessively. On examination, the boy's weight is greater than the 95th percentile for age, but otherwise he appears to be a healthy African American child.

Questions

1. What types of angular deformities affect children's lower extremities?
2. How does children's age help determine whether they have physiological or pathologic angular deformities?
3. What clinical measurements can help distinguish physiological from pathologic angular deformities?
4. To what extent are x-rays used in the routine assessment of angular deformities?

With normal growth and development, the angular alignment of children's legs progresses through a series of developmental stages—from relative bowlegs to knock-knees and eventually straight legs. Rotational problems such as in-toeing and out-toeing are deformities in the transverse plane that occur when a bone rotates either internally or externally along its long axis (Figure 90-1). Angular deformities such as bowlegs and knock-knees are deformities in the frontal plane. The legs distal to the knees are angled or tilted toward the midline in bowleg deformity, whereas they are tilted away from the midline of the body in knock-knee deformity (Figure 90-2). Variations in the knee angle that fall outside the normal range (eg, more than ±2 standard deviations of the mean) are referred to as genu varum for bowlegs and genu valgum for knock-knees (Dx Box). Appreciation of the normal developmental sequence in conjunction with a careful history and physical examination can help pediatricians identify pathologic cases of bowlegs and knock-knees and initiate prompt treatment.

Epidemiology

Bowlegs and knock-knees are common in infants and children. While babies are all born bowlegged, parents usually don't appreciate this finding until infants begin to walk. Knock-knees occur less frequently than bowlegs. Knock-knees are seen more often in females

and are commonly associated with generalized ligamentous laxity. Pathologic cases of bowlegs and knock-knees are uncommon and are defined by the degree of the angulation.

Figure 90-1. Select body reference and rotational planes. Rotational problems are deformities in the transverse plane. Angular deformities are in the frontal plane.

Figure 90-2. Varus and valgus deformities of the lower extremities. A. Bowleg deformity. B. Knock-knee deformity.

Clinical Presentation

Children with **bowlegs** have a characteristic wide-based stance with increased distance between the knees. They may walk with a waddling gait. In-toeing may be noted as a result of associated internal tibial torsion. When the distance between the knees (intercondylar distance) is more than 10 cm when children are lying supine with their hips and knees in extension and their medial malleoli just touching, they require evaluation for pathologic bowlegs.

Severe **knock-knees** may produce an awkward gait with the knees rubbing. Children may walk with both feet apart in an effort to avoid knee-to-knee contact. They may need to place one knee behind the other to stand with both feet together. When the distance between the ankles (intermalleolar distance) is more than 10 cm when children are lying supine with their hips and knees in extension and their knees just touching, they warrant evaluation for pathologic knock-knees.

Pathophysiology

The normal variation in the angular alignment of the lower extremities changes with age. During the first 2 years of life, relative bowing of the legs is common. Although physiological bowing of the lower leg may be appreciated at birth, it is most prominent during the second year of life, when it most commonly involves both the tibia and the femur. When associated with internal tibial torsion, the deformity may appear more striking. Physiological knock-knees develop between 3 and 4 years of age. The knock-knee stage resolves somewhere between 5 and 7 years of age, when normal adult alignment develops. A slight knock-knee appearance remains in normal adults. Bowlegs or knock-knees that develop outside of this sequence require further evaluation for pathologic causes.

The **tibiofemoral angle,** the angle between the long axis of the femur and the long axis of the tibia, is used to assess the angular

---

Dx **Pathologic Bowlegs and Knock-Knees**

- Asymmetrical deformity
- Inconsistency with the normal sequence of angular development
- Stature less than the fifth percentile for age
- Severe deformity (>10 cm intermalleolar or intercondylar distance)
- History of rapid progression
- Presence of other musculoskeletal abnormalities

alignment of the leg. At birth the tibiofemoral angle is approximately 15 degrees varus, and it decreases to 0 between the ages of 18 and 24 months. By 3 to 4 years, the angle peaks at about 10 degrees of valgus angulation. Then between 5 and 7 years it decreases to the normal range of about 7 to 9 degrees in girls and 4 to 6 degrees in boys (Figure 90-3).

Differential Diagnosis

The most common causes of genu varum and genu valgum are presented in Box 90-1. Physiological bowlegs and knock-knees are usually bilateral, and they occur in a sequence that follows the normal developmental pattern. Lateral bowing of the tibia is commonly noted during the first year of life. Bowlegs (involving both the femur and the tibia) are pronounced during the second year, and knock-knees become prominent between 3 and 4 years of age. This is the normal sequence of angular development. Most cases of bowlegs are the result of normal physiological processes, Blount disease (tibia vara), and rickets. Common causes of pathologic knock-knees are severe renal rickets and "old" fractures of the proximal tibia.

Box 90-1. Common Causes of Genu Varum and Genu Valgum

Genu Varum
- Physiological bowlegs
- Rickets (vitamin D deficiency [nutritional] or vitamin D resistance [hereditary])
- Blount disease (tibia vara)
- Achondroplasia
- Metaphyseal dysplasia
- Trauma, infection, or tumor of the proximal tibia (resulting in malunion or partial physeal arrest)
- Excessive prenatal fluoride ingestion

Genu Valgum
- Physiological knock-knees
- Rickets (renal osteodystrophy)
- Trauma, infection, or tumor of the distal femur or proximal tibia (resulting in malunion or partial physeal arrest)
- Paralytic conditions (eg, myelodysplasia, polio, cerebral palsy) leading to contracture of the iliotibial band
- Osteogenesis imperfecta
- Rheumatoid arthritis of the knee

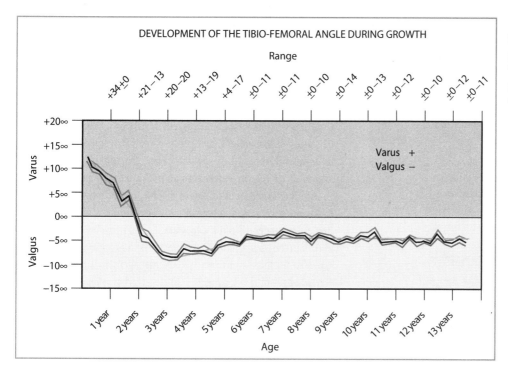

Figure 90-3. Development of the tibiofemoral angle. (Reproduced with permission from Salenious P, Vankka E. The development of the tibiofemoral angle in children. *J Bone Joint Surg.* 1975;57A:259–261.)

Blount disease, a growth disturbance involving the posterior-medial aspect of the proximal tibia (physis, epiphysis, and metaphysis), is the most frequent cause of pathologic bowlegs. The cause is unknown but related to undergrowth of the medial side of the tibia. Both infantile and juvenile forms of the disease are more common in African Americans. The infantile form, initially classified by Langenskiöld, affects children 1 to 3 years of age. Usually bilateral, it is associated with internal tibial torsion. The etiology is believed to involve mechanical stress on the growth plate, thus converting physiological bowlegs to pathologic varus. Affected children are often obese, in the upper growth percentiles, and early walkers, which puts early stress on the growth plate. Blount disease produces a sharp angulation at the proximal tibia, whereas physiological bowlegs lead to a gradual curvature of the legs involving both the femur and the tibia. Six stages of x-ray progression based on the degree of epiphyseal depression and metaphyseal fragmentation at the proximal tibia have been identified (Langenskiöld staging). It may be difficult to distinguish between early stages of Blount disease and physiological bowlegs.

The less common juvenile form of Blount disease occurs in older children and adolescents. Knee pain, rather than deformity, is the most common presenting sign. Usually unilateral, it is more common in males than females. Affected children are generally obese and have a normal height. Although the etiology is unclear, it is believed that in predisposed obese adolescents, the decreased growth of the medial tibial physis is due to the repetitive trauma of excessive weight bearing.

Rickets, a disease of the growing skeleton, produces inadequate mineralization of the bone. The disorder is due to a disturbance in calcium and phosphorus metabolism. Rickets takes several forms, including vitamin D–deficient (nutritional) rickets, vitamin D–resistant (hereditary) rickets (the most common form), and severe renal osteodystrophy. Signs of rickets include short stature, poor muscle tone, joint pain, and angular deformities of the lower extremities. Nutritional rickets may occur in infants who are exclusively breastfed and not supplemented with Vitamin D. The alignment at the time of onset of disease determines the direction of angulation. For example, vitamin D–deficient or vitamin D–resistant rickets generally has an early onset and is more often associated with bowlegs. Children with rickets and bowlegs, unlike those with Blount disease, are late walkers and often have evidence of growth impairment. Renal osteodystrophy, which usually has a later onset, results in a valgus deformity.

Pathologic processes, including trauma (fractures), infections, and tumors, involving the proximal tibia, are additional potential causes of both bowlegs and knock-knees. Overgrowth or malunion following fractures of the proximal tibial metaphysis most commonly results in genu valgum rather than genu varum.

Evaluation

History

A family history; a description of the deformity; its progression, impact, and prior treatment; and an assessment of the child's growth and nutritional history (Questions Box) should be obtained from the parents or caregivers. A dietary history is also important, particularly whether the infant was exclusively breastfed.

Physical Examination

Physical examination begins with a general screening of children's nutritional growth and developmental status. Children's growth parameters (height, weight, head circumference) should be measured and plotted on standard growth curves. The rotational status of the lower limb should be assessed because internal tibial torsion is

Questions

Pathologic Bowlegs and Knock-Knees

- When was the deformity first noticed?
- Has it changed? If so, how fast?
- Has the problem been treated in any way?
- Does the problem seem to affect how the child walks?
- Has the child had any recent illness or trauma in the affected leg?
- Does anyone else in the family have a similar problem?
- Aside from this condition, is the child growing and developing normally?
- Has the infant been exclusively breastfed?
- Does the child eat a well-balanced diet?
- Does the child have any chronic medical problems such as kidney disease?

often associated with bowleg deformity (see Chapter 89). Children should be observed both standing and ambulating to determine the alignment of the legs. The intercondylar and intermalleolar distances can be measured with the child supine to determine the presence of excessive bowlegs or knock-knees (see Clinical Presentation). The intercondylar and intermalleolar distances should be followed every 6 months to monitor the progression of the deformity.

Laboratory Tests

Most children with physiological angulation do not require any laboratory studies. A general metabolic screening, including hemoglobin, calcium, phosphorus, creatinine, and alkaline phosphatase, may be ordered if a systemic or metabolic abnormality is suspected.

Imaging Studies

X-rays are usually performed in the evaluation of bowlegs or knock-knees if pathology is suspected, such as if the deformity is unilateral, painful, very asymmetrical, or progressing at an accelerated rate. If obtained, x-rays should include the entire leg so that the alignment of the femur and tibia may be assessed. Children should be standing, and a single radiograph of both legs should be taken, if possible. Pathologic conditions such as rickets (osteoporosis, metaphyseal fraying, cortical thinning, widening of the growth plates), Blount disease (beaking of the medial metaphysis of the femur and tibia), various bone dysplasias, and forms of dwarfism can usually be ruled out by x-rays. An increased uptake of the proximal medial aspect of the tibia on bone scan may help differentiate early infantile Blount disease from extreme physiological bowlegs.

Management

Angular deformities within normal developmental limits should be managed with continual observation and reassessment. The severity of the deformity should be documented, and children should be followed at 3- to 6-month intervals until the condition resolves. Physicians should **reassure parents** that bowlegs and knock-knees are normal developmental variations that will correct spontaneously

with time. Special diets, braces or shoe wedges, arch supports, and bars are generally best avoided; they have not been shown to affect the normal developmental sequence.

Children with physiological varus may be followed clinically until 18 months to 2 years of age. Pathology should be suspected if correction has not begun by this time or if the lesion is progressive. Children with more than 10 degrees of valgus (or an intermalleolar distance >10 cm) after 8 to 9 years of age may require further evaluation. Children with suspected cases of pathologic bowlegs and knock-knees require **referral to an orthopedist** for evaluation.

Although treatment of Blount disease in children younger than 3 to 4 years may consist of **bracing** if the deformity is mild and identified early, **surgery** is often necessary. Surgery involves an osteotomy to realign the tibia. Failure to do so may result in damage to the medial aspect of the knee over time. Medical management, such as administration of vitamin D for nutritional rickets, is of primary importance in the treatment of the various forms of rickets. Surgical correction, such as osteotomies to correct varus or valgus deformities, should be reserved until medical management has been maximized because even severe deformities may resolve with conservative management.

Prognosis

Physiological bowlegs and knock-knees spontaneously resolve without further sequelae. Although knock-knees are primarily a cosmetic problem, degenerative arthritis may rarely be a late complication. Surgical correction may be required for adolescents with severe deformity to prevent such late complications.

CASE RESOLUTION

The boy described in the case history should be evaluated for pathologic causes of genu varum, especially Blount disease, for the following reasons: (1) his age is at the upper limit of normal for bowlegs and his deformity is severe, (2) he is African American, (3) he has a history of early walking, and (4) he is obese. A standing x-ray of the lower extremities should be obtained, and the boy should be referred to an orthopedist for further evaluation and management.

Selected References

Bruce RW. Torsional and angular deformities. *Pediatr Clin North Am.* 1996;43:867–881

Eggert P, Viemann M. Physiologic bowlegs or infantile Blount's disease. Some new aspects on an old problem. *Pediatr Radiol.* 1996;26:349–352

Henderson RC. Tibia vara: a complication of adolescent obesity. *J Pediatr.* 1992;121:482–486

Kling TF. Angular deformities of the lower limbs in children. *Orthop Clin North Am.* 1987;18:513–527

Mankin KP, Zimbler S. Gait and leg alignment: what's normal and what's not. *Contemp Pediatr.* 1997;14:41–70

Scherl SV. Common lower extremity problems in children. *Pediatr Rev.* 2004;25:52–61

Scoles PV. Lower extremity development. In: *Pediatric Orthopedics in Clinical Practice.* 2nd ed. Chicago, IL: Year Book Medical Publishers; 1988:82–121

Wilkins KE. Bowlegs. *Pediatr Clin North Am.* 1986;33:1429–1438

Orthopedic Injuries and Growing Pains

Sara T. Stewart, MD

CASE STUDY

A 6-year-old boy has a 1-week history of leg pains. He wakes up at night and cries because his legs hurt; yet during the day he is fine, with no pain or movement limitations. He has no history of trauma, fever, or joint swelling. The family history is negative for rheumatic or collagen-vascular disease. The boy's height and weight are at the 50th percentile for age, he is afebrile, and the physical examination is unremarkable.

Questions

1. What is the differential diagnosis of leg pains in school-aged children?
2. What laboratory or radiographic studies are appropriate for children with leg pains?
3. How do musculoskeletal injuries in children differ from those in adults (eg, the type of injury sustained, the location of the injury, etc)?
4. How does one decide the extent of the diagnostic workup in a child with extremity pain?
5. What physiological factors cause musculoskeletal injury patterns to change with age?

Children by nature are active and explorative. They experience cuts, scrapes, minor injuries, and pain routinely. Because primary care physicians are often the first to examine children with injuries, they play an important role in making the preliminary diagnosis and assessment regarding the need for further evaluation and treatment. The more common complaints and injuries seen in the pediatrician's office are discussed in this chapter: growing pains; nursemaids' elbow; and fractures, including growth plate injuries. The evaluation of children with limp is discussed in Chapter 93.

Epidemiology

The term **growing pains** is somewhat misleading because there is no evidence that these pains are associated with growth. The period of middle childhood, when growing pains are diagnosed, is not the period of most rapid growth in the child. *Leg aches* or *idiopathic leg pain* may be better terms, but *growing pains* is the most widely used term.

Growing pains occur in 15% to 30% of all children. They are seen most commonly in children between the ages of 3 and 12 years; the reported age range is infancy to 19 years. Girls are affected more frequently than boys.

Nursemaids' elbow, pulled elbow, or radial head subluxation is the most common joint injury in childhood. It occurs most commonly in children 1 to 4 years of age, with a peak incidence between 2 and 3 years of age. Other ligament and tendon injuries are relatively uncommon in prepubertal children due to the relative strength of these structures in comparison to the growth plate of the adjacent developing bone. Most commonly, fractures involving the growth plate occur before ligamentous injury. When joint dislocations and ligamentous injury occur in children (with the exception of nursemaids' elbow), they are usually due to significant trauma.

Trauma and injury are significant causes of morbidity and mortality in childhood. Injuries are the most common reason for hospitalization in children and adolescents younger than 18 years and are the leading cause of death beyond the first year of life. Musculoskeletal problems account for 15% of all injuries and most commonly occur in the upper extremity. Fractures are perhaps the most common significant form of musculoskeletal injury in children who present to physicians for evaluation and treatment.

Clinical Presentation (Dx Box)

Children with growing pains typically present with a history of intermittent, poorly localized pain in the bilateral lower extremities that occurs at night over a long period. The pain most commonly involves the calves and anterior thighs, never the joints. Symptoms usually resolve over several minutes, and in the morning the child has normal activity.

Nursemaids' elbow is characterized by a sudden onset of elbow pain associated with the traumatic event and subsequent decreased use of the arm. At the time of presentation for medical care, a child

Dx Growing Pains and Orthopedic Injuries

Growing Pains

- Age between 3 and 12 years
- Normal growth and development
- Intermittent pain or aches in the legs
- Occurrence of symptoms at night
- Pain poorly localized to the anterior thighs, calves, and behind the knees; absence of joint involvement
- Absence of limp, disability, or inflammation
- Response to supportive measures such as heat and massage

Nursemaids' Elbow

- Age between 1 and 4 years
- Elbow pain of acute onset
- History of sudden longitudinal traction on an extended and pronated arm
- Forearm held in a position of flexion and pronation
- Lack of spontaneous movement of the elbow

Fractures

- Obvious deformity
- Swelling or tenderness over the fracture site
- Limited range of movement or absence of movement of the affected extremity

Localized swelling, tenderness, and limited range of movement may all be signs of a fracture.

Pathophysiology

Growing pains are recurrent aches or pains localized to the muscles of the legs. The pain is located deep within the extremity and not in the joints. The etiology is unclear. Rapid growth, emotional and psychological stress, and myalgias secondary to exercise or physical activity have all been implicated.

Nursemaids' elbow is a subluxation of the radial head caused by a rapid and forceful extension and pronation of the forearm. This mechanism most commonly occurs when a caretaker pulls a child toward himself or herself and the child resists, wanting to go in the other direction. As illustrated in Figure 91-1, the subluxation occurs due to tearing of the annular ligament, with trapping of the ligament between the radius and the capitellum. This injury is seen primarily in young children because the attachment of the ligament to the bone becomes thicker with age and growth.

Because of anatomical and physiological differences (eg, presence of cartilaginous growth plate as well as thicker periosteum and greater plasticity of the skeleton), fracture patterns seen in children often differ from those in adults. Additionally, fractures may influence long-term growth and development of the affected limb in a growing child.

Fractures are classified based on anatomical location, type of fracture, and degree of angulation or displacement. Fracture location may be described as diaphyseal, metaphyseal, or epiphyseal/growth plate depending on the portion of the bone involved (Figures 91-2 and 91-3). Fractures may be either open or closed. In closed fractures, the skin over the fracture site is intact, whereas in open fractures, the skin is broken. Fractures in which the 2 bone fragments are displaced relative to each other are described as angulated or displaced; the direction and degree of displacement are based on the distal fragment.

with nursemaids' elbow typically appears well, aside from a refusal to use the affected arm. The child typically holds the arm close to the body with the elbow in slight flexion and the forearm pronated. There is usually no gross deformity, swelling, or overlying skin trauma, and the child typically refuses to supinate the forearm during examination. There may also be point tenderness laterally over the radial head.

An underlying **fracture** is strongly indicated by obvious deformity or lack of spontaneous movement in the extremity in question.

Figure 91-1. Nursemaids' elbow. The sudden traction on the outstretched arm pulls the radius distally, causing a tear in the annular ligament at its attachment to the radius. A portion of the ligament becomes trapped within the joint as the traction is released and the arm recoils. **A.** Mechanism of injury. **B.** Pathology. **C.** Method of reduction (hyperpronation).

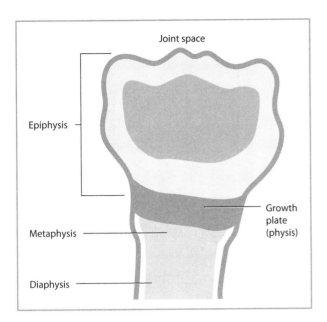

Figure 91-2. **Anatomy of a long bone.**

Table 91-1. Long Bone Fracture Patterns Seen in Children	
Type	*Description*
Non-Epiphyseal Plate Fractures	
Complete	Both sides of the bone fractured; type depends on direction of fracture line
Transverse	Perpendicular to long axis of the bone
Oblique	At an angle to long axis of the bone
Spiral	Zig-zag course around the bone
Comminuted	Fractures with 3 or more fragments (rare in children)
Buckle or torus	Bone compression causes it to bend or buckle rather than break; occurs at junction of metaphysis and diaphysis
Greenstick	Cortex broken on tension side but intact on compression side
Bowing	Deformation of bone due to bending without fracturing
Classic metaphyseal lesion	Fracture of distal, poorly mineralized metaphysis, perpendicular to long axis of bone; previously termed bucket-handle or chip fracture
Epiphyseal Plate Fractures (Salter-Harris Classification)	
Type I	Horizontal fracture through the physis
Type II	Fracture through the physis, extending into the metaphysis
Type III	Fracture through the epiphysis, extending into the physis
Type IV	Fracture through the epiphysis, physis, and metaphysis
Type V	Crush injury of the physis

The Salter-Harris classification is used most commonly to classify growth plate injury (Table 91-1, Figure 91-4). Approximately 15% of all fractures in children involve the growth plate. Type I and II fractures are the most common fractures involving the growth plate. Type III and IV fractures are intra-articular. Type V fractures are uncommon and are due to a crush injury to the growth plate. Initial x-rays in type I and V fractures may appear normal, because bone fragments are not displaced. Due to involvement of the growth plate, there is a risk of growth arrest with any physis injury. The risk is variable, however, depending on the type of injury.

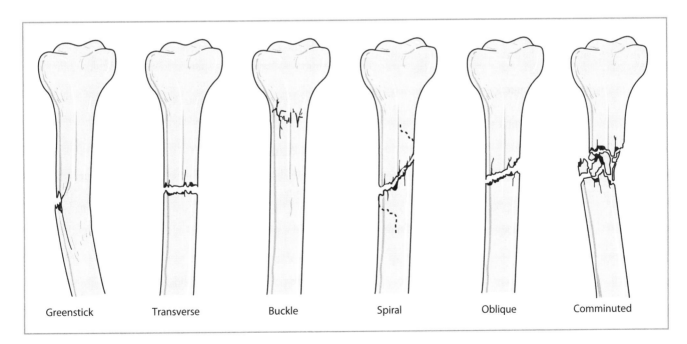

Greenstick   Transverse   Buckle   Spiral   Oblique   Comminuted

Figure 91-3. **Non-epiphyseal plate fractures.**

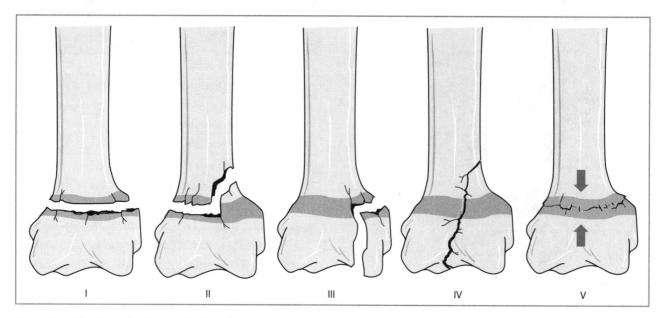

Figure 91-4. Salter-Harris classification of epiphyseal plate fractures.

Differential Diagnosis

The diagnosis of **growing pains** is one of exclusion. Leg pain in children has many causes (Box 91-1). If they are limited to vague pains in the legs at night with no associated limp or signs of inflammation, the differential diagnosis may be limited to growing pains, general systemic diseases such as leukemia, benign bone tumors such as osteoid osteoma, and perhaps fibromyalgia. Leukemic infiltration of the bones may cause leg pain before systemic signs such as fever, weight loss, and adenopathy are present. Osteoid osteoma, a benign bone tumor that most commonly occurs in adolescent boys, characteristically causes pain that is worse at night and is usually relieved by anti-inflammatory medications. The pain may be localized in one place, however, unlike with growing pains. Fibromyalgia, which is probably underdiagnosed in the pediatric population, is a well-recognized cause in adults of chronic, generalized limb pain without a clear, organic source. It is seen more commonly in adolescents than in younger children. This benign, intermittent musculoskeletal pain syndrome is associated with multiple tender "trigger points," stiffness, fatigue, and a non-restorative sleep pattern.

When evaluating for **nursemaids' elbow,** an elbow fracture should be ruled out. Certain fractures and specific features of fractures deserve mention (see Figure 91-3). Fractures that often occur during childhood include clavicular fractures (the most common childhood fracture and most commonly fractured bone from birth trauma) and spiral fractures of the distal tibia—the "toddler's fracture." The toddler's fracture typically occurs in children who have not been walking long, those between 9 months and 3 years of age. It is thought to be due to a rotational force on the lower leg, which could occur as an ambulatory child falls in a twisting motion. Often, when the child presents for medical care the parents are unaware of a history of trauma and the chief complaint is that the child refuses to bear weight on the affected leg. Elbow fractures occur commonly due to a fall directly on the elbow, or due to a fall on an outstretched hand. These fractures require careful attention to neurovascular status because of the risk of associated injury to the median or radial nerve, or brachial artery, leading to Volkmann ischemic contracture. A Monteggia fracture is a dislocation of the radial head in association with an ulnar shaft fracture. Long bone fractures in pre-ambulatory children, rib fractures, classic metaphyseal lesions, and the presence of multiple fractures in one child are all concerning for non-accidental trauma and should prompt a more thorough evaluation of possible physical abuse (see Chapter 115).

Because of the relative weakness of the physis compared with the surrounding ligaments, trauma sustained near joints may be more likely to cause a type I Salter-Harris growth plate fracture rather than ligamentous injury (eg, sprain or strain). Therefore, it is important to include this type of fracture in the differential diagnosis of children with point tenderness near the end of a long bone because this injury does require cast immobilization.

Evaluation

Accurate diagnosis of pediatric orthopedic injuries is often challenging because children may be not only poor "historians" but also uncooperative with examinations, especially if they are experiencing pain.

History

A thorough history is essential for the accurate diagnosis of growing pains and orthopedic injuries (Questions Box: Growing Pains and Questions Box: Orthopedic Injuries). A complete history of the events related to the injury, including what happened after the injury was sustained, should be obtained.

Box 91-1. Common Causes of Leg Pain in Children

Growing Pains (Leg Aches, Idiopathic Leg Pains)

Trauma

- Fracture
- Compartment syndromes
- Soft tissue injury
- Muscle strain/sprain

Infection

- Cellulitis
- Soft tissue abscess
- Myositis
- Osteomyelitis
- Septic arthritis

Neoplasia

- Malignant bone tumors (eg, osteogenic sarcoma, Ewing sarcoma)
- Leukemia
- Metastatic disease (eg, lymphoma, neuroblastoma)

Benign Bone Lesions

- Osteoid osteoma
- Bone cysts
- Histiocytosis X

Collagen-Vascular Disease

- Juvenile rheumatoid arthritis
- Dermatomyositis
- Fibromyalgia
- Rheumatic fever

Other Musculoskeletal Causes

- Legg-Calvé-Perthes disease
- Slipped capital femoral epiphysis
- Osgood-Schlatter disease
- Transient synovitis of the hip
- Osteochondritis dissecans
- Patellofemoral stress/chondromalacia patellae
- Generalized ligamentous laxity and joint hypermobility

Miscellaneous Causes

- Sickle cell disease pain crisis
- Psychosomatic conditions

Questions

Growing Pains

- When (ie, what time of day) does the pain typically occur?
- How long has the pain been occurring?
- Does the pain resolve and then recur in any predictable manner?
- Where is the pain? Does it change location?
- Does anything make the pain better or worse?
- Is the child sick in any other way?
- Does the pain interfere with the child's activities?
- Does the parent notice any changes such as swelling or redness in the child's legs?

Questions

Orthopedic Injuries

- How did the injury occur?
- How long ago was the injury sustained? When did the symptoms begin?
- Was the incident witnessed by an adult?
- How strong was the injuring force? What direction did it come from?
- What was the position of the affected extremity at the time of the injury?
- Did the child experience any head trauma or loss of consciousness?
- What, if any, first aid was administered at the scene?
- Has the child been able to move the affected extremity since the injury occurred?

Physical Examination

The physical examination of children with suspected **growing pains** should include evaluation for signs of systemic disease such as fever, lymphadenopathy, hepatosplenomegaly, abnormal growth, and generalized weakness or fatigue. Leg length and circumference should be measured. The legs should be palpated and range of motion assessed in the hip, knee, and ankle.

Children with suspected **nursemaids' elbow** should be observed for how they hold the affected arm compared with the unaffected arm. They should be evaluated for limited active motion at the elbow and resistance to attempts at passive movement, especially supination. No swelling should be present, but there may be tenderness over the radial head. The shoulder and wrist should also be well examined.

It is important to undress children with suspected **fractures** and perform a complete physical examination. Simply examining the involved extremity is insufficient. The presence of a deformity, point tenderness, or limitation of motion supports the diagnosis of a fracture. All long bones should be palpated, and the presence of bruises and scars should be noted because these may indicate child abuse. The examination of the involved extremity includes inspection of the overlying skin for swelling, lacerations, or punctures. The degree of active and passive motion and strength compared with the uninvolved side should be noted. In cases of suspected leg injuries, the child's gait should be observed, if possible. Assessment of neurovascular function distal to the injury includes evaluation of capillary refill, peripheral pulses, and motor and sensory function.

Laboratory Tests

A complete blood count and erythrocyte sedimentation rate (ESR) may be considered for children with leg pains that do not resolve. Rheumatologic screening tests can be ordered based on abnormalities in these tests (eg, elevated ESR or white blood cell count). Routine laboratory studies are not necessary in the evaluation of nursemaids' elbow or fractures. However, because fractures of the femur are often associated with significant blood loss, it is important to monitor the hematocrit in these patients.

Imaging Studies

If leg pains persist and interfere with routine activity, x-rays or a bone scan of the legs may be considered. Radiographic evaluation is not required for children with nursemaids' elbow if presentation is typical and reduction is successful. X-rays, if taken in such children, are usually completely negative because the dislocation is often corrected during positioning for x-rays. However, x-rays should be obtained in children with suspected fractures. Fractures involving the growth plate, especially type I and V Salter-Harris fractures, may be particularly difficult to diagnose radiographically because the growth plate is primarily cartilaginous and, hence, radiolucent. A bone scan or follow-up x-ray may be used to diagnose suspected fractures when initial x-rays are negative.

Management

Parental education and reassurance regarding the benign nature of **growing pains** are important. The pains themselves usually respond to **supportive measures** such as heat, massage, and analgesia. Stretching exercises for the legs have also been recommended. Referral to an orthopedist should be considered if the pain is severe and persistent and physical examination and laboratory workup fail to reveal a specific diagnosis.

Nursemaids' elbow is one of the few medical conditions that has a dramatic, immediate cure. To treat the elbow, the annular ligament must be reduced back to its anatomical position, and there are 2 common methods of reduction. In both methods the elbow is stabilized with application of pressure laterally over the radial head with the thumb of the medical provider. In the first method, there is rapid, firm hyperpronation of the forearm. In the second, the forearm is firmly supinated then the elbow is flexed. A click may be heard or felt as the radial head is reduced, and relief of pain is usually immediate for those children treated shortly after the injury. Return of function may require up to 30 minutes, however. If treatment is delayed, such rapid relief of symptoms may not be seen. Following reduction, the parents should be advised that the child may need mild pain medication. Some providers recommend short-term immobilization in a sling or splint to facilitate soft tissue healing.

Most **fractures** should be referred to an orthopedic surgeon for evaluation and treatment unless the primary care physician is experienced in reducing and casting fractures. Several techniques are used in fracture management. **Closed reduction** is the nonoperative reduction or realignment of fracture fragments. **Open reduction** implies that an incision has been made to expose the fracture and proceed with manipulating the bone fragments into place. Fixation, or stabilization of the fracture with any type of device, may be required following the reduction. This is termed **internal fixation** if the device is under the skin and **external fixation** if the device begins outside of the skin but passes through the skin to bone. Indications for open reduction include failure of closed reduction, need for precise anatomical reduction, and complex multisystem trauma.

Certain fractures are common in pediatrics. Most clavicular fractures do not require reduction and can be treated with immobilization in a sling for 4 to 8 weeks. Elbow fractures (eg, lateral condyle and supracondylar humeral fractures) are serious and often necessitate open reduction to achieve anatomical reduction. Distal forearm fractures are usually managed with closed reduction and casting, but forearm fractures in the middle and proximal thirds of the bone may be harder to reduce in the office setting. Stable metacarpal and phalangeal fractures can be either splinted in an aluminum splint or be taped to an adjacent finger ("buddy taping"). The metacarpophalangeal joints should be maintained in 50 to 90 degrees of flexion, and the interphalangeal joints should be in about 20 degrees of flexion to minimize stiffness. Unstable finger fractures may require open reduction and pin fixation.

Femoral shaft fractures in infants and children can be managed with closed reduction and spica cast placement. As children become older, a fixation device may be required in addition to the closed reduction. Open reduction is necessary on rare occasions. Closed reduction and cast immobilization are usually used in the management of tibial shaft fractures. Short cast immobilization may be required for metatarsal fractures, and buddy taping is used for stable toe fractures.

Because of the potential for infection, open fractures are orthopedic emergencies that require immediate attention. Careful debridement of the wound is required. Antibiotics should be administered, and tetanus immunization may be given based on a review of the immunization history.

Prognosis

Growing pains resolve over time without sequelae. Recurrence of nursemaids' elbow is common, occurring again in up to a third of patients. Therefore, parents should be cautioned regarding pulling children's arms or lifting them by one hand. Fractures in children generally heal faster and remodel (the spontaneous correction of deformity) better than equivalent fractures in adults. Vascular and nerve injuries and growth disturbances are potential complications of fractures and their management. Compartment syndrome, a potentially serious vascular injury, may also develop.

Growth plate injuries require special attention because of the potential for subsequent growth abnormalities of the affected bone. Prognosis of growth plate fractures depends on the type of injury sustained. Salter-Harris type I and II fractures generally have a good prognosis for long-term healing and growth. The severity of the injury and the accuracy of reduction determine the prognosis of type III and IV fractures. Growth arrest is common following type V fractures because the physis itself is injured.

CASE RESOLUTION

The child presented in the opening scenario has the benign condition commonly referred to as growing pains. Management involves parental education and reassurance. Local heat, massage, and analgesia (using ibuprofen) may be recommended.

Selected References

American Academy of Pediatrics Council on Sports Medicine and Fitness. *Sports Shorts*. www.aap.org/family/sportsshort.htm

Anderson SJ. Lower extremity injuries in youth sports. *Pediatr Clin North Am.* 2002;49:627–641

Carson S, Woolridge DP, Colletti J, Kilgore K. Pediatric upper extremity injuries. *Pediatr Clin North Am.* 2006;53:41–67

Eiff MP, Hatch RL. Boning up on common pediatric fractures. *Contemp Pediatr.* 2003;20:30–59

Gladden PB, Wilson CH, Suk M. Pediatric orthopedic trauma: principles of management. *Semin Pediatr Surg.* 2004;13:119–125

Hutson AM, Rovinsky D. Casts and splints. In: Reichman EF, Simon RR, eds. *Emergency Medicine Procedures.* New York, NY: McGraw-Hill; 2004:669–689

Mitchell S, Monsell F. Growing pains: making an accurate diagnosis. *Practitioner.* 2006;250:28, 31–32, 34

Soprano JV. Musculoskeletal injuries in the pediatric and adolescent athlete. *Curr Sports Med Rep.* 2005;4:329–334

Tse SML, Laxer RM. Approach to acute limb pain in childhood. *Pediatr Rev.* 2006;27:170–179

Sports-Related Acute Injuries

Monica Sifuentes, MD

CASE STUDY

A 15-year-old female basketball player complains of 6 months of intermittent pain in her left knee. Occasionally the knee gives out while she is playing ball. The teen denies any associated swelling or erythema over the joint. She is able to walk with no problem and reports no history of direct trauma to the area. She is otherwise healthy.

On physical examination, she is a well-developed, well-nourished teenaged female in no acute distress. The examination is normal except for mild pain to direct palpation of the left patella. No swelling, erythema, or effusion of the knee joint is evident, and the left hip, knee, and ankle have full range of motion. The back is straight.

Questions

1. What are some of the most common orthopedic complaints in adolescent patients, and why do they occur in this age group?
2. What is the pathophysiology of overuse syndromes?
3. What is the purpose of the preparticipation sports physical examination?
4. What conditions disqualify adolescents from participation in competitive sports?
5. What are the current recommendations for the treatment and rehabilitation of acute soft tissue injuries?

Many adolescents with varying degrees of athletic ability participate in sports during their junior high and high school years. Some choose to continue this participation at the college level. Regardless of the ultimate goal, team sports are an important means by which children and adolescents can experience both winning and losing. Individuals learn the importance of group participation and develop interactive skills with other team members. They are exposed to the concept of physical fitness, which can improve body image as well as self-esteem.

Participation in athletics carries significant risks, however. Injuries, inappropriate coaching, and aggressive training sessions are not uncommon occurrences that may have long-term sequelae for young athletes. Primary care practitioners are responsible not only for the evaluation of children prior to their participation in sports but also for the diagnosis, treatment, and prevention of athletic injuries.

Epidemiology

Estimates indicate that as many as 7 million adolescents per year participate in organized sports activities in the United States. Several studies have attempted to quantify the overall injury rate associated with athletic participation. In general, the rate of injury for 13- to 19-year-olds is 7% to 11%. Approximately 20% of those injured sustain a significant injury. The sport with the highest injury rate in all age groups for boys is football, followed by basketball and soccer. Gymnastics leads to the most injuries in girls. Gender differences between boys and girls have been found in some studies depending on the sport. Overall, boys tend to have more shoulder-related injuries, whereas girls tend to have more knee and ankle injuries and more problems with overuse syndromes. Reports also indicate that girls tend to have more injuries requiring surgical correction.

Preparticipation Physical Evaluation

The goal of the preparticipation physical evaluation (PPE) is the identification of any physical conditions or abnormalities that may predispose young athletes to injury. Examples include a history of concussion with head trauma or an incompletely healed sprain.

The PPE consists of 2 parts: (1) a review of the patient's current health; medical history, including sports injuries; and pertinent family history pertaining to participation in strenuous activities and (2) a complete physical examination with a focus on the musculoskeletal system. Known as a "2-minute orthopedic examination," the musculoskeletal examination is a detailed assessment of all muscle groups, assessing their strength, tone, and function. Congenital or acquired deformities are also noted. The American Academy of Pediatrics (AAP) has developed a form specifically for the PPE visit (see Chapter 24).

Disqualification from participation in specific sports is appropriate in certain situations. Competitive sports are classified according to their degree of contact or impact and how strenuous they are. Recommendations differ depending on the adolescent's medical condition and the type of sport the athlete desires to play. For details of these recommendations, see Selected References. Fortunately, many young athletes are healthy and rarely need to be restricted from participation.

Clinical Presentation

Older children and adolescents with sports-related injuries usually present to the practitioner with specific complaints of pain or swelling in a particular joint (Dx Box). In addition, they may complain of nonspecific musculoskeletal pain occurring in certain areas such as the lower back or shoulder. Other complaints may include a limp, decreased range of motion of an extremity, or an inability to participate in a desired activity without pain.

Dx Orthopedic Injury

- Joint pain or swelling
- Tenderness to palpation of the affected joint
- Decreased range of motion of the affected joint or extremity
- May or may not have associated bruising of the skin overlying the injury

Pathophysiology

Adolescents, unlike adults, are particularly susceptible to injury because their bones and joints are developing. Most injuries during adolescence involve the epiphysis, which is the weakest point of the musculoskeletal system. In addition, the presence of congenital anomalies such as leg length discrepancies or hip rotation abnormalities puts the young athlete at further risk for injury. Biomechanical and neuromuscular factors, hormonal influences, and anatomical differences also have been proposed for the higher rates of some injuries in young female athletes over young male athletes.

Most orthopedic injuries are the result of either macrotrauma or microtrauma. Sprains are an example of macrotrauma, whereas overuse syndromes can be considered microtrauma. **Macrotrauma** occurs from complete or partial tearing of muscle, ligaments, or tendons and is often associated with acute injuries. In contrast, **microtrauma** is usually produced by chronic repetitive trauma to a particular area, leading to inflammation and ultimately to pain. This most commonly occurs in soft tissues such as the muscle and tendon but can occur in the bone as well.

Definitions

A **sprain** is a stretching injury of a ligament or the connective tissue that attaches bone to bone. A **strain** is a stretching injury of a muscle or its tendon, which is the connective tissue that attaches muscle to bone. **Tendinitis** is an inflammation of the tendon. **Apophysitis** is an inflammation of the apophysis, which is the site of ligament or tendon attachment to growth cartilage (eg, Osgood-Schlatter disease [apophysitis of the tibial tubercle], Sever disease [calcaneal apophysitis]). A **stress fracture** is an incomplete fracture often occurring in the bones of the legs and feet from repetitive trauma to the area. It is believed that the pain associated with shin splints may be due in part to atypical stress fractures of the distal tibia.

Overuse syndromes occur from repetitive microtrauma to the musculoskeletal system secondary to excessive or biomechanically incorrect activity. They are usually the result of training errors in which athletes are "trying to do too much too fast." Common syndromes in adolescents include Osgood-Schlatter disease, shin splints, and patellofemoral syndrome (chondromalacia patellae).

Grading of Sports Injuries

Sprains can be classified according to the degree of injury and most commonly occur in the knee or ankle. Assigning a grade that describes the injury is useful when considering the prognosis of a particular injury. Consultants also find these grades helpful. Grade I through III is the usual classification used for sprains. Stability of the joint, range of motion, and degree of pain and swelling determine the grade of the sprain. The grading system for strains, on the other hand, is based on an assessment of strength. Because strains do not usually cause joint instability, criteria for grading strains are different than for sprains and may be more subjective. A general description of these 2 grading systems appears in Table 92-1.

Differential Diagnosis

The differential diagnosis of orthopedic conditions depends on the anatomical site of the injury or complaint and the mechanism of injury. Box 92-1 lists some of the more common orthopedic conditions by location. Anomalies of skeletal development such as congenital angular deformities of long bones and soft tissue abnormalities like Ehlers-Danlos syndrome also should be considered as possible etiologies for overuse syndromes. Other non-orthopedic conditions such as collagen-vascular diseases, infections, and tumors may present with joint or bone symptomatology.

Table 92-1. General Classification of Sprains and Strains					
	Joint	Range of Motion	Weight Bearing	Pain	Swelling
Sprains					
Grade I	Stable	Normal	Normal	+	+
Grade II	Stable	↓	↓	++	++
Grade III	Unstable	↓↓	↓↓	+++	+++
	Strength	Palpable Defect	Pain		
Strains					
Grade I	>4/5	–	+		
Grade II	3/5–4/5	+/–	++		
Grade III	<3/5	+/–	+++		

Box 92-1. Differential Diagnosis Based on the Site of Injury

Back Injuries

- Muscle strain
- Spondylolysis
- Epiphyseal injury
- Herniated disks

Injuries to the Upper Extremity

- Acromioclavicular sprains
- Sternoclavicular sprains
- Glenohumeral dislocation
- Glenohumeral subluxation
- Impingement syndrome
- Acute elbow injuries
- Olecranon bursitis
- Lateral epicondylitis
- Flexor-pronator tendinitis
- Wrist sprains
- Navicular fractures
- Hamate fractures
- Finger injuries

Injuries to the Lower Extremity

- Iliac crest contusion
- Iliac apophysitis
- Quadriceps contusion
- Femoral stress fracture
- Medial/lateral ligament sprains
- Anterior cruciate ligament sprain
- Posterior cruciate ligament sprain
- Patellar dislocation/subluxation
- Prepatellar bursitis
- Patellofemoral stress syndrome
- Patellar tendinitis
- Osgood-Schlatter disease
- Shin splint syndrome
- Ankle sprains
- Achilles tendinitis
- Calcaneal apophysitis
- Plantar fasciitis

Evaluation

History

The history should focus on the musculoskeletal system and how the injury occurred (Questions Box).

Questions

Sports-Related Injuries

- What is the acuity of the injury?
- What activity or sport was the patient engaged in at the time of the injury?
- How often has the patient engaged in this sport or particular activity in the past?
- Were there any new additions to the routine this time?
- Did the pain begin after a single injury or after repetitive activity?
- If the injury is related to a repetitive activity, does the pain occur at a specific time during this activity?
- What was the mechanism of injury?
- Is the pain incapacitating?
- Has a similar injury ever occurred in the past?
- How was the injury treated?
- Was there any pain following the previous injury?
- Does the patient feel as if he or she has completely recovered?
- How was this current injury managed acutely?
- Has the patient altered daily activity in any way to compensate for this problem?

Physical Examination

The physical examination should focus on the musculoskeletal system. If, however, teenagers have not had a physical examination within the past year, a complete physical examination should first be performed to exclude any systemic condition that might manifest itself initially as bone or joint pain. This is especially important in adolescents with chronic or systemic complaints, such as intermittent extremity pain associated with swelling of an affected joint and fever.

In general, any pain or swelling of the affected joint or muscle should be noted. If adolescents have a history of acute trauma, an area of ecchymosis may be seen. The affected joint should be tested for range of motion and joint laxity that would differentiate a grade I from a grade II or III sprain. Various maneuvers for testing ligamentous laxity at each joint can be used (Figure 92-1).

The most common method is the drawer test for anterior and posterior movement of the knee joint. Muscle spasms and diminished range of motion in an adjacent joint also should be noted because this may indicate a strain injury. Strength of the strained muscle(s) and any pain on palpation or contraction of the muscle(s) should be assessed. A palpable defect of the muscle suggests complete rupture of the muscle, whereas muscular contusions are associated with

Figure 92-1.   Maneuvers used to determine stability of the knee joint. A. Anterior drawer test: Anterior force is applied. B. Posterior drawer test: Posterior force is applied. C. Medial ligament stability: Lateral force is applied.

localized pain, soft tissue swelling, or hematoma. Pinpoint tenderness over a particular bone may indicate a fracture or, if at the site of a tendon insertion, inflammation. Reviewing the mechanism of injury and the timing of the symptoms is often helpful in differentiating between a fracture and tendinitis.

Laboratory Tests

A complete blood count and erythrocyte sedimentation rate may be helpful in adolescents with a history of chronic joint pain or swelling. If the results are abnormal, further workup is indicated to distinguish between a collagen-vascular disease such as systemic lupus erythematosus, an infection such as osteomyelitis or, rarely, an arthritic disorder such as juvenile idiopathic arthritis.

Imaging Studies

A plain radiograph of the involved joint or bone is often the only necessary diagnostic study to perform. Other plain radiographs of joints above and below the symptomatic area are sometimes useful. In general, advanced diagnostic tests such as computerized tomography scanning have limited value in the evaluation of an acute soft tissue injury. Magnetic resonance imaging may be indicated for the injury that does not improve despite adequate treatment and rehabilitation. See Chapter 93 for a discussion of imaging studies to help in the diagnosis when limp is the presenting complaint.

Management

With soft tissue injuries, the aim of acute management is to limit the extent of bleeding and inflammation that occur in the first 48 to 72 hours following the injury. The mnemonic **RICE** (rest, ice, compression, elevation) is helpful. Rest should be explained as "relative rest" because the athletes should be allowed to do whatever they want as long as they are pain-free during or within 24 hours of the activity. Ice should be placed in a plastic bag and applied directly to the skin for a continuous 20 minutes. Longer periods of icing are discouraged because this can result in peripheral nerve palsy from cryoinjury. Patients should ice the injury 3 to 4 times a day for the first 48 hours, and then at least once daily until the swelling or pain is gone. Compression is especially important and should be started as quickly as possible distal and proximal to the injured area. Elevation of the injured extremity should occur as often as possible. The use of this plan for soft tissue injuries facilitates early healing and allows rehabilitation to proceed quickly.

Anti-inflammatory or analgesic medications such as ibuprofen, aspirin, and naproxen are useful in controlling the symptoms of pain and swelling. For adolescent patients, dosages are similar to those used in adults: aspirin, 650 to 1,000 mg every 6 hours; ibuprofen, 400 to 800 mg every 6 to 8 hours; naproxen, 500 mg twice daily. To minimize gastrointestinal side effects, the medication should be administered with a snack or milk. Ideally, these drugs should be used for 7 to 10 days. Corticosteroids, either oral or parenteral, are not indicated in the management of overuse injuries.

After this acute phase, therapy is aimed at resolution of any edema and hematoma and at rehabilitation (Box 92-2). Athletes should slowly begin range-of-motion exercises as tolerated. Full tissue healing may take 6 to 8 weeks, but most young athletes do not have to wait that long to return to athletic activity.

Box 92-2. Principles of Rehabilitation

- Resolution of hematoma
- Resolution of edema
- Regain full range of motion or flexibility
- Regain full muscle strength and endurance
- Regain agility and coordination
- Regain cardiovascular endurance

Modified activity, depending on the degree of tissue damage, should initially be recommended in athletes who have suffered from overuse syndromes. Complete rest is rarely indicated. Participation in another sport such as swimming or cycling is often preferable to complete immobilization. In addition to the use of anti-inflammatory agents, physical therapy is another important therapeutic modality. Cryotherapy, whirlpool, or alternating heat and ice treatments can be helpful. Reconditioning should be continued after 3 to 12 weeks of modified activity, depending on the degree of recovery. This entails gradual strengthening and flexibility training as well as a reevaluation of previous modes of training to minimize the risk of reinjury (Box 92-3).

Box 92-3. Rehabilitation of Musculoskeletal Injuries[a]

Four Phases of Rehabilitation

1. Limit additional injury and control pain and swelling (RICE mnemonic).
2. Improve strength and flexibility (range of motion) of the injured structures.
3. Progressively improve strength, flexibility, proprioception, and endurance training until near-normal function is attained.
4. Return to exercise and sports symptom-free.

[a]Modified and reproduced with permission from Hergenroeder AC. Prevention of sports injuries. *Pediatrics.* 1998;101:1060–1061.

Prevention

Injury prevention is an important aspect of sports medicine with which the primary practitioner should be familiar. Because most injuries are the result of "trying to do too much too soon," proper physical **training and conditioning** are essential, no matter how fit the athlete appears. Stretching, warm-up and cool-down exercises, and the type of equipment used for the sport should be reviewed with the athlete during the sports physical visit. The type of sport to be played should also be reviewed and, if participating in a contact sport, the adolescent should be **matched with other athletes** based on weight and pubertal development rather than age. Some studies suggest that such matching will greatly reduce the risk of injury to the smaller, less mature athlete. Because an old or incompletely healed injury is a significant risk factor for reinjury, all **previous injuries should receive proper treatment and rehabilitation** before the athlete returns to play. **Protective equipment,** especially for collision and contact sports, as well as for those involving a ball or racquet, also should be emphasized to athletes and their parents. In addition, the AAP recommendation of **avoiding strength and weight training** until the athlete reaches sexual maturity rating (Tanner stage) 5 of pubertal development, to prevent the risk of serious injury, should be endorsed. **Education regarding the hazards of anabolic steroid use** also may be indicated.

Prognosis

Orthopedic injuries in young athletes and active adolescents have a great capacity for healing if given the opportunity. Early medical intervention to prevent irreversible tissue damage ensures complete recovery in most cases. Long-term sequelae are associated with repeated trauma, incompletely treated cases, and chronic inflammatory changes. Some conditions, however, such as Osgood-Schlatter disease, will resolve even without treatment and do not lead to any permanent damage to the joint.

CASE RESOLUTION

In the case presented at the beginning of the chapter, the teenager has symptoms and physical findings consistent with patellofemoral pain syndrome (traditionally referred to as chondromalacia of the patella). Because plain radiographs are usually not helpful in confirming the diagnosis, none are necessary at this time. Management should include strength training for the quadriceps muscles, activity modification, nonsteroidal anti-inflammatory medication, and ice compresses after activity.

Selected References

Brenner JS, Council on Sports Medicine and Fitness. Overuse injuries, overtraining, and burnout in child and adolescent athletes. *Pediatrics.* 2007;119:1242–1245

Dyment PG, ed. Sports medicine. *Pediatr Ann.* 1997;26:13–64

Group on Science and Technology, American Medical Association. Athletic pre-participation examinations for adolescents. Report of the Board of Trustees. *Arch Pediatr Adolesc Med.* 1994;148:93–98

Hergenroeder AC. Acute shoulder, knee, and ankle injuries, part 2: rehabilitation. *Adolesc Health Update.* 1996;8:1–8

Hergenroeder AC. Prevention of sports injuries. *Pediatrics.* 1998; 101:1057–1063

Mankin KP, Zimbler S. Foot and ankle injuries: solving the diagnostic dilemmas. *Contemp Pediatr.* 1996;13:25–45

Metzl JD. Preparticipation examination of the adolescent athlete: part 1. *Pediatr Rev.* 2001:22:199–204

Metzl JD. Preparticipation examination of the adolescent athlete: part 2. *Pediatr Rev.* 2001;22:227–235

Risser WL. Sports medicine. *Pediatr Rev.* 1993;14:424–431

Rodenberg RE, Cayce K, Hall S. Your guide to a dreaded injury: the ACL tear. *Contemp Pediatr.* 2006;23:26–39

Rome ES. Sports-related injuries among adolescents: when do they occur, and how can we prevent them? *Pediatr Rev.* 1995;16:184–187

Ryu RKN, Fan RS. Adolescent and pediatric sport injuries. *Pediatr Clin North Am.* 1998;45:1601–1635

Stricker PR. *Sport Success Rx! Your Child's Prescription for the Best Experience.* Elk Grove Village, IL: American Academy of Pediatrics; 2006

Sullivan JA, Anderson SJ. *Care of the Young Athlete.* Rosemont, IL: American Academy of Orthopaedic Surgeons, American Academy of Pediatrics; 2000

Evaluation of Limp

Paul Bryan, MD

CASE STUDY

A 6-year-old boy who has a 2-day history of right knee pain and limp is brought to the office. No history of knee trauma, swelling, redness, or associated fever is present. The medical history is unremarkable. The boy is afebrile, and his height and weight are at the 10th percentile for age. Examination of the right leg reveals decreased abduction and internal rotation of the hip; the knee is normal. The boy limps when he walks and favors his right leg.

Questions

1. What is the differential diagnosis of painful and painless limp in children?
2. What is the differential diagnosis of knee pain in children?
3. What laboratory and radiographic tests are indicated in the evaluation of children with limp?
4. What is the appropriate management of children with suspected infectious causes of limp?

A limp is a gait disturbance that occurs when an effort is made to minimize weight bearing on an affected leg so that pain and instability are reduced. The disturbance may be secondary to muscle weakness, deformity, pain, or a combination thereof. Muscle weakness may be due to primary muscle disease, neurologic conditions, or disuse atrophy. Structural causes of limp include leg length discrepancy and joint stiffness, while painful causes of limp include trauma, synovitis, infection (ie, bone, joint, or soft-tissue), or neoplasm. A limp can be a sign of significant underlying disease, and accurate diagnosis and appropriate management are essential to prevent potentially serious morbidity, including long-term disability.

Epidemiology

A limp may be due to pain originating in a leg or to pain referred from the abdomen or spine. Age often defines the diagnostic possibilities because certain disorders are seen more frequently in particular age groups. Infectious causes of limp occur more frequently in infants and young children, and noninfectious causes are more common in school-aged children and adolescents (Box 93-1).

Clinical Presentation

A painful limp usually has an acute onset and may be associated with systemic signs such as fever or irritability, especially when the etiology is infectious. Toddlers may simply refuse to walk or walk with a slow cautious gait when they are in pain rather than limp. Non-painful limp often has an insidious onset and is commonly due to weakness (eg, muscular dystrophy) or deformity (eg, leg length discrepancy).

Pathophysiology

Normal gait has 2 phases: stance and swing. During the stance phase, either one or both feet are on the ground; during the swing phase, one foot is not touching the ground as the limb is moved forward. Stance phase is shortened in limp to decrease the amount of time spent in bearing weight on the affected side or to minimize instability.

Normal adult gait is smooth and efficient, requiring the coordinated actions of the muscles of the legs and pelvis. Normal gait in children varies according to age and developmental maturity. Toddlers typically walk with a broad-based, tiptoe, "bouncing" gait with arms abducted for balance. They may initiate the stance phase with either toe or heel strike. By 2 years of age, children should initiate the stance phase consistently with heel strike. Children who are 3 to 4 years of age should exhibit normal adult gait with reciprocating arm swing most of the time.

Several types of abnormal gaits are recognized. A shortened stance phase due to pain is characteristic of an **antalgic gait.** Weakness of the hip abductors (gluteus medius) leads to a **Trendelenburg gait,** where the pelvis dips down during stance phase, producing a swaying type of gait. A tiptoe or **toe-to-heel gait** is normal in children for several months after they learn to walk. Persistence of such a gait beyond 2 years of age is abnormal and may result from either idiopathic heel-cord contracture or contracture secondary to cerebral palsy.

Differential Diagnosis

Trauma is a frequent cause of limp in children and adolescents. Toddlers may simply refuse to walk and have an occult fracture, such as a **toddler's fracture.** This is an oblique or spiral fracture of the middle or distal tibia, which occurs after a fall or jump involving

Box 93-1. Differential Diagnosis of Limp in Children	
Children Ages 1 to 3 Years	***Painless Limp***
Painful Limp	• LCPD (chronic phase)
• Septic arthritis/osteomyelitis	• Developmental hip dysplasia
• Transient synovitis	• Neuromuscular disease (cerebral palsy, muscular dystrophy)
• Intervertebral diskitis	• Leg length discrepancy
• Juvenile idiopathic arthritis (JIA)	
• Neoplasia (leukemia, metastatic disease)	***Children and Adolescents Ages 11 Years and Older***
• Trauma (toddler's fractures)	***Painful Limp***
• Child abuse	• Trauma
	• Septic arthritis/osteomyelitis
Painless Limp	• Slipped capital femoral epiphysis (SCFE)
• Developmental hip dysplasia	• Osgood-Schlatter disease
• Neuromuscular disease (cerebral palsy)	• JIA
• Leg length discrepancy	• Sickle cell pain crisis
	• Neoplasia (leukemia, primary bone tumor, metastatic disease)
Children Ages 4 to 10 Years	
Painful Limp	***Painless Limp***
• Septic arthritis/osteomyelitis	• SCFE
• Transient synovitis	• Leg length discrepancy
• Trauma	• Neuromuscular disease (cerebral palsy, muscular dystrophy)
• Legg-Calvé-Perthes disease (LCPD) (acute phase)	• Scoliosis
• Intervertebral diskitis	
• JIA	
• Sickle cell pain crisis	
• Neoplasia (leukemia, primary bone tumor, metastatic disease)	

a twisting motion. Toddlers are at risk for such injuries because of their unsteady gait. Standard anteroposterior (AP) and lateral x-ray views can initially be normal, and oblique views may be helpful. Follow-up x-rays or a bone scan may be necessary to make the diagnosis. Older children will usually be able to recall a specific injury and localize pain to a specific area. X-rays are usually obtained to determine if a fracture is present. Individuals who have tenderness over open growth plates should be splinted and warrant close follow-up even with normal x-rays, as there is a possibility of a Salter-Harris type I fracture, which occurs through the growth plate and may not be radiographically apparent.

Painless limp in toddlers may be due to **developmental hip dysplasia, cerebral palsy,** or **leg length discrepancy** (anisomelia). As a result of developmental hip dysplasia, children may have a Trendelenburg gait secondary to leg length discrepancy or to weakness of the hip abductors. Children with spastic cerebral palsy often walk on their toes because of increased tone or heel-cord contractures. Functional or apparent leg length discrepancies may result from pelvic obliquity or spinal deformity. Children with true leg length inequality compensate by either walking on tiptoe on the shorter side or bending the knee on the longer side; in either case, their gait is abnormal. Limb discrepancies may be managed with orthotics (eg, heel lifts) for mild cases, and surgical lengthening or shortening procedures may be necessary for more severe cases.

Transient synovitis of the hip is a benign self-limited inflammatory process involving the synovial lining and is one of the most common causes of limp in the young child. The exact cause of the inflammation is not known. There has been an association with certain upper respiratory infections, but no infectious agent has been identified. Trauma has also been implicated as a potential factor in initiating the inflammatory response because the contusion triggers a chemical synovitis. Age varies, but it typically affects children 3 to 8 years old. Individuals usually present with acute onset of unilateral hip pain associated with a limp. There can be referred pain to the anterior thigh or knee. Most children are either afebrile or have low-grade temperatures (<38.5°C [101.3°F]). The leg may be held in a position of abduction, flexion, and external rotation to reduce intracapsular pressure and associated pain. Symptoms are usually unilateral, but in up to 5% of cases there is bilateral involvement, often with one side being more symptomatic than the other.

Laboratory evaluation typically consists of complete blood count (CBC), erythrocyte sedimentation rate (ESR), and C-reactive protein (CRP). The laboratory results are usually within normal limits or slightly elevated. X-rays are often obtained, which are usually normal or show signs suggestive of an effusion. An ultrasound is often performed to look for the presence of an effusion within the joint, which is often present in this condition. If an arthrocentesis is performed, the fluid in transient synovitis usually has a white blood cell (WBC) count of less than 50,000/mm³ and a negative Gram stain. Individuals with normal laboratory values or with a fluid aspirate not suggestive of septic arthritis (when arthrocentesis has been performed) are typically managed with supportive care and close follow-up within

24 to 48 hours. Rest and nonsteroidal anti-inflammatory agents are the mainstays of therapy. Virtually all children recover within 3 to 10 days with no significant sequelae. Recurrence rates vary from 4% to 17% within the first 6 months following an episode of synovitis.

Septic arthritis occurs when there is an infection within the joint space. In children, this usually occurs in the face of bacteremia, with hematogenous spread to the highly vascular synovium. It can also occur from contiguous spread of an adjacent infection (eg, osteomyelitis) or by direct inoculation (eg, surgery or penetrating trauma). *Staphylococcus aureus* remains the most common pathogen identified across all age groups, with increasing incidences of community-acquired methicillin-resistant strains. Infants younger than 2 months of age can also be infected by neonatal pathogens, such as *Streptococcus agalactiae* (eg, group B streptococcus [GBS]) and gram-negative enteric organisms (eg, *Escherichia coli*). *S aureus*, *Streptococcus pyogenes*, *Streptococcus pneumoniae*, and *Kingella kingae* are the main organisms identified in the 2-month to 5-year age group. Children older than 5 years will usually have infections caused by *S aureus* or *S pyogenes*. *Neisseria gonorrhoeae* infections can be seen in sexually active adolescents.

Infants and children will often present with fever, decreased use of the affected extremity, limp, and refusal to walk. The most commonly affected joint is the hip, which is classically held in a position of abduction, flexion, and external rotation to reduce intracapsular pressure and associated pain. Passive range of motion typically elicits significant discomfort and resistance. Parents of infants may notice considerable crying with manipulation of the legs with activities such as diaper changing.

Subtle or early cases can often present a diagnostic challenge because there can be significant clinical and laboratory overlap with transient synovitis. Unfortunately there is no highly sensitive or specific laboratory test that can readily distinguish these 2 entities. Fever higher than 38.5°C (101.3°F) was shown to be the single best predictor of septic arthritis in one study, with no children diagnosed with transient synovitis having a temperature above 38.5°C. Other predictors include refusal to bear weight, ESR greater than 40 mm/h, a CRP greater than 2.0 mg/dL, and serum WBC count greater than 12,000/mm³. Unfortunately, with the exception of high fevers, one or more of these factors can also occur with transient synovitis. The presence of one of these 5 factors was associated with a probability of having septic arthritis of around 37%, while the presence of all 5 factors was associated with a probability of 98%. Imaging often consists of x-rays and ultrasound. X-rays usually are non-diagnostic but may demonstrate joint-space widening suggestive of an effusion. Ultrasound will usually demonstrate the presence of an effusion.

Analysis of synovial fluid remains the gold standard for the diagnosis of septic arthritis, and arthrocentesis of any effusion under sedation or anesthesia is indicated if there is a clinical suspicion of septic arthritis. A WBC count greater than 50,000/mm³ within the fluid aspirate is generally considered diagnostic of septic arthritis; however, elevated counts can be seen in certain rheumatologic conditions. The presence of bacteria on Gram stain of joint aspirate regardless of WBC count suggests infection. Routine cultures of joint aspirate as well as peripheral blood cultures should be sent. In addition, with the increasing recognition of *K kingae* as a causative agent in septic arthritis, joint aspirations should be directly inoculated into blood culture bottles to enhance isolation because this organism is difficult to recover with standard culture techniques. In most studies, only around 50% of joint aspirate cultures grew out an identifiable pathogen. In one recent study, close to 50% of the aspirates that were sterile on standard culture media grew out *K kingae* from blood cultures.

Complications occur in 10% to 25% of all cases, increasing when delays of 5 days or more have passed before initiation of therapy. These complications include abnormal bone growth, permanent limp, unstable articulation of the affected joint, and decreased range of motion.

Osteomyelitis is an infection of the bone that is typically caused by a bacterial organism. Close to 50% of pediatric cases of osteomyelitis occur in children younger than 5 years. Most cases of osteomyelitis in children occur from hematogenous deposition of bacteria into the bone marrow during a transient episode of bacteremia. Other cases may be caused from contiguous spread of an adjacent infection or direct inoculation. Osteomyelitis most commonly begins in the highly vascularized metaphysis of long bones of young children. The femur, tibia, and humerus account for most cases. As with septic arthritis, *S aureus* remains the most common organism identified across all age groups. Other organisms include *S pyogenes*, *S pneumoniae*, and *K kingae*. Young infants can also be infected by neonatal pathogens such as GBS and enteric gram-negative organisms. Individuals with sickle-cell disease are commonly infected with *Salmonella*. Individuals who have suffered a puncture wound through the foot can be infected with *Pseudomonas aeruginosa*, resulting in osteochondritis.

Children often present with fever and pain at the affected site. Younger children may present with limp or refusal to bear weight. If there is subperiosteal spread, there may be erythema, warmth, and swelling at the affected site.

Laboratory tests can be supportive of a diagnosis of osteomyelitis, but are usually not specific. Typically a serum CBC, ESR, and CRP are obtained along with blood cultures. Leukocytosis may be present, but in more than half the cases, the WBC count can be normal. Inflammatory markers are elevated in up to 90% of cases. Blood cultures are positive in up to 55%. X-rays are often normal or show only soft-tissue changes early in the course of the disease. Periosteal reactions and lytic lesions are usually not present until day 10 to 21 into the disease. Bone scans can be helpful in the preverbal child or in individuals who cannot localize their pain. Magnetic resonance imaging (MRI) has become the study of choice, with a reported sensitivity of 97%. It is very useful for distinguishing between bone and soft-tissue infections.

Diskitis refers to an inflammatory process involving the intervertebral disks. This disease typically occurs in children younger than 5 years. It occurs almost exclusively in the lumbar region, causing progressive limp, back pain, and refusal to walk. Most children are afebrile. It is thought to occur in younger children because of the presence of vascular channels in the cartilaginous region of the disk space as well as an abundant intraosseous arterial anastomoses. These vascular channels disappear with age. Laboratory studies are often nonspecific, with slight elevations in the peripheral WBC count and ESR. X-rays are abnormal in most cases (75%), with decreased vertebral disk space and erosion of adjacent vertebral endplates being the most common abnormalities seen. Bone scans will demonstrate nonspecific increased marker uptake in the affected area. Computed tomography scans rarely provide a specific diagnosis and are not generally used. Magnetic resonance imaging will demonstrate characteristic inflammatory changes and allow for differentiation from other conditions, such as vertebral osteomyelitis.

The exact etiology of diskitis is not known, and the treatment is somewhat controversial. Several authors propose that it is the result of an infectious process and warrants antibiotic therapy. Others propose that it is simply a benign self-limited disease because most cultures are sterile and patients can recover without any antimicrobial therapy.

Legg-Calvé-Perthes disease (LCPD) is an idiopathic avascular necrosis of the femoral head. The exact etiology is unclear but involves some disruption in the vascular supply of the capital femoral epiphysis. This is most commonly seen in children 3 to 12 years old (median age 7 years). It is usually unilateral, but can be bilateral in up to 15% of cases. Children typically present with a chronic intermittent limp that can be either painful or painless. It is not uncommon for the child to be symptomatic for months before a diagnosis is made. Pain is usually worsened with internal rotation and abduction.

Laboratory tests are usually normal. X-rays early in the course of the disease may either be negative or show widening of the joint space. In later stages, radiographic findings include an increased density and decreased size of the femoral head (necrosis), patchy areas of radiolucency near the epiphysis (fragmentation), and flattening of the femoral head (reconstitution).

Slipped capital femoral epiphysis (SCFE) is a displacement or slipping of the femoral head from the neck of the femur through the open physis (growth plate). This is the most common hip disorder affecting adolescents. It is more common in boys than girls and occurs more frequently among African Americans and Hispanics than whites. Typical age of onset is 11 to 14 years. Individuals who are often noted to be overweight present with a chief complain of knee pain. They will often have an antalgic gait. The foot is noted to be externally rotated in severe slips but may be neutral or intoed in mild slips. The examination of the knee will be normal without discomfort, despite the complaint of knee pain. Passive flexion of the hip will often result in obligate external rotation. There will usually be pain with internal rotation. Laboratory testing is not indicated. X-rays of the hip in the AP and frog-leg positions reveal the diagnosis in approximately 80% of the cases. Both hips should be viewed because up to 20% of SCFEs are bilateral. Ultrasound in experienced hands has been shown to be an effective diagnostic tool (sensitivity of 95%). Computed tomography scan and MRI can both reveal the

presence of a slip. The MRI is much more sensitive and can detect physeal widening in the pre-slip condition.

Osgood-Schlatter disease (OSD), or traction apophysitis of the tibial tubercle, is an overuse injury of the knee seen most commonly in adolescent athletes. Repetitive microtrauma causes partial avulsion of the patellar tendon at its insertion on the tibia. Individuals will typically present with a localized bony prominence, swelling, and tenderness over the tibial tubercle at the insertion of the patellar tendon. X-rays are commonly performed to rule out other pathology and will typically demonstrate soft tissue swelling/edema of the skin and tissues, as well as ossific fragments within the tendon. Computed tomography, MRI, and ultrasound will show characteristic changes consistent with OSD, but are generally not indicated.

A limp can also result from certain systemic disease processes, such as **juvenile idiopathic arthritis, sickle cell disease** (SCD), and **neoplastic disease.** Juvenile idiopathic arthritis may involve multiple joints, and there is usually evidence of inflammation (eg, warmth, swelling/effusion, redness). The pain is usually worse in the morning and improves throughout the day. **Sickle cell disease** is now detected on newborn screen, and most patients know of their diagnosis. Acute pain crises with SCD can affect multiple areas, resulting in significant discomfort, limp, and refusal to walk. Careful consideration for infectious etiologies (ie, osteomyelitis) is necessary in the highly febrile or ill child with SCD who presents with a limp or bone pain. In addition, SCD patients are at risk of avascular necrosis of the hip secondary to vasoocclusive episodes. Neoplastic disease processes such as leukemia or primary bone tumors (eg, Ewing sarcoma or osteosarcoma) can present with bone pain and limp. The presence of pallor, petechiae, disseminated lymphadenopathy, or hepatosplenomegaly may suggest the presence of leukemia. The peripheral CBC will usually show the presence of blasts and varying degrees of involvement of the various cell lines (ie, anemia, thrombocytopenia). Primary bone tumors may present with bony deformities or overlying soft-tissue swelling. X-rays will often reveal characteristic bony lesions, which may require an MRI to ascertain involvement. Computed tomography scans may be necessary to look for metastases. Individuals may require referral to an orthopedist for biopsy to ascertain a definitive diagnosis and possibly for amputation. Referral to an oncologist will be necessary to initiate appropriate therapy, including possibly chemotherapy or radiation.

Evaluation

History

The history should focus on the time of onset of the limp, its chronicity, and the degree of disability it produces. Often a history of trauma is provided, even when a non-traumatic cause is present. Young toddlers are often falling as they learn how to walk, and parents will frequently relay some trivial or unrelated injury. Delayed motor development may be a sign of neuromuscular disease such as cerebral palsy, whereas a history of loss of motor milestones may indicate muscular dystrophy or spinal cord tumor. It is important to remember that pelvic pathology may be referred to the hip, and hip pathology is often referred to the knee or thigh.

Physical Examination

Physical examination begins with observation for any overt deformities (eg, leg length discrepancy, deformity, joint swelling). All joints should be palpated, and the presence of swelling, tenderness, erythema, or warmth should be noted. A thorough evaluation of the hips is essential in children with knee pain. The type of gait abnormality may be determined by observing children walk or run.

Children should also be examined both supine and standing, if possible. Standing children can be assessed for pelvic obliquity and spinal deformities. Range of motion of the hips, knees, ankles, and feet can be checked in supine children, comparing the affected side with the non-affected side. Deep tendon reflexes and muscle strength should be assessed, and leg length measurements should also be made as indicated. Children should be supine for a true measurement of leg length, taken as the distance from the anterosuperior iliac spine to the medial malleolus. A discrepancy of more than 2 cm is considered significant in adults. The significance of discrepancies can be confirmed by imaging studies.

Laboratory Tests

Laboratory procedures are usually necessary in children with an acute onset of limp. Complete blood count, CRP, and ESR are useful markers of systemic disease or significant inflammation. There can be significant overlap between the differing etiologies, and no single screening test reliably distinguishes between the various inflammatory and infectious causes of limp. Blood and local cultures (eg, joint or bone fluid) may be useful in the evaluation of suspected infectious entities. Additional testing for rheumatologic causes may be clinically indicated, such as antinuclear antibody or rheumatoid factor (see Chapter 130).

Imaging Studies

X-rays are the most commonly used imaging study. Usually 2 views are obtained. Examination of the hip involves imaging in the AP view as well as the frog-leg position. Both hips should be x-rayed for comparison and to assess for the presence of bilateral disease. Ultrasound is helpful if there is concern about an effusion within the joint space and can also be used to guide diagnostic and therapeutic interventions (eg, arthrocentesis). Computed tomography scan can sometimes provide useful information, but MRI is being used with increasing frequency because of its superior resolution and lack of radiation. Bone scans may be helpful in the early stages of disease when x-rays are typically normal or when there is difficulty establishing a localized area of involvement.

Management

The management depends on the etiology. Management of septic arthritis consists of surgical drainage and intravenous (IV) antibiotics. Empiric therapy typically consists of a semisynthetic

penicillinase-resistant penicillin (eg, nafcillin or oxacillin). If there are high rates of community-acquired methicillin-resistant strains of *S aureus* in the region, then clindamycin or vancomycin may be necessary until sensitivities can be performed. The addition of a third-generation cephalosporin is indicated in the newborn period pending gram stain and culture results or when *N gonorrhoeae* is suspected in adolescents. Length of therapy is typically 2 to 4 weeks of IV antibiotics. Prognosis is generally good with prompt diagnosis and management within 4 days of symptom onset.

Management of osteomyelitis also consists of IV antibiotics. Occasionally surgery may be indicated, particularly if there is a subperiosteal or soft-tissue abscess or sequestra are present. Empiric antibiotic therapy consists of a semisynthetic penicillinase-resistant penicillin (eg, nafcillin or oxacillin). In areas where community-acquired methicillin-resistant organisms are of concern, clindamycin or vancomycin may be necessary. Neonates and individuals with SCD require the addition of a third-generation cephalosporin pending culture results. In individuals with a presumed pseudomonal infection, an extended spectrum β-lactam (eg, ceftazidime, cefepime, or piperacillin/tazobactam) plus an aminoglycoside are indicated. Four to 6 weeks of antibiotic therapy is recommended. Some studies have shown that switching to an oral antibiotic may be acceptable following a week of parenteral therapy if good compliance is likely, an organism has been identified, clinical improvement is noted, the patient is afebrile, and the inflammatory markers have begun to normalize. Oral dosages 2 to 3 times those normally recommended for non-bony infections are often used for β-lactam antibiotics. Other oral antibiotics (eg, clindamycin, trimethoprim-sulfamethoxazole, fluoroquinolones) have excellent bioavailability, and the usual oral dosages may be used. Consultation with an infectious disease specialist is often indicated.

Supportive measures with nonsteroidal anti-inflammatory agents are generally indicated for the management of diskitis. Most patients recover without any complications.

Prompt referral to an orthopedist is indicated in cases of LCPD. The goal of treatment of LCPD is to maintain full joint mobility and prevent deformity of the femoral head. Bed rest and immobilization decrease the pain and help restore range of motion. Traction and abduction casts/braces are used to contain the femoral head within the acetabulum in an effort to maintain its spherical shape. Surgical correction of gross deformities of the femoral head may be necessary in severe cases.

Treatment for SCFE consists of surgical reduction and stabilization with placement of screws through the epiphysis. The screws are typically left in place and do not need to be removed. Non–weight bearing is maintained until early callus is seen on the posterior-inferior metaphysis and the pain has resolved. Gradual and progressive weight bearing is allowed, and progression to full weight bearing usually occurs 3 to 4 months after fixation. No running or jumping is allowed until the physis closes.

Treatment of OSD consists of rest, ice, nonsteroidal anti-inflammatory agents, and strengthening exercises of the quadriceps and hamstring muscles. Surgical treatment is rarely indicated and is reserved for those patients who do not respond to conservative therapy.

Prognosis

The prognosis depends on the etiology of the limp.

The prognosis is good in most cases of septic arthritis and osteomyelitis if the infection is diagnosed early and treated appropriately. Prognosis of osteomyelitis is usually good, with less than 2% of patients who receive at least 3 weeks of antibiotic therapy developing chronic osteomyelitis. Treatment of chronic disease can be difficult, often necessitating prolonged courses of antibiotics (up to 6–12 months) and multiple surgeries for debridement. Rare complications include disturbances in bone growth, limb length discrepancies, arthritis, abnormal gait, and pathologic fractures. Prognosis is also good if diagnosis occurs at a young age (<8 years old). The main complication is degenerative arthritis of the hip.

Prognosis of LCPD is related to the degree of femoral head involvement and age at onset of the disease. Children younger than 6 years have the best prognosis. The risk of development of degenerative arthritis in adulthood increases in children whose disease is more extensive and whose condition is diagnosed later (ie, after 8 years of age).

If patients with SCFE are untreated, the potential for further slipping of the femoral head remains until the growth plate closes. Potential treatment-related complications of SCFE include chondrolysis of the femoral head and acetabulum, avascular necrosis, and fracture at the site of pin placement. In general the prognosis is good and is based on the degree of slippage. The main complication is the development of avascular necrosis of the femoral head, which typically leads to degenerative hip disease later in life. This occurs in up to 15% of slips and is more common in an unstable SCFE. An SCFE is stable when the individual can walk with or without crutches, an unstable SCFE occurs when the child cannot walk. Only 7% of patients in the moderate-slip category have a poor outcome compared with 24% of patients in the severe-slip category.

In about 5% to 10% of cases, OSD may become chronic, with persistent swelling and tenderness. In such cases an x-ray may show the formation of an ossicle over the tibial tubercle; this ossicle may require surgical resection.

Selected References

Caird MS, Flynn JM, Leung YL, Millman JE, D'Itallia JG, Dormans JP. Factors distinguishing septic arthritis from transient synovitis of the hip in children. *J Bone Joint Surg.* 2006;88:1251–1257

Dahl MT. Limb length discrepancy. *Pediatr Clin North Am.* 1996;43:849–865

Do TT. Transient synovitis as a cause of painful limps in children. *Curr Opin Pediatr.* 2000;12:48–51

Fernandez M, Carrol CL, Baker CJ. Discitis and vertebral osteomyelitis in children: an 18-year review. *Pediatrics.* 2000;105:1299–1304

Frank G, Mahoney HM, Eppes SC. Musculoskeletal infections in children. *Pediatr Clin North Am.* 2005;52:1083–1106

Gutierrez K. Bone and joint infections in children. *Pediatr Clin North Am.* 2005;52:779–794

Henrickson M, Passo MH. Recognizing patterns in chronic limb pain. *Contemp Pediatr.* 1994;11:33–62

Hurley JM, Betz RR, Loder RT, Davidson RS, Alburger PD, Steel HH. Slipped capital femoral epiphysis. The prevalence of late contralateral slip. *J Bone Joint Surg.* 1996;78:226–230

Kocher MS, Mandiga R, Zurakowski D, Barnewolt C, Kasser JR. Validation of a clinical prediction rule for the differentiation between septic arthritis and transient synovitis of the hip in children. *J Bone Joint Surg.* 2004;86:1629–1635

Koop S, Quanbeck D. Three common causes of childhood hip pain. *Pediatr Clin North Am.* 1996;43:1053–1066

Lehman CL, Arons RR, Loder RT, Vitale MG. The epidemiology of slipped capital femoral epiphysis: an update. *J Pediatr Orthop.* 2006;26:286–290

Loder RT. Controversies in slipped capital femoral epiphysis. *Orthop Clin North Am.* 2006;37:211–221

Luhman SJ, Jones A, Schootman M, Gordon EJ, Schoenecker PL, Luhman JD. Differentiation between septic arthritis and transient synovitis of the hip in children with clinical prediction algorithms. *J Bone Joint Surg.* 2004;86:956–962

MacEwen GD, Dehne R. The limping child. *Pediatr Rev.* 1991;12:268–274

Renshaw TS. The child who has a limp. *Pediatr Rev.* 1995;16:458–465

Reynolds RAK. Diagnosis and treatment of slipped capital femoral epiphysis. *Curr Opin Pediatr.* 1998;11:80–83

Schmit P, Glorion C. Osteomyelitis in infants and children. *Eur Radiol.* 2004;14:L44–L54

Shah SS. Abnormal gait in a child with fever: diagnosing septic arthritis of the hip. *Pediatr Emerg Care.* 2005;21:336–341

Vazquez M. Osteomyelitis in children. *Curr Opin Pediatr.* 2002;14:112–115

Yagupsk P. *Kingella kingae:* from medical rarity to an emerging pediatric pathogen. *Lancet.* 2004;4:358–367

CASE RESOLUTION

In the case described at the beginning of the chapter, the child's history and physical examination seem to be consistent with Legg-Calvé-Perthes disease. The child's knee pain is actually secondary to hip pathology. The diagnosis may have been missed if the physician had not examined the hips and noted the abnormality in range of motion. Both anteroposterior and frog-leg x-rays of the hips were taken, which showed widening of the joint space. Orthopedic consultation was obtained, and hospitalization for bed rest and ensured immobilization were recommended.

Musculoskeletal Disorders of the Neck and Back

Carol D. Berkowitz, MD

CASE STUDY

A 4-week-old male infant is brought to the office by his mother, who complains that her son always holds his head tilted to the right. She reports that he has held it in this position for about 1 week and prefers to look mainly to the left. The infant is the 8-lb, 8-oz product of a term gestation born via forceps extraction, and he had no complications in the neonatal period. He is feeding well on breast milk and has no history of fever, upper respiratory symptoms, or vomiting and diarrhea.

On examination, the head is tilted toward the right side with limited lateral rotation to the right and decreased lateral side bending to the left. Except for the presence of a small mass palpable on the right side of the neck, the examination is within normal limits.

Questions

1. What laboratory or radiologic studies are indicated in infants with torticollis?
2. What is the differential diagnosis of torticollis in infants?
3. What are some of the common musculoskeletal abnormalities that may be seen in association with torticollis?
4. What are other common musculoskeletal problems in children and adolescents?
5. What is the current recommended management of children and adolescents with idiopathic scoliosis?

Children with disorders of the spine can present with deformity, back pain, or occasionally both. Non-traumatic congenital and developmental deformities of the spine are frequently encountered in pediatric practice. Torticollis and scoliosis are 2 of the most common disorders in children that present as spinal deformity. **Torticollis,** or wry neck, is a positional abnormality of the neck resulting in abnormal tilting and rotation of the head. **Scoliosis** refers to any lateral curvature of the spine that measures more than 10 degrees as determined by an anteroposterior x-ray of the spine. Scoliosis can be divided into 3 categories: infantile (birth–3 years), juvenile (3–10 years), and adolescent. **Back pain** is a far less common complaint in children than in adults. When such pain occurs in children, it usually signals the presence of organic disease. In adolescents, musculoskeletal strain is a common etiology.

Epidemiology

Some degree of spinal asymmetry is seen in about 2% to 5% of the population.

The most common type of **torticollis** seen in children is congenital muscular torticollis. The incidence of this common neonatal orthopedic complaint is increased in breech presentations and difficult deliveries. It is associated with developmental dysplasia of the hip (DDH) in as many as 10% to 20% of affected infants. Family history may be positive in up to 10% of cases.

Acquired torticollis, usually secondary to infectious or traumatic causes, is much more common in older children. Episodes of benign paroxysmal torticollis, which often begin in the first year of life and generally resolve by 5 years of age, may have a familial basis. An association with benign paroxysmal vertigo and migraines has been noted.

Infantile scoliosis is rare in the United States and usually spontaneously resolves. The prevalence of juvenile **scoliosis** among school-aged children is 3% to 5%. A right thoracic single curve is the most common curve seen by physicians. Seventy-five percent to 80% of cases of structural scoliosis are idiopathic, 10% are due to neuromuscular causes, 5% are congenital, and the remaining 5% to 10% are due to trauma or miscellaneous causes. Scoliosis that begins in childhood affects boys and girls equally, and affected boys actually outnumber girls during the first 3 years of life. Idiopathic scoliosis that develops after the age of 10 years is seen more frequently in girls than in boys, however. The ratio is approximately 5 to 7:1. In children with cerebral palsy, the incidence of scoliosis is increased, and it is found in about 20% of all cases.

Back pain is quite uncommon in preadolescent children. In most cases of back pain in children, it is possible to determine the etiology, unlike in adults, where it is often difficult to identify the cause.

Clinical Presentation

Although **torticollis** may be noted at birth, it usually manifests at 2 to 4 weeks of age. Infants with congenital muscular torticollis present with a characteristic head tilt toward the affected side and the chin pointing toward the opposite side secondary to unilateral fibrosis and contracture of the sternocleidomastoid muscle (Figure 94-1). Unrecognized or untreated cases of torticollis may present as plagiocephaly (see Chapter 58) or facial asymmetry during infancy. Benign paroxysmal torticollis of infancy may present as recurrent episodes of head tilt that may be associated with vomiting, ataxia, agitation, or malaise (Dx Box).

Figure 94-1. Torticollis. Infant with congenital muscular torticollis showing head tilt.

Dx

Torticollis and Scoliosis

Torticollis
- Head tilt
- Limited range of motion of the neck
- Contracture of the sternocleidomastoid muscle
- Plagiocephaly (congenital torticollis)
- Firm, non-tender, mobile mass within the body of the sternocleidomastoid muscle (congenital torticollis)

Scoliosis
- Lateral curvature of the spine
- Some pain
- Back or truncal asymmetry

No obvious deformity may be noted in mild **scoliosis.** Asymmetry of shoulder heights, scapular prominence or position, and waistline or pelvic levelness may all be signs of scoliosis (see Dx Box) (Figure 94-2A). Back pain is reported in 25% of adolescents with idiopathic scoliosis. Scoliosis may be detected during school-based screening programs or preparticipation sports physicals.

When pain is present, further examination for some other cause (eg, bone tumors, spondylolysis, spondylolisthesis) is warranted.

Preverbal children with **back pain** may present with limp or refusal to bear weight or walk.

Figure 94-2. Scoliosis. A. Child with scoliosis (rear view). B. Child with scoliosis performing bend test.

Pathophysiology

Torticollis may be either congenital or acquired. The etiology of congenital muscular torticollis is unknown. It is believed to be due to intrauterine positioning or trauma to the soft tissues of the neck during delivery, with resulting ischemia of the sternocleidomastoid muscle secondary to venous occlusion. This leads to edema and degeneration of the muscle fibers with eventual fibrosis of the muscle body. Deformities of the face and skull may result if the condition is left untreated. Plagiocephaly (cranial asymmetry), with flattening of the face on the affected side and flattening of the occiput on the contralateral side, is seen most commonly.

Scoliosis is a lateral curvature of the spine, unlike kyphosis and lordosis, which are curves in the anteroposterior plane. Scoliosis can be either functional (nonstructural) or structural. Because no fixed deformity of the spine is associated with functional scoliosis, the apparent curvature disappears on lying down or forward flexion. Individuals with leg length discrepancies appear to have scoliosis but have no spinal abnormality. Structural scoliosis may be idiopathic or caused by various underlying disorders. The cause of idiopathic scoliosis is unknown, and there seems to be a higher incidence of scoliosis in other family members. In addition, there are reports of lower levels of melatonin in patients with scoliosis, compared with age-matched controls. This finding has not been confirmed and its relationship to the scoliosis is unclear. Abnormalities of fibrillin have also been seen in some patients with scoliosis, a finding also reported in patients with Marfan syndrome. In structural scoliosis, as the spine curves laterally, it forces the vertebrae to rotate, resulting in deformity of attached structures. For example, a "rib hump" may be produced due to scoliosis in the thoracic spine (see Figure 94-2B). Pelvic obliquity or flank prominence may be produced when the curvature is in the lumbar spine.

Differential Diagnosis

The differential diagnosis of congenital and acquired **torticollis** is presented in Box 94-1. Congenital muscular torticollis is the most common cause of congenital torticollis. Torticollis may appear in association with nystagmus and head nodding, a condition referred to as spasmus nutans. Acquired torticollis is seen primarily in older infants and children. Cervical lymphadenitis is a common cause in children 1 to 5 years of age, whereas trauma to the soft tissues or muscles of the neck is seen more frequently in school-aged children. Acute episodes (eg, benign paroxysmal torticollis of infancy) must be differentiated from chronic conditions (eg, Sandifer syndrome, rheumatoid arthritis).

Box 94-1. Common Causes of Torticollis

Congenital
- Congenital muscular torticollis
- Pterygium coli (skin web)
- Occipitocervical spine anomalies (eg, Klippel-Feil syndrome)

Acquired
- Infectious
- Cervical lymphadenitis
- Retropharyngeal abscess
- Osteomyelitis of cervical vertebrae
- Traumatic
- Atlanto-occipital, atlas-axis (C1–C2), or C2–C3 subluxation
- Cervical musculature injury (spastic torticollis)
- Cervical spine fractures
- Neurologic
- Tumors (posterior fossa or cervical cord)
- Dystonic drug reactions
- Syringomyelia
- Ocular disturbances (strabismus, nystagmus)
- Other
- Spasmus nutans
- Sandifer syndrome (hiatal hernia with gastroesophageal reflux)
- Benign paroxysmal torticollis of infancy
- Rheumatoid arthritis
- Hysteria
- Soft tissue tumors of the neck

Box 94-2. Common Causes of Scoliosis

Functional Scoliosis
- Poor posture
- Leg length discrepancies
- Muscle spasm
- Herniated disk
- Back injury

Structural Scoliosis
- Idiopathic
- Congenital
- Neuromuscular
- Miscellaneous
- Trauma (eg, fractures or dislocations of the vertebrae)
- Intraspinal tumors
- Metabolic disorders (eg, juvenile osteoporosis, osteogenesis imperfecta, mucopolysaccharidosis)
- Neurocutaneous syndromes (eg, neurofibromatosis)
- Marfan syndrome

Functional or nonstructural **scoliosis** may be secondary to poor posture, leg length discrepancies, or muscle spasm. Structural scoliosis can be classified into idiopathic, congenital, neuromuscular, and miscellaneous forms (Box 94-2). Idiopathic scoliosis, which is by far the most common type of structural scoliosis, may be divided into 3 categories based on age: infantile (0–3 years), juvenile (3–10 years), and adolescent (>10 years). The adolescent form occurs most frequently.

Congenital scoliosis results from anomalies of the spine such as hemivertebrae or failure of vertebral segmentation. The incidence of cardiac and renal anomalies is increased. Although neuromuscular scoliosis is most often seen in children with spastic cerebral palsy, it may also be apparent in other conditions such as poliomyelitis, meningomyelocele, muscular dystrophy, Friedreich ataxia, and spinal muscular atrophy. The miscellaneous causes of scoliosis are uncommon and include trauma, metabolic disorders, and neurocutaneous diseases.

The most common causes of **back pain** in children may be classified into 5 categories (Box 94-3). Because the spine of children is smaller and has greater flexibility and ligamentous strength, children have a higher tolerance to trauma and a lower risk of injury than adults do. Infection (eg, diskitis) and neoplasia are perhaps more common in children. Common causes of back pain in adults, such as herniated disks or musculoskeletal low back pain (usually secondary to muscle strain), are uncommon in children. Only about 2% of all herniated disks occur in children. Predisposed individuals often experience their first episode of musculoskeletal low back pain during adolescence or young adulthood.

Box 94-3. Common Causes of Back Pain in Children

Infectious
- Myalgias (eg, influenza)
- Diskitis (more common in children <5 years of age)
- Vertebral osteomyelitis (pyogenic, tuberculosis [Potts disease])
- Referred pain (pyelonephritis, pneumonia)

Inflammatory
- Rheumatologic diseases (juvenile rheumatoid arthritis, ankylosing spondylitis)
- Crohn disease/ulcerative colitis/psoriatic arthritis
- Disk space calcification

Neoplastic
- Primary vertebral and spinal tumors (eg, Ewing sarcoma, osteosarcoma, neuroblastoma)
- Metastatic disease (eg, neuroblastoma)
- Benign tumors (eg, eosinophilic granuloma, osteoid osteoma)

Developmental
- Spondylolysis, spondylolisthesis (adolescents)
- Scheuermann kyphosis (adolescents)

Traumatic
- Herniated nucleus pulposus (disk herniation)
- Ligamentous or muscle strain (eg, overuse syndromes)
- Compression fracture of vertebrae

Other
- Sickle cell crisis
- Osteoporosis (eg, rickets, osteogenesis imperfecta)
- Child abuse
- Psychogenic

Evaluation

History

A careful history may provide clues to diagnosis and etiology (Questions box). Back pain is reported in about 25% of adolescents with scoliosis.

Physical Examination

In children with suspected **torticollis,** a thorough examination with specific attention to the head and neck region should be performed. Limited head rotation toward the affected side with decreased lateral side bending to the opposite side may occur. During the first 4 to 6 weeks of life, a firm, non-tender mobile mass, which gradually regresses by 6 months of age, may be palpated within the body of the sternocleidomastoid muscle. The hips should be examined for stability because of the association of torticollis with DDH.

In addition, a neurologic examination should also be performed to look for any neurologic deficits that may be signs of an underlying tumor. Fever or signs of inflammation point to infectious causes. Because torticollis may be secondary to visual disturbances such as strabismus, a careful eye examination is warranted. The presence of nystagmus or head nodding suggests spasmus nutans.

Questions

Torticollis, Scoliosis, and Back Pain

Torticollis
- Is there any family history of torticollis?
- What type of delivery did the mother have (eg, cesarean or vaginal)? Were forceps required?
- When was the head tilt first noticed?
- Does the infant move his or her neck in all directions, or does he or she always prefer to look in one direction?
- Does the infant have any recent history of trauma to the head or neck area?
- Is the head tilt persistent or does it come and go?
- Has the infant been sick or febrile?
- Does the child have nystagmus or head bobbing?

Scoliosis
- Is there a family history of scoliosis?
- Have the parents noticed the curvature of the spine? If so, how old was the child when the condition was first noted?
- Has the curvature increased since it was first noticed?
- Does the child have any back pain?
- Has the child had any previous treatment for the condition?
- (If appropriate) Has the child begun menstruating?

Back Pain
- How long has the child had the pain?
- Where is the pain localized?
- Is the pain persistent or does it come and go?
- Does the pain radiate anywhere (eg, down the legs)?
- Is the child limping or having difficulty walking?
- Has the child lost any motor milestones (eg, skills such as walking or standing that he or she could previously perform)?
- What makes the pain better? What makes it worse?
- Has there been any recent history of trauma or has the child begun participating in a new sport or physical activity?
- Has the child had a fever?
- Has the child had any problems with bowel or bladder function?
- Is the child taking any medication?

Screening for **scoliosis** should be part of the routine health maintenance examination of school-aged children and adolescents. Children should be examined with the back fully exposed. The posture should be observed. The presence of any skin lesions such as café-au-lait spots should be noted. Any midline skin defects such as dimples or hair patches should also be noted because they are often associated with underlying spinal lesions. The spine should be palpated for any signs of tenderness, and a complete neurologic examination should be performed.

The back should be observed for asymmetry of the shoulders, scapulae, or pelvis. Physicians should have children bend forward at the waist to an angle of 90 degrees. This maneuver accentuates the curvature of structural scoliosis and emphasizes the rotational deformity of the spine. For example, in thoracic scoliosis, a characteristic rib hump is apparent on the convex side of the curve. A scoliometer can be used to determine the degree of scoliosis. More than 7 degrees of angulation as measured by a scoliometer, felt to correlate with a Cobb angle of 20 degrees, warrants referral to an orthopedist.

Scoliosis is described in terms of the primary or major curve, which is predominantly thoracic. The major curve may be single or compensated by a secondary or minor curve, which is predominantly lumbar. The location is defined by the apical vertebra (eg, T2–T11 = thoracic, T12–L1 = thoracolumbar), the direction of the curvature by the side of convexity, and the severity indicated by the degree of curvature as measured on the spinal radiograph. Curves greater than 15 degrees are abnormal. Mild scoliosis is defined as curvature of less than 20 degrees, moderate as 20 to 40 degrees, and severe as greater than 40 to 45 degrees.

The evaluation of **back pain** begins with observation of children's posture and gait. Any midline skin lesions should be noted. A thorough general physical examination is important because referred pain (eg, pancreatitis, pyelonephritis, nephrolithiasis) may be causing the symptoms in the back. The spine should be palpated for any signs of tenderness. A complete neurologic examination should be performed, and any motor or sensory deficits should be noted. The motor examination should emphasize evaluation of the hips and the lower extremities, including range of motion and strength.

Laboratory Tests

In cases of **congenital torticollis,** laboratory studies are rarely necessary. In acquired torticollis, if any infection is suspected, a complete blood count (CBC) and blood and local cultures may aid in the diagnosis.

No specific laboratory tests are required in the evaluation of idiopathic **scoliosis.** Specific laboratory studies may be performed in the evaluation of other forms of scoliosis as indicated by the history and physical examination (eg, a urine metabolic screen for suspected metabolic disturbances).

Laboratory assessment for **back pain** depends on the history and physical examination. A CBC, blood culture, and erythrocyte sedimentation rate may be useful in the evaluation of suspected infectious etiologies. Rheumatologic studies such as a rheumatoid factor or human leukocyte antigen typing may help in the diagnosis of inflammatory conditions. If the back pain is of acute onset, studies such as a urinalysis or serum amylase would help establish that the pain is referred.

Imaging Studies

X-rays are generally not useful in children with suspected **torticollis** unless bony anomalies are suspected. Magnetic resonance imaging (MRI) of the sternocleidomastoid muscle mass may be considered if an underlying condition (eg, a branchial cleft cyst) is suspected. Computed tomography scan or MRI of the head or cervical spinal cord would be indicated if a neurologic tumor is suspected.

Routine x-rays are not required in the evaluation of all children with mild scoliosis (ie, minor degrees of curvature noted on physical examination). It may be best to obtain x-rays after orthopedic evaluation is complete. A standing anteroposterior spine x-ray is used to determine the location and direction of the curvature, measure the degree of asymmetry (Cobb angle), and evaluate the vertebrae. Repeat x-rays of the spine are used to follow the progression of the curvature over time. Because the risk of curve progression before skeletal maturity is a primary concern, hand and wrist x-rays should be taken to assess bone age in prepubertal children with scoliosis. Magnetic resonance imaging is recommended in individuals with rapid progression of their curve at more than 1 degree per month. Magnetic resonance imaging should include cervical, thoracic, and lumber spine to identify deformities such as an Arnold-Chiari malformation or a tethered cord.

As with scoliosis, routine x-rays are not indicated in all cases of **back pain.** Various radiologic studies may be ordered depending on the suspected diagnosis. X-rays may be useful in the evaluation of suspected vertebral abnormalities such as spondylolysis and spondylolisthesis. However, these conditions may represent incidental findings and not be the source of the back pain. If diskitis is suspected, a bone scan may be more appropriate than x-rays. Similarly, a bone scan or MRI is useful in the evaluation of suspected vertebral tumors.

Management

Treatment of congenital muscular **torticollis** consists of **passive stretching exercises** of the neck. With the neck in a neutral position (ie, not hyperextended), the head is bent to one side so that the ear on the side opposite to the contracted muscle is brought to the shoulder, or the chin is lowered to touch the shoulder on the affected side. In addition, **changing the placement of the crib** in relation to the nursery door and **repositioning toys and mobiles** in the crib stimulate children to look toward the side opposite the preferred gaze. Torticollis resolves spontaneously in most infants. When the deformity persists beyond the age of 1 to 2 years, **surgical release** of the contracted muscle may be indicated.

Management of acquired torticollis depends on etiology. The evaluation and treatment of many of these conditions can be complex and often require consultation with specialists in head and neck surgery, neurology, and orthopedic surgery.

Management of **scoliosis falls into 3 groups: observation, bracing, and surgery. Observation** involves **close follow-up** with careful repeat examinations and radiographic studies. Children who have not undergone their rapid growth phase are at greatest risk of marked progression of their curve. The Risser sign is used to assess the degree to which skeletal maturation has progressed. The sign is based on the degree of ossification of the iliac apophysis, with a Risser 0 signifying no ossification and a Risser 5 representing full ossification. An initial consultation with an orthopedic surgeon is generally advisable, even in minor degrees of curvature. The goal of follow-up is early detection of curvature with implementation of treatment to prevent or reduce curve progression. Children with curves less than 20 to 25 degrees should be monitored for progression. Curves between 25 to 45 degrees do not require bracing in skeletally mature individuals

(Risser 4 or 5) but should be braced (eg, with Milwaukee brace) in growing children. The goal of **bracing** is not to correct any existing curvature but to prevent further curve progression. The efficacy of bracing is determined by adherence to the regimen. **Surgery** (eg, the Harrington rod or posterior spinal fusion) may be indicated for children with curves greater than 40 to 45 degrees. These curves have a high likelihood of progression regardless of the patient's age and skeletal maturity. The development of pedicle screws has advanced the process of spinal fusion.

Although the management of **back pain** is diagnosis dependent, **rest** and **immobilization** are principles of treatment that apply in many instances. In the management of diskitis, antistaphylococcal antibiotics may be necessary in addition to immobilization. If spondylolisthesis and spondylolysis do not respond to rest and immobilization, operative stabilization may be required. In adolescents with low back pain related to muscular injury, conservative treatment including bed rest, heat, and anti-inflammatory medications may be tried for 1 to 2 weeks followed by a gradual return to normal activity. It is not advisable to institute such treatment in younger children without pursuing a more extensive evaluation or consultation with an orthopedic surgeon because the risk of serious disease is significant in this age group.

Prognosis

Congenital muscular **torticollis** responds to conservative management in about 90% of infants. The asymmetry of the face and skull also corrects over time once the contracture of the sternocleidomastoid resolves. Spasmus nutans, a condition that develops between 4 and 12 months of age, resolves spontaneously by 3 years of age.

The direction and location of the curvature in **scoliosis** do not change with age, but the degree of curvature may remain stable or progress. Factors associated with a high risk of curve progression include female gender, positive family history for scoliosis, younger age at diagnosis (especially before the adolescent growth spurt), and a larger curve at the time of diagnosis. In addition, a double curve is more likely to progress than a single curve, and a thoracic curve is more likely to progress than a lumbar curve. Left untreated, severe scoliosis can produce cardiopulmonary impairment or cosmetic deformity, which may lead to low self-esteem and poor body image. Decreased exercise tolerance has been reported in individuals with curves as small as 20 degrees. Individuals with infantile and juvenile scoliosis experience increased mortality from pulmonary and cardiac conditions during their 40s and 50s.

Most cases (80%–90%) of low **back pain** in adolescents and young adults resolve spontaneously in 2 to 8 weeks. It is important for patients to learn how to prevent recurrence by improving posture, learning how to lift heavy objects appropriately, and instituting a program of exercises to help strengthen the abdominal and back muscles.

CASE RESOLUTION

The history of the infant presented in the opening case scenario is consistent with congenital muscular torticollis. Physical examination helps confirm the diagnosis. The hips should be evaluated thoroughly because of the association of congenital muscular torticollis with congenital hip dysplasia. A program consisting of neck stretching exercises and repositioning of interesting toys and objects in the infant's crib to the side opposite the preferred gaze should be instituted. The infant can be reevaluated in 2 to 3 weeks to monitor progress.

Selected References

Ballock RT, Song KM. The prevalence of nonmuscular causes of torticollis in children. *J Pediatr Orthop.* 1996;16:500–504

Boachie-Adjei O, Lonner B. Spinal deformity. *Pediatr Clin North Am.* 1996;43:883–897

Cheng JCY, Au AWY. Infantile torticollis: a review of 624 cases. *J Pediatr Orthop.* 1994;14:802–808

Epps HR, Salter RB. Orthopedic conditions of the cervical spine and shoulder. *Pediatr Clin North Am.* 1996;43:919–931

Glancy GL. Advances in idiopathic scoliosis in children and adolescents. *Adv Pediatr.* 2007;54:55–66

Kautz SM, Skaggs DL. Getting an angle on spinal deformities. *Contemp Pediatr.* 1998;15:111–128

Lenke LG, Betz RR, Harms J, et al. Adolescent idiopathic scoliosis: a new classification to determine extent of spinal arthrodesis. *J Bone Joint Surg Am.* 2001;83A:1169–1181

Lowe TG, Edgar M, Marguiles JY, et al. Etiology of idiopathic scoliosis: current trends in research. *J Bone Joint Surg Am.* 2000;82A:1157–1168

Payne WK, Ogilvie JW. Back pain in children and adolescents. *Pediatr Clin North Am.* 1996;43:899–917

Ramirez N, Johnston CE, Browne RH. The prevalence of back pain in children who have idiopathic scoliosis. *J Bone Joint Surg Am.* 1997;79:364–368

Stewart DG Jr, Skaggs DL. Adolescent idiopathic scoliosis. *Pediatr Rev.* 2006;27:299–306

Gastrointestinal Disorders

95. Vomiting 575

96. Gastroesophageal Reflux 581

97. Gastrointestinal Bleeding 587

98. Diarrhea 595

99. Constipation 601

100. Abdominal Pain 607

101. Jaundice 613

102. Infectious Hepatitis 621

Vomiting

George Gershman, MD

CASE STUDY

A 6-week-old male infant who has been vomiting after each meal for 3 days is brought to the office. He is breastfed, afebrile, and otherwise well. The history of the pregnancy and birth are normal. His birth weight was 3,500 g, and his current weight is 4,500 g. The physical examination is unremarkable. The mother nurses the infant in the office. Although he feeds hungrily and well, he vomits about 5 minutes after the feeding. The vomiting is projectile, and the vomitus shoots across the room. The vomitus contains curdled milk. On reexamination of the abdomen, a small mass is felt in the right upper quadrant.

Questions

1. What is the mechanism of vomiting, and how does it differ from regurgitation and rumination?
2. What are the common causes of vomiting in infants?
3. What are the common causes of vomiting in older children?
4. What is the significance of bilious vomiting?
5. What are the unique features of vomiting related to increased intracranial pressure?
6. What are some strategies for the management of vomiting in older children?

Vomiting is a common complaint of infants and children, and led Thomas Phaire to write, "Many times the stomake of ye child is so feble that it cannot retayne eyther meate or drynke" (*The Boke of Chyldren,* 1553). **Vomiting** is defined as the forceful ejection of the stomach contents through the mouth. The mechanism involves a series of complex, neurologically coordinated events under the control of the central nervous system (CNS). In contrast, **regurgitation** is the effortless bringing up of 1 or 2 mouthfuls of food without distress or discomfort. This is a frequent symptom of gastroesophageal reflux (GER) in infants (see Chapter 96). **Rumination,** a form of autostimulation, is the voluntary induction of regurgitation. It is most often noted in infants between the ages of 3 and 6 months. Rumination occurs in infants with developmental retardation or with a disturbed mother-infant relationship. It is said that affected infants always smell like vomitus, which is on the clothing, but that the vomiting is rarely seen because the presence of another person provides distraction.

Rumination should be considered in infants from deprived environments (eg, neglectful homes). Cases of rumination have been described in premature infants who were maintained in a neonatal intensive care unit after they no longer needed vigilant care from the nursing staff. Incubators, which were cut off from the outside environment, contributed to the isolation and subsequent rumination. The condition resolved once the infants were held and nurtured.

Epidemiology

Fifty percent of infants have spitting up or vomiting as an isolated complaint and less than 5% of these infants have significant underlying disease. Vomiting occurs less frequently in older children, who often experience acute, self-limited illnesses such as gastroenteritis.

Clinical Presentation

Infants and children may present with vomiting as an isolated complaint or in association with other symptoms, including faintness, diaphoresis, sweating, pallor, tachycardia, fever, anorexia, abdominal pain, or diarrhea (Dx Box). When vomiting has persisted over a period, weight loss or failure to thrive (FTT) may occur. Neurologic symptoms, including headache and gait disturbances, may be noted in children with CNS problems. Other neurologic symptoms of altered muscle tone, lethargy, seizures, or coma in young infants suggest inborn errors of metabolism.

Dx Vomiting

- Vomiting
- Nausea
- Abdominal pain
- Anorexia
- Diarrhea
- Headache
- Fever
- Lethargy

Pathophysiology

Vomiting is a reflex reaction that occurs in response to numerous stimuli: enteric infections, toxins, drugs, chemotherapy, radiation, etc. The final common pathway involves expulsion of food from the relaxed stomach into the mouth due to coordinated contraction of the abdominal wall, respiratory muscles, increased intra-abdominal and thoracic pressure, and relaxation of the lower and upper esophageal sphincters.

Anything that delays gastric emptying may be associated with vomiting. Gastric emptying may be retarded by a high-fat meal, swallowed mucus (eg, maternal mucus after birth, nasal mucus with an upper respiratory infection), fever, infection, and malnutrition. Delayed gastric emptying may develop with long-standing diabetes mellitus.

Vomiting can be divided into 3 phases: nausea, retching, and emesis. However, nausea may occur without retching and vomiting, and retching may occur without vomiting.

Nausea is a significant and difficult to define discomfort related to the sensation of a need to vomit. It can be produced by various stimuli (eg, bacterial toxins, drugs, intestinal distention, visceral pain, unpleasant memories, labyrinthine stimulation, noxious odors, visual stimulations, unpleasant taste, and increased cerebral pressure). **Peripheral receptors** in the stomach and the small and large intestines detect emetic stimuli; distention and contractions are recognized by mechanoreceptors and toxins are sensed by chemoreceptors. Emetic stimuli may also originate from the obstructed or inflamed bile ducts, peritoneal inflammation, mesenteric vascular occlusion, the pharynx, and the heart. Vagal pathways mediate emetic responses to a variety of peripheral stimuli. Most afferent vagal fibers project to the nucleus tractus solitarius and some to the area of postrema or the dorsal vagal motor nucleus. The serotoninergic pathway plays the central role in nausea induced by peripheral stimuli.

The area postrema on the dorsal surface of the medulla close to the fourth ventricle is considered the **chemoreceptor trigger zone** to a variety of neurochemical stimuli. Bacterial toxins, drugs, toxic products of metabolic disorders, and radiation therapy may induce nausea by stimulation of numerous central receptors: dopamine D_2, muscarinic M1, histaminergic H_1, serotoninergic 5-HT3, and vasopressinergic subtypes located in the area postrema. However, afferent excitation of multiple brain sites, including nucleus tractus solitarius, the dorsal vagal and phrenic nuclei, the medullary nuclei controlling respiration, the hypothalamus, and the amygdala, is responsible for coordinated activities of various organs and muscles and the induction of retching and emesis.

Retching is the second phase of vomiting. It is produced by concurrent contractions of inspiratory thoracic, diaphragmatic, and abdominal muscles against the closed glottis. The generated high positive intra-abdominal pressure forces gastric contents into the esophagus and herniates the gastric cardia into the thorax. At this phase, the high negative thoracic pressure prevents emesis of gastric fluids.

Emesis is the final stage of vomiting. Synchronous contractions of the inspiratory and expiratory muscles generate high positive intrathoracic pressure sufficient to produce expulsion of gastric contents into the mouth. Oral propulsion of the vomitus is facilitated by the elevation of the hyoid bone and larynx. Airways are protected from aspiration by glottis closure. Elevation of the soft palate prevents passage of the vomitus into the nasal cavities. Hyperventilation may occur before emesis. During vomiting, breathing is suppressed.

With emesis, retrograde giant contractions originate from the middle of the small intestine. Intestinal contents move into the stomach causing enterogastric reflux. Within the stomach, the fundus remains flaccid, but the antrum and pylorus contract. Relaxation of the lower esophageal sphincter also occurs.

In children with pyloric stenosis, enterogastric reflux is prevented by hypertrophy of the pylorus. Projectile vomiting is facilitated by giant, often-visible contraction of the antrum and relaxation of the proximal stomach and low esophageal sphincter. No nausea is associated with the vomiting of pyloric stenosis, and affected infants are frequently eager to eat immediately after vomiting. Vomiting induced by increased intracranial pressure (ICP) is also not associated with nausea. In addition, such vomiting frequently occurs first thing in the morning on awakening and on an empty stomach. Regurgitation, which may be misdiagnosed as vomiting, is often related to GER (see Chapter 96 for a more detailed discussion).

Differential Diagnosis

Vomiting may be related to various different gastrointestinal (GI) or extraintestinal (parenteral) conditions. Some conditions respond to medical management, and others mandate surgical intervention (Box 95-1). The presence of bile in the vomitus, referred to as **bilious vomiting,** is a serious sign, usually indicative of intestinal obstruction distal to the major duodenal papilla and of the need for surgical intervention. Bilious vomiting can also occur in children with pseudo-obstruction syndrome or acute pancreatitis and other conditions leading to paralytic ileus.

Box 95-1. Differential Diagnosis of Vomiting in Infancy

Medical Conditions

- Gastroenteritis
- Ingestion of maternal blood or mucus
- Overfeeding
- Food allergies

- Inborn errors of metabolism
- Congenital adrenal hyperplasia
- Parenteral infections (eg, otitis media, urinary tract infection)

Surgical Conditions

- Atresia/stenosis of gastrointestinal tract
- Pyloric stenosis
- Ulcers

- Intussusception
- Volvulus
- Appendicitis

The presence of blood in the vomitus is another ominous sign and is discussed in Chapter 97. In acute gastroenteritis, the most common cause of vomiting, the infectious agent may be a virus, such as enterovirus or rotavirus, or a bacterium, such as salmonella. Acute gastroenteritis is discussed in greater detail in Chapter 98. In cases that are not related to gastroenteritis, considering the age of the patient is the best approach to the differential diagnosis of vomiting.

Infants

Vomiting in neonates may be associated with the ingestion of irritants such as maternal **blood** or **mucus.** Either of these substances delays gastric emptying. **Structural anomalies of the GI tract** may also cause vomiting in neonates. The onset of symptoms is directly related to the level of obstruction: The higher the structural obstruction, the earlier the onset of vomiting. Lesions of the esophagus, such as esophageal atresia, may be evident in the delivery room, with an unsuccessful attempt to pass a nasogastric tube. Lower GI lesions, such as ileal atresia, may not present for several days. These lesions usually require surgical intervention. Infants with atretic lesions may also have a history of polyhydramnios or a single umbilical artery.

Overfeeding is the most common reason for spitting up in young infants. Frequently, infants who present with vomiting are actually experiencing spitting up or regurgitation. Overfeeding is less likely to occur in breastfed infants, because they have better control of their satiation. Mothers of bottle-fed infants may feel that the volume of formula consumed by their infants is insufficient. Nursing mothers, on the other hand, cannot "unscrew" their breasts from their bodies to determine how much milk their infants have consumed. Some non-nursing mothers feel the need to reinsert a nipple in the infant's mouth, and infants who are still interested in sucking (nonnutritive sucking) continue to feed, often exceeding the capacity of the stomach. Vomiting then results. The physician should approach breastfed infants who are vomiting with care and concern.

Food allergies are another eating-related problem. Infants with cow's milk formula intolerance may experience vomiting. At least 30% of these infants are also allergic to soy protein. Associated symptoms such as diarrhea, rhinorrhea, eczema, and growth failure frequently occur.

Gastroesophageal reflux is a common cause of regurgitation. It is described in detail in Chapter 96.

Achalasia is defined as an absence of effective esophageal peristalsis and coordinated relaxation of the low esophageal sphincter. Ingested food that is unable to pass into the stomach may be regurgitated. Children with achalasia usually do not present until later in childhood, although they may have a prenatal history of polyhydramnios, a sign suggesting an abnormal swallowing pattern, even in utero.

Metabolic disorders, including inborn errors of metabolism and endocrine problems, may also be associated with vomiting. For example, children with galactosemia may present with vomiting as well as with jaundice, dehydration, cataracts, and hepatomegaly. Other inborn errors of metabolism include methylmalonic acidemia, disorders of the urea cycle, phenylketonuria, maple syrup

urine disease, renal tubular acidosis, hypercalcemia, and diabetes insipidus. Some of these disorders induce symptoms suggestive of sepsis, such as lethargy and seizures.

Male infants with **congenital adrenal hyperplasia (CAH)** may present with vomiting and electrolyte disturbance, symptoms indicative of adrenal insufficiency. Affected male infants usually present at about 10 to 14 days of age with vomiting and hyperkalemia (which should not be attributed to hemolysis of the specimen); hyponatremia develops later. In females, CAH is usually detected in the newborn nursery because of ambiguous genitalia. Diagnosis of this potentially lethal condition is critical to ensure the institution of replacement therapy and survival of affected infants.

Vomiting may be symptomatic of **infection** in parts of the body other than the GI tract. Most notably, urinary tract infections (UTIs) of young male infants may cause projectile vomiting, a symptom highly suggestive of pyloric stenosis. These infants are usually febrile, and may be jaundiced, and the diagnosis is considered when the urinalysis or culture is positive. Otitis media may also be associated with vomiting.

Vomiting, especially if unrelated to meals, may occur with **increased ICP.** In young infants, this suggests the possibility of an intracranial hemorrhage as occurs with inflicted, non-accidental head trauma.

Pyloric stenosis, a condition caused by hypertrophy of the muscle surrounding the pyloric channel, is the most common surgical condition associated with vomiting in infancy. The condition affects males much more frequently than females and usually appears in infants between the ages of 2 weeks and 2 months. Factors that are known to increase risk of pyloric stenosis include being firstborn, male, a greater birth weight, and early exposure to erythromycin.

The emesis is projectile, non-bilious, and frequently contains curdled milk, which reflects delayed gastric emptying, a problem caused by failure of the hypertrophied pylorus to relax.

Affected infants have an intact appetite and are eager to eat. In some infants, starvation leads to few bowel movements and constipation; in others there may be small, frequent, mucus-laden stools (starvation diarrhea) that represent succus entericus. If pyloric stenosis is not diagnosed promptly, infants may fail to gain weight or may exhibit FTT. Symptoms suggestive of pyloric stenosis may result from an antral web or duplication of the GI tract.

Children

Vomiting in children is frequently associated with **gastroenteritis.** Infections elsewhere in the body, particularly UTIs, streptococcal pharyngitis, and otitis media, are also associated with vomiting. Labyrinthitis presents with vomiting associated with dizziness. Older children with new-onset **diabetes mellitus** may present with vomiting. Vomiting may also appear in children who are already known to be diabetic. This is particularly true when ketosis is present. Slow gastric emptying (gastroparesis) is a complication of longstanding diabetes mellitus. Vomiting is also a component of peptic ulcer disease, which is described in more detail in Chapter 100.

Vomiting may be a major symptom of **CNS-related problems,** such as tumors, infections, hydrocephalus, malformations, and other causes of increased ICP. As previously noted, vomiting in CNS-related conditions is often unrelated to meals and may not be associated with nausea. Autonomic epilepsy and migraine headaches are also associated with vomiting. **Cyclic vomiting** is an unusual condition characterized by recurrent episodes of vomiting with intervals of complete wellness between attacks. Emotional upset can precipitate events, and there may be a history of migraine headaches.

Vomiting is one of the hallmarks of **Reye syndrome,** a disorder that involves an encephalopathy in association with fatty infiltration of the liver. The etiology of the condition is unclear, but the root of the disorder seems to be related to mitochondrial dysfunction. Affected children usually have a history of an antecedent viral illness, most commonly influenza or chickenpox. Following a period of recovery, they experience altered consciousness with vomiting. Hepatic enzymes and serum ammonia are elevated. Aspirin, which uncouples oxidative phosphorylation, is apparently linked to Reye syndrome, both epidemiologically as well as theoretically. There has been a marked reduction in the incidence of Reye syndrome related to the decrease in the use of aspirin and vaccination of children against varicella and influenza.

Certain **medications,** including theophylline, erythromycin, and digitalis, may also be associated with vomiting. Some of these medications cause transient relaxation of the lower esophageal sphincter and others affect the chemoreceptor trigger zone.

Familial **dysautonomia,** Riley-Day syndrome, a rare condition that affects Jewish individuals, results in vomiting. The disorder is inherited in an autosomal-recessive manner and consists of an imbalance in the autonomic nervous system. Children experience intractable vomiting in addition to excess perspiration, inability to produce tears, difficulty swallowing and chewing, and cold hands and feet. They also have hyperpyrexia and hypertension. These children require fluid replacement and management with antiemetics.

Surgical conditions such as appendicitis, gall bladder disease, and twisted ovarian cysts are discussed in Chapter 100.

Adolescents

Vomiting during the adolescent years may be caused by any of the previously mentioned conditions. In addition, adolescents may develop vomiting in association with intentional **ingestion of illicit drugs or alcohol.** Many adolescents have incorrect notions of the sexual activity needed to initiate pregnancy. Teenage girls, who have been vomiting, especially for a time, should be evaluated for **pregnancy,** regardless of their disclosed sexual activity status.

Adolescents with **eating disorders,** particularly bulimia, vomit but may not disclose their vomiting. They may ingest emetics, such as ipecac, to help control their weight (see Chapter 120).

Evaluation

History

A complete history is essential for correct diagnosis (Questions Box). A positive family history of vomiting may suggest a diagnosis of migraine, peptic ulcer disease, or familial dysautonomia.

Questions

Vomiting

- What is the nature of the vomiting (projectile, bilious, non-bilious)?
- How long has the child been vomiting?
- Are any symptoms such as fever, diarrhea, dizziness, or lethargy associated with the vomiting?
- What is the relationship of the vomiting to meals?
- Does the vomiting occur at night, indicating possible hiatal hernia and gastroesophageal reflux?
- Is there a family history of vomiting?
- Is the child taking any medications?
- Have any measures been taken to relieve the vomiting?

Physical Examination

The examination shows the impact of vomiting on children's growth. The weight may provide evidence of the chronicity of the process; weight loss suggests a protracted course. Evidence of other infections, such as otitis media or pneumonia, may also be apparent. An abnormal neurologic examination would suggest a CNS process or an inborn error of metabolism. The fundi of the eyes should be assessed for the presence of papilledema or retinal hemorrhages. Nystagmus may be noted in children with labyrinthitis or CNS disturbances. The examination of the abdomen may show masses or signs of obstruction and a surgical condition. Distention of the abdomen may be present with an obstruction. Peristaltic waves are an abnormal finding characteristic of pyloric stenosis.

Laboratory Tests

The laboratory assessment is determined by the differential diagnosis. If gastroenteritis is suspected, an examination of the stools for leukocytes and occult blood is appropriate. Specimens for bacterial or viral cultures or viral antigen detection can be submitted. A complete blood count may support the diagnosis of infection or reveal signs of anemia. In neonates, vomited blood should be evaluated using the Apt Downey test to determine whether it came from the mother or infant.

Electrolytes should be obtained in infants or children with a history of significant vomiting, and may confirm dehydration, acid-base imbalance, or electrolyte disturbance. Infants with pyloric stenosis who vomit stomach contents develop a hypochloremic-hypokalemic alkalosis. A urinalysis also may show evidence of dehydration as well as signs of a UTI. Tests for inborn errors of metabolism, such as urine for amino acid analysis, are appropriate if this is suspected.

Imaging Studies

Radiographic procedures, such as x-rays, are the procedure of choice for diagnosis of esophageal and duodenal atresia and intestinal malrotation. An abdominal ultrasound is the most effective in diagnosis of pyloric stenosis. A flat plate of the abdomen may show stomach distention, a "double bubble" (air in the stomach and duodenum), or a paucity of intestinal air in cases of high-level obstruction. Consultation with a pediatric gastroenterologist may lead to additional diagnostic tests, such as endoscopic evaluation.

Management

The initial step in the management of vomiting infants or children is to ensure adequate hydration and integrity of the cardiovascular bed. This may require the administration of intravenous fluids. **Oral rehydration** is the mainstay of therapy in infants and children whose vomiting is related to gastroenteritis. Small, frequent feedings with clear fluids are better tolerated than large, infrequent feedings, although the latter may be necessary in infants with diarrhea because each feeding may result in a bowel movement. Antiemetics such as phenothiazines are discouraged in children because of the high incidence of side effects, including dystonic posturing. Drugs commonly used in pediatric practice include antihistamines, dopamine D_2, and serotonin 5-HT3 receptor antagonists.

Further management depends on the diagnosis. Infections should be treated with the appropriate antibiotics. Surgical conditions, such as pyloric stenosis or intussusception, should be managed operatively. Inborn errors of metabolism require consultation with a geneticist and dietary manipulation. Congenital adrenal hyperplasia should be managed in consultation with an endocrinologist. This condition necessitates replacement hormonal therapy.

Prognosis

Most cases of acute vomiting resolve spontaneously or are readily managed once the underlying condition is diagnosed. The overall prognosis is therefore quite good.

Protracted vomiting may result in starvation and FTT, however. Severe vomiting may cause tears in the esophagus and lead to hematemesis. Obstructive causes of vomiting in infants respond to surgical intervention.

CASE RESOLUTION

The infant in the case history exhibits the signs and symptoms consistent with pyloric stenosis. The boy is a healthy, vigorous breastfed infant, and his weight gain of 1,000 g in 6 weeks (average: 25 g/d) is normal. The vomitus is curdled indicating that it has been in the stomach for more than 3 hours. Gastric emptying is delayed. The presence of a mass in the right upper quadrant is also consistent with the diagnosis. An ultrasound would confirm the finding. It would be equally appropriate to feed the infant nothing by mouth, start intravenous fluids, and obtain surgical consultation.

Selected References

Chelimsky G, Czinn SJ. Peptic ulcer disease and gastritis. In: Lifschitz CH, ed. *Pediatric Gastroenterology and Nutrition in Clinical Practice.* New York, NY: Dekker; 2002:501–515

Chong SKF. Gastrointestinal problems in the handicapped child [gastroenterology and nutrition]. *Curr Opin Pediatr.* 2001;13:441–446

Gordon N. Recurrent vomiting in childhood, especially of neurologic origin. *Dev Med Child Neurol.* 1994;36:463–470

Gershman G. Approach to the child with gastroesophageal reflux. In: Osborn LM, DeWitt TS, First LR, Zenel JA, eds. *Pediatrics.* Philadelphia, PA: Mosby; 2005:658–665

Murray KF, Christie DL. Vomiting. *Pediatr Rev.* 1998;19:337–341

Sondheimer JM. Vomiting. In: Walker WA, Goulet OJ, Kleinman RE, et al, eds. *Pediatric Gastrointestinal Disease, Pathophysiology, Diagnosis, Management.* 4th ed. Vol 1. Philadelphia, PA: B. C. Decker; 2004:203–209

Gastroesophageal Reflux

Jeremy Screws, MD

CASE STUDY

A 22-month-old boy presents with a history of vomiting small amounts of food twice weekly. The emesis occurs most often after meals or periods of being very active. There does not seem to be any pain or discomfort with the vomiting. He has been otherwise healthy, with an uneventful course as an infant, good weight gain, and no hospitalizations. He has had mild respiratory symptoms beginning at 6 months with some nighttime cough and occasional wheezing. There is no history of pneumonia, dysphagia, or abdominal pain. Physical examination is normal, with no anemia or urinary tract disease noted on laboratory assessment.

Questions

1. What are the characteristics of gastroesophageal reflux (GER)?
2. What is the difference between GER and gastroesophageal reflux disease (GERD)?
3. What groups of children are at risk for GER?
4. What is the appropriate workup for an infant with suspected GER?
5. What is the appropriate management of infants and children with GER and GERD?
6. What is the natural history of GER in children?

Gastroesophageal reflux (GER) includes a spectrum of disease from physiological phenomena to pathologic disease. It involves the retrograde movement of gastric contents into the esophagus. Reflux episodes often follow meals and are brief. Gastroesophageal reflux may manifest as **regurgitation** to the oral pharynx with re-swallowing or vomiting with expulsion from the mouth. Gastroesophageal reflux is common in infants beginning at 2 to 3 months of age and resolving in most individuals by the second year of life.

Although this process is common in the first year of life, it typically does not pose a problem unless it fails to resolve by 18 to 24 months. In contrast, gastroesophageal reflux disease (GERD) denotes a more severe pattern involving injury to the esophagus as well as the presence of extra-intestinal disease. This term is used when there are symptoms present such as pain, feeding or swallowing difficulties, cough, wheezing, or poor weight gain. Complications including pneumonia or esophagitis are also part of reflux disease. While GER may require only anticipatory guidance and monitoring, GERD necessitates further evaluation and medical therapy. Although GER and GERD are defined separately, there is sometimes confusion in the medical community. It must be emphasized that GERD involves symptomatic disease.

Epidemiology

Gastroesophageal reflux has a heterogeneous presentation, making it difficult to study longitudinally. Although GER and GERD are not synonymous, the distinction between these terms is not well emphasized among pediatricians. Most infants with either condition who are brought for medical care will present by 6 months of age. Regurgitation occurs at least once daily in half of infants younger than 3 months and in nearly two-thirds of infants by 4 months. By 12 months only 5% of infants will continue to have symptoms. Gastroesophageal reflux disease is considerably less common, with the prevalence depending on the type of symptom studied. It is reported at less than 10%. Most infants with reflux will need little to no medical intervention.

Patients with neurologic injury have a higher prevalence of GERD. The management of these individuals requires a more aggressive approach. They are more likely to have esophagitis or aspiration, and anti-reflux surgery should be considered early in the treatment regimen. Infants who have undergone repair of esophageal atresia also have more severe disease, with at least one-half requiring anti-reflux surgery. Chronic respiratory disease such as cystic fibrosis is associated with GERD. It is described in two-thirds of patients with asthma, but this association is controversial. It is not clear whether the altered physiology of these diseases causes reflux, or if reflux exacerbates the pulmonary dysfunction. Similar triggers for asthma and GERD are described, so it may be that they are coexisting and unrelated. Recent studies with intraluminal impedance monitoring (see Evaluation) show that non–acid reflux occurs frequently in asthmatics. This would help to explain the lack of success of therapy aimed at acid suppression in this group of patients.

Clinical Presentation

The most frequent presentation for infants with GER is recurrent vomiting that is non-forceful and small in volume (Dx Box). Vomiting typically occurs after feeding and does not seem to disturb the patient. Some parents report a link between fussiness or crying with feeding. Further symptoms such as poor weight gain, anemia, or swallowing difficulties are characteristic of GERD. Nighttime cough, asthma, and recurrent pneumonia are respiratory presentations that may be seen. Older children can have recurrent emesis but may also complain of chest or abdominal pain. Sandifer syndrome is a rare presentation in infants, with paroxysmal movements involving arching of the back that may be mistaken for seizures.

Dx Presenting Signs and Symptoms of Gastroesophageal Reflux Disease

- Regurgitation
- Vomiting
- Fussiness or sleep disturbance
- Poor weight gain
- Hematemesis or anemia
- Odynophagia or dysphagia
- Asthma/apnea/aspiration

Pathophysiology

There are many factors felt to be involved in the pathophysiology of reflux disease. Many of these change as the child grows. Motility and pressure differentials between the esophagus and stomach control the flow of gas and liquid across the lower esophageal sphincter (LES). Refluxate is allowed into the distal esophagus multiple times daily in all ages by transient lower esophageal relaxations. Increased frequency or duration of these relaxations, rather than low LES pressure, is felt to be a major cause of GERD. Transient lower esophageal relaxations are mediated by a brain stem reflex involving the vagal nerve and the release of nitric oxide.

The position of the gastroesophageal junction and its relationship to the diaphragmatic crura play an important role. The opposed crura have a "pinchcock" action that works with the esophagogastric angle, or angle of His, to prevent reflux. As this angle becomes more open or obtuse, reflux may increase. Disruption of this anatomical association, as seen with hiatal hernia, predisposes individuals to reflux.

Relaxations of the LES that are too frequent or prolonged expose the esophageal mucosa to noxious material. Secretions from the esophagus and salivary glands neutralize the refluxate and sweep it into the stomach. Appropriate peristalsis of the esophagus is therefore necessary for clearance. Inflammation in the distal esophagus exacerbates this process by decreasing peristalsis. Position influences gravity, with the upright position favoring anterograde movement. The composition of the refluxate influences the damage that can occur. Hydrochloric acid, pepsin, bile acids, and pancreatic enzymes have all been implicated in mucosal injury. The mucosa must combat this exposure with its own defense.

Before food or secretions can move out of the esophagus, the stomach must be ready to accept it. The fundus normally relaxes without an increase in pressure. Dysfunction of this **fundic accommodation**

or delay in gastric emptying can increase pressure in the stomach and exacerbate reflux. The volume of ingested feedings is noted to be a factor in infants. Based on the size of their stomachs, infants typically take twice the volume of older children. This leaves more material in the stomach at any given time, potentially increasing intragastric pressure.

Differential Diagnosis

A diverse group of symptoms, each with its own list of potential diagnoses, are associated with reflux disease. Regurgitation and vomiting are the most commonly reported symptoms. Many of the causes of vomiting in the newborn can be separated from reflux with a history and physical examination (Box 96-1). Forceful, bilious, or bloody emesis is not typical of reflux. Fussiness and crying are nonspecific symptoms with etiologies ranging from infantile colic to meningitis. Esophagitis has many other etiologies of which eosinophilic esophagitis must be considered. This condition presents more typically in the atopic child with dysphagia. It may also present with food impaction in the esophagus. However, the pain and vomiting may mimic GERD.

Box 96-1. Common Non-Reflux Causes of Vomiting[a]

Infections
- Sepsis
- Meningitis
- Urinary tract infection
- Otitis media

Obstruction
- Pyloric stenosis
- Malrotation
- Intussusception

Gastrointestinal
- Eosinophilic esophagitis
- Peptic ulcer disease
- Achalasia
- Gastroparesis
- Gastroenteritis
- Gall bladder disease
- Pancreatitis
- Celiac disease
- Pill esophagitis
- Crohn disease

Metabolic/Endocrine
- Galactosemia
- Fructose intolerance
- Urea cycle defects
- Diabetic ketoacidosis

Toxic
- Lead poisoning

Neurologic
- Hydrocephalus and shunt malfunctions
- Subdural hematoma
- Intracranial hemorrhage
- Tumors
- Migraine

Allergic
- Dietary protein intolerance

Respiratory
- Post-tussive emesis
- Pneumonia

Renal
- Obstructive uropathy
- Renal insufficiency

Cardiac
- Congestive heart failure

Other, Seen in Adolescents
- Recreational drugs
- Alcohol
- Pregnancy

Other
- Overfeeding
- Self-induced vomiting

[a]Adapted from Michail S. Gastroesophageal reflux. *Pediatr Rev.* 2007;28:101–110.

Evaluation

Separating the mildly symptomatic "happy spitter" from the child with very apparent, painful erosive esophagitis may not prove difficult. However, deciding how much vomiting is too much may prove vexing. The presence of certain risk factors in the initial history should prompt further evaluation. These factors include poor weight gain, food avoidance, respiratory disease, unexplained anemia or frank hematemesis, or significant chest or abdominal pain.

History

Targeted questions about the timing and volume of feedings and their relationship to regurgitation can help build the case for reflux. Specific attention should be paid to respiratory symptoms such as nighttime cough or previous episodes of pneumonia. Difficulties with feeding and swallowing should be outlined carefully. Gagging or dysphagia with different consistencies should be noted. Family history of reflux, especially as an infant, may be helpful. A history of atopy in the family, including asthma and food allergies, will assist when considering eosinophilic esophagitis. Clinical questionnaires, including the Infant Gastroesophageal Reflux Questionnaire, have been validated but are more useful in the research setting.

Physical Examination

One should perform a full physical examination, including an observance of feeding. Neurologic deficits or delay should be noted. The abdomen should be carefully palpated for masses or distension. Growth parameters should be reviewed longitudinally and the child's body habitus, particularly the presence or absence of subcutaneous tissue, should be noted.

Laboratory Tests

Most patients with reflux will need no laboratory testing. Children with large volume emesis or weight loss should be assessed for acidosis or other electrolyte abnormalities. Markers of kidney and liver function are reasonable to obtain. If anemia is suspected based on the physical examination or the presence of hematemesis, hematologic studies should be obtained.

Intra-esophageal pH Monitoring

Currently measurement of the intra-esophageal pH for periods of 24 to 48 hours is considered the gold standard for the diagnosis of GERD. This is performed by placing a catheter transnasally into the distal esophagus to measure the intraluminal pH as the patient records the symptoms of interest, such as cough and pain. Meals are also recorded. pH monitoring can be performed safely in all age groups, and certain parameters of this study do correlate with esophagitis. It does not detect non–acid reflux, making its utility in linking respiratory disease to GERD questionable. It may be combined with multichannel sleep studies to investigate apnea or nighttime symptoms. A wireless device that attaches to the esophageal mucosa has been used in children. The device can be placed with or without endoscopy, but the size of the capsule may prohibit its use in smaller children.

Upper Gastrointestinal Series (UGI)

Contrast radiography of the upper gastrointestinal (GI) tract is often employed early in the evaluation of reflux. The utility of the test is not for screening; however, its sensitivity and specificity are both low. The brief duration of the examination misses episodes of reflux. Conversely, if episodes are seen it must be noted that the positioning of the patient and the pressure applied to the abdomen are not physiological. This test should be used only to identify anatomical anomalies that could cause vomiting, such as malrotation, esophageal or intestinal webs, pyloric stenosis, or hiatal hernia. Large volumes of refluxate to the level of the proximal esophagus or pharynx, if seen, are more likely to indicate GERD.

Scintigraphy

Nuclear medicine studies may be employed in the evaluation of reflux. In general they involve the administration of an age-appropriate feeding of technetium-labeled food. For infants this would be labeled formula at a volume that approximates a typical feeding. For older children this would include a mixed meal of liquids and solids. Scans are taken serially to mark the location of the tracer. There are 3 questions that can be answered with these studies. The first use of this method is to quantify the rate at which the stomach empties. This may be expressed as half time ($T_{1/2}$), which refers to the time taken to empty 50% of the tracer from the stomach. Alternatively, it may be expressed as percentage emptied at 90 minutes. For children younger than 1 year the $T_{1/2}$ should be less than 60 minutes for liquids. For older children a $T_{1/2}$ of 90 minutes has been accepted. The second use for scintigraphy is measurement of tracer in the esophagus, indicating a reflux episode. Shorter intervals between scans are required, and both acid and non–acid reflux are measured. As with the UGI, this test has a low sensitivity for reflux disease, making it unacceptable as a screening examination. However, the specificity is higher and multiple episodes may be supportive for the diagnosis of GERD. The third use for this modality is detection of aspiration. Delayed scans up to 24 hours later may be employed, which can show tracer in the pharynx or lung fields. This use is also limited due to low sensitivity. However, a positive test is helpful in linking reflux to pulmonary pathology.

Endoscopy With Biopsy

Endoscopy of the upper GI tract is moderately invasive but allows direct visualization of the esophagus. The presence and severity of esophagitis can be documented. Other disease processes causing esophagitis, including infection, eosinophilic infiltration, and Crohn disease, can be diagnosed. Biopsies should always be taken, even in the absence of macroscopic findings, as histologic esophagitis may be responsible for symptoms. Basal zone hyperplasia and increased papillary length are found in reflux esophagitis. Eosinophilic esophagitis may have specific endoscopic findings of linear or circular furrowing or white specks. However, the location and number of eosinophils on biopsy are necessary to separate this diagnosis from GERD. Traditional pH monitoring catheters or wireless devices can be placed at the time of endoscopy.

Multichannel Intraluminal Impedance

Impedance monitoring is increasing in clinical use as smaller, less expensive equipment becomes available. This technology involves the placement of a catheter transnasally into the distal esophagus, similar to traditional pH monitoring. However, these catheters have multiple sensors arranged from proximally to distally that can detect the flow of liquid or gas and determine the direction of movement of this bolus. Liquids moving from the distal catheter to the proximal (retrograde) catheter are noted to be reflux. Typically a pH sensor at the distal end is included so that boluses may be described as acid or non-acid. This study is especially attractive in small infants where frequent feedings buffer acidity and in respiratory diseases where non–acid reflux has been implicated. Normal values for all pediatric age groups are not available at this time.

Management

Infants that are thriving with no symptoms other than regurgitation or vomiting will benefit primarily from alleviation of parental anxiety. Discussion involving the normal course and benign nature of GER may be all that is required. The infant should be followed for changes in feeding, weight, or respiratory complaints and the regurgitation should begin to resolve by the end of the first year. When the regurgitation is problematic or associated with symptoms described earlier, further therapy should be initiated.

Lifestyle Changes

Life in recumbency has its disadvantages for infants, namely allowing the esophagus and stomach to reside at the same level. This concept has led to the use of positioning in infants. There are multiple positions used including prone, prone at a 30-degree angle, or supine at a 30-degree angle. The only proven position seems to be prone. Unfortunately this position has been associated with a higher rate of sudden infant death syndrome (SIDS) in infants. The practitioner must balance the risk of GERD with that of SIDS in the individual patient. The 30-degree supine position does not seem to be more effective in decreasing reflux than the flat supine position, but there is conflicting evidence on this point.

Infants with reflux are often put through "formula roulette." Cow's milk or soy-based formulas are employed and some progress to partially digested or elemental formulas. There is a select group of infants with regurgitation that have cow's milk protein intolerance who may respond to a 2-week trial of hypoallergenic formula. This is more likely in the patient with a family history of atopy. Nearly half of infants intolerant of milk protein will also exhibit symptoms with soy, thus protein hydrosylate formulations may be of more use. There is no indication for lactose-free cow's milk formulas in this patient population. Rice cereal may be used as a thickening agent. This does not change findings on esophageal pH monitoring, but it may decrease the frequency of regurgitation. Patients with poor weight gain will benefit from the increased caloric density of the thickened formula. One tablespoon of rice cereal per 2 ounces of formula will increase the content from 20 to 27 cal/oz. Increasing amounts of rice cereal will increase the viscosity and caloric density, but this also increases osmolarity. Excessively concentrated formulas may worsen vomiting. Nipples used with thickened formula will need to be tailored by crosscutting, but this may lead to increases in coughing or gagging.

Environmental and dietary factors have been studied in the older child and teenager. Currently only caffeine, chocolate, and spicy foods *that provoke symptoms* should be avoided. Obesity and exposure to tobacco smoke have also been implicated.

Medications

The pharmacologic agents that are used in reflux disease are generally safe and, therefore, sometimes used empirically without diagnostic confirmation (Table 96-1). This may be helpful when the symptoms of interest are mild and clearly delineated so that a response to medication can be followed. Acid suppression is the mainstay of treatment. The goal is to reduce exposure of the esophagus to acid. There are 3 main types of drugs that can be used: antacids, histamine-2 receptor antagonists (H2RA), and proton pump inhibitors (PPI). The only clinically effective antacids are those that contain aluminum, which is contraindicated in infants because of its toxicity. Histamine-2 receptor antagonists inhibit acid production in the gastric parietal cell. They are effective in the healing of esophagitis; however, tachyphylaxis has been seen as early as 1 week after initiation. Cimetidine and famotidine have the most evidence for use in pediatrics. Proton pump inhibitors bond and deactivate hydrogen, potassium-adenosinetriphosphatase pumps and reduce meal-induced acid production. They should be taken 30 minutes prior to a meal so that the drug is in the bloodstream in the largest concentration at mealtime. Omeprazole and lansoprazole have been studied the most in children. Proton pump inhibitors may be used as the initial drug, or following failure by H2RAs. There are 2 approaches that are used in initiating these medications. **Step-up** therapy involves beginning with H2RAs or low-dose PPI and escalating therapy until symptoms have improved. **Step-down** therapy progresses from high-dose PPI to resolve symptoms then low-dose PPI or H2RA to maintain remission. Healing of esophagitis at higher doses takes 4 to 8 weeks, with symptoms resolving in this time frame. Histamine-2 receptor antagonists are more effective than PPIs in the fasting state. Therefore, they may be effective for nighttime symptoms that persist through high-dose PPI therapy when taken at bedtime.

Prokinetic agents are indicated in the patient with evidence of delayed gastric emptying. Effects on LES tone and esophageal peristalsis seem to be less important than accelerated gastric emptying. Cisapride, a mixed serotonergic agent, was the model drug for this class. It has been shown to improve reflux symptoms and pH parameters in infants. However, it has been associated with QT prolongation and arrhythmia with some deaths. The use of cisapride has been severely restricted since 2000. Other drugs in the group are less likely to improve reflux but are still widely used. Metoclopramide also has mixed serotonergic effects, in addition to anti-dopaminergic and cholinomimetic actions. Adverse effects including central nervous system complications limit the use of this drug. Erythromycin is a

Table 96-1. Pharmacologic Agents Used for Reflux Disease		
Drug	*Pediatric Dose*	*Adverse Effects*
Cimetidine	20–40 mg/kg/d, divided 3–4 times per day	Hypotension, gynecomastia, reduced hepatic metabolism of other drugs, neutropenia, agranulocytosis, thrombocytopenia
Famotidine	0.5–1 mg/kg/d divided every day to twice per day	Headache, dizziness, constipation, diarrhea
Omeprazole	0.7–3.3mg/kg/d divided every day to twice per day	Headache, diarrhea, abdominal pain, nausea, rash, vitamin B_{12} deficiency, constipation
Lansoprazole	15 mg (weight <30 kg) 30 mg (weight >30 kg)	Headache, nausea, constipation, diarrhea, abdominal pain, proteinuria, hypotension, elevated transaminases
Metoclopramide	0.1mg/kg/dose 4 times per day before meals	Drowsiness, restlessness, dystonia, gynecomastia, galactorrhea
Erythromycin	3–5 mg/kg/dose 3–4 times per day before meals	Diarrhea, vomiting, cramps, antibiotic effect, pyloric stenosis

motilin receptor agonist that is also used less commonly in GERD. There is evidence that its use in pregnancy or in young infants may increase the risk of pyloric stenosis. Many interactions have been seen with this macrolide antibiotic, which also limits is use.

Barrier agents include sodium alginate, which is not readily available in the United States, and sucralfate, which contains aluminum. The former is not effective in most cases of GERD and the latter should be reserved for short-term treatment of erosive lesions in the esophagus.

Anti-Reflux Procedures

Patients that continue to have reflux on maximum medical therapy or those that have serious extra-esophageal manifestations such as recurrent aspiration or Barrett esophagus should be considered for surgery. Patients requiring long-term drug therapy may also be selected for surgery. The most popular procedure is the Nissen fundoplication. The laparoscopic approach to fundoplication is used widely and entails a full wrap of the fundus of the stomach around the esophagus to increase LES tone and create a more acute angle of His. More than 90% of patients remain symptom-free up to 11 years postoperatively. Complications including gas bloat, dumping syndrome, and dysphagia are reported at variable frequencies. Failure rates are higher in neurologically impaired children and those with esophageal atresia repair. There are several other fundoplication procedures that have variable degrees of wrapping.

Significant delay in gastric emptying may require an additional surgical procedure at the gastric outlet. Antroplasty or pyloroplasty enlarges the exit from the stomach. There is some theoretical concern that fundoplication itself results in accelerated gastric emptying. The additive effects of pyloroplasty might result in dumping of gastric contents into the duodenum too rapidly. This has not been shown to be a significant problem, and this procedure should be given strong consideration in infants or children with moderate or severe gastric-emptying delay noted clinically or by scintigraphy.

Endoscopic anti-reflux procedures have mixed results in adults. Endoscopic transesophageal plication involves placing sutures through the gastroesophageal junction, pleating the mucosa and reducing the size of this opening. This procedure has yet to be used in children. Endoluminal application of radiofrequency energy has been used to remodel the tissue of the LES to reduce reflux episodes. This has been used in only 2 pediatric trials with some success. Other options include endoscopic placement of inert barriers into the tissue of the LES. All of these endoluminal techniques need further clinical data, especially in children, before they can be recommended broadly.

Prognosis

Complications arising from untreated GERD include esophagitis, Barrett esophagus, strictures, and esophageal adenocarcinoma. However, most infants with GER have a more favorable outcome. Regurgitation resolves in most children by 18 months and is absent by 24 months in 98%. There is some evidence that a portion of patients that become asymptomatic will continue to have abnormal histology in the esophagus at follow-up endoscopy. Therefore, it is unclear if the disease process continues into later childhood. Future studies that follow infants with reflux longitudinally into adulthood will be of great benefit. There is much to be learned in the area of non–acid reflux and its role in respiratory disease as intraluminal impedance becomes more widely used.

Children with persistent reflux symptoms into later childhood have a worse prognosis. Patients with a history of esophageal atresia repair or severe neurologic injury may have a poor prognosis, often requiring high-dose medication or anti-reflux surgery. They are more likely to suffer from complications of GERD.

CASE RESOLUTION

This toddler continues to have frequent emesis at almost 2 years of age with extra-esophageal manifestations including wheezing. He should be referred to a pediatric gastroenterologist for evaluation of gastroesophageal reflux disease. He is unlikely to have spontaneous symptom resolution at this age.

Selected References

Michail S. Gastroesophageal reflux. *Pediatr Rev.* 2007;28:101–110

Orenstein S, Khan S. Gastroesophageal reflux. In: Walker WA, Goulet O, Kleinman RE, Sherman PM, Shneider BL, Sanderson IR, eds. *Pediatric Gastrointestinal Disease: Pathophysiology, Diagnosis, Management.* 4th ed. Hamilton, Ontario, Canada: BC Decker Inc.; 2004:384–399

Rudolph CD, Mazur LJ, Liptak GS, et al. Guidelines for evaluation and treatment of gastroesophageal reflux in infants and children: recommendations of the North American Society for Pediatric Gastroenterology and Nutrition. *J Pediatr Gastroenterol Nutr.* 2001;32(suppl 2):S1–S31

Vanderplas Y. Gastroesophageal reflux. In: Wyllie R, Hyams JS, Kay M, eds. *Pediatric Gastrointestinal and Liver Disease.* 3rd ed. Philadelphia, PA: Elsevier Inc.; 2006:305–325

Gastrointestinal Bleeding

George Gershman, MD

CASE STUDY

A 4-year-old boy is evaluated for intermittent passing of bright red blood from the rectum for 2 weeks. Blood either coats the stool or appears as a spot after a bowel movement. The mother reports no vomiting, diarrhea, loss of appetite, weight loss, fever, or abdominal pain. The boy has no history of constipation, straining, or pain with defecation and is taking no medications. The family has no pets and has not traveled recently.

On physical examination, the boy is a well-appearing, energetic, interactive youngster. Weight and height are at the 75th percentile for age. The abdomen is soft, flat, and non-tender, and bowel sounds are normally active. No organomegaly or masses are evident. No rashes, bruising, or hemangiomas are present. No tags, fissures, or fistulas are seen on close visual inspection of the perianal area. Digital rectal examination reveals normal sphincter tone,

and a small, mobile, pea-like mass is palpable in the rectal vault. A film of bright red blood is present on the glove after the examination. A complete blood count with platelet count and a prothrombin/partial thromboplastin time determination yield normal results.

Questions

1. What is involved in the assessment of children with gastrointestinal (GI) bleeding?
2. How are upper and lower GI tract bleeding differentiated?
3. What conditions usually account for upper and lower GI tract bleeding?
4. What management options are available for GI bleeding?
5. How does the physician decide what type of management is appropriate for each individual patient?

Bleeding from the gastrointestinal (GI) tract in infants and children is always stressful and frightening for patients and their parents and challenging for a physician, especially if bleeding is severe.

Fortunately, life-threatening GI bleeding is rare in pediatric practice. However, a pediatrician or emergency department (ED) physician should be prepared to initiate effective resuscitation and diagnostic workup focusing on common age-specific causes of GI bleeding.

The primary goal of this approach is a reduction of morbidity associated with significant hemorrhage.

Epidemiology

The incidence of bleeding from the upper GI tract (upper GI bleeding) among infants and children is unknown. Clinical experience suggests that the incidence in children is significantly less than in adults. It is supported indirectly by epidemiological data from the United Kingdom and United States, which indicate that the incidence of upper GI bleeding in adults younger than 29 years is approximately 18 to 23 per 100,000 adults per year, which is almost 4 to 5 times lower than among older age groups. However, the risk of upper GI bleeding is higher (between 6.2% and 10.2%) in infants and children admitted to pediatric intensive care units.

Despite the fact that rectal bleeding is quite common in pediatric practice, the epidemiology of this problem is not well established.

According to published data, rectal bleeding was a chief complain of 0.3% of all visits to a tertiary ED during a 10-month period.

Clinical Presentation

There are 4 presentations of blood loss from the GI tract: hematemesis, melena, occult bleeding, and hematochezia.

Hematemesis is the term that applies to the vomiting of bright-red "fresh" blood or "coffee ground" emesis of dark-brown "old" blood exposed to hydrochloric acid. Usually hematemesis reflects acute bleeding from the esophagus, stomach, or proximal duodenum. Swallowing of maternal blood in neonates, and epistaxis in older children, should be ruled out to avoid unnecessary invasive procedures.

Melena is defined as liquid, coal black, shiny, sticky, tarry, foul-smelling stool. It suggests bleeding from the upper GI tract. Occasionally the site of bleeding can be located in the ileum or right colon. However, in this case stool is black but not tarry. Melena suggests a minimum loss of 50 to 100 mL in adults or 2% of blood volume in children. Stool may remain black or tarry for a few days after massive hemorrhage even though active bleeding has ceased.

Occult bleeding implies the presence of an invisible quantity of blood in stool detected by a special technique. It is a synonym for chronic, recurrent losses of small amounts of blood, which often lead to severe microcytic anemia. The most commonly used technique for detection of blood in stool is the hemoccult stool test. This test is based on the chemical reaction of a dye (guaiac) with peroxidase-containing substances and hydrogen peroxide. It is not specific for presence of blood (hemoglobin) in stool.

False-positive results could be secondary to peroxidase activity in food products such as cantaloupe, radishes, bean sprouts, cauliflower, broccoli, grapes, and red meat or iron preparations. False-negative results of the hemoccult test are associated with prolonged colonic transient time and bacterial degradation of hemoglobin to porphyrin, which does not have peroxidase activity.

Hematochezia is the passage of bright red or maroon-colored blood from the rectum. This may be pure blood, bloody diarrhea, or blood mixed with stool. As a rule, it is a sign of lower GI bleeding from the distal colon or less frequently from the right colon or the distal ileum. Rarely hematochezia may occur in children with massive bleeding from the duodenum.

Pathophysiology

Compensatory responses to acute bleeding facilitate a restoration of depleted intravascular volume, maintenance of a normal cardiac output (CO) and adequate oxygenation of vital organs (brain, heart, lungs, and adrenal gland), and mobilization of internal energy stores.

Two parameters determine the degree of compensation: volume of blood loss and velocity of bleeding.

Mild Blood Loss (<15% of Circulatory Volume) or Class 1 Bleeding

Relatively slow blood loss of less than 15% of blood volume triggers (1) redistribution of depot blood from the venous system to systemic circulation and (2) shift of extracellular fluids into the vascular space. Adequate CO without changes in heart rate and blood pressure is maintained and there are no hemodynamic abnormalities. However, a rapid blood loss (even <10% of blood volume) may compromise CO and trigger tachycardia and other compensatory mechanisms to restore normal blood circulation.

Moderate Blood Loss (Between 15%–30% of Circulating Volume) or Class 2 Bleeding

Blood loss of more than 15% of blood volume leads to tachycardia, an increased systemic vascular resistance (SVR) due to activation of the sympathetic nervous system and hypothalamic-pituitary-adrenomedullary axis. In children, CO depends on heart rate rather than stroke volume due to smaller ventricular mass. With hemorrhage, tachycardia is the principal mechanism for maintenance of an adequate CO in pediatric patients; however, prolonged tachycardia increases myocardial oxygen demand and decreased diastolic-dependent coronary perfusion. This eventually leads to cardiovascular decompensation if fluid resuscitation is delayed or insufficient.

Normal blood pressure and adequate perfusion of vital organs in children with moderate bleeding is maintained by increased SVR and redistribution of blood from skin, muscle, splanchnic organs, and kidney to the brain, heart, lungs, and adrenal gland due to local production of adenosine, nitric oxide, and prostaglandins. Therefore, blood pressure is a poor indicator of cardiovascular homeostasis in children with moderate GI bleeding. In contrast, persistent tachycardia is the red flag of pending cardiovascular collapse.

Severe Blood Loss (>30% of Circulating Volume) or Class 3 Bleeding

Failure of compensatory mechanisms and decreased CO leads to hypotension and tissue hypoxia. Compensatory tachypnea contributes to respiratory alkalosis in the initial phase of severe bleeding. Tissue hypoxia compromises mitochondria functional capacity to generate energy as adenosine triphosphate. This leads to metabolic acidosis due to excessive production of lactic acid and cellular death.

Hypoperfusion of the kidney causes acute spasm of the preglomerular arterioles and acute tubular necrosis and renal failure. Hypoxia and excessive cytokine production can induce liver failure: sudden onset of jaundice due to hepatocellular necrosis, elevation of transaminases, coagulopathy, hypoglycemia, and encephalopathy. Myocardial ischemia is a common consequence of severe bleeding. Sepsis, thrombotic microangiopathy, and a systemic inflammatory response syndrome may occur in the late stages of uncontrolled or inadequately treated severe hemorrhage.

Evaluation

Initial assessment of the child with suspected GI bleeding should be focused on hemodynamic stability and clues for etiology of bleeding. Four major questions must be answered promptly:

1. Is the patient stable?
2. Is the bleeding real?
3. Where is the source of bleeding?
4. What is the best approach to hemostasis?

The first and the most important step in the initial assessment of the child with suspected GI bleeding is determination of hemodynamic stability.

A prompt assessment of estimated blood loss and the degree of hemodynamic instability should be done using objective criteria, such as mental status, skin color, capillary refill, pulse, blood pressure, and orthostatic maneuvers (Table 97-1). Special attention should be focused on tachycardia and narrowed pulse pressure, which are the earliest signs of impending shock. Hypotension usually occurs in the late phase of shock in children and is an ominous finding. The value of the initial hematocrit may not accurately reflect the severity of blood loss. First, the hematocrit does not fall immediately with hemorrhage due to proportionate reductions of plasma and red cell volumes. Second, the hematocrit begins to fall due to compensatory restoration of the intravascular volume by the shift of extravascular fluids into the vascular bed. This process begins shortly after the onset of bleeding; however, it is not complete for 24 to 72 hours. At this point, plasma volume is larger than normal and the Hct reaches its true nadir assuming that bleeding has stopped.

Symptoms and Signs	Blood Loss		
	<15%	*15%–30%*	*>30%*
Normal appearance	+	−	−
Anxiety	−	+	+
Disorientation	−	−	+
Lethargy	−	−	+
Tachycardia	−	++	+
Pallor	−	+	++
Livedo reticularis	−	+	++
Cold extremities	−	+	+
Capillary refill >2 seconds	−	+	+
Hypotension	−	−	+
Narrowed pulse pressure	−	+	+
Elevated diastolic pressure	−	+	−
Low diastolic pressure	−	−	+

Table 97-1. Clinical Manifestations of Gastrointestinal Bleeding According to Blood Loss Volume

Differential Diagnosis

There are 3 essential components of the diagnosis of GI bleeding
- Confirmation that bleeding is real
- Allocation of the bleeding area to the upper versus lower GI tract
- Detection of the specific cause of bleeding

Red staining of emesis or stool can be induced by cranberries, cranberry juice, cherries, strawberries, beets, tomatoes, candies, amoxicillin, phenytoin, and rifampin. Bismuth preparations, activated charcoal, iron, spinach, blueberries, and licorice can simulate bleeding by staining emesis and coloring stool black. An appropriate history, a normal physical examination, and guaiac-negative stool are sufficient to rule out a true bleeding episode.

It is important to remember that hematemesis and/or melena can be secondary to epistaxis. History of recent tonsillectomy and adenoidectomy, nasal allergies, dry environment, or nose-picking habits increases the probability of epistaxis. Thorough examination of the nose and oropharynx can help to establish the right diagnosis.

Detailed history and physical examination help narrow the diagnostic workup. For example, treatment with nonsteroidal anti-inflammatory drugs (NSAIDs) is a risk factor for acute gastric ulcers and bleeding from the stomach. Jaundice, hepatomegaly, spider hemangiomata, prominent vessels of the abdominal wall, or ascites are the signs of chronic liver disease and suggestive of portal hypertension. However, GI bleeding in an acutely ill, febrile child with jaundice could be secondary to coagulopathy and acute ulceration of the stomach or the duodenum due to sepsis.

Careful assessment of the perineum can reveal fissures, fistulas, or perianal inflammation as causes of blood in the stool.

If the source of bleeding is not obvious, the placement of a nasogastric tube is very useful. A tube with the largest bore tolerable should be placed for adequate gastric lavage: a 10F to 12F sump tube is a reasonable choice for small children; 14F to 16F for older patients. Room temperature saline is the optimal fluid for irrigation. Iced saline lavage is no longer recommended because it compromises platelet function at the bleeding site and may induce hypothermia (especially in infants) with subsequent clinically significant arrhythmia. A bloody or coffee ground aspirate indicates upper GI bleeding, if epistaxis was ruled out. The absence of blood in the stomach does not exclude upper GI bleeding because the source of hemorrhage can be in the duodenum. The presence of coffee ground fluid in gastric aspirate, which promptly clears by gastric lavage, suggests that bleeding has stopped. Ineffective gastric lavage indicates ongoing bleeding.

The results of blood tests give some clues to the nature of bleeding. Low hemoglobin and hematocrit with normal mean corpuscular volume (MCV) are typical for acute blood loss. An elevated blood urea nitrogen (BUN) suggests volume depletion and absorption of the blood proteins in the small intestine, which support the diagnosis of upper GI bleeding. Very low hemoglobin, hematocrit, and MCV in a hemodynamically stable patient is consistent with chronic GI blood loss.

Knowledge of common causes of GI bleeding in an age-specific group of children helps with the diagnostic strategy (Table 97-2).

In general, endoscopy is the method of choice for the diagnosis of the specific causes of acute and chronic GI bleeding related to mucosal and submucosal lesions of the GI tract. The choice of the particular type of endoscopic procedure is related to suspected pathology. Upper and lower GI endoscopy and enteroscopy are routine methods for diagnosis of such diseases as acute or peptic ulcers, esophagitis, gastritis, esophageal varices, vascular malformations, ulcerative colitis, Crohn disease, polyps, and other causes of GI bleeding. Capsule endoscopy is the new method with the unique ability to assess the entire small intestine. It is used for diagnosis of GI bleeding of obscure origin usually after negative results of conventional endoscopic procedures.

X-ray and abdominal ultrasound are useful for diagnosis of structural abnormalities such as intussusception, necrotizing enterocolitis, and malrotation.

Technetium (Tc)-99m pertechnetate scan is the diagnostic procedure of choice in children with suspected Meckel diverticulum. It is 85% sensitive and 95% specific.

A tagged red blood cell scan and angiography are alternative methods used to diagnose children with active GI bleeding of obscure origin, especially when vascular anomalies or hemobilia are suspected.

Age-Associated Causes of GI Bleeding

Neonates

In the first few days of life, coffee ground emesis or bloody stools in otherwise healthy and hemodynamically stable neonates are most likely caused by swallowed maternal blood either during delivery or breastfeeding. In such cases, the Apt-Downey test should be

Table 97-2. Common Causes of Gastrointestinal (GI) Bleeding in Children

Age	Upper GI Bleeding	Lower GI bleeding
Neonates (0–30 days)	• Swallowed maternal blood • Stress ulcers/sepsis • Hemorrhagic gastritis • Hemorrhagic disease of the newborn	• Necrotizing enterocolitis • Midgut volvulus • Hirschsprung disease • Vascular malformation
Infants (30 days–6 mo)	• Cow's milk or soy protein allergy • Esophagitis • Prolapse gastropathy	• Anal fissure • Allergic proctitis or enterocolitis • Nodular lymphoid hyperplasia • Intussusception
Infants and children (6 mo–6 y)	• Epistaxis • Esophagitis • Prolapse gastropathy • Portal hypertension • Drug-induced ulcers • Gastritis • Mallory-Weiss tear	• Anal fissures • Intussusception • Meckel diverticulum • Nodular lymphoid hyperplasia • Polyps • Infectious colitis • Hemolytic uremic syndrome • Henoch-Schönlein purpura
Children and teenagers (7–18 y)	• Epistaxis • Drug-induced gastropathy and acute ulcers • Peptic ulcer • Esophagitis • Gastritis • Portal hypertension	• Infectious colitis • Ulcerative colitis • Crohn disease • Anal fissure • Polyps

performed to differentiate between maternal and infant blood. The test is based on the chemical reaction of adult hemoglobin with sodium hydroxide, which leads to a color change from bright red to yellow or crusty brown. Fetal hemoglobin is resistant to hydroxylation, and blood from the infant remains bright red.

Acute gastric or duodenal ulcers should be suspected in sick premature or full-term asphyxiated or septic newborns or patients with intracerebral bleeding, raised intracranial pressure, congenital heart disease, respiratory failure, or hypoglycemia. The typical scenario includes sudden onset of hematemesis or melena and signs of hemodynamic instability. Occasionally, severe upper GI bleeding can occur in healthy full-term neonates within the first few days of life.

Gastrointestinal bleeding is a common manifestation of necrotizing enterocolitis (NEC).

The warning signs of NEC are abdominal distention, feeding intolerance with increased gastric residuals, mild diarrhea, and hematochezia or stool positive for occult blood.

Plain x-rays show either nonspecific distribution of bowel gas, pneumatosis intestinalis, or gas in the portal vein, reflecting the degree of bowel ischemia.

Rare causes of GI bleeding in the first month of life include Hirschsprung enterocolitis, midgut volvulus, duplication cyst, vascular malformation, and hemorrhagic disease of the newborn, particularly in breastfeeding neonates who did not receive vitamin K.

Infants Up to First 6 Months of Age

One of the leading causes of GI bleeding in infants younger than 6 months is cow's milk or soy protein allergy. The spectrum of symptoms includes recurrent vomiting, hematemesis, failure to thrive, and diarrhea with guaiac-positive stools or hematochezia.

Exclusively breastfeeding infants may develop similar symptoms on rare occasions. Elimination of cow's milk, eggs, peanuts, fish, and tree nuts from maternal diet may lead to resolution of allergic symptoms in the breastfeeding infant. For infants with persistent symptoms or whose mothers are unable to restrict their diet according to current recommendations and for formula-fed infants with cow's milk protein allergy, hypoallergenic (extensively hydrolyzed and free amino acid–based) formulas can be used to relieve the symptoms. Most infants with GI manifestations of cow's milk protein allergy will improve within the first 2 weeks of treatment.

An anal fissure is another common cause of bleeding in infants. The diagnosis is made by careful examination of the anus.

Intermittent rectal bleeding with streaks of frank blood mixed with normal-appearing stool can be secondary to nodular lymphoid hyperplasia of the colon or terminal ileum. During endoscopy, multiple hemispheric smooth nodules of less than 4 mm can be found in clusters or diffusely throughout the GI tract. It is considered an excessive reaction of the GI tract lymphatic tissue (lymphoid follicles and Peyer patches) to food-related or other antigens. Spontaneous regression of lymphoid follicles is quite common. In addition to parental reassurance, an elimination diet for breastfeeding mothers is a reasonable initial treatment. Feeding with extensively hydrolyzed protein formula is the next therapeutic step. Corticosteroid therapy is restricted to infants with a severe form of this disease: recurrent abdominal pain, significant anemia, persistent rectal bleeding, diarrhea, and failure to thrive. In such cases, immunodeficiency has to be excluded.

Esophagitis should be suspected as a cause of bleeding in infants with a history of recurrent emesis and interrupted feeding patterns associated with crying, irritability, or arching. The patients with repaired esophageal atresia with or without tracheoesophageal fistula are at higher risk of severe reflux disease and esophagitis. Bleeding induced by esophagitis is usually recurrent and not intensive. The patients may have hematemesis with streaks of blood or guaiac-positive stool.

Infants or older children can develop minor bleeding due to prolapse of gastric mucosa into the esophagus through the gastroesophageal junction (prolapse gastropathy). This condition is manifested by recurrent emesis with food and appearance of brown flecks of denatured blood at the end of vomiting. The presence of frank blood or clots at the end of recurrent emesis suggests a more serious problem such as Mallory-Weiss tear.

Infants and Children Younger Than 7 Years

Several diseases have a high incidence in this age group.

The signs and symptoms of **portal hypertension** are a large-volume hematemesis; history of omphalitis secondary to catheterization of the umbilical vein; presence of splenomegaly or hepatosplenomegaly; and other stigmata of chronic liver disease such as jaundice, spider angiomas, caput medusa, and ascites. Esophageal varices are the most common site of bleeding in children with intrahepatic-sinusoidal and extrahepatic-presinusoidal forms of portal hypertension. Two-thirds of children with portal hypertension will bleed before 5 years of age. The diagnosis is based on the presence of esophageal or gastric varices or hypertensive gastropathy during an upper GI endoscopy.

Intussusception, which is common in the first 2 years of life, is strongly considered in infants and children with sudden onset of severe, cramping abdominal pain intercepted with pain-free episodes and currant jelly stools. A lead point is often present in children older than 2 years. Diagnosis is confirmed by ultrasonography (positive: "concentric circles" or the "target-shaped" sign) or barium enema. Hydrostatic reduction of intussusceptions is successful in more than 90% of children.

Meckel diverticulum is the most common congenital anomaly in children. It is estimated that approximately 2% of infants have a remnant of the omphalomesenteric duct. However, less than 5% of children will develop complications, including GI bleeding. Of those who become symptomatic, half do so in the first 2 years of life. The predominant location of Meckel diverticulum is the distal ileum (40–60 cm above the ileocecal valve). Ectopic tissue is present in up to 80% of symptomatic patients. Gastric mucosa is the most common type of ectopia. The cause of bleeding is peptic ulceration at the junction of the ectopic gastric mucosa and normal ileum, the so-called marginal ulcer. Bleeding can be massive, but it may cease spontaneously secondary to contraction of the splanchnic vessels in response to hypovolemia. This phenomenon explains the intermittent nature of bleeding from Meckel diverticulum. Bleeding is usually painless, but sometimes coincides with recurrent abdominal pain.

The diagnostic procedure of choice is a Tc-99m pertechnetate scan.

Juvenile polyps may occur in as many as 1% of children, with peak incidence from 2 to 5 years of age. The common clinical presentation is recurrent, painless bleeding with a small amount of blood on formed stool. Diarrhea and tenesmus can occur when the polyp is large and located in the left colon.

Typical juvenile polyps are smooth, rounded, and red. Polyps of less than 1 cm are usually sessile; polyps larger than 1 cm have short or long stalks. Juvenile polyps are composed of normal and cystically dilated crypts embedded in an abundant lamina propria. Colonic mucosa adjacent to the large polyp has distinguished, so-called chicken skin appearance. Colonoscopy is indicated due to the high incidence (almost 50%) of coexisting polyps in the descending and more proximal portions of the colon.

Endoscopic polypectomy is the treatment of choice. There is a general consensus that a single juvenile polyp is not a premalignant condition. Therefore, removal of a solid juvenile polyp is curative. Surveillance colonoscopy is not indicated unless the child develops a new episode of rectal bleeding.

Hemolytic uremic syndrome (HUS) should always be suspected in infants and toddlers with bloody diarrhea, present in three-quarters of children with epidemic HUS. In two-thirds of these children, *Escherichia coli* 0157:H7 can be isolated. Bloody diarrhea in HUS results from hemorrhagic colitis caused by the presence of endothelial damage produced by verotoxin and Shiga toxin and submucosal hemorrhages. Tenesmus is common. Diffuse, severe abdominal pain with peritoneal signs can occur.

The presence of the so-called thumbprinting sign on a barium enema or a computed tomography scan reflects a submucosal hemorrhage of the colon. Colitis-related symptoms last no longer than a week, followed by signs of hemolytic anemia and oliguria. Known GI complications of HUS are intussusception, pancreatitis, and intestinal obstruction. Small or large bowel perforation may occur during peritoneal dialysis, which may be performed to manage the acute renal failure that can accompany HUS.

Henoch-Schönlein purpura is most common in children younger than 7 years. The median age is 4 years. Henoch-Schönlein purpura should be suspected in children with sudden onset of severe diffuse abdominal pain, vomiting, and hematochezia following a viral illness during the winter and early spring and about a week after the appearance of purpuric-type skin lesions on the buttocks or lower extremities.

On rare occasions, GI manifestations may precede the skin rash. Severe anemia is uncommon. The small and large bowels have different degrees of hemorrhagic lesions. These may be apparent on a small bowel x-ray series or barium enema with coarsening of folds and thumbprinting. Abdominal pain and hematochezia are self-limited. Treatment with corticosteroids is controversial, although it may shorten the course of GI symptoms of abdominal pain by 1 or 2 days.

Children 7 Years and Older

The common causes of GI bleeding in these patients are listed in Table 97-2. Drug-induced gastritis or acute ulcer should be strongly suspected in children treated with NSAIDs or oral steroids. The degree of bleeding ranges from mild to moderate. The usual clinical presentation is the sudden onset of abdominal discomfort followed by hematemesis or melena. Hemorrhage usually originates from the stomach. Two types of lesions are seen: gastropathy or acute gastric ulcers due to alteration of both the mucosal microcirculation and the mucosal cytoprotection related to suppression of local synthesis of prostaglandins. The incidence of NSAID-related GI bleeding is much higher in patients with *Helicobacter pylori* gastritis. Therefore, eradication of *H pylori* infection is recommended before long-term therapy with NSAIDs.

Although peptic ulcer disease (PUD) is relatively rare in pediatric patients, it accounts for at least a third of the cases of upper GI bleeding in school-aged children. Most bleeding ulcers are located in the duodenal bulb. At least 80% of bleeding episodes from duodenal ulcers cease spontaneously. However, if the bleeding is arterial, it may recur and become life-threatening. Urgent endoscopy is necessary as soon as the patient becomes more stable after fluid resuscitation.

The risk factors for recurrent bleeding are large ulcer (>2 cm), location of the ulcer on the posteroinferior wall of the duodenal bulb, blood spurting from the base of the ulcer, a visible vessel, or an adherent clot. In these circumstances the risk of recurrent bleeding is high even after initially successful endoscopic hemostasis and acid suppression with intravenous (IV) infusion of proton pump inhibitors. These high-risk patients require a second-look endoscopy 24 hours after the initial endoscopy and careful observation in an intensive care unit. The most critical time for re-bleeding is the first 3 days following the initial hemostasis. The risk of recurrent bleeding is minimal in children with a clear base ulcer or a pigmented spot sign, a small flat thrombus in the center of an ulcer. Endoscopic hemostasis is not indicated in these cases. Hemodynamically stable children without the endoscopically identified risk factors can be managed safely on an outpatient basis.

Colitis is the most common cause of rectal bleeding in older children and teenagers. Infectious colitis is by far more common than inflammatory bowel disease.

In general, bacterial colitis is an acute, self-limited disorder manifested by sudden onset of fever, tenesmus, and bloody diarrhea lasting from 5 to 7 days.

Chronic diarrhea (lasting ≥2 weeks) is usually associated with chronic inflammatory bowel disease. Rare causes of chronic infectious colitis are *Yersinia enterocolitica,* tuberculosis, *Entamoeba histolytica, Strongyloides stercoralis,* and opportunistic infections in immunocompromised patients.

Clostridium difficile colitis should be ruled out, especially in children treated with antibiotics or hospitalized patients. Ulcerative colitis usually presents with insidious onset of diarrhea, nocturnal diarrhea, and subsequent hematochezia. Clinical manifestations of moderate to severe forms of ulcerative colitis include bloody diarrhea, abdominal cramps, urgency to defecate, malaise, anorexia with weight loss, intermittent low-grade fever, and some degree of anemia and hypoalbuminemia. Crohn disease has a more indolent onset associated with abdominal pain, diarrhea, poor appetite, and weight loss. Diarrhea is not grossly bloody unless there is bleeding from an anal fistula or colitis that is diffuse or left-sided.

Differentiation between bacterial colitis and the early stage of chronic inflammatory bowel disease is always a challenge. A high index of suspicion and negative bacterial stool culture results, including *Yersinia* species and other rare pathogens, are essential parts of early diagnosis. The definitive diagnosis of chronic inflammatory bowel disease is based on the results of upper and lower GI endoscopy including multiple biopsies.

Management

Resuscitation

It is imperative to initiate resuscitation of the hemodynamically unstable patient almost immediately before any diagnostic procedure is considered. Two large-bore peripheral IV lines or a central line should be placed and secured. Blood has to be typed and crossmatched and sent for baseline laboratory assessment of hemoglobin, hematocrit, MCV, platelet count, electrolytes, creatinine, BUN, liver enzymes, and clotting factors. Oxygen supplementation and large boluses of saline target restoration of circulation and tissue oxygenation. The volume of isotonic solution should be sufficient to improve tachycardia and reverse narrow pulse pressure. Blood transfusion is indicated for patients with

- Persisted tachycardia, abnormal pulse pressure, or orthostatic hypotension after replacement of 15% to 20% of blood volume with isotonic solution
- Estimated blood loss of 30% or more
- Hemoglobin 6g/dL or less
- Uncontrolled bleeding
- Hemorrhagic shock
- Hemoglobin of 7g/dL to 9g/dL in children with chronic heart and lung diseases and signs of hypoxia

Packed red cells are the product of choice for replacement of blood loss. Matched whole blood is preferred for patients with massive bleeding. Fresh-frozen plasma is indicated for children with suspected or documented clotting factor deficiency including those with acute or chronic liver disease. Platelet transfusion is indicated in rare cases of severe bleeding with estimated blood loss of more than 50% of the patient's blood volume or children with active hemorrhage and platelet count less than 50,000/mm³. Early blood transfusion is reasonable for children with active bleeding and known chronic heart or lung diseases. Monitoring of vital signs is a more accurate way to assess the effect of blood transfusion than monitoring of hematocrit soon after transfusion. It is reasonable to wait 6 hours before checking a posttransfusion hematocrit.

Octreotide (a synthetic somatostatin analogue) is effective adjuvant medical therapy of severe bleeding from esophageal or gastric varices. It should be given to the child with active hemorrhage and any evidence of chronic liver disease or previously diagnosed portal hypertension. The initial bolus of 1µg/kg of IV octreotide is followed by continuous infusion of octreotide 1µg/kg/h. The dose can be increased every 6 hours up to 5 µg/kg/h.

The definitive therapy of moderate to severe upper GI bleeding related to PUD or varices (esophageal or gastric) and lower GI bleeding from polyps or vascular malformation relies on endoscopic hemostasis.

Although few conditions require surgery (eg, Hirschsprung disease, Meckel diverticulum), operative procedures should be considered for children who are bleeding severely or for those with undiagnosed, persistent bleeding (Box 97-1).

Box 97-1. Procedural Management of Gastrointestinal Bleeding

Endoscopic Hemostasis of Non-Variceal Bleeding

Indications

- Active bleeding from a gastric or duodenal ulcer
- Stigmata of recent bleeding: a non-bleeding visible vessel in the ulcer base and a densely adherent clot
- Bleeding arteriovenous malformation
- Bleeding after polypectomy

Methods

- Injection of vasoconstrictive agent
- Thermal coagulation
  - Bipolar coagulation
  - Heater probes
  - Argon plasma coagulation device
- Metal clips

Endoscopic Hemostasis of Variceal Bleeding

Indications

- Active bleeding from esophageal or gastric varices
- History of bleeding secondary to portal hypertension
- Failure of shunting procedure

Techniques

- Sclerotherapy
- Endoscopic variceal ligation

Polypectomy

Indication

- Juvenile polyps less than 3 cm
- Multiple polyps less than 2 cm

Prognosis

The prognosis for infants and children with GI bleeding depends on the condition causing the bleeding. Early, aggressive treatment of the consequences of blood loss is essential to decreasing morbidity and mortality. Generally the prognosis is good, and overall mortality is less than 5%.

CASE RESOLUTION

The young child in the case history with episodic, painless rectal bleeding has a juvenile polyp. No associated nausea or vomiting is present. The polyp is palpable on digital rectal examination. Full colonoscopy and therapeutic polypectomy are performed. In addition, the polyp is evaluated for dysplasia. The polyp is benign as are most polyps found in children.

Selected References

Ament ME. Diagnosis and management of upper gastrointestinal tract bleeding in the pediatric patient. *Pediatr Rev.* 1990;12:107–116

Chaibou M, Tucci M, Dugas MA, Farrell CA, Proulx F, Lacroix J. Clinically significant upper gastrointestinal bleeding acquired in a pediatric intensive care unit: a prospective study. *Pediatrics.* 1998;102:933–938

Gilger MA. Upper gastrointestinal bleeding. In: Walker WA, Goulet OJ, Kleinman RE, Sanderson IR, Sherman RM, Shneider BL eds. *Pediatric Gastrointestinal Disease: Pathophysiology, Diagnosis and Management.* 4th ed. Hamilton, Ontario, BC; BC Decker; 2004:258–265

Goyal A, Treem WR, Hyams JS. Severe upper gastrointestinal bleeding in healthy full-term neonates. *Am J Gastroenterol.* 1994;89:613–616

Lacroix J, Nadeau D, Laberge S, Gauthier M, Lapierre G, Farrell CA. Frequency of upper gastrointestinal bleeding in a pediatric intensive care unit. *Crit Care Med.* 1992;20:35–42

Lacroix J, Nadeau D, Laberge S, Gauthier M, Lapierre G, Farrell CA. Frequency of upper gastrointestinal bleeding in a pediatric intensive care unit. *Crit Care Med.* 1992;20:35–42

Stringer MD, Howard ER. Longterm outcome after injection sclerotherapy for esophageal varices in children with extrahepatic portal hypertension. *Gut.* 1994;35:257–259

Teach SJ, Fleisher GR. Rectal bleeding in the pediatric emergency department. *Ann Emerg Med.* 1994;23:1252–1258

Diarrhea

George Gershman, MD

CASE STUDY

An 8-month-old male infant is evaluated for a 2-day history of fever and blood-streaked, mucus-laden stools. His appetite is reduced, and he is only taking sips of diluted apple juice. He has had a single episode of vomiting. There are no ill contacts. On examination, the patient is irritable with a temperature of 102.2°F (39.0°C), a pulse of 180/min, a respiratory rate of 58/min, and a blood pressure of 90/65. The mucous membranes are dry, the fontanelle is depressed, and the skin turgor is reduced. The abdomen is somewhat scaphoid, and bowel sounds are active.

Questions

1. What are the 4 major categories of diarrhea?
2. What are the common infectious agents that cause diarrhea in infants and children?
3. What are the characteristics of diarrheal stools caused by different etiologies?
4. What conditions lead to prolonged diarrhea in infants and children?
5. How is diarrhea managed in infants and children?

The word *diarrhea* is derived from Greek and means "to flow through." Diarrhea is characterized by increased volume of stool, which is associated with a looser consistency and an increased frequency of bowel movements. The frequency of defecation and consistency of stool vary from individual to individual. For example, wide variations in frequency of bowel movement may be seen under certain conditions such as breastfeeding. Some breastfed infants have a bowel movement every 1 to 2 weeks, whereas others may pass stool 12 to 15 times a day.

Diarrhea has several causes, which include infection; inflammation; and exposure to foods, drugs, and hormones that affect the absorption of water from the small and large intestines.

Epidemiology

Acute diarrhea is very common throughout the world. In the United States, acute gastroenteritis is second in frequency only to upper respiratory infections. According to the World Health Organization, 2.5 million children in Latin America, Asia, and Africa die annually from dehydration secondary to diarrhea. In contrast, approximately 400 children die from this condition in the United States each year. These children often come from lower socioeconomic classes.

In the United States, each child experiences an average of 0.9 episodes of diarrhea per year unless enrolled in a child care facility. In that case, the number increases to up to 3.2 episodes per year, a figure similar to that of children in developing nations. The leading cause of diarrhea in children in developing nations is infection with viruses, bacteria, or parasites. The severity of the infection is influenced by the underlying state of nutrition. An episode of acute gastroenteritis can precipitate severe malnutrition in marginally intact children. The fecal-oral route is the major path for the spread of infectious diarrhea. In developing nations, poor sanitation and contaminated drinking water perpetuate the problem. In the United States, contaminated food supply, such as the contamination of eggs and poultry with *Salmonella,* is associated with the spread of bacterial gastroenteritis. Puppies have been found to be a reservoir of *Campylobacter.*

Definitions

Diarrhea is defined as stool mass more than 10 g/kg in infants and more than 200 g in older children.

Acute diarrhea comprises 2 criteria: (1) sudden onset and (2) resolution of diarrhea within 2 weeks.

Persistent diarrhea implies an acute onset of diarrhea that lasts at least 14 days. The definition is based on acute onset diarrhea that continues beyond the expected duration of an infectious etiology.

Chronic diarrhea is defined as diarrhea lasting at least 14 days and associated with specific causes (eg, celiac disease or inflammatory bowel diseases).

Clinical Presentation

The presenting symptoms include frequent, watery stools, which may contain blood or mucus. Affected children may experience fever, vomiting, bloating, and abdominal pain. Signs and symptoms of dehydration such as decreased skin turgor, dry mucous membranes, depressed fontanelle, diminished tearing, and tachycardia may be present. Persistent diarrhea may be associated with weight loss and failure to gain weight at an appropriate rate (Dx Box).

Dx   Diarrhea

- Liquid stools
- Frequent stools
- Blood in stool
- Mucus in stool
- Fever
- Poor weight gain or weight loss
- Dehydration
- Vomiting
- Abdominal pain

Pathophysiology

The consistency of stool depends on the stool's water content. The movement of water through the wall of the intestine is always related to the movement of electrolytes, because no active transport of water occurs. The absorption of water is associated with the active transport of sodium, and the secretion of water is associated with the electrogenic transport of chloride. Regulatory mechanisms of water and electrolyte transport across the intestine require integration of the enteric nervous system, cells in the lamina propria, and epithelial cells. This complex system works through the generation of hormone peptides, active amines, arachidonic acid metabolites, and nitric oxide. The bulk of absorbed water crosses the intestinal epithelium between the cells (tight junctions) following the osmotic gradient generated by the transport of nutrients and electrolytes. Thus diarrhea is the reversal from the normal status of absorption to exaggerated secretion. This can be induced by 2 processes: (1) excessive osmotic load generated by ingestion of nonabsorbable sugars such as lactulose or malabsorption of lactose, or other nutrients, which generates an abnormal osmotic pressure inside the lumen of the intestine and water leak into the gut and (2) active secretion of enterocytes secondary to direct action of viral or bacterial products/toxins and different substances on the cells, particularly in the crypt areas.

Osmotic diarrhea occurs whenever digestion and/or absorption are impaired. In general, it is relatively small-volume diarrhea, which is dependent on oral intake and abolished with fasting. The most common causes of osmotic diarrhea are (1) malabsorption of carbohydrate due to excessive consumption (eg, concentrated formulas or carbonated beverages) or decreased production of brush-border enzymes or the presence of non-absorbable substances such as lactulose, sorbitol, or magnesium salts in the intestinal lumen; (2) decreased absorptive capacity of the intestine due to acute or chronic inflammation of the small bowel mucosa (eg, acute viral gastroenteritis, cow's milk protein allergy, bacterial overgrowth, giardiasis, or celiac disease); (3) lack of pancreatic enzymes or bile acid; and (4) decreased absorptive capacity of the small intestine secondary to congenital or acquired short bowel syndrome. In general, nonabsorbed nutrients create an osmotic load that stimulates water leak into the intestinal lumen across the tight junction. In addition, unabsorbed nutrients, such as carbohydrates, are the substrate for fermentation by colonic bacteria with liberation of short-chain organic acids, which create a secondary osmotic load in the large intestine and exacerbation of osmotic diarrhea.

Secretory diarrhea can be induced by any process, which creates a state of active intestinal secretion. In general, secretory diarrhea is associated with intestinal loss of large volumes of fluids, which continues despite cessation of eating. Secretory diarrhea can be induced by bacterial, viral (eg, rotavirus and human immunodeficiency virus [HIV]), or protozoon (*Cryptosporidium parvum* in immunocompromised children) infection or excessive secretion of several hormones and neuropeptides such as serotonin, histamine, cholecystokinin, etc. Secretory diarrhea is also seen with certain tumors, such as ganglioneuroblastoma, and congenital disorders of fluid and electrolyte metabolism, such as congenital chloridorrhea. The classic example of secretary diarrhea is infection with enterotoxigenic *Escherichia coli* and *Vibrio cholerae*. Both bacteria produce toxins that bind to specific enterocyte membrane receptors and activate adenyl cyclase, and production of cyclic adenosine monophosphate (by cholera toxin and heat-labile toxin from enterotoxigenic *E coli*) or cyclic guanosine monophosphate (by heat-stable toxin produced by *E coli*). The ultimate pathway involves the opening of chloride channels and massive water loss. Secretory diarrhea is particularly common in the developing nations, where it is related to infection with organisms such as enterotoxin *E coli* and *V cholerae*. In the United States, the most common cause of secretory diarrhea is rotavirus infection. Vasoactive intestinal peptide-secreting tumors such as ganglioneuroma and neuroblastoma must be considered in the diagnosis in children with persistent secretory diarrhea.

In reality, both osmotic and secretory components are present in many cases of diarrhea.

Motility disorders such as Hirschsprung disease or pseudo-obstruction syndrome can be associated with persistent nonspecific diarrhea.

Inflammatory diarrhea occurs acutely with certain infections or chronic inflammatory bowel disease. **Steatorrhea** refers to the presence of an excessive amount of fat in the stools. Approximately 95% of the fat content of food should be absorbed. In infants younger than 12 months, 10% of ingested fat may appear in the stool. Fat malabsorption occurs with problems of the small intestine, including giardiasis, chronic liver and pancreatic disorders such as biliary atresia, and cystic fibrosis.

Differential Diagnosis

Acute Diarrhea

The major cause of diarrhea in children and infants is **acute gastroenteritis,** most commonly with a **viral infection.** The most common virus is rotavirus, which usually occurs during the winter months. The disorder was referred to as *winter vomiting syndrome.* Infants present with a history of antecedent mild upper respiratory symptoms, followed by fever and vomiting. Watery diarrhea, which is usually free of blood or mucus, then occurs. About 10% of infected infants have signs of otitis media. Dehydration may also occur secondary to rotavirus infection. It is typically mildly hypernatremic, with serum sodium values of about 150 mEq/L. Enteric adenovirus is the second most common viral pathogen causing diarrhea. In the summer months, enteroviral infections may produce similar pathology.

The most common **bacterial agents** associated with gastroenteritis in the United States are *Shigella, Salmonella,* and *Campylobacter. Aeromonas,* a common pathogen in developing countries, is recovered in less than 1% of cases of diarrhea in the United States.

Campylobacter produce signs of colitis, with blood and mucus in the stools. Patients are usually febrile and experience abdominal cramps. As a rule, children infected with *Shigella* are sicker, with higher levels of fever and more marked leukocytosis. In addition, infants and toddlers are particularly prone to seizures. Infection with *Salmonella* may also be associated with high fever. Stools may be mucus-laden, and inflammation of the small intestine may be evident. Parasitic infections, particularly with *Giardia lamblia, Entamoeba histolytica,* and *Cryptosporidium parvum,* may be associated with diarrhea and may follow a more protracted course. Infestation with these organisms does not usually result in fever.

Infectious conditions that do not affect the gastrointestinal (GI) tract (otitis media and urinary tract infection) may also be associated with diarrhea. Sixty percent of children with hepatitis A develop diarrhea in the first week of illness. Other conditions may also result in diarrhea. In newborns, infection with *E coli* may produce epidemic outbreaks of large, explosive, watery, green stools without blood. These outbreaks may result in closure of newborn nurseries. Watery stools may herald the onset of **necrotizing enterocolitis**; blood is usually present, however. Necrotizing enterocolitis most often affects preterm infants with respiratory distress syndrome. The pathogenesis of necrotizing enterocolitis remains largely unknown. One of the risk factors appears to be hypoxia and ischemia related to pulmonary immaturity. The mechanism of disease production seems to be related to hypoxia of the intestinal mucosa. Enterocolitis may also occur in infants with Hirschsprung disease. Feeding intolerance, bloody stools, pneumatosis intestinalis, and air in the portal vein are the hallmarks of the disorder. Adrenal insufficiency, as well as certain inborn errors of metabolism such as galactosemia, may lead to diarrhea. In general, other symptoms such as vomiting occur. Infants may present in shock because of hypovolemia related to dehydration.

Food intolerance may result in diarrhea in infants as well as in older children. Overfeeding or the ingestion of large quantities of fruit juices, dried fruits, or sorbitol-containing products can produce osmotic diarrhea. Food allergies may also be associated with malabsorption. In infants, cow protein intolerance can produce diarrhea, growth retardation, anemia, hypoproteinemia, edema, respiratory symptoms, and eczema. Eosinophilia and elevated levels of immunoglobulin E (IgE) are uncommon in infants with cow's milk protein allergy. Because 25% to 50% of cow protein–allergic children are also soy protein–allergic, symptoms of diarrhea may not abate when soy formula is offered. However, soy formula does help infants with lactase deficiency. Congenital lactose intolerance is an extremely rare disorder. Acquired lactase deficiency is fairly common, especially in certain racial groups; it is reported in 10% of whites, 70% to 80% of African Americans, and 90% of Asians. The disorder is associated with diarrhea, cramping, bloating, and abdominal pain after consumption of lactose. The stool has an acid pH, floats because it contains air, and is positive for reducing substances. Lactase deficiency may occur following an episode of acute gastroenteritis, when the brush border of the small intestine has been disrupted.

Persistent Diarrhea

Infants and children may have a protracted course of loose stools following an episode of acute gastroenteritis.

Risk factors for persistent diarrhea are
- Caloric and protein malnutrition
- Vitamin A and zinc deficiency
- Prior infection such as measles
- Male gender and young age between 6 and 24 months
- Young maternal age

In most cases, no cause for persistent diarrhea can be detected, but infestation with *Shigella* or enterotoxigenic *E coli* may be a contributing factor. The possibility of infection with HIV should be considered in infants and children with protracted diarrhea, especially in geographic areas where disease prevalence is high. Certain children with acute diarrhea have such a modified diet (eg, clear fluids) that they develop starvation stools. These slimy, dark green or golden stools represent succus entericus, the secretion of the small intestine. Starvation stools do not have a fecal odor. Insufficient fat in the diet may contribute to starvation diarrhea.

Chronic Diarrhea

Inflammatory bowel disease, which occurs more commonly in older children and adolescents, is associated with chronic diarrhea. Ulcerative colitis presents with infiltration of the lamina propria with inflammatory cells, distortion of the glands, and crypt abscesses. Fever, weight loss, and anorexia are often present. Diarrhea is the hallmark of the disease, and patients experience tenesmus as well as mucus-laden and bloody stools. Inflammation always affects the rectum. It can be localized in the left colon (left-side colitis) or spread out through the entire large intestine (pancolitis).

Crohn disease may also lead to chronic diarrhea, although lower abdominal pain aggravated by defecation may be a more prominent part of the medical history. Affected individuals frequently experience extraintestinal manifestations of the disease, such as fever, anorexia, weight loss or growth retardation, recurrent stomatitis, uveitis, arthralgia and arthritis, and clubbing. Perianal disease, such as fistulas, may be noted in 30% of patients.

Irritable bowel syndrome may lead to chronic diarrhea in infants and children. Affected children do not suffer from diarrhea at night, which is the sign of infectious or secretory diarrhea. Partially formed first stool in the morning and increased frequency during the day is the classic history. Stooling tends to occur after each meal, suggesting a prominent gastrocolic reflex. Children may have 3 to 10 stools per day, which may be mucus-laden and contain undigested vegetable fiber. Alternating periods of constipation may occur. Affected children appear well throughout this illness, without weight loss, growth impairment, fever, leukocytosis, steatorrhea, or protein malabsorption. Their appetite remains good. Treatment of this type of chronic diarrhea involves the use of a high-residue diet to add bulk to the stool and thereby prevent small, frequent stools. Other conditions that lead to chronic diarrhea include intestinal polyposis; the use of certain medications, such as antibiotics; and the use of heavy metals, such as iron.

Chronic diarrhea may also be associated with **maldigestion,** as with cystic fibrosis, or **malabsorption,** as with celiac disease or gluten enteropathy.

Newborns with **cystic fibrosis** may present with meconium ileus or rarely with acute appendicitis. Failure to thrive is common among patients with cystic fibrosis despite the fact that many of them have voracious appetites. Stools are large, bulky, and foul-smelling secondary to the steatorrhea. Isolated GI complaints are reported in 15% to 20% of patients with cystic fibrosis, but most affected children are also prone to pulmonary infections. Rectal prolapse is another complication.

Celiac disease is related to an allergy to the gliadin portion of the wheat protein, gluten. This protein is also found in barley, rye, and oat. Characteristically, villous flattening is apparent on small intestinal biopsy. This flattening restricts the absorptive capacity of the intestine and leads to malabsorption. Children with the classic form of celiac disease have short stature, pale skin, sparse hair, protuberant abdomen, and wasted buttocks. In recent reports, subtle signs of celiac disease have been recognized and usually reflect the growth failure or anemia. Symptoms appear a few months after grains are introduced into the diet, usually between the ages of 9 and 12 months. Stools are mushy, bulky, and foul-smelling. Fat content in the stool may be 2 to 3 times the normal level.

Evaluation

History

A careful history should be obtained (Questions Box).

Physical Examination

Children should be assessed for the presence of dehydration as evidenced by altered vital signs, delayed capillary refill, decreased skin turgor, a sunken fontanelle, dry mucous membranes, and reduced tearing. Skin changes in the perianal area or evidence of diaper dermatitis would indicate the irritative nature of the stools. Perianal fissures may be present in Crohn disease. Evidence of growth retardation should be determined by assessing the growth parameters, particularly weight. Failure to gain weight over a period of months should trigger the workup of GI disorders such as chronic inflammatory bowel disease, celiac disease, or cystic fibrosis.

Laboratory Tests

Stool assessment, a major component of the evaluation, involves 4 steps. First, the stool is evaluated for its quantity as well as its gross appearance. Undigested pieces of fruits and vegetables in the stool of toddlers are often a sign of poor chewing. Small, thread-like

Questions

Diarrhea

- How long has the diarrhea been present?
- How frequent is the stooling?
- What is the consistency of the stools?
- Is stooling related to eating, which is a sign of osmotic diarrhea, or does it occur even if the child does not eat, which is a sign of secretory diarrhea?
- Do the stools contain any blood or mucus, which suggests a bacterial or parasitic infection?
- Is the child febrile?
- Does the child have any symptoms associated with the stooling problems?
- Does the child have a recent history of travel or exposure to animals?
- Is anyone at home ill?
- Has the child experienced any change in the frequency of urination, which is an important measure of the state of hydration?
- What is the child's diet now? What has it been?

bodies that resemble worms are concretions of bile and are common in the stool of infants. The change in stool volume with fasting can also be checked. Reduced volume in the face of fasting is consistent with osmotic diarrhea.

Second, the stool is subjected to chemical and microscopic analyses to detect the presence of unabsorbed nutrients such as carbohydrates and fats. The presence of carbohydrates may be detected using a small amount of stool liquefied in about 1mL of water. A Clinitest tablet is added to the sample, and a change in color from blue to green or orange is indicative of the presence of undigested carbohydrate. If the main source of dietary sugar is sucrose, as determined by the history, the specimen must be hydrolyzed by heating with hydrochloric acid. If the specimen sits around for too long, the presence of bacteria in the stool may break down the carbohydrate and lead to a false-negative result. The presence of fat can be determined both qualitatively and quantitatively. The stool may be examined under a microscope with just water or using a Sudan or Carmine red stain. If there are 10 or more globules of fat per high-power field, a quantitative fat analysis over a 3-day period should be undertaken. Ten percent of children with abnormal stool fat on microscopic assessment have a normal 3-day quantitative stool fat value.

Third, the stool is examined for the presence of blood and leukocytes. Blood may be present in the stool but originates from excoriations in the diaper area rather than from the GI tract. To assess for leukocytes in the stool, the mucous component of the stool should be smeared on a glass slide and stained with methylene blue. More than 2 to 4 leukocytes per high-power field is abnormal and suggests a bacterial infection. The sensitivity of the fecal leukocyte test is 85% but the specificity is only 50% to 60%. Absence of leukocytes or erythrocytes in the stool signifies a very low probability of an invasive bacterial infection (predictive value of a negative test is 95%). A stool specimen should be submitted for culture and may be evaluated for ova and parasites. Stool analysis using Rotazyme will detect rotavirus. Fourth, stool is assessed for levels of sodium and potassium and stool osmolality to calculate the so-called ion gap (ion gap = stool osmolarity – [(Na+K) × 2). Ion gap exceeding 100 mOsm/kg and low sodium concentration in stool (<40 mEq/L) is typical for osmotic diarrhea. On the contrary, ion gap equal to or lower than 100 mOsm/kg and sodium concentration in stool higher than 70 mEq/L is consistent with secretory diarrhea.

Additional studies, especially in the face of dehydration or fever, include serum electrolytes, complete blood count, urinalysis, and urine culture. Upper GI endoscopy with a small bowel biopsy is indicated for diagnosis of such diseases as celiac disease or other causes of persistent or chronic malabsorptive diarrhea. Colonoscopy should be considered after consultation with a gastroenterologist if inflammatory bowel disease or familial polyposis is suspected.

Management

Initial management of children with gastroenteritis involves **adequate hydration and replacement of any fluid or electrolyte deficits** (see Chapter 54). Bolus therapy may be necessary in children with significant dehydration. Children with significant dehydration may require admission to the hospital and the administration of intravenous fluids. Less severely affected children may be managed as outpatients using oral rehydrating solutions such as Pedialyte or Infalyte. Alternatively, parents can be advised to make oral rehydrating solutions by using water (1 liter), sugar (4–8 teaspoons), and salt (1/2 teaspoon).

Dietary manipulation in the treatment of diarrhea is somewhat controversial. Traditionally, affected children have been placed on clear fluids for 1 or 2 days, with a gradual return to a more regular diet with time. A **BRAT diet** (bananas, rice or rice cereal, applesauce, tea or toast) was often recommended because of the intrinsic binding properties of the particular food. Recent studies recommend a full resumption of a normal diet, including dairy products, as the way to ensure adequate nutrition during the acute illness. A high-fat, low-carbohydrate diet accelerates improvement. A lactose-free diet is beneficial for infants and children with persistent diarrhea.

Antimicrobial therapy is indicated for infection with certain pathogens such as *Campylobacter, E histolytica, G lamblia,* and *Shigella.* Antimicrobial agents are used to treat *Salmonella* infection in certain populations such as neonates, immunodeficient children, and children with sickle cell anemia. **Antidiarrheal agents** are not usually recommended for the management of diarrhea in children. Diarrhea is believed to be the body's way of eliminating a toxic substance that has been ingested. In addition, the diarrhea often progresses in spite of the medication, which has its most binding effect after the illness has subsided, leading to constipation.

Children with chronic diarrhea secondary to a specific condition should be managed as dictated by the particular disorder.

Prognosis

Most cases of diarrhea in infants and children in the United States are self-limited and resolve without problems. More chronic cases may lead to malnutrition. Enteral feedings or hyperalimentation may be used to ensure a good outcome. Some children require consultation with a pediatric gastroenterologist.

CASE RESOLUTION

In the case history, the presence of blood and mucus in the stool suggests a bacterial etiology. The stool should be examined microscopically for leukocytes using methylene blue. Their presence supports a bacterial etiology. A stool specimen as well as a blood specimen should be sent for culture. Because the infant appears dehydrated (ie, sunken fontanelle, poor skin turgor, tachycardia), admission to the hospital should be considered to allow for rehydration and the administration of parenteral antibiotics.

Selected References

Gastanaduy AS, Beque RE. Acute gastroenteritis. *Clin Pediatr.* 1999;38:1–12

Guandalini S. Acute diarrhea. In: Walker WA, Goulet OJ, Kleinman RE, et al, eds. *Pediatric Gastrointestinal Disease, Pathophysiology, Diagnosis, Management.* 4th ed. Philadelphia, PA: B.C. Decker; 2004:166–179

Guarino A, De Marco G. Persistent diarrhea. In: Walker WA, Goulet OJ, Kleinman RE, et al, eds. *Pediatric Gastrointestinal Disease, Pathophysiology, Diagnosis, Management.* 4th ed. Philadelphia, PA: B.C. Decker; 2004:180–193

Limbos MA. Approach to the child with diarrhea. In: Osborn LM, DeWitt TG, First LR, Zenel JA, eds. *Pediatrics.* Philadelphia, PA: Mosby; 2005:627–633

Richards L, Claeson M, Pierce NE. Management of acute diarrhea in children: lessons learned. *Pediatr Infec Dis J.* 1993;12:5–9

Sondheimer JM. Office stool examination: a practical guide. *Contemp Pediatr.* 1994;Suppl:5–14

Talusan-Soriano K, Lake AM. Malabsorption in childhood. *Pediatr Rev.* 1996;17:135–142

Walker-Smith JA. Chronic diarrhea. In: Lifschitz CH, ed. *Pediatric Gastroenterology and Nutrition in Clinical Practice.* New York, NY: Dekker; 2002:685–700

Constipation

Doron D. Kahana, MD, and George Gershman, MD

CASE STUDY

A 6-year-old child is brought to the office by her mother who reports 6 months of episodic belly pain. The mother states that the child complains mostly in the afternoon and evening and rarely at night or morning. She notes that her daughter vomited once and had soiled her underwear on a few occasions. She believes the child goes to the bathroom every day but has not asked her directly. She reports that the toilet was plugged a few times after the child defecated. The child has a great appetite and eats an age-appropriate diet that is high in pastas, breads, and cheese. The child is "very gassy" and sometimes looks bloated. Otherwise the child is healthy, growing and developing normally, and is in first grade. On examination, her vital signs are normal, she is at the 75th percentile in height and 90th percentile in weight. On questioning the child as to the specific location of her pain, she points to her umbilicus. On deep palpation there is a firm mass in the left lower quadrant; it is non-tender and the abdomen is otherwise soft. A rectal examination reveals hard, dry stool in the vault. The rest of the examination is normal.

Questions

1. What is the definition of constipation?
2. How is the stooling pattern related to diet?
3. What diseases and medical conditions are associated with constipation?
4. How do familial factors influence stooling patterns?
5. How is functional constipation managed?

Constipation refers to the ease of passage of stool. It is defined by stools that are dry, hard, and difficult to pass. Reduced frequency of stooling is a characteristic of constipation, but infrequent passage of soft stool is not a characteristic of constipation. The guidelines of the North American Society for Pediatric Gastroenterology, Hepatology and Nutrition define constipation as "a delay or difficulty in defecation, present for two or more weeks and sufficient to cause significant distress to the patient." Normal stooling frequency ranges from an average of 4 per day during the first weeks of life to 2 per day at 1 year of age. After age 4 and into adulthood, normal stool frequency ranges from 3 per day to 3 per week.

Many factors influence the frequency of stooling in normal infants and children, including diet, familial pattern of intestinal motility, personal sensitivity, hydration, stressors, and medications. For example, exclusively breastfed asymptomatic infants may have long intervals (up to 14 days) between soft to loose bowel movements.

Functional constipation is defined as constipation in the absence of disease; however, it is important to note that chronic constipation is also a condition that begets disease and, thus, must be treated.

In infancy, peristaltic motility may be weak. In addition, the lack of physical mobility may require the infant to exert a physiological effort (eg, Valsalva maneuver) to facilitate the passage of stool. This is often misinterpreted by parents as a sign of constipation. In early childhood, parent-child interactions around the time of toilet training may be associated with resistance on the part of the child, resulting in stool withholding. A painful evacuation can lead to resistance as well. School-aged children may withhold because of fear of going to the toilet in school or because of social stressors. Assessment of the etiology of constipation requires a careful medical history to determine the age of onset and the presence of contributing factors. After all, a regular pattern of defecation is considered by many to be a sign of good health.

Epidemiology

Prevalence of constipation is low (<3%) in infants. Constipation usually appears between the age of 2 and 4 years. It coincides with toilet training and decreased frequency of defecation due to change in diet and increased colonic transient time. Longer transit allows for colonic fermentation and salvage of micronutrients as well as absorption of water but is associated with harder, drier stools that may trigger abdominal and rectal discomfort associated with bowel movements and lead to withholding behavior.

Fecal soiling or encopresis is reported in one-third of the girls and half of the boys with constipation. Although prevalence of constipation and soiling is equal in male and female infants and toddlers, it becomes 3 times more frequent in boys than in girls 5 years and older (see Chapter 42).

Clinical Presentation

Infants often present with infrequent stooling. Some parents report facial grimacing and grunting during defecation as well as apparent discomfort or fussiness with bowel movements. History of recurrent vomiting or poor weight gain indicates the need for further evaluation. Toddlers usually present complaining of pain related to hard or large stools. Preschool-aged children may present with fecal soiling, which often represents overflow incontinence. Parents will report that the child maintains a withholding posture where the legs are clamped together and the gluteal muscles are contracted in an effort to suppress defecation (Figure 99-1). About 60% of constipated children experience recurrent abdominal pain. Poor appetite, periodic vomiting, or poor growth may be noted in severe cases secondary to a persistent sense of fullness from a dilated and impacted colon. Hydronephrosis, urinary tract infections, and enuresis are also associated with chronic constipation and an impacted colon.

Figure 99-1. Child exhibiting retentive posture.

Pathophysiology

What Is the Colon?

The colon is a muscular organ that reabsorbs more than 90% of the water that enters it and prepares stool for excretion (Figure 99-2). Moreover, the colon is full of hundreds of species of bacteria and other microflora. Food products entering the colon undergo the process of fermentation, which produces gas (eg, hydrogen, methane) and short-chain fatty acids. Short-chain fatty acids provide colonocytes with readily available fuel (via butyric acid) and enter the portal circulation for calorie salvage in the liver (eg, propionic and acetic acids). The fermentation process may release other micronutrients and vitamins and is thus an important component of gastrointestinal (GI) function.

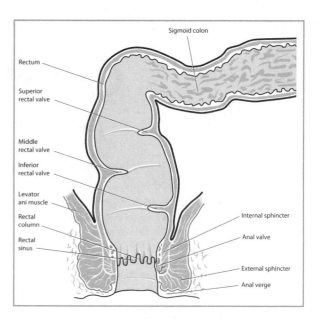

Figure 99-2. Diagram of anus, rectum, and sigmoid colon.

Normal Physiology

Digested food normally takes about 2 hours to reach the cecum from the duodenum. This occurs via peristaltic waves called the migrating motor complex. Once in the cecum, the chyme may take several hours to several days to be expelled as stool. The more prolonged the transit time, the more extensive the water resorption and fermentation process and the more likely it is for the stool to be formed and hard. The rectosigmoid is the sensing organ that initiates the process of defecation and can store stool while furthering water resorption. Contraction and emptying of the descending colon and rectosigmoid is stimulated by eating, a process called the *gastrocolic reflex*. In the rectum, the pelvic floor muscles (levator ani, puborectalis) regulate fecal retention and defecation. The puborectalis suspends the rectosigmoid and imposes constraints that facilitate voluntary stool retention (continence). Continence is also promoted by contraction of the internal and external anal sphincters.

Defecation

The urge to defecate is signaled by the propulsion of feces from the sigmoid colon to the rectum. Distention of the rectum causes relaxation of the internal anal sphincter; the external anal sphincter and puborectalis must voluntarily relax under parasympathetic conditions. The pelvic floor muscles descend, permitting straightening of the anus and rectum (see Figure 99-2). Thus defecation is facilitated by squatting or sitting and by increasing intra-abdominal pressure (ie, Valsalva maneuver). The urge to defecate can be consciously repressed by voluntary contraction of the external anal sphincter and likely subconscious sympathetic reflex inhibition and contraction of the puborectalis muscle. The process of defecation is learned early in childhood and remains spontaneous throughout life. The spontaneity of this process may be lost for a variety of reasons, including secondary to trauma, pelvic floor dysfunction (dyssynergia), pseudo-obstruction, or surgical resection.

The Vicious Cycle of Constipation

If the urge to defecate is suppressed for some time, the rectosigmoid and eventually the entire colon will become dilated and impacted, and defecation may become difficult. The increase in the caliber of the colon makes contractions less powerful and less effective in propagating stool. Moreover, the constipated child may become desensitized to rectal distention and further delay defecation. Eventually, delayed defecation leads to formation of very hard, bulky stool, which makes defecation extremely difficult and painful. As a result, the child learns to tighten the external anal sphincter and the gluteal muscles, which push feces higher in the rectal vault and suppress the urge to defecate. This is the vicious cycle of constipation. In children, the initiating event may be a painful passage of stool, possibly after an acute illness. Intentional and prolonged suppression of defecation is an important factor in the pathogenesis of constipation. In school-aged children it is common for a child to suppress the urge to defecate during school hours. A similar phenomenon occurs for toddlers during toilet training.

Familial Factors

Some families are predisposed to constipation. Concordance for constipation is 4 times more common in monozygotic twins than dizygotic twins. It may be related to increased absorption of water in the colon leading to drier, harder stools. In other cases, the bowel is unusually long or poorly motile. In some families, sensitivity to critical rectal volumes seems to be decreased, or particularly large rectal volumes are necessary for initiation of the process of defecation.

Differential Diagnosis

The differential diagnosis of constipation can be divided into the following etiologic categories: congenital or acquired, anatomical, neurologic, hormonal, infectious or toxic, drug-induced, or functional (Box 99-1). Functional constipation is supported by a characteristic history including poor hydration, diet, and stool withholding behavior as well as a normal examination. A recent illness in which the child may have been dehydrated (eg, febrile illness, pharyngitis, upper respiratory infection) may have lead to constipation or a painful bowel movement. A dietary history may reveal high consumption of milk (>24 oz/d), cheese, or sugary fruit juice, as well as poor intake of fruits, vegetables, and whole grains. Stool withholding is most commonly seen in preschool-aged and early school-aged children and often is a product of a stressful environment such as a new sibling, a move, parental struggles, or a new school environment.

Chronic constipation that is resistant to medical therapy should not be ignored. Especially in infants and toddlers, several conditions, such as Hirschsprung disease and congenital intestinal malrotation, can present past the neonatal period and lead to intestinal devastation (ie, ischemia) if not recognized early.

Several conditions are particularly important to consider when evaluating constipation in infants, including Hirschsprung disease, hypothyroidism, anal stenosis/atresia, meningomyelocele, and cerebral palsy. Failure to pass or a delay in passage of meconium (meconium ileus) of more than 24 hours should also raise a suspicion for Hirschsprung disease and cystic fibrosis.

Hirschsprung disease is an intestinal motility disorder resulting from aganglionosis of the myenteric plexus that usually affects the rectosigmoid colon. However, the entire colon can be involved. The severity of the disease and complexity of surgical treatment is directly proportional to the length of the affected colon. When ganglion cells are missing in the very distal portion of the rectum, the disorder may resemble chronic idiopathic constipation, oftentimes resistant to medical therapy. The prevalence of Hirschsprung disease is about 1 in 5,000 live births and accounts for 3% of all constipated children referred to a gastroenterologist. Physical examination of a patient with Hirschsprung disease may reveal some degree of abdominal distention and an empty rectal vault. In infants, a rectal examination frequently induces explosive stool due to distention of the internal anal sphincter. Early recognition of this condition is important to prevent the development of toxic megacolon and enterocolitis, a condition that carries high morbidity and mortality. Hirschsprung disease may be seen in conjunction with syndromes such as trisomy 21, Smith-Lemli-Opitz, and Waardenburg syndromes, and several genetic mutations in the receptor tyrosine kinase gene *RET* have been described as the inciting event.

Box 99-1. Differential Diagnosis of Constipation

Anatomical	Neurologic	Hormonal	Other	Infectious/Toxic	Drug-Induced/ Metabolic	Functional
• Anal stenosis	• Hirschsprung disease	• Hypothyroidism	• Cystic fibrosis	• Post-infectious ileus	• Analgesics (opioids)	• Dehydration
• Imperforate anus	• Cerebral palsy	• Panhypopituitarism	• Celiac disease	• Botulism	• Antacids	• Stool withholding
• Ectopic anus	• Hypotonia	• Multiple endocrine neoplasia	• Cow's milk protein allergy		• Anticholinergics (eg, pseudoephedrine)	• Stress
• Postsurgical stricture	• Spina bifida (occulta)	• Pheochromocytoma			• Bismuth	• Anxiety
	• Meningomyelocele				• Iron	• Fear of painful evacuation
	• Sacral agenesis				• Cholestyramine	
	• Intestinal pseudo-obstruction syndrome				• Hypocalcemia	
					• Hyperkalemia	

Infants with hypothyroidism secondary to hypopituitarism may also present with constipation and are not diagnosed through the newborn screening process because of normal (ie, low) levels of thyroid-stimulating hormone. These children may either appear clinically normal or display some of the features of hypothyroidism (eg, large fontanels, umbilical hernia, coarse facies, macroglossia).

Anal stenosis, imperforate anus with a perineal fistula, or an anteriorly displaced anus may not be recognized immediately in the newborn period because the condition may be subtle. Anorectal malformations occur in about 1 in 7,000 live births, which enforces the need for a perianal and rectal examination with every constipated child.

Constipation that begins prior to toilet training is more suggestive of an organic etiology such as Hirschsprung disease, malrotation, or pseudo-obstruction syndrome. Pseudo-obstruction may also present in older children who may have a history of abdominal distention, pain, and intestinal paresis. Onset of constipation around the time of toilet training, when stooling has been normal in the past, suggests functional constipation.

Constipation may develop in some children in association with the use of medications such as iron or bismuth (Pepto-Bismol), codeine or other narcotics, chemotherapeutic agents (eg, vincristine), and agents with anticholinergic properties (eg, pseudoephedrine, imipramine).

Evaluation

History

Commonly associated historical signs and symptoms of constipation include abdominal pain, especially during or after meals, abdominal distention and excessive flatulence, bright-red blood in toilet water or on toilet paper, toilet plugging, and enuresis (Questions Box). Overflow incontinence may lead to a history of chronic diarrhea or fecal soiling, although a good physical examination in such a setting should reveal an impacted colon or rectum. It is important to ask about recurrent mouth sores, rashes, joint pain, weight loss, bloody stools, incomplete evacuations, and tenesmus (rectal spasm and strong urge to defecate usually with the passing of blood and/or mucus). A family history of inflammatory bowel disease should also be noted with every child presenting with abdominal pain.

Physical Examination

The physical examination is usually normal. If the child is experiencing discomfort, ask the child to indicate with one finger the area of greatest pain. Most often, the child will point to the periumbilical area or not be able to localize a specific area. A firm stool mass may be palpable in the left lower quadrant of some patients and is usually non-tender. A rectal examination should be performed on every child with constipation. The consistency and color of the stool in the rectum will vary, but a hard, dry stool will strongly support the diagnosis. A rectum empty of stool, followed by the explosive passage of liquid stool, suggests

> ## Questions
>
> ### Constipation
>
> - What is the child's stooling pattern? How often does the child have a bowel movement? What is the appearance and consistency of the stool?
> - What was the child's age when the problem began?
> - What makes up the child's diet?
> - Does the child take any medications?
> - Does the child have any symptoms associated with constipation, such as recurrent abdominal pain? If so, how long have these been occurring?
> - Has the child been sick recently with any illnesses that might cause constipation?
> - Has the child recently experienced any changes in routine that could cause constipation?
> - Is there a family history of constipation?
> - How old was the child when he or she was toilet trained?
> - Is there any bleeding with stooling?
> - Is there pain with stooling?
> - Have any remedies such as laxatives, enemas, or suppositories been used to relieve the symptoms?

Hirschsprung disease. The back of the child should be inspected for a sacral dimple or a hair tuft, especially in infants because this may be a sign of occult spinal cord anomaly.

It is important to note whether pallor, mouth sores, hepatosplenomegaly, arthritis, and rashes are present because these findings may point to a more severe underlying disease process.

Laboratory Tests

If malnourishment is a concern, suggested by either the history or physical examination, a complete blood count with red cell indices should be ordered. Iron-deficiency anemia may be an early sign of poor nutritional intake. A chemistry panel may reveal hypocalcemia or hypoalbuminemia. Thyroid function studies and stool test for botulinum toxin may be ordered if these conditions are suspected.

Imaging Studies

Flat plates of the abdomen or any other x-ray studies are not indicated for children with functional constipation. Although it may reveal an impacted and/or dilated colon, normal images are not standardized and the variability of the size of a normal colon may be great. Anatomical studies such as a barium upper GI series or enema may help rule out malrotation or establish the diagnosis of an imperforate anus or Hirschsprung disease. It is suggested that a barium enema be attempted without prior clean-out to better document the presence of a transitional zone between dilated colon and the rectum.

Further Tests

Anorectal manometry and a suction rectal biopsy may be carried out by a gastroenterologist to help diagnose Hirschsprung disease; however, only a full-thickness rectal biopsy will confirm the presence or absence of aganglionosis and must be performed by a surgeon. Colonic manometry can also measure colonic peristaltic waves and help diagnose pseudo-obstruction.

Management

In the Primary Care Setting

Most cases of constipation can be evaluated and managed by primary care physicians. In functional constipation, the mainstay of management involves dietary manipulation and behavioral modification. Diets that predispose to constipation are rich in simple carbohydrates (ie, sugar), refined and processed carbohydrates (eg, pasta), and dairy (specifically milk and cheese) and low in fruits, vegetables, and whole grains. It may be a real challenge to change a child's diet; however, good parenting technique may allow for elimination of some items with the introduction of others. Prune juice and fruit nectars (eg, pear, peach, and apricot) are well tolerated and effective. Certain fruits, including papaya, cantaloupe, and grapes, are very high in fiber. Popcorn is a readily acceptable and effective bulking food but should not be given to young children due to the risk of choking. All dried fruits (eg, raisins, cranberries) are mildly cathartic. It is important to keep introducing new vegetable options. Often a child will welcome 1 or 2 vegetables (eg, carrots, corn, peas), but the parent must be persistent. Introduction of whole grain breads and brown rice may require some adjustment but will render lifelong benefits to the child.

Behavioral modification can be challenging but it is also absolutely essential to break the vicious cycle of constipation. Introducing the concept of "toilet hygiene" to the child should be done in a firm and consistent manner. The parent should engage the child with a daily star or sticker chart, and the child must sit on the toilet every day at least once, normally after a meal (to use the natural gastrocolic reflex), for 8 to 10 minutes (not much longer, as this may lead to fissure formation). However, even if the child does not have a bowel movement with each toilet sitting, good toilet hygiene will make the experience a routine and hopefully help prevent further reluctance to use the toilet. Biofeedback may be useful, especially in children with encopresis and/or paradoxical contraction of their external anal sphincter.

Medications are generally safe and now mostly over the counter (eg, milk of magnesia). Lactulose, a nonabsorbable, high molecular weight sugar, and PEG-3350 (MiraLAX), a nonabsorbable synthetic polymer, both help retain fluid in the colon and thus prevent the complete solidification of the stool. This allows for softer stools. Lactulose can undergo fermentation in the colon, which may lead to gassiness and bloating in some patients. A glycerin suppository or Fleet enema may be indicated with severe impaction but is generally not necessary. Mineral oil is effective in reducing the pain associated with hard stools; however, it may leak and stain the underwear and in infants has been associated with aspiration and chemical pneumonitis. Other medications, such as Dulcolax or Senokot, are less effective. Dietary fiber supplements such as psyllium husk (Metamucil)

or guar gum (Benefiber) may help some patients but may also be a difficult habit to maintain with children.

The most important element in the management of functional constipation is persistence and chronicity. Several months (eg, 3–6) of MiraLAX or lactulose therapy are often needed and considered safe and non–habit forming. Dietary changes and toilet hygiene should be incorporated into lifestyle and practiced into adulthood.

When to Refer to a Gastroenterologist

Constipation that is resistant to medical therapy should not be ignored. Anatomical disease (eg, malrotation) may present late, as can Hirschsprung disease and pseudo-obstruction, and can lead to toxic megacolon or mid-gut volvulus with intestinal ischemia and devastation. These conditions will require surgical intervention and long-term follow-up and thus should be referred to a specialist.

Special attention should be paid to infants with persistent constipation because of the high risk of serious conditions such as Hirschsprung disease, internal rectal sphincter achalasia, or malrotation.

Prognosis

The prognosis varies with the etiology. Functional constipation is usually amenable to routine management, although treatment failures are reported in 20% of children with functional fecal retention. Long duration of symptoms, poor self-esteem, and prior sexual abuse are associated with a poorer prognosis. Even in these cases, functional retention is uncommon after the age of 12 years. With appropriate surgical treatment, the prognosis for children with Hirschsprung disease or anatomical abnormality is excellent.

CASE RESOLUTION

The child in the case scenario has functional constipation. The belly pain is visceral and related to gas distention and stool retention. The relation of her pain to meals is a reflection of the gastrocolic reflex. A single episode of vomiting may be coincidental and is not overly concerning. Soiling may occur with overflow incontinence. It is surprising how often the parents are unaware of their children's toileting habits. Gassiness is simply the reflection of stool fermentation in the colon. It is essential to note that the child has maintained normal appetite and growth parameters. The rectal examination confirms the diagnosis. No further tests are necessary at this point, and therapy should be initiated by the primary care physician.

Selected References

Abi-Hanna A, Lake AM. Constipation and encopresis in children. *Pediatr Rev.* 1998;19:23–31

Baker SS, Liptak GS, Colletti RB, et al. Constipation in infants and children: evaluation and treatment. A medical position statement of the North American Society for Pediatric Gastroenterology and Nutrition. *J Pediatr Gastroenterol Nutr.* 1999;29:612–626

Biggs WS, Dery WH. Evaluation and treatment of constipation in infants and children. *Am Fam Physician.* 2006;73:469–477

Constipation Guideline Committee of the North American Society for Pediatric Gastroenterology. Evaluation and treatment of constipation in infants and children: recommendations of the North American Society for Pediatric Gastroenterology, Hepatology and Nutrition. *J Pediatr Gastroenterol Nutr.* 2006;43:e1–e13

Croffie JM, Fitzgerald JF. Idiopathic constipation. In: Walker WA, Goulet OJ, Kleinman RE, et al, eds. *Pediatric Gastrointestinal Disease.* Hamilton, Ontario, BC: Decker; 2004:1000–1015

Johanson JF. Geographic distribution of constipation in the United States. *Am J Gastroenterol.* 1998;93:188–191

Loening-Baucke V. Prevalence, symptoms and outcome of constipation in infants and toddlers. *J Pediatr.* 2005;146:359–363

Rubin G. Constipation in children. *Clin Evid.* 2004;11:385–390

Wald A. Evaluation and management of constipation. *Clin Perspect Gastroenterol.* 1998;1:106–115

Abdominal Pain

George Gershman, MD

CASE STUDY

An 8-year-old girl has a 3-month history of intermittent abdominal pain. The pain is present prior to eating and is intensified by food. Vomiting often follows and relieves the pain. The pain also occurs at night. As a result of her symptoms, the child has missed 1 to 2 days of school each week. The family moved to the area 6 months ago, and initially the child seemed to be adjusting to her new school and environment. In addition, the girl has a history of a 5-lb weight loss. She has a positive family history of abdominal pain; her father has been diagnosed with a peptic ulcer. On physical examination, the vital signs are normal. The weight is at the fifth percentile and the height is at the 25th percentile. There are no abnormal physical findings, and the patient is quiet and cooperative. The rectal examination is normal, and the stool is negative for occult blood.

Questions

1. What are the different types of abdominal pain?
2. What characteristics distinguish functional from organic abdominal pain?
3. What are the common organic causes of recurrent abdominal pain in children?
4. What are 2 etiologies for functional pain?

Abdominal pain is a common pediatric complaint. Pain may be acute or occur on a recurrent basis. Most children with acute abdominal pain have self-limiting conditions such as viral or bacterial gastroenteritis. However, a sudden onset of abdominal pain can be caused by serious, life-threatening conditions (eg, acute appendicitis, intussusception, or hemolytic uremic syndrome). Traditionally, recurrent abdominal pain is defined as pain that has occurred on 3 or more occasions in a 3-month period and interferes with the patient's activity. This definition is applicable to so-called functional abdominal pain or abdominal pain related to organic disorders. The criteria for functional abdominal pain were modified recently: symptom duration was decreased from 3 to 2 months and a frequency of "at least once per week" was added. Functional abdominal pain is the most common type of abdominal pain in children. It should be considered in patients without any evidence of anatomical, metabolic, infectious, inflammatory, and neoplastic processes. The term *functional abdominal pain* should not suggest that affected children are malingerers or their symptoms are fictitious.

An organic etiology is found in less than 10% of school-aged children with recurrent abdominal pain (RAP). However, failure to recognize and/or delayed therapy can have devastating effects.

Epidemiology

Abdominal pain, one of the most common symptoms of childhood, is often fleeting and, therefore, not brought to medical attention. Acute pain may be related to multiple etiologies, which occur with variable frequency in different age groups. Recurrent abdominal pain, also a common problem, is reported in 10% to 25% of school-aged children. Primary peptic ulcers, which affect 4 to 8 million adults, are uncommon in children. Even large pediatric centers see only 5 cases per year.

Pathophysiology

There are 3 main reasons for acute or chronic organic abdominal pain: inflammation, distention of the viscera, and ischemia.

Abdominal pain can originate from abdominal viscera (visceral pain), parietal peritoneum, abdominal wall, retroperitoneal skeletal muscles (somatic pain), and extra-abdominal sites (so-called referred pain). Impulses of visceral pain are carried out primarily by small, unmyelinated, slow-conducting afferent C fibers incorporated into the autonomic sensory pathways. Each visceral organ receives dual sympathetic and parasympathetic innervations. Sensory fibers associated with the sympathetic nervous system traverse both prevertebral (celiac, superior and inferior mesenteric ganglion) and paravertebral ganglion and terminate in the spinal cord. Sensory fibers contained in the vagus and pelvic nerves (parasympathetic branch of the autonomic nervous system) terminate in the brain stem and lumbosacral spinal cord respectively. Sensory fibers from visceral organs that connect with the spinal column terminate within the 4 to 5 spinal segments. This explains why visceral pain is poorly localized and often perceived along the midline as a dull or aching sensation. For example, the onset of acute appendicitis is usually manifested by pain in the periumbilical or epigastric areas before the pain migrates to the right lower quadrant. It is frequently accompanied by symptoms of autonomic disturbance (eg, nausea or pallor).

Somatic pain is induced by irritation of parietal peritoneum and supportive tissue. The signals from the pain receptors (nociceptors) are transmitted for the most part by rapid conducting myelinated

A-delta fibers responsible for tactile, thermal, and chemical stimulation and discrimination of location and intensity of stimuli. As a result, somatic pain is well localized, intense, and sharp. The important characteristic of somatic pain is aggravation by movement. Therefore, the child with somatic abdominal pain is likely to lie still in contrast to the restless patient with visceral pain.

The classic example of referred pain is abdominal pain induced by inflammation of parietal pleura at the onset of pneumonia as the result of shared central projections of the parietal pleura and abdominal wall.

The location of abdominal pain is determined by the level of spinal cord connection with the corresponding visceral organs through the afferent sensory fibers. The structures of the foregut origin such as distal esophagus, stomach, duodenum, liver, and pancreas are innervated by the nerves that enter the spinal cord at the level T5 to T9 segments. Pain from these organs is perceived between the xiphoid and umbilicus. The structures related to the primitive midgut (small intestine, appendix, and right colon) project the afferent fibers to the T8 to T9 segments of the spinal cord. As a result, the associated pain affects the periumbilical area. The structures related to the embryonic hindgut, including the left colon and the rectum, share the innervation, which involve the spinal segments T10 to L1 and allocate the pain between the umbilicus and symphysis pubis.

Radiation of the pain may be helpful in diagnosis (eg, pain related to acute cholecystitis or biliary colic often refers to the area just under the inferior angle of the right scapula or above the right clavicle). Another example of referred pain is pain between the scapulas and middle back region in patients with pancreatitis.

The pathophysiology of functional abdominal pain is different from acute or chronic organic abdominal pain. The genesis of functional abdominal pain is related to abnormalities in the enteric nervous system and dysregulation of the brain-gut interaction. It is now believed that children with functional abdominal pain may have abnormal responses to the normal physiological functions related to meals as well as intestinal distention during peristalsis, associated hormonal changes, and psychological conditions like anxiety and parental separation.

Research data suggest that visceral hyperalgesia is the key element in the pathophysiology of functional abdominal pain. This theory implies sensitization of the various receptors associated with afferent innervation of the gastrointestinal (GI) tract by an infectious or allergic process or abnormal processing of afferent signals by the central nervous system.

Clinical Presentation

Children who experience abdominal pain may present with pain that may be characterized as persistent or intermittent, waxing and waning or steady and unrelenting, sharp or dull, and worsened or unaffected by movement. They may have associated complaints, including vomiting, diarrhea, constipation, fever, weight loss, headache, and anorexia (Dx Box).

Dx **Abdominal Pain**

- Abdominal pain
- Abdominal wall rigidity
- Abdominal tenderness
- Vomiting
- Alterations in bowel sounds
- Diarrhea or constipation
- Anorexia
- Fever

Pain from distention of smooth muscle also waxes and wanes, is poorly localized, and is unaffected by motion. Distention of any hollow viscus, including the stomach, intestines, biliary tree, fallopian tubes, or ureters, can result in such symptomatology. A classic example of such pain is renal colic, where the patient is writhing because of the discomfort.

Differential Diagnosis

In assessing the possible disease entities that may account for abdominal pain, patient age and duration of symptoms are the key differential components. The location of the pain may provide a clue to the etiology. Disease affecting the stomach is usually appreciated in the epigastrium. Duodenal problems are noted between the xiphoid and the umbilicus, small intestinal pathology is appreciated in the periumbilical area, and cecal inflammation may be felt from the epigastrium to McBurney point. Disease in the colon is less specifically noted but is usually felt in the hypogastrium. Bladder and colon problems may be suprapubic or sacral. Pain may also be referred to the back. Renal colic is also noted in the back, but more in a lateral or costovertebral angle (CVA tenderness) site.

Acute and Recurrent Abdominal Pain

Young Infants: Medical Conditions

A unique disorder of infants, **colic** has been referred to as paroxysmal fussiness of infancy (see Chapter 35). The onset of symptoms is usually between 2 and 4 weeks of age, with resolution by 3 to 4 months. Although recurrent abdominal pain seems to be present, abdominal pain has never been established as the cause of colic. Colic is characterized by fussiness and crying. Symptoms usually appear after feeding, particularly late in the day around dinnertime. Infants cry, clench their fists, and flex their legs. A gas-cry–air-swallowing cycle seems to occur. The symptoms may respond to a number of measures, including rhythmic motion and anti-gas medications. Infants with colic usually appear well otherwise and often have accelerated weight gain secondary to repeated feeding made in efforts to quiet them.

Abdominal pain may also occur with **food allergy,** particularly cow's milk protein allergy. Generally, symptoms such as vomiting, diarrhea, Hemoccult-positive stools, failure to thrive, rhinitis, eczema, pallor, irritability, and a positive family history of allergies are associated with food allergies. Disaccharidase deficiency may result in abdominal pain, but diarrhea is also usually present.

Young Infants: Surgical Conditions

Intussusception occurs in infants between the ages of 6 and 24 months. Children may have been previously well or have experienced a recent bout of diarrhea. Vomiting is reported in about 50% of patients, and pallor is frequently present. Lethargy is not an uncommon associated symptom. An etiology is noted in less than 2.5% of affected infants, although a lead point (lymphoma or Meckel diverticulum) may be found in 5% to 10% of older children. The intussusception most often involves the area around the ileocecal valve. Compression of the vessels within the bowel wall may lead to necrosis and gangrene. The presence of blood and mucus in the stools gives a "currant jelly" appearance, although the initial stool is often normal, having been the stool that was present in the rectum prior to the intussusception.

The abdominal examination of affected children may be benign except for pain over the area of the intussusception or may reveal the presence of a mass. Bowel sounds may be increased secondary to the obstruction. The rectal examination may reveal blood and the presence of a mass. Fever and leukocytosis may also be noted. A flat plate of the abdomen may show an obstructive pattern, with distended loops of bowel and air fluid levels. Intussusception is diagnosed by abdominal ultrasound or barium enema. Hydrostatic reduction is the treatment of choice of intussusception. It is successful in almost 90% to 95% of children. Failure of hydrostatic reduction or associated complications are related to delayed diagnosis and severe edema and necrosis of the affected bowel.

School-Aged Children: Medical Conditions

Peptic ulcers may develop in children in 3 situations. (1) Acute infantile ulcers may occur in newborns secondary to stress and hypoxia. (2) Stress ulcers may occur in children who are the victims of trauma, including burns and hypoxia (eg, after submersion). The routine use of histamine H$_2$ receptor antagonists has reduced the incidence of ulcers in hospitalized critically ill children. (3) Adult or chronic primary ulcers may develop in children with no apparent precipitating factors. A positive family history of peptic ulcer disease is reported in 25% to 50% of children. Unlike the classic ulcer symptoms of adults, in which pain occurs on an empty stomach and is relieved by eating, younger children may find that ulcer-related pain is exacerbated by eating and relieved by vomiting. Hematemesis and Hemoccult-positive stools are clues to the diagnosis. There is clear evidence linking ulcer disease and infection with *Helicobacter pylori* in adults. The relationship between *H pylori* and peptic ulcer disease in children is not so strong, though one third of pediatric patients with endoscopic evidence of peptic ulcer disease have infection with *H pylori*. Ulcers may also develop in children taking both nonsteroidal anti-inflammatory drugs and corticosteroids.

Primary peritonitis is secondary to infection with *Streptococcus pneumoniae* and is seen in children with nephrotic syndrome, cirrhosis, and sickle cell disease, and in young girls with fever, abdominal pain, and vaginal discharge.

Mesenteric adenitis may produce symptoms indistinguishable from appendicitis, although affected children may not be so ill-appearing. Nausea and vomiting and a history of an antecedent upper respiratory infection are often present.

Parenteral infections such as tonsillitis or pneumonia may present with fever and abdominal pain. In addition, hepatitis may result in pain and tenderness localized to the right upper quadrant in association with anorexia. Hepatitis in children is usually due to hepatitis A, and many infected young children are anicteric (see Chapter 102).

Pancreatitis produces abdominal pain that is often referred to the back. In the past, mumps was the most common cause of pancreatitis. Other infections such as hepatitis B, Epstein-Barr virus and Coxsackievirus B, and *Mycoplasma pneumoniae* are the common infectious etiologies of acute pancreatitis.

Currently certain medications (eg, steroids, chemotherapeutic agents) induce pancreatitis as a side effect. Familial and recurrent forms of pancreatitis are also reported. Trauma, particularly from injuries sustained as a result of an impact against handlebars of bicycles, is a common cause. In children with pancreatitis and no apparent etiology, trauma related to child abuse should be considered.

Parasitic infestations, particularly with *Giardia lamblia,* may produce abdominal pain, often with bloating and diarrhea.

Genitourinary problems may result in abdominal pain. An abnormal urinalysis provides clues to the etiology. Renal stones occur infrequently in children, and boys are more often affected than girls. In two thirds of affected children, stones are detected incidentally or in association with a urinary tract infection (UTI). Stones may be composed of calcium phosphate or oxalate, magnesium, uric acid, cystine, or xanthine. In addition to flank or abdominal pain, patients may also experience hematuria, fever, recurrent UTI, and persistent pyuria.

Hematologic and vascular disorders such as sickle cell disease, rheumatic fever, and Henoch-Schönlein purpura may also present with abdominal pain. Sickle cell anemia should be considered in African American children with abdominal pain. Pain may be related to vaso-occlusive events including bowel ischemia and splenic infarction or cholecystitis. Henoch-Schönlein purpura, which is also referred to as anaphylactoid purpura, is characterized by a hemorrhagic skin rash, joint pain, and renal abnormalities in addition to abdominal pain. This pain may result from a number of processes, including vasculitis and ischemia of the bowel wall, edema of the bowel wall, and intussusception of the small intestine. The intussusception that occurs in 10% of affected children may be difficult to diagnose because the colon is unaffected and a barium enema is normal.

Diabetes mellitus may lead to abdominal pain secondary to cramping of accessory muscles of respiration during a bout of ketoacidosis.

Acute intermittent porphyria is an uncommon cause of abdominal pain in children. The pain is often colicky and may be associated with constipation, nausea, and vomiting. Neurologic symptoms such as pain or paresthesia in the extremities may be present. Often symptoms are precipitated by the ingestion of medications (eg, barbiturates, sulfa drugs). Some antispasmodic medications, such as Donnatal elixir, contain phenobarbital and can precipitate an attack. The diagnosis is made by evaluating the urine for the presence of protoporphyrins.

School-Aged Children: Surgical Conditions

Appendicitis is the most common surgical condition that produces abdominal pain in school-aged children. Appendicitis may even occur in newborns, where it is seen in association with conditions such as cystic fibrosis and Hirschsprung disease that lead to diminished passage of stool. The condition is frequently difficult to diagnose in children younger than 3 or 4 years for 2 reasons: (1) examination of such young children for pain is difficult and (2) symptoms are similar to those of acute gastroenteritis (ie, fever, abdominal pain, anorexia). Classically, patients complain of periumbilical pain that localizes to the right lower quadrant in 1 to 5 hours. They often have a low-grade fever, with a temperature of 100.4°F (38°C). Vomiting and increased urinary frequency may occur. Stooling is variable.

The physical examination may reveal guarding and localized pain as well as rebound tenderness. A positive psoas or obturator sign may be present, indicating inflammation of these muscles. Tenderness may also be noted on rectal examination. Leukocytosis over 10,000/μL is also usually present. An x-ray of the abdomen may reveal 1 of 4 signs: a fecalith in the appendix (appendicolith), air in the cecum (sentinel loop), blurring of the shadow of the psoas muscle, or edema of the abdominal wall on the right side. A chest x-ray is also useful to rule out the presence of pneumonia, which may produce symptoms that mimic appendicitis.

Meckel diverticulum may be responsible for abdominal pain in a number of ways. It may serve as the lead point for an intussusception, cause symptoms of ulcer disease (pain or hemorrhage) secondary to the presence of ectopic gastric mucosa, or become acutely inflamed as in appendicitis. Meckel diverticulum follows the rule of 2s: it affects 2% of the population, is 2 feet from the ileocecal valve, is 2 inches in length, and is 2 times more common in males than in females.

Adolescents

In female adolescents, **gynecologic problems** such as torsion of the ovary, mittelschmerz, dysmenorrhea, and pelvic inflammatory disease must be considered as causes of abdominal pain (see Chapter 86). In addition, pain may result from gall bladder disease secondary to cholelithiasis or cholecystitis. Cholelithiasis is also a consideration in previously pregnant adolescent patients with abdominal pain and fatty food intolerance.

Recurrent Abdominal Pain

As noted previously, most children with RAP do not have a diagnosable condition that accounts for their pain. Much has been written about the family dynamics of these children and the reactions of families to children's pain. Pain in these children is functional rather than structural. According to the clinical presentation, functional abdominal pain can be subdivided into 4 categories: isolated paroxysmal abdominal pain, abdominal pain associated with functional dyspepsia, abdominal pain associated with altered bowel pattern, and abdominal migraine. Children with isolated paroxysmal abdominal pain do not have any association of pain with eating, defecation, menses, or exercise. It is often triggered by new environment, difficulties at school, or domestic problems. The pain is usually periumbilical and quite severe. It can be recurrent or continuous and may affect daily activity. Children with functional dyspepsia experience ulcer-like or dysmotility-like symptoms. The dominant feature of non-ulcer dyspepsia is epigastric pain before a meal or at night. The pain is often relieved by food or medical inhibition of gastric secretion. Children with dysmotility-like symptoms suffer more from nausea, early satiety, postprandial fullness, retching, vomiting, and a sense of bloating. Although many children seem to outgrow the pain, some investigators believe that a percentage of these children experience irritable bowel syndrome (IBS) as adults.

Abdominal migraine is characterized by an acute onset of incapacitating, non-colicky, midline abdominal pain lasting for hours and is accompanied by pallor, anorexia, photophobia, headache, vomiting, and fever and limb pain. There is an increased incidence of maternal migraine in children with abdominal migraine.

As mentioned previously, an organic etiology is found in less than 10% of school-aged children with RAP. The alarming symptoms and signs of organic diseases are persistent right upper and right lower quadrant pain, pain that wakes the child from sleep; dysphagia; persistent vomiting; arthritis; perirectal disease; GI blood loss; nocturnal diarrhea; involuntary weight loss; deceleration of linear growth; delayed puberty; unexplained fever; and family history of inflammatory bowel disease, celiac disease, or peptic ulcer disease.

Evaluation

History

A thorough history should be obtained (Questions Box). A detailed description of pain may suggest a specific etiology. For example, pain worsened by eating can occur in children with gastroesophageal reflux disease, gastritis, cholecystitis, or pancreatitis. Nocturnal pain or pain relieved by a meal is more common in children with peptic ulcer disease. Pain relieved by defecation is suggestive of IBS. Pain aggravated by defecation raises suspicion of chronic inflammatory bowel disease. Localization of abdominal pain is an important additional diagnostic clue; functional abdominal pain is usually localized along the midline or periumbilical area. Associated symptoms such as fever, weight loss, anorexia, vomiting, diarrhea, leukocytosis, and an elevated sedimentation rate also suggest an organic etiology.

Physical Examination

The physical examination should include an assessment of the severity of the pain. Children should be observed when they do not suspect that they are being watched. For example, a child who stands up and hops around when the physician leaves the room may have pain with a psychosomatic basis. Detection of abdominal tenderness may be ascertained during auscultation of the abdomen by pressing down with the stethoscope. In young children suspected of having an acute abdomen, sedation may be necessary to assess the presence of tenderness. Sedated children with an acute abdomen awaken with palpation of the abdomen.

A rectal examination is also an integral part of the evaluation. In prepubescent girls with genitourinary symptoms or adolescent females, a genital assessment should be included.

Growth parameters should be evaluated for evidence of impairments, especially in children with RAP. Abnormal findings such as abdominal masses or perianal skin tags are clues to an organic etiology. Children who appear vigilant and keep their eyes open during the examination often have organic problems.

Laboratory Tests

The laboratory assessment is determined by the differential diagnosis. In general, laboratory tests include a complete blood count, a urinalysis, and an erythrocyte sedimentation rate (ESR) (in recurrent cases). In children with suspected lactose intolerance, a hydrogen breath test is recommended by some physicians, although a trial of dietary manipulation or use of exogenous lactase (eg, Lactaid) may be more cost-effective. Other laboratory tests, such as serum amylase or liver function studies, are appropriate if pancreatitis or hepatitis is suspected. Detection of *H pylori* antigen in the stool supports the diagnosis of *H pylori*. Stool evaluation for occult blood and parasites is also helpful. Consultation with a gastroenterologist should be considered in patients suspected of having ulcer disease or inflammatory bowel disease. Specialists may order diagnostic procedures such as endoscopy to arrive at the diagnosis.

Imaging Studies

In general, a flat plate of the abdomen should be obtained, especially if an acute surgical condition is suspected. A chest x-ray may also be ordered in children with acute symptoms consistent with appendicitis. Abdominal ultrasound and a barium enema are indicated to diagnose intussusception. Technetium scans help detect Meckel diverticulum if ectopic gastric mucosa is present. Ultrasonography is useful in suspected cases of cholelithiasis and cholecystitis. It may also detect pancreatic edema or pseudocyst, hydronephrosis, or abdominal masses.

Management

Management depends on the suspected cause of the abdominal pain. Medical conditions warrant treatment with **pharmacologic agents.** Peptic ulcer disease requires H_2 blockers such as cimetidine, proton pump inhibitors such as omeprazole, or cytoprotective agents like sucralfate. Infection with *H pylori* is managed with a triple therapy including proton pump inhibitor, amoxicillin, and clarithromycin. Urinary tract infections should be treated with antibiotics. Conditions such as appendicitis mandate **surgical intervention.**

The management of children with RAP is challenging. A 3-tiered empiric trial has been suggested for children in whom no distinct cause is identified. First, a high-fiber diet should be implemented. This helps alleviate the abdominal pain symptoms of children with IBS. Second, antacids, H_2 blockers or proton pump inhibitors are used empirically to see if symptoms respond to decreased acid levels. Third, a trial of Lactaid or a lactose-free period may also be implemented. A low dose of tricyclic antidepressant (eg, amitriptyline 0.1mg/kg–0.2 mg/kg) has been used successfully in children with functional abdominal pain.

Prognosis

In general, the prognosis for children with acute abdominal pain is good, although it varies depending on the condition. In 30% to 50% of children with RAP, the symptoms resolve within 2 to 6 weeks of diagnosis. Thirty percent to 50% of affected children experience abdominal pain as adults, although the pain does not limit their activities. As adults, these individuals may experience IBS or other chronic nonspecific complaints, such as headache, backache, and chronic pelvic pain.

CASE RESOLUTION

In the case history, the girl has the classic symptoms of peptic ulcer disease. Her symptoms are exacerbated by eating and relieved by vomiting. In addition, the family history is positive. Further evaluation may include a serologic test for *Helicobacter pylori,* an upper gastrointestinal series, or consultation with a gastroenterologist. Management involves the institution of H_2 blockers.

Selected References

Boyle JT. Abdominal pain. In: Walker WA, Goulet OJ, Kleinman RE, et al, eds. *Pediatric Gastrointestinal Disease: Pathophysiology—Diagnosis—Management.* 4th ed. Philadelphia, PA; B. C. Decker

Hamilton AB, Zeltzer LK. Visceral pain in infants. *J Pediatr.* 1994; 125:S95–S102

Hyman PE, Milla PJ, Benninga MA, Davidson GP, Fleisher DF, Taminiau J. Childhood functional gastrointestinal disorders: neonate/toddler. *Gastroenterology.* 2006;130:1519–1526

Rasquin A, Di Lorenzo C, Forbes D, Guaraldes E, et al. Childhood functional gastrointestinal disorders: child/adolescent. *Gastroenterology.* 2006;130:1527–1537

Walker LS, Guite JW, Duke M, Barnard JA, Greene JW. Recurrent abdominal pain: a potential precursor of irritable bowel syndrome in adolescents and young adults. *J Pediatr.* 1998;132:1010–1015

Jaundice

Melissa Egge, MD

CASE STUDY

A 2-month-old male infant is brought to the office for a routine well-child checkup. He was the product of a full-term, normal, spontaneous vaginal delivery, with a birth weight of 3,600 g. He has been feeding well, exclusively at the breast. Loose stools follow each feeding. On physical examination, the infant weighs 4,900 g. The examination is normal except that the boy appears jaundiced. On further questioning, the mother states that her son has been jaundiced since shortly after birth, and she feels that his appearance has not changed. The color of the stool is yellow.

Questions

1. What are the common causes of unconjugated hyperbilirubinemia in young infants?
2. What are the common causes of conjugated hyperbilirubinemia in young infants?
3. What are the usual causes of jaundice in older children and adolescents?
4. What is the appropriate management of hyperbilirubinemia in breastfed infants?

Jaundice is a condition that occurs when bilirubin reaches a level in the blood that makes it visibly apparent. In newborn infants, this level is 5 mg/dL. In older children and adolescents, jaundice becomes apparent at serum bilirubin levels of 2 mg/dL. The term **physiological jaundice** is used to denote the jaundice that normally occurs following birth. In full-term infants, bilirubin reaches its peak of about 6 mg/dL between the second and fourth days of life. Levels above 10 mg/dL are probably not physiological. Bilirubin generally returns to a normal level (<1 mg/dL) by 12 days of age. Premature infants experience their peak level of bilirubin, which may be up to 10 to 12 mg/dL, between the fifth and seventh days of life. Levels over 14 mg/dL are probably not physiological. Levels may be elevated in premature infants for up to 2 months.

Although physiological jaundice, a benign finding, affects all infants, other more serious disorders may present with similar symptomatology. The physician must be able to differentiate between these conditions to ensure appropriate intervention and management. New-onset jaundice in older children and adolescents is caused by other disorders.

Epidemiology

Jaundice is nearly universal in neonates because of the rapid turnover of red blood cells and the relative immaturity of the liver. Breast milk jaundice affects about 1% of breastfed infants. Various illnesses, particularly bacterial infections, also may precipitate jaundice in newborns. Neonatal cholestasis (conjugated hyperbilirubinemia), which is seen in a small number of cases of neonatal jaundice, is due to neonatal hepatitis or extrahepatic biliary atresia 45% of the time. Genetic and metabolic diseases now comprise approximately 45% of the cases of neonatal cholestasis that were previously known as idiopathic. Jaundice occurs much less frequently in the post-neonatal period and is most often secondary to viral hepatitis (see Chapter 102).

Clinical Presentation

Children with jaundice have yellow skin, conjunctiva, and mucous membranes. In newborns, the coloration may not be appreciated by parents because of its gradual onset and the parents' inexperience. The finding may be apparent in otherwise asymptomatic infants during routine health maintenance visits. In addition to the yellow color, children with jaundice may also present with symptoms related to the cause of the jaundice, including vomiting, anorexia, failure to thrive, acholic (white) stools, dark urine, fatigue, and abdominal pain or fullness (Dx Box).

 Jaundice

- Yellow skin, mucous membranes, and conjunctiva
- Tenderness in the right upper quadrant of the abdomen
- Hepatomegaly
- Anorexia
- Acholic stools
- Vomiting
- Pruritus

Pathophysiology

Bilirubin, a yellow pigment found primarily in bile, forms from the breakdown of heme-containing compounds, mainly hemoglobin, but also muscle myoglobin, cytochromes, catalases, and tryptophan pyrrolase. Blockage along any point in the physiological or anatomical pathway may result in increased levels of bilirubin and the appearance of jaundice (Figure 101-1). After the breakdown of hemoglobin, unconjugated bilirubin is taken up by the hepatocyte plasma membrane carrier, bilitranslocase. Once within the hepatocyte, bilirubin is bound to intracellular proteins (Y proteins or ligandin). Uptake depends on hepatic blood flow and the presence of the necessary binding proteins. Once in the liver, unconjugated bilirubin is conjugated by the enzyme glucuronyl transferase. Conjugated bilirubin, which is water-soluble, can be eliminated through the kidneys. Following conjugation, bilirubin passes into the bile through the bile canaliculi. It then moves to the gastrointestinal (GI) tract, where some of it may be reabsorbed (enterohepatic circulation), or be acted on by bacteria to form urobilinogen and stercobilinogen, which may appear in the urine or stool, respectively.

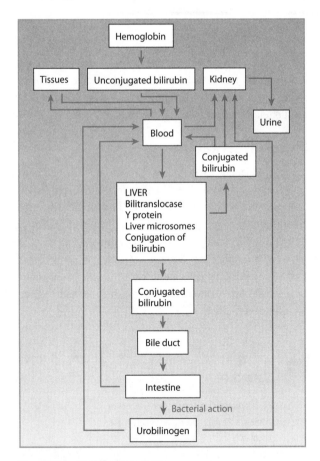

Figure 101-1. **The bilirubin pathway.**

In neonates, a number of factors contribute to physiological jaundice. Increased destruction of red blood cells occurs because the red blood cell survival in infants is only 70 to 90 days, as opposed to 120 days in older children. Hepatic uptake is lower, perhaps as a result of decreased levels of hepatic proteins as well as decreased hepatic blood flow. Levels of glucuronyl transferase do not reach adult values until the second week of life. These decreased levels of glucuronyl transferase mean that conjugation of bilirubin occurs at a slower rate. In some infants, glucuronyl transferase levels remain low; these individuals remain prone to jaundice at times of illness, stress, and starvation (Gilbert syndrome). Some breastfed infants also experience prolonged jaundice. Jaundice in breastfed infants may be related to poor caloric or fluid intake, weight loss, slow passage of meconium, or the type or number of bacteria in the intestine. It is believed that some unknown substance in the mother's milk, perhaps pregnanetriol, blocks glucuronyl transferase. (See Chapter 15 for more information about breastfeeding.) Reabsorption of bilirubin is increased through the enterohepatic circulation because of the diminished number of bacteria in the GI tract in young infants.

In older children, similar mechanisms may act to cause an increase in the bilirubin level. Hemolytic anemias (eg, glucose-6-phosphate dehydrogenase [G6PD] deficiency or pyruvate kinase deficiency [PKD]) may lead to increased red blood cell destruction. Inflammatory or infectious processes involving the liver, such as hepatitis, may impair the ability of the liver to excrete bilirubin. Pharmaceutical and toxicological agents may also interfere with the ability of the liver to metabolize bilirubin.

Differential Diagnosis

The differential diagnosis of jaundice in children involves 3 criteria: (1) age; (2) the type of hyperbilirubinemia (conjugated or unconjugated); and (3) if the hyperbilirubinemia is conjugated, the nature of the obstruction (intrahepatic or extrahepatic). The latter 2 factors are particularly important in determining the etiology of jaundice in young infants. A diagrammatic representation of the differential diagnosis of jaundice in children is shown in Figures 101-2, 101-3, and 101-4.

Infants Younger Than 8 Weeks of Age

Unconjugated Hyperbilirubinemia

Jaundice occurs universally in all newborns, but marked elevation of bilirubin levels or presence of jaundice in the first 24 hours of life or beyond 2 weeks of age warrants assessment. When less than 15% of the total bilirubin is direct, unconjugated hyperbilirubinemia is present. This is best determined by measuring the levels of total and direct bilirubin in the blood. **Physiological jaundice** is associated with unconjugated hyperbilirubinemia. The hematologic workup of affected infants is normal. Jaundice related to breastfeeding is called *breastfeeding jaundice,* which may resemble physiological jaundice and occurs during the first week of life, or *breast milk jaundice,* where bilirubin levels rise during the second week of life when physiological jaundice is improving. In breastfed infants, levels may reach as high as 25 to 30 mg/dL. Breast milk jaundice usually peaks by the age of 4 weeks and can last up to 12 weeks.

Conditions associated with slow intestinal transit time and increased enterohepatic circulation, such as hypothyroidism, also

Figure 101-2. Differential diagnosis of jaundice in neonates (during the first 8 weeks of life). Unconjugated hyperbilirubinemia. Abbreviations: Hgb, hemoglobin; SGA, small for gestational age; IDM, infant of diabetic mother; G6PD, glucose-6-phosphate dehydrogenese.

may result in jaundice. As with physiological and breast milk jaundice, the hematologic workup is normal. High intestinal obstructions, such as pyloric stenosis, duodenal atresia, annular pancreas, and jejunal atresia, may lead to jaundice, perhaps because of starvation and decreased levels of glucuronyl transferase.

Crigler-Najjar syndrome type I involves an absence of glucuronyl transferase in which bilirubin levels can approach 50 mg/dL at birth. An indirect hyperbilirubinemia on the order of 20 mg/dL that persists beyond 2 weeks in the absence of hemolysis is indicative of the type II version of this syndrome. Because of very high bilirubin levels, type I disease may lead to kernicterus unless managed with exchange transfusion. Phototherapy, cholestyramine, and eventual liver transplantation are additional therapies. The disorder is inherited in an autosomal-recessive manner and is extremely rare.

Hematologic problems may also produce jaundice in the neonatal period. Such problems are most often associated with blood group (usually Rh or ABO) incompatibility between mothers and infants, but some minor blood group determinants can precipitate similar problems. Jaundice occurs in affected infants because of the rapid destruction of red blood cells. Other infants may have a hemolytic anemia such as spherocytosis. Jaundice may also occur if excess blood is present in the infant's system. Situations in which elevated

hemoglobin is associated with jaundice include maternal-infant or twin-twin transfusions, infants who are small for gestational age, delayed clamping of the umbilical cord, infants of diabetic mothers, and infants with hyperviscosity syndrome.

Conjugated Hyperbilirubinemia

When more than 15% of the total bilirubin is direct, the jaundice is categorized as conjugated hyperbilirubinemia. Conjugated hyperbilirubinemia is always pathologic. Total parenteral nutrition is the most common cause of conjugated hyperbilirubinemia in the neonatal intensive care unit but does not usually present a diagnostic dilemma. The institution of oral feedings helps reverse the process. In other cases, determination of whether the problem is intrahepatic or extrahepatic is the major consideration. Some conditions of intrahepatic involvement represent a spectrum involving progression from inflammation of bile canaliculi (hepatitis) to their destruction (biliary atresia).

Inflammation of the hepatocytes is hepatitis. This disease may be caused by an infection in the liver or elsewhere in the body (eg, sepsis and urinary tract infections [UTIs] in young infants). Urinary tract infections are usually caused by *Escherichia coli*. The hepatic involvement resolves with appropriate antibiotic therapy of the primary infection.

Primary liver infection may be due to **TORCHS** (toxoplasmosis, other agents, rubella, cytomegalovirus [CMV], herpes simplex virus [HSV], syphilis) agents, the most common culprits being CMV and HSV. Infants infected prenatally often have low birth weights, hepatosplenomegaly, petechial rashes, and ocular findings such as cataracts and chorioretinitis. Hepatitis A may cause an acute infection, but rarely manifests as jaundice in neonates. Hepatitis B is a possible etiology of neonatal cholestasis, and hepatitis C is usually an asymptomatic infection. **Other infectious causes** include enteroviruses, reovirus 3, parvovirus B19, adenovirus 2, *Listeria monocytogenes,* and tuberculosis. Differentiating among these conditions is usually done on the basis of culture, polymerase chain reaction, or serology. Certain physical and epidemiological findings may help to distinguish these entities, however. Syphilis is more common in the developing nations of the world. Jaundice may appear within the first 24 hours of life or be of later onset. Infection with *L monocytogenes* infection may be associated with the presence of focal granulomas on the posterior pharynx. Similar granulomas in the liver are evident.

Metabolic diseases and **inborn errors of metabolism** may also lead to hepatitis. Most of these conditions are inherited in an autosomal-recessive manner. In addition to jaundice, infants may present with vomiting, irritability, lethargy, anorexia, hepatomegaly, hypoglycemia, failure to thrive, bleeding, or cataracts. Galactosemia may

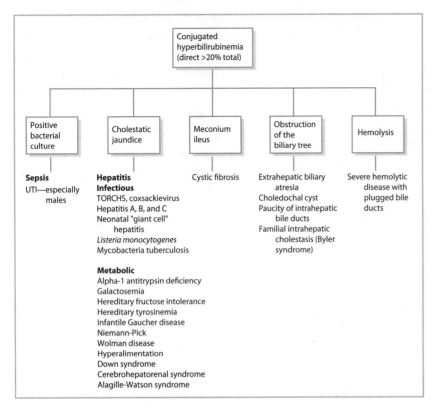

Figure 101-3. Differential diagnosis of jaundice in neonates (during the first 8 weeks of life). Conjugated hyperbilirubinemia. Abbreviation: UTI, urinary tract infection.

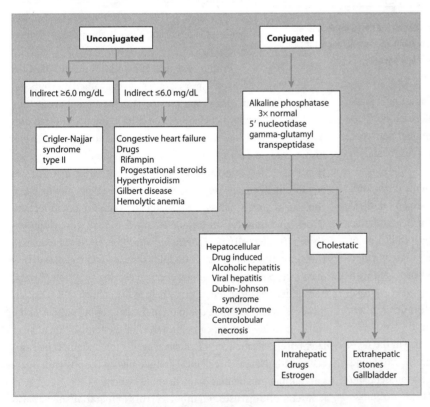

Figure 101-4. Differential diagnosis of jaundice in older infants, children, and adolescents.

be detected through neonatal screening or may present earlier as *E coli* sepsis. Infants with hereditary fructose intolerance present after exposure to fructose, sucrose, or sorbitol. α_1-antitrypsin deficiency may account for 20% to 30% of cases of idiopathic neonatal liver disease and for 10% of neonatal cholestatic disease. Inborn errors of metabolism generally present with a direct hyperbilirubinemia, while inborn errors of erythrocyte metabolism (PKD or G6PD) present with an indirect hyperbilirubinemia.

Genetic conditions that lead to jaundice in newborns include hereditary tyrosinemia, infantile Gaucher disease, Niemann-Pick disease, and Wolman disease. Cystic fibrosis may also cause cholestatic jaundice because of the presence of inspissated bile in the bile canaliculi. Fifty percent of these infants have meconium ileus, meconium peritonitis, or intestinal atresia. "Plugged" bile ducts may be seen with severe hemolytic anemia where bilirubin production is markedly elevated. Drugs may also induce intrahepatic cholestasis. A number of syndromes are associated with persistent intrahepatic cholestasis. Alagille syndrome, (arteriohepatic dysplasia) is characterized by unusual facies, skeletal and cardiovascular anomalies, and a paucity of intralobular bile ducts. The incidence is 1 in 100,000 live births. Progressive familial intrahepatic cholestasis and bile acid synthetic defect, together with Alagille syndrome comprise 10% of neonates with cholestasis. Not surprisingly, as the etiologies for more of these cases are identified through genetic and pathologic testing, fewer cases are labeled *idiopathic neonatal hepatitis*.

Extrahepatic biliary atresia accounts for about 25% of cases of cholestasis in newborns. Obliteration of the biliary tree is apparent. Infants are often well until 3 to 6 weeks of age, when they develop conjugated hyperbilirubinemia. The incidence is 1 in 14,000 live births. It has been postulated that some primary viral infections such as CMV and HSV may incite biliary atresia. Choledochal cysts appear as dilatations of the biliary tree and obstruct the passage of bile.

Older Infants, Children, and Adolescents

The approach to the differential diagnosis of jaundice in older infants and children is similar to the process in young infants. Unconjugated hyperbilirubinemia is usually due to hemolysis, and the level of indirect bilirubin helps clarify the differential diagnosis. Patients whose indirect bilirubin is greater than 6 mg/dL may have **Crigler-Najjar syndrome type II** and respond favorably to phenobarbital. Patients with levels under 6 mg/dL may have hemolytic anemia. **Congestive heart failure (CHF)** and **hypothyroidism** may also produce unconjugated hyperbilirubinemia. **Gilbert disease,** a benign condition in which the bilirubin rises to about 5 mg/dL in response to stress and starvation, may result in jaundice. The prevalence of Gilbert syndrome, an autosomal-recessive disease, is 5%. **Drugs,** including rifampin and birth control pills, may also be associated with unconjugated hyperbilirubinemia.

Conjugated hyperbilirubinemia may result from 2 different processes: (1) cholestasis and (2) hepatocellular inflammation or injury. Signs of cholestasis are high levels of alkaline phosphatase (3 times normal), mildly to moderately elevated transaminases, and increased γ-glutamyl transpeptidase. Cholestatic jaundice, related to drugs (estrogens) and alcohol, may occur on an intrahepatic basis. **Byler syndrome** is a familial disorder characterized by intrahepatic cholestasis. Extrahepatic cholestasis is seen with cholelithiasis or other obstructions of the biliary tree. Cholelithiasis may occur in individuals with hemolytic anemia and in adolescents who are overweight or postpartum. Hepatocellular injury most often results from hepatitis (see Chapter 102), including infectious, alcoholic, and drug-induced hepatitis. Rarer disorders include Dubin-Johnson syndrome and Rotor syndrome. Metabolic diseases such as Wilson disease, α₁-antitrypsin deficiency, and cystic fibrosis should be considered in the differential diagnosis of every older child presenting with conjugated hyperbilirubinemia.

Evaluation

History

A careful history must be obtained (Questions Box).

> ## Questions
> ### Jaundice
> - What associated symptoms are present?
> - How long have the symptoms been present?
> - Does the child have a fever, which may suggest the presence of an infection?
> - What is the color of the stools (acholic stools suggest obstruction)?
> - Does the child have a family history of jaundice or consanguinity?
> - What makes up the child's diet? If the child is an infant, is he or she breastfed or bottle-fed?
> - When did the parents first notice the jaundice?
> - Has the child been jaundiced previously?
> - Has the child been vaccinated against hepatitis A and B?
> - Is there a history of foreign travel or shellfish ingestion?

Physical Examination

Patients should be evaluated for evidence of organomegaly, ocular anomalies, rashes, hearing deficits, and unusual facial features. The unique facial features are pathognomic for certain genetic disorders such as Byler or Alagille syndromes. Rashes and lymphadenopathy are associated with certain infectious conditions, including congenital infections (TORCHS) in newborns and infectious mononucleosis in adolescents. Patients should also be checked for the presence of any cardiac anomaly, which may suggest a genetic syndrome or CHF.

Laboratory Tests

In the newborn nursery, noninvasive methods are used to measure the level of jaundice. The "jaundice meter" uses reflectance spectrophotometry to determine the skin color and correlates highly with serum bilirubin levels. An icterometer is another noninvasive method, which uses an acrylic plastic color chart that is placed against an infant's nose.

The aim of the laboratory assessment is to discover where the bilirubin metabolism is abnormal. The total bilirubin as well as the fractionated bilirubin levels should be determined. The presence of elevated levels of direct-reacting bilirubin represents conjugated hyperbilirubinemia. The demonstration of a yellow color to the foam of a shaken specimen of urine is a rapid test for conjugated hyperbilirubinemia. Urine test strips also readily detect conjugated bilirubin in the urine.

In children with unconjugated hyperbilirubinemia, a complete blood count with reticulocyte count and evaluation of the peripheral smear confirm hemolytic anemia. Serum haptoglobin levels are diminished in hemolytic disorders. In neonates, the Coombs test should be performed, and infant and maternal blood types should be determined. The hemoglobin should also be determined. A normal or low hemoglobin may be seen in the face of hemolytic anemia. An elevated reticulocyte count or an abnormal peripheral blood smear indicates hemolysis. Hemolytic anemias with abnormal peripheral smears include spherocytosis, elliptocytosis, stomatocytosis, and pyknocytosis (see Chapter 71).

In children with conjugated hyperbilirubinemia, tests should be performed to determine if infections such as bacteremia, UTI, congenital infection, or hepatitis are present. Evaluation for metabolic diseases should also be obtained by assessing the urine for the presence of reducing substances, organic acids, and bile acid metabolites. A sweat test and α₁-antitrypsin level should be considered. The status of liver function can be determined by evaluating aspartate aminotransferase, alanine aminotransferase, γ-glutamyl transpeptidase, or alkaline phosphatase. To assess synthetic liver function, one should test prothrombin time, total protein, albumin, glucose, cholesterol, and ammonia.

Imaging Studies

The anatomy of the biliary tree can be evaluated using ultrasound. Choledochal cysts may be visualized using this modality. When a "triangular cord sign" is seen on ultrasound, the diagnosis of biliary atresia is almost certain. A triangular-shaped echogenicity demonstrates the atretic ductal remnant in the area cephalad to the portal vein bifurcation. Other imaging tests, including excretion studies (radioisotope scans) and cholangiogram, can be used to help differentiate hepatitis from biliary atresia. Consultation with a pediatric gastroenterologist may be appropriate.

Liver Biopsy

A histologic evaluation may be necessary if laboratory results have not defined an etiology. Detailed review by an experienced pathologist may be diagnostic and save the infant from an exploratory surgery.

Management

The management of jaundice depends on the cause of the condition. Physiological jaundice and jaundice secondary to breastfeeding frequently require no intervention. Primary prevention is the best strategy to combat breastfeeding jaundice. Educate the mother to initiate breastfeeding within 1 hour of life with continuous rooming-in, breastfeed every 2 to 3 hours, promptly respond to hunger cues, and prohibit supplementation with water or sugar water. However, if bilirubin levels are greater than 20, interrupting breastfeeding for 24 to 48 hours will successfully lower bilirubin levels, but support and counseling are mandatory to ensure that breastfeeding resumes. Studies suggest that the use of a casein hydrolysate formula such as Nutramigen may lead to a greater degree of reduction in the level of bilirubin than the use of a whey-predominant formula such as Enfamil. Some practitioners use **bilirubin-reducing lights,** but other clinicians believe that breastfed infants can tolerate bilirubin levels as high as 25 to 30 mg/dL without danger of kernicterus. Newer phototherapy techniques involve the use of woven fiberoptic pads that can be used in the home. Increasing the exposure of the infant to phototherapy by using standard phototherapy above and a fiberoptic pad below is more effective than either modality alone. Clinical trials are demonstrating the efficacy of a single intramuscular dose of Sn-mesoporphyrin in treating and preventing neonatal hyperbilirubinemia. Sn-mesoporphyrin, a **metalloporphyrin,** blocks heme oxygenase, the first step in the production of bilirubin. Sn-mesoporphyrin may be especially helpful in situations when blood transfusions are prohibited by the parents for religious reasons or when known hemolytic disease will put the infant at risk for kernicterus. Infants who are preterm, ill, or have jaundice as a result of hemolysis may be at a greater risk from elevated bilirubin levels. **Exchange transfusion** may be indicated in addition to placement under bilirubin-reducing lights. A rule of thumb: Preterm infants should receive exchange transfusions when the bilirubin reaches the infant's weight (eg, 11 mg/dL in a 1,100-g infant). Intravenous immunoglobulin may prevent the need for exchange transfusion in babies with hemolysis due to blood group incompatibility.

Diet and nutrition can be an integral part to supporting an infant with conjugated hyperbilirubinemia. Medium-chain triglyceride formulas such as Pregestimil or Alimentum allow for absorption independent of bile acids. Supplementation with fat-soluble vitamins A, D, E, and K is also beneficial. If galactosemia is suspected, switch to soy formula pending results of the newborn screen.

Medications play a limited role in the management of jaundice. **Phenobarbital** may speed up the liver's excretion of bilirubin, even in cases of hemolytic anemia. This drug is also useful in the management of jaundice due to certain genetic conditions such as Crigler-Najjar syndrome type II. The appropriate **antibiotics** should be used to combat infections associated with jaundice. For relief of pruritus, ursodeoxycholic acid (15–30 mg/kg/d) or rifampicin may be offered.

Infants with biliary atresia may require **surgery.** Surgery links the surface of the liver to the intestinal tract, allowing for passage of bilirubin directly into the lumen of the small intestine. Adolescents with gallbladder disease may also require surgical intervention (ie, a cholecystectomy).

Prognosis

Most infants with elevated bilirubin levels have physiological jaundice or breast milk jaundice. The prognosis is excellent in these children. In recent years, concern has arisen about a recrudescence of kernicterus, including cases in breastfed, healthy term infants. Early discharge from the nursery and late follow-up may have contributed to this debilitating complication. Physicians should pursue an appropriate assessment of hyperbilirubinemia in jaundiced infants and not ascribe the symptoms to breastfeeding. Conditions other than physiological jaundice or breast milk jaundice may be less amenable to therapy and may require ongoing medical or surgical intervention. Children with metabolic abnormalities usually require lifelong nutritional intervention, those with hepatic disease may succumb to their hepatic dysfunction, and those treated with surgical correction of biliary atresia may have recurrent episodes of cholangitis leading to cirrhosis and the eventual need for liver transplantation.

In contrast, older infants, children, and adolescents with jaundice often have self-limited conditions that spontaneously resolve.

CASE RESOLUTION

In the case history, the infant is breastfed, which raises the possibility of breast milk jaundice. Fractionated bilirubin and hemoglobin determination are appropriate to assess the bilirubin level and confirm the absence of hemolysis. One approach to the diagnosis of breast milk as the etiology of the jaundice is to stop breastfeeding for a day or two to see if the bilirubin level decreases. (Sometimes an infant may not resume breastfeeding.) Biliary atresia or metabolic or infectious hepatitis should also be considered because of the infant's age.

The presence of normal-colored stools is reassuring, however, and makes biliary atresia less likely. The urine should be checked for the presence of reducing substances, which is a noninvasive way of evaluating the infant for galactosemia. The birth record should be obtained. Knowledge of the maternal and infant blood types would allow evaluation for mother-infant blood group incompatibility.

Selected References

Balistreri WF, Bezerra JA. Whatever happened to "neonatal hepatitis"? *Clin Liver Dis.* 2006;10:27–53

Burton BK. Inborn errors of metabolism in infancy: a guide to diagnosis. *Pediatrics.* 1998;102:e69

Farrant P, Meire HB, Mieli-Vergani G. Ultrasound features of the gall bladder in infants presenting with conjugated hyperbilirubinemia. *Br J Radiol.* 2000;73:1154–1158

Gourley GR. Bilirubin metabolism and kernicterus. *Adv Pediatr.* 1997;44:173–229

Haber BA, Russo P. Biliary atresia. *Gastroenterol Clin North Am.* 2003;32:891–911

Kappas A. A method for interdicting the development of severe jaundice in newborns by inhibiting the production of bilirubin. *Pediatrics.* 2004;113:119–123

Maisels MJ. Neonatal jaundice. *Pediatr Rev.* 2006;27:443–454

Pashankar D, Schreiber RA. Jaundice in older children and adolescents. *Pediatr Rev.* 2001;22:219–225

Suchy FJ. *Liver Disease in Children.* St Louis, MO: Mosby; 1994

Infectious Hepatitis

Monica Sifuentes, MD, and ChrisAnna M. Mink, MD

CASE STUDY

A 15-year-old boy is brought to the office with a 1-week history of intermittent fever, vomiting, diarrhea, and diffuse abdominal pain. His mother reports the appearance of "yellow eyes and skin" on the day before the visit. Her son was previously in good health. He is taking no medications and has no known ill contacts. He has no history of recent travel outside the United States and denies any unusual food ingestions. Mom reports that he frequently eats at a local fast-food restaurant with his soccer team, but his family does not eat there. He denies sexual activity, drug use, piercing, or tattooing.

The physical examination is significant for a temperature of 101.4°F (38.6°C), pulse of 100/min, and blood pressure of 110/63. The teen is a well-developed, well-nourished male with yellow skin and sclera. The abdomen is soft, with mild diffuse tenderness, most notably over the right upper quadrant, and normal bowel sounds. The

liver edge is palpated 5 cm below the right costal margin, and no splenomegaly is present. The rectal examination is normal, with guaiac-negative stool.

Questions

1. What conditions could account for symptoms of jaundice and gastrointestinal upset?
2. What is the appropriate evaluation for children with suspected hepatitis?
3. What are the most common causes of hepatitis in children?
4. What complications are associated with viral hepatitis?
5. What treatments are currently available for viral hepatitis, and how does treatment differ depending on the specific etiology?

Hepatitis is an inflammation of the liver that can occur as the result of an exposure to a toxin, such as a chemical or drug, or an infectious agent. Viruses are the most common cause of hepatitis in children, and most cases are the result of hepatitis A or B infection. With the advent of routine immunization for pediatric and adolescent age groups, the incidence of both hepatitis A and hepatitis B has dramatically declined, 88% and 67% respectively. Routine immunizations have reduced illness, as well as complications and long-term consequences, especially for hepatitis B. Other common viruses that can cause hepatitis in children are Epstein-Barr virus (EBV), varicella-zoster virus (VZV), adenovirus, enteroviruses, and herpes simplex virus (HSV); however, their contribution to the overall morbidity and mortality associated with infectious hepatitis is minimal.

Epidemiology

In 2005 more than 10,000 cases of viral hepatitis were reported in the United States to the Centers for Disease Control and Prevention. Most cases were due to hepatitis A or B, and fewer than 700 were identified as due to hepatitis C virus (HCV). This reflects a nearly 80% decline from the peak incidence in 1995, with the introduction of immunization against hepatitis A and B. The total number of hepatitis cases is probably underestimated as a result of under-recognition and underreporting.

Children younger than 15 years have the highest incidence of infectious hepatitis, though the incidence rates of both hepatitis A

and B are declining with use of routine immunizations. Both genders are equally affected. Certain situations are associated with increased risk for infection with hepatitis A. These include crowded living conditions, chronic care facilities, military institutions, prisons, child care centers, travelers to endemic areas, and high-risk sexual practices (eg, commercial sex workers and men who have sex with men). Poor personal hygiene and inadequate sanitation are also risk factors. In approximately 50% of hepatitis A cases, however, the source of infection is unknown. Hepatitis A is found worldwide, but specific locations are associated with an increased incidence of the disease, including Central and South America, Africa, the Mediterranean region, and Asia.

Groups at high risk for hepatitis B virus (HBV) infection include illicit parenteral drug users, commercial sex workers, men who have sex with men, heterosexuals with multiple sexual partners, health care workers, recipients of hemodialysis, household contacts of carriers of HBV, and immigrants from HBV-endemic areas. Individuals who live in crowded environments with poor hygienic standards, such as institutions for the developmentally disabled or correctional facilities, are at risk for HBV infection. No risk factors are identified in 40% of cases. Areas with the highest incidence of hepatitis B include Southeast Asia, most of Africa, the Pacific Islands, China, and parts of the Middle East.

Approximately 10% to 15% of primary infections with HBV result in a chronic carrier state. The younger children are when they are infected with HBV, the more likely they are to become chronic carriers. Between 70% and 90% of infants born to infected mothers become carriers, and at least 50% of children infected before the age of 5 years become carriers. Boys have a greater risk of becoming carriers than girls.

Hepatitis C accounts for 20% to 40% of all viral hepatitis in all age groups. High-risk individuals are recipients of transfusions of blood or blood products, recipients of organ or tissue transplants, intravenous (IV) drug users, health care workers with blood exposure, hemodialysis patients and, infrequently, sexual or household contacts of infected persons. No identifiable source can be found in at least 35% of cases. In the pediatric population, recipients of blood and blood products before 1992, clotting factor concentrates before 1987 (eg, hemophiliacs), dialysis patients, institutionalized children, and high-risk infants (eg, maternal history of IV drug abuse, sexually transmitted infections [STIs], human immunodeficiency virus [HIV] coinfection) are most likely to be at risk for hepatitis C.

Because hepatitis D only occurs as a coinfection with hepatitis B, high-risk groups are the same, with the exclusion of health care workers and homosexual males. High prevalence rates occur in Eastern Europe, Central Africa, southern Italy, and the Middle East.

No cases of hepatitis E acquired in the United States have been reported. The infection is endemic in developing countries such as Mexico, Central and Southeast Asia, North Africa, China, and India. In these regions, hepatitis E is the most common cause of symptomatic hepatitis in children. Young and middle-aged adults are most commonly affected, and this infection is especially severe for pregnant women.

Clinical Presentation

Children with acute hepatitis generally present with complaints suggestive of a "flu-like" illness, including fever, malaise, decreased appetite, nausea, and vomiting. They may also report diffuse abdominal pain. Unlike adults in whom jaundice is a common finding, pediatric patients, particularly infants and young children, are frequently anicteric. Hepatomegaly is often found on physical examination though not universally, and there may be varying degrees of right upper quadrant discomfort (Dx Box). A nonspecific macular rash, papulovesicular acrodermatitis (Gianotti-Crosti syndrome), and arthralgias can also occur in the course of hepatitis B.

Dx **Hepatitis**

- Diffuse abdominal pain
- Nonspecific symptoms (fever, malaise, anorexia, nausea, and vomiting)
- Jaundice (not necessarily in all cases)
- Dark urine and light-colored stool
- Pain or tenderness over the liver area
- Hepatomegaly

Pathophysiology

Hepatitis A

Hepatitis A is caused by a picornavirus composed of single-stranded RNA with only one serotype. The most common modes of transmission are through close personal contact and contaminated food and water. This generally occurs by fecal contamination and oral ingestion. Shellfish, such as raw oysters, clams, and mussels, are a frequent source of infection. Infected food handlers may also transmit the disease.

The average incubation period for hepatitis A is 28 to 30 days (range: 15–50 days). Peak viral secretion occurs before the onset of jaundice. The virus is shed in the stool 2 to 3 weeks before the onset of jaundice and up to 1 week after its appearance. Most young children, however, are anicteric, so infections often go unnoticed during this highly contagious period (Figure 102-1). The duration of illness is usually 2 to 4 weeks. A prolonged course or relapse occurs in 10% to 20% of adult cases. A chronic carrier state for hepatitis A does not exist, although fulminant infections can occur. Lifelong immunity is conferred after a single infection. Mortality is rare, especially in children.

Hepatitis B

Hepatitis B is caused by a double-stranded DNA virus in the *Hepadnaviridae* family. The disease is usually spread by contact with infected blood or blood products, but it can also occur through close interpersonal contact. Although hepatitis B surface antigen (HBsAg) is found in numerous body secretions (blood and blood products, feces, urine, tears, saliva, semen, breast milk, vaginal secretions, cerebrospinal and synovial fluid), only serum, semen, vaginal secretions, and saliva have been proven contagious. No fecal-oral transmission occurs. Transmission is facilitated through percutaneous inoculation (eg, tattooing, IV drug use) and exposure of cuts in the skin

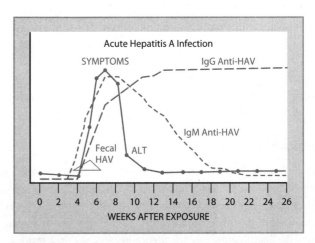

Figure 102-1. Course of acute hepatitis A infection. Abbreviations: 1g, immunoglobulin; HAV, hepatitis A virus. (Reproduced with permission from Tabor E. Etiology, diagnosis and treatment of viral hepatitis in children. In: Aronoff SC, Hughes WT, Kohl S, Speck WT, Wald ER, eds. *Advances in Pediatric Infectious Diseases.* Chicago, IL: Year Book Medical Publishers; 1988.)

and mucous membranes to contaminated fluids on objects such as razors and utensils. Sexual transmission occurs via semen, vaginal secretions, and saliva. Perinatal vertical transmission occurs in mothers who are acutely infected or chronic carriers. Although the exact mode of transmission is unclear for household contacts, postnatal infection from household exposure is reported.

The average incubation period for hepatitis B is 3 to 4 months (range: 1–6 months). Figure 102-2 depicts the typical course of acute hepatitis B, along with the course of the chronic carrier state.

Hepatitis C

Hepatitis C results from infection with a single-stranded RNA virus in the *Flavivirus* family, and it is able to mutate rapidly, thus escaping detection by the host's immune system. Like HBV, HCV can be spread through contact with contaminated blood and blood products. Conditions associated with hepatitis C infection in children include hemoglobinopathies such as thalassemia and sickle

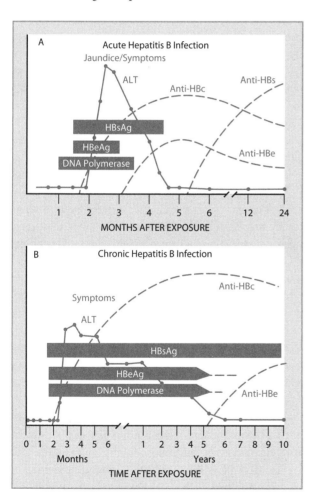

Figure 102-2. Course of hepatitis B infection. A. Acute hepatitis B infection. B. Chronic hepatitis B infection. Abbreviations: ALT, alanine aminotransferase; HBc, hepatitis B core; HBs, hepatitis B surface; HBsAg, hepatitis B surface antigen; HBeAg, hepatitis B e antigen; HBe, hepatitis B e. (Reproduced with permission from Tabor E. Etiology, diagnosis and treatment of viral hepatitis in children. In: Aronoff SC, Hughes WT, Kohl S, Speck WT, Wald ER, eds. *Advances in Pediatric Infectious Diseases.* Chicago, IL: Year Book Medical Publishers; 1988.)

cell disease, hemophilia, a history of malignancy, administration of hemodialysis or solid organ transplantation, and IV drug use. Vertical transmission can occur, but seems to be infrequent (~5% of infants born to HCV-infected mothers). Contaminated immunoglobulin (Ig) administered between April 1, 1993, and February 23, 1994, has been implicated as a source of hepatitis C. Transmission of infection via household and sexual contact has been demonstrated as well.

The incubation period is variable, ranging from 2 weeks to 6 months, and averages 6 to 7 weeks. Most affected children are anicteric as well as asymptomatic. If symptomatic infection is present, it is usually mild, insidious, and indistinguishable from hepatitis A or B. Jaundice occurs in only 25% of patients. Fulminant hepatitis is extremely uncommon.

Hepatitis D

Acute delta hepatitis, or hepatitis D, is caused by a distinct single-stranded RNA virus that requires HBsAg for replication. Both the virus and a delta antigen are enclosed in an envelope of HBsAg. Transmission is similar to hepatitis B, but vertical transmission is uncommon. Hepatitis D occurs either as a coinfection with HBV or a superinfection in a chronic carrier of HBV. Acute disease is usually more severe and carries a higher risk of fulminant hepatitis than hepatitis B infection alone.

Hepatitis E

Hepatitis E is caused by an enterically transmitted RNA virus. Transmission is primarily through contaminated drinking water and fecal-oral spread, especially during rainy or monsoon seasons in endemic areas.

The incubation period ranges from 2 to 9 weeks, with most cases of acute infection being self-limited. Mortality is low in endemic populations, except in pregnant women. Nearly all cases of hepatitis E infection in the United States have been in travelers to endemic areas.

Differential Diagnosis

The differential diagnosis of hepatitis depends on the patient's age, possible exposures, and immunization history. Possible infectious causes in neonates include overwhelming bacterial sepsis, VZV, and congenital infections (TORCHES [toxoplasmosis, rubella, cytomegalovirus (CMV), HSV, HIV, enteroviruses, and syphilis]), in addition to hepatitis B. Perinatal transmission of hepatitis A virus is rare. Genetic disorders and anatomical abnormalities causing biliary obstruction (eg, biliary atresia) should also be considered (see Chapter 101).

In older infants and children, in addition to hepatitis A and B, other viral etiologies include EBV, CMV, enteroviruses (including coxsackieviruses), adenovirus, VZV, HSV and, less commonly, rubella, rubeola, and HIV. Acute or chronic anemias such as sickle cell disease can also cause hepatomegaly and jaundice. Noninfectious conditions to consider include drug-induced hepatitis (eg, treatment with isoniazid, phenytoin); toxin ingestion (eg, acetaminophen, herbal remedies); and conditions such as cystic fibrosis, α$_1$-antitrypsin deficiency, Wilson disease, and other congenital disorders such as Caroli disease (intrahepatic dilation of the bile ducts).

In adolescents, viral etiologies to consider are similar to those listed for children. Other infectious processes to consider in the adolescent age group include biliary tract infections, bacterial sepsis, Fitz-Hugh–Curtis syndrome (liver inflammation associated with pelvic infections, especially with *Chlamydia* and gonorrhea), and *Mycoplasma*. The list of prescribed and illicit drugs that may cause liver toxicity is extensive and includes oral contraceptives, seizure medications, alcohol, inhalants, acetaminophen, and tetracycline.

Evaluation

History

A comprehensive history should be obtained in children of all ages (Questions Box). A dietary and travel history is essential, especially when considering hepatitis A or E.

Questions

Hepatitis

- Does the child have any history of fever, malaise, anorexia, or weight loss?
- Has the child experienced any vomiting or diarrhea?
- Is any abdominal pain or discomfort present? If so, in what location?
- Are yellow eyes or any changes in skin color apparent? If so, for how long?
- Is the color of the urine dark and the stool light?
- What is the child's recent travel history?
- Has the child ingested any shellfish in the previous 1 to 2 months?
- Has the child been in contact with any individuals with hepatitis or jaundice (including sexual contacts)?
- Is the child taking any medications (eg, isoniazid)?
- Does the child have a history of transfusion with blood or blood products?
- Is the adolescent sexually active, or has the adolescent had any known exposure to sexually transmitted infections (STIs)?
- Does the adolescent have a history of intravenous (IV) drug use?
- Does the mother have a history of hepatitis, IV drug use, STIs, or multiple sexual partners?

For young infants, a complete maternal and obstetrical history should be obtained and include the following questions: Does the mother have any history of IV drug use? Does the mother come from an area where hepatitis is highly endemic, such as Southeast Asia? Did the mother receive prenatal care? Was hepatitis B screening performed prenatally or at delivery? Did the mother have any known sexual contacts with hepatitis B–infected individuals, or did she have multiple sexual partners?

The physician should ask adolescents about sexual activity, STIs, and the number of sexual partners. In addition, it is important to inquire about parenteral drug use and tattoos.

Physical Examination

Most children with viral hepatitis are asymptomatic and generally do not present for medical evaluation. For symptomatic children, there are no clues on examination to aid in differentiating the causes. However, a complete physical examination should be performed to help rule out other etiologies. All vital signs should be recorded. The temperature is important, especially if children have a recent history of fever. In children who are vomiting, signs of dehydration (eg, tachycardia, evidence of orthostatic hypotension, dry mucous membranes, tenting of the skin, sunken eyes, and lethargy) should be noted. Growth parameters, particularly weight, should be obtained and compared with previous measurements if available.

The skin should be examined for jaundice; evidence of pruritus (eg, excoriations), which may be associated with elevated bilirubin; or a nonspecific rash. Icterus of the sclera, tympanic membranes, and palate should also be noted. The abdomen should be palpated for tenderness and organomegaly, particularly hepatomegaly. The liver span should also be determined by percussion because it will help monitor the patient's progress. Splenomegaly, which is not typically found in hepatitis, indicates a different diagnosis, such as leukemia, or another infectious cause, such as EBV or CMV. A rectal examination should also be performed to look for masses or blood in the stool, which may suggest a neoplastic etiology.

A neurologic examination is important to document any signs of encephalopathy from hyperammonemia, which occurs more commonly in chronic liver disease or fulminant hepatic failure.

Laboratory Tests

The initial laboratory tests needed are directed by the severity of illness in the child at presentation. At a minimum, these include liver function tests (LFTs) (alanine aminotransferase [ALT], aspartate aminotransferase, γ-glutamyltransferase, and total and direct bilirubin) and coagulation studies (prothrombin time [PT]/partial thromboplastin time). A PT is particularly useful because of its rapid turnaround time and predictive utility; if the value is greater than 3 seconds above the upper limit of normal (international normalized ratio >1.5), the prognosis is poor. Serologic testing for hepatitis A (hepatitis A virus [HAV]-IgM and HAV-IgG) and hepatitis B panel (HBsAg, HBs antibody, hepatitis B e antigen [HbeAg], HBe antibody, and hepatitis B core antibody) should also be performed.

In patients at high risk for hepatitis C, serum antibody to HCV (anti-HCV) should be sent. A confirmatory test such as a recombinant immunoblot assay, which measures antibody to various regions of the HCV genome, is always run after a screening enzyme immunoassay is performed. Both assays detect IgG anti-HCV antibody; IgM tests are not available. Hepatitis C virus polymerase chain reaction can also be considered in some situations. Serologic markers for hepatitis D (IgM and IgG anti-hepatitis D virus [HDV]) can be sent when concurrent HBV infection is evident. Isolation of the hepatitis D antigen in the liver, however, is the gold standard test for diagnosis of hepatitis D. Other serologic testing may be performed as indicated by history (eg, testing for syphilis with rapid plasma reagin for sexually active teens). A complete blood count and comprehensive metabolic panel may be needed in ill-appearing children, especially with signs of dehydration. A urinalysis for bilirubin should be done.

Management

For most cases of acute hepatitis A, B, and C, therapy consists of general **supportive care.** These illnesses are usually self-limited, and no specific therapy is indicated. Adequate nutrition and hydration are of primary importance. Therefore, the **intake of sufficient food and fluids** should be ensured. A low-protein diet during the acute phase of the illness may be considered. The use of **antipyretics** such as acetaminophen or ibuprofen for fever usually does not pose a problem in patients with mild disease and acutely elevated LFTs. However, because it is metabolized by the liver, it is preferable to limit the use of acetaminophen. Physical activity should be limited until patients feel better and LFTs return to normal. Children and adolescents can return to school when they are no longer jaundiced; they can resume a normal diet at that time.

In children with more severe symptoms, IV hydration and an antiemetic, such as promethazine (eg, Phenergan), may be indicated. Hospitalization is required for children who are moderately to severely dehydrated, are unable to tolerate fluids, or have evidence of fulminant liver failure. Treatment is aimed at correcting any metabolic abnormalities or electrolyte disturbances, including hypoglycemia. Coagulopathies should be corrected with vitamin K, fresh frozen plasma, and cryoprecipitate. Total parenteral nutrition may be required to maintain caloric needs. Consultation with a pediatric gastroenterologist is important for children with acute fulminant liver failure or chronic, active hepatitis.

Treatment of chronic, active hepatitis B and C with recombinant interferon (IFN) α-2b has been effective in adults. Approximately 40% to 50% of patients have responded with normalization of LFTs, particularly ALT, and histologic improvement. Only 10% to 15% of patients, however, have a sustained biochemical response. Currently no approved treatments exist for children. Although limited numbers of clinical trials of IFN in children show response rates similar to those in adults, IFN is not approved by the US Food and Drug Administration for use in individuals younger than 18 years. Fortunately, most pediatric patients with chronic HCV infection are asymptomatic.

Patients with hepatitis C should be counseled to avoid hepatotoxic medications and alcohol. Their parents should be informed of the possibility of transmission to others, and patients should refrain from donating blood, organs, tissue, or semen. Specifically, sexually active adolescents should be informed of the possible risk to sexual partners. Toothbrushes and razors should not be shared among household contacts. Children with HCV should not be excluded from child care centers because of their infection.

All children should routinely receive immunizations for hepatitis A (starting at 12 months of age) and hepatitis B (starting as early as birth). For older children and adolescents, review of their immunization records should be performed at all encounters, and catch-up doses of hepatitis A and B vaccine should be provided. Because children with chronic HCV infection are at risk for the development of serious liver disease, they should be followed regularly by their physician in conjunction with a pediatric gastroenterologist experienced in caring for children with HCV.

Prevention

Hepatitis A

Routine **immunization** for children starting at the age of 12 months has been recommended by the Advisory Committee on Immunization Practices and American Academy of Pediatrics since late 2006. In 1995 target groups were given hepatitis A vaccine, which led to a more than 85% decline in disease incidence. **Hand washing** by food handlers, medical personnel, and child care workers is a primary method for prevention of the spread of hepatitis A. **Contact precautions** should be used for hospitalized patients. Active immunization with hepatitis A vaccine and passive immunization with Ig is recommended as postexposure prophylaxis for all people who have had intimate exposure to infected individuals. The hepatitis A vaccine and Ig may be administered at the same time in different sites. Postexposure Ig is indicated for all susceptible household and child care contacts but not routinely for contacts at school or work. The dose is 0.02 mL/kg within 48 hours of exposure, given no later than 2 weeks after exposure. Immune globulin is 80% to 90% effective in prevention of clinical HAV disease. Pre-exposure prophylaxis with vaccine and/or Ig is recommended for travelers to endemic areas. If the stay is less than 3 months, the dose is 0.02 mL/kg; for longer stays, the dose is 0.06 mL/kg every 5 months. Two inactivated hepatitis A vaccines have been licensed for use in the United States. Both have been approved for children 12 months of age and older, as well as for adults. The 2 licensed vaccines seem to be interchangeable. Two doses of the vaccine are recommended and should be given initially and 6 to 12 months later.

In addition to routine childhood immunization, specific other groups for whom hepatitis A vaccine is recommended include travelers older than 12 months, individuals with chronic liver disease, men who have sex with men, users of injection and illicit drugs, and those at occupational risk of exposure. Other potential recipients include child care center staff and attendees, hospital personnel, food handlers, and individuals with hemophilia.

Hepatitis B

Preventive strategies for hepatitis B include universal immunization of all infants beginning shortly after birth and pre-exposure and postexposure prophylaxis. In addition, the vaccination of all adolescents, especially those at high risk, and other selected individuals at increased risk is recommended.

Hepatitis B immunoglobulin (HBIG) (passive immunization) is recommended for infants born to known HBsAg-positive mothers or mothers whose status is unknown. Passive immunization is also recommended for susceptible individuals who are sexual partners of persons with acute hepatitis B infections, household contacts (including children <1 year who have received <2 doses of vaccine), and those who experience mucosal or percutaneous exposure to HBsAg-positive blood. Unimmunized victims of sexual assault or abuse should receive HBIG if the offender is known to be HBsAg-positive. Simultaneous active immunization with the hepatitis B vaccine is recommended in these cases.

Immunization with the hepatitis B vaccine (active immunization) is currently recommended for all infants, adolescents not previously immunized, IV drug users, men who have sex with men, children receiving blood or blood products regularly (eg, hemophiliacs), children in chronic care facilities, household contacts of chronic carriers, and health care professionals. The schedule consists of 3 doses. Infants should receive the first dose before discharge from the nursery or shortly thereafter, the second dose 1 to 2 months later, and the third dose at 6 to 18 months of age. Intervals for other individuals should be similar.

Perinatal vertical transmission of hepatitis B can be prevented by giving newborns HBIG (0.5 mL intramuscularly) within 12 hours after birth and hepatitis B vaccine concurrently (at a different site) prior to discharge. This practice prevents approximately 90% of chronic infections in infants born to mothers with HBsAg and HBeAg. Post-immunization serologic screening is recommended, however, for these infants at 1 year of age because approximately 5% become carriers despite appropriate preventive vaccination. Special schedules for active and passive immunizations against hepatitis B should be consulted for premature infants.

Hepatitis C

No vaccine exists for the prevention of hepatitis C infection. Because Ig is manufactured from plasma that is anti-HCV–negative, it is not recommended for prophylaxis.

Current recommendations include screening individuals with risk factors for HCV infection (see Pathophysiology); infants born to HCV-infected women, recipients of Ig between April 1993 and February 1994, and children with clinical hepatitis found not to have hepatitis A or B.

Hepatitis D

Prevention of HBV infection through universal vaccination is the most important means of controlling HDV infection.

Prognosis

The prognosis for children with viral hepatitis depends on etiology as well as age at the time of infection. For hepatitis A, the outcome is generally good, with an uneventful recovery. Infants and children infected with hepatitis B, on the other hand, are at high risk of becoming chronic carriers, especially if infected at a young age. Approximately 25% of carriers develop chronic, active hepatitis, which often progresses to cirrhosis. In addition, the risk of

developing hepatocellular carcinoma is 12 to 300 times higher in these patients compared with the rest of the population.

Chronic hepatitis also occurs with hepatitis C, though it is unknown whether chronic infection and subsequent complications are higher for neonates. Autoimmune complications such as arthritis, serum sickness, and erythema multiforme are common, however, with chronic disease. Approximately 70% of patients with acute disease later develop chronic hepatitis, and 10% to 20% progress to cirrhosis and hepatic failure. Hepatocellular carcinoma has also been described in a small proportion of patients.

Likewise, complications of hepatitis D, such as cirrhosis and portal hypertension, are not uncommon. They occur more frequently than with hepatitis B, however, and progress more rapidly. Infection with hepatitis E does not result in a chronic condition. Fatal hepatitis A is a rare occurrence. The overall mortality associated with hepatitis B, C, and E is also low (approximately 1%–2%). For hepatitis D, however, it is more variable, ranging from 2% to 20%. Figures increase to 30% for hepatitis B with coinfection with hepatitis D. In addition, hepatitis E can be fatal in 20% of infected pregnant women.

CASE RESOLUTION

In the case history, the teen has a classic presentation of viral hepatitis despite no history of travel to an endemic area. Because he does not appear to be dehydrated or seriously ill, he can be managed as an outpatient. Statistics point to probable infection with hepatitis A. Serologies for both hepatitis A and B should be performed, in addition to liver function tests (LFTs) and coagulation studies. The parents should be informed of the probable diagnosis and all household contacts receive prophylaxis with immunoglobulin and hepatitis A vaccine. They should also be educated regarding the infectivity of the disease and counseled about supportive therapy. The boy should be scheduled for a follow-up visit in a few days for repeat LFTs and coagulation tests. The prognosis is good.

Selected References

Advisory Committee on Immunization Practices, Fiore AE, Wasley A, Bell BP. Prevention of hepatitis A through active or passive immunization: recommendations of the Advisory Committee on Immunization Practices (ACIP). *MMWR Recomm Rep.* 2006;55(RR-07):1–23

American Academy of Pediatrics. Hepatitis A. In: Pickering LK, Baker CJ, Long SS, McMillan JA, eds. *Red Book: 2006 Report of the Committee on Infectious Diseases.* 27th ed. Elk Grove Village, IL: American Academy of Pediatrics; 2006:326–335

American Academy of Pediatrics. Hepatitis B. In: Pickering LK, Baker CJ, Long SS, McMillan JA, eds. *Red Book: 2006 Report of the Committee on Infectious Diseases.* 27th ed. Elk Grove Village, IL: American Academy of Pediatrics; 2006:335–355

American Academy of Pediatrics. Hepatitis C. In: Pickering LK, Baker CJ, Long SS, McMillan JA, eds. *Red Book: 2006 Report of the Committee on Infectious Diseases.* 27th ed. Elk Grove Village, IL: American Academy of Pediatrics; 2006:355–361

American Medical Association. *Prevention, Diagnosis, and Management of Viral Hepatitis A.* Kader HH, Balistreri WF, eds. Chicago, IL: American Medical Association; 1995

Centers for Disease Control and Prevention. Recommendations for prevention and control of hepatitis C virus (HCV) infection and HCV-related chronic disease. *MMWR Recomm Rep.* 1998;47(RR-19):1–39

Curry MP, Chopra S. Acute viral hepatitis. In: Mandell GL, Bennett JE, Dolin R, eds. *Mandell, Douglas, and Bennett's Principles and Practice of Infectious Diseases.* 6th ed. Philadelphia, PA: Elsevier; 2005:1426–1441

Fishman LN, Jonas MM, Lavine JR. Update on viral hepatitis in children. *Pediatr Clin North Am.* 1996;43:57–74

Goldstein ST, Alter MJ, Williams IT, et al. Incidence and risk factors for acute hepatitis B in the United States, 1982–1998: implications for vaccination programs. *J Infect Dis.* 2002;185:713–719

Kim WR. The burden of hepatitis C in the United States. *Hepatology.* 2002;36:S30–S34

Krugman S. Viral hepatitis: A, B, C, D, and E—infection. *Pediatr Rev.* 1992;13:203–212

Krugman S. Viral hepatitis: A, B, C, D, and E—prevention. *Pediatr Rev.* 1992;13:245–247

Lee MA, Meissner HC. Hepatitis in adolescents. *Adolesc Med State Art Rev.* 1991;2:499–507

Mast EE, Weinbaum CM, Fiore AE, et al. A comprehensive immunization strategy to eliminate transmission of hepatitis B virus infection in the United States: recommendations of the Advisory Committee on Immunization Practices (ACIP) part II: immunization of adults. *MMWR Recomm Rep.* 2006;55(RR-16):1–33

Nowicki MJ, Balistreri WF. The Cs, Ds, and Es of viral hepatitis. *Contemp Pediatr.* 1992;9:23–42

Schwimmer JB, Balisteri WF. Transmission, natural history, and treatment of hepatitis C virus infection in the pediatric population. *Semin Liver Dis.* 2000;20:37–46

Shapiro CN. Epidemiology of hepatitis B. *Pediatr Infect Dis J.* 1993;12:433–437

Shapiro CN, Hadler SC. Hepatitis A and hepatitis B virus infection in day-care settings. *Pediatr Ann.* 1991;20:435–441

Stevens CE, Toy PT, Taylor PE, Lee T, Yip HY. Prospects for control of hepatitis B virus infection: implications of childhood vaccination and long-term protection. *Pediatrics.* 1992;90:170–173

Tovo PA, Lazier L, Versace A. Hepatitis B virus and hepatitis C virus infections in children. *Curr Opin Infect Dis.* 2005;18:261–266

Wasley A, Miller JT, Finelli L, Centers for Diseases Control and Prevention. Surveillance for acute viral hepatitis—United States, 2005. *MMWR Surveill Summ.* 2007;56:1–24

Neurologic Disorders

103. Hypotonia.. 631

104. Headaches 637

105. Tics.. 643

Hypotonia

Kenneth R. Huff, MD

CASE STUDY

A 6-month-old girl is brought to the office because she does not reach for her toys anymore. The pregnancy was full term, but the mother remembers that the fetal kicking was less than with an older brother. Delivery was uncomplicated, and the infant fed well. The girl began to show visual attention at 2 to 3 weeks, smiled socially at 1 month, and pushed up while prone at 2 months. Although she turned over at 4 months, she has not done this in the last month. She no longer reaches up to the mobile over her crib.

On examination, the girl lies quietly on the table and watches the examiner intently. Her growth parameters, including head circumference, are normal. After she has been undressed, it is apparent that she "seesaw" breathes (ie, abdomen rises with inspiration) and has a "frog-leg" posture. Her cranial nerve examination is normal except for head-turning strength. When she is pulled to a sitting position, her head lags far behind and her arms are straight at the elbows. She cannot raise her arms off the table. When a rattle is placed in her hands, she manipulates the toy, which she regards from the corner of her eye. Her deep tendon reflexes are absent, but her pain sensation is intact.

Questions

1. How is the level of nervous system involvement determined in infants with hypotonia? What levels of the nervous system are usually involved in the infant with hypotonia?
2. What is the significance of the loss of developmental milestones or abilities?
3. How are clinical management issues related to prognosis?
4. When is genetic counseling appropriate for children with hypotonia?

Infants with decreased tone are referred to as hypotonic or "floppy." Hypotonia is most simply defined as lower than normal resistance to passive motion across a joint, but is also suggested by abnormal posture. Although the lack of resistance may have other components (such as connective tissue abnormalities suggested by an unusual range of joint mobility, blue sclera, hyper-elastic skin, or Down syndrome features), muscle strength is a key component. Tone can be used as a surrogate indicator of strength in infants who cannot cooperate with testing. Weakness can also be inferred from the inability to sustain limbs against gravity or the lack of a withdrawal response of a limb to a painful stimulus. Identification of the level of the nervous system affected (eg, upper motor neurons, spinal cord, anterior horn cell, peripheral nerve components, myoneural junction, or muscle fibers) is most important in determining the etiology of hypotonia in infants and children. Only after this localization is the likely pathology defined in most cases.

Epidemiology

Hypotonia is not unusual in neonates, and non-neuromuscular causes of hypotonia are more common than neuromuscular conditions. Non-neuromuscular causes include hypoxic-ischemic encephalopathy and brain lesions related to premature birth, such as intraventricular hemorrhage and periventricular leukomalacia. Spinal muscular atrophy (SMA) is a common genetic condition with an incidence similar to cystic fibrosis, about 1 in 5,000. Duchenne muscular dystrophy is the most common neuromuscular condition in childhood, with an incidence of 1 in 1,700 to 1 in 3,500 male births. The Duchenne gene has been found to spontaneously mutate in approximately 50% of the cases. Among nongenetic disorders, the incidence of acute postinfectious polyneuritis or Landry–Guillain–Barré syndrome is 2 to 8 per 100,000.

Clinical Presentation

Hypotonia in infants often presents as an unusual posture of the infant, diminished resistance to passive movements of limbs or trunk, or an excessive range of joint mobility. Hypotonic infants have delayed motor milestones, decreased movements, and poor head and trunk control (Figure 103-1). Older children may have decreased ability to resist with strength testing of individual muscle groups as well as impaired functional strength in sitting, standing, walking, climbing, or running (Dx Box). Swayback posture in standing may indicate hip girdle or proximal weakness. Pointed toes in the supine position may indicate an upper motor cause.

Figure 103-1. Hypotonic infant being pulled into sitting position. Arms are completely extended, head control is poor, and legs are abducted at the hip.

Pathophysiology

Tone is a product of connective tissue structural elements, including ligaments, tendons, and joint capsules; muscle fiber number and integrity; and nerve fiber input to muscle. Nerve input to the muscle includes the number and myelination of axon fibers, trophic factors from the nerve, and the frequency of action potentials depolarizing the muscle membrane. The control of tone through the anterior horn cell is complex and involves more than just corticospinal tract (upper motor unit) influences. Lesions of the neuromuscular apparatus (lower motor unit), which includes muscle, nerve, nerve sheaths, and anterior horn cell, can most directly decrease tone, but lesions of any of the other structures at many levels of the nervous system can also affect tone. The final common pathway of upper or lower motor unit modification of tone is through the gamma loop (fusimotor) system. Gamma motoneurons within the anterior horn of the spinal cord innervate the contractile muscle portions on each end of the intrafusal fiber and enhance the sensitivity of the sensory endings to stretch, which in turn transmit signals back to the alpha motoneurons in the anterior horn innervating the rest of the muscle. It is through their effect on the gamma motoneuron that different levels of the central nervous system (CNS) (motor cortex, thalamus, basal ganglia, vestibular nuclei, reticular formation, and cerebellum) can modify tone.

The nature of the lesion at any level of the nervous system may be quite variable. Ultrastructural abnormalities occur in congenital myopathies, including those related to respiratory chain defects. Anterior horn cell apoptosis occurs in SMA and may also occur with ischemic insults. Stripping of myelin by macrophages occurs with acute postinfectious polyneuritis.

Dx Hypotonia

- Decreased resistance to passive movement of a joint
- Muscular weakness in older children
- Etiologic diagnosis related to the nervous system level of the lesion

Differential Diagnosis

Distinguishing clinical features in determining the level of the lesion in the nervous system include pattern of weakness, activity of muscle stretch reflexes, presence of fasciculations or sensory loss, cerebrospinal fluid findings, serum muscle enzyme levels, **electromyography (EMG)** pattern, nerve conduction studies, and histologic appearance of the muscle and/or nerve biopsy. It is useful when assessing the hypotonic child to separate upper motor neuron or brain causes from neuromuscular causes (Table 103-1). The former include perinatal hypoxia-ischemia, intracranial hemorrhage, and cerebral dysgenesis. These problems may present with hypotonia in infancy but later present as a static encephalopathy. A child with a central cause may have a below normal level or range of attention and may lack age-appropriate social skills. Seizures or hemiparesis also signify a likely CNS cause. Fine motor coordination, quality and repertoire of movements, and language may be affected in an older child. The deep tendon reflexes may be brisk or easily elicited. The Babinski

Table 103-1. Differential Diagnosis of Infantile Hypotonia	
Level	*Specific Lesion*
Cerebral hemisphere	• Static encephalopathy related to perinatal or prenatal insults • Dysgenesis (eg, Down syndrome) • Degenerative conditions (eg, storage disease)
Spinal cord	• Traumatic transection • Dysraphism or other malformation
Anterior horn cell	• Spinal muscular atrophy • Poliomyelitis
Peripheral nerve	• Leukodystrophy • Type III hereditary sensorimotor neuropathy • Acute polyneuritis (rarely occurs in infancy)
Myoneural junction	• Myasthenia gravis • Toxin (botulism or "mycin" antibiotic)
Muscle	• Congenital structural myopathy • Congenital myotonic dystrophy • Congenital muscular dystrophy • Mitochondrial myopathy
Systemic	• Amino and organic acidopathies, hypercalcemia, renal acidosis, rickets, scurvy, celiac disease, hypothyroidism, collagen disease, congenital heart disease

reflex may be dorsiflexor. In infants, fisting of the hands, scissoring of the extended legs on vertical suspension, and movement through postural reflexes such as the asymmetrical tonic neck reflex are clues to an upper motoneuron process. Enzymes, EMG, nerve conduction, and muscle biopsy will all be normal. However, neuromuscular causes include congenital myopathy, SMA, muscular dystrophy, and acute postinfectious polyneuritis. A child with a neuromuscular cause for the hypotonia may have an interested and visually attentive facial appearance in the presence of severe weakness that allows only sparse or nearly absent limb movements. Deep tendon reflexes may be difficult to elicit or absent in many neuromuscular lesions.

Older children may display a pattern of weakness that gives a clue to the level of involvement. If the weakness is preferentially in upper extremity extensor and lower extremity knee flexor, ankle dorsiflexor, and ankle everter muscle groups, the lesion may involve the upper motoneuron. Static bilateral hemiparesis may suggest severe hypoxemic-ischemic insult; diplegia may suggest periventricular leukomalacia in a former prematurely delivered infant. This differential weakness from CNS causes may be present and contribute to hypotonia for a long period before spasticity intervenes and affects tone. If the weakness involves limb agonist and antagonist muscles equally, however, it may represent a neuromuscular process. It should also be remembered that hypotonia can result from disorders with combined lesions in levels above the lower motoneuron and in the motor unit. Examples include Krabbe leukodystrophy, Pompe disease, and hypoxic-ischemic insults involving both the upper motoneuron and the anterior horn cell during the acute phase.

Evaluation

A methodical assessment using clinical and laboratory features in children to localize the lesion to a level of the nervous systems can help anatomically narrow a wide differential diagnosis (Table 103-2).

History

Particular areas of the history are especially important (Questions Box). Level of fetal movements relative to other pregnancies and possibilities of toxic or infectious fetal exposures should be obtained. Relatively decreased fetal movements may signify an early

degenerative condition. Polyhydramnios can signal prenatal interference with swallowing. Birth events should be investigated for sources of possible trauma to the neonatal nervous system, such as prematurity or birth asphyxia. The physician should determine whether any developmental skills have been lost. Any associated loss of tone or strength could signify a progressive condition rather than a static problem as would occur with a birth injury. The acuity of the developing weakness also is an important clue in the differential diagnosis. Immediate-onset hypotonia accompanied by constipation, poor feeding, and other bulbar involvement may suggest botulism. Acute losses of tone and strength may also occur with enteroviral poliomyelitis, Landry–Guillain-Barré syndrome, myasthenia, and myositis. Relapsing-remitting courses of hypotonia may be seen with myasthenia, metabolic myopathies, and periodic paralysis in the older child. A progressive deterioration in intellectual functions might point to a leukodystrophy, storage disorder, or other degenerative disorders, such as Leigh syndrome, particularly if ataxia, brain stem symptoms, and respiratory dysfunction subsequently develop.

Questions

Hypotonia
- Were the fetal movements of the child abnormal or less than those of previous pregnancies?
- Was the pregnancy full term? Was the delivery complicated?
- Does the mother, any siblings, or other family members suffer from a similar weakness?
- Has the child lost any developmental skills? Is the problem getting worse?
- If the weakness is worsening, how rapidly is it progressing?

In addition, the family history should be determined. The presence of weakness or hypotonia in other family members, or the presence of early unexplained neonatal deaths in the family, may indicate a genetic or maternal basis for the patient's hypotonia.

Physical Examination

Dysmorphic features should be noted in developmentally delayed children with hypotonia because they may suggest cerebral dysgenesis in some instances (eg, the characteristic stigmata of Down

Table 103-2. Approach to the Diagnosis of Hypotonia

Clinical Feature	Anatomical Site				
	Cerebrum	Spinal Cord	Anterior Horn Cell	Neuromuscular Junction	Muscle
Alertness	Decreased	Normal	Normal	Normal	Normal
Cry	Decreased	Normal	Normal/weak	Weak	Normal/weak
Eye movements	Sometimes abnormal	Normal	Normal	Abnormal	Normal
Tongue fasciculations	Absent	Absent	Present	Absent	Absent
Muscle bulk	Normal	Normal	Decreased	Normal	Decreased
Deep tendon reflexes	Normal/increased	Decreased/increased	Absent	Normal	Normal/decreased

syndrome) or neuromuscular conditions in other instances (eg, hypoplastic mandible, high-arched palate, thin ribs with deformed rib cage, or pectus excavatum). Poor feeding with small male genitalia in the neonate may suggest Prader-Willi syndrome. A large tongue with decreased growth parameters may point to hypothyroidism. Hepatomegaly may be seen with Niemann-Pick and Zellweger syndromes. Signs of brain dysfunction, such as lethargy, unresponsiveness to the environment, and lack of social skills, should be noted. The neonate who acutely develops signs of sepsis along with generalized hypotonia may have an inborn error of metabolism that is decompensating and requires emergent intervention. Age-appropriate cognitive abilities should be assessed as a measure of cerebral function. This assessment may range from primarily observation of visual attention in very young infants to evaluation of language and academic skills in older children. Cranial nerve examination with regard to eye movements, facial strength, and presence of tongue fasciculations is important, especially in the differential diagnosis of many neuromuscular conditions. Ocular muscle involvement may be part of mitochondrial myopathies, myotubular myopathy, and myotonic dystrophy. Blindness and hyperacusis may suggest Tay-Sachs disease. Facial muscle involvement is common in some congenital myopathies and myotonic dystrophy but not a part of SMA. Sucking and swallowing difficulty is a feature of SMA, congenital myotonic dystrophy, myotubular and nemaline myopathies, neonatal myasthenia, and Prader-Willi syndrome, in addition to birth asphyxia.

Tone and strength should be examined carefully in both trunk and limbs with the head in the midline. Passive pronation, supination, flexion, extension, and gentle shaking of hands and feet can demonstrate hypotonia, as can the traction maneuver for head control, horizontal prone suspension for trunk tone, scarf sign and axillary suspension for shoulder girdle tone, and popliteal angle for lower extremity tone. In premature infants there is normally a caudal-rostral progression of tone development, particularly flexor tone, with age up to term. Individual joint movements should be observed and agonist-antagonist strengths should be tested bilaterally to look for asymmetries and focal discrepancies. There may be a paucity of spontaneous limb movements, and breathing may be paradoxical with chest lowering and stomach rising due to primarily diaphragmatic strength. Severe respiratory compromise along with profound hypotonia may be features of neonatal spinal cord injury as well as congenital myopathies. The plantar response should be obtained. The presence of contractures is common in congenital muscular dystrophy and congenital myotonic dystrophy. The older child may have developed scoliosis from gravity effects on a weak spine. The presence of deep tendon reflexes and percussion myotonia should also be carefully noted. Sensory testing is important in suspected neuropathies, radiculopathies, and myelopathies. The responses to be observed are latency, limb movement (more than stereotyped triple flexion), facial grimace and cry, and habituation. In the case of the hypotonic neonate, the mother may also need to be examined for the presence of signs of myotonic dystrophy or myasthenia gravis.

Observation rather than formal neuromuscular testing is often easier and more revealing, particularly in infants and preschool-aged children. Useful activities to observe include walking, running, climbing stairs or stepping onto a stool, lying on the floor and coming to a standing position unassisted, smiling, closing the eyes tightly, and speaking. The ambulatory child may have waddling gait, genu recurvatum, or talipes planus. Arising from a prone position on the floor the child may demonstrate the Gower sign by getting to the hands and knees, then walking the feet forward to the hands, then walking the hands up the trunk to gain an upright position.

Laboratory Tests

One purpose of laboratory tests in children with neuromuscular conditions is to confirm the level of the nervous system involved (Table 103-3). **Serum creatine phosphokinase (CPK),** a screen for muscle fiber necrosis, should be requested when the history suggests a degenerative condition or the examination indicates the cause of the hypotonia is in the neuromuscular unit. Creatine phosphokinase is 10 to 100 times higher than normal in children with muscular dystrophy, and it may also be mildly elevated in female carriers of the mutant dystrophin gene in their first 3 decades of life. The serum CPK level may be less markedly elevated in children with inflammatory myopathies, such as dermatomyositis and polymyositis, and to some extent following muscle trauma. Severe hypotonia at birth can be a result of inborn errors of metabolism, such as peroxisomal disorders, non-ketotic hyperglycinemia, congenital lactic acidosis, organic acidemias, fatty acid oxidation disorders, maple syrup urine disease, molybdenum cofactor deficiency, and hyperammonemic syndromes, which can be screened using blood or plasma tests. The evaluation of the hypotonic depressed neonate should include an evaluation for infection (complete blood count and appropriate cultures) as well

Table 103-3. Laboratory Tests Useful in the Diagnosis of Hypotonia Caused by Neuromuscular Lesions

| Test | Anatomical Site | | |
	Anterior Horn Cell	Neuromuscular Junction	Muscle
Muscle enzymes	Normal	Normal	Normal/increased
Tensilon test	Normal	Abnormal	Normal
Electromyography	Neuropathic	Decremental/incremental	Myopathic
Muscle biopsy	Group atrophy	Normal	Myopathic

as an assessment of pH; blood gas; glucose; electrolytes; liver function tests; ammonia; amino acids of blood; and sugars, organic acids, and ketones of urine. Spinal fluid examination is sometimes helpful if there is an increase in white cells related to possible infection or inflammation or if there is an increased level of protein as seen in immune, storage, or necrotizing CNS conditions.

Useful information about the presence of neuropathic, myopathic, and neuromuscular junction disorders can be obtained from the **nerve conduction velocity** and EMG. Demyelinating neuropathies slow nerve conduction or produce signs of a segmental conduction block. If the problem is a motor neuropathy, an axonal neuropathy may have depressed amplitude of the nerve action potential or fibrillation potentials on EMG. In some myopathies, bizarre or small amplitude potentials and myotonia may be seen on EMG. Decremental response to stimulation and other abnormalities are evident with myasthenia gravis and neuromuscular junction blockade caused by the botulinum toxin. An intravenous (IV) edrophonium (Tensilon) test can confirm the diagnosis of myasthenia gravis in children with easy fatigability by history or on examination. Some neuromuscular conditions are associated with cardiomyopathies and, therefore, the electrocardiogram can help in diagnosis as well as bring to light potentially critical problems needing intervention.

When properly handled, the **muscle biopsy** gives useful diagnostic information about neuromuscular disorders that may cause hypotonia. A large portion of the tissue should be frozen for histochemical studies. Histochemistry can differentiate neuropathic changes from myopathic changes related to fiber type specificities as well as disclose structural abnormalities pointing to dystrophy or congenital myopathy. Histochemical stains can also give information about metabolic myopathic disorders. Another portion of the muscle should be fixed in glutaraldehyde for electron microscopy to determine if ultrastructural abnormalities such as those seen in specific congenital or mitochondrial myopathies are present.

Metabolic and molecular genetic studies can sometimes be done on blood or urine samples, such as white blood cell enzymatic assays, very–long-chain fatty acid profiles, plasma amino acid levels, and urine organic acid levels. However, if a genetic disorder is preferentially expressed in muscle tissue and direct gene analysis is not feasible, a muscle biopsy specimen must be analyzed. Tissue can be subjected to specific analyses such as dystrophin protein levels, glycolytic enzyme activity, respiratory chain enzyme complex assays, carnitine levels, or fatty acid transport assays to confirm the diagnosis. Tissue or blood sample molecular techniques, including use of specific nucleic acid probes, restriction fragment length polymorphism analysis, and linkage analysis can sometimes be used to help make specific diagnoses for genetic disorders (eg, Duchenne or other X-linked muscular dystrophies, myotonic dystrophies, mitochondrial cytopathies, and SMA). Cytogenetic analysis may be useful when Down syndrome or Prader-Willi syndrome is suspected as a cause of non-paralytic hypotonia. Thyroid function tests should be run if there has not been a universal screen or clinical suspicion persists for the diagnosis.

Imaging Studies

A magnetic resonance imaging scan is often helpful in at least 4 situations: (1) when deficits in mental status, cognitive function, or attention are apparent in children with hypotonia; (2) when the neurologic examination suggests an upper motoneuron component to the weakness or hypotonia such as active deep tendon reflexes or persistent ankle clonus; (3) when a progressive congenital muscular dystrophy is suggested by both myopathic signs and CNS signs; and (4) when children have hypotonia as part of a multiorgan system dysgenesis such as with a chromosomal aberration, because of the relatively higher likelihood of a CNS component to the dysgenesis. A computed tomography scan is also sometimes helpful in evaluating the presence of calcification in brain structures as might occur in metabolic abnormalities and necrotizing brain insults if these are part of the clinical differential.

Management

Specific management depends on diagnosis but ranges from supportive respiratory measures to anti-inflammatory therapies to physical and orthopedic therapy and devices to improve function. The potential for recovery is an important factor sometimes in determining the degree of aggressiveness in the management of children with neuromuscular conditions. An infant with a congenital myopathy may gradually increase in strength and should, therefore, receive intensive supportive care including long-term ventilatory support and gastrostomy feeding. On the other hand, the family of an infant with a degenerative terminal condition such as the severe infantile type of Werdnig-Hoffmann anterior horn cell disease may elect not to undertake respiratory support after they understand the course of the disease and lack of curative therapy. Such families benefit from the information provided by the physician and the support of paramedical personnel and lay groups. Affected children can benefit from palliative therapies and hospice care.

Children with profound weakness easily succumb to respiratory infections and have difficulty with recovery from anesthesia; therefore, they require vigilance and early intervention because they may need intense **respiratory support.** Children with long-term neuromuscular weakness can sometimes benefit from **orthopedic** procedures to improve limb function by joint stabilization or equalizing of muscle strengths across joints. **Physical and occupational therapy** can accelerate recovery after procedures and maximize function.

Children with acquired acute hypotonic weakness (Box 103-1) may require therapies more directed at the underlying pathophysiological process. Acute postinfectious polyneuritis requires careful, frequent monitoring of respiratory status and artificial ventilation when significant loss of vital capacity has occurred. In addition, children should be considered for **plasmapheresis** when their condition rapidly worsens early in the course of the disorder. **Intravenous immunoglobulin** is an alternative therapy that may be particularly useful in a child too small for the venous access required for pheresis. Specific antisera are used for botulinum intoxication. Dysimmune myasthenia can be treated with anticholinesterase medication, IV immunoglobulin, and/or thymectomy when it is resistant or only partly responsive to immunosuppressive medication. In addition to the more acute disorders, chronic relapsing polyneuritis and myositis can be treated effectively with anti-inflammatory agents such as prednisone and immunoglobulin during periods of exacerbation. Suspected metabolic disorders can be managed with focused therapy such as stopping a toxic nutrient; using a high-energy nutrient (glucose); treating hyperammonemia with benzoate, phenylbutyrate, or arginine; dialysis; administering insulin to control hyperglycemia; reducing catabolism; and providing vitamins and carnitine. Metabolic myopathies are still often empirically treated with thiamine, riboflavin, nicotinamide, coenzyme Q10, biotin, l-carnitine, succinate, vitamins C or K, and medium-chain triglyceride oil, using these in some cases based on tissue analysis.

Box 103-1. Specific Etiologies of Hypotonia Caused by Acute Generalized Weaknesses

- Acute postinfectious polyradiculoneuritis (Landry–Guillain-Barré syndrome)
- Postinfectious myositis
- Enteroviral poliomyelitis
- Acute myasthenia gravis
- Infantile botulism
- Tick paralysis
- Periodic paralysis (hyperkalemic, hypokalemic, and normokalemic)
- Metabolic myopathy

Treatment and care of children with muscular dystrophy is presently directed individually toward maintaining mobility and preventing contractures through physical therapy, bivalved casts, braces, and surgical repair. Inactivity increases disability. Adjunctive corticosteroid therapy is useful in children with Duchenne dystrophy, but beneficial effects are temporary and must be weighed against steroid toxicity. Many new hardware technologies (eg, long leg braces, electric wheelchairs, battery-operated ventilators, and noninvasive positive-pressure ventilation for some cases of respiratory insufficiency) have allowed affected children to overcome previously insurmountable disabilities.

Prognosis

The course of many genetic conditions can be quite variable and is related to different alleles at the disease gene locus or other loci that may have a modifying effect on either disease gene expression or the pathophysiology of the disease. For example, both the SMA and dystrophin genes have multiple abnormal modes of expression with different prognostic implications for rapidity of progression. Spinal muscular atrophy type I, over a couple of years, and Duchenne muscular dystrophy, over 15 to 20 years, generally progress to death, however. The weakness of congenital myopathies sometimes improves slowly. Toxin-mediated infant botulism and immune-mediated disorders, particularly Landry–Guillain-Barré, generally have a good outcome.

CASE RESOLUTION

The 6-month-old girl in the case history was judged to have hypotonia caused by a neuromuscular condition, in part because of her alert appearance and absent deep tendon reflexes. Neuropathic abnormalities on electromyography and muscle biopsy were also present. A blood test for the survival motor neuron genes did not detect any normal sequences, confirming the diagnosis of spinal muscular atrophy type I. The family received genetic counseling, became involved in a support group, and eventually reached a decision to forego intubation for the eventuality of respiratory failure for their daughter. The physician coordinated hospice services for the family.

Selected References

Dubowitz V. *Muscle Disorders in Childhood.* 2nd ed. Philadelphia, PA: W. B. Saunders; 1995

Fenichel GM. *Clinical Pediatric Neurology.* 5th ed. Philadelphia, PA: W. B. Saunders; 2005:149–170

Huff K. Approach to the child with weakness or paralysis. In: Osborne L, DeWitt T, First L, Zenel J, eds. *Pediatrics.* Philadelphia, PA: Elsevier; 2006

Iannaccone S. Rehabilitation for pediatric neuromuscular patients. *Semin Pediatr Neurol.* 1998;5:77–131

Leonard JV, Morris AA. Diagnosis and early management of inborn errors of metabolism presenting around the time of birth. *Acta Paediatr.* 2006;95:6–14

Sarnat H, Menkes J. Diseases of the motor unit. In: Menkes J, Sarnat H, Maria B, eds. *Child Neurology.* Philadelphia, PA: Lippincott; 2006

Swaiman K. Muscular tone and gait disturbances. In: Swaiman K, Ashwal S, Ferriero D, eds. *Pediatric Neurology Principals and Practice.* 4th ed. Philadelphia, PA: Elsevier; 2006

Volpe J. Neonatal hypotonia. In: Jones HR, Devivo D, Darras B, eds. *Neuromuscular Disorders in Childhood and Adolescence.* Philadelphia, PA: Butterworth Heinemann; 2003

Headaches

Kenneth R. Huff, MD

CASE STUDY

A 12-year-old girl is brought in with a history of headaches. Although she has been sent home from school twice in the last 6 weeks, she has experienced headaches for at least a year. The last episode, 1 week ago, was typical. The headache began as a dull feeling over both eyes, radiated up to the top of her head, and eventually became pounding. She had no preliminary visual symptoms or other warning signs prior to the head pain. The episode began during an afternoon class after she had been outside on a hot, sunny day for physical education. The headache worsened after she walked home from school. Once she got home, she went to her room, drew the curtains, and lay down on her bed. She experienced some nausea and loss of appetite but no vomiting. She did not get up for dinner. She denied diplopia, vertigo, ataxia, or limb weakness, and her speech was observed to be articulate and coherent. She took two 80-mg children's acetaminophen tablets without significant relief but eventually fell asleep. The following morning she felt fine.

Between headaches, her behavior has not changed, and she has continued to make above-average grades. She has not experienced any major changes in her home environment. When initially questioned, her mother denied having migraines, but she admits to needing to lie down because of headaches about once a month. A detailed **neurologic examination of the girl is completely normal.**

Questions

1. What are the major types of headache?
2. How do the symptoms help differentiate the types?
3. How does family history influence the etiology and help in the management of the headache ?
4. What is the appropriate treatment for the problem headache?

Headaches, which are very common in adolescents and older children, frequently prompt parents to bring their children to the physician's attention. The physician must differentiate headaches that are symptomatic of a progressive intracranial process from those that may possibly be intermittently disabling but do not necessitate surgery. The cornerstone of this determination is obtaining key historical information and noting abnormalities on examination of the nervous system. Decisions about management strategies are most influenced by etiology and, if it has become a chronic problem, the impact the headaches are having on the child's life.

Epidemiology

The contribution of "symptomatic" headaches (those related to tumors, vascular abnormalities, or meningitis) to the overall prevalence of headache is relatively small. Chronic recurrent headaches in children that are not related to a self-limited condition are frequently lumped together as migraine, which includes classic and common migraine. The prevalence of migraine that comes to a physician's attention is about 3% to 10% for all children, but as many as 30% of children by age 15 admit to having experienced a headache in the last year. Although initial headache symptoms begin most often between ages 6 and 12 years, many patients come to medical attention for the first time during adolescence, especially girls whose headache prevalence is double that of boys. Headaches are also commonly associated with trauma, acute intercurrent infection, or systemic illness. A multigenerational family history of "sick headaches" is a frequent finding in the child with migraine. This history must be specifically elicited by the physician, however, because its significance is often discounted by the parents.

Clinical Presentation

Parents must interpret the nature and severity of their child's experience and symptoms, which may be difficult especially in younger children. Younger children may complain of head pain or stomachache or present with nausea or vomiting. Adolescents may report persistent, dull, aching, or pounding head pain. It may be increasing in intensity or frequency and be associated with neurologic signs, suggesting an intracranial mass lesion, or the pain may be episodic, stable in frequency, and similar to that experienced by other family members either presently or in the past (Dx Box). Classic migraine, which is relatively unusual in children, is distinguished from common migraine by the presence of an aura and sensory symptoms that precede the headache. Both types of headache may be associated with lethargy, slowness of movement and response, intolerance of intense sound or light, and loss of appetite.

Pathophysiology

Pain fibers are carried in the trigeminal nerves from the scalp, skull, meninges, and vessel walls within the brain. Traction on these fibers or inflammation at the endings produces the pain that is associated with mass lesions or meningeal inflammation. The usual distinction between migraine and tension headache pathophysiology is more difficult to make in the younger child and may involve the types of trigger factors (Box 104-1) that occur at different ages. Several different mechanisms that involve one or many environmental factors may trigger headache in genetically predisposed individuals. The migraine generator probably resides in the brain stem and has input to the trigeminal nucleus. The pathogenic neurotransmitter at the nerve endings may be serotoninergic (perhaps emanating from platelet stores), but release may be precipitated by a cascade of local cytokines, substance P, calcitonin gene-related peptide, and histamine in and around vessel walls leading to changes in vascular permeability and local swelling. The relative roles of genetic susceptibility and environmental agents are subjects of active investigation.

Differential Diagnosis

Acute Headaches

Emergent causes should be considered if headaches have an abrupt onset, develop rapidly, or are especially severe or if children describe them as a "thunderclap" or "the worst of my life." **Intracranial hemorrhage** from a ruptured aneurysm, an arteriovenous malformation or, rarely, as a secondary effect of hypertension is foremost on the list of such causes. If children have a condition that may potentially

---

Box 104-1. Triggers of Migraine

- Glare, dazzle, bright sunlight, or fluorescent lighting
- Physical exertion, fatigue, lack of sleep, hunger
- Change in ambient temperature or humidity
- Allergic reactions, pungent odors
- Certain foods, alcoholic beverages, and cold foods or beverages
- Anxiety, stress, and worry
- Head trauma
- Menstruation and oral contraceptives
- Refractive errors (rare)

---

lead to stroke, such as coagulopathy, hemoglobinopathy, or heart disease, the stroke may become hemorrhagic and produce acute, severe headache.

Non-hemorrhagic meningeal irritation, such as the inflammation produced by bacterial or viral meningitis, may also cause acute headaches. These conditions may render patients confused and lethargic while still conscious and are often associated with fever. Both types of meningitis produce signs of meningeal irritation: nuchal rigidity (stiff neck) and Kernig and Brudzinski signs.

Chronic Progressive Headaches

Children with brain tumors, brain abscesses, or a block in cerebrospinal fluid (CSF) flow producing hydrocephalus frequently have a "crescendo" history of increasing severity or frequency of headaches. The headache may be consistently localized or may awaken the patient from sleep, presumably related to relative shift in intracranial traction forces due to gravity and the horizontal position. Many other children with brain tumors do not complain of a localized headache and may present with vomiting without headache as a prominent symptom. Idiopathic intracranial hypertension most often presents with headaches, and papilledema will be present when the eyes are examined. Standard imaging studies are normal, but CSF pressure is high when measured during a lumbar puncture. There may be a relationship to intracranial venous sinus obstruction in some cases. A serious sequela of idiopathic intracranial hypertension is an enlarging blind spot in visual fields and eventual loss of vision if pressure is not relieved. Therapies include CSF withdrawal, diuretics such as Diamox, and optic nerve fenestration or CSF diversion surgically.

Chronic Recurrent Headaches

The pain of **migraine headaches,** the most common chronic headache type, is dull in character, and if headaches are severe, patients shun other intense sensory stimuli. **Sinus infection** may be a cause of either chronically recurring headaches or acute headaches, especially if children relate that the pain is more facial than cranial. Symptoms of chronic nasal congestion, allergies, and postnasal drip may be associated with sinus headaches. Children with asthma also have recurring headaches possibly triggered by sinus involvement, generalized cytokine release, cerebrovascular smooth muscle reactivity, or medication side effect susceptibility.

Other types of headaches may recur. **Chronic daily headaches** (more than 15 headache days per month) in some cases may be transformed migraine or rebound headache due to abortive medication overuse. In other cases the history, though suggestive of migraine, is more consistent with **tension headaches** characterized by a feeling of a tightening band around the head; occurrence late in the day; and association with anxiety, depression, or a stressful environment. Adolescents, if they are susceptible individuals, may also have frequently recurring headaches due to irregular lifestyles such as not eating regularly or getting adequate sleep. **Posttraumatic headaches** may recur with gradually decreasing severity up to several months following head trauma. **Cluster headaches** are associated with lancinating pain, unilateral tearing, nasal stuffiness, and nighttime pacing, but are exceedingly rare in children.

Evaluation

History

Information should be obtained from patients, parents, and other caregivers concerning the quality, intensity, and location of the headache as well as other associated symptoms before and during the headache (Questions Box). The duration, clinical course, and conditions that evoke, intensify, or alleviate the pain are also important. It is useful to have children describe a typical episode (perhaps the most recent), including the circumstances of when and where the headache began and how it affected activities at the time. The degree to which the headache problem affects the child's lifestyle influences the management plan for chronic recurrent headaches.

Questions

Headaches

- Where is the child, what time of day is it, and what is the child doing when a typical headache or the last recalled headache begins?
- Where is the pain located? How severe is the pain? How long does the pain last?
- Is nausea, vomiting, or photophobia associated with the headache?
- What does the child do after getting the headache? Does the episode require cessation of activities?
- Does the child take any medication for the pain? If so, was it successful? What else, if anything, allows the child to feel better?
- How long ago did the first headache occur? Are the headaches becoming more frequent or severe?
- Have headaches ever awakened the child at night?
- Have there been any changes in speech, vision, gait, or personality, or any loss of skills or abilities between headaches?
- Does the child have any warning symptoms before the pain? Does unilateral visual loss, weakness or numbness, diplopia, confusion, or loss of consciousness occur with the headache?
- How often does the child miss school because of a headache?
- Do other members of the family have headaches? Do they ever need to lie down or do they take medicine for these headaches?

Physical Examination

The blood pressure should be noted even though primary hypertension is an unusual cause of headaches in children. A thorough neurologic examination is needed to determine if findings suggest an emergent problem such as meningitis or potential neurosurgical condition such as intracranial hemorrhage, or brain tumor. The examination should assess for the presence of sinus tenderness by palpation, nuchal rigidity, funduscopic abnormalities such as papilledema or hemorrhages, and any focal neurologic signs. A brain tumor or other space-occupying lesion may present with ataxia and cranial nerve signs for a posterior fossa lesion; loss of visual fields or hypothalamic dysfunction (endocrine abnormalities) for a suprasellar

or third ventricular region lesion; and hemiparesis, hemisensory deficit, or language dysfunction for a cerebral hemispheric lesion. Personality changes or developmental regression should be especially noted. Increased intracranial pressure (ICP) may lead to papilledema, loss of upgaze, general hypertonicity, leg weakness, positive Babinski sign, spastic gait, loss of continence, or confusion or stupor owing to blockage of CSF by the tumor.

Rarely, children in the midst of a migraine headache may display confusion, aphasia, unilateral numbness or, less commonly, weakness, hemianopsia, or ophthalmoplegia. In these circumstances, the diagnosis of complicated migraine or a migraine syndrome is reached only after other diagnostic tests have eliminated more emergent conditions.

Laboratory Tests

If stiff neck is present and focal or lateralized neurologic signs are absent, an immediate CSF examination is indicated to diagnose the cause of meningeal inflammation. When hemorrhagic fluid is encountered, it is often useful to centrifuge a specimen to check for xanthochromia and to count cells in a subsequent sample to differentiate a traumatic spinal tap from subarachnoid hemorrhage.

Imaging Studies

Recent trauma, persistent vomiting, depressed alertness, crescendo history, change in pattern, or possibly even just recent onset of the headaches all may be indications for an immediate head magnetic resonance imaging (MRI) or computed tomography (CT) scan. Such decisions are also influenced by reliability of follow-up and ease of communication level with the child's caretaker. If signs or symptoms of increased ICP are apparent, a CT or MRI scan must be obtained to diagnose the etiology of the headaches. New focal or general neurologic signs also indicate the need for a CT or MRI scan. Cerebral angiography may be necessary in rare cases to locate a focal source of subarachnoid hemorrhage. Less emergent radiologic studies, but also including CT or MRI, are helpful with the diagnosis of chronic or recurrent sinus headaches.

Management

If a careful assessment has revealed no acute or progressive conditions, pain is not severe, frequency is low, duration is short, and effect on lifestyle or daily activities is minimal, the appropriate management is often just **reassurance.** Frequently, parental anxiety about a potential mass or hemorrhage far outweighs the morbidity produced by the headache symptom itself. Sometimes placing the child's headache problem in context with the parent's or other family member's headaches will help with reassurance, and sometimes in milder cases, non-pharmacologic or nonprescription medication strategies can be agreed on as a management plan. Education and sometimes a headache diary or log helps patients and their families take control and own their own problem (discern triggers and track intervention efficacy).

However, it may be apparent that the headaches have produced significant discomfort or an affect on lifestyle for the child and symptomatic or prophylactic treatment, or a combination, is warranted (Table 104-1). Interventions should weigh side effects against effectiveness of treatment. A goal is a reduction in headache frequency, severity, duration, or disability with improved quality of life. Both pain and nausea may need treatment. **Symptomatic treatment** should begin as soon after the onset of prodromal or headache symptoms as possible, and often begins with an adequate trial of **acetaminophen or nonsteroidal anti-inflammatory drugs.** Headaches in adolescents are often helped by **isometheptene mucate.** For severe, recurrent headaches, serotonin receptor agonists are useful, and **sumatriptan and other triptans** have relatively mild side effects but patients need to be informed about them as with any new medication. Dihydroergotamine or sumatriptan given intranasally are also effective abortive treatments and work faster than the tablets, but they may have a disagreeable taste if they enter the oropharynx. Refractory very severe headaches may respond to Compazine or intravenous (IV) **dihydroergotamine** or **dexamethasone along with a bolus of IV fluids.**

The decision to begin a **prophylactic medication** should be based on the frequency and severity of the headaches. Again, the benefits of potentially controlling headache-related symptoms must be weighed against the risk of daily side effects. Anticonvulsants such as **diphenylhydantoin and carbamazepine** have been found to be successful anti-migraine agents, as have **valproic acid and topiramate.** The beta-blockers, including **propranolol,** have demonstrated efficacy as prophylactic agents. The antihistamine **cyproheptadine** has also been successful in many patients. **Amitriptyline** is an effective preventive treatment in older children and adolescents; a single bedtime dose should be used at first. A 1- to 2-week trial is necessary before concluding the initial treatment has been ineffective. Amitriptyline can be combined with propranolol if necessary. Calcium channel blockers, such as **verapamil,** and serotonin reuptake inhibitors, such as **fluoxetine,** may also be useful in older children and adolescents. Chronic daily headaches may be successfully treated with education, use of prophylactic medication, avoidance of analgesics because of rebound potential, and helping the children work their way back into a functional daily routine. Healthy lifestyle changes have been beneficial, particularly in adolescents, and biofeedback-assisted relaxation training has had mixed results. If severe environmental stressors or psychological trauma is present as an ongoing headache trigger, patients may benefit from psychotherapy.

Table 104-1. Drugs Useful in Childhood Headaches	
Abortive (Symptomatic)	
Acetaminophen, PO	325–975 mg every 4 h (15 mg/kg/dose) (max: 5 doses/24 h)
Ibuprofen, PO	200–800 mg every 6 h (10 mg/kg/dose) (max: 40 mg/kg/24 h)
Naproxen, PO	5–7 mg/kg/dose every 8–12 h (max: 15 mg/kg/ 24 h [age >2 y])
Sumatriptan, SC, IN, or PO	6 mg SC or 5–20 mg IN or 25–100 mg PO (may repeat after 1 h SC, 2 h IN and PO) (max: 2 doses/24 h)
Ergotamine, PR	¼ rectal suppository (2 mg), repeat ¼ suppository every 30 min as needed (max: 4 mg/d [older children and adolescents])
Rizatriptan, PO	5–10 mg orally disintegrating or regular tablets (may repeat after 2 hours) (max: 3 doses/24 h)
Isometheptene mucate with dichloral-phenazone and acetaminophen, PO	1–2 caps at onset (may repeat every 1 h to 3–5 caps/d [adolescents])
Dihydroergotamine, IN or IV	4 mg IN (1 spray each nostril, repeat once after 15 min) or 0.25–1 mg at onset and 1 mg/h × 2 (max: 6 mg/wk [older children and adolescents])
Dexamethasone, IV	4–16 mg single dose (0.25 mg/kg) or rapidly tapering every 6 h
Prophylactic	
Diphenylhydantoin	2–4 mg/kg/dose twice a day (max: 5 mg/kg [follow serum level])
Propranolol	10–40 mg 2–4 times a day (max: 40–80 mg/24 h if ≤35 kg;
	120–160 mg/24 h if >35 kg; no more than 320 mg/24 h)
Cyproheptadine	1–4 mg 2–4 times a day (0.25–0.5 mg/kg/24 h) (max: 16 mg/24 h)
Amitriptyline	10–75 mg at bedtime (max: 150 mg/24 h [older children and adolescents])
Verapamil	40 mg every 8 h (age 1–5 y); 40–80 mg every 8 h (age >5 y) (max: 240 mg/24 h)
Valproic acid	10–15 mg/kg/d initial, 30–60 mg/kg/d maintenance, divided twice a day or every day if ER (max: 60 mg/kg/d [follow clinical signs of toxicity and serum level])
Topiramate	50–200 mg/d divided twice a day after ramping from 25 mg twice a day over a few weeks
Fluoxetine	10 mg every morning initial (max: 40 mg/d [adolescents])

Abbreviations: PO, orally; SC, subcutaneously; IN, intranasally ; PR, rectally; IV, intravenously; ER, extended release.

Prognosis

Many children with headaches have a good prognosis and do not require ongoing intervention after families are reassured of the benign nature of the problem. For the remainder of children, symptomatic medications are frequently effective. Prophylactic medication is necessary in a few cases. For patients receiving prophylactic therapy, periodic withdrawal of the medication should be attempted to establish its continued necessity. Pediatric patients frequently experience remission of their headaches by late adolescence, and by adulthood, the incidence of headaches is decreased, particularly for males.

CASE RESOLUTION

In the case history, the child's symptoms and the circumstances of the headache suggest a diagnosis of migraine. No laboratory tests or imaging studies are necessary. The girl is begun on amitriptyline and instructed to keep a calendar of headache occurrences. She has 2 headaches in the first 2 weeks, which are aborted effectively with ibuprofen. Following these episodes, she has no further recurrences, and the amitriptyline is withdrawn successfully after 3 months.

Selected References

Ball AK, Clarke CE. Idiopathic intracranial hypertension. *Lancet Neurol.* 2006;5:433–442

Diamond S. *Diagnosing and Managing Headaches.* 2nd ed. Caddo, OK: Professional Communications, Inc.; 1998

Forsyth R, Farrell K. Headache in childhood. *Pediatr Rev.* 1999;20:39–45

Landy S. Migraine throughout the life cycle: treatment through the ages. *Neurology.* 2004;62(suppl 2):S2–S8

Lewis D. Headaches in infants and children. In: Swaiman K, Ashwal S, Ferriero D, eds. *Pediatric Neurology Principals and Practice.* Philadelphia, PA: Elsevier; 2006

Mack KJ. An approach to children with chronic daily headache. *Dev Med Child Neurol.* 2006;48:997–1000

Rothner AD. Pediatric headaches. *Semin Pediatr Neurol.* 2001;8:1–51

Solomon GD. The pharmacology of medications used in treating headache. *Semin Pediatr Neurol.* 1995;2:165–177

Tics

Kenneth R. Huff, MD

CASE STUDY

An 8-year-old boy has unusual recurring behaviors that began 2 to 3 months ago. He stretches his neck or raises his eyebrows several times a day. Sometimes he is able to suppress these actions. The boy's parents report that in the last 2 years he has displayed several repetitive behaviors, including blinking, grimacing, rubbing his chin on his left shoulder, making a "gulping" sound, and sniffing. Originally they thought the sniffing was related to hay fever, but the boy has no other allergic symptoms. He does not use profane words. In conversations, he sometimes repeats the last phrase of a sentence that was just used whether by himself or someone else. In addition, he must touch each light switch in the hallway every time he leaves his room, and he must retie his shoelaces several times until they are exactly the same length. Although his schoolwork has not deteriorated, he has always had trouble completing tasks and finishing homework. Both his teacher and his best friend have asked about his strange behavior. His mother has a "psychological" problem with her son's gulping sounds (ie, they recur in her own mind), and she recalls that her father had a habit of frequently looking over one shoulder for no apparent reason.

Although during examination the boy does not exhibit any unusual behaviors, he raises his eyebrows twice and places his hand over his crotch several times while his parents are interviewed. Except for mild fine motor incoordination, the neurologic examination is normal.

Questions

1. What are the characteristics of tics?
2. What are the social implications of tics?
3. Should pharmacologic treatments be part of the management of tic disorders?
4. What other problems are associated with the tic disorder that also should receive intervention?

Tics are brief, abrupt, non-purposeful movements or utterances. They occur in a background of normal activity and are repetitive and involuntary but can be suppressed. Tourette syndrome is a common etiology of tics in children. It is defined by multiple types of tics displayed over time. These include both motor tics and vocal tics produced by some sudden movement of air or saliva within the larynx, nasopharynx, or oropharynx, causing a perceptible sound. Tourette syndrome frequently is associated with other neurobehavioral problems, which may include attention-deficit/hyperactivity disorder (ADHD), obsessive-compulsive disorder, mood and rage disorders, anxiety, and personality and conduct difficulties that may be more disabling than the tics.

Epidemiology

Tics are relatively common in children but often go unrecognized as movement disorders. The onset of tics associated with Tourette syndrome is generally between 5 and 12 years of age but can be as late as 21 years of age. The prevalence of tics is 5 times higher in males than in females. By some estimates, Tourette syndrome incidence estimates vary between 1 in 83 and 1 in 10,000, but many cases of Tourette syndrome are familial, and other family members may have symptoms so mild that they never seek medical attention. In addition, some family members may have only non-tic manifestations of the syndrome, such as obsessive-compulsive symptoms. The prevalence in the general population may be 0.1% to 3.0%.

Clinical Presentation

Children with tics display sudden repetitive movements of the face, neck, shoulders, or hands in the context of normal behaviors. Sometimes these actions can be suppressed for periods, such as when they would be embarrassing or during a time of intense physical activity, but they also may be worsened by stress or strong emotional feelings. Tics associated with Tourette syndrome will vary in their manifestations over periods of weeks to months. Some examples of tics are blinking, eye rolling, grimacing, neck stretching, head turning or shaking, shoulder shrugging, and wrist flicking. Tics may either mimic normal, sometimes complex, movements or involve a series of orchestrated simple movements such as sequential finger flexing, wrist bending, and arm stretching.

Tics may include sudden repetitive sounds from the vocal apparatus (Dx Box). The sounds may include throat clearing, sniffing, sucking, or blowing. In addition, children with Tourette syndrome may also have socially inappropriate words or gestures or repeat what they have just said or heard. Children may have learning problems of distractibility and inability to finish schoolwork or may have intrusive repetitive thoughts, unfounded fears, or ritualistic actions that may involve touching, cleanliness or neatness, counting and exactness, symmetry or evenness, or irrational checking.

Dx   Tics

- Sudden, brief uncontrolled movements
- Repetitive sounds from the vocal apparatus
- Behaviors occurring in the context of or mimicking normal behaviors but having no purpose

Classifications of tics as part of Tourette syndrome have been described (Box 105-1). Clonic tics are brief and dystonic tics are more sustained movements. In addition to simple tics, patients may rarely have other unusual behaviors (complex tics) including echopraxia (repetitive gestures), copropraxia (obscene gestures), and coprographia (obscene writing). Unusual speech patterns include irrelevant or nonsense words, palilalia (repeating one's own words), echolalia (repeating another's words), and coprolalia (obscene speech). Many affected children describe a sensory tic, which is an indescribable, uncomfortable feeling that is relieved by a motor tic. Diagnosis is often delayed because of misunderstandings about the common and uncommon manifestations of Tourette syndrome (Box 105-2).

Pathophysiology

Tics are thought to be generated from a functional abnormality in deep brain nuclei that might include the striate nuclei, the globus pallidus, the subthalamic nuclei, and the substantia nigra. The frontal cortex, thalamus, and limbic systems may also be involved.

Dopaminergic neurotransmission within these structures is likely to be part of the abnormal function because of one type of medication worsening the symptoms and another type effective as a treatment. In patients with Tourette syndrome, the cerebrospinal fluid

---

Box 105-1. Types of Tics Seen in Children With Tourette Syndrome

Simple Tics
- Clonic
- Dystonic

Complex Tics
- Series of different or similar simple tics
- More complicated coordinated movement
- Copropraxia and coprographia

Vocal Tics
- Oropharyngeal, nasopharyngeal, or laryngeal sounds
- Consonants or syllables
- Meaningless or nonsense words or phrases
- Coprolalia
- Palilalia and echolalia

Sensory Tics

Box 105-2. Misconceptions in Diagnosing Tourette Syndrome

- Attributing the unusual tic symptom to attention-getting or emotionally based behavior
- Diagnosing the episodic behavior as a seizure on the basis of inadequate historical information
- Attributing a vocal tic to an upper airway, sinus, or allergic condition
- Attributing an ocular tic to an ophthalmologic problem
- Requiring tics to be observed in the office before making the diagnosis
- Waiting for coprolalia to be present before making the diagnosis
- Assuming severe tics are necessary for the diagnosis, or assuming tics are a normal developmental phase

contains low baseline levels of homovanillic acid, a dopamine metabolite, which could result from a hypersensitive dopamine receptor. In addition, amphetamines and methylphenidate increase dopamine release, and in some instances, these agents precipitate tic symptoms. Haloperidol, an effective tic-suppressing medication, blocks the dopamine receptor and, therefore, may block a potentially hypersensitive receptor for dopamine. The observations of good clinical response with low doses of haloperidol and the finding of increased homovanillic acid levels remaining high long after disappearance of the neuroleptic drug due to receptor desensitization both support this hypothesis. Other transmitters are probably involved as well because effective medications in other classes are also useful.

Recently an autoimmune hypothesis has been generated to explain an association of the sudden onset of tics and/or obsessive-compulsive symptoms with preceding group A streptococcal infections of the pharynx. This association has been termed *PANDAS* (pediatric autoimmune neuropsychiatric disease associated with streptococcus). It is intriguing that a clear relationship has been known for some time between the same bacteria and another movement problem, Sydenham chorea, but the evidence is somewhat conflicting for the bacteria's role in common neuropsychiatric disease such as Tourette syndrome or obsessive-compulsive disease and, therefore, routine screening has not been recommended.

Differential Diagnosis

The duration, frequency, and appearance of the movement and circumstances of occurrence of tics help distinguish them from several other episodic movement disorders. Myoclonus is a lightning-like, non-suppressible jerk of a small group of muscles, and chorea involves nearly constant, small amplitude movements of the fingers, hands, and feet that are often accompanied by grimacing movements of the face. Tremor is an oscillatory movement of an extremity or the head. Hemiballismus is an uncontrollable episodic throwing movement of an extremity. Hyperexplexia is a hyperactive startle response provoked by touch or sudden noise. Torticollis, or neck writhing, may be paroxysmal but is part of either a benign transient disorder or a chronic degenerative disorder, such as dystonia musculorum deformans. Paroxysmal kinesigenic choreoathetosis, an unusual episodic condition precipitated by a sudden movement, is characterized by a twisted trunk and limb posture lasting a few seconds and not accompanied by loss of consciousness. Hypnagogic jerks and bruxism are persistent normal variant behaviors that occur in sleep.

Other repetitive behaviors are sometimes confused with tics. Compulsions are complex actions that are done against one's will or better judgment. Stereotypies are persistent repetitive senseless movements. Perseverative behaviors are continued activity after the cause for it has ceased. Self-injurious behaviors are usually biting or banging of a body part during periods of agitation. Addictive behaviors occur with psychological dependence due to a reward system. Habits are fixed practices established by repetition. Mannerisms are stereotyped movements or habits peculiar to an individual and part of their personality. Anger outbursts are sudden emotion-generated behaviors occurring with relatively little provocation.

Tic disorders are sometimes divided into 3 groups: (1) **simple transient tics,** which are monomorphic (always the same appearance over a period of months), last less than 12 months, and may be caused by particular environmental situations or psychological states; (2) **chronic tics,** which last longer than 12 months but are a single type; and (3) the **tics of Tourette syndrome** (Box 105-3). However, all 3 types of tic disorders are sometimes found in the same family.

> **Box 105-3. Conditions Necessary for Diagnosis of Tourette Syndrome**
> - Multiple motor and vocal tics variably manifested over time
> - Tics present for at least 1 year
> - Onset of tics before 21 years of age
> - Tics not due to another known condition or substance

Evaluation

History

A thorough history should be taken when evaluating children with potential tic disorders. The physician should find out as much as possible about the duration, circumstances of occurrence, and frequency of the movements (Questions Box). Parents may imitate the behavior or, if possible, bring in a videotape of the child's behavior. This may give the physician more telling information than verbal descriptions.

> **Questions**
> **Tics**
> - How long and how often has the child been displaying the unusual behaviors?
> - In what circumstances do the unusual behaviors occur? For example, do the behaviors occur when the child is eating or sleeping, engrossed in an activity, or excited? Or do they occur when attention is on the child or after a startle or other triggering behavior?
> - Can the parents or other caregivers imitate the child's unusual behavior?
> - Is the child having difficulty at school (cognitively or socially)?

The physician should describe suggested tic behaviors because the parent may not be aware these behaviors may be tics.

Physical Examination

Frequently tics are not seen by the physician when confronting the child directly, but the physician may still be able to see the child's tics. The physician might be able to observe the child unobtrusively while the child and family are still in the waiting room, and the child should be observed for tics "out of the corner of one's eye" during the course of the parent interview and physical examination. A screen of cognitive abilities and fine-motor coordination should be included in the examination because of the high comorbidity of ADHD and other learning disabilities.

Laboratory Tests

There are no definitive diagnostic or supportive laboratory tests for Tourette syndrome or for confirming the presence of tics. Children with atypical movement disorders should be screened for potential metabolic abnormalities, including routine determinations of calcium, magnesium, glucose, liver function enzymes, and ceruloplasmin levels (for Wilson disease). Thyroid function tests may also be requested if there are signs or symptoms of thyroid dysfunction, because treatable endocrine hormone problems can produce tic-like movements.

Imaging Studies

Magnetic resonance imaging (MRI) of the brain may be helpful in considering metabolic abnormalities symptomatic of a movement disorder that might produce a characteristic image or rarely a structural lesion in the basal ganglia producing a tic-inducing movement disorder. Otherwise, imaging has been largely used in research evaluations of Tourette syndrome male populations where it has demonstrated volumetric increases in primarily right frontal white matter and the anterior parts of the corpus callosum in MRI studies, reduced right basal ganglia activity in single-photon emission computed tomography studies, and during tic suppression increased right caudate and frontal cortex activity in functional MRI studies.

Management

Goals of management should include (1) reduction in the frequency of tics during critical circumstances with a minimum of medication side effects and (2) attention to the other coexisting learning or behavioral disabilities. Before physicians prescribe drug treatment, they must consider the severity of the tic disorder and its potential for possible psychosocial effects. Some children do not need medication for the movement disorder, and they and their families can be reassured by an understanding of the problem. Other patients may experience remission for weeks or months, during which they can reduce or discontinue their medications. Several classes of drugs are useful in the treatment of tic disorders. A first-line medication because of its relatively good efficacy, side-effect profile, and convenience is the **Catapres** transdermal skin patch containing clonidine, an α_2-adrenergic agonist. Dosage is titrated using the minimally effective size and strength of the patch. The atypical antipsychotics, particularly **risperidone,** have also been effective with sometimes less sedation or potential for extrapyramidal side effects than tranquilizing dopamine blockers. Another useful medication is the neuroleptic **Pimozide** (Orap). An electrocardiogram is recommended before beginning this medication because it has been associated with prolonged QTc. Concomitant use of inhibitors of CYP3A liver metabolism should not be given. **Haloperidol** has been useful in divided doses starting as low as 0.5 mg/d up to 2 to 6 mg/d. Children should begin with a low dose that is then titrated up to maximum efficacy or development of intolerable side effects. A potential disadvantage of haloperidol and other antipsychotics is cognitive sedation and the small possibility of tardive dyskinesia. Other medications that may be beneficial include the α_2-adrenergic agonist **guanfacine** and the neuroleptic **fluphenazine. Botulinum toxin type A** injections may be useful for isolated persistent tics occurring in needle-accessible locations. Behavioral approaches including habit reversal training may be viable medication alternatives in some cases.

Treatment for children with Tourette syndrome should be multimodal and prioritize, address, and monitor all problematic aspects of the syndrome (Box 105-4). Children with Tourette syndrome should be assessed for learning disabilities including ADHD. Interventions may include organizational aids, homework time management, reduction in potential environmental distractions, and more **individualized instruction. Pharmacologic therapy** may include the Catapres patch, a tricyclic antidepressant, atomoxetine, or a stimulant. Long-acting methylphenidate or mixed amphetamine salt preparations are not necessarily contraindicated in children with Tourette syndrome; these drugs do not worsen tics in all patients. Children with Tourette syndrome are also susceptible to obsessive-compulsive symptoms. **Fluoxetine, sertraline,** and **clomipramine** are most useful for this comorbid problem.

Children with Tourette syndrome and their families also frequently benefit from **lay educational materials** about the disorder. **Support groups** composed of other families that have children with the syndrome and local chapters of the Tourette's Syndrome Association may help. Referral for psychological or psychiatric counseling for patients and their families may be necessary because in its severe form, Tourette syndrome may be socially devastating and may provoke secondary frustrations, low self-esteem, depression, and other emotional problems as well as the primary psycho-behavioral difficulties.

Prognosis

The prognosis in most children with tics is good. Less than 20% of adults and older children who were symptomatic in grade school manifest clinically impairing tic symptoms of Tourette syndrome. A few symptomatic children may not, however, have a productive educational experience or appropriate peer relationships. Therefore, the physician must individualize the management strategy to optimize the prognosis in more difficult cases. Because the movements may change or even remit over long periods, the psychological adjustments become very important in the long-term prognosis.

Box 105-4. Therapies Useful in Tourette Syndrome

Tics
- Clonidine (Catapres transdermal patch): α_2-adrenergic agonist
- Haloperidol (low dose): dopamine receptor blocker
- Pimozide (Orap): dopamine receptor blocker
- Fluphenazine: dopamine receptor blocker
- Guanfacine (Tenex): α_2-adrenergic agonist

Attention-Deficit/Hyperactivity Disorder and Learning Disability
- Clonidine (Catapres transdermal patch): α_2-adrenergic agonist
- Methylphenidate: if tics are not worsened
- Atomoxetine: norepinephrine transporter inhibitor
- Desipramine: tricyclic antidepressant
- Education interventions: individualized or small-group instruction

Obsessive-Compulsive Disorder
- Fluoxetine (Prozac): serotonin uptake inhibitor (non-tricyclic)
- Clomipramine (Anafranil): tricyclic antidepressant

Depression and Adjustment Problems
- Psychotherapy (individual and family)
- Imipramine: tricyclic antidepressant
- Support group

CASE RESOLUTION

The boy in the case history is diagnosed as having Tourette syndrome. After a discussion with his family about the disorder, he is treated with Catapres patches. A questionnaire is sent to his teacher concerning attention-deficit/hyperactivity disorder symptoms at school. At a 6-week follow-up visit, he has fewer tics and is doing better in school (classroom situation of 15 students for most of the day).

Selected References

Coffey B, Shechter R. Treatment of co-morbid obsessive compulsive disorder, mood, and anxiety disorders. *Adv Neurol.* 2006;99:208–221

Comings DE, Comings BG. A controlled family history study of Tourette syndrome. I. Attention deficit hyperactivity disorder, learning disorders and dyslexia. *J Clin Psychiatry.* 1990;51:275–280

Dale R. Post-streptococcal autoimmune disorders of the central nervous system. *Dev Med Child Neurol.* 2005;47:785–791

Denckla M. Attention-deficit hyperactivity disorder (ADHD) comorbidity: a case for "pure" Tourette syndrome? *J Child Neurol.* 2006;21:701–703

Erenberg G. The relationship between Tourette Syndrome, attention deficit hyperactivity disorder, and stimulant medication: a critical review. *Semin Pediatr Neurol.* 2006;12:217–221

Huff K. Approach to the child with movement disorders. In: Osborn L, Dewitt T, First L, Zenel J, eds. *Pediatrics.* Philadelphia, PA: Elsevier; 2005:770–777

Leckman JF, Bloch MH, Scahill L, King RA. Tourette syndrome: the self under siege. *J Child Neurol.* 2006;21:642–649

Piacentini J, Chang S. Behavioral treatments for tic suppression: habit reversal training. *Adv Neurol.* 2006;99:227–233

Robertson M. Tourette syndrome, associated conditions and the complexities of treatment. *Brain.* 2000;123:425–462

Singer HS. Neurobiologic issues in Tourette's syndrome. *Brain Dev.* 1994; 16:353–364

Snider LA, Swedo SE. PANDAS: current status and directions for research. *Mol Psychiatry.* 2004;9:900–907

Zinner S. Tourette disorder. *Pediatr Rev.* 2000;21:372–383

Dermatologic Disorders

106. Acne 651

107. Disorders of the Hair and Scalp 657

108. Diaper Dermatitis 663

109. Papulosquamous Eruptions 667

110 Maculopapular Rashes 673

111. Vesicular Exanthems 679

Acne

Monica Sifuentes, MD

CASE STUDY

A 15-year-old adolescent male comes to your office for a preparticipation sports physical. He is healthy and he has no questions, complaints, or concerns.

The adolescent is well developed and well nourished, with normal vital signs, including blood pressure. The physical examination is entirely normal except for the skin. Erythematous papules and pustules are present across the hairline and over both cheeks. Scattered blackheads are located over the nose and cheeks as well. The chest and back are clear, with no lesions.

Questions

1. What is the pathogenesis of acne vulgaris?
2. What are some contributing factors in the development of acne?
3. What are the different types of acne lesions?
4. What management options are available for the treatment of mild, moderate, and severe acne in adolescents?
5. What are the indications for the use of isotretinoin (Accutane)?
6. What is the prognosis for adolescent patients with acne?

Acne vulgaris is a common condition that most frequently occurs in adolescents. The spectrum of disease varies from individual to individual and may be caused by a variety of factors. Regardless of the etiology and extent of acne, the disease can be devastating to adolescents both physically and psychologically. Primary care physicians should, therefore, acknowledge acne as a medical problem, even when patients do not mention it, and should treat the condition accordingly.

Epidemiology

Most cases of acne that require treatment occur in individuals 9 to 19 years of age, although the condition can also affect young infants and young adult women. Boys and girls are equally affected, but the condition is usually more severe in boys. Certain individuals may be genetically susceptible to acne. White teens are more likely to have acne than African American and Asian teens. Certain cultural practices, such as the use of oily grooming agents by some African Americans, also can lead to a specific pattern of lesions. Estimates indicate that more than 85% of adolescents in the United States are affected with acne and that more than $124 million dollars is spent annually on acne treatments. And although acne is generally believed to be a pubertal event, a fair number of young adults continue to develop lesions after 25 years of age.

Several factors contribute to the development of acne-like eruptions. Internal agents include endogenous hormones (eg, androgens, progesterone) and specific drugs (eg, progestin-only contraceptives, isoniazid, phenytoin, corticosteroids, anabolic steroids, lithium-containing compounds). External agents include skin bacteria, especially *Propionibacterium acnes*; industrial chemicals (eg, petroleum,

animal and vegetable oils); oil- or wax-containing cosmetics; greasy sunscreen or suntan preparations; and local pressure from objects such as headbands, shoulder pads, or helmets. Excessive perspiration and emotional stress can also aggravate acne. Specific foods such as chocolate, caffeine-containing soda, pizza, and French fries have not been shown to cause or worsen acne.

Clinical Presentation

The lesions of acne vulgaris primarily affect the face, especially the cheeks, forehead, and chin; the chest; the back; and the shoulders. Lesions can be non-inflamed or inflamed (Dx Box). Non-inflamed lesions, or comedones, can be opened or closed to the environment. Closed comedones (whiteheads) are small, flesh-colored bumps, and open comedones (blackheads) contain central, dark material. Inflamed lesions are typically erythematous papules or pustules and may be more cystic in appearance.

Dx Acne

- Occurrence predominantly during puberty
- Lesions more severe in males
- Location on face, chest, back, and shoulders
- Non-inflamed, open comedones (blackheads) or closed comedones (whiteheads)
- Inflamed papules or pustules
- Nodules or cysts may be present
- Possible exacerbation around menses or related to stress

Lesions are generally concentrated in the centrofacial areas or "T-zone" early in the course of acne. The T-zone includes the forehead, nose, and chin areas, which are rich in sebaceous glands. Over time, lesions can develop in other areas of the body such as the neck, chest, shoulders, and back.

Pathophysiology

Although the exact etiology of acne remains unclear, the pathogenesis of acne involves certain processes.

1. **Abnormal follicular keratinization.** The earliest change in the formation of acne occurs in the horny cells that line the sebaceous follicle. A disturbance in the differentiation of these cells leads to excessive shedding of the cells into the lumen. Impaction of the follicle occurs as these horny cells stick together.

2. **Overproduction of sebum.** The sebaceous gland is highly responsive to hormonal stimulation, namely androgens. With the rise in androgens during puberty, hypertrophy of the sebaceous gland occurs, and the production of sebum is increased. The flow of sebum is obstructed by the above follicular hyperkeratosis, resulting in retention of all material.

3. **Proliferation of *P acnes.*** The overproduction of sebum in acne provides a ripe environment for the proliferation of *P acnes,* an anaerobic diphtheroid that, along with *Staphylococcus epidermidis* and *Pityrosporum ovale,* is part of the microflora of the sebaceous follicle. In addition, *P acnes* possesses a lipase that hydrolyzes sebum triglycerides into free fatty acids. These acids irritate the follicular wall and cause inflammation.

4. **Inflammation.** The expulsion of sebum into the dermal layer of the skin occurs as a result of the rupture of the pilosebaceous follicle. This initiates an inflammatory process and the formation of inflammatory lesions such as pustules and cysts. In addition, *P acnes* produce biologically active extracellular materials, which increase the permeability of the follicular epithelium. The bacterium also produces chemotactic factors that are responsible for the migration of inflammatory cells to the area.

5. **Comedones.** The above processes can lead to a number of noninflammatory and inflammatory lesions (Table 106-1). Comedones are early noninflammatory lesions made up of sebum, horny cells, and bacteria. They can be closed or open. A **closed comedo,** or **whitehead,** is a dilated plugged sebaceous follicle that is closed to the surface of the skin. An **open comedo,** or **blackhead,** occurs as a result of dilatation of the follicular orifice at the surface of the skin and open communication with the outside environment. The dark color at the surface of the skin is believed to result from melanin in the horny cells, not dirt.

6. **Pustules** and **papules** are inflammatory lesions. Pustules lie in the superficial epidermal layer of the skin, and papules occur in the lower dermal layer. Because of their deeper location, they are often accompanied by a more severe inflammatory reaction, and scarring may result. **Nodules** or **cysts** are suppurative inflammatory lesions located deep within the dermis. Associated with the most severe form of acne, nodules are the result of deep pustules that rupture and then become lined with epithelium. When nodules are present, significant scarring is a major problem.

Evaluation

History

The primary historical issues to explore in patients with acne vulgaris are both medical and psychological (Questions Box). From a medical standpoint, practitioners should determine how long the acne has been present and if the condition has ever been treated. Psychological aspects should include questions to assess the patient's overall self-esteem. Expectations regarding treatment and recovery should also be assessed at the initial visit before therapy is begun.

Table 106-1. Classification of Acne	
Category	*Physical Findings*
Grade I	Noninflammatory acne → open and closed comedones
	Closed comedones then lead to any of the next 3 levels of inflammatory acne
Grade II	Early inflammatory acne → presence of comedones and papules (obstructed follicles)
Grade III	Moderate, localized inflammatory acne → pustules or larger, more inflamed papules
Grade IV	Severe, more generalized inflammatory acne → cystic, nodular lesions

Questions

Acne

Medical Aspects
- How long has the adolescent had acne?
- Has the adolescent ever received treatment for acne?
  — How long did treatment continue?
  — What treatment methods were used?
  — For what reasons was the therapy discontinued?
- Is the adolescent currently using any treatment products?
  — Do the lesions seem to be getting better or worse?
- If the acne has never been treated, is treatment desired?
- Do any activities, medications, or environmental agents seem to exacerbate the lesions?
- Does the adolescent have a family history of acne?
- Is the adolescent taking any oral medications?

Psychological Aspects
- Is the adolescent bothered by the lesions?
- Is the adolescent embarrassed about his or her appearance? If so, does this embarrassment prevent the adolescent from participating in certain activities?
- Is the adolescent ever ridiculed by his or her peers because of the acne?

Physical Examination

The physical examination should focus on the primary sites of acne: face, chest, back, and shoulders. The entire skin should be inspected closely at the first visit, however. Individual lesions should be checked for signs of inflammation and infection at each follow-up visit. Their distribution also should be recorded along with their response to treatment. The presence or absence of scarring should be assessed as a measure of the severity of acne and a predictor of outcome. Young women with very irregular menses and obesity should be examined for hirsutism, which might indicate excessive adrenal or ovarian androgen production as a cause of acne.

Laboratory Tests

In general, no laboratory studies are needed either at the time of the initial evaluation or during the treatment of mild to moderate acne. If there is a history of abnormal menses and evidence of hirsutism or virilization in the adolescent female, a total serum testosterone, early morning cortisol and 17-hydroxyprogresterone, and serum dehydroepiandrosterone sulfate levels are indicated to differentiate between the various causes of hyperandrogenism. In the case of severe acne when isotretinoin is indicated, several pretreatment studies are necessary. A complete blood count, liver function tests, and a fasting lipid profile are recommended. In addition, a pregnancy test must be performed within 2 weeks of starting isotretinoin in sexually active female adolescents. These studies should be obtained in consultation with a dermatologist, who is generally responsible for prescribing isotretinoin.

Management

The general management of acne begins with counseling and should include patient education regarding the pathophysiology of the condition to dispel any myths regarding its etiology and treatment. In addition, the patient's motivation should be assessed to better individualize therapy. Realistic expectations regarding duration of therapy and likely outcome of treatment should be reviewed with the teenager. Parental involvement is optimal in cases of severe acne. All adolescents with acne should follow these general recommendations:

1. Wash skin with mild soap and water once or twice daily.
2. Use cosmetics sparingly or switch to oil-free products that indicate they are noncomedogenic.
3. Avoid picking and excessive scrubbing, especially with abrasive cleansers.
4. Note that dietary modifications are not indicated.
5. Restrict ultraviolet therapy.
6. Follow the prescribed regimen carefully (Table 106-2).

The specific therapies prescribed depend on the severity and duration of the acne, the type of lesions, and patients' ability to comply with the proposed treatment. The patient's skin type should be taken into consideration when selecting the appropriate vehicle for the active ingredient, such as a cream, gel, lotion, solution, or ointment. Oily skin types tend to respond better to gels or solutions, whereas creams, lotions, and ointments are better for dry skin. The

Table 106-2. Treatment of Acne[a]	
Classification	*Recommended Treatment Regimen*
Grade I (mild)	Benzoyl peroxide 2.5%–5% every other day or at bedtime
	May increase to twice a day, if tolerated, and/or retinoic acid at bedtime
Grade II (mild-moderate)	Benzoyl peroxide and/or retinoic acid as above plus topical antibiotics once or twice a day if inflammation present
Grade III (moderate)	Benzoyl peroxide in the morning and/or retinoic acid at bedtime *plus* oral antibiotics
Grade IV (severe)	Above treatment for grade III acne, *plus* referral to a dermatologist for consideration for treatment with isotretinoin

[a]Modified with permission from Strasburger VC. Acne: what every pediatrician should know about treatment. *Pediatr Clin North Am.* 1997;44:1514.

most effective regimens include topical products such as benzoyl peroxide, retinoic acid, and antibiotics; systemic antimicrobials; hormonal agents; and isotretinoin. Most often, however, combination therapy is used and later modified according to patients' responses. Physicians should remember and discuss with the adolescent that the acne often looks worse before it gets better. Noticeable improvement usually takes at least 4 to 6 weeks.

Topical Therapy

Several topical products are available for the treatment of acne. **Benzoyl peroxide** is bactericidal for *P acnes* and acts as a comedolytic agent as well. It should be considered as the first line of therapy for the management of both comedonal and inflammatory acne. Although over-the-counter lotions are available, the more effective gel preparations are preferable. The lowest concentration possible should be used initially. Higher concentrations should be used in cases in which the trunk or back are involved.

Therapy should be initiated gradually, especially if used in combination with retinoic acid, because benzoyl peroxide is inherently irritating and drying. Initially, a thin application should be made once a day every other day, and the frequency should be increased as tolerated. Allergic contact dermatitis rarely develops, but if it does, treatment must be discontinued. A nonacnegenic, noncomedogenic sunscreen is recommended as well to protect against the photosensitivity associated with benzoyl peroxide usage.

Tretinoin or retinoic acid (Retin-A, Avita) is the mainstay of therapy for noninflammatory or comedonal acne. This vitamin A derivative reduces microcomedo formation by normalizing follicular keratinization and decreasing the adhesiveness of horny cells shed into the follicular lumen. It is available by prescription as a gel, cream, or liquid in several different concentrations. Recently, microsphere technology has become available, which is less irritating and allows the medication to be delivered slowly at higher concentrations. It seems to be as effective as the older formulations.

Like benzoyl peroxide, retinoic acid can be very irritating and may cause some erythema and peeling. Therefore, therapy should be initiated cautiously with a cream or gel, which is less potent and drying than the liquid preparation. To further reduce irritation, patients should be instructed to wash with a mild soap no more than 2 times a day and to wait at least 20 to 30 minutes for the skin to dry completely before applying the product. Physicians often recommend that patients apply retinoic acid before bedtime rather than in the mornings, which tend to be more hectic for the average teenager. A small, pea-sized dot of tretinoin should be used each time and divided into 3 smaller dots on the skin before rubbing it gently into the area. Patients also should be cautioned against excessive sun exposure while using retinoic acid because this agent lowers the sunburn threshold. Alternate daily treatment with benzoyl peroxide is warranted in cases of inflammatory acne.

Adapalene (Differin) and tazarotene (Tazorac) are 2 relatively new third-generation topical retinoids that have been used in the treatment of acne. Adapalene is less irritating and has been shown to be more photostable than tretinoin. It is available in an alcohol-free gel, cream, or solution. Tazarotene, originally created for the treatment of psoriasis, is the most effective of the topical retinoids, but is more expensive and irritating than the other retinoids, and there are concerns about its teratogenicity. It is therefore not widely prescribed for the treatment of acne.

Azelaic acid (Azelex), a naturally occurring derivative from wheat, has both antibacterial and anti-keratinizing activity. It inhibits the growth of *P acnes* and has an antiproliferative effect on keratinocytes. Although less potent than tretinoin, azelaic acid may be useful in patients with mild to moderate acne who cannot tolerate topical tretinoin or benzoyl peroxide because it seems to be less irritating. Pruritus, burning, stinging, tingling, and erythema have been reported, however. It is available by prescription as a 20% cream and should be applied twice daily.

Antibiotic Therapy

Both topical as well as systemic antibiotics can be used in the treatment of inflammatory acne. The choice of which to use usually depends on the extent of skin involvement and severity of inflammation. **Topical antibiotics** are often useful in patients with inflammatory lesions that are unresponsive to benzoyl peroxide or retinoic acid alone. Such antibiotics act by inhibiting the growth of *P acnes* and reducing the number of comedones, papules, and pustules. Erythromycin, tetracycline, and clindamycin are available as topical preparations. The **erythromycin gel** is most popular; the recommended dosage is twice daily. Allergic reactions from topical formulations rarely occur. Compared with systemic antibiotics, topical preparations have fewer systemic side effects because of decreased absorption. Topical antibiotics alone are not recommended as monotherapy because resistance generally develops with prolonged use and the therapeutic response can take a while. Both erythromycin and clindamycin are available in combination with benzoyl peroxide and are very effective against *P acnes*.

Systemic antibiotics are the mainstay of therapy in patients with nodular or cystic inflammatory acne and in patients who have not responded to topical antibiotics. However, systemic agents have not been shown to be effective with comedonal acne. The success of oral antimicrobial therapy relates to the suppression of *P acnes* and the inhibition of bacterial lipases. As a result, free fatty acids and other by-products are reduced, thereby decreasing inflammation.

Tetracycline and its derivatives (**doxycycline and minocycline**) are the preferred first-line oral antibiotics for the treatment of moderate to severe inflammatory acne. Other systemic antibiotics such as erythromycin have been used in the past; however, antibiotic resistance is now a problem. In addition, clindamycin is used much less frequently because of its associated side effects like pseudomembranous colitis. Doxycycline and minocycline are particularly beneficial when lesions fail to respond to tetracycline. However, tetracycline and doxycycline are not recommended in children younger than 9 years or in pregnant females. The most common side effects include candidal vaginitis, especially in females who also take oral contraceptives (OCPs), gastrointestinal (GI) disturbances, and photosensitivity. The ultimate goal of oral antibiotic therapy is use of the minimum dose to control lesions and minimize side effects. Most patients require prolonged or frequent intermittent courses of antibiotics, however, before remission occurs. In general, the dose of the antibiotic and the dosing interval should not be reduced before a significant clinical effect is seen, which may take 6 to 8 weeks. At that time the dose of the oral antibiotic may be gradually tapered and topical antibiotic treatment may be substituted.

Hormonal Therapy

Hormonal therapy is indicated in menstruating females who are unresponsive to other forms of treatment and who may or may not be candidates for isotretinoin. Oral contraceptives antagonize the action of circulating androgens by increasing the production of sex-binding globulin, which decreases biologically active free testosterone. In addition there is decreased androgen production by the ovaries through feedback inhibition of pituitary gonadotropin secretion. Clinical improvement in inflammatory lesions has been reported with ethinyl estradiol (35 µg) and the progestin norgestimate (Ortho Tri-Cyclen) and ethinyl estradiol/drospirenone (Yasmin). In general, OCPs must be taken for 2 to 4 months before any improvement is seen, with relapses occurring if treatment is discontinued. Ortho Tri-Cyclen and Estrostep have been approved by the US Food and Drug Administration specifically for their antiandrogen effects, although other OCPs have shown similar efficacy in reducing acne lesions.

Low-dose glucocorticoids (dexamethasone) are indicated in females with acne accompanied by virilization or any other evidence of excessive androgens. These agents work by decreasing adrenal androgen production. Low-dose glucocorticoids in combination with OCPs also can be extremely effective.

Systemic Therapy

Because sebaceous glands are androgen-dependent, antiandrogens such as spironolactone can reduce sebum production, and therefore improve acne. Doses range from 100 to 200 mg/d; however, lower doses may also be effective. Several months of spironolactone therapy are needed for maximum benefit, with prolonged therapy often required. Gynecomastia occurs not infrequently. Agranulocytosis is a rare complication.

Isotretinoin Therapy

Isotretinoin (Accutane), a systemic oral analog of vitamin A, is currently the most effective treatment available for severe nodulocystic acne that is resistant to conventional therapy. This agent is also useful in patients with a propensity for scarring. It influences all aspects of acne formation: sebum secretion, follicular keratinization, and inflammatory responses.

Because isotretinoin has numerous potentially serious side effects, referral to a dermatologist is strongly recommended for patients who require isotretinoin therapy. The most significant of these side effects is teratogenicity, although other issues include dryness and chapping of the skin and mucous membranes, musculoskeletal effects, GI issues, neurologic problems, and hematologic abnormalities. Therefore, isotretinoin should be used cautiously in women of childbearing age, and the drug should not be prescribed in pregnant or breastfeeding women. Compliance with 2 forms of effective contraception must be established before the initiation of treatment. Isotretinoin can also elevate triglyceride levels, particularly in patients with diabetes mellitus, obesity, alcohol abuse, and familial hyperlipidemia. There also are concerns regarding isotretinoin use and its possible association with mood disorders. To date, however, this has not been confirmed. However, to ensure informed consent as well as avoid potential complications, patients must receive careful instructions prior to the initiation of therapy and must be followed closely during the course of their treatment.

Prognosis

Fortunately, most uncomplicated cases of acne (approximately 90%) resolve in the third decade of life. For those individuals with nodulocystic lesions, however, acne and significant scarring can continue to be a problem. Therefore, aggressive treatment is imperative.

CASE RESOLUTION

In the case history, the adolescent should be offered treatment for his acne. This may include benzoyl peroxide, retinoic acid (Retin-A), and oral antibiotics. The common side effects of the medications (eg, dry skin, peeling) should be reviewed, and the teen should be instructed to use a noncomedogenic sunscreen. A follow-up appointment should be arranged after 3 to 4 weeks to assess compliance with and tolerance of the treatment regimen.

Selected References

Goldsmith LA, Bolognia JL, Callen JP, et al. American Academy of Dermatology Consensus Conference on safe and optimal use of isotretinoin: summary and recommendations. *J Am Acad Dermatol.* 2004;50:900–906

Koblenzer CS. The emotional impact of chronic and disabling skin disease: a psychoanalytic perspective. *Dermatol Clin.* 2005;23:619–627

Krowchuk DP. Managing adolescent acne: a guide for pediatricians. *Pediatr Rev.* 2005;26:244–255

Krowchuk DP, Lucky AW. Managing adolescent acne. *Adolesc Med.* 2001;12:355–374

National Campaign to Control Acne. Secaucus NJ: Thomas Professional Postgraduate Services; 2003

Paller AS, Mancini AJ. *Hurwitz Clinical Pediatric Dermatology: A Textbook of Skin Disorders of Childhood and Adolescence.* 3rd ed. Philadelphia, PA: W. B. Saunders; 2006

Smith JA. The impact of skin disease on the quality of life in adolescents. *Adolesc Med.* 2001;12:343–353

Strasburger VC. Acne: what every pediatrician should know about treatment. *Pediatr Clin North Am.* 1997;44:1505–1523

Witchel SF. Hyperandrogenism in adolescents. *Adolesc Med.* 2002;13:89–99

Yan AC. Current concepts in acne management. *Adolesc Med.* 2006;17:613–637

Disorders of the Hair and Scalp

Kathy K. Langevin, MD, MPH, and Noah Craft, MD, PhD

CASE STUDY

A 6-year-old child presents with a 1-month history of a swelling on the right side of her scalp that is associated with hair loss. She has previously been in good health, and she has no history of fever. On examination, she is afebrile, has normal vital signs, and appears well. An area of non-tender, boggy swelling 2 × 2 cm with associated alopecia is apparent over the scalp in the right temporal area. Small pustular lesions are scattered over the involved area. Generalized scaling of the scalp and occipital adenopathy are evident.

Questions

1. What are the common causes of circumscribed hair loss in children?
2. What are the common causes of diffuse hair loss in children?
3. What are the common causes of scalp scaling in children?
4. What features distinguish tinea capitis from alopecia areata?
5. What is the treatment for tinea capitis? Is there a role for topical antifungal agents?

Disorders of the scalp may be either congenital or acquired during childhood or adolescence. Conditions may be further classified according to the presence or absence of hair loss (alopecia), whether the hair loss is diffuse or circumscribed, and whether the hair loss results in scarring of the scalp.

Epidemiology

Acquired circumscribed hair loss is more commonly seen than diffuse hair loss. Most cases of acquired circumscribed hair loss result from tinea capitis, alopecia areata, or trauma due to traction or trichotillomania.

Tinea capitis is a fungal infection of the scalp most often caused by the dermatophytes *Microsporum canis* or *Trichophyton tonsurans*. *T tonsurans* accounts for most cases in the United States, but in a given geographic area, the etiologic fungus may change over time. Tinea capitis, which is less common in infants and postpubertal adolescents, is seen primarily in school-aged children between the ages of 3 and 7 years. Prevalence is estimated to be between 3% to 13% in the pediatric population. Boys are affected more often than girls with *M canis*, though both are affected equally in epidemics caused by *T tonsurans*. African American and Latin American children are more vulnerable to infection. Human-to-human transmission is more common with *T tonsurans*, an anthropophilic fungus. Children who handle dogs or cats, which harbor *M canis*, a zoophilic

fungus, are susceptible to infection. Carriers are most commonly adults exposed to affected children, and carriers are considered contagious. Up to 60% of affected children are asymptomatic. Tinea capitis can result in localized patches of hair loss and can result in scarring if the infection becomes inflammatory.

Alopecia areata is believed to be an organ-specific autoimmune disorder with a prevalence of 158 per 100,000 persons, occurring equally in males and females. Family history is positive in 10% to 50% of affected patients. Although alopecia areata may develop at any age, it is rare before the age of 1 year and 40% to 50% of cases develop alopecia areata before the age of 21 years. It may be seen in association with atopic dermatitis, Down syndrome, and other autoimmune diseases.

Trichotillomania, or compulsive pulling at the hair, may be seen in association with other impulse disorders such as thumb sucking and nail biting (see Chapter 40). It results in hair loss due to self-induced trauma. Usually the scalp hair is involved, but eyebrows or eyelash hair may also be affected. Although trichotillomania may be seen at any age, onset is usually between the ages of 5 to 12 years. It is more commonly seen in girls and women rather than boys and men and in children rather than adults. **Traction alopecia** is more commonly seen in females whose hair-grooming practices result in excessive tension and trauma to the hair.

Clinical Presentation

Children may present with specific complaints, including localized baldness, pruritus, scaling, or inflammation (Dx Box). Occasionally, lymphadenopathy, particularly in the occipital area, is the major presenting symptom.

Dx Disorders of the Hair and Scalp

- Circumscribed or generalized hair loss (alopecia)
- Scaling
- Pruritus
- Erythema of the scalp
- Localized or generalized swelling of the scalp
- Occipital adenopathy

Pathophysiology

An understanding of the physiology of the normal hair growth cycle helps in the evaluation of hair and scalp disorders. The scalp of an average human being contains about 100,000 hairs. Individuals with blonde hair generally have 10% more hairs and those with red hair have 10% less. Healthy terminal hair grows an average of 0.3 mm per day or approximately 1 cm per month.

The hair follicle is responsible for most disturbances of hair growth because the hair shaft itself is a nonliving structure. Normal hair growth is a cyclical process composed of 3 stages. The anagen phase, the period of active hair growth, lasts for an average of 3 years (range: 2–6 years). Normally, about 85% to 90% of scalp hair is in this phase at any one time. The catagen phase, the transition period, lasts for about 10 to 14 days. The telogen phase, the final resting phase, lasts for about 3 to 4 months. About 13% of scalp hairs are in this phase at one time. The average individual loses about 100 to 150 telogen hairs per day. The normal hair cycle results in replacement of each scalp hair every 3 to 5 years.

Tinea capitis is a communicable infection and can be acquired via interpersonal contact, contact with infected animals, and via fomites. There are 3 patterns of hair invasion. In endothrix infections (eg, *T tonsurans*), the fungus produces chains of spores within the hair shaft. In ectothrix infections (eg, *M canis*), spores are present around the exterior of the hair shaft. Favus, the most severe form of tinea capitis, demonstrates hyphae and air spaces within the hair shaft. This is usually caused by *Trichophyton schoenleinii*, a less common etiologic organism. Though dermatophytes have a relatively short incubation period (up to 3 weeks) they are viable in fomites for months. Subcutaneous invasion in conjunction with an exaggerated host response can result in kerion. Alopecia areata is thought to be due to aberrant expression of class I human leukocyte antigens on early anagen follicles resulting in T lymphocyte recognition of these normally immune hairs. There follows an immunologic attack causing premature telogen. The hairs then break easily at the surface of

the scalp. The hairs at the margins of alopecia are easily plucked and they have an "exclamation mark" appearance with the proximal end thinner than the distal end.

Differential Diagnosis

Scalp Disorders Without Associated Hair Loss

These conditions are divided into those disorders seen most often in neonates and young infants and those seen more frequently in children and adolescents (Box 107-1). **Caput succedaneum,** a generalized edema involving the soft tissues of the scalp, and **cephalhematoma,** a subperiosteal hematoma, are 2 of the most common lesions of the scalp that occur during the neonatal period. A cephalhematoma does not extend beyond the suture lines of the affected bone, which distinguishes it from caput succedaneum. Both conditions result from birth trauma and generally resolve spontaneously within a few weeks to months without further complications.

Box 107-1. Common Disorders of the Scalp Without Associated Hair Loss

Neonatal Period and Early Infancy
- Birth trauma to the scalp (eg, caput succedaneum, cephalhematoma)
- Scalp abscess (at fetal scalp electrode site)
- Herpes simplex infection
- Cradle cap/seborrheic dermatitis
- Atopic dermatitis[a]
- Scabies

Childhood and Adolescence
- Seborrheic dermatitis[a]
- Atopic dermatitis[a]
- Head lice (pediculosis capitis)
- Psoriasis[a]

[a]May occur with or without associated hair loss.

Other neonatal scalp conditions include infections such as **scalp abscess** and **herpes simplex virus (HSV) infection.** Scalp abscess, a self-limited condition that occurs most commonly as a complication of scalp electrode placement, has an incidence of 0.4% to 4.5%. The infectious agents are usually flora of the cervix and vagina. Management depends on the severity of the infection (eg, associated cellulitis or signs of systemic involvement). Herpes simplex virus infections of the scalp are not uncommon in neonates; 85% of neonatal HSV infections occur at time of delivery and the scalp usually has the longest contact with the cervix, one of the sites for transmission of infection. Herpes lesions are typically vesicular, but petechial, purpuric, or bullous lesions may also be apparent. Skin lesions typically develop at 1 week of life but may be present at birth or develop as late as 3 weeks later.

Seborrheic dermatitis is a greasy, scaly eruption that occurs mainly on the scalp, face, and postauricular and intertriginous areas (see Chapter 109). It is often seen in infants younger than 2 years.

Additionally, the nongreasy scale often termed *dandruff* in children 2 to 10 years is usually seborrheic dermatitis. Cradle cap, involving the scalp of neonates, is usually noninflammatory, diffuse, greasy scaling of the scalp and usually develops during the first several months of life. Unlike atopic dermatitis, seborrheic dermatitis is generally non-pruritic. Occasionally the inflammatory process is severe enough to result in diffuse hair loss. Psoriatic lesions of the scalp and Langerhans cell histiocytosis can mimic seborrheic dermatitis. Skin biopsy may be required for definitive diagnosis. It is often seen in conjunction with adenopathy of the head and neck without associated tinea infection.

Atopic dermatitis and **seborrheic dermatitis** are the 2 most common diagnoses of scalp scaling among infants and children younger than 10 years. Atopic dermatitis is characterized by erythema and scaling of the scalp that can become papular. Rubbing and scratching produces the secondary effects of crusting and lichenification. Severe atopic and seborrheic dermatitis, as well as psoriasis, can result in **tinea amiantacea** (not a fungal infection), in which thick white or gray crust can be localized over the scalp, often with resultant temporary alopecia.

Head lice (pediculosis capitis) are an extremely common childhood infestation that affects girls more often than boys and is most common in children aged 3 to 11 years. Lice are spread by direct contact with infected individuals or infested clothing, combs, or other hair accessories. Pruritus is the primary symptom along with erythema and scaling, with secondary impetigo common. The viable ova or nits may be visible as small, oval, tan to brown specks found most commonly in the hair above the ears and the nape of the neck. Hatched eggs are clear to white. Generally, only the ova closest to the scalp are viable. They are difficult to remove.

Scabies, a pruritic infestation commonly seen in children, generally does not affect the scalp, except in infants, the elderly, and the immunocompromised. On the scalp of infants, 2- to 3-mm erythematous papules are seen, with overlying excoriations and, often, secondary bacterial infection.

Scalp Disorders Associated With Hair Loss

Box 107-2 lists the common scalp disorders associated with hair loss. When evaluating hair loss in children, it is important to determine whether the loss is diffuse or circumscribed.

Nevus sebaceus is a common cause of congenital circumscribed hair loss, occurring in about 3 of 1,000 neonates. The lesions are solitary, well-circumscribed plaques on the scalp, yellow-orange in color, and ovoid to linear in shape. They can sometimes occur on the head and neck as well. They are usually alopecic. They may be a component of the epidermal nevus syndrome when associated with multiple neurologic abnormalities. They are benign lesions with a 10% to 30% possibility of a low-grade malignancy developing within them after puberty. **Aplasia cutis congenita** is a congenital skin defect with localized areas of epidermal, dermal, and subcutaneous tissue loss. Lesions can occur anywhere on the body, but most are found along the midline of the scalp. At birth, the lesions usually appear as

> ### Box 107-2. Common Disorders of the Scalp With Associated Hair Loss
>
> *Circumscribed Hair Loss*
> **Congenital**
> - Aplasia cutis congenita
> - Nevus sebaceous
> - Epidermal nevus
>
> **Acquired**
> - Tinea capitis
> - Alopecia areata
> - Traction alopecia
> - Trichotillomania
> - Discoid lupus erythematosus
> - Secondary syphilis
> - Herpes simplex virus
> - Lichen planus
>
> *Diffuse Alopecia*
> **Congenital**
> - Congenital hypothyroidism
> - Hair shaft defects (eg, Menkes syndrome, monilethrix)
> - Ectodermal dysplasias and other genetic syndromes
>
> **Acquired**
> - Seborrheic dermatitis
> - Psoriasis
> - Telogen effluvium
> - Anagen effluvium (secondary to toxins or chemicals)
> - Endocrine (eg, diabetes mellitus)
> - Hypothyroidism-hypoparathyroidism-hypopituitarism
> - Medication-induced (isotretinoin)
> - Androgenic alopecia (eg, male pattern baldness)
> - Loose anagen syndrome
>
> **Other**
> - Nutritional (eg, acrodermatitis enteropathica, malnutrition, iron deficiency, rickets)
> - Systemic lupus erythematosus

punched out round or oval defects with a thin glistening membrane. Erosion, ulceration, or a scar due to healing in utero can also be seen. A "hair collar" often surrounds the lesion. Etiology is unknown, and it can be an isolated defect or in association with other congenital defects such as cleft lip or palate, syndactyly, or multiple other anomalies. Small defects generally heal well, whereas larger defects may require surgical excision and eventual skin grafting. Preoperative imaging studies may be required.

Tinea capitis, a fungal infection of the scalp, is one of the most common causes of acquired hair loss in children. This condition is characterized by patchy alopecia with broken-off hairs and scaling of the scalp. *T tonsurans* infection sometimes appears as a series of black dots within the affected area due to the presence of fragmented hairs. The diagnosis can be difficult in children with either diffuse scalp scaling or a diffuse pustular eruption without significant alopecia. Occasionally, an intense hypersensitivity response may result in a boggy swelling of the scalp known as a **kerion.** The surface of the kerion may be smooth or covered with small pustules, mimicking a bacterial infection. Uncomplicated tinea capitis leaves no scars, but kerions or favus may result in permanent, scarring hair loss.

Alopecia areata, which frequently leads to hair loss, is characterized by well-defined areas of complete hair loss without associated scaling, irritation, or inflammation of the scalp. Hairs at the periphery of bald patches can usually be easily plucked. Patchy alopecia is most common, characterized by scattered round or oval patches. An ophiasis pattern shows a band-like pattern of hair loss along the periphery of the temporal and occipital scalp or a sisaipho pattern with opposite pattern of loss to ophiasis. A reticular variant has diffuse patchy loss and may represent another disorder altogether. Associated nail defects, including nail pitting (most common) and ridging, may be seen. Occasionally, alopecia totalis (loss of all scalp hair) or alopecia universalis (loss of all body and scalp hair) may result.

Common traumatic causes of alopecia in children are traction alopecia and trichotillomania. **Traction alopecia** often occurs along the margins of the hairline secondary to having the hair pulled back in tight ponytails or braids. Short, broken hairs and follicular papules may be seen. Chronic, prolonged traction can result in permanent, scarring alopecia. **Trichotillomania** is a self-induced form of traction alopecia in which children twist or pull out their hair either consciously or subconsciously (see Chapter 40). Hair pulling is generally believed to occur in a younger population and usually resolves with minimal or no intervention needed. Trichotillomania is now classified in *Diagnostic and Statistical Manual of Mental Disorders, Fourth Edition,* in the habit and impulse disorders category. Hair is generally plucked in a wave-like fashion across the scalp or centrifugally from a starting point. The occiput is generally spared. Trichotillomania may mimic other types of alopecia, but the diagnosis can usually be made on the basis of the bizarre patterns of hair loss with hairs broken at differing lengths. Children occasionally eat the hairs as they are pulled out, resulting in the formation of a **trichobezoar** (hair ball) in the stomach.

Discoid lupus erythematosus, lichen planus, and **secondary syphilis** are uncommon causes of localized hair loss from the scalp in children. The patches of alopecia in discoid lupus erythematosus often appear hypopigmented with hyperpigmentation at the periphery. Because adnexal structures are involved in discoid lupus, scarring alopecia is commonly seen. Lichen planus, an idiopathic inflammatory disease of skin and mucous membranes, can result in both scarring and non-scarring alopecia. Secondary syphilis lesions appear as "moth-eaten" patches of alopecia that are non-scarring.

A variety of structural defects, endocrine and metabolic disorders, and toxins may be associated with diffuse loss of scalp hair (see Box 107-2). **Intrinsic structural defects of the hair** may cause hairs to break, thus resulting in failure of hair growth. In some forms of

ectodermal dysplasia, the number of hair follicles is reduced or the follicles are altogether absent, giving the appearance of sparse or thinning hair. Many of the ectodermal dysplasias have abnormalities of the teeth, nails, and sweat glands. **Monilethrix** is an autosomal-dominant condition that can appear in isolation or in association with other anomalies. Microscopic evaluation of hairs show a "beads on a string" appearance due to alternating nodes and internodes resulting in fractures between the nodes. Pili torti can be seen in several syndromes including **Menkes syndrome (kinky hair syndrome).** Affected patients have twisted hair leading to premature breakage and, thus, chronically short hair. There is often baldness at sites of friction.

Telogen effluvium is a common cause of diffuse hair loss that may occur 2 to 4 months after a variety of events, including pregnancy, discontinuation of oral contraceptives, severe febrile illness, medications, severe diets, or significant emotional stress. Hair loss results from the abrupt conversion of numerous scalp hairs from the anagen (growth) phase to the telogen (resting) phase. Loss of more than 150 hairs per day is considered abnormal. Patients may complain of losing several hundred hairs a day, but the occurrence of clinically significant baldness is rare. Estimates indicate that individuals must lose about 25% of their hair before thinning becomes clinically apparent. The hair loss may continue for several weeks, but complete regrowth usually occurs within 6 to 12 months. **Anagen effluvium** results in the loss of growing hairs due to a sudden cessation of the growing phase. It occurs most commonly after systemic chemotherapy.

Loose anagen syndrome is a disorder in which the anagen hair follicle is anchored improperly, resulting in easy, painless plucking of the hairs. This can result in patchy diffuse hair loss or focal areas of alopecia. This is a familial condition, with fair-haired females more commonly affected. Oftentimes, these children will not need a haircut through early childhood. The hair may spontaneously become normal by the teenage years without treatment.

Evaluation

History

The age of the child guides the differential diagnosis, because some lesions are more common at one age than another (Questions Box).

Physical Examination

The scalp should be examined to see if the hair loss is diffuse or circumscribed and whether scalp hairs can be plucked easily. Signs of irritation, inflammation, or scaling of the scalp should also be noted, as well as the presence of adenopathy, nail changes, or hair loss elsewhere on the body.

Wood light examination of the scalp for fungus is helpful if positive. A negative examination does not rule out the possibility of fungal infection, however, because *T tonsurans,* the most common cause of tinea capitis in the United States, does not fluoresce. *M canis* fluoresces yellow-green under the Wood light.

Disorders of the Hair and Scalp

- Is the child losing any hair?
- If so, is the child losing hair from all over the scalp or only from localized areas on the scalp?
- Has the child lost any body hair (eg, eyebrows, eyelashes) in addition to the scalp hair?
- How long has the child been losing hair?
- Is the scalp pruritic or scaling?
- Have the parents noticed the child twisting or pulling the hair?
- Is the child's hair often in ponytails or braids?
- Has there recently been any significant stress in the child's life?
- Do any pets live in the home?
- Is the child taking any medications?
- Is anyone else in the home or anyone in close contact with the child having similar symptoms?

Laboratory Tests

Laboratory assessment is useful in some cases. If fungal infection is suspected, a KOH examination should be performed by the primary care physician. Scales and broken hairs can be obtained from involved areas by brushing, scraping (eg, with a No. 15 scalpel blade), plucking, or rubbing a moistened 4 × 4 gauze over affected areas and then removing broken hairs and scale from the gauze with forceps. The scrapings should be placed on a glass slide, dissolved in KOH solution, heated gently, and examined under the microscope. Hyphae and spores within the hair shaft (eg, *T tonsurans* infection) or surrounding the hair shaft (eg, *M canis* infection) should be noted.

In addition to microscopic examination, many dermatologists recommend routine fungal cultures in all cases of suspected tinea capitis. Brushings using either a moistened sterile cotton swab or a sterile brush as used in Pap smears will yield the most reliable results. Hair or scalp scrapings are inoculated onto Sabouraud agar or dermatophyte test medium (DTM). Within 5 to 14 days, a distinctive growth seen on the Sabouraud agar or a color change from yellow to red in the DTM confirms the diagnosis. A negative KOH examination in addition to a lack of inflammation and scaling may be required for differentiating trichotillomania or alopecia areata from tinea capitis.

The diagnosis of telogen effluvium is usually suggested by the history and counting the number of hairs lost each day. If the diagnosis is in question, the patient may be referred to a dermatologist for examination of the involved hair roots via biopsy and determination of the anagen-telogen ratio, which is usually about 85:15. A telogen count of more than 25% is considered to be diagnostic of telogen effluvium. The ratio of anagen to telogen hairs is normal in trichotillomania.

A more extensive laboratory workup may be required if the hair loss is persistent or the history or physical examination is suggestive of systemic disease (see Box 107-2). Studies that may be considered include liver function tests, thyroid function studies, a serum Venereal Disease Research Laboratory test, antinuclear antibodies, and serum electrolytes.

Management

Management depends on the diagnosis. Herpetic infection in a newborn requires immediate attention and systemic antiviral therapy because the risk of systemic infection is significant. Scalp electrodes and vacuum-assisted vaginal deliveries should be avoided in neonates with mothers known to have HSV infections because these can increase the rate of infection transmission. Currently cesarean section delivery remains the standard of care, though most cases of herpes simplex in infants are in those born to mothers without known infection at time of delivery.

Children suspected of nevus sebaceus should be referred to a dermatologist. Early identification is important because 10% to 30% of lesions undergo secondary neoplastic changes during puberty or adulthood. However, early excision, which used to be the mainstay of therapy, has decreased in favor of watchful observation because most of the neoplasms are low-grade. The patient can then make an independent decision after puberty whether to have the lesion excised.

Seborrheic dermatitis can persist into the pubertal years, contrary to previously held belief. Cradle cap, the greasy form of seborrheic dermatitis, can be treated with simple skin care measures such as bathing and the use of moisturizing emollients. Gentle shampoos, low-potency corticosteroids and, if needed, 2% ketoconazole cream can resolve most cases. Past infancy, seborrheic dermatitis may be treated with **shampoos containing tar, pyrithione zinc, ketoconazole, or selenium** in rotation. Topical, mild corticosteroid solutions can be used if pruritus is significant.

Head lice may be treated with **pyrethrin products** such as permethrin 1% cream rinse (Nix) or the prescription 5% cream typically used for scabies. Other medications such as malathion and ivermectin can also be effective. All topical medications should be used twice, 1 week apart, regardless of package insert information. A fine-toothed comb or tweezers may be required after rinsing to remove the ova or nits of head lice. Other alternative treatments have been unsubstantiated, such as using mayonnaise or petroleum jelly. Heat, such as that associated with blow-drying the hair, also kills a large percentage of the lice.

Five percent permethrin cream is the preferred scabicide. It should be applied from head to toe in infants, and from neck to toe past infancy, for 8 to 12 hours, washed off, and repeated in 1 week. For both scabies and lice, the treatment of fomites is also important.

Oral griseofulvin administered for at least 8 weeks has been the long-held treatment of choice for **tinea capitis.** Although griseofulvin can have many side effects, including gastrointestinal disturbances, hepatotoxicity, and leukopenia, it is generally well tolerated by children and is available in suspension form. Hematologic, renal, and liver function studies can be monitored in children on high doses or prolonged treatment. Higher dosing is occasionally required due to increasing resistance. Care should be made to use proper dosing when using micronized or ultra-micronized griseofulvin. Newer antifungal agents are also being used with great success, often for shorter durations than griseofulvin, which can increase compliance. **Itraconazole** can be given as either continuous or pulse therapy and is also available as a solution. **Fluconazole,** also available as solution, is usually administered for 4 to 6 weeks or at a higher dose once weekly for 4 to 6 weeks. **Terbinafine,** available in tablet form, has also been effective at shorter treatment times than griseofulvin. Monitoring of blood counts and liver and renal function are recommended monthly before and during treatment. Ketoconazole is contraindicated in this population due to its potential for adverse effects, especially in light of other available agents. Generally, longer courses of treatment are needed for *M canis* infection. Topical antifungal agents are not effective on the scalp for treatment of tinea capitis because the hair follicle must be penetrated, requiring the use of systemic therapy. Twice-a-week shampooing with povidone iodine and selenium sulfide shampoos has been shown to reduce carriage of spores and reduce infectivity. A course of oral **prednisone** may be required in conjunction with an oral antifungal if a kerion is present to minimize itching; discomfort; and permanent, scarring hair loss. Children with kerions are often misdiagnosed as having a bacterial infection of the scalp and treated with oral antibiotics. However, the pustules in kerions are generally sterile, and even when secondary bacterial infection is present (eg, about 30%–50% of patients), antibiotics do not alter the course of the condition.

Children believed to have alopecia areata should be referred to a dermatologist immediately. Therapy for **alopecia areata** consists of **both topical and intralesional corticosteroids,** topical anthralin, or minoxidil. Topical immunotherapy with a sensitizer such as squaric acid or dinitrochlorobenzene has also been used for the treatment of extensive alopecia areata. Occasionally oral steroids can be tried for extensive or rapidly progressing disease. Many psychosocial factors should be considered when treating children with this condition. Children with severe forms of the disease may benefit psychologically from wearing a wig. The National Alopecia Areata Foundation is available as a support group for affected children and their families.

Prognosis

Common disorders of the scalp such as seborrheic dermatitis, head lice, and tinea capitis generally respond well to treatment and rarely result in long-term sequelae. The course and prognosis of alopecia areata is quite variable and may be difficult to predict. Generally, the prognosis for regrowth is good if hair loss has occurred in only a few patches. The prognosis is usually poorer with younger age at onset, positive family history, nail involvement, and an ophiasis pattern of hair loss. It is important to pursue further workup if a condition does not respond to therapy because it is critical that a condition such as Langerhans cell histiocytosis, a mimicker of seborrheic dermatitis, not be missed. Many of the hair disorders are a result of syndromes that will not respond to therapy and, thus, education for patients and their families is important.

CASE RESOLUTION

The child presented in the case scenario exhibits physical findings of a kerion. Diagnosis can be made clinically on the basis of the appearance of the lesion. The diagnosis is established by microscopic evidence of hyphae and culture confirmation. Treatment with oral antifungals and possibly oral steroids should be initiated. Carriers should also be identified and treated. The child should be examined in 4 weeks to ascertain the response to therapy and check for any adverse reactions.

Selected References

Harrison S, Sinclair R. Optimal management of hair loss (alopecia) in children. *Am J Clin Dermatol.* 2003;4:757–770

Honig PJ. Treatment of kerions. *Pediatr Dermatol.* 1994;11:69–71

Hordinsky M. Alopecias. In: Bolognia JL, Jorizzo JL, Rapini RP, eds. *Dermatology.* St Louis, MO: Mosby; 2003:1033–1050

James WD, Berger TG, Elston DM. *Andrews' Diseases of the Skin.* 10th ed. Toronto, Ontario, Canada: Elsevier, Inc.; 2006:298–299, 483–485, 749–751

Koot RW, Reedijk B, Tan WF, De Sonnaville-De Roy van Zuide. Neonatal brain abscess: complication of fetal monitoring. *Obstet Gynecol.* 1999;93:857

Meinking TL, Burkhart CN, Burkhart CG. Infestations. In: Bolognia JL, Jorizzo JL, Rapini RP, eds. *Dermatology.* St Louis, MO: Mosby; 2003:1321–1326

Möhrenschlager M, Seidl HP, Ring J, Abeck D. Pediatric tinea capitis: recognition and management. *Am J Clin Dermatol.* 2005;6:203–213

Nield LS, Keri JE, Kamat D. Alopecia in the general pediatric clinic: who to treat, who to refer. *Clin Pediatr.* 2006;45:605–612

Pierson D, Randel C, et al. Benign epidermal tumors and proliferations. In: Bolognia JL, Jorizzo JL, Rapini RP, eds. *Dermatology.* St Louis, MO: Mosby; 2003:1711–1712

Sybert VP, Zonana J. Ectodermal dysplasias. In: Bolognia JL, Jorizzo JL, Rapini RP, eds. *Dermatology.* St Louis, MO: Mosby; 2003:906–913

Williams JV, Eichenfield LF, Burke BL, Barnes-Eley M, Friedlander SF. Prevalence of scalp scaling in prepubertal children. *Pediatrics.* 2005;115:e1–e6

Diaper Dermatitis

Kathy K. Langevin, MD, MPH, and Noah Craft MD, PhD

CASE STUDY

A 6-month-old infant has a 3-day history of a rash in the diaper area. The mother has been applying cornstarch, but the rash has gotten worse and has spread to the inner thighs and the abdomen. The infant has no history of fever, upper respiratory tract symptoms, vomiting, or diarrhea. He was seen in the emergency department 1 week ago for acute gastroenteritis, which has since resolved. On examination, a poorly demarcated, shiny, erythematous rash is noted over the convex surface of the buttocks, lower abdomen, and genitalia, with relative sparing of the intertriginous creases. The rest of the physical examination is within normal limits.

Questions

1. What are the common causes of rashes in the diaper area (diaper dermatitis)?
2. What are the features that distinguish one type of diaper dermatitis from another?
3. What systemic diseases may present with diaper dermatitis?
4. What are some common treatments for diaper dermatitis?

Diaper dermatitis is used to describe a wide variety of skin disorders that present with a rash in the area covered by the diaper. The most familiar form of diaper rash, irritant contact diaper dermatitis, is one of the most common skin disorders of infants and young children. Other infectious and inflammatory processes in the diaper area can also result in dermatitis. Successful management requires making the correct diagnosis and identifying the etiology and associated factors.

Epidemiology

Diaper dermatitis is the most common dermatologic disorder in infancy, with a peak incidence at 9 to 12 months of age, though some reports have shown a high incidence in the first month of life. Prevalence in infants is estimated at anywhere from 7% to 35%. This disorder is not limited to infants and small children but to any individuals who wear diapers, though the incidence in adults is unknown.

Clinical Presentation

The lesions of diaper dermatitis primarily affect the skin of the buttocks, gluteal cleft, lower abdomen, perineal area, and proximal thighs. Irritant contact dermatitis, the most common type of diaper dermatitis, appears as erythema and scaling papules and plaques or poorly demarcated, glistening erythema over the convex surfaces, with relative sparing of the intertriginous folds (Figure 108-1A). Candidal infection is characterized by a beefy red, sharply demarcated plaque with small, satellite papules and pustules along the margins. Candidal infections are primarily concentrated within the skin folds (Dx Box) (Figure 108-1B). Other etiologic causes of

Figure 108-1. Diaper dermatitis. A. Diaper dermatitis secondary to contact. Convex surface areas are affected. B. Diaper dermatitis secondary to *Candida*. Intertriginous areas are affected, and satellite lesions are present.

diaper dermatitis can be challenging to distinguish from one another but can usually be differentiated by their distribution and response to therapy.

Diaper Dermatitis

- Urinary or fecal incontinence requiring diaper wearing
- Erythematous rash over anogenital region
- Associated gastroenteritis, antibiotic therapy, or oral thrush

Pathophysiology

Many factors are involved in the pathophysiology of irritant diaper dermatitis. Prolonged contact with moisture, urine, feces, or irritating chemicals plays an important role in the initiation of these disorders. Friction generated as the infant tries to move around may further aggravate the condition and lead to maceration of the skin. Secondary infection, most often with *Candida albicans,* may be seen in many cases.

Ammonia produced by bacterial breakdown of urea is no longer believed to be the causative factor in cases of irritant diaper dermatitis. The cause is multifactorial, with prolonged exposure to moisture resulting in fragile skin and a compromised protective barrier, leading to increased irritant penetration and potential growth of microorganisms. Fecal enzymes (proteases, lipases, and urease) also weaken this barrier. Friction from a diaper can easily abrade this fragile skin. Diapers clearly play a role in this disorder; societies where diapers are not worn do not see this condition.

Differential Diagnosis

Technically, any rash that occurs in the area covered by the diaper can be called diaper dermatitis, but certain rashes occur primarily in this area in infants and young children. The differential diagnosis of diaper dermatitis is presented in Box 108-1.

Irritant contact dermatitis, the most common cause of diaper dermatitis, is most prominent on the skin of the buttocks, perineal area, lower abdomen, and proximal thighs. The skin of the creases is relatively unaffected. Exposure to proteolytic enzymes and irritant chemicals in the face of excessive heat or moisture is believed to lead to this condition. Friction with the diaper at sites of contact may aggravate it. Such a rash is poorly demarcated and can give the skin a glistening, red appearance. **Granuloma gluteale infantum** is a possible complication of diaper dermatitis, presenting with violaceous nodules and plaques on the buttocks, vulva, scrotum, and perianal area. Though alarming in appearance, these are benign and will resolve once the dermatitis is cleared, though scarring can result.

Candidiasis, due to infection with *C albicans,* typically begins in the creases (intertriginous areas) and then spreads to other surfaces. Sometimes associated with oral thrush, it is also a common sequelae to systemic antibiotic therapy. The rash appears as bright,

Box 108-1. Differential Diagnosis of Diaper Dermatitis

Most Common Causes
- Irritant contact dermatitis
- Candidiasis
- Seborrheic dermatitis

Less Common Causes
- Allergic dermatitis
- Impetigo
- Perianal streptococcal disease
- Congenital syphilis
- Atopic dermatitis
- Psoriasis
- Zinc deficiency, including acrodermatitis enteropathica
- Biotin deficiency
- Langerhans cell histiocytosis

beefy red plaques with sharp, raised borders and many small satellite papules, vesicles, and pustules along its margins, often with desquamation. *C albicans* can be a cause of secondary infection of already inflamed skin as well as a primary causative factor in some cases of diaper dermatitis. Recurrent candidal diaper dermatitis can be associated with candidal colonization of the gut and oral cavity.

Seborrheic diaper dermatitis, like candidal diaper dermatitis, also primarily affects the intertriginous areas of the groin. The lack of pruritus, manifest as sleeping and feeding well, distinguishes it from atopic dermatitis. The rash has a characteristic salmon-colored, greasy appearance with a yellowish scale, though can be acutely inflamed. Satellite lesions can be seen. Seborrheic dermatitis of the face, scalp (including postauricular areas), neck, trunk, and proximal extremities is usually seen in association with seborrheic dermatitis of the diaper area.

A less common cause of diaper dermatitis is **allergic dermatitis.** True **allergic contact dermatitis** in the diaper area is rare in the first 2 years of life, though it can be due to some ingredients in baby wipes such as benzalkonium chloride and fragrance. Irritation caused by harsh soaps or cleansing agents may be commonly seen.

Impetigo, especially bullous impetigo, is a not uncommon eruption in the diaper area. It is more commonly observed in neonates, often as epidemics. Bullous impetigo is caused by *Staphylococcus aureus* and is toxin-mediated. The rash presents as vesicles on the diaper area, as well as the trunk and face. These enlarge into 3- to 5-cm bullae that easily rupture, leaving superficial erosions with thick, honey-colored crusts. There can be associated systemic symptoms of fever and diarrhea.

Perianal streptococcal disease due to group A beta-hemolytic streptococcus manifests as well-demarcated, tender perianal patches of erythema. Rectal bleeding and painful defecation may also be noted.

Congenital syphilis can present with diaper dermatitis findings in 30% to 60% of those born with this infection. Initially, there is usually a bright erythematous morbilliform eruption that fades to a coppery color, often with scaling. Pustules can develop later. Buttocks, face, extremities, palms, and soles are generally affected.

Diaper rashes that seem to persist despite seemingly adequate therapy should raise suspicion for other systemic diseases. Though less common, these include psoriasis, atopic dermatitis, zinc deficiency, biotin deficiency, and Langerhans cell histiocytosis. **Psoriasis** may occur anywhere on the body, but lesions typically occur on the scalp, face, elbows, and knees. In infants, generally between 2 to 8 months of age, psoriasis may involve the diaper area. Unlike lesions elsewhere on the body, which are typically well-circumscribed, erythematous plaques with a thick, silvery scale, psoriatic lesions in the diaper area may be difficult to differentiate from seborrheic dermatitis or candidal infection. Plaques are brightly erythematous and sharply demarcated. Psoriasis should be considered in the differential diagnosis of a diaper rash that persists despite seemingly adequate therapy. Skin biopsy, family history of psoriasis, or nail involvement may help confirm the diagnosis.

Atopic dermatitis is rare in the diaper area, even in infants who have lesions elsewhere on the body. The relative sparing of the diaper area is perhaps a result of the increased moisture of the skin in this area (see Chapter 109 for a discussion of atopic dermatitis).

Zinc deficiency is oftentimes discovered as infants are weaned off breast milk, and can be due to **acrodermatitis enteropathica,** a rare, autosomally recessive inherited disorder of zinc metabolism or an acquired deficiency. These infants present with diarrhea, failure to thrive, and skin lesions involving the distal extremities and perioral and perineal areas. Erythematous bullous and pustular lesions can be seen, as well as dry, red, scaly patches. Lesions in the diaper area are often mistaken for candidiasis, though candidal and *S aureus* superinfection can occur. The etiology of acrodermatitis enteropathica is usually impaired gastrointestinal zinc uptake. Acquired zinc deficiency is usually seen in premature infants being weaned off breast milk, though full-term infants with higher zinc requirements and those with malabsorption syndromes, such as cystic fibrosis, can also present with these skin findings. Treatment consists of oral zinc supplementation. Biotin deficiency, as well as several other nutritional deficiencies, can present with identical skin findings, and treatment is with supplementation of the deficient nutrient.

Langerhans cell histiocytosis refers to a group of disorders characterized by proliferation of histiocytes, a progenitor cell in the bone marrow. Members of this group include Letterer-Siwe disease and Hand-Schüller-Christian disease, eosinophilic granuloma, and congenital self-healing reticulohistiocytosis. Skin lesions may involve the scalp and flexural areas of the perineum, axilla, and neck. The lesions appear as small, pink to tan scaling papules and pustules that can coalesce; ulceration may be apparent in the inguinal crease with secondary impetiginization (honey-colored crusting caused by *S aureus* superinfection). The rash is most often confused with that of seborrheic dermatitis. Diagnosis can be confirmed by skin biopsy.

Evaluation

History

A thorough history should be obtained (Questions Box). Candidal

> **Questions**
>
> **Diaper Dermatitis**
> - When did the rash begin?
> - Does the rash resolve and then recur?
> - Is the rash pruritic?
> - Is the infant feeding, sleeping? Is he/she irritable?
> - Have any home remedies or previous treatments been used? Which ones?
> - Does the child have a family history of atopic dermatitis or psoriasis?
> - Is the child taking antibiotics now or has the child used them recently?
> - What type of diapers are used?
> - How frequently are the diapers changed?

diaper dermatitis should be suspected if oral antibiotic therapy has recently been used.

Physical Examination

On physical examination, the presence of skin lesions elsewhere on the body should be noted. This is particularly important in the case of a persistent, resistant, or recurrent diaper rash, where systemic diseases such as psoriasis must be considered. The distribution of the rash within the diaper area itself may provide clues to the diagnosis. Candidal and seborrheic dermatitis occur primarily in the creases, whereas irritant contact dermatitis usually affects the convex areas of the skin with relative sparing of the intertriginous areas. Streptococcal disease manifests primarily as marked perianal erythema.

Laboratory Tests

Although the diagnosis of candidal diaper dermatitis is usually evident clinically, microscopic examination of skin scrapings with KOH may be performed to establish the diagnosis. Typically, budding yeast with hyphae and/or pseudohyphae is seen. The diagnosis of perianal streptococcal disease or bullous impetigo may be confirmed by bacterial cultures from the perianal area or bullous lesions, respectively. Biopsies may be warranted for recalcitrant diaper dermatitis. Other laboratory studies may be carried out to investigate for suspected nutritional deficiencies.

Management

The mainstay of therapy is prevention, requiring **good hygiene,** which involves keeping the diaper area clean and dry. Gentle but thorough cleansing of the diaper area with water alone or water and a mild soap is usually sufficient. The area should then be patted dry and allowed to air-dry completely if possible or dry with the use of cotton balls. Too frequent cleansing with harsh soaps or scrubbing too vigorously can actually aggravate skin that is already damaged and inflamed.

In addition, the diaper should be **changed frequently.** The diaper area should be exposed to as much air as reasonably possible (eg, by allowing the infant to sleep without a diaper). Cloth and regular disposable diapers are not as effective as superabsorbent gel diapers in decreasing moisture. Although **dusting powders** such as cornstarch or talc minimize friction and talc does not enhance the growth of yeast on skin, concern about pulmonary effects from inhalation precludes their routine use even in the absence of any skin inflammation. **Moisture-resistant barrier ointments or creams** such as zinc oxide or petrolatum are usually not needed if the above hygiene measures are carried out routinely. However, use after bathing can help minimize irritation from excessive moisture. The role of hygiene in all forms of diaper dermatitis cannot be overemphasized. Topical application of medicated creams and ointments is not effective in the presence of poor hygiene.

Irritant contact dermatitis usually responds to hygienic measures and the application of barrier ointments and low-potency **topical corticosteroids** such as 0.5% or 1% hydrocortisone ointment or cream. Seborrheic dermatitis usually resolves spontaneously but can also be treated with low-potency topical corticosteroids. Candidal diaper dermatitis responds to **topical antifungal creams** such as nystatin, miconazole, or clotrimazole. In addition, a low-potency corticosteroid may be required if inflammation is severe. Oral antifungal therapy is usually not indicated, though may be needed in cases of recurrent candidiasis. Oral penicillin or erythromycin usually clears perianal streptococcal disease, but the relapse rate is high. The topical antibiotic mupirocin may be used to treat bullous impetigo only if the lesions are superficial, few, and isolated. Oral antibiotics (eg, erythromycin, cephalexin, amoxicillin/clavulanate) may be required for more extensive bacterial infections. Combination topical medications containing both a corticosteroid and an antifungal should not be recommended routinely because they usually contain high-potency corticosteroids. When topical steroids and antifungals are used in conjunction with barrier ointment, the medication should be applied before the barrier ointment.

When the more common causes of diaper dermatitis, such as irritant contact dermatitis, *Candida,* or seborrheic dermatitis, do not respond to conventional therapy, further workup must be initiated because there may be an underlying systemic disease manifesting as diaper dermatitis; some of these can be life-threatening.

Prognosis

Although recurrence of diaper dermatitis is common, the usual varieties respond well to measures aimed at keeping the diaper area clean and dry and to medicated creams.

CASE RESOLUTION

The infant presented in the case scenario has irritant contact dermatitis. He has a recent history of gastroenteritis, and stool is known to be particularly irritating to the skin. Treatment includes keeping the diaper area clean and dry with frequent diaper changes, use of superabsorbent diapers, and fastidious toilet, as well as topical application of a low-potency corticosteroid ointment or cream and a barrier ointment such as zinc oxide after bathing.

Selected References

Fritsch PO, Reider N. Other eczematous eruptions. In: Bolognia JL, Jorizzo JL, Rapini RP, eds. *Dermatology.* St Louis, MO: Mosby; 2003:216–217

James WD, Berger TG, Elston DM. *Andrews' Diseases of the Skin.* 10th ed. Toronto, Ontario, Canada: Elsevier, Inc.; 2006:360–361, 483–485

Scheinfeld N. Diaper dermatitis: a review and brief survey of eruptions of the diaper area. *Am J Clin Dermatol.* 2005;6:273–281

Ward DB. Characterization of diaper dermatitis in the United States. *Arch Pediatr Adolesc Med.* 2000;154:943–946

Papulosquamous Eruptions

Kathy K. Langevin, MD, MPH, and Noah Craft, MD, PhD

CASE STUDY

A 6-month-old female infant presents with an erythematous, confluent, slightly raised and scaly rash on the cheeks. The extremities are also covered with a fine papular rash. The infant has had some scaling behind the ears and on the scalp since early infancy, but the symptoms have recently increased. The mother has been applying baby oil to the scalp to relieve the scaliness. Except for some intermittent rhinorrhea, the infant has otherwise been well. Immunizations are deficient; she received only the first set when she was 2 months old. The family history is positive for bronchitis. The infant's weight is at the 75th percentile, and the height is at the 50th percentile.

Vital signs are normal. The physical examination is normal except for the presence of the rash.

Questions
1. What are the characteristics of papulosquamous eruptions?
2. What are the common conditions associated with papulosquamous eruptions in children?
3. What are the appropriate treatments for the common papulosquamous eruptions?
4. When should children with papulosquamous eruptions be referred to a dermatologist?

Rashes, a common problem in children, can be classified in ways that help to establish a diagnostic approach. First, rashes are assessed in terms of appearance, whether macular (flat), papular (raised), squamous (scaly), vesicular (fluid-filled), or bullous (large, fluid-filled). Next, the extent of the rash is determined. Rashes may be described as generalized or localized. Location is also important. The site of a localized rash may be consistent with certain diagnoses, for instance, diaper dermatitis. Pruritus is an important distinguishing feature. Other systemic symptoms must also be taken into consideration. Rashes may be a primary skin condition or may be a manifestation of an underlying infection or reaction to a precipitating agent.

Papulosquamous eruptions, the subject of this chapter, are rashes characterized by scaly papules and plaques. Eczema is a poorly defined group of skin disorders characterized clinically by scale, and histologically by spongiosis, and makes up a large component of the papulosquamous disorders. The etiology of many papulosquamous eruptions is unknown, and the clinical appearance of lesions is the reason they are classified together.

Epidemiology

Although a large number of conditions may cause papulosquamous eruptions in children, a select number of diagnoses account for most problems. One of the most common causes of papulosquamous eruptions in children is atopic dermatitis. Atopic dermatitis has become increasingly more common, and the prevalence in school-aged children in the United States is estimated to be between 10% to 20%. Positive family history is often elicited. Climate (cold and dry), urbanization, and higher socioeconomic status may be contributing

factors. Though the severity of atopic dermatitis generally improves with age, lifelong dry, itchy skin, in varying degrees of severity, is not uncommon. Seborrheic dermatitis is another common eczematous skin rash seen in the pediatric population. Though most commonly described in infants younger than 3 or 4 months, it can occur in all pediatric age groups. It is estimated to have a prevalence of up to 5%, encompassing both the pediatric and adult populations, though higher in adults with males more commonly affected. It is generally more severe during the winter months.

Scabies is likely the most common cause of worldwide papulosquamous eruptions and is frequently encountered in both general pediatric and dermatology settings. The prevalence is much greater in developing countries and in situations where populations are forced into close proximity (eg, during wars or incarcerated individuals). Family members and close contacts are at greatest risk of infection.

Clinical Presentation

Papulosquamous eruptions consist of skin-colored to erythematous raised, scaly papules and plaques that may involve the face, trunk, or extremities. The lesions can be pruritic, and scratching may lead to crusting or secondary infection. Sometimes multiple family members are affected (Dx Box). Chronicity and, thus, repeated manipulation, may lead to thickening or lichenification of involved skin.

Pathophysiology

The pathophysiology of atopic dermatitis has not been definitively established. Recent evidence suggests that mutations in the filaggrin gene, which is responsible for much of the skin barrier function,

Dx

Dx — Papulosquamous Eruptions

- Raised, scaly papules and plaques
- Pruritus
- Afebrile, unless secondary infection is present
- Allergic personal or family history
- Intertriginous rash

may play a large role in atopic dermatitis. However, it seems to be a multifactorial disease with variable expression, influenced by environmental factors. Inheritance of this disease is associated with atopy, made up of the triad of atopic dermatitis, allergic rhinitis, and asthma. The disorder is attributed largely to skin barrier function; however, immune dysfunction and reactivity of nerves and blood vessels may also be involved. Initially, the disease is characterized by Th1 cytokine predominance, but later in chronic disease, there is activation of the Th2 immune pathway with a resultant synthesis of cytokines, including IL-4 and IL-5, causing elevated immunoglobulin (Ig) E levels, eosinophilia, and diminished cell-mediated immunity. Elevated IgE is reported in 43% to 82% of patients with atopic dermatitis.

Like atopic dermatitis, the etiology of seborrheic dermatitis remains unclear. Individuals with seborrheic dermatitis seem to have some sort of immune dysfunction, as the condition is routinely severe in individuals with uncontrolled human immunodeficiency virus (HIV) and acquired immunodeficiency syndrome. There is believed to be an association with the yeast *Malassezia furfur*, though whether this organism is causative has not been established. It is widely accepted that this yeast has some role in seborrheic dermatitis, which is further substantiated by the improvement of this skin condition with antifungal agents.

The inflammatory response in scabies is triggered by an infestation with a mite, *Sarcoptes scabiei*. The adult female burrows under the skin and lays 60 to 90 eggs. After 2 weeks, the eggs become adults. Affected individuals may be asymptomatic on first exposure. Up to 2 to 6 weeks after infestation, the host's immune system becomes sensitized to mites or scybala (mite feces), resulting in systemic pruritus and rash. In most individuals the rash associated with scabies is an allergic phenomenon and does not represent mites at each eruptive papule on the body.

Differential Diagnosis

Most conditions that are associated with papulosquamous eruptions in children include atopic dermatitis, seborrheic dermatitis, contact dermatitis, psoriasis, pityriasis rosea, lichen planus, lichen striatus, scabies, and fungal infections of the skin.

Eczema is a general term that is used to denote a type of papulosquamous eruption. The most common eczematous conditions seen in children are atopic eczema or dermatitis, seborrheic dermatitis, and contact dermatitis. **Atopic dermatitis** is a disorder of infancy and childhood, but commonly persists into adulthood. More than half of affected individuals are symptomatic by 1 year, and 90% of cases have their onset by 5 years of age. The area of involvement changes with age. In infancy, the face, scalp, and extensor surfaces are involved, often in areas where the infant can relieve itching by rubbing, and the diaper area is often spared (Figure 109-1A). By childhood, the more typical pattern seen in adulthood becomes prominent with involvement of the neck and antecubital and popliteal fossae. Adults tend to have greater extremity involvement, along with the head and neck. Clinically, xerosis (dry skin), erythema, and a pruritic papular eruption are apparent. Scratching and rubbing lead to crusting, weeping, and eventually lichenification. Changes in coloring, including hypopigmentation and hyperpigmentation, may also occur. Hypopigmented areas with fine scale that are usually noted on the face are called pityriasis alba (considered to be the mildest form of atopic dermatitis). Xeroderma, or dry skin, is a frequent coexisting condition. Ichthyosis vulgaris, characterized by dirty-appearing

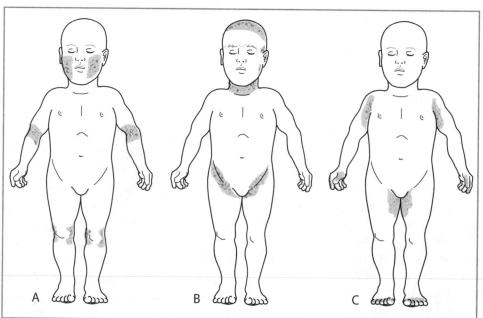

Figure 109-1. Typical distribution of papulosquamous eruptions in children. **A. Atopic dermatitis:** usually located on cheeks, creases of elbows, and knees. **B. Seborrheic dermatitis:** usually located on scalp, behind ears, thigh creases, and eyebrows. **C. Scabies:** usually located on axillae, webs of fingers and toes, and intragluteal area.

excessive scaling and hyperlinear palms, is seen in half of patients affected with atopic dermatitis. Lesions around mucosa (Dennie-Morgan lines in the infraorbital fold under the eye and cheilitis around the mouth) may also be seen. Symptoms of other allergic conditions, such as rhinorrhea, wheezing, or food-related allergies, will occur in many of these patients.

Seborrheic dermatitis, which frequently develops during the first 3 months of life, is characterized by scaly papules or confluent scaly plaques, particularly of the scalp. Scalp eruptions in infancy are referred to as cradle cap. Seborrheic dermatitis has a predilection for areas with a high density of sebaceous glands, such as the scalp, face, ears, presternal chest, penis, and intertriginous areas, including the folds of the diaper region (Figure 109-1B). The red or pink papules and plaques may have a greasy quality. Secondary infections may occur with *Candida,* particularly in the intertriginous areas. Seborrheic dermatitis is usually not exceedingly pruritic, and this feature can be used to distinguish between it and atopic dermatitis. The intertriginous involvement and the onset shortly after birth also differentiate these 2 types of dermatitis. Severe seborrheic dermatitis can be associated with an immune deficiency, most commonly in HIV-infected patients.

Irritant or allergic contact dermatitis occurs when individuals come into physical contact with an irritant or a specific allergen, respectively. Irritant dermatitis is caused by direct cytotoxic effect, while allergic contact dermatitis is a delayed type IV hypersensitivity response to an allergen. Though their etiologies are different, they typically have a similar clinical appearance. Individuals usually develop well-defined erythematous vesicles, papules, or plaques, often with scale, and can have oozing and subsequent lichenification. Diaper dermatitis is one of the most common types of irritant dermatitis in the pediatric population (see Chapter 108). Rhus dermatitis (poison ivy/oak) and nickel allergy are 2 common types of allergic contact dermatitis seen in this population. It remains controversial whether atopic dermatitis is a risk factor for allergic contact dermatitis. However, children with atopic dermatitis may have more exposure to sensitizers, in conjunction with a damaged epithelial barrier, putting them at risk.

Plaque-type psoriasis, a chronic papulosquamous skin condition manifested most commonly as well-defined erythematous papules and plaques with silvery scale, is not an uncommon disease of childhood, with females more frequently affected. About 40% of adult patients with psoriasis report having the disease in childhood. It most commonly affects the scalp in the pediatric population as well as the face and intertriginous areas. There is controversy whether psoriasis of the diaper area is a true psoriasis. Guttate psoriasis has smaller scaly papules and is usually precipitated by group A streptococci infection. Pruritus is variable, but not prominent. Classically, psoriatic lesions can develop at sites of trauma (scratches and cuts), known as the Koebner phenomenon.

Pityriasis rosea is a self-limited papulosquamous eruption that is frequently seen in adolescents by both pediatricians and dermatologists. The lesions tend to be round or ovoid and classically have a symmetrical distribution on the trunk extending downward from the midline at a 45-degree angle. Classically, there is a larger "herald patch" preceding the eruption by a few days to weeks. It should be duly noted that the classic presentation is not always present—many patients cannot recall a herald patch and the pattern over the trunk is commonly haphazard. It is generally self-limited and resolves in 1 to 2 months. It is pruritic in about one-quarter of those affected. Though the etiology is unknown, recent evidence suggests that human herpesvirus 7 infection is associated with most cases, and some patients may have a viral prodrome preceding the rash.

Lichen planus is an uncommon papulosquamous eruption in the pediatric population. It is characterized by pruritic, polygonal, pink to purplish flat-topped papules overlying Wickham striae; white scale can be seen. Etiology is also unknown, though hepatitis C, as well as other viruses, as a causative factor has been proposed. Flexor surfaces are usually affected and these lesions can Koebnerize.

Lichen striatus is an asymptomatic lichenoid eruption consisting of flat-topped papules that are skin color to slightly hyperpigmented. The lesions develop along the lines of Blaschko and spontaneously resolve over months to years. It is mostly commonly seen between 9 months to 9 years of age. The etiology is unknown.

Scabies may resemble atopic or seborrheic dermatitis in infants and young children. The lesions may be papules, pustules, or vesicles. The characteristic burrow, which is only 1- to 10-mm long, is often difficult to appreciate unless certain diagnostic maneuvers are undertaken. The lesions are most often noted on the skin of the hands and feet, including the palms and soles in infants and young children. Intertriginous areas such as the intragluteal region, groin, and finger webs are commonly infected (Figure 109-1C). In infants, the face and head may be involved. Scratching and secondary infection may alter the appearance of the rash. Reddish-brown nodules may be characteristic of more chronic infection. In institutionalized or immunosuppressed individuals, extensive mite infection can occur, resulting in thick, greasy-appearing, yellowish scale and crusts over the extremities and trunk, a condition referred to as *crusted scabies*.

Fungal infections (tinea corporis and tinea pedis) commonly appear as papulosquamous eruptions. Commonly, the lesions assume a characteristic distribution, with scaly papules grouped in a circle or coalesced into a plaque with central clearing.

Evaluation

History

A thorough history should be obtained (Questions Box). The presence of a rash in other family members suggests a contagious condition such as scabies or a familial disorder such as atopic dermatitis. An onset in the first few weeks of life is consistent with seborrheic dermatitis. It is important to determine if any medications have been used because these may modify the appearance of the rash. In addition, certain medications can cause a rash themselves, though these tend to be more morbilliform in appearance (see Chapter 110).

Questions

Papulosquamous Eruptions

- How long has the child had the rash?
- What did the rash look like when it first appeared?
- Are other family members affected?
- Have any medications been used to treat the rash or any been given prior to the onset of the rash?
- Is pruritus present?
- Does the child have any other symptoms such as wheezing or rhinorrhea?
- Does the child have a history of any contact between the affected skin and any irritating substance?
- Has the child been febrile?

Pruritus should be noted. Asking about lesions developing at sites of previous trauma can aid in diagnosing eruptions that Koebnerize, such as psoriasis and lichen planus.

Physical Examination

The physical examination helps define the exact nature of the eruption and its distribution, which is often the clue to its etiology. The entire body should be examined, and particular attention should be paid to the intragluteal region and web spaces between fingers and toes. Certain rashes have characteristic appearances. For example, a circular cluster of scaly papules with central clearing signifies tinea corporis or the herald patch of pityriasis rosea. The presence of burrows characterizes scabies. Burrows appear as a 3- to 10-mm grayish-white line (only about 1 mm wide). Vesicles, pustules, and nodules may also be present in scabies.

It is also important to distinguish if any secondary lesions, such as linear excoriations, are present. The lesions of lichen planus, though often itchy by history, will often not appear to have been excoriated because affected individuals tend to rub these lesions more than scratch at them. Secondary infections are also important to diagnose and treat because they can complicate many of the papulosquamous eruptions.

Associated symptoms can also aid in diagnosis. Hyperlinear palms, keratosis pilaris (erythematous 1–2-mm folliculocentric papules often on lateral upper arms, anterior thighs, and cheeks), and perioral/periocular lichenified papules are often seen in children with atopic dermatitis.

Overall health, height, and weight should also be measured. Failure to thrive in conjunction with eczematous skin changes should raise the suspicion for an immunodeficiency.

Laboratory Tests

Certain diagnostic tests may help clarify the etiology. Skin or radio-allergosorbent testing is recommended by some to identify offending food allergies (see Chapter 68). There is mixed information on the impact of dietary restriction on atopic dermatitis, though restricting egg exposure in egg-allergic patients has been found to be beneficial,

and communication with an allergist can aid in diagnosis and treatment. Patch testing may identify allergens causing contact dermatitis. Some immunologists consider the presence of elevated IgE to be required for a diagnosis of true atopic dermatitis.

The burrow of the mite that causes scabies may not be readily apparent. Scrapings with mineral oil are most commonly done today to help identify the mite, eggs, or feces (scybala)—any of which are diagnostic. Multiple burrows or web spaces are scraped. Scrapings of skin also assist in diagnosing candidal or tinea infections. These scrapings should be mixed with 10% to 20% KOH, which facilitates the dissolution of epithelial debris and allows for identification of the spores or hyphae.

If a secondary bacterial infection is suspected, cultures of the skin are indicated. Most of the papulosquamous eruptions are diagnosed clinically and no other specific diagnostic tests, short of a skin biopsy, assist in the diagnosis.

Management

The management is determined by the diagnosis.

Management of atopic dermatitis hinges on skin barrier function and the reduction of dryness and irritation with **vigilant skin care.** There has been debate whether frequent short baths daily versus bathing infrequently is more beneficial. It is most crucial that these patients bathe for short times only, applying cleansers only to the face, groin, and other soiled areas. The cleanser should be soap-free or the soap should be nonirritating, nondrying, and perfume- and dye-free. Children should pat dry after bathing with immediate application of either emollient or medication. Thick emollients such as petroleum jelly or other greasier ointments are preferable. In general, moisturizer from a jar tends to be more hydrating than that from a pump. For school-aged children, using greasier emollients at night under pajamas and then thinner emollients during the day may increase compliance. Sunflower seed oil is an inexpensive emollient that can be used after morning bathing for daytime use. Avoiding scratchy clothing such as wool can be helpful, as can humidifiers in the winter to prevent excessive dryness. The humidifiers should be cleaned regularly to prevent mold buildup, and a cool mist is considered safer to prevent burns.

Topical steroids are used to treat various papulosquamous eruptions, especially during flares. These drugs are the mainstay of therapy designed to minimize inflammation. The agents usually prescribed in cases of atopic as well as seborrheic dermatitis are triamcinolone 0.025%, 0.1%, and hydrocortisone 1% creams or ointments. Though ointments allow for better penetration and, often, less irritation, they are often disliked for their greasy texture, minimizing its usefulness because they are not applied regularly. The weaker hydrocortisone should be used for the face and groin and the higher strengths in areas of thicker skin. Chronic use should be discouraged to avoid skin atrophy. Parents can be educated on applying the medication to the appropriate areas for 1 to 2 weeks for flares, with maintenance use on weekends or 2 days per week. Sometimes brief courses of systemic steroids may be needed during more severe exacerbations, but if a patient is requiring oral steroids regularly, a referral to a dermatologist may be needed to consider other treatments such as systemic immunomodulators or ultraviolet (UV) therapy, both used for atopic dermatitis and psoriasis. Oral steroids may be required for rhus contact dermatitis, one of the more common forms of allergic contact dermatitis, and should be given for 2 to 3 weeks to prevent flaring.

For scaly scalp psoriasis, seborrheic dermatitis, and atopic dermatitis, several treatments can be used. For pruritus and inflammation, a topical steroid in gel, liquid, or foam vehicle can be applied. Mineral oil can help loosen scale, but needs to be washed out using an anti-seborrheic shampoo to prevent buildup. It should be massaged gently onto the scalp and allowed to sit for several minutes before rinsing. Fluocinolone oil or steroid shampoos can be used effectively for scalp psoriasis as well.

Steroid-sparing agents: Tacrolimus and pimecrolimus are topical calcineurin inhibitors, which can be used as steroid-sparing agents, most often in mild cases of atopic dermatitis, seborrheic dermatitis, and inverse psoriasis (intertriginous). As of January 2006, a black box warning was placed on these 2 medications because there have been rare cases of skin cancer and lymphoma among patients using these drugs. The causal relationship for this warning was not well defined and, thus, many dermatologists still prescribe these medications in conjunction with steroids for their patients. As stand-alone agents, they are not as effective as steroids for more severe cases and are substantially more expensive.

In psoriasis, topical steroids are often used in conjunction with **calcipotriene** ointment. **Tar** and **anthralin** are still used today as adjunctive topical treatments, though are falling out of favor due to their messy quality and more favorable alternatives.

Antihistamines may play a role in reducing the pruritus, especially at bedtime due to their sedating effect. Hydroxyzine and diphenhydramine work well in the evenings. For daytime, fexofenadine, cetirizine, or loratadine are non-sedating choices. Regular use of antihistamines during a flare can help to break the itch-scratch cycle often observed in children with atopic dermatitis. The other conditions can have variable degrees of pruritus for which antihistamines can be useful. Clipping fingernails decreases the risk of skin trauma after scratching.

Antibiotics are indicated if secondary infection is present. The most common pathogen involved is *Staphylococcus aureus.* Staphylococcal antigens also exacerbate the inflammation of atopic dermatitis. Treatment with antistaphylococcal systemic antibiotics such as cephalosporins may be needed for more widespread secondary infections. Topical antibiotics such as mupirocin may be used in localized secondary infections. Streptococcal-associated guttate psoriasis should be treated with either penicillin or erythromycin for 4 weeks.

Seborrheic dermatitis is generally treated with a combination of products including topical keratolytics, corticosteroids, and antifungals (see also Chapter 107). The seborrheic dermatitis of infancy can be treated with topical shampoos containing selenium sulfide and gentle sloughing of the scaly lesions using a soft brush or cloth.

Topical calcineurin inhibitors have anti-inflammatory properties without skin atrophy side effects, but are generally reserved for periorbital or recalcitrant cases due to the cost of the medications.

If children with atopic dermatitis develop infection with herpes simplex (eczema herpeticum), they should be treated with **acyclovir.** Involvement of the nasal tip is concerning for eye involvement and warrants an ophthalmology consult. If involvement is severe, the patient may need to be hospitalized for intravenous antiviral therapy. Children with atopic dermatitis are also prone to viral infections resulting in warts and molluscum contagiosum, and these should be managed accordingly.

Coinfection with *Candida,* which occurs with seborrheic dermatitis and psoriasis, requires the use of topical medications such as **nystatin, clotrimazole, or miconazole.** Antifungal shampoos may also help in reducing the scaling due to fungal agents such as *Pityrosporum.* Tinea corporis also responds to topical antifungal agents. Tinea capitis will require systemic antifungals (see Chapter 107).

The treatment for pityriasis rosea remains controversial, especially because it is a self-resolving condition. There are several studies demonstrating effectiveness of **acyclovir** or **erythromycin** or **UV therapy** to speed recovery.

There are several medications used to treat scabies. The current preferred product is 5% **permethrin** cream. It has few adverse effects across the age spectrum. It should be applied from head to toe in infants and from neck to toe in small children and adults, left on for 8 to 12 hours, then rinsed off. **Lindane,** which has been used for more than 50 years and previously used worldwide, is a 1% cream. Because of concern about the percutaneous absorption of lindane and its potential neurotoxicity, it is no longer widely used and is not available in some areas. Oral **ivermectin** is also a successful scabicide. Two hundred to 400 µg/kg, repeated in 1 week, can be used in children weighing more than 15 kg and women who are not pregnant or breastfeeding. All scabicides should be re-administered 7 days after initial treatment. The effective elimination of scabies necessitates that all affected household members be treated simultaneously and that bed linens and clothing be washed in hot water. Patients should be warned that the pruritus of scabies often takes several weeks to subside and can be treated supportively with topical steroids and antihistamines.

Prognosis

In general, the prognosis for children with papulosquamous eruptions is excellent with appropriate management, which is contingent on accurate diagnosis. Both atopic dermatitis and seborrheic dermatitis tend to improve as children get older. However, chronic problems such as hand dermatitis, which can be exacerbated by occupational exposures, can become a significant problem. Children with significant atopic dermatitis should be counseled against careers with frequent wet work, such as hairdressers, hospital workers, or food service. It is also critical to counsel families that maintaining atopic dermatitis with the prevention of flares is the primary goal and is more important than having perfect skin. Families of children with severe atopic dermatitis can have difficulty in maintaining quality of life for these patients, and the entire family structure can suffer as chronic care can be challenging. Children with atopic dermatitis frequently face remissions and exacerbations, particularly associated with seasonal changes. Prevention and maintenance must be stressed. It is advisable that patients with recalcitrant eczema have further workup with an allergist to eliminate triggers.

Many of these eruptions, such as lichen striatus and pityriasis rosea, are self-limited and only need symptomatic treatment. Psoriasis has a more chronic course, and early diagnosis and treatment can help to reduce the disease severity and progression. Chronic disease such as atopic dermatitis and psoriasis can be psychologically challenging for children because they can often be ridiculed at school and excluded from activities for unfounded fears of contagiousness. The teachers may need to be educated as well and emotional and psychological support provided for these children.

Scabies and tinea will improve with appropriate management and education to prevent recurrence.

CASE RESOLUTION

The infant's presentation in the case history is characteristic of atopic dermatitis. The baby experienced the onset of symptoms as a young infant (most atopic patients develop symptoms after 2 months of age). Atopic dermatitis can often affect the head and face of young patients. Xerosis is also apparent.

The most important discussion with the mother should be on good skin care. The mother should be advised that although she may use the baby oil to loosen the scale on the scalp, she should shampoo afterward with a mild antiseborrheic shampoo to prevent buildup. A mild topical steroid, such as hydrocortisone 1% ointment, may also be recommended though chronic use should be dissuaded. If skin scrapings reveal secondary infection with *Candida,* an antifungal cream should be added to the regimen; if a secondary bacterial infection is suspected, a culture should be taken and treatment with either topical or systemic antibiotics initiated. Short baths with a mild cleanser and regular application of emollients is critical.

The mother should also be educated on potential flares with vaccinations and infections, as well as with climate changes. It is important that the infant catch up on her vaccinations, but cautioning the mother about a potential flare can prevent distress.

Selected References

Clayton TH, Wilkinson SM, Rawcliffe C, et al. Allergic contact dermatitis in children: should pattern of dermatitis determine referral? *Br J Dermatol.* 2006;154:114–117

Eichenfield LF, Friedlander SF. Coping with chronic dermatitis. *Contemp Pediatr.* 1998;15:53–66

Gupta AK, Bluhm R, Cooper EA, et al. Seborrheic dermatitis. *Dermatol Clin.* 2003;21:401–412

Kang K, Postr AM, Nederost ST, et al. Atopic dermatitis. In: Bolognia JL, Jorizzo JL, Rapini RP, eds. *Dermatology.* St Louis, MO: Mosby; 2003:199–214

Lewkowicz D, Gottlieb AB. Pediatric psoriasis and psoriatic arthritis. *Dermatol Ther.* 2004;17:364–375

Nelson JS, Stone MS. Update on selected viral exanthems. *Curr Opin Pediatr.* 2000;12:359–364

Peterson CM, Eichenfield LF. Scabies. *Pediatr Ann.* 1996;25:97–100

Sidbury R, Poorsattar S. Pediatric atopic dermatitis: should we treat it differently? *Dermatol Ther.* 2006;19:83–90

Williams JV, Eichenfield LF, Burke BL, Barnes-Eley M, Friedlander SF. Prevalence of scalp scaling in prepubertal children. *Pediatrics.* 2005;115:e1–e6

Morbilliform Rashes

Kathy K. Langevin, MD, MPH, and Noah Craft, MD, PhD

CASE STUDY

A 10-month-old infant girl is brought to the office with a history of rhinorrhea, cough, and fever for 3 days prior to the onset of a confluent, erythematous rash. The rash started on her face. She has been irritable, and her eyes are red and teary. Her immunizations include 3 sets of diphtheria, tetanus, and acellular pertussis (DTaP), polio, *Haemophilus influenzae* type b, conjugated pneumococcal, and hepatitis B vaccines. No one at home is ill. The girl was seen in the emergency department 2 weeks before because she caught her finger in a car door. On physical examination, the girl's temperature is 102.2°F (39°C). A confluent eruption of erythematous macules and papules is evident on the face, trunk, and extremities. Rhinorrhea and conjunctivitis are also present.

Questions

1. What are the common causes of febrile maculopapular or morbilliform rashes in children?
2. What features distinguish one disease from another?
3. How does a child's nutritional status affect their reaction to certain exanthem-inducing viruses?
4. What are the public health considerations concerning viral exanthems in children?

Exanthems are skin findings resulting from an underlying disease. More than 50 different viruses, in addition to bacteria and *Rickettsia*, have been identified, though viruses tend to be the leading cause. In children, these exanthems are most commonly macular, papular, or mixed. The rash of measles is described as morbilliform, and this adjective is used to describe similar-appearing maculopapular rashes. Frequently this is seen in conjunction with fever, and additional symptoms include myalgias, rhinorrhea, conjunctivitis, headache, gastrointestinal (GI) complaints, and lymphadenopathy. The exanthems of various underlying viruses can also be seasonal. Although many of the common childhood illnesses of the past are now prevented by immunizations, not all segments of the population are adequately immunized. In addition, some children are not eligible for immunization because of their young age. Allergic reactions to medications, particularly antibiotics, may also result in similar eruptions and can be accompanied by symptoms of low-grade fever and pruritus. Differentiating viral exanthems from allergic reactions may be difficult in febrile children who have been empirically started on antimicrobial agents.

Epidemiology

In most children, the viruses that cause exanthems produce mild disease without significant morbidity or long-term sequelae. Of greater concern is that some diseases are a public health risk because of potential spread through the population. Morbilliform eruptions are a common presenting complaint, particularly in certain age groups and at certain times of the year.

Measles, also known as rubeola, is caused by a paramyxovirus, an RNA virus, and has markedly decreased in the United States since the live vaccine was introduced in 1963. It is transmitted by direct contact with infectious droplets or by airborne spread. In temperate climates, it is most frequently seen in the winter and spring. In the pre-vaccine era, measles was a significant cause of morbidity and mortality. Periodic resurgences have occurred, particularly among unimmunized preschoolers, older adolescents, and young adults. In addition, young infants are also at risk because of decreased levels of passively transferred maternal immunity related to lack of maternal natural infection or immunization. Vaccine-related immunity apparently wanes more rapidly in mothers than does naturally acquired immunity. Because of the increased number of cases in preschoolers and in children with primary vaccine failure who received the vaccine appropriately, the 2-dose recommendation by the American Academy of Pediatrics was implemented in 1989, though there continue to be cases each year. Measles is no longer endemic in the United States but continues to be imported. The incubation period of measles is about 10 days. Individuals are infectious from about 3 to 5 days before the onset of rash until 4 days following its appearance.

Rubella is also caused by an RNA virus and now rarely occurs, with fewer than 25 cases annually in the United States. Sporadic outbreaks are reported, generally in foreign-born or underimmunized persons, but about 10% of US-born individuals older than 5 years are considered to be susceptible. The peak incidence is in the late winter to spring, and it is likely transmitted via direct or droplet contact from nasopharyngeal secretions. Historically, adolescents and young adults had been considered to be at greatest risk for the disease though that risk has decreased. Congenital rubella syndrome may develop in the offspring of pregnant women who have rubella, with the greatest risk of congenital defects during the first trimester. The incubation period is 14 to 23 days.

Erythema infectiosum, also called fifth disease, is most commonly seen in children 4 to 10 years of age during late winter to early spring. Most adults have antibodies indicating previous infection. The disease is caused by an acute infection with parvovirus B19, a DNA virus, and spread through respiratory secretions, percutaneous exposure to blood or blood products, and vertical transmission from mother to fetus. The incubation period is generally 4 to 14 days but may be up to 21 days.

Roseola infantum, also known as exanthem subitum, may affect children from 6 months to 2 years of age, as maternal antibodies are protective until the age of 6 months. The illness is due to infection with human herpesvirus (HHV) 6 or 7, though HHV-6, a DNA virus, is most commonly the etiologic agent. The virus is shed in the saliva, even among healthy, previously infected infants. All children are seropositive by the age of 4. Reinfection is possible, and there is no seasonal pattern. The incubation period for HHV-6 is likely 5 to 15 days and is unknown for HHV-7.

Enteroviruses are the most common cause of exanthems in the summer and fall. Sixty-nine different types of enteroviruses are recognized. They are all RNA viruses of the picornavirus group and include coxsackieviruses (groups A and B), echoviruses, and enteroviruses. Infection is spread through fecal-oral and respiratory routes as well as via fomites. There is also vertical transmission. Infection is more common in young children and in those with poor hygiene. The incubation period is usually 3 to 6 days.

Kawasaki disease is of uncertain etiology, although an infectious cause is suspected. Epidemics occur usually in the winter and spring. Most patients are between 18 and 24 months of age, and children older than 8 are rarely affected. Males outnumber females by a ratio of 1.5:1. The incidence of the disorder among Asians is higher than in other populations. The incubation period is unknown.

Gianotti-Crosti syndrome, also known as papular acrodermatitis of childhood, has historically been associated with hepatitis B infection. In the United States, it is believed to be a host response to multiple viral infections including, but not limited to, hepatitis A and B, Epstein-Barr virus (EBV), measles, and the enteroviruses. It is seen most frequently in children 1 to 6 years of age.

Scarlet fever is a cutaneous reaction to several erythrogenic exotoxins produced by group A streptococcus (GAS) via delayed-type hypersensitivity. It is transmitted through respiratory secretions. Scarlet fever is usually seen in young children between 1 to 10 years with pharyngitis. It occurs most commonly in cooler climates during the late fall, winter, and early spring. The incubation period is 2 to 5 days.

Rocky Mountain spotted fever (RMSF) is caused by *Rickettsia rickettsii*, an intracellular organism. Infection is transmitted by the bite of *Ixodes* ticks, which are both reservoirs and vectors of the organism. It can be seen throughout the United States, with most cases seen in the southern states. Children younger than 15 years are most commonly infected. Highest incidence of infection is seen between April and September. The incubation period lasts from 2 to 14 days.

Clinical Presentation

Maculopapular or morbilliform eruptions may involve the face, trunk, or extremities. The eruption is usually erythematous, and the lesions are flat or slightly raised. Occasionally, lesions within the mouth, referred to as enanthems, are evident. Most children are febrile (Dx Box) and may have other symptomatic complaints.

Dx **Morbilliform Rashes**

- Macular, papular, or combined rash
- Fever
- Enanthems (lesions in the mouth)
- Lymphadenopathy
- Respiratory symptoms
- Gastrointestinal symptoms

Pathophysiology

The mechanism for development of a rash is variable. In some cases, the rash is the reaction of the body to infection or to the presence of a toxin. In general, the sequence involves exposure to an infectious agent and then acquisition of the agent most commonly through droplet infection or fecal-oral contamination. The agent, usually a virus, then replicates, perhaps in the reticuloendothelial system. Lymph nodes enlarge, reflecting the involvement of the reticuloendothelial system. Associated viremia may be present.

In Kawasaki disease, vasculitis affects multiple organ systems. Various cytokines and autoantibodies play a role in the inflammatory response. In a toxin-mediated rash (eg, scarlet fever), previous exposure to the toxin is believed to sensitize the individual.

Differential Diagnosis

Morbilliform exanthems are associated with several diseases, such as measles, rubella, erythema infectiosum, roseola, enterovirus infections, Gianotti-Crosti syndrome, Kawasaki disease, scarlet fever, and RMSF. Drugs can also cause eruptions similar to those caused by the aforementioned diseases.

The rash associated with **measles** is preceded by the 3 "Cs" of cough, coryza, and conjunctivitis in addition to fever, which last for several days before the eruption of the exanthem. Lesions on the buccal mucosa, called Koplik spots, are well-circumscribed white-gray papules (Figure 110-1) that appear 2 to 3 days after the prodrome and resolve after 2 to 3 days. This enanthem, though rare, is pathognomonic for measles. The measles rash itself usually begins on the head, particularly behind the ears and around the margin of the scalp, and then spreads cephalocaudally. After 2 to 3 days, the rash becomes confluent and copper-colored, and then desquamation occurs.

Measles is not generally associated with systemic lymphadenopathy. The major complications of measles in children in developed nations are pneumonia, encephalitis, and secondary bacterial

Figure 110-1. Koplik spots.

infections. In developing nations, death usually results from respiratory and neurologic complications, often in those with marginal nutritional status. In individuals who were initially immunized with killed measles vaccine (1963–1968), acquisition of measles results in atypical measles, characterized by acute high fever, myalgias, and cough, followed a few days later by a papular or vesicular eruption that may be hemorrhagic. Lobar pneumonia is usually present, and associated findings include hepatosplenomegaly and weakness.

Rubella produces a relatively minor illness in children, although adults, particularly women, may experience a painful arthritis. Up to half of infections are asymptomatic. There can be a prodrome of fever, headache, conjunctivitis, and upper respiratory symptoms. The rash consists of fine macules and papules, starting on the face and progressing caudally, resolving after 3 days. Lymphadenopathy, particularly of the postauricular or suboccipital nodes, is characteristic of the disease. Forschheimer spots are pinpoint rose-colored macules that can develop on the soft palate in patients with this infection. Congenital rubella syndrome results in multisystem anomalies that can result from maternal infection and is part of the TORCH congenital infections (toxoplasmosis, other agents, rubella, cytomegalovirus, herpes simplex).

Erythema infectiosum (EI) is characterized by a distinctive rash that may be preceded by mild prodromal symptoms including low-grade fever, headache, myalgias, and malaise. The rash generally occurs 7 to 10 days after the prodrome. The facial rash consists of erythematous patches on the cheeks with sparing of the nasal bridge and periorbital areas. This slapped-cheek appearance generally fades after several days. If involved, the extremities may develop a lacy reticulated rash of macules and papules that can be pruritic. This usually lasts about a week but may have recurrences over several months with triggers such as activity, sunlight, emotional stress, and hot baths. Most children are only mildly ill and may attend school, but children with underlying hematologic disorders may experience

aplastic crises because of the affinity of parvovirus B19 for developing red blood cells. Immunocompromised children are also at risk for chronic anemia. Pregnant females may transmit this infection to their fetuses, which can result in fetal hydrops, growth retardation, isolated pleural and pericardial effusions, and fetal loss. Adults with parvovirus infection frequently develop arthritis, though only 10% of children experience this symptom. Neurologic disturbances including encephalitis and neuropathies may follow parvovirus infection, though this is rare. **Papular-purpuric gloves and socks syndrome (PPGSS)** is a self-limited acute eruption linked to parvovirus B19 infection. It occurs usually in the spring and summer, characterized by often-painful edema and erythema and progressing to purpuric macules and papules with a sharp line of demarcation at the wrists and ankles. A nonspecific enanthem of petechiae and erosions can occur. Symptoms of myalgias, lymphadenopathy, anorexia, and fatigue may follow the rash. The exanthem generally resolves after 1 to 2 weeks with no residual sequelae.

Roseola infantum usually causes a fairly mild illness in children, though there can be associated complications. Defervescence usually accompanies the rash, which consists of fine, non-pruritic, blanchable, pink macules or papules with a surrounding halo that generally appear first on the trunk, then spread centrifugally. Periorbital edema can also be seen. On average, the rash evolves over 12 hours and usually resolves by 2 days. Infants may appear sickest during the prodromal phase, when the fever is high (temperature: often ≥103°F [39.5°C]), and infants are irritable as a result. Fever generally lasts 3 to 5 days and can be accompanied by upper respiratory symptoms and lymphadenopathy. Seizures during the febrile period can occur in up to 15% of primary infections. Workup to rule out sepsis is often warranted.

The rashes associated with **enterovirus infections** are highly variable. They may resemble measles or rubella or may be distinct and characteristic, such as hand-foot-and-mouth disease (HFMD), most commonly associated with coxsackievirus A16 and enterovirus 71. There is a brief prodrome of low-grade fever, malaise, abdominal pain, anorexia, and sore mouth. Patients can have either the exanthem or enanthem, though most have both. The exanthem of HFMD usually follows the enanthem and consists of erythematous macules and papules with central gray vesicles. They crust and heal without scarring in 5 to 10 days. Though called HFMD, the buttocks are also frequently affected. Oral lesions are more frequently seen on the hard palate, tongue, and buccal mucosa. These progress from erythematous macules and papules to vesicles, and then ulcerate, resolving in about 1 week. Neurologic complications associated with enteroviral infections include aseptic meningitis and encephalitis and have been reported in infections with coxsackievirus B and enterovirus 71. Other systems affected by enteroviral infections include respiratory, GI, ophthalmic, and cardiac.

The rash of **Kawasaki disease** is also highly variable; it may be morbilliform, urticarial, scarlatiniform, or resemble erythema multiforme. During the first week of illness, there is desquamation of the perineum. The diagnosis of Kawasaki disease requires fever (generally >39°C [lasting at least 5 days] and 4 out of the 5 following findings: (1) bilateral non-purulent conjunctivitis; (2) changes in the oropharyngeal mucosa including fissured lips, oral erythema, and strawberry tongue; (3) changes in the extremities such as erythema/edema or desquamation; (4) cervical lymphadenopathy with one node measuring at least 1.5 cm in diameter; and (5) the exanthem described previously. Irritability, abdominal pain, and diarrhea are not uncommon. Incomplete Kawasaki disease can be diagnosed when only 2 of the additional criteria are met, thus the practitioner should consider this diagnosis when persistent high fever and only 2 or 3 of the above symptoms are present. The major complication of Kawasaki disease is coronary artery abnormalities and can be seen in 20% of patients not treated within 10 days of onset of symptoms. Males, infants younger than 12 months, and children older than 8 years are at increased risk of coronary artery aneurysms.

The exanthem of **Gianotti-Crosti** syndrome consists of monomorphic, pink- to skin-colored, usually non-pruritic papules on the face, buttocks, and extremities, with sparing of the trunk. There is often a prodrome of fever and upper respiratory symptoms with associated generalized lymphadenopathy and hepatosplenomegaly. The exanthem fades after 2 to 3 weeks but can last up to 2 months.

Scarlet fever is primarily a disease of childhood. Onset is marked by sudden high fever, headache, vomiting, malaise, and sore throat. Within 12 to 48 hours, erythema develops on the neck, chest, and axillae. The rash quickly becomes generalized to a sandpaper-like rash of fine red papules on an erythematous background. Linear accentuation in the axillary, antecubital, and inguinal folds is known as Pastia lines. The face is flushed, except around the mouth (circumoral pallor). There is pharyngeal injection with exudate developing after a few days. The tongue is initially white with prominent red papillae (Figure 110-2), known as strawberry tongue. As the scarlet fever rash resolves, desquamation begins in 7 to 10 days, lasting up to 6 weeks.

Figure 110-2. Strawberry tongue.

The rash of **RMSF** begins as blanching pink macules or papules that evolve into petechial or purpuric non-blanching lesions. They begin on the wrists and spread centripetally. The palms and soles are almost always involved. The exanthem is preceded by symptoms of fever, headache, and malaise. Gastrointestinal symptoms such as nausea, vomiting, and diarrhea can be present. The rash generally develops 2 to 3 days after the prodrome.

Morbilliform rashes are the most common type of cutaneous **drug eruption.** They generally begin as erythematous macules and papules on the trunk that then spread to the extremities symmetrically. There is usually concurrent eosinophilia. Pruritus and low-grade fever can also be present, often confounding the diagnosis. In general, most drug rashes begin 1 to 2 weeks after starting the drug, but it is possible to have an eruption develop after a drug has been discontinued. After stopping the offending medication, the rash usually resolves over 1 to 2 weeks, but there can be progression to Stevens-Johnson syndrome or toxic epidermal necrolysis. The underlying pathogenesis of many of these drug rashes continues to be unknown; however, current studies indicate that T cells play a large role. Drug-specific CD4+ T cells cause inflammation of the skin via the release and induction of cytokines and chemokines, which then contribute to eosinophilia.

Infection with **EBV** is associated with rash in young children and in adolescents on antibiotics, usually ampicillin or amoxicillin. The eruption is morbilliform, and the lesions may be erythematous or copper-colored. Fever, upper respiratory symptoms, lymphadenopathy, hepatosplenomegaly, and facial and peripheral edema, including unilateral periorbital edema, may be noted. A case of PPGSS has been reported in a patient taking trimethoprim-sulfamethoxazole, suggesting that viral or drug-related antigens are responsible for an immune response resulting in rash.

Evaluation

History

A thorough history should be obtained (Questions Box).

Questions

Morbilliform Rashes

- What does the rash look like? Has a similar rash occurred before?
- What symptoms, if any, are associated with the rash or occurred before the onset of rash?
- How long has the child had these symptoms?
- Is the child taking any medications (antibiotics)?
- Does the child have any ill contacts?
- What is the child's immunization status?

Physical Examination

The focus of the physical examination is to help define the characteristics of the eruption such as location, extent, and degree of coalescence. The presence of any associated physical findings such as fever, lymphadenopathy, enanthem, desquamation, rhinorrhea, conjunctivitis, organomegaly, or central nervous system (CNS) symptomatology should be determined.

Laboratory Tests

Laboratory assessment may be helpful in certain conditions, though most of these diagnoses are made clinically. Serologic testing is most valuable for defining a community outbreak of a specific disease such as measles. In most viral exanthems, the results of serologic studies are not available until the condition has resolved and the patient has recovered. Tests may include acute and convalescent titers for specific viruses. Alternatively, immunoglobulin (Ig) M levels of antibodies against certain infections may be used to document that the infection was recent. However, presence of IgM is unreliable for detecting recent infection in roseola infantum. Newer modalities such as polymerase chain reaction may expedite the identification of enterovirus. Viral cultures can be used to detect many of the viruses, but are costly and are not usually obtained unless aseptic meningitis is diagnosed. Because neutropenia and lymphocytosis characterize many viral illnesses, such findings are not helpful in differentiating specific causal agents. Lymphocytosis, with characteristically atypical lymphocytes, distinguishes EBV infection. Although a mononucleosis spot test is usually positive in older children and adolescents, it may be nonreactive in young children, where infection is documented by specific EBV serology.

Pregnant women with suspected parvovirus B19 infection should have IgM and IgG levels drawn. If infection is confirmed, serial ultrasounds should be performed to monitor for symptoms of hydrops fetalis.

Kawasaki disease is associated with specific laboratory abnormalities, including thrombocytosis, elevated erythrocyte sedimentation rate, and C-reactive protein. Sterile pyuria is noted in 70% of the cases. Scarlet fever is characterized by leukocytosis. Eosinophilia can also be seen after a few weeks in up to 20% of patients. Laboratory confirmation, either via rapid streptococcal test or throat culture, should be done to confirm that the pharyngitis is due to GAS, not a virus. If the pharyngitis has resolved, serologic studies such as antistreptolysin O or anti-deoxyribonuclease provide evidence of the recent infection.

A 4-fold or greater change in titer between acute and convalescent serum as determined by indirect immunofluorescent antibody assay is diagnostic for RMSF. Many patients will have thrombocytopenia, leukopenia, anemia, and hyponatremia. In general, any child presenting with headache, fever, and possible exposure to tick bite should be evaluated for this disease.

Imaging Studies

Ultrasound, if performed in children with suspected Kawasaki disease who present with symptoms of an acute surgical abdomen, may reveal hydrops of the gallbladder in 15% of patients. An echocardiogram to check for evidence of coronary artery aneurysm is a mandated part of the evaluation in this disorder, both during the acute phase and 6 to 8 weeks after onset of symptoms. Long-term cardiac management is required for those with identified coronary artery abnormalities.

Management

The management of most viral exanthems is supportive and symptomatic. Hydration is critical because GI complaints of diarrhea are often associated. Antihistamines should be used for symptoms of pruritus in addition to regular use of emollients. Painful oral lesions can be treated with topical analgesics. In cases where complications such as encephalitis or pneumonia develop, hospitalization is indicated. Spread of infection such as measles to susceptible contacts can be reduced through the use of vaccine within 72 hours of exposure, or Ig within 6 days. Immunoglobulin is given in a dose of 0.25 mL/kg intramuscularly (0.5 mL/kg in immunocompromised children) with a maximum dose of 15 mL. Measles vaccine should be administered 5 months after the Ig in children who received the lower dose and after 6 months in children who received the higher dose. Human immunodeficiency virus infection is not a contraindication to measles vaccination. In developing nations, administration of vitamin A is recommended to all children with measles if vitamin A deficiency is present in the community and mortality from measles is 1% or greater. Antibiotic therapy should be initiated if bacterial coinfection is suspected but should not be started empirically. The management of Kawasaki disease includes the administration of intravenous immune globulin (IVIG), which should be started within 10 days of onset of fever. The current recommendation is to administer a single dose at 2 g/kg given as an infusion over 10 to 12 hours, though the optimal dosage remains unclear. Aspirin is initially administered at 80 to 100 mg/kg divided 4 times a day until several days after defervescence to prevent coronary thrombosis. Dosage is reduced to 3 to 5 mg/kg until 6 to 8 weeks after onset of illness if no coronary artery abnormalities have been found and continued indefinitely if present. Periodic echocardiograms are also required in these patients with close monitoring by a cardiologist. Measles and varicella vaccinations should be deferred for 11 months in any patient receiving IVIG.

If there is a concern for hepatitis in patients with Gianotti-Crosti syndrome, workup should be initiated.

Control measures are important because most morbilliform exanthems are due to infectious agents. Children with postnatal rubella should be kept from school or child care facilities for 1 week after onset of rash. Those with congenital rubella syndrome are considered contagious for 1 year, and caregivers must be educated. Females receiving rubella vaccine should not become pregnant for 28 days following vaccination. Hand hygiene is an important control measure that should be used to minimize spread of many of these viruses.

Vigilant education about the importance of immunizations is vital to reducing the impact of diseases such as measles and rubella. Though the number of cases in the United States is low, importation of these viruses from other countries mandates continued widespread vaccination.

Pregnant women infected with parvovirus B19 with ultrasound suggestive of hydrops fetalis should be referred to a tertiary care facility because intrauterine blood transfusions have proven successful. Routine exclusion of pregnant women from the workplace where erythema infectiosum has been identified is not recommended because the virus is transmitted before the onset of rash and is, thus, unlikely to be effective. Patients with aplastic crisis and chronic parvovirus infection may be contagious for extended periods and require longer periods of precautions. In addition, patients with PPGSS are considered potentially infectious when clinical symptoms of their eruption are present. Patients with aplastic crises may need transfusions, and IVIG has been used successfully in immunocompromised patients with chronic infection. However, most cases of EI do not require absence from school or treatment beyond supportive care.

Treatment with doxycycline is the drug of choice for infection with *R rickettsii*. Penicillin within 10 days of onset of symptoms is used to treat scarlet fever as a result of GAS pharyngitis to prevent the development of rheumatic fever. Erythromycin can be used in patients allergic to penicillin.

Prognosis

The prognosis for most morbilliform or maculopapular rashes of childhood is generally good, with full resolution of symptoms unless children are very young, have congenital disease, have an underlying condition, or develop long-term complications. In some young infants, viruses that cause exanthems may produce severe complications such as pneumonia and encephalitis. Subacute sclerosing panencephalitis is a late-onset, rare, and serious degenerative CNS disease that occurs as a complication of measles infection. Some patients with roseola may develop chronic neurologic sequelae, but most cases are benign. The prognosis for Kawasaki disease is usually favorable with appropriate management, though 2% to 4% of children will develop coronary artery aneurysms despite therapy. Kawasaki disease is the leading cause of acquired heart disease in children in the United States. In patients with severe infection with RMSF, long-term neurologic complications can be seen.

CASE RESOLUTION

The infant in the case scenario has the classic symptoms of measles. Normally such a young infant would not yet have received immunization against measles because the first dose is administered at 12 to 15 months of age with the second dose at 4 to 6 years of age. Immunoglobulin will likely not modify the disease in this patient because her rash is near confluent, suggesting exposure more than 6 days ago. She should be evaluated for evidence of complications, including pneumonia. Unimmunized household contacts, as well as pregnant women and other contacts younger than 1 year, should receive immunoglobulin. Treatment is supportive.

Selected References

American Academy of Pediatrics. *Red Book: 2006 Report of the Committee on Infectious Diseases.* 27th ed. Pickering LK, Baker CJ, Long SS, McMillan JA, eds. Elk Grove Village, IL: American Academy of Pediatrics; 2006

Berger JR, Chumley W, Pittman T, Given C, Nuovo G. Persistent coxsackie B encephalitis: report of a case and review of the literature. *J Neurovirol.* 2006;12:511–516

Blume JE, Levine EG, Heymann WR. Bacterial diseases. In: Bolognia JL, Jorizzo JL, Rapini RP, eds. *Dermatology.* St Louis, MO: Mosby; 2003:1119–1120

Gable EK, Liu G, Morrell DS. Pediatric exanthems. *Prim Care.* 2000;27:353–369

Mancini J. Exanthems in childhood: an update. *Pediatr Ann.* 1998;27:163–170

Mancini AJ, Shani-Adir A. Other viral diseases. In: Bolognia JL, Jorizzo JL, Rapini RP, eds. *Dermatology.* St Louis, MO: Mosby; 2003:1255–1269

Meissner HC, Strebel PM, Orenstein WA. Measles vaccines and the potential for worldwide eradication of measles. *Pediatrics.* 2004;114:1065–1069

Nelson JS, Stone MS. Update on selected viral exanthems. *Curr Opin Pediatr.* 2000;12:359–364

Newburger JW, Takahashi M, Gerber MH, et al. Diagnosis, treatment, and long-term management of Kawasaki disease: a statement for health professionals from the Committee on Rheumatic Fever, Endocarditis, and Kawasaki Disease, Council on Cardiovascular Disease in the Young, American Heart Association. *Pediatrics.* 2004;114:1708–1733

Scott LA, Stone MS. Viral exanthems. *Dermatol Online J.* 2003;9:4

Yawalkar N. Drug-induced exanthems. *Toxicology.* 2005;209:131–134

Zaoutis T, Klein JD. Enterovirus infections. *Pediatr Rev.* 1998;19:183–191

Vesicular Exanthems

Kathy K. Langevin, MD, MPH, and Noah Craft, MD, PhD

CASE STUDY

A 2-year-old toddler is evaluated for a 2-day history of fever (temperature: 103°F [39.5°C]), runny nose, decreased appetite, and a rash over the abdomen. The boy has had no previous known exposures to chickenpox (varicella) and no history of varicella vaccination. He attends child care daily. No one at home is ill. The boy is currently taking no medications except for acetaminophen for fever, and he has no history of dermatologic problems. On physical examination, the heart rate is 120/min, the respiratory rate is 20/min, and the temperature is 100.4°F (38.0°C). The toddler's overall appearance is nontoxic. The skin examination is significant for a few scattered erythematous vesicular lesions over the abdomen and one erythematous papule on the back. The rest of the examination is normal.

Questions

1. What are the most likely causes of vesicular exanthems in febrile children?
2. How can types of vesicular rashes be differentiated on the basis of patient history?
3. What are the key historical questions to ask?
4. What is the natural course of varicella?
5. What treatment options are available for children with varicella? What options are available for other vesicular exanthems?

Exanthems are generalized, erythematous rashes that are due to an underlying disease. They are most frequently caused by viral or bacterial infections, though they can also be due to noninfectious etiologies. Infectious eruptions are most commonly morbilliform in the pediatric population, but they can have protean manifestations, including vesicular, bullous, petechial, and purpuric. Vesicles are elevated, fluid-filled lesions that measure 1 cm or less in diameter. Bullae are quite similar, only larger in size. Vesicles often lose their initial morphology quickly because they can break spontaneously or coalesce into bullae. They can arise de novo or from macules or papules. Vesicles may be discrete, grouped, generalized, or linear, depending on their etiology, and their specific distribution is often helpful in formulating a differential diagnosis.

Epidemiology

Epidemiological factors can help differentiate infectious from noninfectious etiologies. Patient age, season of the year, presence or absence of similar cases in the community, regular attendance at child care or school, and lower socioeconomic class, which may contribute to exposure, should all be considered. Gender and ethnicity are usually less informative but can help distinguish certain diseases causing exanthems.

Primary varicella-zoster virus (VZV), or chickenpox, is one of the most common vesicular exanthems seen in childhood. In the pre-vaccine era, 90% of children in the United States were infected before the age of 10, with 3 to 4 million cases annually. The peak incidence is in late winter and early spring. Males and females are equally affected. Most reported cases are in children younger than 10 years, although the percentage of infections in adolescents and young adults has increased with the routine administration of the varicella vaccine at 1 year of age. It is transmitted person to person by direct contact with vesicular fluid, by airborne spread of respiratory secretions, from contact with zoster lesions, and vertically from mother to fetus. It is extremely infectious because transmission to susceptible household contacts approaches 90%. The incubation period ranges from 10 to 21 days, but varicella can develop between 1 to 16 days of life in newborns delivered to mothers with active disease around the time of delivery.

Herpes simplex virus (HSV) is a DNA virus with HSV-1 infections generally occurring above the waist and HSV-2 infections in the genitalia and below the waist. Neonatal infection is generally acquired at delivery or in utero from an infected mother who is often unaware of her infection. Herpes simplex virus-1 is typically transmitted by direct contact with oral secretions or lesions and HSV-2 from direct contact with infected genital secretions. The incubation for HSV infections is 2 days to 2 weeks beyond the neonatal period.

Hand-foot-and-mouth disease (HFMD), as well as herpangina, are due to enteroviral infections. Hand-foot-and-mouth disease is most commonly due to infection with coxsackievirus A16 and enterovirus 71 (See Chapter 110). Coxsackieviruses A1 through A6, A8, A10, and A22, as well as B1 through B4, and echoviruses, have been implicated in herpangina. Enteroviral infections occur most commonly in summer and early fall. Children younger than 10 years tend to develop HFMD while younger children develop herpangina. The incubation period for most enteroviruses is between 3 to 6 days.

Bullous impetigo is a less common cause of impetigo than nonbullous forms. It is most frequently seen in the summer and is transmitted by direct person-to-person contact. It is caused by coagulase-positive *Staphylococcus aureus*, mostly due to phage group 2, and is a localized reaction to exfoliative toxin released by the bacteria. It affects mostly neonates, infants, and younger children.

Infections caused by scabies or fungi can cause vesicular eruptions as well. Scabies is transmitted during prolonged close contact with an infested individual. Scabies has an incubation period of 4 to 6 weeks in patients without previous exposure. Reexposed patients develop symptoms a few days after repeat exposure. Tinea pedis is a common infection worldwide, though less so in children. It is acquired via contact with infected skin scales and in damp areas where the fungi reside. Tinea capitis, a common fungal infection in children (See Chapter 107), does not result in a vesicular rash, but like tinea pedis, can result in a dermatophytid or id reaction. The incubation period of fungi is unknown.

Dyshidrotic eczema is a disease that can occur in children with chronic eczematous dermatitis or atopic dermatitis, but can occur in unaffected children as well. It is similar in appearance to an id reaction though the latter tend to be unilateral. Rhus dermatitis is the prototypical allergic contact dermatitis, which develops about 1 to 3 days after exposure. Linear papules and vesicles are seen at points of contact between the antigen and the skin.

Clinical Presentation

Vesicular exanthems are eruptions of distinctive lesions that are raised and fluid-filled (Dx Box). They may be located anywhere on the child's body and, depending on the etiology, may or may not be pruritic. Other symptoms that may accompany such rashes include fever, upper respiratory symptoms, and gastrointestinal and central nervous system (CNS) involvement.

Dx Vesicular Exanthems

- Raised, fluid-filled vesicles on the skin
- Lesions may be pruritic
- Possible associated fever, upper respiratory infection symptoms, myalgias
- History of affected contacts
- Lesions on mucous membranes

Pathophysiology

Vesicles and bullae arise from a cleavage at various levels of the skin either within the epidermis (intraepidermal) or at the epidermal-dermal junction (subepidermal). Sometimes the 2 types of lesions can be differentiated based on the amount of pressure required to collapse the lesion, especially if the lesion is a large bulla. In addition, the thickness of the wall of a bulla can be estimated by its translucency or flaccidity. A biopsy of the lesion, however, is the only way to reliably differentiate between the 2 areas of separation, though this will not necessarily provide the diagnosis. Specific changes occur in the epidermis depending on the etiology of the vesicular exanthem.

For example, with certain viral infections such as herpes simplex, varicella, and herpes zoster, a "ballooning degeneration" of epidermal cells occurs.

In bullous impetigo, the vesicles and bullae are caused by staphylococcal toxins, which cause the keratinocytes in the granular layer of the epidermis to split apart. There are no bacteria seen within the blister cavity and a few inflammatory cells can be present.

The rash due to scabies infection is the result of a hypersensitivity reaction to the proteins of the parasite. In vesicular lesions, there is spongiosis, or intercellular edema, in the spiny layer of the epidermis caused by the mite, which can result in a vesicle. Spongiosis also leads to vesicle formation in dyshidrotic eczema, though the pathogenesis of this disease is not known. This is similar to id reactions and allergic contact dermatitis. Dyshidrotic is a misnomer because this disease is not related to sweat gland dysfunction or occlusion.

Differential Diagnosis

Primary VZV infection (chickenpox) consists of an average of 300 vesicles generalized throughout the body, with lesions in various stages of resolution, progressing from erythematous macules and papules that then evolve into vesicles and, eventually, pustules that then crust and heal normally without scarring. Characteristically, the vesicle has been described as a "dewdrop on a rose petal." There can be associated mild fever. Symptoms tend to be more severe in older patients. Fetal infection during the first or early second trimester can result in fetal demise or in congenital varicella syndrome, consisting of limb hypoplasia, cutaneous scarring, ophthalmic abnormalities, and CNS defects. Fetal infection acquired from 5 days pre-partum to 2 days postpartum can also be fatal. Bullous varicella can result when *S aureus* infects the vesicles of chickenpox, with greater chance for scarring.

Herpes zoster, a reactivation of a latent infection with the VZV, can also cause a vesicular rash. The virus resides in neuronal cells that travel along the nerves when reactivated and become released into the skin. It is generally a disease of older people because only 5% of patients with herpes-zoster are younger than 15 years. In zoster, the lesions are grouped in the distribution of 1 to 3 sensory dermatomes. It can be quite painful, and postherpetic neuralgia can last for months. In immunocompromised patients, the rash of zoster can become disseminated.

Disseminated HSV in an infant is usually due to HSV-2, is very severe, and is often unaccompanied by skin findings. In children and adolescents, HSV-1 gingivostomatitis and perioral vesicles are the most common clinical findings. There can also be an ulcerative enanthem. Herpes simplex virus persists for life and, when reactivated, results in single or grouped vesicles, often on the vermilion border with an erythematous base. Genital lesions are more frequently due to HSV-2, but the prevalence of infection due to HSV-1 is increasing.

Hand-foot-and-mouth disease is associated with a brief, mild prodrome of fever, malaise, and mouth pain. The enanthem tends to appear first and can consist of erythematous macules, papules, or vesicles that then ulcerate. They resolve in about 1 week. The exanthem consists of erythematous macules and papules with a central gray vesicle. Generally, the hands, feet, and buttocks tend to be involved. In herpangina, patients acutely develop fever, malaise, headache, and neck pain. There is an enanthem of small grayish-white vesicles on the anterior tonsillar pillars, soft palate, uvula, and tonsils. These ulcerate with a surrounding red halo. Usually no exanthem is seen.

Impetigo is the most common bacterial skin infection in children. In bullous impetigo, there can be associated fever, weakness, and diarrhea, though there are often no systemic symptoms. Small vesicles enlarge rapidly into flaccid bullae that easily rupture. These lesions can be generalized and can arise from normal-appearing skin.

Parasites such as the tiny mite *Sarcoptes scabiei* can cause an intensely pruritic, generally papular eruption, though vesicular lesions can occur. Commonly, secondary excoriations are seen (see Chapter 109). In older children and adults, interdigital folds, flexor wrists, waistline, trunk, and genital area are more commonly affected. A linear burrow is pathognomonic but often difficult to identify clinically. Patients younger than 2 years have involvement predominantly of the head, neck, palms, and soles. In this population, the eruption is more likely to be vesicular (Box 111-1). Arthropod bites can also result in isolated and scattered vesicles.

Fungal pathogens that cause tinea pedis include *Trichophyton rubrum, Trichophyton mentagrophytes, Trichophyton tonsurans,* and *Epidermophyton floccosum.* Infection can directly cause a scaly or vesicular rash or can result in a hypersensitivity reaction to the fungi,

---

Box 111-1. Common Causes of Acute Vesicular Exanthems

Infectious

Viral
- Varicella-zoster virus
- Herpes simplex virus
- Enterovirus

Bacterial
- *Staphylococcus aureus*

Fungal
- *Trichophyton rubrum*
- *Trichophyton mentagrophytes*
- *Trichophyton tonsurans*
- *Microsporum canis*
- *Epidermophyton floccosum*

Infestations
- *Sarcoptes scabiei*
- Arthropod bites

Noninfectious
- Allergic contact dermatitis
- Dyshidrotic eczema
- Id reaction

---

presenting as vesicles on the palms, soles, sides of the fingers, and occasionally on the extremities and trunk. *T mentagrophytes* can cause vesicles and bullae on the medial foot. It is associated with an id reaction, in which deep-seated pruritic vesicles develop secondary to tinea infection elsewhere. An id reaction, most commonly on the hands, face, and trunk, can also result from tinea capitis, usually caused by *T tonsurans* and *Microsporum canis,* though it does not cause a vesicular exanthem on its own.

The clinical appearance of dyshidrotic eczema can be identical to that of an id reaction or fungal infection and consists of "tapioca," pearl-like, deep-seated vesicles frequently on the palms and soles, as well as the lateral sides of the fingers that are extremely pruritic. Secondary impetiginization (bacterial superinfection) is common. Though many cases are acute and preceded by infections (including fungal, as seen in id reaction), contact reactions, and stress, there can also be chronic cases.

A delayed type 4 hypersensitivity reaction secondary to contact with plants of the genus *Toxicodendron* is a common cause of allergic contact dermatitis. The main allergen in these plants are catechols. Rhus dermatitis causes a classic linear vesicular rash (see Chapter 109). Contact with other allergenic substances may also produce a vesicular rash and include nickel, rubber compounds, fragrances, and preservatives in cosmetics.

The differential diagnosis of acute vesicular exanthems can also be organized according to the distribution of the lesions. Distinctive locations as well as specific patterns are important to consider in each individual case. The presence or absence of fever can assist in developing the appropriate differential (Figure 111-1). Epidemiological, as well as historic, information may suggest the diagnosis. For example, known exposure to VZV (chickenpox) 10 to 21 days prior to a vesicular eruption facilitates diagnosis of this disease. A history of hiking, camping, or other outdoor activities suggests possible contact with poison ivy or poison oak.

In addition, the presence of a specific prodrome can often be elicited with primary or recurrent herpes simplex. Pain on swallowing often occurs with enteroviral infection. A history of similar lesions lessens the likelihood of acute primary infection and suggests a chronic condition such as the recurrent disorder pompholyx (dyshidrotic eczema).

Evaluation

History

A thorough history should be obtained (Questions Box). Practitioners must inquire about the current state of general health, as well as the specific details about the eruption.

Physical Examination

Although the physical examination focuses on the skin, other aspects of the examination are helpful diagnostically. Vital signs should be taken to verify the presence or absence of fever. The oropharynx should be examined closely for any lesions on the tongue, gingiva,

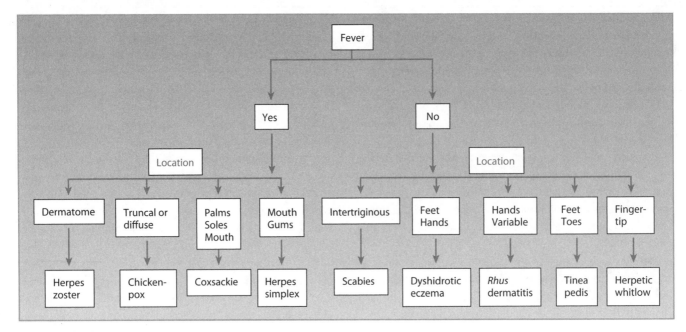

Figure 111-1. Approach to the evaluation of vesicular eruptions.

buccal mucosa, anterior tonsillar pillars, and posterior pharynx. The lips should also be examined for any evidence of vesicular lesions that may occur with a primary or recurrent herpes simplex infection.

Patients should be completely unclothed to permit a thorough examination of the skin. The distribution of the lesions should be noted. Physicians should determine whether the vesicles are grouped in a particular dermatomal distribution, as with zoster (shingles), or more generally distributed and in various stages of development, as with varicella. A linear distribution may suggest contact with poison ivy or poison oak. Physicians should also note the following: Do the lesions include or exclude the palms and soles? Are the buttocks involved? Are the lesions concentrated on one specific part of the body, such as the feet and toes or the hands? Are the sizes of the lesions uniform? If not, are other larger bullous-like lesions present in addition to vesicles?

Questions

Vesicular Exanthems

- How long has the child had the rash? Where is it located?
- Does the child have associated symptoms such as fever, runny nose, cough, or sore throat?
- Does the child have nonspecific symptoms such as decreased appetite?
- If the child has any symptoms accompanying the rash, did these develop at the same time as the rash?
- Is there any reason to suspect that the patient is relatively immuno-compromised from chronic steroid use, chemotherapy, or an acquired immunodeficiency?
- Does the child have a history of similar lesions?
- Does anyone else in the family have a similar rash?
- Has the child been camping or hiking in the woods?
- Are there pregnant contacts?

It is also helpful, if at all possible, to examine the skin of family members for similar lesions.

Laboratory Tests

Few, if any, laboratory studies are usually needed in healthy children with vesicular eruptions because the diagnosis is often made clinically. A Tzanck smear showing multinucleated giant cells that contain intranuclear viral inclusions may be useful in making a preliminary diagnosis of HSV or VZV, but serologies, culture, or polymerase chain reaction can be more accurate. Serologies are not helpful in neonates with HSV infection but are indicated in immunocompromised patients with an unknown history of varicella and a definite exposure to the virus. This information may be helpful when considering prophylaxis with varicella-zoster immune globulin (VZVIG) (see Chapter 23).

Definitive confirmation of scabies can be made by microscopic examination of skin scrapings from suspicious lesions. The presence of the adult mite or ova, larvae, nymphs, or feces (scybala) is diagnostic. For children with suspected tinea pedis, a skin scraping mixed with potassium hydroxide can be performed and examined under the microscope. Fungal cultures can also be taken.

Management

The mainstay of treatment for most vesicular eruptions is parent and child education as well as reassurance. Conditions are usually self-limited and require only **supportive therapy.** For example, most varicella, HSV, gingivostomatitis, HFMD, and herpangina infections are self-limited and no treatment except parental reassurance and education regarding adequate hydration is necessary. Depending on the etiology of the vesicular rash, immunocompromised children such as those with human immunodeficiency virus or acquired immunodeficiency syndrome and patients who are receiving chemotherapeutic agents or systemic corticosteroids may require specific intervention.

Topical agents such as calamine lotion, oatmeal soaks, or Aveeno baths should be used in children with intense pruritus or multiple lesions. Topical products, which are potentially sensitizing (eg, diphenhydramine-containing agents) should be used cautiously and discontinued if the condition is not improving. Cool, wet compresses with plain water or aluminum acetate (Burow solution) can be quite soothing in cases of *Rhus* dermatitis, scabies, or tinea pedis. Wet compresses may also be helpful with open, macerated lesions of dyshidrotic eczema, though they are often poorly tolerated in small children.

Antipyretics (acetaminophen, ibuprofen) may be used to treat otherwise healthy children with varicella. Aspirin-containing medications should be avoided in children with varicella because of the association with Reye syndrome. Oral analgesics may also be indicated for symptomatic relief of pain associated with herpetic gingivostomatitis or enterovirus mouth lesions.

Oral antihistamines (diphenhydramine or hydroxyzine) may be used in children with varicella or scabies for treatment of pruritus. These drugs are also helpful in allergic contact dermatitis (*Rhus* dermatitis) and dyshidrotic eczema. Though the sedating antihistamines are generally more effective, non-sedating antihistamines can also be used in the daytime, particularly for the more chronic dyshidrotic eczema.

Steroids may be effective in the control of some vesicular rashes; however, the practitioner must first be certain the lesions are not secondary to varicella or herpes simplex. Topical steroids can be used for outbreaks of vesicles of dyshidrotic eczema, reserving oral steroids for severe outbreaks. In severe cases of *Rhus* dermatitis, a course of systemic steroids, such as prednisone, 1 to 2 mg/kg/d, may be warranted and generally requires at least 2 to 3 weeks of therapy. Use of an oral histamine-2 blocker such as ranitidine or famotidine can help prevent gastritis as a complication of oral prednisone.

Oral acyclovir is not recommended routinely for the treatment of uncomplicated varicella in otherwise healthy children, but should be considered when the risk of developing moderate to severe disease is increased. According to the American Academy of Pediatrics (AAP) Committee on Infectious Diseases, acyclovir is indicated in patients older than 12 years of age; those with chronic cutaneous or pulmonary disorders; those receiving chronic or short, intermittent courses of corticosteroids (systemic or aerosolized); or those receiving salicylates long term. Oral or intravenous (IV) acyclovir may also be warranted in pregnant women infected with varicella. Acyclovir is most effective if initiated within the first 24 hours of the exanthem though the impacts on symptoms may be minimal. (See the AAP 2006 *Red Book* for further details and specific recommendations regarding immunocompromised children and the role of VZVIG.) A live attenuated varicella vaccine has been licensed for use in the United States since 1995 and is available and recommended for all nonimmune individuals (see Chapter 23).

Additional recommendations for children with varicella include keeping fingernails short in young children to prevent superinfection of lesions from scratching. Children should drink plenty of fluids to avoid dehydration. Patients are considered contagious from 1 to 2 days prior to the onset of the rash until the lesions are all dried and crusted (usually 5–7 days after the rash develops), at which time they may return to school. In children with persistent or recurrent fever, secondary complications should be considered. A significant association between primary varicella injection and invasive group A beta-hemolytic streptococcal infection has been recognized and should be considered in the child with fever on or beyond the fourth day of the illness. In infants greater than 28 weeks' gestational age born to mothers with varicella infection 5 days pre-partum, disease severity can be mitigated by VZVIG maternal antibody.

Treatment for zoster, or shingles, is primarily symptomatic and should consist of pain medications. Acyclovir can be considered if the eruption becomes generalized or affects immunocompromised patients. It is possible that the varicella vaccine may reduce the risk of developing zoster. Though 1 dose of varicella vaccine is routine, there is currently a recommendation for 2 doses of varicella vaccine as immunity appears to wane and sporadic outbreaks occur.

Herpetic whitlow is an HSV infection on the fingertip as a result of direct autoinoculation from oral or genital lesions. Treatment is not usually indicated. Herpes gladiatorum is a cutaneous HSV infection on the skin seen in wrestlers. While it does not require treatment with antiviral agents such as acyclovir, athletes should not be engaged in person-to-person contact when herpes lesions are present. Eczema herpeticum is HSV infection in children with underlying atopic dermatitis or other underlying skin disease that results in rapidly progressive widespread vesicles that then erode and crust. There can be significant fever and irritability, and severe infection may warrant hospitalization for treatment with IV acyclovir.

Localized bullous impetigo in otherwise healthy patients can be treated with topical mupirocin 2% ointment. More widespread or complicated infections require **oral antistaphylococcal therapy** with agents such as amoxicillin and clavulanate (Augmentin), erythromycin, or cephalexin (Keflex). Recurrent disease should warrant workup for carriage and treatment if needed. Local knowledge of methicillin-resistant *S aureus* rates and bacterial cultures should be considered. For the treatment of tinea pedis, topical **antifungal agents,** in powder, cream, or ointment formulations, can be effective when applied twice daily until clear. Discomfort can be alleviated with cool water or Burow solution soaks. Tinea pedis can be difficult to control. Its treatment is centered on meticulous foot hygiene. Because careful foot care is often not a priority for most patients, complete eradication is not realistic. Patients should be instructed to wash their feet and change their socks when they return from school, dry their feet completely, avoid occlusive shoes, and wear open-air shoes or sandals whenever possible. Topical antiperspirants may be needed (aluminum chloride). Cotton socks are recommended. In severe or refractory cases, an oral antifungal preparation such as griseofulvin may be prescribed for an extended period, generally 4 weeks. Tinea capitis also requires oral antifungal therapy (see Chapter 107). For the treatment of scabies, see Chapter 109.

Prognosis

Overall, the prognosis for vesicular exanthems is good, with most children recovering in 1 to 2 weeks, depending on the etiology. Secondary infections can occur with varicella, however, and should be suspected in children with persistent or recurrent fever. Additional complications in non-immunosuppressed patients include bacterial superinfection of the skin, pneumonia, CNS involvement, Reye syndrome, glomerulonephritis, and arthritis. Complications from HSV infections include conjunctivitis, keratitis, and encephalitis.

Secondary infections with skin flora can be a complication of any of these skin conditions because denuded lesions allow for superinfection. In addition, many of these rashes can be pruritic, resulting in open, excoriated skin.

CASE RESOLUTION

In the case presented at the beginning of this chapter, the toddler has a classic presentation of primary varicella (chickenpox). Management should include symptomatic treatment with acetaminophen and antihistamines, along with topical preparations such as calamine lotion and oatmeal baths. The parent should be instructed regarding the natural course of this infection and be informed that the infection is highly contagious. In addition, symptoms indicating possible complications, such as persistent or recurrent fever, circumferential redness or swelling of the lesions, and shortness of breath, should be reviewed with the parents.

Selected References

American Academy of Pediatrics Committee on Infectious Diseases. *Red Book: 2006 Report of the Committee on Infectious Diseases.* 27th ed. Elk Grove Village, IL: American Academy of Pediatrics; 2006

American Academy of Pediatrics. Varicella-zoster infections. In: Pickering LK, Baker CJ, Long SS, McMillan JA, eds. *Red Book: 2006 Report of the Committee on Infectious Diseases.* 27th ed. Elk Grove Village, IL: American Academy of Pediatrics; 2006:711–725

Dyer JA. Childhood viral exanthems. *Pediatr Ann.* 2007;36:21–29

Frieden, IJ. Childhood exanthems. *Curr Opin Pediatr.* 1995;7:411–414

Lopez AS, Guris D, Zimmerman L, et al. One dose of varicella vaccine does not prevent school outbreaks: is it time for a second dose? *Pediatrics.* 2006;117:e1070–e1077

Mancini AJ, Bodemer C. Viral infections. In: Schachner LA, Hansen RC, eds. *Pediatric Dermatology.* St Louis, MO: Mosby; 2003

Scott LA, Stone MS. Viral exanthems. *Dermatology Online J.* 2003;9:4

The New Morbidity

112. Autism Spectrum Disorders 687

113. Attention-Deficit/Hyperactivity Disorder 695

114. Psychopharmacology in Children 701

115. Physical Abuse 707

116. Sexual Abuse 711

117. Failure to Thrive 717

118. Infants of Substance-Abusing Mothers 723

119. Substance Abuse 729

120. Eating Disorders 737

121. Body Modification: Tattooing and Body Piercing 745

122. Childhood Obesity 753

123. Divorce. 759

124. School-Related Violence 763

125. Disaster Preparedness 767

126. Adolescent Depression and Suicide 771

Autism Spectrum Disorders

Robin Steinberg-Epstein, MD

CASE STUDY

The mother of 18-month-old twin boys is concerned because one twin is not talking as much as his twin sibling. They are both very active. She feels that even though the child is quiet, he is very smart. He likes to figure out how things work. He seems very sensitive to sounds and covers his ears around loud noises. He loves music and even knows which CD his favorite song is on. He will play with his sibling, but doesn't seem interested in other children.

In your office both boys are very active. It is difficult to get an adequate examination, because this child is screaming the whole time. While both children have stranger anxiety, the twin about whom the mother is concerned seems to have extreme stranger anxiety. He otherwise appears well.

Questions

1. What are autism spectrum disorders (ASDs)?
2. How do ASDs differ from language delay?
3. How do you evaluate a child for ASDs?
4. Where can a clinician refer a patient with an ASD?
5. What types of treatment are available?
6. Should a child suspected of having an ASD receive further immunizations?

Autism spectrum disorders (ASDs) are characterized by impairment in communication, social interaction, and odd behaviors/interests. According to the *Diagnostic and Statistical Manual of Mental Disorders* (4th edition), a person with autistic disorder must meet 6 of 12 possible criteria across 3 primary domains: social interaction, communication, and restrictive or repetitive behaviors. These disturbances must originate prior to age 3 and cause significant degrees of impairment (Box 112-1).

Autism spectrum disorders include autistic disorder, Asperger syndrome, Rett syndrome, and pervasive developmental disorder not otherwise specified. While the criteria differ somewhat, all of these disorders have in common an impairment in social communication

---

Box 112-1. *Diagnostic and Statistical Manual of Mental Disorders (DSM-IV)* Diagnostic Criteria for Autistic Disorder[a]

A. A total of six (or more) items from (1), (2), and (3), with at least two from (1) and one or more from (2) and (3):

    (1) qualitative impairment in social interaction, as manifested by at least two of the following:

        i. the use of multiple nonverbal behaviors such as eye-to-eye gaze, facial expression, body postures, and gestures to regulate social interaction

        ii. failure to develop peer relationships appropriate to developmental level

        iii. a lack of spontaneous seeking to share enjoyment, interests, or achievements with other people

        iv. lack of social or emotional reciprocity

    (2) qualitative impairment in communication as manifested by at least one of the following:

        i. delay in, or total lack of, the development of spoken language (not accompanied by an attempt to compensate through alternative modes of communication such as gesture or mime)

        ii. in individuals with adequate speech, marked impairment in the ability to initiate or sustain a conversation with others

        iii. stereotyped and repetitive use of language or idiosyncratic language

        iv. lack of varied, spontaneous make-believe play or social imitative play appropriate to developmental level

    (3) restrictive repetitive and stereotyped patterns of behavior, interests, and activities, as manifested by at least one of the following:

        i. encompassing preoccupation with one or more stereotyped and restricted patterns of interest that is abnormal either in intensity or focus

        ii. apparently inflexible adherence to specific, nonfunctional routines or rituals

        iii. stereotyped and repetitive motor mannerisms (i.e. hand or finger flapping or whole body movements)

        iv. persistent preoccupation with parts of objects (i.e. wheels, doors, lights)

These symptoms result in significant or abnormal functioning in at least one area (social interaction, social language, or symbolic/imaginative play) with onset prior to age 3.

[a]Reprinted with permission from American Psychiatric Association. *Diagnostic and Statistical Manual of Mental Disorders.* 4th ed. Washington, DC: American Psychiatric Association; 2000.

and repetitive or unusual interests of varying degrees. Because these disorders require similar management and treatment, and there is some subjectivity in assessing the level of impairment, many choose to use the term *ASD* to incorporate all those who are significantly effected by its symptomatology.

Epidemiology

As recently as 1999 the prevalence of this disorder was thought to be 1 in 2,500. More recent numbers from the Centers for Disease Control and Prevention (2007) cite 1 in 150 children. This amounts to 1.5 million Americans. The incidence is rising by almost 15% a year. Autism is considered the fastest-growing developmental disability. This increase is, in part, the result of an understanding of a broader phenotype. Boys are affected approximately 4 times as often as girls, but affected girls are often more impaired.

Clinical Presentation

Autism spectrum disorders are truly a spectrum of social communication deficits. While there is a certain set of behaviors that defines the disorder, any child may have any combination of the symptoms that lead to the same result—severe and incapacitating social deficits. Furthermore, the challenges that face this population are more than just developmental delays. Their behaviors are aberrant and odd.

Many children with autism have difficulty with eye contact and body posture. Even those that have some eye contact often do not use their eyes to convey a social message. They may look out of the corner of their eyes, focus only on the lips of the speaker, or only look infrequently. In other words, they may make eye contact, but at the wrong time. They may talk to you with their bodies facing away from you. They may not gesture to help clarify intention.

While some children have limited communication, some offer too much information. They may be quick to talk to you about things they are interested in, but are not able to talk to you about your interests. They seem socially insensitive. As younger children they are often entertained by their own interests for long periods. They do not need, nor do they care for, the company of others. While many of these children are nonverbal, some repeat or echo what they hear from movies, television, or nearby conversation. Others seem able to converse, but have trouble with social banter. It is important not to be deceived by a child who interacts or hugs, but only on his own terms.

Autistic children often have a fascination with patterns. The pattern may be in the form of household routines, or patterns within a particular subject area. This may manifest in an obsession for sameness and resistance to change or in an obsessive need to know everything about a particular topic. Many know all there is to know about such favorite topics as Thomas the Tank Engine or dinosaurs from the Jurassic period, but cannot answer a question such as, "How are you?" or "What is your name?" They may be upset by a road detour or a furniture rearrangement. Some of these children, out of an incredible ability to recognize patterns, will be able to read as early as 2, even though they are unable to speak functionally and cannot comprehend what they read.

A significant portion of children have difficulty with sensory processing. This takes the form of problems with smells, tastes, sounds, sights, and touch. This symptom may be manifest in the need to taste everything including nonfood items, covering ears in loud situations, or an inability to tolerate tags in clothing.

There is a huge variation in cognitive ability. The severity of autism is independent of cognitive ability. While a significant portion of those with autism are mentally retarded, many are of normal intelligence and even gifted.

Parents often raise behavioral concerns. It is important to recognize red flags and behaviors that demand further evaluation (Boxes 112-2 and 112-3). In other words, there are certain classic symptoms, but be mindful of the child that is just unable to connect with others. Clinicians should rely on their own instinct. Inconsistent symptoms are the hallmark of this disorder. Some parents of children with autism describe a phenomenon whereby the children are developing normally until 12 to 15 months of age and then suddenly lose skills or stop progressing. This is particularly concerning.

Pathophysiology

There are numerous proposed etiologic possibilities for the origins of autism, from the inbreeding of computer "wizzes" to exposure to microwaves. However, no consistent explanation or pattern has emerged. We do know that the structure of the brain is different, but why?

Box 112-2. Red Flags (Common Aberrant Behaviors Associated With Autism)
• Decreased eye contact (common, but NOT universal)
• Only wants to be cuddled on his terms
• Areas of unusual knowledge—recognizes entire alphabet by 2, all types of dinosaurs by 4, names of all Thomas trains, interest in fans or spinning items
• More interested in how things work than with playing
• Unusual sensitivities—oversensitive to hearing, bright lights, shirt tags, new foods, new places
• Smelling or licking nonfood items
• Repeating words instead of answering questions or answering off topic
• Difficulty interacting with other children
• Plays amongst children, not with them
• Resistance to change, "very independent"
• "In his own world"
• Lines things up
• Unusual hand movements or jumping when emotional
• Things have to be a certain way
• Odd tone of voice (prosody)
• Increased pain tolerance

Box 112-3. Absolute Indications for Referral[a]

- Not babbling or gesturing (pointing, waving) by 12 months
- No single words by 16 months
- Absence of 2-word non-echolalic phrases by 24 months
- ANY loss of ANY language or social skills at ANY age requires immediate evaluation.

[a]Filipek PA, Accardo PJ, Baranek GT, et al. The screening of autism spectrum disorders. *J Aut Dev Discord.* 1999; 29:439–484.

Box 112-4. Medical Conditions Associated With Autism

- Epilepsy
- Fragile X
- Tuberous sclerosis
- Prader-Willi syndrome
- Visual or auditory impairment syndrome
- Down syndrome
- Cerebral palsy
- Neurofibromatosis
- Congenital rubella

Box 112-5. Disorders That May Mimic Autism

- Hearing impairment
- Global developmental delay
- Tourette syndrome and comorbidities
- Selective mutism
- Reactive attachment disorder
- Lead ingestion
- Sensorimotor integration dysfunction
- Severe auditory processing/language deficit
- Severe anxiety
- Severe attention-deficit/hyperactivity disorder
- Brain trauma
- Childhood onset schizophrenia

Box 112-6. Disorders That Can Occur With Autism

- Tuberous sclerosis
- Congenital blindness
- Global developmental delay
- Chromosomal abnormalities (Down syndrome, fragile X syndrome, Prader-Willi syndrome, etc)
- Phenylketonuria
- Epilepsy
- Elevated lead level
- Congenital infections
- Brain trauma
- Bipolar disorder
- Neurofibromatosis
- Congenital profound hearing loss
- Tourette syndrome
- Landau-Kleffner syndrome
- Inborn errors of metabolism
- Anemia
- In utero exposure to drugs/alcohol
- Depression/anxiety
- Attention-deficit/hyperactivity disorder

Up to 10% of those with autism have another medical condition (Box 112-4) that might have led to this disorder. However, this leaves 90% without an etiology.

Genetics seems to play a role in the development of autism. There is a risk of the disorder among siblings of up to 6%, which is more than 10 times the risk in the normal population. Family members are more likely to exhibit social deficits, anxiety, or depression than are family members who do not have a relative with the disorder. Several candidate chromosome, including X and 22, have been suggested as being associated with this disorder.

It is also important to realize that up to 30% of children with autism have abnormalities on electroencephalogram (EEG). This may point to the structural abnormalities in the autistic brain but does not seem to account for the disease itself. The epileptiform changes should be evaluated by a neurologist to determine if medication is indicated.

Several environmental markers have also been suggested as being linked to autism, but none have proved credible. Major epidemiological studies both within the United States and internationally have examined the role of either the measles, mumps, rubella vaccination or thimerosal preservative in the development of this disorder. None of these studies have found proof to support these theories.

Differential Diagnosis

Very few entities present with impairment in the same 3 domains as those that are affected by autism. There are a limited number of disorders that mimic autism (Box 112-5). On the other hand, there are several disorders that commonly co-occur with autism (Box 112-6) and, if not identified, will make treatment more difficult.

Evaluation

There is not one diagnostic test, blood or otherwise, that will confirm the diagnosis of autism. The diagnosis is based on history and the interaction with the child.

History

Regular developmental surveillance and screening should be part of every well-child evaluation, especially between ages 9 and 30 months. The American Academy of Pediatrics recently suggested adding a 30-month visit for developmental screening in an attempt to capture atypical development to target for early intervention. Special attention should be given to a child who has a sibling with autism or a child whose parent or caregiver has expressed concern. Several screening tools can be used, including the Parents' Evaluation of Developmental Status (PEDS), Ages and Stages Questionnaire (ASQ), or the Brigance. The Modified Checklist for Autism in Toddlers (M-CHAT) is another excellent screening tool (moderate sensitivity and high specificity) to identify both developmental and social competency skills which, when deficient, may be associated with autism. These screening tools are quick and easy and can be filled out by the parent in the waiting area or with minor assistance from office personnel.

Once you suspect that a child has a developmental difference, it is important to gather as much information as possible. Thorough birth and medical histories are important in helping to understand if early experiences may predispose this child to any deficits.

Family history is also important because this disorder is presumed to be genetic. Furthermore, it may help to consider other etiologies. Family structure will help to determine if abuse, neglect, or maternal depression play any role in the child's delay. However, autism is NOT due to poor parenting.

Developmental history is the most important part of the history. It is important to probe all 4 areas of developmental milestones: fine motor, gross motor, language, and social development (see Chapter 18). Again, we expect more significant delays in language and social interaction, but you may see delays in all components of development. Additionally, probing for abnormal behaviors specific to autism helps distinguish this disorder from others. See the Questions Box for some suggestions that may help elicit information relevant to a diagnosis of autism in a toddler, but you must adjust the history depending on the age of the child. Always include early language milestones. Be aware that children with autism tend to have splinter skills. These are skills that may be normal or above developmental level for age. Don't let these skills distract you from probing areas of suspected delay.

Finally, parents and physicians often fall victim to common myths and excuses regarding development (Box 112-7) because it is not easy for many parents to discuss or admit delays. These myths, while they sound plausible, are not substantiated and only serve to further delay onset of intervention.

Physical Examination

A thorough physical examination with special attention directed to the growth parameters, neurologic examination, dysmorphic features, and neurocutaneous stigmata are essential to a complete evaluation. Height, weight, and head circumference should be plotted. Keep in mind that 25% of children with autism have a head circumference greater than the 97th percentile. That is not to say that everyone with a large head has autism, only that it is an associated feature. Those with Rett syndrome have a head circumference that may arrest by 5 months of age. Of course, in utero infections may predispose to a small occipitofrontal circumference and developmental concerns.

Questions

Autism

Questions to Ask Parents

- Does he seem to hear you? Did he have a hearing test in the neonatal period?
- Does he make noises? If so, what kind?
- When did he say his first word after "mama" and "dada"? Does he have 2-word phrases?
- Are there any other behaviors that concern you?
- Can he scribble? Has he lost any skills? Does he line things up?
- When did he first walk? What does he like to play with?
- Do tags on the back of clothes bother him?
- Is he interested in other children? What does he do if he sees another child in a park?
- When do you first remember him pointing with one finger?
- Does he play peek-a-boo? Will he try to engage you?
- Does he talk into a play phone?
- Does he eat a variety of foods?
- Does he turn when you call him?

Questions to Ask Yourself as the Clinician

- Are there any complicating historical factors that may predispose this child to a developmental problem?
- Is this merely personality variation, or does this represent delays and aberrant behavior?
- Is this a language delay or are you concerned about more social or odd behaviors?
- What should be done to evaluate?
- What types of intervention would be helpful?

Box 112-7. Common Excuses for Unusual Behaviors

1. We speak 2 languages at home. (By age 3 in a bilingual home, language should follow a normal progression. Social and unusual behaviors should always follow a normal trajectory.)
2. He is a boy. (This is accounted for in the range of normal.)
3. He is a twin. (If one twin is autistic, the other twin has a great risk of being autistic or delayed.)
4. He is the first child. (No evidence that firstborns speak late.)
5. He is the baby. (No evidence that last borns speak late.)
6. He is having a bad day.
7. He watches too much television. (Neglect can lead to delays, but these children still need intervention.)

These are NOT reasons to delay evaluation!

Detecting subtle physical signs such as clinodactyly, simian crease, or a high-arched palate, while not diagnostic, are somewhat helpful in raising suspicion for neurodevelopmental delays.

A series of dysmorphic features like a thin upper lip, flat philtrum, and upturned nose might suggest a syndrome such as fetal alcohol syndrome. Hypotonia is a common finding amongst children with autism, but might suggest an inborn error of metabolism. One must also check reflexes because degenerative disorders, such as muscular dystrophy, can present with language delay.

One of the most useful examinations in the office is to simply have a conversation with an older child or to play with a younger child. Bring out bubbles and engage in a popping game. Watch the child's eyes and his interaction with you and with his parent. Pretend the otoscope is a phone that rings, pick it up, talk briefly, and pass it to the child. Watch his response. Does he play with you or just with the bubbles or neither? Does he display repetitive flapping when excited?

Laboratory Tests

No single laboratory or radiologic evaluation will make the diagnosis. However, some tests are helpful to rule out comorbid conditions. If the child has not had an audiological evaluation, then this is step one. However, do not wait for the audiology results before referring the patient for help. From a medical perspective, laboratory studies should include a high-resolution karyotype and a DNA test for fragile X. In those with global developmental delay or regression (or when indicated), consider a lead level, acyl carnitine level, serum amino acids, urine organic acids, thyroid evaluation, and vision evaluation. The yield is expected to be low, but if positive, they aid in the diagnosis of a specific disorder.

Imaging Studies

If there is a history of regression or the presence of focal findings, consider a magnetic resonance imaging (MRI) test. Otherwise, obtaining an MRI is considered low yield. Children with regression, more significant involvement, or behavior suspicious of a seizure should receive an EEG. While positron emission tomography and single-photon emission computed tomography scans will show abnormalities, they are not considered specific enough for either diagnosis or to direct care. There are no present indications for their use in an individual child with autism. They are used primarily in the research setting.

Management

Making the diagnosis is sometimes challenging, but early diagnosis is critical in changing ultimate outcomes. Early diagnosis and intervention can reduce cost of lifelong care by two-thirds.

For children younger than 3 years, refer to the local governmental agency. In most states there exists a government-sponsored early intervention program for children 0 to 3. This agency is responsible for the evaluation and behavioral/educational/therapeutic interventions for children with suspected delays. This should lead to a comprehensive diagnostic evaluation and placement in an intensive intervention program. Therefore, once a hearing test has been completed, a referral to such an agency is the next step. It takes on average 6 months from the time a child is seen in a physician's office to when those services are obtained. Therefore, it is important to identify children before age 2 ½ years. Make that referral!

For children older than 3 years, the responsibility belongs to the local school system. So even though a child is not yet school-aged, their local school district is responsible for both the evaluation and interventions necessary to appropriately remediate this child. However, the clinician should check with local resources to ensure that such a system exists in the respective state. Be aware that between ages 3 and 21 years, each child is entitled to a free and appropriate education guaranteed under the federal mandate known as the Individuals with Disabilities Education Act. This program should be comprehensive and individualized to each child's needs. After a thorough assessment, the school will meet with the parents to develop an Individualized Education Plan.

Most children with autism require at least speech and language services, occupational therapy, and social skills training. Many require a one-on-one aide in a mainstream class, and others benefit from special education services in the form of pullout or a special day class. Augmentation can be created privately. Some states have mandated that medical insurance support these additional, yet necessary, services, but in others it is the sole responsibility of the parent.

Interventions

Autism is a neurologic condition that improves with intensive **multimodality interventions.** This improvement is slow. There are no quick solutions, magic medications, or diets to "cure" autism. Behaviors like impulsive aggression, repetitive behaviors, resistance to change, and obsessive behaviors are frequently targeted by systematic interventions. Furthermore, some basic social learning behaviors can be shaped with different types of intervention. There are a number of different techniques (Box 112-8) based on different psychological principles that may be used to help improve the difficulties associated with autism.

Speech and language services are a vital component of intervention. The initial goal is to help establish communication. In higher-functioning children who already have established language, this service is vital for the establishment and development of prosocial language—eye contact, inferences, understanding jokes, and the more subtle aspects of language. Social skills groups are often used to teach appropriate social responses in a semi-naturalistic environment.

Occupational therapy is often necessary to help with both fine motor skills and the processing of sensory information. This can be helpful in easing transitions. There is not a great deal of research to support its use for sensory concerns, but it is a widely accepted premise that sensory exposure helps children who have either an oversensitive or an undersensitive sensory system.

Special education in the form of an aide, classroom pullout, or special day class is often necessary to help with commonly associated learning disabilities. Children with autism can have a full array of learning difficulties. Commonly associated learning difficulties are in reading comprehension, written expression, specific math disability, and auditory comprehension.

Under the law, these services should occur in the least restrictive and most appropriate environment.

Box 112-8. Techniques Used for Treatment

Floor Time

This intervention uses personal relationships and play in the child's area of interest to draw the child through increasingly complex developmental tasks.

Applied Behavioral Analysis

Applied behavioral analysis strives to achieve pre-learning skills such as eye contact, imitation, sitting, and following simple directions using the principles of conditioning and behavioral psychology. In a 1:1 fashion a child is trained to respond in a predetermined way using a specific curriculum and reinforcers.

Behavioral Analysis

This method uses close study of behaviors, determining antecedent triggers and consequences, such as a tantrum. The goal is to substitute acceptable responses, such as using words, and increases rewards for substituted behaviors.

Pivotal Response Training

This strategy uses principles of behavior analysis but also uses the child's interests and internal drives to motivate. The hope is to generalize the skills from a therapy room to a variety of environments. Children with autism often have difficulty performing the same previously mastered skill in a new setting.

Picture Exchange Communication System

This system uses pictures that the nonverbal child can use to show a caregiver what they want.

Treatment/Education of Autism and Communication Handicapped Program

This is a complete program that incorporates the child into a large autism community. The goal is toward autonomy and uses many methods based on cognitive therapeutic principles.

Social Stories

These are often used as a complementary strategy. These stories describe in detail basic social skills in different scenarios.

Pharmacotherapy

The mainstay for treatment of autism remains behavioral. Medications do not seem to help the core symptoms of autism. However, almost 2 of 3 of these children receive medications for behaviors that, despite intensive behavioral intervention, continue to obstruct progress or become dangerous.

Only one drug is US Food and Drug Administration–approved for use in this population; Risperidone is approved for the agitation associated with this disorder. On the other hand, there are many other targeted behaviors for which medications are used. The choice to use medication is not a simple one. It should be directed toward the emotion or psychological function causing the symptom. The most common medications include selective serotonin reuptake inhibitors and stimulants. However, research and clinical experience tells us that children with autism are more sensitive to side effects and at lower doses. Therefore, the choice and direction of medication management in this population is often best guided by a developmental-behavioral pediatrician, neurologist, or child psychiatrist (see Chapter 114).

Alternative Treatments

A variety of alternative treatments have been suggested. Secretin injections, dietary restrictions, chelation, high-dose vitamins, antifungals, and neuron injections are just some of the interventions considered in this realm. Some of these methods reported anecdotal improvement; others are dangerous and have resulted in death. None of these methods are considered traditional or the standard of care because there are minimal empiric data to support their use.

Prognosis

Many children show dramatic improvements with early intervention. Unfortunately, others show minimal improvement. Therefore, all children need intensive interventions. Some prognostic indicators such as IQ, early and intensive interventions, and a supportive family forebode well. Obtaining an accurate IQ is often challenging. The major determinant of ultimate outcome seems to be progress in a comprehensive, early intervention program for 2 years, prior to age 5. Having little or no language by age 6 is a poor prognostic indicator. Therefore, the goal remains focused on early identification, intensive treatment, and advocacy for children to receive such interventions with ongoing support.

The intensive early intervention programs have only been available since about 1995. Autistic children have now moved into the mainstream. In spite of receiving early intervention, these children continue to have problems with transitions, more complex social interactions, and higher-level organization tasks. Therefore, physicians must continue to advocate for and support these families through the years.

Many adults with autism also continue to require significant support. They may require sheltered living and work environments, safety monitoring, ongoing medical support and, depending on severity, institutionalization.

Another significant portion of autistic children attend college, get married, and have children. This portion is difficult to quantify because these numbers are changing very rapidly and the true number of children with this disorder has yet to be realized.

CASE RESOLUTION

The child described in the vignette was evaluated by a developmental pediatrician and the local governmental agency where he received a comprehensive assessment by a multidisciplinary team. The diagnosis was confirmed and his brother was also noted to have a language delay. They were both placed into an early intervention program. The primary patient was placed in a one-on-one structured teaching environment for 4 months. After significant improvement, he was moved to a therapeutic preschool setting that emphasized generalization of his newly acquired skills, speech therapy, occupational therapy, and social skills. His brother received speech therapy 2 times a week. Both are due to start a regular kindergarten class in the fall with ongoing speech and social support. The primary patient has been placed on a stimulant medication to control hyperactivity and problems with attention.

Selected References

Aman MG. Treatment planning for patients with autism spectrum disorders. *J Clin Psychiatry.* 2005;66(suppl 10):38–45

American Academy of Pediatrics Council on Children With Disabilities, Section on Developmental Behavioral Pediatrics, Bright Futures Steering Committee, Medical Home Initiatives for Children With Special Needs Project Advisory Committee. Identifying infants and young children with developmental disorders in the medical home: an algorithm for developmental surveillance and screening. *Pediatrics.* 2006;118:405–420

American Psychiatric Association. *Diagnostic and Statistical Manual of Mental Disorders.* 4th ed. Washington, DC: American Psychiatric Association; 1994

Autism Society. www.autism-society.org

Barbaresi WJ, Katusic SK, Voigt RG. Autism: a review of the state of the science for pediatric primary health care clinicians. *Arch Pediatr Adolesc Med.* 2006;160:1167–1175

Courchesne E, Carper R, Akshoomoff N. Evidence of brain overgrowth in the first year of life in autism. *JAMA.* 2003;290:337–344

Filipek PA, Accardo PJ, Baranek GT, et al. The screening of autism spectrum disorders. *J Aut Dev Discord.* 1999;29:439–484

Jarbrink K, Knapp M. The economic impact of autism in Britain. *Autism.* 2001;5:7–22

Madsen KM, Hviid A, Vestergaard M, et al. A population-based study of measles, mumps, and rubella vaccination and autism. *N Engl J Med.* 2002;347:1477–1482

MMWR. Surveillance Summaries. February 9, 2007. Vol 56. No. SS-1/ Prevalence of Autism Spectrum Disorders—Autism and Developmental Disabilities Monitoring Network, Six Sites, United States 2000; Prevalence of Autism Spectrum Disorders—Autism and Developmental Disabilities Monitoring Network, 14 Sites, United States, 2002; and Evaluation of a Methodology for a Collaborative Multiple Source Surveillance Network for Autism Spectrum Disorders _ Autism and Developmental Disabilities Monitoring Network, 14 Sites, United States, 2002

Richardson A, Montgomery P. The Oxford-Durham study: a randomized, controlled trial of dietary supplementation with fatty acids in children with developmental coordination disorder. *Pediatrics.* 2005;115:1360–1366

Attention-Deficit/ Hyperactivity Disorder

Allison Golnik, MD, MPH, and Iris Wagman Borowsky, MD, PhD

CASE STUDY

A 9-year-old boy is seen in the emergency department after nearly colliding with a car while riding his bicycle. He sustained only minor abrasions from a fall. The boy's mother states that her son is impulsive and frequently engages in risky behaviors. She reports that he is extremely active and has a short attention span. He is in the fourth grade and an average student, but he has a hard time following directions and is easily distracted in class. In addition, he tends to have trouble keeping friends. In the examining room, the boy is quiet but answers questions appropriately. Except for a few scrapes, his physical examination is entirely normal.

Questions

1. What are the primary symptoms of attention-deficit/ hyperactivity disorder (ADHD)? What other conditions should be considered in the differential diagnosis of ADHD?
2. What other psychiatric disorders or neurodevelopmental disabilities commonly coexist with ADHD?
3. What is the appropriate evaluation of children with suspected ADHD?
4. What treatment modalities are useful in the management of ADHD?

The core symptoms of attention-deficit/hyperactivity disorder (ADHD) are inattention, impulsivity, and hyperactivity. The *Diagnostic and Statistical Manual of Mental Disorders, Fourth Edition (DSM-IV)* diagnostic subtypes of ADHD are (1) predominantly inattentive type, (2) predominantly hyperactive/impulsive type, and (3) combined type. Most children and adolescents with the disorder have the combined type, exhibiting symptoms of both inattention and hyperactivity/impulsivity.

For diagnosis of predominantly inattentive or hyperactive/impulsive ADHD, documentation of at least 6 of 9 behaviors from either the inattentive or hyperactive/impulsive subtype *DSM-IV* domains is necessary (Box 113-1). For combined type, 6 or more criteria of both subtypes are necessary. Symptoms of ADHD must appear (by history) before 7 years of age, be present in at least 2 major settings of a child's life (eg, home and school), and persist for at least 6 months. The behaviors must be more frequent and severe than those typically seen in normally developing children of the same age and must impair the child's learning and/or social interactions. The symptoms should not be better explained by another mental disorder (such as anxiety).

Epidemiology

Attention-deficit/hyperactivity disorder is the most common neurobehavioral disorder in children. An estimated 4% to 12% of school-aged children have ADHD, and there is a 3:1 predominance of boys in community samples. Over the past 2 decades, ADHD diagnoses have increased, but without population-based studies, it is uncertain whether this represents a true increase in incidence. Proposed explanations for the debated increased incidence of ADHD include overdiagnosis, cultural and gender biases, and environmental neurotoxins.

Clinical Presentation

Children with ADHD have problems with selective attention. They may make careless mistakes or fail to pay attention to details. In addition, they may be easily distracted and have difficulty concentrating on tasks long enough to complete them. Difficulties following instructions and organizing tasks and activities are also characteristic of ADHD. Poor impulse control manifests as difficulty waiting one's turn, frequently blurting out answers, and interrupting or intruding on others. Symptoms of hyperactivity include fidgetiness, difficulty remaining seated or playing quietly, and subjective feelings of restlessness in adolescents (Dx Box). Difficulties with social

Dx Core Symptoms of Attention-Deficit/ Hyperactivity Disorder

- Inattention
- Impulsivity
- Hyperactivity

Box 113-1. *DSM-IV* Criteria for Attention-Deficit/Hyperactivity Disorder[a]	
Diagnostic Criteria for ADHD	

A. Either 1 or 2

1) Six (or more) of the following symptoms of **inattention** have persisted for at least 6 months to a degree that is maladaptive and inconsistent with developmental level:

Inattention

a) Often fails to give close attention to details or makes careless mistakes in schoolwork, work, or other activities

b) Often has difficulty sustaining attention in tasks or play activities

c) Often does not seem to listen when spoken to directly

d) Often does not follow through on instructions and fails to finish schoolwork, chores, or duties in the workplace (not due to oppositional behavior or failure to understand instructions)

e) Often has difficulty organizing tasks and activities

f) Often avoids, dislikes, or is reluctant to engage in tasks that require sustained mental effort (such as schoolwork or homework)

g) Often loses things necessary for tasks or activities (eg, toys, school assignments, pencils, books, or tools)

h) Is often easily distracted by extraneous stimuli

i) Is often forgetful in daily activities

2) Six (or more) of the following symptoms of **hyperactivity-impulsivity** have persisted for at least 6 months to a degree that is maladaptive and inconsistent with developmental level:

Hyperactivity

a) Often fidgets with hands or feet or squirms in seat

b) Often leaves seat in classroom or in other situations in which remaining seated is expected

c) Often runs about or climbs excessively in situations in which it is inappropriate (in adolescents or adults, may be limited to subjective feelings of restlessness)

d) Often has difficulty playing or engaging in leisure activities quietly

e) Is often "on the go" or often acts as if "driven by a motor"

f) Often talks excessively

Impulsivity

g) Often blurts out answers before questions have been completed

h) Often has difficulty awaiting turn

i) Often interrupts or intrudes on others (eg, butts into conversations or games)

B. Some hyperactive-impulsive or inattentive symptoms that caused impairment were present before 7 years of age.

C. Some impairment from the symptoms is present in 2 or more settings (eg, at school [or work] or at home).

D. There must be clear evidence of clinically significant impairment in social, academic, or occupational functioning.

E. The symptoms do not occur exclusively during the course of a pervasive developmental disorder, schizophrenia, or other psychotic disorder and are not better accounted for by another mental disorder (eg, mood disorder, anxiety disorder, dissociative disorder, or personality disorder).

Code Based on Type

314.01 Attention-Deficit/Hyperactivity Disorder, Combined Type: if both criteria A1 and A2 are met for the past 6 months

314.00 Attention-Deficit/Hyperactivity Disorder, Predominantly Inattentive Type: if criterion A1 is met but criterion A2 is not met for the past 6 months

314.01 Attention-Deficit/Hyperactivity Disorder, Predominantly Hyperactive, Impulsive Type: if criterion A2 is met but criterion A1 is not met for the past 6 months

314.9 Attention-Deficit/Hyperactivity Disorder Not Otherwise Specified

[a]Reprinted with permission from American Psychiatric Association. *Diagnostic and Statistical Manual of Mental Disorders.* 4th ed. Washington, DC: American Psychiatric Association; 2000.

relationships and low frustration tolerance are also commonly seen in children with ADHD.

Pathophysiology

The etiology of ADHD is unknown. Genetic, neurologic, and prenatal/perinatal factors may play a role. Family studies indicate that first-degree relatives of children with ADHD have a risk of ADHD that is 5 times greater than normal controls. In addition, measures of behavior and attention are more alike in monozygotic twins than in same-gender dizygotic twins. The most widely confirmed gene association with ADHD is the 7-repeat allele of the D_4 dopamine receptor gene that, while found in about 30% of the general population, is found in 50% to 60% of those with ADHD.

Attention-deficit/hyperactivity disorder may be the result of neurologic factors. Patients with frontal lobe disorders exhibit inattention, hyperactivity, and impulsivity. The frontal and prefrontal regions of the brain seem to be involved in selective attention, distractibility, inhibition, planning, and organization. Brain imaging studies have shown that prefrontal circuits that control attention are smaller, are less active, and have altered electroencephalogram (EEG) activity in individuals with ADHD. Dopamine and norepinephrine are thought to be prominently involved in ADHD. The prefrontal cortex is rich in catecholamine receptors, and psychostimulants that are effective in the treatment of ADHD alter catecholamine metabolism. Stimulants are presumed to increase synaptic dopamine in the striatum (involved in planning and execution of behavior) by binding to the dopamine transporter. Subsequently, the striatum influences the prefrontal cortex to enhance executive functioning. Executive functions include organizing, planning, paying attention, curbing impulsivity, ability to "stick to a plan" yet change it when it is not working (set maintenance), the ability to self-talk through internal rules, and working memory.

Prenatal and perinatal risk factors that have been associated with ADHD include in utero exposure to alcohol or cigarettes, or brain injury.

Differential Diagnosis

The symptoms of ADHD can be seen in a variety of other conditions (Box 113-2). Sensory deficiencies, especially hearing impairment, can imitate attention deficits. Inattention is often a component of autism spectrum behaviors, but autistic children exhibit impaired social interactions and communication and stereotypical, restricted, and repetitive behaviors. Iron deficiency anemia and low-level lead poisoning also may have detrimental effects on behavior and development. Seizure disorders, such as petit mal (absence) or partial complex seizures, may be misdiagnosed as predominantly inattentive-type ADHD. Possible side effects of certain medications, such as phenobarbital or theophylline, may mimic ADHD. Hyperthyroidism can cause the hyperactive symptoms of ADHD, but other signs of increased metabolism, such as elevated heart rate, tremors, or weight loss, should be apparent. Exposure to alcohol or drugs in utero has been associated with subtle difficulties with learning and attention as the child develops. Congenital infections, central nervous system infections in early childhood, and traumatic brain injuries may produce behaviors similar to those seen in ADHD. In addition, psychosocial problems, such as family stresses (eg, marital discord, unemployment, poverty, substance abuse) or ineffective parenting (eg, inconsistent discipline) must be considered in the differential diagnosis of ADHD.

Children with ADHD have an increased prevalence of comorbid conditions, including oppositional defiant disorder (35%), conduct disorder (26%), depression (18%), anxiety disorder (26%), and many developmental disorders such as speech and language delays and learning disabilities. In adolescents and young adults, conduct disorder (aggression, delinquency, and other antisocial behaviors) and substance abuse are often seen together with attention deficits. These conditions can magnify the symptoms of children with ADHD.

Evaluation

All children and adolescents with symptoms of inattention, hyperactivity, and impulsivity deserve an evaluation for ADHD.

History

The diagnostic evaluation of ADHD should begin with a description and examples by caregivers of the child's problem behaviors and a comprehensive history (Questions Box). The clinician should find out how parents handle their child's behavioral problems; this provides insight into their parenting style. Family stresses should be evaluated. Interviewing the child alone provides an opportunity for the child to describe his or her thoughts and feelings. The clinician

---

Box 113-2. Differential Diagnosis of Attention-Deficit/Hyperactivity Disorder

Developmental Delay

- Learning disability
- Language disorder
- Sensory deficiencies (especially hearing impairment)
- Autism
- Seizure disorder
- Iron deficiency
- Environmental toxins (lead)
- Side effects of medication (eg, phenobarbital)
- Hyperthyroidism
- Congenital infection
- In utero exposure to drugs or alcohol
- Previous brain insult (trauma, infection)
- Family stresses
- Ineffective parenting
- Psychiatric disorders
  — Conduct disorder
  — Oppositional disorder
  — Anxiety disorders
  — Affective disorders (depression, bipolar illness)
  — Personality disorders (aggression, antisocial behavior)
  — Substance abuse

---

should inquire about the child's difficulties and coping strategies at home and school. Additionally, information from the child's teacher is necessary, including descriptions of the child's behavior and report cards.

Questions

Screening for Attention-Deficit/Hyperactivity Disorder

- How is your child doing in school?
- Are there any problems with learning that parents or the teacher have seen?
- Is your child happy in school?
- Has your child been held back in any grade, suspended, dropped out, or considered dropping out?
- Does your child have any major problems controlling his or her behavior at home, in school, or with friends? Does your child have problems completing class work or homework?
- Is behavior management difficult at home?
- What are the problem behaviors?

Historical information should cover the *DSM-IV* diagnostic criteria of inattention, hyperactivity, and impulsivity (see Box 113-1). Parents and teachers may report the child's behaviors using an ADHD-specific questionnaire or rating scale that includes all of the 18 behaviors (eg, Vanderbilt scales), which can be found in the

American Academy of Pediatrics (AAP) toolkit *Caring for Children With ADHD: A Resource Toolkit for Clinicians*. Although broad developmental screening tools are useful in other circumstances, non–ADHD-specific developmental tools are not recommended in the ADHD diagnostic assessment because their sensitivity and specificity for ADHD are too low for diagnostic purposes.

The clinician should evaluate for coexisting conditions that would warrant further investigation. This is where broad screening tools, such as the Child Behavior Checklist and Behavior Assessment for Children, can be used to screen for coexisting conditions. For example, frequent sadness or isolation would suggest depression, and persistent negative, hostile, and defiant behavior toward authority would suggest oppositional-defiant disorder. The AAP toolkit for clinicians includes both a scale specific to ADHD behaviors and a broader scale for possible coexisting conditions.

Physical Examination

The child's weight, height, and head circumference should be plotted on a growth curve and the pattern of growth evaluated. Children should be examined for minor congenital anomalies or dysmorphic features such as the facies associated with fetal alcohol syndrome. A neurologic examination should include an assessment of the child's affect, speech, hearing, and vision.

Observing the child's behavior during the office visit is important, but most children with ADHD do not display hyperactivity in the office. Interaction between the child and his or her parents should be observed. The clinician should note whether the child listens to parental instructions and how parents deal with any misbehavior. Does the child cooperate with the examination? How well does the child relate to adults? The clinician should watch the child play (eg, draw, play with toys) and note the child's organization of activities, attention span, distractibility, and motor activity.

Laboratory Tests

Diagnostic tests, such as computerized attention tasks or specific psychological measures, are not a routine part of the ADHD evaluation, unless indicated by findings on the history and physical examination. Referral for further evaluation of speech, hearing, and vision should be done if indicated. Blood tests, such as hematocrit, lead level, and thyroid hormone, likewise, are only indicated if there are relevant signs or symptoms. Additionally, continuous performance tests of the child's behavior, such as testing vigilance or distractibility, have low sensitivity and specificity of less than 70% when differentiating children with ADHD from controls. Psychometric testing may be used to determine whether a discrepancy exists between the child's learning potential (intelligence quotient) and academic progress (academic achievement scores), indicating a learning disability.

Brain imaging studies, including magnetic resonance imaging, single photon emission computed tomography scans, and EEG, should not be routinely used to diagnose ADHD. While children with ADHD have been found to differ from controls in brain morphology and EEG interpretations, these differences do not reliably discriminate between children with and without ADHD. An EEG is indicated if absence or partial complex seizures are suspected.

Management

Treatment of ADHD must be multifaceted and long term, recognizing that ADHD is a chronic disorder. Family education should emphasize the strengths of children and families, and address parental concerns. Families should be aware that children with ADHD often experience functional impairments in academic achievement, self-esteem, social skills, peer status, unintentional injuries, and family functioning. The clinician can ease parents' guilt by explaining the neurologic basis of ADHD and assuring that ADHD is not the result of insufficient parenting. Children who discover that their problems are not their fault may feel that a heavy burden has been lifted from their shoulders. However, both parents and children may find it difficult to accept that the child has a chronic disorder. Support groups such as Children and Adults with ADHD (CHADD) (www.chadd.org) may be helpful for families. Clinicians should work together with the child, family, and school personnel to specify appropriate target outcomes. They should then monitor the child for target behaviors and adverse effects. If target outcomes are not met, the clinician should reevaluate the initial diagnosis, use of available treatments, adherence to the plan, and potential for coexisting conditions.

Behavior Management

The goals of behavior management are to modify the child's physical and social environment at home and school in order to change behavior. Behavioral techniques include rewards for the target outcome behaviors (eg, verbal praise; hugs; points or stars on a chart that can be traded for material objects or a desired activity, such as a game or special time with a parent) and punishments for unacceptable behaviors (eg, time out, loss of a privilege, extra chores, or reduction in allowance). Acceptable and unacceptable behaviors should be clearly defined and measurable, and rewards and punishments should be spelled out in a contract drawn up with the child. The strongest behavioral interventions follow immediately after a behavior (eg, immediate praise when a child follows a command after the first time it was given). If rewards or punishments are used over time, parents and teachers must be creative in periodically varying the rewards and penalties. Management of overactive children who have difficulty focusing attention, following rules, and controlling impulses can be challenging for both parents and teachers. The best results come from praising and reinforcing positive behaviors and ignoring negative behaviors unless they are dangerous or intolerable. Using praising and ignoring in combination can be very successful. Parent commands should be clear and countable (eg, "You need to go upstairs to brush your teeth before the egg timer goes off in 3 minutes."). Because children with ADHD can have difficulty carrying out multistep commands, it is best to set them up for success by giving clear, doable, single-step commands. Behavior management in combination with medication management can be extremely effective. Potential benefits of behavioral therapy when used concurrently with medication include improved scores on some academic measures, improved behavior, and decreased anxiety symptoms. Interventions such as play therapy, psychotherapy, and cognitive therapy have no documented efficacy in managing core ADHD symptoms.

Educational Interventions

The pediatric practitioner can aid in the child's educational experience by contacting the child's teachers and attending school conferences. While most children with ADHD can be managed in the regular classroom, special education in a smaller, more focused setting may be indicated for behavioral or academic difficulties. Teachers can use specific strategies to help children with ADHD focus their attention and follow directions in the classroom (Box 113-3). Behavioral therapy should be integrated into the classroom. Teachers should focus on children's strengths and be careful not to embarrass them. Teachers who are most successful in working with children with ADHD are able to set firm limits and discipline children without anger or frustration, while at the same time remaining flexible enough to recognize when a change in tactics is necessary. Children with ADHD may be able to get needed classroom accommodations through Section 504 of the Americans with Disabilities Act, and children whose ADHD symptoms lead to significant learning deficits may qualify for an Individualized Education Plan (IEP) through the Individuals with Disabilities Educational Act (IDEA).

Box 113-3. Strategies for Managing Children With Attention-Deficit/Hyperactivity Disorder in the Classroom

- Seat children in the front of the classroom, where distractions can be minimized and teachers can see whether children are paying attention.
- Cue children secretly to remind them to refocus their attention.
- Give clear instructions and repeat them frequently.
- Shorten work periods by allowing children to get up and move around (eg, handing out papers, cleaning chalkboard).

Because children with ADHD are easily provoked into misbehavior and are prone to clashes with peers, they can also benefit from closer supervision in unstructured school areas such as the playground, cafeteria, halls, and bus. Programs designed to improve social competence and peer relationships (eg, group social skills training, therapeutic recreational activities) may also be helpful.

Pharmacotherapy

Research has shown that psychostimulant medication with and without behavioral therapy is efficacious in reducing the core symptoms of ADHD. Furthermore, there is some evidence that these effects translate into an increased ability to follow rules, improved classroom behavior, and improved relationships with peers and parents. Effects of stimulant medication on learning are not well studied. Caution should be exerted in treating children younger than 5 years with stimulant medication because effects on early brain development are unknown, efficacy is unpredictable, and adverse effects

are more frequent.

Psychostimulants are the most commonly used agents for ADHD and, by far, the most evidence-based. Currently available stimulants include short-acting (3–6 hours), intermediate-acting (6–8 hours), and long-acting (10–12 hours) formulations of methylphenidate and amphetamines (Box 113-4). Pemoline (Cylert) is rarely used because of the potential for fatal hepatotoxicity. Studies have found few, if any, differences between the efficacy of methylphenidate and dextroamphetamine, but some children will respond better to one or the other.

Stimulants affect behaviors within 30 minutes and affect attention (eg, for a school subject like math) within 1.5 hours after adminis-

Box 113-4. Stimulant Medications

Methylphenidate
- Short (Ritalin, Metadate, Methylin)
- Intermediate (Ritalin SR, Metadate ER, Methylin ER)
- Extended release (Concerta, Metadate CD, Ritalin LA, Focalin XR, and methylphenidate patch [Daytrana])

Amphetamine
- Short (Dexedrine, Dextrostat)
- Intermediate (Adderall, Dexedrine)
- Extended release (Adderall-XR)

tration. There is little evidence of tolerance to stimulants over time, but short-term tolerance occurs so that blood levels must increase during the day to maintain efficacy. Long-acting stimulants, such as Concerta, produce increasing plasma concentrations throughout the day, eliminate the need to take medication at school, and may persist during after-school homework time. A transdermal delivery system (Daytrana) is now available for children aged 6 to 12 years.

The most common side effects of stimulant medications are decreased appetite, stomachaches, headaches, delayed sleep onset, and jitteriness, occurring in 4% to 10% of children. Transient motor tics may occur while on the medication. At higher doses, stimulants may negatively influence height velocity. Dosing of stimulant medication is not based on weight, but rather on individual variation for optimal effects and minimal side effects. Researchers have found that children do considerably better on an optimal dose of stimulant medications, rather than the lowest dose that shows a clinical effect. For this reason, it is recommended that clinicians try multiple dosages of a single agent using a systematic method. For example, try Concerta 18, 36, 54 or Adderall XR 10, 20, 30 in 1-week blocks, and have the teacher and parent complete *DSM*-based scales, such as the Vanderbilt or Conners scales, at the end of each week. The clinician can then use these scales to develop a medication management plan with the family.

Once the medication dosage is stable, follow-up should occur at least every 3 months, with particular attention to improvement in targeted problems caused by ADHD symptoms, interim history, weight, height, blood pressure, and scales of clinical response from caregivers and teachers.

If a particular stimulant is not efficacious, the clinician should systematically try 1 or 2 other stimulants because more than 80% of children will respond to at least one of the stimulants tried. If 2 or 3 psychostimulants are not effective or produce unacceptable side effects, other medications can be used. Atomoxetine (Straterra) is a non-stimulant medication that selectively inhibits the norepinephrine transporter. Recent studies found that atomoxetine reduced ADHD symptoms, but not as effectively as extended-release stimulants. Atomoxetine is approved for children older than 6 years, has once-daily dosing, and often takes 1 to 6 weeks to produce effects. Tricyclic antidepressants and bupropion have shown some positive effects on ADHD symptoms. Modafinil is a non-stimulant wakefulness-promoting agent that has been shown to diminish symptoms of ADHD, but is not yet approved by the US Food and Drug Administration for ADHD because of concerns about Stevens-Johnson syndrome.

Complementary and alternative medicines, such as vitamins, dietary restrictions, and occupational therapy, are used by 54% of parents, but only 11% discuss these with their child's clinician. The Feingold diet eliminates artificial flavors, colors, or preservatives. While there is increasing recognition of subclinical neurobehavioral toxicity with low doses of environmental toxins, particularly in developing children, recommendations should emphasize prevention and additional research is necessary. Studies of self-regulation through biofeedback are promising, but again, further research is needed.

Prognosis

Attention-deficit/hyperactivity disorder is a chronic condition, persisting into adolescence in 60% to 80% of children. Studies have shown that, overall, adults who had childhood ADHD complete less schooling, hold lower-ranking occupations, have lower self-esteem and more social-skill deficits, and exhibit more antisocial behavior and alcohol and drug abuse. However, ADHD does not preclude attaining high educational and vocational goals, and more than half of adults with childhood ADHD no longer meet the full *DSM-IV* criteria. Hyperactivity usually greatly diminishes or resolves in high school or early adulthood. Attention problems and impulsivity may continue to varying degrees. Adults with ADHD can choose occupations that match their strengths and minimize reliance on weaker areas. While some adults with ADHD choose to continue medication, others may function well without medication.

CASE RESOLUTION

In the case history presented at the beginning of this chapter, the boy's mother expresses concerns about her son's behavior. She describes symptoms of attention-deficit/hyperactivity disorder. The boy is referred to his primary care clinician for diagnostic evaluation, which should include a full history, physical examination, and an assessment from his teachers at school.

Selected References

American Academy of Pediatrics Committee on Quality Improvement, Subcommittee on Attention-Deficit/Hyperactivity Disorder. Clinical practice guideline: diagnosis and evaluation of the child with attention-deficit/hyperactivity disorder. *Pediatrics.* 2000;105:1158–1170

American Academy of Pediatrics Subcommittee on Attention-Deficit/Hyperactivity Disorder, Committee on Quality Improvement. Clinical practice guideline: treatment of the school-aged child with attention-deficit/hyperactivity disorder. *Pediatrics.* 2001;108:1033–1044

American Psychiatric Association. *Diagnostic and Statistical Manual of Mental Disorders.* 4th ed. Washington, DC: American Psychiatric Association; 1994

Brown RT, Amler RW, Freeman W, et al. Treatment of attention-deficit/hyperactivity disorder: overview of the evidence. *Pediatrics.* 2005;115:e749–e757

Chan E, Rappaport LA, Kemper KJ. Complementary and alternative therapies in childhood attention and hyperactivity problems. *J Dev Behav Pediatr.* 2003;24:4–8

Khan SA, Faraone SV. The genetics of ADHD: a literature review of 2005. *Curr Psychiatry Rep.* 2006;8:393–397

MTA Cooperative Group. A 14-month randomized clinical trial of treatment strategies for attention-deficit/hyperactivity disorder. The MTA Cooperative Group. Multimodal Treatment Study of Children with ADHD. *Arch Gen Psychiatry.* 1999;56:1073–1086

Reiff MI, Stein MT. Attention-deficit/hyperactivity disorder evaluation and diagnosis: a practical approach in office practice. *Pediatr Clin North Am.* 2003;50:1019–1048

Rushton JL, Fant KE, Clark SJ. Use of practice guidelines in the primary care of children with attention-deficit/hyperactivity disorder. *Pediatrics.* 2004;114:e23–e28

Schneider H, Eisenberg D. Who receives a diagnosis of attention-deficit/hyperactivity disorder in the United States elementary school population? *Pediatrics.* 2006;117:e601–e609

Spencer TJ, Biederman J, Wilens TE, Faraone SV. Overview and neurobiology of attention-deficit/hyperactivity disorder. *J Clin Psychiatry.* 2002;63(suppl 12):3–9

Stein MT, Perrin JM. Diagnosis and treatment of ADHD in school-age children in primary care settings: a synopsis of the AAP practice guidelines. *Pediatr Rev.* 2003;24:92–98

Wilens TE. Mechanism of action of agents used in attention-deficit/hyperactivity disorder. *J Clin Psychiatry.* 2006;67(suppl 8):32–38

Wilens TE, Prince JB, Spencer TJ, Biederman J. Stimulants and sudden death: what is a physician to do? *Pediatrics.* 2006;118:1215–1219

Wolraich ML, Wibbelsman CJ, Brown TE, et al. Attention-deficit/hyperactivity disorder among adolescents: a review of the diagnosis, treatment, and clinical implications. *Pediatrics.* 2005;115:1734–1746

Psychopharmacology in Children

Robin Steinberg-Epstein, MD, and Kenneth W. Steinhoff, MD

CASE STUDY

An 8-year-old girl has been diagnosed with high-functioning autism. The local developmental-behavioral pediatrician has recommended treating her anxiety and inattention with atomoxetine. The girl's mom is very hesitant. She trusts you and wants your opinion.

Questions

1. How does one assess the safety and appropriateness of psychotropic medications?
2. What kind of blood tests are used to maximize safe administration and how often are they performed?
3. What is the evidence that psychotropic medications are overprescribed?
4. What are the usual side effects of commonly used psychotropic medications?

Psychopharmacologic agents are now used with greater frequency in the pediatric population. Approximately 10% of children and adolescents carry a psychiatric diagnosis. Unlike antibiotics or other medications used in children, psychopharmacologic agents are used daily and for extended periods. Furthermore, it is important to recognize that there is a dearth of evidence-based information supporting the use of many medications in children, including psychotropics. Therefore, most of these medications are used in an **off-label** fashion. The medical community must then rely on published data (often in adult subjects), clinical experience, and expert consensus to guide medication choice, dose, and management. This often provokes parental anxiety and sparks numerous concerns from families who don't understand that the US Food and Drug Administration (FDA) label limits claims a manufacturer can make but does not limit a medication's use. Furthermore, families are often anxious because clinicians rely almost exclusively on history and structured behavioral observation, which is the most important "test" for most of these disorders. Unfortunately, there is a national shortage of pediatric subspecialists trained to choose, monitor, and manage these medications for children. It is, therefore, necessary for pediatricians to be familiar with the various medication classes and the controversies facing families of affected children.

Pediatricians need to understand the principles guiding the use of these medications and to become familiar with some of the more frequently used psychopharmacologic agents. The most used classes of medication in children include **stimulants, selective norepinephrine reuptake inhibitors (SNRIs), selective serotonin reuptake inhibitors (SSRIs),** and **atypical neuroleptics,** also known as **serotonin-dopamine antagonists (SDAs).** This information can also be useful in helping families navigate this confusing maze.

The decision to use psychopharmacologic agents should not be made without considerable thought. Medication should be an integral part of a comprehensive treatment program that addresses the academic, behavioral, medical, and developmental needs of the child. The decision to place a child on any agent should be based on significant dysfunction as well as discussion and full disclosure of potential risks and benefits with both parents and child. Rating scales should be employed and target symptoms identified as a means of monitoring medication benefit. A medication trial, once undertaken, should be carefully monitored, methodically addressing both adverse events and effectiveness. It is generally best to change one agent or dose at a time, followed by structured observation (eg, rating scale[s]) to determine the effect of the change. Therefore, one usually begins with **monotherapy,** optimizes the dose, and assesses risks and benefits before developing a more complex regimen. Such a trial necessitates frequent visits and discussion with the administering physician. Given current scientific information and clinical experience, the use of psychopharmacologic agents in young children (<5 years) should be reserved for extraordinary circumstances.

It should come as no surprise that children are not little adults. Pharmacokinetics in children is affected by increased rates of metabolism in their relatively larger livers, a faster glomerular filtration, and variable fatty tissues. Some children, therefore, require a larger dose than those used for adults. Conversely, perhaps due to size, fat distribution, and other explanations, a much smaller, and seemingly ineffective, dose may be enough. There is little correlation between blood level and treatment response for most agents. Furthermore, some medications have a duration of effects that well exceed their **half-life** (atomoxetine), but for others (such as stimulants) their effect diminishes despite having a significant blood level. Additionally, for most agents (such as stimulants and SDAs) there is no correlation with milligrams per kilogram. Frequent clinical monitoring and communication with parent and family are vital to understanding medication benefit and adherence.

Psychostimulants

Psychostimulants (see Chapter 113) are the most studied psychotropics used in pediatrics. These medications are used to treat the hyperactivity, inattention, and impulsivity seen with **attention-deficit/hyperactivity disorder (ADHD),** and disturbances of attention seen in other disorders (**autism, traumatic brain injury, depression,** etc). Stimulants are also used in the treatment of **narcolepsy.** Over the past decade many new delivery systems have been developed with differing durations of action, which help to cater to the specific lifestyle needs of the patient. Much work has been done to determine optimal blood level delivery leading to the most consistent effect. Overall, the duration of action and clinical efficacy are more relevant than the blood level in this class of medication.

The mechanism of action of these agents is to increase **dopamine** and **norepinephrine** in the synapse. Overall, this enhances activity in the **prefrontal cortex** of the brain responsible for attention, focus, and **executive function** (organization and planning).

There is substantial evidence in multisite, double-blind, placebo-controlled studies (eg, Multimodal Treatment Study of Children With Attention-Deficit/Hyperactivity Disorder) to support the first-line use of these medications in the treatment of school-aged children, adolescents, and adults with ADHD. There is evolving evidence (Preschool ADHD Treatment Study) to support the use of these drugs in preschoolers. There is a growing body of evidence to support their use in autism, albeit at lower doses and with a lower threshold for side effects.

Parents have a variety of concerns related to stimulants, much of which is propagated by the media; however, NOT treating ADHD results in significant comorbidities and risks for negative outcomes. Substance abuse has long been linked with stimulant medication. In reality it is ADHD that is linked with substance abuse. Large, reproducible studies show that using medication during adolescence reduces the risk for substance abuse from more than 3 times normal to only slightly elevated compared with controls without ADHD. The potential is that treatment with medication will reduce a whole host of other potential negative outcomes.

Nonetheless, several areas of controversy exist, and often become a primary focus for hesitant parents. Understanding the facts can help to demystify these medications for parents. For example, it had been suggested that stimulants were responsible for an increase in sudden unexpected deaths. This would obviously raise discomfort for any parent. However, scrutiny over these statistics by the FDA actually revealed a lower incidence of sudden unexpected deaths in those

on stimulants compared with the unmedicated population. Those who died tended to have an underlying cardiac defect. This led to the FDA recommendation (2006) that those persons with **preexisting cardiac conditions** not use stimulants and those families with a history of cardiac structural defects or sudden unexpected death receive an echocardiogram and cardiac clearance prior to starting medication. **Height suppression** has also historically been raised as a concern with these medications. Numerous studies have tried to answer this question. Unfortunately, the jury remains undecided. But parents can be reassured that if there is height suppression it seems to be minimal, in the range of 1.5 cm. It is better to have a high school graduate who is slightly shorter than a taller dropout. Finally, parents believe that their children will be "zombies" on medication. Children who are overmedicated can appear glassy-eyed and overly passive, but good communication and interaction between families and doctors will quickly alleviate this problem. Additional information regarding these medications may be found in Chapter 113.

Selective Norepinephrine Reuptake Inhibitors

The SNRIs presently include one medication that is frequently used in children: **atomoxetine** (Strattera). Atomoxetine is used in both the treatment of ADHD and for the **inattention** and **anxiety** associated with autism.

The mechanism of action for atomoxetine is to block the reuptake of norepinephrine in the synapse. This may have a direct effect on enhancing the signal-to-noise ratio in the brain and may also ultimately lead to an increase in dopamine in the prefrontal cortex of the brain. Unlike stimulant medications, atomoxetine avoids the nucleus accumbens so that it has no abuse liability.

Atomoxetine was originally studied as an antidepressant, but early investigation did not yield robust antidepressant effects. Marketed as providing "continuous symptom relief," a careful duration of action study shows little effect on core ADHD symptoms after 9 hours, but some possible other small effects (compliance) may last slightly longer. Its attractiveness stems from its identity as an FDA-approved non-stimulant. Although usually less effective than stimulants, it has a different side-effect profile and may show slight mood benefits.

Research shows that this medication, which is FDA approved for ADHD, is effective in treating symptoms of this disorder for a given individual, but in groups of people is not as effective as the stimulant medications. Atomoxetine generally has a 60% response rate (measured by 25% reduction in ADHD ratings) compared with a 70% to 80% response (measured by 30% reduction in ADHD ratings) found in stimulant medications. Furthermore, 3 different head-to-head studies with stimulants have demonstrated atomoxetine as less effective on average; however, some individual patients do well with this medication. It should especially be considered in cases of stimulant failure (poor tolerance and/or poor effect of a trial on a methylphenidate preparation and a trial on an amphetamine preparation), worries about substance use and diversion, exacerbation of tic disorder with stimulants, and the presence of comorbid anxiety or autism.

This medication is not without **side effects.** Response to this medicine is more like that to an antidepressant, in that it may take 4 to 6 weeks to see the full impact of a particular dose. The dosage range is 0.5 mg/kg to 1.8 mg/kg. Those on the autistic spectrum tend to respond at lower doses and with a lower threshold for adverse side effects.

There have been 2 reports of a serious **idiosyncratic reaction** suggesting liver failure. Both patients were on FDA-approved doses of atomoxetine for several months. Both had vomiting and elevated liver enzymes. These findings resolved off medication and returned with reexposure to the drug. This led to an FDA warning to consider potential liver failure in a vomiting patient on atomoxetine.

In consideration of both the stimulants and SNRIs, the American Academy of Pediatrics and the American Academy of Child and Adolescent Psychiatry recommend stimulants and SNRIs as first-line treatments for ADHD. There is no indication that blood or urine tests need to be monitored for either class of medication. Improvement, adverse event, and adherence monitoring using rating scales should occur regularly—at least every 3 months (once dose and agent have been optimized). Stimulants and SNRIs have their best results when administered 7 days a week and without large breaks. Longitudinal studies suggest that while some symptoms may resolve over time, significant impairment from even a small number of symptoms persists into adulthood for 80% to 90% of those diagnosed with ADHD. Therefore, many people will continue on medication for a number of years. Annually, it is beneficial to reoptimize doses and agents. As children grow larger they often need higher doses. However, as compensatory mechanisms develop and some symptoms subside, some patients may require less medication. The value of "holidays" from medications has no established intrinsic value on their own and should be undertaken for children with significant medication side effects such as substantial weight loss. If a parent is requesting a **drug holiday** it is a signal that the parent is not convinced of the value of the medication (usually outside of the academic setting), and careful discussion should ensue as to whether the parent is discounting the value of the medication, the patient is having subtle yet troubling side effects, or the medication at any dose is not helpful with concerning symptoms. A drug holiday should be offered for one period a year to ensure that the medications are still required. Atomoxetine, once stopped, needs time to rebuild in the system.

Selective Serotonin Reuptake Inhibitors

The SSRIs (Table 114-1) are frequently used in children and adolescents to treat a variety of depression- and anxiety-based symptoms (Box 114-1). Similar to the SNRIs, the SSRIs block reuptake of serotonin after it is released into the synapse, thereby enhancing serotonin activity in the synapse. Empirical evidence has established their benefit in the treatment of depressive disorders and anxiety disorders.

Medication is NOT a substitute for therapeutic support. As a matter of fact, most clinical guidelines recommend psychotherapy as first-line treatment for most anxiety and depressive disorders. Biological intervention should only be undertaken if psychotherapy progress is minimal or impairment severe. Empirical evidence suggests that children and adolescents generally do best when both forms of treatment are in place. **Obsessive-compulsive disorder** (OCD) is a unique anxiety disorder that typically requires higher doses of SSRIs but is also responsive to a specific form of cognitive-behavioral therapy that includes exposure response prevention.

Medications are chosen based on side-effect profile and half-life. Due to a significant placebo effect and a lack of multiple, large, highly powered studies in children, only a few have any FDA approval in children (Table 114-1). There are numerous studies that may not meet strict scientific criteria, but taken together with vast clinical experience and consensus imply reasonably well-tolerated and beneficial effects of these medications. Studies have consistently found SSRIs to be more effective and safer than the tricyclic antidepressants as a treatment for depression.

These drugs are metabolized via the liver through the **cytochrome P450 system.** There are individual enzyme variations that lead to variable metabolism of any of the many medications that travel through these pathways. Overwhelming this system may lead

---

Box 114-1. Disorders Treated by Selective Serotonin Reuptake Inhibitors

- Depression
- Obsessive-compulsive disorder
- Generalized anxiety disorder
- Separation anxiety disorder
- Panic disorder
- Selective mutism
- Post-traumatic stress disorder
- Autism
- Bulimia

Table 114-1. Selective Serotonin Reuptake Inhibitors

Generic	Product	FDA Pediatric Approval	Suggested Pediatric Dose, mg	Half-life	Time Steady State
Fluoxetine	Prozac	Depression/OCD	2.5–60	4–6 d	28–35 d
Sertraline	Zoloft	OCD	12.5–200	26 h	5–7 d
Fluvoxamine	Luvox	OCD	12.5–100 bid	15 h	5–7 d
Paroxetine	Paxil	None	5–30	21 h	5–10 d
Citalopram	Celexa	None	5–40	36 h	7 d
Escitalopram	Lexapro	None	2.5–20	27–32 h	7 d

Abbreviations: FDA, Food and Drug Administration; OCD, obsessive-compulsive disorder; bid, twice a day.

to inhibition and buildup of medications or facilitated rapid metabolism of others. Thus monitoring of all medications metabolized via this pathway is necessary. Reduced metabolism of the SSRIs may lead to **serotonin syndrome**—a relatively rare response to a flood of serotonin—presenting with confusion, hypomania, restlessness, diaphoresis, shivering, tremor, hyperreflexia, and diarrhea. This syndrome often goes unrecognized and these patients may find their way to a pediatrician's office or emergency department (ED). Occasionally, the combination of an SSRI with an SDA or stimulant may precipitate such a response.

Many children with anxiety or depression go on to experience intermittent exacerbations throughout life. This does not mean that they should stay on these medications forever. Present recommendations support an initial 6- to 12-month treatment period with the SSRI that provided response. If the symptoms return after discontinuation, the next trial should last 2 years. Finally, if the symptoms again return, then this suggests longer-term treatment. Occasionally, symptoms will not respond the next time the same agent is used.

Selective serotonin reuptake inhibitors are generally well tolerated with mild transient side effects such as gastrointestinal symptoms, headache, increased motor activity, or insomnia. One needs to monitor for less common side effects like disinhibition, a phenomenon of increased impulsive behaviors in association with SSRIs that is usually dose related. Those with autism are particularly susceptible to this response.

There are no specific recommendations on dose other than to start low and go slow. Typically effects may be seen between 1 and 4 weeks. The value of increasing the dose (except in the case of OCD) versus continuing on at the same dose versus changing agents is not clear until a patient has been treated for at least a month. See suggested dosage ranges in Table 114-1.

Some have suggested that these medications are **addictive.** This relates to the appearance of withdrawal symptoms on sudden cessation. Stopping medications such as paroxetine and sertraline that have a shorter half-life abruptly may lead to flu-like symptoms including body aches and vomiting. A child may present to their primary care provider with flu-like symptoms, not recognizing a connection between the symptoms and having skipped their medications for several days. The onset and severity of symptoms is proportional to the dose and duration of use and inversely proportional to the half-life. Occasionally, these children end up hospitalized for vomiting and dehydration. Simply readministering their skipped dose alleviates the symptoms. A planned taper should take 4 to 6 weeks.

Again, controversy follows these medications. In 2004 the FDA created a black box warning advising that children and adolescents on SSRIs should be monitored for worsening depression, agitation, and suicidality, particularly in the early stages of treatment. This warning came out of an FDA meta-analysis showing an increased risk of suicidal ideation in depressed teens soon after starting the medications. No completed suicides occurred. This prompted an FDA recommendation to see children placed on SSRIs weekly for a month,

then bimonthly for a month, then monthly and, ultimately, at longer regular intervals. It is important to recognize that the overall rates of suicide have only decreased since the introduction of these medications and are now increasing with their decreased use. It is important to monitor each individual patient carefully, but the potential for benefit usually outweighs the risks. These concerns should NOT detract from the importance of these medications. An increase in suicidality has not been noted in adolescents with isolated anxiety or autism. Selective serotonin reuptake inhibitors serve a vital role in helping children paralyzed by anxiety, obsession, and depression to lead near normal lives.

Atypical Antipsychotics (Serotonergic Dopamine Antagonists)

The **atypical antipsychotics** or **second-generation antipsychotics** (Table 114-2), also known as **SDAs,** are medications with dopamine D2 and serotonin 5-hydroxytryptamine type 2 antagonism. These newer medications offer a lower risk of both **extrapyramidal side effects** like **dystonia, akathisia**—a feeling of restlessness, tremor, tardive dyskinesia, and hyperprolactinemia compared with the conventional antipsychotics.

Table 114-2. Serotonin-Dopamine Antagonists (Atypical Antipsychotics)			
Generic	*Product*	*FDA Pediatric Approval*	*Dose*
Risperidone	Risperdol	Agitation with autism	.25–10 mg/d
Olanzepine	Zyprexa	None	2.5–20 mg/d
Quetiapine	Seroquel	None	12.5–250 mg bid
Ziprasodone	Geodon	None	20–120 mg/d
Aripiprazole	Abilify	None	2.5–30 mg/d

Abbreviations: FDA, Food and Drug Administration; bid, twice a day.

While often used off-label, these medications are incorporated into best practice clinical guidelines for psychotic depression, schizophrenia, bipolar disorder, oppositional defiant disorder, conduct disorder, agitation in mental retardation, Tourette syndrome, stuttering, and autism. The only diagnosis for which an atypical antipsychotic has pediatric approval is agitation associated with autism. Therefore, while these medications often lack enough empiric evidence to be validated for all the indications mentioned, clinical consensus by experts recommend judicious use in treating children with serious mental illness after other forms of intervention have failed or in cases of severe psychosis or aggression. These medications should NOT be used to promote weight gain, as a sedative or sleep aid, or as a treatment for ADHD.

Medications are chosen based on clinical experience and side-effect profile. These medications are not innocuous. They must be used with full disclosure to parents. The most common side effects are listed in Box 114-2. The severity of some of the side effects deserve discussion. The SDAs, with possibly the exception of aripiprazole,

Box 114-2. Serotonin-Dopamine Antagonists: Potential Side Effects

- Weight gain
- Sedation
- Dizziness
- Hypotension
- Prolongation of QT interval
- Metabolic syndrome (hyper-glycemia and increased lipids)
- Constipation
- Dry mouth
- Headache
- Cataracts (in dogs)
- Increased liver function tests
- Decreased triiodothyronine, thyroxine
- Extrapyramidal side effects
- Akathisia (sense of restlessness)

have caused increases in glucose and lipids, otherwise known as *metabolic syndrome.*

There have been transient elevations of **prolactin** among recipients of these medications. The clinical significance of this increase is unclear. Weight gain frequently accompanies these medications and must be monitored. A prolonged QT interval on electrocardiogram (ECG) is rarely noted and has not been associated with death, but remains a clinical concern.

Risperidone is the best studied medication of its class for children. It has the only pediatric FDA indication among these medications—to treat agitation associated with autism. However, the studies on which its approval hinged exposed side effects, most notably weight gain. Therefore, anticipatory counseling regarding diet management is routinely recommended. Another important finding indicated that a small but significant number of children were successfully able to stop treatment after 6 months, suggesting that a trial off medication may be warranted in those successfully treated for 6 months.

Neuroleptic malignant syndrome is a rare, potentially life-threatening complication of neuroleptics that is extremely unlikely with the newer generation of medication. However, due to its lethality and its potential presentation to a pediatric office or ED this entity should be mentioned. Neuroleptic malignant syndrome is characterized by hyperthermia, autonomic instability, diaphoresis, "lead pipe" rigidity, increased creatine phosphokinase due to rhabdomyolysis, and delirium. It may occur at any point during treatment with these medications.

There is no set agreement on appropriate monitoring of use of these medications in children. Most conservative suggestions include regularly checking complete blood count, liver function tests, triiodothyronine, thyroxine, prolactin, and fasting glucose and lipid levels, especially in overweight children or in families with a history of diabetes mellitus. An ECG prior to starting medications, 1 month after baseline and biannually, are frequently suggested to monitor the QT interval. Children are often sent to the primary care provider to obtain these tests and to monitor for clouding of the cornea, which may occur with use of typical antipsychotics and has been found in dogs on such medications.

As with any medication, psychotropic agents are sometimes misprescribed. By and large, however, psychopharmacologic agents are still underused in the treatment of many disorders. Hopefully, new and ongoing research will help physicians recognize mental illness in children and substantiate and refine the use of such medications in their care.

Careful thought and discussion of target symptoms as well as side effects will help physicians choose the best medication and treatment plan. It will also prepare parents to observe both the positive and negative response to medication.

While this chapter goes into significant detail on side effects, it is critical to understand that the diseases being treated are often incapacitating. Informed consent and parent/child involvement are vital in medication choice. Pediatricians have an extremely influential voice in supporting compliance. Therefore, knowledgeable guidance is crucial in helping parents make an uncomfortable and difficult decision that may ultimately lead to dramatic improvements in quality of life.

CASE RESOLUTION

You empathize with the parents over this decision but are able to explain that this medication is a reasonable and safe one to try. The patient starts the medication and experiences some nausea in the first few days. With your reassurance, this resolves. Her mom calls a few weeks later to thank you for your advice and to let you know that while her daughter still has difficulties from the autism, she seems to be somewhat less anxious and is functioning better at school.

Selected References

American Academy of Pediatrics Subcommittee on Attention-Deficit/Hyperactivity Disorder and Committee on Quality Improvement. Clinical practice guideline: treatment of the school-aged child with attention-deficit/hyperactivity disorder. *Pediatrics.* 2001;108:1033–1044

Filipek PA, Steinberg-Epstein R, Book TM. Intervention for autism spectrum disorders. *NeuroRx.* 2006;3:207–216

Greenhill L, Kollins S, Abikoff H, et al. Efficacy and safety of immediate-release methylphenidate treatment for preschool children with ADHD. *J Am Acad Child Adolesc Psychiatry.* 2006;45:1284–1293

March J, Silva S, Petrycki S, et al. Fluoxetine, cognitive-behavioral therapy, and their combination for adolescents with depression: Treatment for Adolescents With Depression Study (TADS) randomized controlled trial. *JAMA.* 2004;292:807–820

McCracken JT, McGough J, Shah B, et al. Risperidone in children with autism and serious behavior problems. *N Engl J Med.* 2002;347:314–321

MTA Cooperative Group. A 14-month randomized clinical trial of treatment strategies for attention-deficit/hyperactivity disorder. *Arch Gen Psychiatry.* 1999;56:1073–1086

Pediatric OCD Treatment Study (POTS) Team. Cognitive-behavior therapy, sertraline, and their combination for children and adolescents with obsessive-compulsive disorder: the Pediatric OCD Treatment Study (POTS) randomized controlled trial. *JAMA.* 2004;292:1969–1976

Pliszka SR. AACAP Workgroup on Quality Issues: practice parameters for the assessment and treatment of children and adolescents with attention deficit hyperactivity disorder. *J Adolesc Child Psychiatry.* 2007;46:894–921

Sadock B, Sadock V. *Kaplan and Sadock's Synopsis of Psychiatry.* 9th ed. Philadelphia, PA: Lippincott Williams & Wilkins; 2003

www.fda.gov/ohrms/dockets/ac/06/slides/2006-4212S1-01-01-FDAMannheim.ppt

Physical Abuse

Sara T. Stewart, MD

CASE STUDY

A 6-month-old male infant arrives at the emergency department after becoming limp and nonresponsive at home. The mother states that her son was fine when she left him in the care of her boyfriend before going to the store for cigarettes. When she returned 1 hour later, he was asleep, but then he seized and stopped breathing. The infant is being ventilated by bag-valve-mask ventilation. On examination, the infant is pale and limp. The heart rate is 100/min and the blood pressure is 90/30 mm Hg. The only abnormality is the presence of bilateral retinal hemorrhages.

Questions

1. What are the major lethal injuries associated with physical abuse of children?
2. What are the types of injuries seen in physically abused children?
3. What are the presenting complaints of children with head injuries?
4. What are the legal obligations of physicians in the area of child abuse?

Physical child abuse was first described in the pediatric literature in 1962 by Kempe et al in their classic paper on the **battered child syndrome.** Child abuse or maltreatment takes many forms, including physical abuse; **failure to thrive** (Chapter 117); **sexual abuse** (Chapter 116); **emotional abuse; prenatal exposure to substances** such as drugs and alcohol (Chapter 118); and **Munchausen syndrome by proxy,** a complex disorder in which parents confabulate or create a medical condition in their children.

The nature and extent of inflicted injuries are variable and may include **bruises, burns, fractures, lacerations, internal hemorrhage,** and **ruptures.** Physicians must be aware of the legal obligations related to the suspicion of child abuse. They must assess the nature of the injuries, initiate appropriate medical therapy, and determine if the history offered is consistent with the medical findings.

Epidemiology

It is estimated that the rate of childhood victimization in the United States is 12 per 1,000, and that approximately 15% to 20% of these children suffer some form of physical abuse. Certain factors are associated with physical abuse. Most victims are young children; two-thirds are younger than 3 years and one-third are younger than 6 months. Caring for young children is frequently demanding, so crying infants and toilet-training toddlers are particularly at risk for abuse. Factors such as **lower socioeconomic class, substance abuse, poor parenting skills,** and **domestic violence** place children at increased risk for abuse.

Clinical Presentation

Children who have been physically abused present with injuries that range from non-severe to lethal (Dx Box). Visible bruises, **bites,** and burns may be noted. Children may also have symptoms related to fractures, such as crying or refusal to walk or move an extremity. More severely injured children may present with seizures, apnea, shock, or cardiopulmonary arrest.

Dx Physical Abuse

- Bruises
- Bites
- Burns
- Fractures
- Intracranial hemorrhage
- Intraabdominal hemorrhage
- Retinal hemorrhage
- History that changes
- Injuries not explained by history

Pathophysiology

Injuries in children who experience physical abuse are the result of direct trauma inflicted on the children. Abusive parents often have unrealistic expectations of their children, leading to frustration and abuse when the child does not meet the expectations. Parents who have often been victims of abuse themselves know only corporal punishment as a disciplinary modality. These parents often exhibit poor impulse control; they do not intend to harm their children but desire to alter their children's behavior. As a result, sometimes the outcome is unexpected.

Head injuries, the most deadly form of abuse, may result from either a direct blow to the head or from rotational head movement (eg, shaking). Classically, a crying infant is vigorously shaken and suffers **diffuse axonal injury** or **intracranial hemorrhage.** In particular, subdural hemorrhage may occur from rupture of the bridging veins. The infant may also become apneic either during or after the trauma. Seizures, cerebral edema, hypoxic brain injury, and retinal hemorrhages may also occur. Such injuries are frequently associated with a fatal outcome or long-term damage to the central nervous system.

Abdominal trauma is the second most common cause of fatal child abuse and is typically due to a direct blow to the abdomen. Skeletal fractures result from multiple different types of traumatic forces to the bones. Rib fractures are most classically associated with the head trauma of shaking and are due to compression of the ribs by the hands that are holding the infant or child.

Differential Diagnosis

When evaluating children with physical injuries, the major differentiation is the distinguishing of injuries that are **intentional** or **abuse-related** from those that are **unintentional.** Practitioners should be suspicious of changing histories, histories that are inconsistent with the injuries sustained, and histories that do not match the developmental capabilities of the child. Unwitnessed injuries in young children, particularly pre-ambulatory infants, should also be suspect.

Bruises, burns, and fractures may be intentional or unintentional. Normal ambulatory children sustain bruises over bony prominences such as the forehead, elbows, and shins with unintentional, accidental trauma. Bruises over soft areas such as the thighs, cheeks, or the pinnae of the ear suggest inflicted trauma. Injuries to the oral mucosa may result from efforts at forced feeding or occlusion of the mouth in an effort to silence crying. **Retinal hemorrhages** in infants most often result from intentional head trauma, such as shaking. They may also be due to other medical conditions that can usually be discerned from the history and physical examination and by consultation with an ophthalmologist (Box 115-1).

Box 115-1. Causes of Retinal Hemorrhages

- Inflicted head trauma
- Unintentional head trauma (rare)
- Birth trauma
- Retinopathy of prematurity
- Blood dyscrasias
- Leukemia/lymphoma
- Meningitis
- Vasculitis
- Papilledema
- Hypertension
- Cytomegalovirus retinitis
- High-altitude illness
- Carbon monoxide toxicity

Children may be intentionally burned by being immersed in hot water or having hot objects such as irons or cigarettes held against them. Children who are immersed in hot water develop circumferential burns that may envelop an entire extremity. Such a burn is usually in a glove or stocking pattern, or in a doughnut pattern on the buttocks. These burns are distinct from splash or spill burns, which take on an irregular drip pattern.

Long bone fractures (especially humerus and femur) should be suspect, particularly in preverbal or pre-ambulatory children. Certain fractures, such as **metaphyseal chip, rib, sternum,** and **scapula fractures,** are highly suggestive of inflicted trauma.

Numerous medical conditions may mimic abuse. Bullous impetigo may resemble burns. A coagulopathy may lead to multiple bruises. Leukemia, thrombocytopenia, and aplastic anemia are also associated with bruising. Osteogenesis imperfecta may result in multiple fractures. Bone cysts and osteoporosis due to inactivity from multiple causes (eg, cerebral palsy, paralysis, and meningomyelocele) may predispose to the development of pathologic fractures.

Evaluation

Children who present with injuries need to be evaluated with a careful history and complete physical examination. Infants with altered mental status, apnea, or seizures should be evaluated in a similar manner because their symptoms may be secondary to intracranial injury.

History

The history should focus on an explanation for the medical findings (Questions Box). Children should be interviewed alone if they are of an appropriate age. Physicians should determine if other risk factors, such as domestic violence or substance abuse, are present.

Questions

Physical Abuse

- What caused the injury?
- Was the child healthy until the injury occurred?
- Has the child sustained similar injuries in the past?
- Is there a family history of any conditions that would account for easy bruisability or fragility of the bones (eg, von Willebrand disease, osteogenesis imperfecta)?
- Is the child developmentally normal? What are the child's motor skills?
- Who was with the child when the injury occurred?
- What was done immediately after the injury? Was medical care sought?

Physical Examination

A child's state of hygiene and growth parameters should be noted, and the physical examination should be comprehensive. The location, color, and size of bruises, abrasions, lacerations, or other skin trauma should be recorded. Dating of bruises is imprecise because the degradation rate of hemoglobin, and therefore the rate of color change, is influenced by the depth and extent of the bruise and by the child's health and nutritional status. Large blue-brown spots, which occur commonly on the back and buttocks in darker-skinned children, are termed *mongolian spots.* These should not be mistaken for bruises.

Medical providers should also note any skin findings that resemble characteristic patterns of inflicted skin trauma, such as slap marks to the face or gag marks around the mouth. Pinch marks can also be seen on the genitalia of a toilet-training toddler. Belts, cords, and blunt objects may leave patterned marks on the skin after a child is hit with the object. Bite marks are composed of indentations, bruises, or breaks in the skin that reflect the configuration of teeth that is unique to the perpetrator (Figure 115-1). Inflicted burns may also assume a characteristic pattern depending on the mechanism of injury (Figure 115-2).

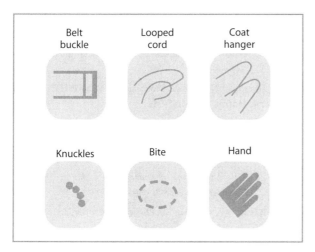

Figure 115-1. Patterned bruises associated with inflicted trauma.

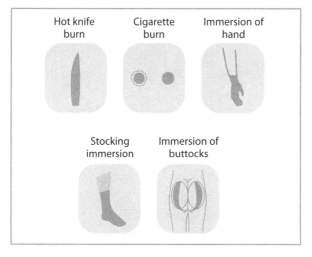

Figure 115-2. Patterned burns associated with inflicted trauma.

The extremities, skull, and ribcage should be carefully examined to detect the presence of skeletal trauma. Findings such as decreased range of movement, tenderness, swelling, redness, or bruising may be associated with an underlying bone fracture. These findings are not always present, however, particularly if the fracture is in its healing stages.

Practitioners should be aware that infants with head or abdominal injuries may also present with no external signs of trauma. Those with head injury may have seizures, apnea, vomiting, increased crying, or altered mental status, often with no explanation as to the etiology. The retina should be evaluated for hemorrhages in these children. Children with abdominal injuries may present in shock or with symptoms such as vomiting, abdominal pain, or distention. They may have a rigid abdomen with guarding and decreased bowel sounds. Inflicted abdominal injuries may include hematomas of the bowel wall, bowel perforations, or trauma to the liver, spleen, pancreas, or kidneys.

Laboratory Tests

Children who present with bruises should have a hematologic assessment with a complete blood count (CBC) and differential (including a platelet count), a prothrombin time, and a partial thromboplastin time. Cultures from lesions may help differentiate infection from burn injury.

Children with suspected abdominal trauma should be evaluated with a CBC, urinalysis, liver function studies, amylase, and lipase. These studies may demonstrate anemia secondary to hemorrhage, hematuria from renal injury, or elevated liver or pancreatic enzymes due to solid organ trauma (see Chapter 51).

Imaging Studies

Children younger than 2 years who are suspected victims of physical abuse are at the highest risk of having an inflicted skeletal fracture. For this reason, this group of patients should be evaluated with a radiographic skeletal survey to identify any acute or healing fractures that may be present. Bone scintigraphy is also useful in detecting occult fractures and may be useful in conjunction with the skeletal survey.

If there is concern that children have suffered non-accidental head trauma, they should be evaluated with a computed tomography (CT) scan and magnetic resonance imaging. The combination of these modalities is particularly helpful in dating intracranial bleeding (see Chapter 52).

Abdominal x-rays may demonstrate air-fluid levels from dysmotility, distended loops of bowel, or free air under the diaphragm. Abdominal and pelvic CT scans may show bowel or solid organ disruption or hemorrhage.

Management

The management of children who are suspected victims of abuse focuses on medical stabilization and psychosocial investigation. Injuries should be treated in the appropriate manner. Children with extensive internal injuries frequently require admission to an intensive care unit. Consultation with appropriate surgical specialists in neurosurgery, orthopedics, or general surgery should be obtained.

The psychosocial assessment of the family often requires the expertise of a social worker. Further assessment may require an in-home evaluation such as that conducted by law enforcement or child protective services. All 50 states require that physicians who suspect child abuse report these suspicions to appropriate agencies. Physicians do not have to be certain of the abuse.

These mandated agencies pursue the investigation. Children may be removed from their homes and placed in foster homes to ensure their safety. Cases of suspected abuse are usually evaluated in court to determine the safety of the children's environment, the ability of parents to care for their children, and the criminal culpability of suspected perpetrators. Physicians may be expected to offer testimony in such hearings.

Prognosis

The prognosis is variable. Some children succumb to inflicted injuries before coming to medical attention, and others sustain permanent neurologic damage. Even in cases in which the physical well-being of children is ensured, their mental and emotional well-being is often significantly impacted, requiring intensive and ongoing mental health care.

Recent longitudinal studies in adults have shown a link between adverse childhood experiences and health problems in adulthood.

CASE RESOLUTION

The case study describes a classic case of non-accidental trauma. The infant was left alone with an individual with limited parenting skills. Most likely, the crying infant was vigorously shaken, resulting in axonal injury, subdural hemorrhage, loss of consciousness, altered mental status, and seizures. The infant is intubated, given anticonvulsants, and admitted to a pediatric intensive care unit. Consultation with neurosurgery, ophthalmology, and social services is obtained. Appropriate imaging studies and skeletal surveys are performed when the infant is sufficiently stabilized.

Selected References

Felitti VJ, Anda RF, Nordenberg D, et al. Relationship of childhood abuse and household dysfunction to many of the leading causes of death in adults: The Adverse Childhood Experiences (ACE) Study. *Am J Prev Med.* 1998;14:245–258

Gerber P, Coffman K. Nonaccidental head trauma in infants. *Childs Nerv Syst.* 2007;23:499–507

Hudson M, Kaplan R. Clinical response to child abuse. *Pediatr Clin North Am.* 2006;53:27–39

Jenny C, American Academy of Pediatrics Committee on Child Abuse and Neglect. Evaluating infants and young children with multiple fractures. *Pediatrics.* 2006;118:1299–1303

Kellogg ND, American Academy of Pediatrics Committee on Child Abuse and Neglect. Evaluation of suspected child physical abuse. *Pediatrics.* 2007;119:1232–1241

Kempe CH, Silverman FN, Steele BF, Droegemueller W, Silver HK. The battered child syndrome. *JAMA.* 1962;181:17–24

Kleinman PR. *Diagnostic Imaging of Child Abuse.* St Louis, MO: Mosby; 1998

Monteleone JA, Brodeur AE. *Child Maltreatment. A Clinical Guide and Reference.* 3rd ed. St Louis, MO: G. W. Medical Publishing, Inc.; 2005

Reece RM, ed. *Child Abuse: Medical Diagnosis and Management.* 2nd ed. Philadelphia, PA: Lippincott Williams & Wilkins; 2001

Sirontnak AP, Grigsby T, Krugman RD. Physical abuse of children. *Pediatr Rev.* 2004;25:264–277

Swerdlin A, Berkowitz C, Craft N. Cutaneous signs of child abuse. *J Am Acad Dermatol.* 2007;57:371–392

Thompson SL. Accidental or inflicted? Evaluating cutaneous, skeletal and abdominal trauma in children. *Pediatr Ann.* 2005;34:373–381

Sexual Abuse

Sara T. Stewart, MD

CASE STUDY

A 4-year-old girl is brought to the emergency department with the complaint of vaginal itching and discharge. Her past health has been good, and she has no medical problems. She lives with her biological parents and her 2-year-old brother.

On physical examination, the vital signs are normal and the child is well except that the genital area is swollen and erythematous and a green vaginal discharge is present. The girl is interviewed briefly but denies that anyone has touched her. The mother states that she has never left her daughter unattended and is angered by the questions.

Questions

1. What are the anogenital findings in prepubescent and postpubescent children who may have experienced sexual abuse?
2. What behavioral problems are common in children who have been sexually abused?
3. What are the pitfalls in disclosure interviews of children who have been sexually abused?
4. What is the significance of sexually transmitted infections in children who have been sexually abused?

Child sexual abuse is the involvement of children and adolescents in sexual activity that they cannot consent to because of their age and developmental level. An age disparity exists between the victims, who are younger, and the perpetrators, who are older. The intent of the abuse is the **sexual gratification** of the older individuals, and the abusive incident(s) may or may not include physical contact. Sexual abuse may include acts of **oral, genital,** or **anal** contact by or to a child and may involve acts such as **exhibitionism** or involvement in **pornography.** It is differentiated from "sexual play" by the difference in the developmental levels of the participants and the coerciveness of the behavior.

Sexual abuse has been recognized with increasing frequency since the 1980s, in part because medical knowledge about the anogenital anatomy in both normal and molested prepubescent children has expanded. Technical advances have altered the manner in which these children are evaluated. In particular, the colposcope, with its potential for magnification and photographic or videotape documentation, has been valuable. Parental awareness and school-based programs have led to increased disclosures about abuse as well as a greater willingness on the part of adults to believe these disclosures.

Patient interviews are another key component of the assessment process that has been shaped by continued research in the field. Non-leading, open-ended questions are asked by interviewers as few times as possible and, when available, these questions are asked by specialized forensic interviewers.

Epidemiology

Approximately 12 in 1,000 children are thought to be victims of child abuse per year in the United States, and 5% to 10% of these are victims of sexual abuse. Exact figures on the prevalence of child sexual abuse are not readily available because they depend on reports of a condition that may not come to medical attention for many years. Anonymous surveys indicate that about 20% to 25% of women and 10% to 15% of men have been sexually abused before reaching adulthood.

Victims of sexual abuse come from all socioeconomic and ethnic groups. Approximately 75% of victims who come to medical attention are girls and 25% are boys. Some investigators believe that the statistics for boys are falsely low because boys are generally reluctant to disclose their abuse. Men are more commonly the perpetrators than women, and at least 20% of perpetrators are adolescents. Frequently, the sexual abuse has been occurring for several years. The mean time from onset of abuse to disclosure is 3 years. Sometimes children are not ready to disclose but the abuse is discovered accidentally because the victims develop symptoms, such as vaginal discharge or functional complaints.

Clinical Presentation

Most cases of child sexual abuse come to the attention of authorities after the child **discloses** the abuse. There may or may not be associated physical or behavioral complaints. Physical symptoms in the anogenital area may include **bleeding, pain, swelling, dysuria, vaginal discharge,** or **difficulty stooling.** More often, however, children have no specific anogenital symptoms. Instead, they have nonspecific complaints such as headache, abdominal pain, or vague systemic symptoms such as fatigue (Dx Box).

Dx **Child Sexual Abuse**

- Anogenital erythema
- Anogenital bleeding
- Genital discharge
- Anogenital scarring
- Behavioral symptoms (eg, encopresis, enuresis)
- Disclosure of abuse
- Somatic complaints (eg, abdominal pain, headache)
- Sexually transmitted infections
- Sexualized behavior
- Pregnancy (adolescents)
- Delinquency, promiscuity (adolescents)

Behavioral changes may also be noted as these children respond to the stress of their victimization and their environments. These changes may include **sleep disturbances, hyperactivity, enuresis, encopresis, decreased appetite,** and **depression.** Sexually abused adolescents may manifest **school failure, delinquency,** and **suicide** attempts. Children may also respond with sexual behavior or sexual knowledge that is considered to be inappropriate or excessive for age.

Psychophysiology

Children suffer sexual abuse after becoming **entrapped.** They may be enticed with promises of rewards or presents, or may be made to feel special or grown-up by being allowed to engage in adult behavior. Some children do not regard the sexual experiences as threatening but rather as a means by which they can obtain the love they crave. Only when they grow older do they realize that these sexual relationships were not normal or appropriate.

Other children are **coerced** into sexual activity with threats of physical harm. Once they have acquiesced, they are maintained in the relationship with threats of reprisal if they disclose the abuse. Children feel both guilty and responsible for what has happened. This sense of responsibility for family disruption is often perpetuated by the legal system, which may remove the children from their families or may place the offending family member in custody.

Lastly, some children enter into sexual relationships out of **curiosity.** They too become entrapped, particularly because they were initially willing to participate.

As a child reacts to an abusive experience, it is common to feel a need for secrecy. As a result, disclosures of abuse are often delayed, and when they do occur, the child often provides the information incrementally over time. Children are also prone to recantation of reported histories of abuse; such recantations are not considered to be reliable indicators of cases where false allegations have been filed.

Differential Diagnosis

A number of medical conditions that involve the anogenital area may be mistaken for acute or chronic changes due to sexual abuse (Box 116-1).

Box 116-1. Conditions Mistaken for Sexual Abuse	
Genital	**Anal**
• Accidental trauma	• Inflammatory bowel disease
• Lichen sclerosus et atrophicus	• Hemorrhoids
• Urethral prolapse	• Anal abscess associated with
• Labial adhesions	neutropenia
• Congenital malformations	• Perirectal abscess
• Hemangioma	• Perianal streptococcal infection

Children may sustain accidental blunt or **penetrating** injuries to the genital area. The most common of these are **straddle injuries** that occur from falls. Pain and bleeding are the most common symptoms with these injuries, and the labia majora, labia minora, or periurethral areas are typically affected. The hymen is unaffected.

Bleeding is also a frequent complaint in girls with **urethral prolapse,** a condition that is reported most often in prepubescent African American girls between 4 and 8 years of age. These girls have a protuberant mass extruding from the urethra. The condition is of uncertain etiology but it is not related to abuse.

Lichen sclerosus et atrophicus is a less common dermatologic condition that can also be confused with the sequelae of sexual abuse. In this condition, there is typically atrophic, hypopigmented skin in a figure eight configuration in the anogenital area with associated macules, papules, and hemorrhagic blisters. The skin changes may be misinterpreted as scarring from prior abuse and because the atrophic skin is easily traumatized, findings may also be confused with recent abuse. One factor that may differentiate this condition from injuries related to sexual abuse is that the hymen is unaffected in lichen sclerosis et atrophicus.

Labial adhesions occur most commonly in toddlers and may be confused with scarring from prior sexual abuse. The adhesions develop as the result of inflammation in the genital area of a prepubertal (hypoestrogenic) female. There can be multiple causes of the inflammation, including poor hygiene, recurrent vulvovaginitis, and trauma. The presence of labial adhesions is not a specific indicator of past sexual abuse.

Congenital malformations may also affect the anogenital area. **Failure of midline fusion** along the median raphe can have the appearance of denuded skin and may be confused with an abrasion or superficial laceration of the area. This failure of fusion is a congenital finding, however, and there is no bleeding as with a traumatic injury. Other congenital malformations include hemangiomas that may bleed and be mistaken for traumatized tissue. These hemangiomas are most often noted in infants younger than 2 to 3 years, and they usually regress with time.

Medical conditions may also affect the perianal area and may be mistaken for abuse. **Crohn disease** may lead to fissures, fistulas, perirectal abscesses, or tags. In general, Crohn disease affects older children and produces other symptoms such as fever, weight loss, and stooling problems, or extraintestinal symptomatology. Perirectal abscesses may occur in patients with neutropenia, sometimes as the presenting complaint of leukemia. Hemorrhoids occur rarely in children, and their presence should raise concern about intra-abdominal venous congestion.

Conditions causing **vaginal discharge** (Box 116-2) may be related to sexual abuse, particularly if they are secondary to sexually transmitted infections (STIs) such as **gonorrhea** or *Chlamydia* infection. Other agents, including *Candida, Shigella,* and **group A beta-hemolytic streptococci,** may produce similar symptoms, yet not be sexually acquired. The streptococci may produce a painful erythematous rash in the perianal area, which is frequently misdiagnosed as secondary to trauma or sexual abuse.

Box 116-2. Conditions Associated With Vaginal Discharge	
• Gonorrhea	• Shigellosis
• *Chlamydia*	• Group A beta-hemolytic streptococcus infection
• *Trichomonas*	
• Bacterial vaginosis	• Vaginal foreign body
• Candidiasis	

Evaluation

The extent and urgency of the evaluation is in part dependent on whether the allegations involve an acute abusive episode or one that occurred in the past. An acute abusive episode (one that has occurred within the previous 72 hours) warrants an immediate assessment.

History

When a child presents with a physical finding, statement, or behavior that raises the concern of possible sexual abuse, it is important for the examiner to ask carefully thought out, non-leading questions to determine whether the level of suspicion has been reached such that the examiner is mandated to report the concern to a child protective services agency. Beyond that, an attempt should be made to minimize the number of times that the child is questioned about the abuse-related incidents. It is also important to establish sufficient medical history to address any pressing clinical issues. Such a history should include a review of systems, menstrual history, sexual activity history, past incidents of abuse, and any prior genital trauma or medical procedures of the anogenital area. A psychosocial history should also be obtained, as behavioral problems, depression, anxiety, suicidality, homicidality, and other issues requiring mental health expertise are common in sexually abused children (Box 116-3).

Because most victims of sexual abuse have a normal physical examination, the history is often of primary importance in the case. As a result, the child must also be interviewed by someone with professional expertise in the areas of interviewing and child sexual abuse.

Box 116-3. Problems Reported in Sexually Abused Children	
• Enuresis	• Sleep disturbances
• Encopresis	• Suicide
• Sexualized behavior	• School failure
• Pseudomaturity	• Delinquency (adolescents)
• Vaginal discharge	• Promiscuity (adolescents)

This individual may be a physician, or it may be a social worker, psychologist, rape counselor, or specialized detective or district attorney. The interview should be structured to include open-ended questions such as, "Tell me what happened" (Questions Box). Interview tools such as drawings or anatomically detailed dolls may be used but are best left to experts with experience in these controversial modalities. Statements that children make should be recorded in the medical record as close to verbatim as possible.

Child Sexual Abuse — Questions

- Can you tell me what happened?
- Has anything like this happened before? If so, what happened the first time?
- Who did this to you?
- Has anyone else done this to you?
- How often has this happened?
- Where were other people (eg, your mother) when this happened?
- Did you tell anyone? Who? What did they do?

Physical Examination

It is helpful for the examiner to be familiar with the normal **anogenital** anatomy of prepubescent children. The anatomy of boys remains constant throughout childhood, except for the increase in size of the penis and testes and the appearance of pubic hair during adolescence. Figure 116-1 shows the normal anogenital anatomy of girls, which changes from infancy through adolescence. All girls are born with a hymen, which is thick and full and covers the hymenal orifice in newborns. As maternal hormones regress, the hymen becomes thinner and more translucent, frequently taking on an annular or crescentic configuration. When puberty begins, the hymen once again becomes thickened, scalloped, and full. Careful examination of the hymen may involve positioning a child in not only the supine frog-leg position, but also the prone knee-chest position (Figure 116-2). For a variety of reasons there are frequently no genital abnormalities noted on examination in victims of sexual abuse. Penetration of the hymen in postpubertal adolescents may result in stretching without tearing of the tissue, and in prepubescent children, hymenal transections may heal with little residual evidence of the trauma. Many types of abuse (eg, orogenital contact, fondling) are not expected to lead to any visible changes. The medical examiner must therefore realize that a normal anogenital examination does not preclude sexual abuse.

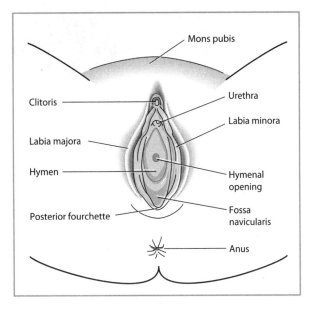

Figure 116-1. **Normal anogenital anatomy of prepubescent girls.**

In cases of acute molestation, evidence of injury may be readily apparent, particularly if the examination is performed with the assistance of magnification such as **colposcopy,** or enhancing agents such as toluidine blue, which is preferentially taken up by exposed endothelium. Injuries that may be noted include **ecchymoses, petechiae, active bleeding, abrasions,** and **lacerations.** Those due to penile penetration commonly involve the hymen in the 6 o'clock position and the area of the posterior fourchette (see Figure 116-1).

The evaluation of children who have been molested in the past or on a chronic basis is more problematic. Many injuries heal with little residual scarring. Scarring that does occur may appear as a notch or concavity in the contour of the hymenal edge. The pattern of blood vessels may also be interrupted, and areas of increased or decreased

vascularity may be apparent. Sometimes a marked reduction in the amount of hymenal tissue is present in an area of prior trauma.

Male genitalia are less often injured by sexual abuse. More often the injuries seen in prepubescent boys, as well as in some girls, involve changes in the perianal area. The incidence of these changes in all children who have been sodomized is unknown but is believed to be low. When changes do occur, they may appear as scars, tags, or irregularities in perianal rugae and anal tone.

Laboratory Tests

When the molestation has occurred within 72 hours of the examination, **forensic evidence** should be collected, as required by law enforcement. This evidence usually involves samples of vaginal washings and dried secretions, which are evaluated for the presence of DNA in an effort to identify the perpetrator. **Forensic packages,** which are referred to as **rape kits,** have specific instructions concerning the appropriate collection of samples.

Approximately 5% of sexually abused children acquire an **STI** as a result of the abuse. Because of this, any child with a history of genital, oral, or anal penetration; a sibling with an STI; an assailant with a history of an infection; or a child, sibling, or assailant with signs or symptoms of an STI must undergo a laboratory evaluation for possible infection. If testing is indicated, cultures should be obtained from the involved body areas (vagina or urethra, rectum, throat). At a minimum, a child with genital discharge should be evaluated for *Neisseria gonorrhoeae, Chlamydia trachomatis*, and *Trichomonas vaginalis*. The presence of these infections in a prepubertal child, in the absence of perinatal transmission, is indicative prior close genital contact. Most frequently this is due to sexual abuse. It is impossible to determine the etiology of vaginal discharge based only on its clinical characteristics.

All tests for STIs in prepubertal children should be evaluated in a reliable laboratory because of the legal implications of venereal

Figure 116-2. **Various positions for an anogenital examination in a prepubescent girl. A. Seated on the mother's lap. B. Supine, frog-leg position. C. Prone, knee-chest position.**

infections in young children. Culture is considered to be the gold standard for diagnosing gonorrhea and *Chlamydia* in this setting because of its specificity. While newer nucleic acid amplification tests may have higher sensitivity in some settings, there are limited data on their use in prepubertal children so they cannot be used as the sole method of evaluation in cases where the information will be used in court.

Testing for human immunodeficiency virus, syphilis, hepatitis B, and hepatitis C should be performed if signs or symptoms of the diagnosis are present, if another STI is detected, if the perpetrator is known to be infected, or if the patient/family wishes to undergo the testing. Genital warts can be diagnosed clinically, and any lesions suspicious for herpes simplex virus types 1 or 2 should be cultured. Lastly, pregnancy testing should be considered in any post-pubertal girl.

Management

The management of children who have been sexually abused has 3 major components.

(1) Any medical problem sustained as a result of the abuse, such as traumatic injuries, must be addressed. In addition, STIs should be managed (Table 116-1). See Chapter 85 for a more extensive discussion of STIs in adolescents. Adolescents who have been the victims of an acute assault should be offered pregnancy counseling, STI prophylaxis, and emergency contraception as medically indicated.

Table 116-1. Management of Sexually Transmitted Infections in Children

Infection	Medication	Dose
Neisseria gonorrhoeae	Ceftriaxone	125 mg IM × 1 dose
	Cefixime (age >8 y, weight ≥45 kg)	400 mg PO × 1 dose
Chlamydia	Azithromycin	20 mg/kg PO x 1 dose (max: 1 g)
	Erythromycin (weight <45 kg)	50 mg/kg/d divided QID × 14 days
	Doxycycline (age >8 y, weight ≥45 kg)	100 mg PO BID × 7 days
Herpes genitalis	Acyclovir	1,200 mg/d divided TID x 7–10 days (max: 80 mg/kg/d)
Trichomonas	Metronidazole	15 mg/kg/d divided TID × 7 days OR 2 g PO × 1 dose (weight ≥45 kg)
Bacterial vaginosis	Metronidazole	15 mg/kg/d divided TID x 7 days OR 2 g PO × 1 dose (weight ≥45 kg)
Syphilis	Benzathine penicillin	50,000 U/kg, single IM dose (max: 2.4 million U)

Abbreviations: IM, intramuscularly; PO, orally; QID, 4 times a day; BID, twice a day; TID, 3 times a day.

(2) The emotional well-being of patients must be ensured. In cases of acute assault, crisis intervention is mandatory. If children have been the victims of chronic or prior sexual abuse, referral to appropriate counseling services should be done.

(3) The physician must report the incident of sexual assault or abuse to the appropriate agencies, as mandated by the laws of the locality in which the physician practices. The physician may be required to testify in court about particular findings and whether abuse occurred. Testifying may be intimidating. It is helpful for the physician to review the medical records ahead of time and to discuss this information with the attorney who issues the subpoena to the physician.

Prognosis

Several factors influence the prognosis in cases of child sexual abuse, including the relationship of the perpetrator to the child, chronicity of the abuse, support following the disclosure, and preexisting psychosocial conditions. Physical injuries are usually nonexistent or minor, and healing occurs with minimal residual evidence. In most cases, psychological counseling is indicated. Such counseling is beneficial, and emotional recovery is not only possible but likely to occur in a supportive environment.

Studies of **adverse childhood experiences** have shown that child sexual abuse may be associated with medical and psychological problems in adulthood.

CASE RESOLUTION

In the case history presented at the beginning of this chapter, the mother claims that no one has access to her child, but the girl's symptoms strongly suggest an infection with *Neisseria gonorrhoeae*. Secrecy about abuse is very common. Both the child and the mother should be interviewed by a skilled person. Cultures for gonorrhea should be carefully collected and sent to the most reliable laboratory. Antibiotic therapy may be initiated if the child is symptomatic. The case may be referred immediately to social services and law enforcement agencies if there is a disclosure. Alternatively, if the child denies the abuse, the referral may be deferred pending laboratory confirmation of the diagnosis.

Selected References

Behrman RE, ed. *The Future of Children: Sexual Abuse of Children.* Palo Alto, CA: Center for the Future of Children, The David and Lucile Packard Foundation; 1994

Centers for Disease Control and Prevention, Workowski KA, Berman SM. Sexually transmitted diseases treatment guidelines, 2006. *MMWR Recomm Rep.* 2006;55:1–94

Chadwick DL, Berkowitz CD, Kerns D, McCann J, Reinhart MA, Strickland S. *Color Atlas of Child Sexual Abuse.* Chicago, IL: Year Book Medical Publishers; 1989

Felitti VJ, Anda RF, Nordenberg D, et al. Relationship of childhood abuse and household dysfunction to many of the leading causes of death in adults: the Adverse Childhood Experiences (ACE) Study. *Am J Prev Med.* 1998;14:245–258

Finkel MA, DeJong AR. Medical findings in child sexual abuse. In: Reece RM, ed. *Child Abuse: Medical Diagnosis and Management.* 2nd ed. Philadelphia, PA: Lippincott Williams & Wilkins; 2001:207–286

Giardino AP, Finkel MA. Evaluating child sexual abuse. *Pediatr Ann.* 2005;34:382–394

Heger A, Emans SJ, Muram D. *Evaluation of the Sexually Abused Child.* New York, NY: Oxford University Press; 2000

Holmes WC, Slap GB. Sexual abuse of boys. *JAMA.* 1998;280:1855–1862

Jenny C. *Medical Evaluation of Physically and Sexually Abused Children. The APSAC Study Guides 3.* Thousand Oaks, CA: Sage Publications; 1996

Kellogg N, American Academy of Pediatrics Committee on Child Abuse and Neglect. The evaluation of sexual abuse in children. *Pediatrics.* 2005;116:506–512

Reece RM, ed. *Treatment of Child Abuse: Common Ground for Mental Health, Medical, and Legal Practitioners.* Baltimore, MD: Johns Hopkins University Press; 2001

Reichert SK. Medical evaluation of the sexually abused child. In: Helfer ME, Kempe RS, Krugman RD, eds. *The Battered Child.* 5th ed. Chicago, IL: The University of Chicago Press; 1997:313–328

Sapp MV, Vandeven AM. Update on childhood sexual abuse. *Curr Opin Pediatr.* 2005;17:258–264

Shapiro RA, Makoroff KL. Sexually transmitted diseases in sexually abused girls and adolescents. *Curr Opin Obstet Gynecol.* 2006;18:492–497

Failure to Thrive

Carol D. Berkowitz, MD

CASE STUDY

A 2-year-old girl is brought to the office because of her small size. She was born at term but weighed only 2,200 g (less than fifth percentile) and measured 43 cm (less than fifth percentile). The mother is a 30-year-old gravida V para IV aborta I who smoked during pregnancy but denies using alcohol or drugs. She received prenatal care for only 2 weeks prior to delivery, and she claims to have felt well.

The child's physical health has been good. She is reported to be normal developmentally but speaks only 4 to 5 single words. She has not yet started toilet training.

The family history for medical problems, including allergies, diabetes, and cardiac and renal disease, is negative. The mother is 5 feet (152 cm) tall, and the father is 5 feet, 4 inches (163 cm) tall. The girl has 3 siblings, aged 5 years, 4 years, and 3 years, who are all normal. The father is no longer in the household. The mother is not employed outside of the home, and she receives public assistance.

She states that frequently there is not enough food in the home, although she receives food stamps.

On physical examination, the girl is less than the fifth percentile in height and weight. Although she is very active, she does not use any understandable words. The rest of the examination is normal.

Questions

1. What are the key prenatal factors that affect the growth of children?
2. How can caloric adequacy of a diet be assessed?
3. How do parental measurements affect their children's stature?
4. What are the behavioral characteristics of infants with environmental failure to thrive?
5. What are some strategies to increase caloric intake of infants and children?

Failure to thrive (FTT) can be defined as the failure of children to grow and develop at an appropriate rate. The term is most often applied to infants and toddlers younger than 3 years. Failure to thrive is not a disease or even a diagnosis but represents a sign that a child's size or rate of growth is below expected. The term *FTT* first appeared in the pediatric literature in 1933 and was used for children whose growth impairment related to a suboptimal environment. Prior to 1933 the condition was referred to as **cease to thrive.** The terms **growth deficiency, growth impairment, undernutrition,** and **inadequate growth** are sometimes used interchangeably. Historically, FTT has been divided into 2 distinct categories, **organic** and **nonorganic.** In organic FTT, an underlying **medical problem,** such as cystic fibrosis or congenital heart disease (CHD), is believed to contribute to the failure to grow at an appropriate rate. In nonorganic FTT, also referred to as **environmental deprivation,** inadequate growth is attributed to lack of nourishment and a non-nurturing home environment. Some clinicians use the term FTT exclusively to mean environmentally related growth impairment. It is important to recognize that many children with growth problems have both organic and environmental components, a condition sometimes referred to as *multifactorial* or *mixed* FTT.

The diagnosis of FTT is entertained when the growth parameters of children as plotted on a standardized curve are below the fifth percentile in height or weight. Children who are above the fifth percentile may also be diagnosed with FTT if the rate of growth has decelerated and 2 major percentiles (eg, decreased from the 75th percentile down to the 10th percentile) have been crossed within 6 months (Dx Box).

Dx Failure to Thrive

- Weight below fifth percentile
- Height below fifth percentile
- Weight for height below fifth percentile
- Rate of growth lower than expected
- Delayed developmental milestones
- Disturbed interactional skills

The challenge for the physician caring for the child with FTT is to determine the etiology of the problem, which may not be readily apparent. Nonspecific, nondirected laboratory tests are not helpful because their yield is low and their cost is high. The evaluation of small, underweight children requires a careful history and physical examination as well as an assessment of mother-infant interactions. A home visit helps because it permits evaluation of the mother-infant relationship in a more natural setting and an assessment of the family's economic and food resources.

Epidemiology

The prevalence of FTT varies in different segments of the population. **Poverty** puts children at risk for **undernutrition,** and 12% of Medicaid recipients are less than the third percentile in weight. **Child neglect** can lead to FTT but is not a necessary component; approximately 60% of cases of child abuse are reported for child neglect. Several other factors may contribute to variations in growth. All of these are not the result of a pathologic process but may reflect variations in individual genetic potential.

Environmental FTT may occur in different family settings. In some families, an **acute depressive episode** in the mother is the key component. Family living conditions are good, and the educational background of the mother is adequate. The depressive episode is most commonly related to a loss that occurred during the pregnancy or shortly after delivery. The mother is too depressed to interact appropriately with her children. In other families **financial resources** are marginal. The mother may be **chronically depressed** and the father involved in alcohol or substance abuse. Domestic violence frequently occurs. Spacing between children is less than 18 months, and the number of children is often the same as the age of the oldest child. The mother is too overwhelmed to meet the needs of the children. A third type of family also involves a mother who is depressed and has experienced losses, usually of a chronic nature. Her financial and educational background are adequate, but she views one of her children (the one who now presents with FTT) as bad or evil and the source of all her problems. As a result, an individual child is singled out, and the neglect is intentional.

Clinical Presentation

Children with FTT present with **low weight, short stature,** or **poor appetite.** Sometimes parents may express concern, and at other times teachers may detect children's growth problems. Some children with FTT are diagnosed during a health maintenance visit or when they are being evaluated for another medical problem, such as a febrile illness.

Pathophysiology

The common pathway for the development of FTT in both organic and nonorganic cases is **insufficient calories** to sustain growth. Caloric intake may be inadequate for several reasons. Some factors are societal, specifically poverty and inadequate access to food. Other factors may involve increased caloric needs. Certain chronic conditions are characterized by increased caloric expenditure (eg, some forms of chronic lung disease) or increased loss of ingested food (eg, diarrhea).

In environmental FTT, a disturbed mother-infant interaction is believed to contribute to reduced caloric intake and any associated gastrointestinal symptoms (ie, vomiting). Although various disturbances in mother-FTT infant dyads have been described, maternal depression is the most common maternal feature noted in environmental FTT. Infants withdraw after unsuccessful attempts to interact with nonresponsive mothers, and infants become apathetic and disinterested in food. Alternatively, overactive mothers, some of whom have a bipolar (manic-depressive) disorder, are out of synchrony with their infants. The infants become agitated, especially during feedings, and cannot feed and frequently vomit. These infants, who may interact with persons other than their mothers, usually do well in other environments.

Older children with long-standing environmental deprivation have **disturbed hypothalamic-pituitary functioning.** The etiology of this dysfunction is uncertain but has been attributed to sleep disturbances.

Differential Diagnosis

The growth of children with FTT may be impaired with regard to weight, height, head circumference, or any combination of growth parameters. If weight is the only abnormal parameter, inadequate caloric intake is probably the major problem. If height is reduced and the weight is appropriate or high for height, the diagnosis may be short stature rather than FTT. Small head circumference in the face of low growth parameters suggests a central nervous system (CNS) basis for the growth delay. It is important to determine if children's skills are developmentally appropriate when determining the etiology of FTT. Affect and interactional skills should also be noted. Environmentally deprived infants are apathetic and noninteractive. They appear hypertonic and may be diagnosed with cerebral palsy or have features suggestive of infantile autism, but their symptoms resolve with a change in surroundings.

The most common causes of short stature include **familial short stature** and **constitutional delay.** Children with familial short stature are small because the parents are short. Except for a deceleration in growth, which usually occurs between the ages of 6 and 18 months, children with constitutional delay appear healthy. They have a delayed bone age that is comparable to their height age (the age when their height is at the 50th percentile), however. In children with either familial short stature or constitutional delay, growth parameters at birth are usually normal.

Children with low growth parameters at birth may have been premature or have suffered from **intrauterine growth restriction (IUGR).** Most studies support the notion that well premature infants exhibit catch-up growth (head circumference by 18 months, weight by 24 months, and height by 40 months). Ill preterm infants may not demonstrate such **catch-up growth,** either because of increased caloric needs related to residual medical problems (eg, bronchopulmonary dysplasia) or impaired nutritional intake resulting from certain conditions (eg, cerebral palsy). Overall, 15% of infants who are classified as IUGR or **small for gestational age (SGA)** do not exhibit catch-up growth.

Children who are **SGA** may have suffered any of several in utero insults that affect postnatal growth, including exposure to cigarettes, alcohol, and illicit drugs. In addition, maternal infection with such diseases as rubella may result in a congenital infection in infants with subsequent growth impairment.

A number of other conditions may lead to disturbed growth, including endocrine disorders, skeletal dysplasias, food allergies, and malabsorption. These conditions occur less frequently and are usually more readily apparent as children undergo the evaluation for the growth problem.

Evaluation

History

Careful questioning about certain topics provides clues to diagnosis in about 95% of cases. The physician should learn about the pregnancy and delivery, children's medical and dietary history, and the family history.

It is important to obtain a history of the pregnancy and delivery (Questions Box: Pregnancy and Delivery). The infant's birth weight and gestational age are key pieces of information. Low birth weight is said to account for 20% to 40% of short children from low-income families. It is helpful to confirm that the neonatal metabolic screen was normal. Recurrent spontaneous abortions suggest that mothers may have an underlying problem such as a balanced chromosomal translocation that leads to fetal wastage. Mothers who have experienced repeated losses may have difficulty bonding with subsequent infants. The physician should determine whether mothers used cigarettes, alcohol, or drugs during the pregnancy by asking mothers questions beginning with the phrase "How much?" Any medications taken by the mother may affect the subsequent growth of the infant.

> ## Questions
> ### Pregnancy and Delivery
>
> - Was the pregnancy planned?
> - How did the mother feel when she learned that she was pregnant?
> - Was the infant wanted?
> - Was prenatal care obtained?
> - How many times has the mother been pregnant?
> - Is there a history of abortions, either spontaneous or therapeutic?
> - How much did the mother drink during the pregnancy, if at all?
> - How much did the mother smoke during the pregnancy, if at all?
> - How much did the mother use drugs (either prescribed or illicit) during the pregnancy, if at all? Which drugs did she use?
> - Did the mother take any medications during the pregnancy?
> - Did the mother have any rashes or illnesses during the pregnancy?
> - Was the infant term or premature?
> - How much did the infant weigh at birth?

A review of children's medical history may also provide a clue to the etiology of FTT (Questions Box: Medical and Family History). It is essential that the physician obtain as many of the previous growth parameters as possible to determine whether children are small but growing at a normal rate or if their rate of growth is too slow. Previous illnesses should be assessed because these events may interrupt growth temporarily. Certain complaints may indicate underlying organic disorders, and recurrent infection raises the possibility of infection with human immunodeficiency virus. A history of easy fatigability may be a clue to CHD. Although most children with CHD

grow normally, growth problems may occur with congestive heart failure, some forms of cyanotic heart disease, and complex atrial septal defects, especially if associated with pulmonary hypertension. Children with urinary incontinence may have renal disease that interferes with their growth. The presence of seizures may be a sign of a CNS problem that makes it difficult to obtain adequate nutrition. Some children with seizures are heavily medicated and are too sleepy to eat.

> ## Questions
> ### Medical and Family History
>
> - Is the child's growth rate normal or slow?
> - Has the child had any previous illnesses (eg, gastroenteritis, recurrent pneumonia)?
> - Does the child tire easily?
> - How tall are the parents?
> - Are there any medical problems that run in the family?

A family history as well as a **social history** is important to obtain. Determination of parental heights, which is best accomplished by measuring the parents, is critical. This is particularly important in children with short stature. Specific **mid-parental height curves** allow the physician to determine if children's height is appropriate given the parental stature.

A nutritional assessment is an essential part of the history. The physician or another member of the health care team, such as a dietician, can perform this assessment. The dietary history can be determined either by using a **24-hour recall** of children's intake during the previous day or a prospective **3-day diary,** in which parents record the kinds and quantities of foods their children eat. This nutritional information can be used to find ways to alter children's diet to ensure adequate and balanced meals.

Physical Examination

The essential component of the physical examination is determination of growth parameters. Calculation of the **body mass index** (BMI = weight [kg] divided by height $[m]^2$) is useful in children older than 2 years. Children with a low BMI are suffering from undernutrition. Short children with a normal BMI are not. Infants younger than 2 years should be plotted on a weight-for-length curve to determine their degree of undernutrition or overnutrition. Measuring arm circumference and triceps skinfold thickness is also useful and provides information about body composition that is not obtained by height and weight. Children should also be evaluated for dysmorphic features. It is important to remember that children with Down syndrome grow at different rates than other children, and separate standardized curves for assessing these children are available (see Chapter 27). The presence of one major congenital anomaly or 2 minor anomalies suggests the existence of other anomalies. The incidence of growth hormone deficiency is reportedly higher in children with cleft lip and palate. Children with heart murmurs may have FTT related to CHD or to a syndrome such as Williams syndrome, in which the heart disease is but one feature.

Infants with environmental FTT exhibit certain **behavioral characteristics** that are easy to recognize. They refrain from making eye contact and exhibit **gaze** avoidance. Infants are not cuddly and do not like being held. When held, they may arch their backs in an effort to avoid the holder. Their muscles seem tense, and they are often considered to be hypertonic. These children may also exhibit specific disabilities including oromotor dyspraxia and sensory-motor disorder, and may demonstrate food texture aversion or difficulty with chewing and swallowing **(sensory food aversion).** Children with neurologic disabilities often exhibit difficulties with oral skills. Children who have negative early experience with eating may have what has been termed *posttraumatic feeding disorder.*

Psychosocial Assessment

The evaluation of children with FTT and their families entails a detailed psychosocial assessment to determine what environmental factors may be affecting children's growth. Such an assessment is helpful even if the FTT has an organic basis, because chronic disease affects family functioning. This evaluation can be carried out by a primary care physician, social worker, or psychologist. The key is to query the caretaker about living conditions, adequacy of food supply, and economic resources.

Laboratory Tests

Routine laboratory tests appropriate for any pediatric health maintenance visit should be obtained in children with FTT if these studies have not been performed recently. Such tests include hematocrit, lead level (screening as determined by risk factors and geographic area), and urinalysis. Other laboratory tests should be determined by the findings on history and physical examination. There is no recommended uniform diagnostic evaluation for FTT. Evaluation for endocrinopathies, such as hypothyroidism or growth hormone deficiency, should be carried out in children whose bone age is less than their height age or who have symptoms of these disorders. Genetic consultation or chromosomal assessment should be performed in children with dysmorphic features or in families with a history of fetal wastage.

Imaging Studies

X-rays to determine bone age are useful in children with short stature that is not related to parental heights. Children with constitutional delay have a bone age that is consistent with their height age.

Management

Any recognized underlying medical problem, for instance nephrogenic diabetes insipidus, should be managed appropriately. Children with IUGR who are not demonstrating catch-up growth may be candidates for growth hormone therapy. Consultation with pediatric endocrinology is warranted.

Adequate Caloric Intake

Ensuring that children receive appropriate caloric intake is essential. The caloric intake, which averages 120 to 150 cal/kg/d for most infants, should be based on children's ideal rather than actual weight (see Chapter 14). For infants on formula, the physician should review the exact preparation of formula with the mother. Overly diluted formula results in an unusually large intake volume with a lack of weight gain. For infants who are breastfed, the physician should observe a feeding session to be certain that mothers have an adequate milk supply and infants are able to suck and swallow appropriately (see Chapter 15). Infants should be weighed before and after feeding. Some infants with FTT have neurologic problems that prevent them from sucking and swallowing consistently without becoming fatigued.

Children who are slow feeders may require **formula concentration** (Table 117-1). These infants may also receive added calories in the form of Polycose (glucose polymer) or oil such as medium-chain triglycerides mixed in the milk. Older children may be placed on supplemental feedings such as PediaSure or instant breakfast drinks. These drinks are a less expensive form of nutritional supplementation than PediaSure and are well tolerated. Up to 24 oz/d of the breakfast drinks can be consumed. They should be mixed with whole milk and given in addition to, not in place of, a balanced diet.

Mothers should be advised that many children preferentially tolerate 6 small meals a day rather than 3 large ones. In addition, parents should be told that access to non-nutritional foods such as cookies adversely affects children's appetites. Excess consumption of fruit juices should also be limited because it decreases the intake of other foods and may induce diarrhea. The physician should inform parents regarding foods that can be added to children's diets to increase caloric intake. These foods include powdered milk, cheese, sour cream, avocado, and peanut butter. Often children have a few favorite foods. Though food variety is appealing to adults, many children prefer a small number of nutritious foods. They should be allowed to consume these foods freely.

Children with neurologic disorders and associated problems with chewing and swallowing may need chronic gavage feeding or be fed through a gastric feeding tube.

Table 117-1. Concentration of Infant Formula to Increase Caloric Intake		
Concentrated Infant Formula (13-oz can)		
Formula (oz)	*Water (oz)*	*Calories (cal/oz)*
13	13	20
13	10	23
13	8	25
Powdered Formula		
Formula (scoops)	*Water (oz)*	*Calories (cal/oz)*
1	2	20
5	8	25

Parenting Issues

Some parents need more help about appropriate child-rearing practices than the physician can provide. They should be enrolled in parenting programs that address multiple aspects of the parenting process. Mothers with substance abuse problems may need to participate in drug treatment programs. Other caregivers may need individual counseling for depression or emotional problems. A nurturing father has an important role in caring for an infant, particularly if a mother is experiencing postpartum depression.

In some middle-class families, mealtime has evolved into a battle of control. Some children find that food is supplied in a manner more conducive to its consumption at school rather than at home. Parents should be counseled about avoiding conflicts about meals with children because the children win simply by closing their mouths. Parents should be encouraged to allow toddlers independence around mealtime.

Families may also require supplementary services to ensure that food supplies are adequate and financial resources are sufficient. Such services include food stamps, Supplemental Food Program for Women, Infants, and Children (WIC), and Temporary Assistance for Needy Families (TANF).

Home Visitation

Home visitation services provide useful diagnostic information and help parents implement advice. Such information may include lack of access to running water, overcrowding, and inadequate food resources. Home visitation may be available in the community through the use of public health nurses or private visiting nurse agencies. These nurses should interact with the primary care physician so that families' compliance with treatment recommendations can be determined.

Child Protective Services

Involvement by **child protective services** (CPS) may be necessary if parents are unable to comply with medical recommendations, if children do not grow, or if there is intentional neglect on the part of families. In some families with children with FTT, the home environment is not safe for the children and they require placement elsewhere. Families in which one child is singled out as "bad" and is intentionally neglected need immediate referral to CPS, and some families overwhelmed by multiple problems including parental substance abuse also need such a referral (see Epidemiology).

Hospitalization

Hospitalization is occasionally necessary if infants with FTT are severely malnourished and food must be given in a controlled environment. These infants may also have intercurrent illnesses that require inpatient care. In addition, health care professionals may determine that the home environment is unsafe and that no other placement, such as foster care, is available.

Children with both organic and nonorganic FTT usually gain weight in the hospital. Thus the hospitalization of children with FTT simply to demonstrate appropriate weight gain in a different environment is considered neither appropriate nor cost-effective. Some insurance companies will not reimburse hospitals for in-patient management of children with FTT. Additionally, some children with environmental FTT do not gain weight in the hospital because they are subjected to many diagnostic tests that interfere with nutritional intake (eg, receiving nothing orally), and they acquire nosocomial infections.

Prognosis

Many children with FTT respond dramatically to change in diet or in environment. Improvement in affect and cognitive functioning frequently follows nutritional improvement. These children grow and achieve and maintain normal stature. With early intervention, cognitive abilities also can be fully realized. Even when intervention has been delayed, catch-up growth and development are expected, although 25% to 30% may have weight and occasionally height below the fifth percentile. Continued monitoring for residual psychosocial or neurodevelopmental disabilities is appropriate even after growth has normalized. School performance and cognitive outcome in children who have experienced FTT is poorer than in children who have not experienced FTT. It is unclear if this association is related to early iron deficiency anemia, lack of calories or other micronutrient deficiencies, or psycho-environmental deficits.

CASE RESOLUTION

In the case scenario presented, the full-term infant had a low birth weight, which suggests intrauterine growth restriction. Although the mother reports using no alcohol or drugs, such denial is not uncommon. The child's growth pattern should be determined to see if the rate of growth has changed recently, and the body mass index should be calculated to check for both undernutrition and short stature. A mid-parental height curve should be used to determine if the child's short stature is related to the parents' short stature. Intervention should involve mobilizing resources for the child and family to ensure adequate food and financial and emotional support.

Selected References

Berkowitz CD. Failure to thrive: a comprehensive approach. *Fam Pract Recertification.* 2004;26:41–59

Cook J, Frank D, Berkowitz C, et al. Food insecurity is associated with adverse health outcomes among human infants and toddlers. *J Nutr.* 2004;134:1432–1438

Drotar D, ed. *New Direction in Failure to Thrive: Research and Clinical Practice.* New York, NY: Plenum Press; 1985

Frank DA, Drotar D. Failure to thrive in child abuse: medical diagnosis and management. In: Reece RM, ed. *Child Abuse: Medical Diagnosis and Management.* Philadelphia, PA: Lea & Febiger; 1994:298–324

Gahagan S. Failure to thrive: a consequence of undernutrition. *Pediatr Rev.* 2006;27:e1–e11

Graham EA. Economic, racial, and cultural influence on growth and maturation of children. *Pediatr Rev.* 2005;26:290–294

Kessler DB, Dawson P. *Failure to Thrive and Pediatric Undernutrition. A Transdisciplinary Approach.* Baltimore, MD: Paul H. Brookes Publishing Co.; 1999

Oates RK, Kempe RS. Growth failure in infants. In: Helfer ME, Kempe RS, Krugman RD, eds. *The Battered Child.* 5th ed. Chicago, IL: The University of Chicago Press; 1997:374–391

Infants of Substance-Abusing Mothers

Sara T. Stewart, MD

CASE STUDY

An infant is born by emergency cesarean section because of abruptio placentae. The mother is a 29-year-old gravida VI para IV aborta II with a history of crack cocaine and heroin abuse during pregnancy. The infant is 36 weeks' gestation. The birth weight is 2,400 g, and the length is 43 cm. The physical examination is normal. The infant does well for the first 10 hours but then develops jitteriness, with irritability, diarrhea, sweating, and poor feeding. A urine toxicology test on the infant and mother are positive for cocaine.

Questions

1. What complications affect infants secondary to maternal substance abuse during pregnancy?
2. What withdrawal symptoms do newborn infants experience as a result of maternal substance abuse during pregnancy?
3. What typical behavioral and learning problems are found in infants and children whose mothers abused illicit substances during pregnancy?
4. What are the appropriate management strategies for infants who have experienced in utero drug exposure?

Maternal substance abuse during pregnancy places infants at risk for a number of medical, psychosocial, and developmental problems. The particular problems experienced by infants depend on the drug (or drugs) to which they have been exposed; many infants have been exposed to multiple drugs in addition to cigarettes and alcohol. The long-lasting effects of alcohol exposure are well established, but the effect of newer drugs is less well defined. Illicit drugs change in their popularity, form of use, and availability at different points in time.

The environment into which children are born also affects their health and eventual development. Environments where substance abuse is common are frequently suboptimal for normal growth and development due to (1) the impact of substance abuse on parenting; (2) fragmentation of families; (3) domestic violence; (4) incarceration of significant family members; (5) illnesses, including human immunodeficiency virus (HIV) infection; (6) limited financial resources; (7) homelessness or substandard housing; (8) unemployment; (9) child abuse and neglect; and (10) limited access to health care. Because of these environmental issues, many drug-exposed infants are cared for by foster parents or nonparental family members. These factors also make it difficult to determine, in a given child, which problems are due to the drug exposure versus the accompanying environmental conditions. This differentiation is of less significance to the practitioner than to the researcher or epidemiologist because the practitioner will care for the problems that drug-exposed children manifest regardless of etiology.

Epidemiology

About 15% of the 56 million women between the ages of 15 and 44 years are substance abusers. While data collected via maternal self-report are typically an underestimate of prevalence, one national survey reported that 5.5% of women used illicit substances while pregnant. The same survey also found that 18% of women reported drinking alcohol and 20% reported smoking cigarettes while pregnant. Meconium analysis has demonstrated not only extensive differences in the prevalence of in utero drug exposure among hospitals, but has also shown differences in the substances of choice in different geographic areas. One high-prevalence area reported that 70% of infants screened were positive for cocaine, yet another study of a suburban hospital revealed a prevalence of 12%. Conversely, recent national data have shown a higher rate of methamphetamine use within the past year for individuals living in small metropolitan or rural communities than among those in metropolitan areas. While studies typically focus on exposure to individual substances, polysubstance abuse is the most common clinical scenario.

Clinical Presentation

Many of the different substances that women use while pregnant can result in similar sequelae in the infant or child. In utero growth restriction, irritability, disordered eating or sleeping, and hypertonicity may be seen in newborns and infants. Older children may have developmental delays, symptoms of attention-deficit/

hyperactivity disorder (ADHD), learning disabilities, or behavioral difficulties such as oppositional or impulsive behavior. Newborns that have been prenatally exposed to opiates such as heroin or methadone may manifest symptoms of neonatal abstinence syndrome (drug withdrawal). These symptoms may include respiratory, gastrointestinal (GI), or nervous system effects such as apnea, tachypnea, emesis, diarrhea, irritability, hypertonicity, tremors, seizures, temperature instability, and sneezing. Symptoms often occur within 72 hours of birth, but due to its long half-life, symptoms may take up to 5 days to develop with methadone exposure.

Alcohol and cocaine have been associated with birth defects as well. Abnormalities such as absent limbs, cardiac defects, genitourinary anomalies, ocular anomalies, and microcephaly have been reported with cocaine exposure. Alcohol has been associated with a spectrum of effects, termed *fetal alcohol spectrum disorders (FASD)*. Within this spectrum, a subset of patients fit the well-defined criteria for a diagnosis of fetal alcohol syndrome (FAS). These criteria include facial dysmorphology, growth deficiency, and neurodevelopmental abnormality. The presence of 3 sentinel features in the facial dysmorphology is the most sensitive and specific diagnostic finding for FAS. These features include a flat philtrum, thin upper lip, and short palpebral fissures. The spectrum of neurodevelopmental problems includes diagnoses such as microcephaly and seizures, as well as many types of developmental, cognitive, and behavioral difficulties. Also included within FASD is a category for alcohol-related birth defects. This category includes anomalies such as congenital heart defects, skeletal deformities, renal anomalies, hearing loss, ophthalmologic abnormalities, and cleft lip and palate.

Pathophysiology

Drugs used by pregnant women may affect infants in 3 different ways: (1) the drugs may be addictive and result in symptoms of withdrawal during the neonatal period, (2) they may be toxic and lead to impaired functioning and neurodevelopmental problems, and (3) they may be teratogenic and cause congenital anomalies and a dysmorphic appearance. The mechanism of action of the various substances on the developing fetus can be understood in terms of their biochemical properties.

In utero exposure to opiates such as heroin and methadone results in physiological addiction. These drugs bind to opiate receptor sites in the brain and GI tract. When the drugs are no longer present after birth, the newborn experiences withdrawal.

Cocaine and its metabolites cross the placenta and concentrate in amniotic fluid. Cocaine is toxic and teratogenic, and it interferes with 3 neurotransmitter pathways in the brain. (1) Cocaine blocks the reuptake of norepinephrine. This is associated with tachycardia, hypertension, diaphoresis, and an increased incidence of preterm labor. Diffuse vasoconstriction may affect the placenta and lead to anomalies such as placental infarcts or abruptio placentae. The fetus may also be affected by the vasoconstriction and its resultant hypoperfusion and ischemia, and may develop anomalies such as atresia of the GI tract, stroke, or absent limbs.

(2) Cocaine decreases the reuptake of dopamine. This effect is apparent in cocaine-using mothers who have decreased appetite and subsequent poor nutrition during pregnancy. Stereotypical behavior, hyperactivity, euphoria, confidence, and heightened sexuality may be associated with sexual promiscuity and increased risk of acquiring HIV and sexually transmitted infections (STIs). (3) Cocaine decreases serotonin reuptake, leading to decreased sleep. The sleep cycle of cocaine-exposed infants is often disrupted.

Methamphetamine is commonly manufactured from ephedrine or pseudoephedrine, and has greater central nervous system (CNS) penetration than its metabolite, amphetamine. It has direct toxic effects on the CNS and causes increased release and decreased reuptake of dopamine, norepinephrine, and serotonin. The neurotransmitter alterations that occur with methamphetamine use result in symptoms that are similar to those described for cocaine. There is very limited published data on the incidence of teratogenesis as a result of in utero methamphetamine exposure.

Direct effects of methamphetamine use are dose- and frequency-dependent in the adult user. It has been shown to have cardiovascular, pulmonary, renal, and hepatic toxicity. Higher dose and increased frequency have also been associated with psychosis and with toxicity to subcortical structures. It is hypothesized that there are toxic effects of methamphetamines on the developing fetus as well, but there are limited data currently.

Reports have documented the occurrence of withdrawal symptoms within days after birth in alcohol-exposed neonates, but the more common effects of prenatal alcohol exposure are direct cellular toxicity and teratogenesis. The specific mechanism by which alcohol and its metabolites damage fetal tissues is unknown, but it has been shown to affect CNS neuronal migration and synaptogenesis. For a given level of alcohol intake, the precise level of fetal exposure to the metabolites is likely to vary among women, depending on maternal genetic makeup and the resulting variability in alcohol metabolisms. The timing of the exposure during different periods of development can also lead to different teratogenic effects on the fetus. Exposure during the first trimester may affect organogenesis or craniofacial development, and exposure in the second and third trimesters can cause poor growth and neurotoxicity. Maternal alcohol use may also be associated with poor nutrition, resulting in poor delivery of nutrients to the fetus.

Phencyclidine (PCP) has sympathomimetic effects, including increases in blood pressure, heart rate, respiratory rate, deep tendon reflexes, and tone. In addition, PCP has cholinergic effects, causing sweating, flushing, drooling, and pupillary constriction. Infants exposed to PCP in utero do not exhibit these symptoms, however, but display neurologic and developmental disorganization.

Differential Diagnosis

The major differential diagnoses relate to the symptomatology produced by the abused substance or substances (Dx Box). Neonates exposed to addictive substances, most commonly opiates such as methadone and heroin, may present with symptoms of withdrawal

(Box 118-1). Irritability and jitteriness may be symptoms of drug withdrawal or direct drug neurotoxicity, but may also be due to hypoglycemia, hypocalcemia, hypomagnesemia, and sepsis. Seizures occur in 1% to 3% of heroin-exposed infants, and the differential diagnosis for neonatal seizures includes intracranial hemorrhage, hypoxic-ischemic encephalopathy, CNS infection, CNS malformation, and metabolic disorders. Gastrointestinal symptoms such as vomiting or diarrhea may be confused with reflux, formula intolerance, obstruction, or infectious gastroenteritis.

Dx **Infants of Substance-Abusing Mothers**

- Symptoms of withdrawal (see Box 118-1)
- Congenital anomalies
- Developmental delay and behavioral disorders
- Growth retardation
- Sexually transmitted infections

Dysmorphic appearance may also be the result of alcohol or drug exposure. Fetal alcohol syndrome is the most clearly defined dysmorphic syndrome related to maternal substance abuse during pregnancy. In making such a diagnosis, other genetic disorders that may have overlapping findings should be considered as well.

Failure to thrive (FTT) may also be a presenting complaint in infants or children with a history of in utero drug or alcohol exposure (see Chapter 117 for a discussion of the differential diagnosis of FTT). It is important to consider maternal substance abuse in all patients who have been diagnosed with FTT, particularly if they were small for gestational age.

Older children may present with a wide range of neurodevelopmental and behavioral problems. Common behavioral complaints include impulsivity, inattention, hyperactivity, and antisocial behavior. While many of these symptoms have been correlated with prenatal drug exposure, postnatal environmental factors such as continued parental substance abuse, violence, inconsistent or poor parenting, and foster care placement are also significant contributors. As a result, it may be difficult to clearly determine the precise etiology of developmental and behavioral problems in a drug- or alcohol-exposed child.

Maternal substance abuse should be considered in all infants who present with STIs such as syphilis, hepatitis B, hepatitis C, and HIV.

Evaluation

History

The possibility of maternal substance abuse should be considered in the face of certain maternal risk factors. These factors include the absence of prenatal care, evidence of poor maternal nutrition, poor maternal weight gain, presence of STIs, symptoms of acute

---

Box 118-1. Symptoms of Neonatal Abstinence Syndrome

• Irritability	• Vomiting
• Jitteriness	• Diarrhea
• Tremors	• Apnea
• Hypertonicity	• Tachypnea
• Seizures	• Sweating
• Sneezing	• Poor feeding
• Hiccups	• Sleeping difficulties

intoxication, abruptio placentae, precipitous delivery, and a history of domestic violence.

Infants who manifest symptoms of withdrawal should be evaluated for the possibility of maternal substance abuse. This assessment involves an appropriate history as well as a toxicological evaluation. Mothers disclose their drug history to varying extents, depending on the circumstances of the interview. If mothers are concerned about the health and well-being of their infants and do not fear legal repercussions, they are more likely to discuss their drug use. An appropriate drug history should be obtained in a nonjudgmental manner (Questions Box). Studies have shown that the use of a structured questionnaire rather than a cursory interview increases the incidence of reported substance abuse by 3- to 5-fold.

Questions

Infants of Substance-Abusing Mothers

- Did the mother use any substances such as alcohol, cigarettes, marijuana, or prescription and illicit drugs during the pregnancy?
- Has she ever used these substances? Is she currently using these substances?
- If so, how much? How frequently? By what route? To what extent is she trying to abstain?
- Is the mother at risk for sexually transmitted infections? Has she ever been tested?
- Did the mother have prenatal care? When did the care start?
- What is the status of other children in the family?
- Does the father abuse alcohol or drugs?

Physical Examination

Infants should be assessed for the common complications related to maternal substance abuse. They should undergo a full physical examination to check for the presence of any anomalies. Growth measurements should be noted, and physicians should determine if intrauterine growth restriction or microcephaly is evident. Premature infants should be monitored for all the problems related to prematurity, such as intraventricular hemorrhage and necrotizing enterocolitis. Signs of neonatal abstinence syndrome should be repeatedly assessed (see Box 118-1). Neurologic and developmental status should be assessed and monitored at each visit. Abnormalities such as hypertonicity, coarse tremors, and extensor leg posture are frequently noted in the newborn period, and disturbances in both fine and gross motor coordination may persist through the toddler years.

Laboratory Tests

In addition to obtaining a toxicological history, screening for drugs should also be performed. The legal guidelines for screening mothers for drugs vary in different localities. In general, infants can be screened on medical grounds without parental consent because the information obtained is important in the care of the infant. Screening of the mother's urine without her consent is more problematic, however, because of the potential legal implications of a positive test.

Some centers have drug panels that screen for the most commonly used illicit substances, such as cocaine, opiates, amphetamines, barbiturates, and marijuana. Most of these tests use immunoassays and require 1 to 2 mL of infant urine. These tests are inexpensive and sensitive, but not very specific. For example, over-the-counter medications containing ephedrine and pseudoephedrine may cause the screen to be positive for amphetamines, and those with dextromethorphan can cause a positive result for opiates. In those cases where a drug screening immunoassay does yield a positive result, confirmatory testing via gas chromatography/mass spectrometry is indicated.

Newer methods check for the presence of illicit drugs or their metabolites in infant hair and meconium. Meconium testing has a high sensitivity and specificity, and may give an indication of drug exposure anytime after 24 weeks of gestation. Hair analysis may reflect exposure in the third trimester. Urine testing is typically able to detect an exposure within the previous 3 days. As a result, a meconium or hair sample may be positive while the urine sample is negative.

Further evaluation in the neonatal period should include an evaluation for the presence of STIs, particularly HIV, hepatitis B, hepatitis C, and syphilis.

Imaging Studies

There is no routine imaging recommended based solely on a history of in utero substance exposure. Instead, imaging should be directed by symptomatology. For example, infants with a heart murmur and a history of prenatal alcohol exposure warrant a cardiac evaluation and possible echocardiography. Also, infants with prenatal drug exposure and abnormal neurologic examinations should have a thorough neurologic evaluation, which may include neuroimaging.

Management

In the neonatal period, the management of drug-exposed infants requires attention to associated conditions such as prematurity, in utero growth restriction, and in utero infection with STIs.

Irritability and crying may occur either from withdrawal or as the result of drug toxicity on the CNS. These infants may respond to swaddling, a soothing voice, or a quiet environment as a means to reduce the symptoms. Some exposed infants may have slow or disordered feeding and may require the same interventions for this problem as well.

Symptoms of neonatal abstinence syndrome may require pharmacologic treatment if they are severe enough. Common medications used for this purpose are paregoric (0.1 mL/kg), phenobarbital (2–8 mg/kg once a day), and methadone (0.05–0.01 mg/kg every 6 hours). Opiates are particularly useful in opiate-exposed infants. Paregoric, once commonly used to treat symptoms of withdrawal, is now used less frequently because of the potential toxic effects associated with the presence of alcohol and benzoic acid in the preparation. Phenobarbital may be preferred in cases of polydrug abuse. Diazepams are useful for symptoms related to alcohol withdrawal or to rapidly reverse symptoms of opioid withdrawal. Problems with using diazepam relate to the presence of sodium benzoate in the preparation, which can displace bilirubin from albumin. Clonidine has a shorter duration of action than phenobarbital, is a non-narcotic, and is still under evaluation for use in the management of neonatal abstinence syndrome. Medications should be tapered over time, allowing infants to outgrow the dosage.

Social service is a key component of management. In many jurisdictions, child protective services must be notified about positive toxicological tests on newborn infants or their mothers. Likewise, infants who display symptoms of neonatal drug withdrawal may also have to be reported to these agencies. These agencies are generally responsible for performing a home assessment and determining the adequacy of the environment. In some cases, infants may be assigned to foster homes. Parents may be ordered to participate in drug treatment programs and parenting classes.

After the newborn period the focus of management is on the provision of **well-child care and developmental monitoring.** Attention should be paid to physical growth and administration of immunizations. If a sensory impairment or neurodevelopmental delay is apparent, children should be referred to appropriate community agencies. Federal programs that operate under the Individuals with Disabilities Education Act provide interventional services for disabled and at-risk children 6 years of age and younger.

Symptoms of ADHD or other behavioral problems in older children may require intervention, with recommendation for specific school programs as well as pharmacologic treatment. Regular assessments of school performance should be obtained from children's teachers. Standardized neurodevelopmental tests should be administered at periodic intervals to ensure appropriate progress.

Prognosis

Many infants, particularly those exposed to alcohol in utero, suffer long-term sequelae and disability. Remedial educational programs help, but do not cure, the problems. Recent studies have shown that for drug-exposed children, the environment in which they are raised is a significant factor affecting their ultimate outcome. A stable, nurturing environment minimizes the many adverse effects of prenatal drug exposure and promotes normal neurodevelopment by enforcing the acquisition of skills and knowledge.

CASE RESOLUTION

The case history presented highlights the typical features of the drug-exposed infant. Management includes testing for hepatitis B, hepatitis C, syphilis, and human immunodeficiency virus and administering medication such as phenobarbital if the irritability does not respond to swaddling or other measures. The situation should be reported to child protective services to ensure an assessment of the infant's home environment.

Selected References

Bar-Oz B, Klein J, Karaskov T, Koren G. Comparison of meconium and neonatal hair analysis for detection of gestational exposure to drugs of abuse. *Arch Dis Child Fetal Neonatal Ed.* 2003;88:F98–F100

Boyle RJ. Effects of certain prenatal drugs on the fetus and newborn. *Pediatr Rev.* 2003;23:17–23

Chiriboga CA, Kuhn L, Wasserman GA. Prenatal cocaine exposures and dose-related cocaine effects on infant tone and behavior. *Neurotoxicol Teratol.* 2007;29:323–330

Davies JK, Bledsoe JM. Prenatal alcohol and drug exposures in adoption. *Pediatr Clin North Am.* 2005;52:1369–1393

Frank DA, Augustyn M, Knight WG, Pell T, Zuckerman B. Growth, development, and behavior in early childhood following prenatal cocaine exposure: a systematic review. *JAMA.* 2001;285:1613–1625

Greene CM, Goodman MH. Neonatal abstinence syndrome: strategies for care of the drug-exposed infant. *Neonatal Netw.* 2003;22:15–25

Koren G, Chan D, Klein J, Karaskov T. Estimation of fetal exposure to drugs of abuse, environmental tobacco smoke, and ethanol. *Ther Drug Monit.* 2002;24:23–25

Osborn DA, Cole MJ, Jeffery HE. Opiate treatment for opiate withdrawal in newborn infants. *Cochrane Database Syst Rev.* 2002;3:CD002059

Osborn DA, Jeffery HE, Cole MJ. Sedatives for opiate withdrawal in newborn infants. *Cochrane Database Syst Rev.* 2005;3:CD002053

Thachray HM, Tifft C. Fetal alcohol syndrome. *Pediatr Rev.* 2001;22:47–55

Substance Abuse

Monica Sifuentes, MD

CASE STUDY

A 17-year-old adolescent male is brought to your office by his father with a chief complaint of chronic cough. You have followed this patient and his siblings for several years and know the family quite well. The father appears very concerned about "this cough that just won't go away." The adolescent is not concerned about the cough, however, and reports no associated symptoms such as fever, sore throat, chest pain, or sinus pain. You ask the father to step out of the room for the rest of the interview and the physical examination.

On further questioning, the patient reports that he smokes a few cigarettes a day and has tried marijuana as well as cocaine. He denies regular use of these substances, but reports exposure to these drugs at parties and when he hangs out with "certain friends." The adolescent is now in the 11th grade, attends school regularly, and thinks school is "OK." His grades are average to above average, but he thinks he might fail history this semester. Although he used to play baseball, he dropped out last year. He hopes to get a part-time job at a local fast food restaurant this summer if his parents let him. Currently he is sexually active and uses condoms occasionally. He denies suicidal ideation and exposure to any firearms.

On physical examination, he appears well developed and well nourished with an occasional dry cough. He is afebrile, and his respiratory rate, heart rate, and blood pressure are normal. Pertinent findings on examination include slight conjunctival injection bilaterally and mild erythema of the posterior pharynx. No tonsillar hypertrophy is apparent. The rest of the examination is within normal limits.

Questions

1. What are the most common manifestations of substance use and abuse in adolescents?
2. What are the risk factors associated with substance abuse in adolescents?
3. What other conditions must be considered when evaluating adolescents with a history of chronic substance abuse?
4. What laboratory evaluation, if any, should be considered in adolescents with suspected substance use or abuse?
5. What are the specific consequences, if any, of short-term and long-term use or abuse of substances such as alcohol, marijuana, cocaine, opiates, and hallucinogens?

Primary care practitioners can become involved in adolescent substance abuse either through prevention and anticipatory guidance or through the identification and treatment of a substance abuse problem in their patients. Ideally, all adolescent patients should be questioned and counseled about the use of illicit drugs, alcohol, and tobacco at each health maintenance visit (see Chapters 5 and 24). Unfortunately, this rarely occurs because most health care professionals often feel uncomfortable opening this Pandora's box. Primary care practitioners thus lose a valuable opportunity to adequately assess adolescents for substance abuse and provide them with the necessary guidance to ensure their future well-being.

Substance use can be defined as the use of or experimentation with illicit drugs, alcohol, or tobacco. Illicit drugs include marijuana; cocaine; amphetamines; hallucinogens such as lysergic acid diethylamide (LSD), mescaline, and psilocybin, which is found in *Psilocybe mexicana* mushrooms; opiates; and phencyclidine (PCP). **Substance abuse** refers to the chronic use of mind-altering drugs in spite of adverse affects. **Addiction** is the term applied to compulsive and continued use of a substance in the face of these adverse consequences. The substance may produce physical dependence or symptoms of withdrawal when it is discontinued.

Epidemiology

Current Trends and Prevalence Rates

A wide range of substances is currently being used by young adolescents in the United States. Alcohol, tobacco, and marijuana are clearly the more common and most popular substances. It is important to remember that most statistics do not include the estimated 15% to 20% of students who drop out of high school before their senior year.

In a recent survey of graduating high school seniors, approximately 80% admitted to **alcohol** use at some time. Just over half (51%) of students reported drinking alcohol during the month preceding the survey, and 3% to 5% admitted that they used alcohol daily. Binge drinking has probably contributed most to the overall morbidity and mortality associated with alcohol use in adolescents. Among high school seniors in the class of 2005, 33% reported having

5 or more drinks in a row at least once during the previous 2 weeks. Although **tobacco** use among adolescents decreased from 1975 to 1993, 2005 data from the Centers for Disease Control and Prevention (CDC) reveal that 23% of teenagers nationwide still report current cigarette use. Eleven percent of adolescents smoked a half a pack or more cigarettes per day in 2005 compared with 19% in 1977. Seven percent of ninth graders also reported smoking on a daily basis, with an equal prevalence among males and females. Nationwide current smokeless tobacco use (eg, chewing tobacco, snuff, or dip) and cigar or cigarillo use is 8% and 14%, respectively. As expected, its use is higher among males than females.

Marijuana is the most commonly used illicit psychoactive substance. In 1993, 35% of high school seniors reported ever having used marijuana, and in 1997, this figure increased to more than 50%. Current estimates from the 2005 Youth Risk Behavior Surveillance System (YRBSS) report this figure to be approximately 48%, with nearly 25% reporting marijuana use one or more times during the month preceding the survey. Daily use of marijuana has been reported in 5% of high school seniors.

The use of other substances among adolescents had generally taken a downward trend in the late 1980s and early 1990s; however, figures are increasing again. Reportedly, approximately 9% of high school graduates in 1997 tried cocaine, with approximately 4% having used it in the previous month. These figures remain unchanged in 2005. The 1991 prevalence rate for LSD usage was 5%, and its use has shown no appreciable decline in the past 10 years. In fact, LSD use among teens has increased significantly and may be more widespread than cocaine among high school students. According to the latest YRBSS 2005 survey, almost 9% of high school seniors nationwide had tried LSD, compared with 12% in 1995. Lifetime amphetamine use among 12th graders was 6% in 2005 and ranged from 2.6% to almost 12% across state surveys. In addition, nationwide ecstasy use was reported as 6.3%.

Concurrently, the reported use of over-the-counter (OTC) nonprescription stimulants that contain caffeine or phenylpropanolamine has increased. Other substances used to "get high," such as inhalants, are often used by younger students (preteens). Nineteen percent of ninth graders surveyed by the CDC in 1997 reported having sniffed or inhaled substances to become intoxicated compared with 14% in 2005. Dextromethorphan is the most recent OTC product to be abused by adolescents secondary to its hallucinogenic effects and easy accessibility. Recent studies report an increasing trend in its abuse, particularly in teens younger than 18 years.

Although not considered an illicit substance by some, anabolic steroids are abused by some adolescents, mostly males, to increase muscle size and strength. In 1997 approximately 3% admitted to using them at some time in their lives. Other studies indicate as many as 5.5% of high school students participating in sports use anabolic steroids (6.6% males, 3.9% females). The 2005 nationwide figure per the CDC is 4%.

Demographics

In general, adolescent males use illicit drugs more than females do, with a few exceptions. Males are more likely to use anabolic steroids, but females reportedly use amphetamines, barbiturates, tranquilizers, and OTC diet pills more than their male counterparts. In addition, although annual prevalence rates for overall alcohol use show little gender difference, adolescent males have a higher rate of heavy or binge drinking. Tobacco usage is essentially the same for both genders.

Non–college-bound adolescents are more likely to use illicit substances than their college-bound counterparts, and these adolescents are also more likely to use drugs more frequently. There is no difference, however, between the 2 groups in the rates of ever having tried illicit substances. The influence of parental education, socioeconomic status, and race or ethnicity on the use and abuse of illicit substances is difficult to determine.

Risk Factors and Risk Behaviors

The strongest predictor of drug use is having friends who use drugs regularly. In addition, it has been shown that the more risk factors identified, the greater the risk of substance abuse.

Several factors are important precursors (risk factors) to drug use during adolescence. These include association with drug-using peers; attitudinal factors, such as favorable attitudes regarding drug use and low religiosity; school failure, beginning in the late elementary years; young age of initiation of alcohol or drug use; environmental factors, such as the prevalence of drug use in a given community; a family history of alcoholism or drug use; poor parenting practices; high levels of conflict within the family; minimal bonding between parents and children; and early and persistent problem behaviors during childhood.

Clinical Presentation

Adolescents who are involved in substance abuse may present to the physician in several different ways. Illicit substance use might be uncovered during the routine interview for an annual health maintenance visit or preparticipation sports physical. Alternatively, the adolescent might have physical complaints including chronic cough, persistent allergies, chest pain, and fatigue. They also recently may have been in a motor vehicle crash, or their parents may complain of frequent mood swings or irritability.

Pathophysiology

Although several theories have been proposed to explain why casual substance use develops into abuse and addiction in some adolescents, the most critical factor seems to be the presence of underlying psychopathology. Adolescents who have major depressive disorders, attention-deficit/hyperactivity disorder (ADHD), or schizophrenia, for example, may use mood-altering substances to treat unpleasant feelings of dysphoria and low self-esteem. Although initially used as a temporary measure, this method of self-medication makes chronic use with some substances more likely.

Differential Diagnosis

The differential diagnosis for symptoms and behaviors associated with substance abuse includes underlying psychiatric disorders. Affective, antisocial conduct and ADHD can be the primary or secondary condition in adolescents who are abusing drugs. Like adults, adolescents may be using illicit drugs to self-medicate. The pharmacology and toxicity of the illicit substances most commonly used by adolescents are summarized in Table 119-1.

Evaluation

History

The interview should be conducted in a private, quiet area with minimal chance of interruptions. If parents have accompanied adolescents, they should be politely asked to leave the room after issues of confidentiality are addressed in the presence of both parties. This avoids further awkward moments when parents may ask what was disclosed during the interview with their teenager. After parents have left the room, issues regarding confidentiality and privacy should be reviewed once again with the patient. Special circumstances, such as a disclosure of sexual or physical abuse and/or possible suicide ideation or homicidal intent, that dictate that confidentiality be broken also should be discussed (see Chapter 5).

The interview should then proceed in a casual, non-pressured fashion. Initial inquiries should cover less-threatening general topics such as school, home life, and outside activities, including activities with friends. **HEADDSSS** (home, education or employment, activities, diet, drugs, sexual activity, suicide or depression, and safety) allows for a thorough review of the essential components of the psychosocial history (see Chapter 5).

Some practitioners prefer to use questionnaires to obtain this background information. A questionnaire is given to patients to fill out while they are waiting to be seen, and the responses are reviewed during the actual visit (Box 119-1). Controversy exists regarding the role of such questionnaires, primarily concerning the truthfulness of answers, because parents may be with the teenager as he or she is attempting to complete the form.

More specific questions related to the use of alcohol and tobacco as well as illicit substances should be asked after general subjects have been discussed (Questions Box). If adolescents seem wary of answering these questions, it may be helpful to initially inquire about their friends. Questions should be phrased with the assumption that the responses will be affirmative (eg, How many beers do you drink in a week?). It is hoped that this less-threatening approach invites more honest answers. An assessment of the risk of suicidal behavior is also indicated. Further questions relevant to substance abuse are given in Box 119-2.

Because many clinicians do not have unlimited time to interview adolescents and obtain all of the details at one visit, another approach has been developed to efficiently screen for drug and alcohol problems using 3 questions: (1) Have you *ever* smoked a cigarette? (2) Have you *ever* had an alcoholic drink? and (3) Have you *ever* used

---

Box 119-1. Questionnaire Items Relevant to Substance Abuse[a]

1. Do you smoke cigarettes?   Y _____ N _____
2. Do you smoke marijuana?   Y _____ N _____
3. Do you often feel "bummed out," down, or depressed?   Y _____ N _____
4. Do you ever use drugs or alcohol to feel better?   Y _____ N _____
5. Do you ever use drugs or alcohol when you are alone?   Y _____ N _____
6. Do your friends get drunk or get high at parties?   Y _____ N _____
7. Do you get drunk or get high at parties?   Y _____ N _____
8. Do your friends ever get drunk or get high at rock concerts?   Y _____ N _____
9. Do you ever get drunk or get high at rock concerts?   Y _____ N _____
10. Have your school grades gone down recently?   Y _____ N _____
11. Have you flunked any subjects recently?   Y _____ N _____
12. Have you had recent problems with your coaches or advisers at school?   Y _____ N _____
13. Do you feel that friends or parents just do not seem to understand you?   Y _____ N _____

[a]Reproduced with permission from American Academy of Pediatrics. *Substance Abuse: A Guide for Professionals.* Schonberg SK, ed. Elk Grove, IL: American Academy of Pediatrics; 1988.

Questions

Adolescent Substance Abuse

- Do any of the adolescent's friends drink alcohol, smoke marijuana or tobacco, or use any other drugs?
- What drugs, including alcohol and tobacco, are currently being used by the adolescent? For how long and how frequently?
- In what environments does the adolescent use these substances?
- Has the adolescent ever blacked out or been arrested while under the influence of drugs or alcohol?
- Has drug or alcohol use ever interfered with school, work, or other social activities?
- Has drug or alcohol use adversely affected relationships with family, friends, or romantic partners?
- Has the patient ever had sexual encounters while under the influence of drugs or alcohol?
- Does the adolescent ever use drugs or alcohol to feel better or to forget why he or she feels sad?
- Do the adolescent's parents use alcohol, tobacco, or illicit drugs?

---

marijuana or any other drug to get high? The thinking is that by using the word "ever" the clinician is asking a clearer question. Additional screening is recommended for any teenager who answers "yes" to

Table 119-1. Pharmacology and Toxicity of Substances Commonly Used by Adolescents[a]

Substance	Pharmacology	Effects	Toxicity
Nicotine	Potent psychoactive drug, acting on receptors in CNS to produce effects: stimulation, relaxation, focuses attention		**Non-tolerant individuals** Weakness, nausea, vomiting Feeling unwell
Marijuana	Active ingredient (Δ^9-tetrahydro-cannabinol) rapidly absorbed into bloodstream from inhaled smoke	**Low dose** Euphoria, relaxation, time distortion, auditory and visual enhancement **High dose/toxic** Mood fluctuations, hallucinations, paranoia, psychosis	**Acute** Panic attacks, psychosis (rare) **Chronic** Short-term memory impairment, amotivational syndrome, reduced sperm counts
Alcohol	Causes nerve cell membranes to expand and become more "fluid"—interfering with neuronal conduction Interference of neurotransmitters	**Mild** Disinhibition, euphoria, mild impaired coordination, mild sedation **Moderate** Increased sedation, slurred speech, ataxia	**Severe** Confusion, stupor, coma, respiratory depression

Cocaine	Increased release and decreased reuptake of biogenic amines causing CNS and peripheral nervous system stimulation
	    Local anesthesia
	    Vasoconstriction
		Produces a sense of well-being and heightened awareness, decrease in social inhibition, intense euphoria	Delirium, confusion, paranoia, hypertension, tachycardia, hyperpyrexia, mydriasis

Stimulants Amphetamines Crystal methamphetamine "Ecstasy"	CNS stimulation (sympathomimetic)	Heightened awareness Restlessness and agitation, decreased appetite Low doses increase ability to concentrate	Hypertension, hyperthermia, seizures, stroke, coma, arrhythmias
Hallucinogens LSD Mescaline Mushrooms	Inhibits release of serotonin	Distortions of reality—perceptual alterations, "synesthesias" common (eg, "hearing" smells)	Paranoia, flashbacks, psychosis, depression
Phencyclidine	Dissociative anesthetic with analgesic, stimulant, depressant, and hallucinogenic properties	Dissociative anesthetic Dose-dependent euphoria, dysphoria, perceptual distortion	Psychoses; aggressive, violent behavior; depression; seizures, rhabdomyolysis
Opiates Opium Heroin Methadone	Binds to opioid receptors in CNS, causing CNS depression	Sedative analgesics Euphoria followed by sedation, somnolence	Respiratory depression, CNS depression, miosis, bradycardia, hypotension, arrhythmia, seizures, rhabdomyolysis
Sedatives Benzodiazepines Barbiturates	CNS depression, binds to specific receptor that potentiates GABA	Sedation Anxiety reduction	Similar to opioid intoxication
Anabolic steroids	Bind to androgen receptors at cellular level, stimulate production of RNA and protein synthesis	Euphoria Increased irritability and aggressiveness Induction of mental changes at high doses	Psychosis
Inhalants	CNS stimulation and excitement, progressing to depression	Euphoria, hallucinations, psychosis	Respiratory depression, arrhythmia, seizures, sudden sniffing death syndrome (sudden death secondary to arrhythmia)

Abbreviations: CNS, central nervous system; LSD, lysergic acid diethylamide; GABA, γ-aminobutyric acid.

[a]Data from Schwartz B, Alderman EM. Substances of abuse. *Pediatr Rev.* 1997;18:206–214, and Joffe A, Blythe MJ, eds. Mental health, psychotropic medications, and substance abuse. *Adolesc Med.* 2003;14:455–466.

Box 119-2. Open-Ended Questions Intended to Provide a Basis for Further Exploration of Advanced Substance Abuse[a]

1. What do your friends do at parties? Do you go to the parties? Do you drink? Get drunk? Get high?

2. Do you drive drunk? Stoned? Have you ridden with a driver who was drunk or stoned? Could you call home and ask for help? What would your parents say? Do?

3. Do you go to rock concerts? Do you drink there? Do you get high? Who drives after the concert?

4. After drinking, have you ever forgotten where you had been or what you had done?

5. Have you recently dropped some of your old friends and started going with a new group?

6. Do you feel that lately you are irritable, "bitchy," or moody?

7. Do you find yourself getting into more frequent arguments with your friends? Brothers and sisters? Parents?

8. Do you have a girlfriend/boyfriend? How is that going? Are you having more fights/arguments with him/her lately? Have you recently broken up?

9. Do you find yourself being physically abusive to others? Your brothers/sisters? Your mother/father?

10. Do you think your drinking/drug use is a problem? Why?

---

[a]Reproduced with permission from American Academy of Pediatrics. *Substance Abuse: A Guide for Professionals.* Schonberg SK, ed. Elk Grove, IL: American Academy of Pediatrics; 1988.

Box 119-3. The CRAFFT Questions[a]

C Have you ever ridden in a **CAR** driven by someone who was "high" or had been using alcohol or drugs?

R Do you ever use alcohol or drugs to **RELAX,** feel better about yourself, or fit in?

A Do you ever use alcohol or drugs while you are by yourself **(ALONE)**?

F Do you ever **FORGET** things you did while using alcohol or drugs?

F Do your **FAMILY** or **FRIENDS** ever tell you that you should cut down on your drinking or drug use?

T Have you ever gotten into **TROUBLE** while you were using alcohol or drugs?

---

[a]From Knight JR, Sherritt L, Shrier LA, Harris SK, Chang G. Validity of the CRAFFT substance abuse screening test among adolescent clinic patients. *Arch Pediatr Adolesc Med.* 2002;156:607–614.

---

any of these 3 initial questions. Six questions, known as the CRAFFT questions, are then reviewed to further screen the adolescent for drug and alcohol problems (Box 119-3). The teen receives 1 point for each "yes" answer; a total score of 2 or more indicates a high risk for a substance abuse problem and the need for additional follow-up as well as a referral to a mental health professional. The validity of this tool with adolescents has been reported in the literature.

Physical Examination

Positive findings on physical examination are rare, especially in adolescents who use alcohol or other substances only occasionally. In adolescents with a history of chronic substance abuse, however, certain physical findings may be present.

All vital signs should be reviewed. Tachycardia and hypertension occur primarily with acute intoxication with cocaine or stimulants such as amphetamines. The current weight also should be recorded and compared with previous values, and any significant loss should be noted. The skin should be examined closely for track marks, skin abscesses, or cellulitis, especially if patients admit to using drugs intravenously. Findings consistent with hepatitis (hepatomegaly and jaundice) may also be present in these individuals. The presence of diffuse adenopathy, thrush, leukoplakia, seborrheic dermatitis, or parotitis should raise the suspicion of human immunodeficiency virus infection. Upper respiratory symptoms such as chronic nasal congestion, long-lasting "colds" and "allergies," and epistaxis can occur with chronic inhalation of cocaine. Signs of nasal congestion,

septal perforation, and wheezing may be noted on examination. In addition, smoking crack cocaine can cause chronic cough, hemoptysis, and chest pain. Smoking marijuana over long periods can result in similar findings. Gynecomastia can be seen with use of anabolic steroids, marijuana, amphetamine, and heroin. In the adolescent female using anabolic steroids, there may be signs of virilization, such as a deep voice, hirsutism, and male pattern baldness. The neurologic evaluation is probably the most important part of the examination. Any abnormalities in memory, cognitive functioning, or affect should be noted. Chronic marijuana use is sometimes accompanied by an amotivational syndrome.

Acute intoxication with some drugs such as cocaine may lead to delirium, confusion, paranoia, seizures, hypertension, tachycardia, arrhythmias, mydriasis, and hyperpyrexia. Acute PCP intoxication produces abnormal neurologic signs, tachycardia, and hypertension. Findings such as central nervous system and respiratory depression, miosis, and cardiovascular effects (eg, pulmonary edema, orthostatic hypotension) are consistent with opiate overdose.

Laboratory Tests

Drug screening in the evaluation of possible substance abuse is not recommended and generally not indicated. Specific laboratory studies should be performed only in those patients who are known substance abusers and enrolled in a drug treatment program or in patients with an acute presentation of altered mental status, intoxication, or abnormal neurologic findings, such as may be seen in an emergency department setting. In the office setting, these symptoms are frequently absent, and urine or serum studies to "check" for drug use are not warranted. If these tests are performed, they require the adolescent's consent. They should not be performed simply to allay parental anxiety or confirm suspicions regarding possible substance abuse.

Urine testing is available to detect marijuana and its metabolites, cocaine, amphetamines, PCP, opiates, barbiturates, and benzodiazepines. Blood levels can be obtained for alcohol, marijuana, cocaine, amphetamines, barbiturates, and benzodiazepines. Although salivary or urinary concentrations of cotinine and nicotine concentrations can also be performed, these measurements are primarily used in research studies.

Testing for specific inhalants is not routinely done. The deleterious effects of these substances on the hematologic, liver, and renal systems can be evaluated by performing a complete blood count, liver function tests, prothrombin time and partial thromboplastin time, and blood urea nitrogen and creatinine.

Management

One of several approaches to the problem of substance abuse can be chosen depending on the degree of risk-taking behavior and drug involvement.

Anticipatory Guidance

If adolescents and their peers are not participating in any high-risk behaviors, pediatricians should provide patients with age-appropriate anticipatory guidance. This should include information regarding safety issues, consequences of alcohol and tobacco use, and exposures to illicit drugs. Adolescents should be encouraged to continue their current behavior but should be invited to return to the office if they have any questions or problems. This may be particularly helpful for adolescents whose daily environment exposes them to high-risk situations.

Early Intervention

Primary care practitioners should provide early intervention guidance to adolescents who are engaging in occasional high-risk behavior but whose substance use does not interfere with or disrupt their daily lives. Such use implies only occasional or casual use of illicit substances by patients or peers. Interventional guidance involves discussing potential risks created by adolescents' current behavior. For example, individuals who drink alcohol or smoke marijuana at parties have an increased risk of involvement in a motor vehicle crash afterward. Another common scenario involves alcohol intoxication and poor judgment with regard to sexual behavior.

Specialized Programs

Adolescents who are routinely using drugs but are clearly motivated to stop can often be managed by primary care physicians. Many of these teenagers began using illicit substances at an older age, have a fairly good relationship with their families, have supportive relationships with friends who do not use drugs, and have continued to do well in school and participate in other outside activities. At first, practitioners should identify the problem and establish that adolescents desire to change their behavior. Then practitioners should meet with families, develop an appropriate strategy, and follow the adolescents periodically in the office. Periodic reinforcement by physicians is necessary, especially in the beginning. Referral to outpatient programs, such as Alcoholics Anonymous or Narcotics Anonymous, also may be indicated.

Mental Health or Treatment Programs

Referral to a mental health or specialized treatment program is indicated for adolescents who continue to use drugs despite office treatment by the primary care practitioner. In addition, those teenagers who are suspected to have a concomitant psychological or psychiatric condition should be referred immediately for psychiatric evaluation. Other criteria for specialty treatment programs include a long history of drug abuse, a serious life-threatening event in conjunction with substance abuse (eg, attempted suicide), familial strife, or persistent involvement with a drug-dependent crowd. Primary care practitioners should become familiar with local inpatient programs and residential substance abuse treatment facilities in the community. Although the selection of a program is often dictated by financial resources, it is very important to select an appropriate one for both the adolescent as well as the family. Guidelines exist to aid practitioners in the selection process. These guidelines include total abstinence, appropriate professionals with expertise in drug abuse, familial involvement in the program, family therapy, and appropriate outpatient follow-up.

Prevention Programs

Prevention programs have been developed to assist and influence the decisions young people make about the use of illicit substances. Current programs focus on multiple aspects of the lives of children and adolescents. Programs may involve individual decision-making, self-esteem, and basic education regarding drugs. They frequently emphasize communication skills, family values and dynamics, parenting skills, and positive peer associations. Structured curricula have also been created for use in the schools, and community outreach programs have been organized by groups such as local police departments. The actual effectiveness of each type of program is a subject of controversy, but they are all aimed at somehow preventing the initial or continued use of illicit substances.

Prognosis

It is difficult to assess the outcome for adolescents who undergo treatment for substance abuse because definitions of success vary. For some teenagers, success implies periods of sobriety, for others it means complete abstinence, and for still others it is abstinence in

---

CASE RESOLUTION

In the case presented, the adolescent is at high risk for substance abuse given his drug-using friends, tobacco use, possible school failure, and recent change in extracurricular activities (ie, dropping out of baseball). The findings on physical examination also are consistent with his smoking history. The physician should review these risk factors with the teenager and acknowledge the difficulty in removing one's self from such an environment. The adolescent's motivation to change his behavior should be assessed, and referrals to special intervention programs can be discussed. Regardless of the outcome, the physician should continue to see the teenager at an agreed-on interval to monitor his behavior.

addition to recovery from other contributing problems. Specific outcome data that are available, however, reveal that abstinence rates are positively correlated with regular attendance in a support group and parental participation in these groups. In addition, general success rates range from 15% to 45%, depending on short- or long-term assessments. As expected, there is a lifetime potential for relapse among all substance abusers.

Selected References

American Academy of Pediatrics Committee on Sports Medicine and Fitness. Adolescents and anabolic steroids: a subject review. *Pediatrics.* 1997;99:904–908

American Academy of Pediatrics Committee on Substance Abuse. Alcohol use and abuse: a pediatric concern. *Pediatrics.* 2001;108:185–189

American Academy of Pediatrics Committee on Substance Abuse. *Substance Abuse: A Guide for Health Professionals.* Schydlower M, ed. Elk Grove Village, IL: American Academy of Pediatrics; 2002

American Academy of Pediatrics Committee on Substance Abuse. Testing for drugs of abuse in children and adolescents. *Pediatrics.* 1996;98:305–307

American Academy of Pediatrics Committee on Substance Abuse. Testing for drugs of abuse in children and adolescents: addendum—testing in schools and at home. *Pediatrics.* 2007;119:627–630

American Academy of Pediatrics Committee on Substance Abuse. Tobacco, alcohol, and other drugs: the role of the pediatrician in prevention and management of substance abuse. *Pediatrics.* 1998;101:125–128

American Academy of Pediatrics Committee on Substance Abuse and Committee on Native American Child Health. Inhalant abuse. *Pediatrics.* 1996;97:420–423

Anderson SL, Schaechter J, Brosco JP. Adolescent patients and their confidentiality: staying within legal bounds. *Contemp Pediatr.* 2005;22:54–64

Barangan CJ, Alderman EM. Management of substance abuse. *Pediatr Rev.* 2002;23:123–131

Bryner JK, Wang UK, Hui JW, Bedodo M, MacDougall C, Anderson IB. Dextromethorphan abuse in adolescence. *Arch Pediatr Adolesc Med.* 2006;160:1217–1222

Eaton DK, Kann L, Kinchen S, et al. Youth risk behavior surveillance—United States, 2005. *MMWR Surveill Summ.* 2006;55:1–108

Fishman M, Bruner A, Adger H Jr. Substance abuse among children and adolescents. *Pediatr Rev.* 1997;18:394–403

Heyman RB, Adger H. Office approach to drug abuse prevention. *Pediatr Clin North Am.* 1997;44:1447–1455

Kaul P, Coupey SM. Clinical evaluation of substance abuse. *Pediatr Rev.* 2002;23:85–94

Knight JR. Adolescent substance use: screening, assessment, and intervention. *Contemp Pediatr.* 1997;14:45–72

Knight JR, Sherritt L, Shrier LA, Harris SK, Chang G. Validity of the CRAFFT substance abuse screening test among adolescent clinic patients. *Arch Pediatr Adolesc Med.* 2002;156:607–614

Levy S, Knight JR. Office management of substance abuse. *Adolesc Health Update.* 2003;15:1–9

MacKenzie RG, Heischober B. Methamphetamine. *Pediatr Rev.* 1997;18:305–309

Schwartz RH. Adolescent heroin use: a review. *Pediatrics.* 1998;101:1461–1466

Schwartz RH. LSD makes a comeback. *Contemp Pediatr.* 1996;13:71–81

Weddle M, Kokotailo P. Adolescent substance abuse. Confidentiality and consent. *Pediatr Clin North Am.* 2002;49:301–315

Werner MJ, Adger H. Early identification, screening, and brief intervention for adolescent alcohol use. *Arch Pediatr Adolesc Med.* 1995;149:1241–1248

Wilson CR, Sherritt L, Gates E, Knight JR. Are clinical impressions of adolescent substance abuse accurate? *Pediatrics.* 2004;114:e536–e540

Eating Disorders

Monica Sifuentes, MD

CASE STUDY

A 16-year-old adolescent female is brought to the office by her mother because she feels that her daughter is too thin. The mother complains that her daughter does not eat much at dinner and always says she is not hungry. Recently the girl bought diet pills that were advertised in a teen magazine. She claims that the pills are supposed to help her gain weight, so she doesn't understand why her mother is so upset. She says she feels fine and considers herself healthy.

The girl is a 10th-grade student at a local public school and attends classes regularly, although her friends are occasionally truant. She is involved in the drill team, the swim team, and the student council. She has many friends who have "nicer" figures than she does. Neither she nor her friends smoke tobacco or use drugs, but they occasionally drink beer at parties. The girl is not sexually active and denies a history of abuse. Her menstrual periods are irregular; the last one was approximately 6 weeks ago.

She currently lives with her mother, father, and 2 younger siblings. Although things are "OK" at home, she thinks her parents are too strict and don't trust her. They have just begun to allow her to date.

Her physical examination is significant for a thin physique and normal vital signs. On the growth chart, her weight is at the 15th percentile and her height at the 75th percentile, giving her a body mass index of 17 (10th percentile). The remainder of her physical examination is unremarkable.

Questions

1. What are the common characteristics of disordered eating in adolescents?
2. What are the important historical points to include when interviewing patients with suspected eating disorders? And which teens are considered at risk?
3. How is the diagnosis of anorexia and bulimia nervosa made?
4. What is the treatment plan for adolescents with eating disorders?
5. What are the medical complications of anorexia and bulimia nervosa?
6. What is the prognosis for these conditions? How can primary care practitioners help improve the outcome?

Eating disorders are complex problems that are sometimes difficult to diagnose based on strict *Diagnostic and Statistical Manual of Mental Disorders, 4th edition (DSM-IV)* criteria (Box 120-1). Adolescents may have partial or atypical forms, a combination of both anorexia and bulimia nervosa, or an underlying affective component that confuses the issue. They may not display a blatant refusal to eat, but may instead exhibit subtle characteristics of disordered eating: constant dieting, obsession with a certain physical exercise, or irregular menstruation. In addition, preoccupation with physical appearance and weight is not uncommon or necessarily pathologic in today's Western society. Both the fashion industry and media promote the idea that thinness and beauty are interrelated. Thus typical adolescents who long to be accepted by peers and who are learning to develop a sense of independence and control are prime targets for the development of eating disorders. The primary care physician is in a unique position to recognize individuals at risk, appropriately screen those teenagers with specific behaviors, and provide early intervention to prevent the development of a full-blown eating disorder (Box 120-2). The overall goal is to decrease the life-long medical and psychological morbidity and mortality associated with this condition in adolescents.

Epidemiology

In general, eating disorders are most common among white females and in more affluent communities. Although they occur in many other settings, in previous years they were nearly unheard of in lower socioeconomic groups. Today they can be seen in all ethnic, cultural, and social backgrounds. In addition, males make up an estimated 5% to 10% of all patients with eating disorders.

Although dieting behavior among adolescents and young adults is not uncommon, true anorexia nervosa has a prevalence of approximately 0.5% to 1% in these individuals. Estimates have ranged from 1% to 10% in high-risk groups such as upper- and middle-class white females. Less than 5% of these cases are males, with a female-male ratio of 9:1. The age of onset is usually during early or middle adolescence (age 12–16 years). However, anorexia has been reported to have a second peak later in adolescence, and it has become increasingly more common for children and younger teens to be dissatisfied with their weight and concerned with body image. Studies have been reported in middle-income elementary school girls where significant body and weight dissatisfaction were noted with increasing grade. Skipping meals and desserts, fasting, and vomiting were all

---

Box 120-1. Diagnostic Criteria for Anorexia and Bulimia Nervosa[a]

Anorexia Nervosa

A. Refusal to maintain body weight at or above a minimally normal weight for age and height

B. Intense fear of gaining weight or becoming fat, even though underweight

C. Disturbance in the way in which one's body weight or shape is experienced, undue influence of body weight or shape on self-evaluation, or denial of the seriousness of the current low body weight

D. In post-menarcheal females, amenorrhea (ie, the absence of at least 3 consecutive cycles)

Bulimia Nervosa

A. Recurrent episodes of binge eating, characterized by the following:

   (1) Eating, in a discrete period, an amount of food that is definitely larger than most people would consume under similar circumstances and in the same period

   (2) A sense of lack of control over eating during the episode

B. Recurrent inappropriate compensatory behavior to prevent weight gain (self-induced vomiting, laxative or diuretic use).

C. Criteria A and B both occur on average at least twice a week for 3 months

D. Self-evaluation is unduly influenced by body shape and weight

E. The disturbance does not occur exclusively during episodes of anorexia nervosa

[a]Adapted and reproduced with permission from American Psychiatric Association. *Diagnostic and Statistical Manual of Mental Disorders (DSM-IV)*. 4th ed. Washington, DC: American Psychiatric Association; 1994.

Box 120-2. *Diagnostic and Statistical Manual for Primary Care (DSM-PC) Child and Adolescent Version* Diagnostic Criteria: Dieting/Body Image Problem[a]

- Dieting and voluntary food restrictions that result in weight loss or failure to gain weight as expected during growth, but behaviors not intense enough to qualify for diagnosis of anorexia nervosa

- Individual becomes obsessed with the pursuit of thinness and develops fears of gaining weight

- Consistent disturbance in body perception, denies dieting or weight loss is a problem

[a]Adapted from Wolraich ML, ed. *The Classification of Child and Adolescent Mental Diagnoses in Primary Care: Diagnostic and Statistical Manual for Primary Care (DSM-PC) Child and Adolescent Version*. Elk Grove Village, IL: American Academy of Pediatrics; 1996.

Box 120-3. Risk Factors for the Development of an Eating Disorder[a]

- Family history of an eating disorder or obesity
- Affective illness or alcoholism in a first-degree relative
- Specific sports: ballet, gymnastics, modeling
- Personality characteristics (eg, perfectionism)
- Parental eating behavior and weight
- Low self-esteem
- Physical or sexual abuse
- Body image dissatisfaction
- History of excessive dieting, frequently skipped meals, compulsive exercise

[a]Adapted from Rome ES, Ammerman S, Rosen DS, et al. Children and adolescents with eating disorders: the state of the art. *Pediatrics*. 2003;11:e100.

---

reported specifically to lose weight. Unfortunately, the goal for many of these young girls is not to be of normal weight, but to be underweight. The prevalence of bulimia nervosa is approximately 1% to 4%, although some studies report that as many as 8% of adolescents and college women and 0.4% of men are bulimic. The age of onset tends to be later than for anorexia, with symptoms beginning during late adolescence (age 17–20 years) and young adulthood. Females outnumber males by a factor of 5.

Several other behavioral and affective disorders have been associated with anorexia and bulimia nervosa. These include major depression and other mood disorders in patients as well as first-degree relatives, alcoholism and substance abuse, other addictive behaviors (eg, laxative abuse), poor impulse control and anxiety disorders, and obsessive-compulsive personality. In addition, suicidal behavior (attempts) is more likely in individuals with bulimia as are increased reports of family members with substance abuse and dependence disorders.

Mild variants of eating disorders, which do not meet full diagnostic criteria, occur in approximately 5% to 10% of post-pubertal females. Additionally, more than half of junior high and high school girls have dieted at some time, many repeatedly.

Clinical Presentation

Patients with eating disorders usually present with complaints related to weight loss or failure to gain weight. Adolescents may also present with secondary amenorrhea. Sometimes an underlying

psychiatric condition such as obsessive-compulsive disorder (OCD) is the grounds for the medical referral. Occasionally patients with eating disorders are hospitalized because of complications such as electrolyte disturbances related to diuretic use or hematemesis from induced vomiting.

Pathophysiology

Anorexia Nervosa

Although several factors predispose individuals to the development of anorexia nervosa, this condition has no single cause (Box 120-3). Longitudinal studies clearly point to a significant role of inappropriate dieting behavior in the pathogenesis of an eating disorder. However, because not all dieters develop an eating disorder, other risk factors must be involved. Current theory suggests that a complex relationship exists among multiple factors, which together contribute to the pathogenesis of anorexia.

Biological Factors

It has been postulated that the normal increase in adipose tissue with the onset of puberty creates a special problem for some females. An eating disorder may develop as an attempt to control or combat this normal pubertal weight gain with the initiation of dieting behavior.

Preexisting hypothalamic dysfunction also has been implicated as a contributing factor to anorexia. In addition, changes in neurotransmitter levels have been shown to occur with initial vomiting or dieting. These changes may then lead to specific psychiatric symptoms that may perpetuate eating disorders. However, recent data with neuroimaging studies have shown that most of the physiological disturbances resolve with normalization of the patient's body weight. In addition, a pre-morbid disturbance in the neurotransmitter serotonin has been speculated to be a risk factor for the development of both anorexia and bulimia. Serotonin controls appetite by creating a sensation of fullness or satiety. In addition, it is known to have an affect on sexual and social behavior, mood, and stress responses. Although further studies are needed to confirm the exact role of this hormone in the development of an eating disorder, it has been shown that decreases in this brain neurotransmitter have been associated with impulsivity, aggression, and depression.

Genetic Factors

A possible genetic predisposition to anorexia has been shown in studies of monozygotic twins. The incidence of the disorder is increased in sisters and other female relatives of patients with anorexia.

Personal Characteristics

In general, patients with anorexia are described as obsessive-compulsive personality types, perfectionists, and overachievers. They also display low self-esteem and high anxiety levels despite their successes. They are the "model daughters" who have never caused any previous problems given their compliant, self-sacrificing, non-assertive nature.

There is an increased association between anorexia and major depression as well, and many studies of women have shown that first-degree relatives of patients with anorexia nervosa have higher rates of depression than the general population. However, many depressive symptoms in patients with anorexia improve with the restoration of body weight. Therefore, some of these clinical features of depression also may be secondary to the adolescent's state of malnutrition or starvation.

Familial Influences

Researchers have noted that certain family dynamics may serve to initiate and perpetuate anorexia nervosa. Typically, the family is overprotective and rigid, with the mother often enmeshed in her daughter's life. Conflict resolution tends to be poor, and an inability to express feelings within the family is often evident. Multiple case-control studies have shown there is a higher rate of both anorexia and bulimia nervosa in relatives of patients with eating disorders. This may be due to inheritance patterns of personality traits as well as comorbid mood and anxiety disorders.

Social/Environmental Pressures

Both the media and Western industrialized societal standards are believed to play a role in "setting the stage" for the development of an eating disorder. Affluent communities are especially at risk for this. Within these social circles, thinness, food, eating, and obsessive exercise can become the prime focus of daily activity.

In addition, young women become caught in what has been labeled a "slender trap" in which thinness is equivalent to attractiveness and success. Food restriction or purging is a means of attaining thinness. An inability to maintain thinness equals failure. Role models in the media, such as fashion models and actresses, also serve as ideals by which young people create their standards.

Other Influences

Involvement in particular extracurricular activities, such as ballet and gymnastics, may contribute to the development of anorexia in females. For male athletes, such influences include participation in sports such as wrestling, in which maintaining a given weight is important and dieting is used to achieve that weight. Chronic medical conditions, such as diabetes mellitus or inflammatory bowel disease (IBD), also may contribute to the development of an eating disorder.

Bulimia Nervosa

Several theories have been proposed to explain the etiology of bulimia nervosa but, similar to anorexia, no single etiology has been confirmed. Most likely multiple factors contribute to the development of this eating disorder, and it is the complex interaction between these factors at a particular developmental point in an older adolescent's life that leads to this condition.

Biological, psychological, familial, and societal influences are thought to contribute to the development of bulimia nervosa in older teenagers and young adults. Among other issues, adolescent and parental obesity are both risk factors for bulimia as are early menarche, early sexual experiences, and a history of childhood sexual or physical abuse that occurs in conjunction with a comorbid psychiatric condition. More importantly, dieting has been documented as an important risk factor in this age group.

Familial dysfunction and high levels of conflict also have been associated with bulimia nervosa. Unlike with anorexia, conflict might be discussed openly but negatively within the family, and there may be an inadequate expression of emotions that may lead to a lack of parental warmth and concern. Thus the relationship between the parent and teenager is distant rather than enmeshed. The adolescent generally has a low level of self-esteem, high impulsivity, and body image dissatisfaction. Additionally, parents and relatives have a high rate of affective and eating disorders as well as alcoholism.

Differential Diagnosis

It is important to differentiate anorexia nervosa from bulimia nervosa, although occasionally this distinction may be difficult to make if patients display behavior consistent with both conditions. In addition, most patients with eating disorders have associated comorbid psychiatric disorders. Major affective disorders to consider include depression, bipolar disorder, and OCD. Anxiety disorders and substance abuse also are commonly seen, although the latter is more strongly associated with bulimia nervosa.

Other diagnoses to consider when evaluating patients for anorexia include IBD, malabsorption, celiac disease, diabetes mellitus, malignancies, Addison disease, hyperthyroidism or hypothyroidism, hypopituitarism, tumors of the central nervous system (CNS), and substance abuse, particularly with amphetamines and crack cocaine. Superior mesenteric artery syndrome is another important condition to consider in the differential diagnosis, however, it also can be a consequence of an eating disorder.

Evaluation

History

A complete medical history should be obtained from all adolescents with suspected eating disorders to rule out the multiple other conditions in the differential diagnosis of weight loss. The primary care provider then should interview the patient alone and focus on establishing the diagnosis of disordered eating by addressing more specific issues related to food, eating behaviors, dieting, exercise, and body image (Questions Box). The severity of both the medical and nutritional aspects of the condition should be determined initially, followed by a psychosocial evaluation. Inquiries should focus on symptoms associated with complications such as dysphagia secondary to esophagitis from recurrent vomiting, constipation from fluid restriction, or muscle weakness associated with emetine toxicity from chronic ipecac use. Although rarely seen by the primary care provider at the initial visit when the diagnosis of an eating disorder is made, recognition of serious medical complications is paramount to determining the urgency of further care. A thorough psychosocial assessment should be performed. The **HEADDSSS** format (home, employment and education, activities, diet, drugs, sexual activity/sexuality, suicide and depression, safety) is useful to direct the psychosocial interview from general topics to more sensitive ones (see Chapter 5). Particular attention should be paid to the adolescent's overall functioning at home, with friends, and at school; the presence of other comorbid psychiatric disorders such as depression or anxiety; and a history of suicidal ideation or sexual/physical abuse. Out-of-control behavior as a result of substance abuse also should be assessed. The use of psychological testing/questionnaires to assess cognition and depression may be beneficial, depending on the comfort level of the primary care practitioner with these tools. Otherwise, consultation with a mental health professional is warranted.

A detailed menstrual history also must be obtained from females because secondary amenorrhea is frequently present in patients as an early sign of anorexia secondary to decreased body fat. Menses may be irregular or absent with bulimia as well. A family history of eating disorders, substance abuse, or psychiatric disease should be reviewed with the teenager and confirmed by the parent.

Physical Examination

In both conditions, the patient should undress, wearing only underwear, for the physical examination. This prevents any bulky clothes from hiding the true body habitus. The height and weight should be plotted on a growth chart, and the body mass index (BMI)

Eating Disorders — Questions

- Have there been any changes in the adolescent's weight? What is the most, and least, the adolescent has ever weighed?
- How does the adolescent feel about how he or she looks?
- Do any particular areas of the body, such as the thighs, lower abdomen, and buttocks, most concern the adolescent?
- How much does the adolescent want to weigh?
- How often does the adolescent weigh himself or herself?
- What did he or she eat yesterday (24-hour dietary recall)?
- Does the adolescent have any food restrictions? Count calories? Binge eat?
- How does the adolescent and his or her friends handle weight control?
- What does the adolescent do when he or she feels "fat"? Does the adolescent vomit to lose weight?
- Has the adolescent or any of his or her friends ever used diuretics, ipecac, enemas, or laxatives to lose weight or compensate for overeating?
- How compulsive is the adolescent about exercise? Is he or she stressed if they miss a workout?
- In what sports, if any, does the adolescent participate?
- For females, are menstrual periods regular? Last menstrual period? Age at menarche?
- Does the adolescent have any other symptoms associated with complications of eating disorders?
- Does the adolescent have any depressive symptoms, such as sleeping problems or fatigue that can accompany eating disorders?

For Patients With Bulimia Nervosa
- When do binges occur?
- What are the precipitating factors?
- What happens specifically during a typical episode?
- Does the adolescent use drugs or alcohol?

---

should be calculated (BMI = weight [kg]/height [m²]). Delayed growth or short stature also should be noted because it can occur with severe malnutrition as well as other systemic conditions. Vital signs, including blood pressure, should be recorded. Evidence of cardiovascular instability can be manifested by tachycardia, bradycardia, or orthostatic hypotension. The patient also may be hypothermic as a result of her overall malnutrition. The general appearance and affect of the patient must be noted. Adolescents with full-blown anorexia nervosa are often emaciated with an obvious loss of subcutaneous tissue, and they may appear apathetic or have a flat affect. Patients with bulimia may be mildly obese or of normal weight with a full-appearing facies secondary to parotid and submaxillary swelling, a complication of frequent purging. In most cases, however, the teen appears "normal" at the initial visit.

Physical findings in patients with **anorexia nervosa** are consistent with a "state of hibernation." Hypothermia, orthostatic hypotension, bradycardia, and lanugo (downy hair) on the arms and back are seen. The palms and soles may be yellow secondary to hypercarotenemia, and pigmentation of the chest and abdomen may be increased as a result of malnutrition. Thinning or loss of pubic and scalp hair as well as dry skin also may be seen. The breasts should be examined carefully for galactorrhea. The presence of galactorrhea, along with a history of amenorrhea, warrants further investigation for a prolactinoma. A cardiac murmur must be noted and further evaluated because one-third of patients with anorexia have mitral valve prolapse. The abdomen should be palpated for tenderness or masses, and may be scaphoid in appearance. Bowel sounds are often decreased in patients with anorexia, and stool may be palpated secondary to constipation. A rectal examination should be performed for any evidence of bloody stool, which is a finding consistent with IBD. The extremities should be evaluated for coldness, mottling, or edema. Finally, a complete neurologic examination, including a mental status evaluation, should be performed to exclude any signs of a CNS lesion or endocrine disorder.

In patients with **bulimia nervosa,** specific physical findings, if any, are often associated with dehydration and electrolyte imbalances that occur as a result of chronic vomiting or laxative abuse. Vital signs should be reviewed for tachycardia, sinus bradycardia, and orthostatic hypotension; their presence indicates hemodynamic instability. The patient also may be hypothermic. The skin should be inspected on the dorsum of the hand over the knuckles for scratches, scars, or calluses from self-induced vomiting (Russell sign). Petechiae and subconjunctival hemorrhages also may be seen as a result of severe retching. The oropharynx should be inspected for dental caries, enamel erosion, or discoloration as well as for parotid hypertrophy. In addition, palatal scratches or mouth sores can be seen. The abdomen should be palpated for epigastric tenderness or mid-abdominal pain. Positive findings may be due to esophagitis, gastritis, or pancreatitis.

From a musculoskeletal standpoint, any muscle weakness or cramping should be appreciated and may indicate an electrolyte abnormality. Edema of the extremities may be seen in laxative abusers and should be noted.

Laboratory Tests

Box 120-4 lists the laboratory studies necessary in the evaluation of patients with **anorexia nervosa.** A complete blood count may be helpful because leukopenia, anemia and, rarely, thrombocytopenia can be found with this disorder. Electrolytes (sodium, potassium, chloride, and carbon dioxide) and blood urea nitrogen are important especially if patients use diuretics, laxatives, or ipecac. Serum calcium and phosphorous must be monitored, especially in the "refeeding" phase of treatment. The erythrocyte sedimentation rate may be low with anorexia and high with IBD or some other inflammatory process. Normal liver function tests aid in excluding other causes of weight loss. Some endocrine tests help differentiate a hormonal problem from anorexia (see Box 120-4). An electrocardiogram allows practitioners to diagnose QTc prolongation, heart block, and arrhythmias.

Laboratory abnormalities in **bulimia nervosa** reflect the type and extent of purging behavior of adolescents. Box 120-4 summarizes the necessary laboratory studies for patients with bulimia.

Radiographic studies, such as computed tomography of the head or magnetic resonance imaging of the brain, are indicated if the

---

Box 120-4. Laboratory Assessment of an Eating Disorder

Anorexia Nervosa
- Complete blood count, erythrocyte sedimentation rate
- Serum electrolytes (Na, K, Cl, CO_2)
- Blood urea nitrogen/creatinine
- Serum glucose
- Serum calcium, phosphorous, magnesium, zinc
- Serum protein, albumin, cholesterol
- Liver function tests
- Endocrine labs (performed in patients who are amenorrheic)
  — Urine pregnancy test
  — Follicle-stimulating hormone
  — Luteinizing hormone
  — Estradiol
  — Thyroid function tests: thyroid-stimulating hormone/T_4/T_3
  — Cortisol
- Urine pH and urinalysis
- Electrocardiogram

Bulimia Nervosa
- Serum electrolytes (Na, K, Cl, CO_2)
- Serum glucose
- Serum calcium, phosphorous, magnesium, zinc
- Blood urea nitrogen/creatinine
- Serum amylase
- Urine pH and urinalysis
- Electrocardiogram

---

diagnosis of an eating disorder is uncertain. The performance of other procedures, however, should be based on the individual case.

Management

It is the role of primary care practitioners to recognize when inappropriate dieting and weight loss become an obsession for adolescents and when abnormal behaviors develop for maintenance of obvious malnutrition. When treating patients with eating disorders, physicians must first establish trust and, in doing this, patients should be assured that practitioners are not attempting to remove all control by trying to make the adolescent "fat." Depending on the severity of symptoms and the comfort level of the physician in monitoring the early medical, nutritional, and psychological issues, the adolescent may be followed by the primary care practitioner in conjunction with a registered dietitian, family therapist, and psychiatrist. Early in the treatment course, the primary physician must be willing to follow the patient frequently (as often as once or twice a week if necessary). If the practitioner wishes to refer the patient to an experienced team of specialists, it is important that the primary provider remain involved in the care of the teenager. Next, a compromise must be reached between the adolescent and pediatrician regarding the minimum acceptable weight given the patient's height. This may be done with the assistance of a registered dietitian who is experienced in working with children and teenagers. Unlike with adults, weight restoration in the adolescent also must take into account normal growth needs. A contract that describes goals of treatment should then be established between the adolescent and the treatment team. Weight gain must be the initial priority, especially in adolescents with anorexia as long as the patient is otherwise medically stable and does not require inpatient hospitalization. Details regarding this nutritional regimen, which includes a stepwise increase in daily caloric intake, amounts of protein to be ingested, daily fat intake, and treatment goal weights, should be developed by the dietitian and reviewed with the adolescent and his or her family.

Family and individual counseling is often indicated and is an important part of the therapeutic plan. The primary care provider must work cooperatively with mental health colleagues to provide the necessary psychological and psychiatric services for their patient. Although extremely difficult, patients must acknowledge the problem and their need for assistance before an effective mental health referral can be made. This allows the adolescent to assert himself or herself and remain in control. Support groups also may be beneficial and frequently are an important component of a day program (partial hospitalization) for those adolescents with eating disorders who require more intensive outpatient care but not an inpatient hospitalization.

Numerous studies have shown that eating disorders are best treated by an interdisciplinary professional team experienced in the care of children and adolescents with eating disorders. This team generally consists of the primary care provider, an adolescent medicine specialist with expertise in caring for patients with eating disorders, a psychologist or psychiatrist, a nutritionist, and a social worker. Ideally, the team is available to offer both inpatient as well as outpatient services, although most cases are managed in an outpatient setting. Criteria for inpatient admission should be established by the team and reviewed with patients and their families.

Medical complications of eating disorders are well known and listed in Box 120-5. Inpatient treatment is required for weight loss greater than 30% below ideal body weight or a BMI less than 16, continued weight loss while on intensive outpatient treatment, or a history of rapid weight loss over 3 months. Other indications include cardiovascular compromise, such as bradycardia (<50 beats/min during the day or <45 beats/min at nighttime), orthostatic hypotension, or altered mental status; evidence of persistent hypothermia (<36°C [96.8°F]); suicidal or out-of-control behavior; electrolyte disturbances or uncompensated acid-base abnormalities; and significant dehydration as evidenced by systolic blood pressure lower than 90. Cardiac arrhythmias, including prolonged QTc, also require inpatient monitoring. Rarely does confirmation of the diagnosis warrant an inpatient stay.

Box 120-5. Medical Complications of Eating Disorders[a]

Associated With Purging Behavior

- Fluid and electrolyte imbalances (from use of laxatives)
- Irreversible cardiac muscle damage (from ipecac use)
- Esophagitis, dental erosions, Mallory-Weiss tears (from chronic vomiting)
- Renal stones (from dehydration)
- Amenorrhea, hypoestrogenemia, osteopenia (from decreased body mass index [BMI])

Associated With Caloric Restrictive Behavior

- Electrocardiogram abnormalities: low voltage, sinus bradycardia, sinus tachycardia segment depression (from electrolyte abnormalities), prolonged QTc
- Cardiac arrhythmias, including supraventricular beats and ventricular tachycardia
- Delayed gastric emptying, slow gastrointestinal motility, constipation, bloating, fullness, abnormal liver function tests (from fatty infiltration of the liver)
- Increased blood urea nitrogen, increased risk of renal stones, total body depletion of sodium and potassium
- Refeeding syndrome (from extracellular shifts of phosphorous)
- Leukopenia, anemia, thrombocytopenia
- Amenorrhea, hypoestrogenism, osteopenia (from decreased BMI)
- Cortical atrophy, seizures

[a]Modified from American Academy of Pediatrics Committee on Adolescence. Identifying and treating eating disorders. *Pediatrics*. 2003;111:207.

Prognosis

Overall, the outcome for patients with eating disorders is variable, with the recovery of some patients after minimal intervention and the development of more chronic problems in others. Binge eating, for example, may replace food restriction. Most studies report the prognosis as more favorable if the patient's condition is identified early and treated aggressively. Predictors of poor outcome for anorexia nervosa include very low body weight at the time of initial treatment, long duration of illness, a concomitant personality disorder, a dysfunctional parent-child relationship, and a compulsion to exercise. For bulimia nervosa, factors found to be predictive of poor outcome include longer duration of illness at presentation, severity of eating pathology and frequency of vomiting, pre-morbid obesity, associated comorbid disorders such as personality disorder or substance abuse, and suicidal behavior. A family history of alcoholism also has been reported as a poor prognostic factor for bulimia.

The mortality rate for anorexia nervosa is approximately 5%. Exact figures for bulimia have not been determined, although it has been quoted as being similar to that of anorexia. The most common cause of death in both disorders is suicide. Medical causes are often due to cardiac arrhythmias from electrolyte abnormalities.

CASE RESOLUTION

In the case history presented at the beginning of this chapter, the girl does not meet the strict criteria for the diagnosis of anorexia nervosa, but her preoccupation with dieting and weight is worrisome. Concerns about her eating and dieting behaviors should be discussed with the teenager alone and then together with her family. When she and her family agree, she should be referred to a mental health professional and nutritionist for further evaluation, with the emphasis on healthy eating and the continued support and involvement of the primary care physician. She should be followed frequently until her weight and eating behaviors have reached the mutually agreed-on goal among all professionals involved in her care.

Selected References

American Academy of Pediatrics Committee on Adolescence. Identifying and treating eating disorders. *Pediatrics.* 2003;111:204–212

Fisher M. Treatment of eating disorders in children, adolescents, and young adults. *Pediatr Rev.* 2006;27:5–16

Fisher M, Golden NH, Katzman DK, et al. Eating disorders in adolescents: a background paper. *J Adolesc Health.* 1995;16:420–437

Fisher M, Golden NH, Jacobson MC, eds. The spectrum of disordered eating: anorexia nervosa, bulimia nervosa, and obesity. *Adolesc Med.* 2003;14:1–173

Hillman JK. 'Just dieting' or an eating disorder? A practical guide for the clinician. *Adolesc Health Update.* 2001;13:1–9

Jamieson MA. Hormone replacement in the adolescent with anorexia and hypothalamic amenorrhea—yes or no? *J Pediatr Adolesc Gynecol.* 2001;14:39–45

Katzman DK. Medical complications in adolescents with anorexia nervosa: a review of the literature. *Int J Eat Disord.* 2005;37:S52–S59

Kriepe RE, Dukarm CP. Eating disorders in adolescents and older children. *Pediatr Rev.* 1999;20:410–421

Levine RL. Endocrine aspects of eating disorders in adolescents. *Adolesc Med.* 2002;13:129–144

Phillips EL, Pratt HD. Eating disorders in college. *Pediatr Clin North Am.* 2005;52:85–96

Rome ES, Ammerman S, Rosen DS, et al. Children and adolescents with eating disorders: the state of the art. *Pediatrics.* 2003;111:e98–e108

Stashwick C. When you suspect an eating disorder. *Contemp Pediatr.* 1996;13:124–153

Steiner H, Lock J. Anorexia nervosa and bulimia nervosa in children and adolescents: a review of the past 10 years. *J Am Acad Child Adolesc Psychiatry.* 1998;37:352–359

Zerbe KJ. Eating disorders: the apple doesn't fall far from the tree. *Contemp Pediatr.* 1996;13:65–78

Body Modification: Tattooing and Body Piercing

Monica Sifuentes, MD

CASE STUDY

A 16-year-old girl comes to your office for her annual physical examination. Although previously healthy, the mother is concerned that her daughter seems irritable and unwilling to participate in recent family events. The adolescent is currently in 10th grade at a local public school, gets As and Bs in most subjects, is a member of the volleyball team, and has just begun working at a movie theater part time. Both of her parents are employed and the adolescent gets along well with her 19-year-old sister, who is currently in college, and her 14-year-old brother. She has many friends in the neighborhood as well as at school.

You interview the adolescent alone and learn that she occasionally smokes marijuana, has tried cocaine on one occasion, and attends parties where many people are drinking alcohol. She has been sexually active in the past but is not currently. She denies depression and describes her mood as generally happy, except when she is forced to spend what she believes is excessive time with her family instead of friends.

On physical examination the adolescent's height and weight are in the 50th percentile for age. Her body mass index is 21. Vital signs are normal. You note a small tattoo at her right hip area. The girl's mother is unaware of its presence according to the teen. She obtained it a few months prior while visiting her sister in college.

Questions

1. What is the epidemiology of body modification in adolescents and young adults?
2. What is the motivation for obtaining tattoos and body piercing in this age group, and is there an association with high-risk behavior?
3. What techniques are used to place tattoos and perform body piercing?
4. What adverse consequences can be seen following body modification, and what should be done to treat them?
5. How can the primary care provider assist an adolescent to make a safe and healthy decision regarding body modification?

Body modification is the practice of permanently altering one's appearance and historically has been practiced in many cultures for thousands of years. This includes tattooing, body piercing, scarification, and branding. Although much less common than tattooing and body piercing, scarification is the use of various techniques to produce scars on the skin. It is described as a more "intense" form of body modification and has been reported to be more appealing to darker pigmented individuals or those seeking a more dramatic result. The practice of body modification should be differentiated from "cutting," which is a disorder of self-mutilation that can be seen in adolescents suffering from anxiety, depression, or abuse and is beyond the scope of this discussion (see Chapter 39).

Although in the past body modification has been associated primarily with the disenfranchised such as criminals, gang members, or psychiatric patients, it is now a common occurrence in mainstream society. **Body art** is seen in most clinical settings serving youth and young adults as well as in middle schools, high schools, and on college campuses. Additionally, it is not uncommon to encounter a teenager with multiple tattoos and body piercings or to evaluate an adolescent for a possible complication of the procedure. Whether described as a rite of passage, expression of their own individuality, or desire to join a particular peer group, obtaining a tattoo or body piercing has become a widespread experience during adolescence and young adulthood and therefore should be added to the primary care provider's list of issues to review during the routine health maintenance visit.

Epidemiology

It is currently estimated that 13% to 25% of the general population has a tattoo in the United States. However, because tattooing was reportedly the sixth fastest-growing retail business in 1996, these figures are probably a gross underestimation. Surveys conducted in outpatient clinics and on school and college campuses confirm that approximately 10% to 13% of teens ages 12 to 18 years have a tattoo. In one particular study of more than 2,000 US high school students, 55% expressed interest in obtaining a tattoo regardless of its permanence or the students' academic success in school. In addition, it has been reported in the literature that half of new tattoos are in women and that many are obtained while in college.

Body piercings are more common in adolescents and young adults, and some experts speculate that this may be because the procedure is not permanent, allowing the individual to remove the jewelry at any time. In one study among college students, 45% had undergone body piercing and 22% had tattoos both with and without piercings. Other studies that include younger adolescents attending an outpatient adolescent clinic report approximately 27% of teens with body piercing and 13% with a tattoo.

The motivation for obtaining body art also has been reviewed in the literature, with most studies confirming the adolescent's search for uniqueness and desire to enhance their independence and self-identity. For some teenagers, it is seen as a form of decoration or it fulfills a desire for peer acceptance and can solidify group membership. Tattoos in particular can be seen as a quest to permanently document a relationship with an individual or group. Despite popular belief, studies do not confirm that most adolescents obtain a tattoo or body piercing impulsively while under the influence of illicit drugs or alcohol. In fact, many older teens and young adults report taking quite a while to decide whether to obtain a tattoo or piercing.

Parental involvement and permission to have a tattoo placed or body piercing performed is variable for many teenagers. In most cases, parents are not consulted prior to the procedure, although in many states parental consent is required by law, and tattooing of minors is prohibited. However, current legislation is not consistently enforced and, in many states, tattooing and body piercing have different regulations.

Clinical Presentation

Tattoos can be found on any area of the body and, depending on the talent of the artist and the desire of the client, can be simple and one color or very elaborate with many colors. In general, amateur tattoos are less intricate and are considered more risky because they are often not performed under ideal circumstances, following antiseptic techniques or with conventional pigments and applicators. Unconventional pigments include charcoal, India ink, and mascara. Pencils, pens, sewing needles, and other sharp objects, including guitar strings, may be used to apply the dye for a self-administered tattoo.

The most common site for piercing is high on the pinna of the ear. Regular lobular ear piercings are not generally included in the context of body modification because they occur commonly at any age. Other body sites that are pierced include the tragus of the ear, eyebrows, tongue, nose, nasal septum, lip, navel, and nipples. Intimate or genital piercings also can be seen in both males and females. The foreskin, penis, scrotum, clitoris, perineum, and labia are all common areas for intimate piercings. Although specific data by gender are not available, it is reported that more men than women tend to obtain genital piercings.

Technique, Application, and Safety Standards

Tattoos

The process for applying a professional or commercial tattoo is fairly standardized, although different tattoo parlors may have their own individual practices. In general, the client selects a design and the tattoo is stenciled or drawn on the skin. The skin is then cleansed with an antiseptic solution, and petroleum jelly is placed on the site. Most professionals use an electric tattoo gun, which is similar to a dental drill, that holds one or several needles in a needle bar that punctures the skin a few millimeters deep and up to several thousand times a minute. The pigment reaches the level of the dermis via the solid bore needle(s), and blood and serosanguineous fluid are wiped away as tattoo placement continues. When the tattoo is completed or the session is finished, an antiseptic ointment is applied, and a bandage is placed over the site.

The client is instructed to remove the dressing in 24 hours and to keep the area moist with an antibiotic ointment. Additionally, clients may place Keri lotion or vitamin E oil over the healing tattoo several times a day. The area should be cleansed with a mild soap and patted dry (not rubbed). If aftercare instructions are followed carefully, most tattoos heal in approximately 1 to 2 weeks.

Ideally the application process uses inks that are poured into one-time use disposable containers and needles that are disposed of after each client. However, although the pigments are subject to US Food and Drug Administration regulation, the tattooing process itself and the use of the inks are not regulated. In addition, certain pigments may not be approved for intradermal use and have been known to contain lead, mercury, and arsenic.

The practice of universal precautions is required by state and local regulatory agencies and advocated by specific educational groups such as the Alliance of Professional Tattooists (APT), a nonprofit organization established in 1992 to promote standards for professional and associate tattooists and develop guidelines for consumers to evaluate the safety of a tattooist. Membership in APT is voluntary and requires that the professional tattooist participate in a health and safety seminar and have at least 3 years of full-time experience at a consistent location. Despite these efforts and standards, however, specific areas of concern regarding the tattoo industry remain and include unlicensed tattoo artists and establishments, the presence of unregulated ingredients in the pigments, inconsistent cleaning of equipment between clients, an inability to reliably sterilize all parts of the equipment despite good efforts, and infrequent inspections of tattoo parlors by regulatory agencies.

Body Piercing

The process for body piercing is generally less complicated than tattooing and depends, in part, on the site to be pierced. The client chooses the jewelry and body part to be pierced, the area is cleaned with a topical antiseptic, and a large hollow needle is brought through the skin. The jewelry is then brought through the hole following the needle and sealed with a bead, bar, or metal disc. Because the procedure is relatively quick, topical anesthetics are usually not required.

While earlobe piercings are relatively straightforward, they are commonly performed using a "piercing gun" at a local mall, cosmetic shop, or kiosk. Because the stud is driven through the earlobe via the gun rather than through a hollow tube manually, the tissue ends up torn rather than pierced. Additional concerns regarding the piercing gun include inconsistent and informal training of personnel, an inability to sterilize all parts of the gun, and embedded earrings and ear backs. The gun cannot be adjusted for the thickness of other tissues, so although it is a popular method for earring placement, this tool is not recommended for sites other than the earlobe.

The immediate aftercare of piercing varies by the site pierced. For example, local skin discoloration and a non-malodorous serous exudate can occur with piercings of the nares or navel. Tongue or lip piercings have been associated with significant swelling for several days following the procedure. In addition, a yellow-white fluid secretion can occur that can mimic an infection to the unfamiliar examiner. Clients with oral piercings are generally instructed to dissolve ice in their mouths immediately post-piercing to help with pain and swelling, treat further discomfort with a nonsteroidal anti-inflammatory agent, and elevate the head when sleeping.

Healing times greatly vary depending on the body site. In general, sites with greater vascularity and exposure, such as the face and tongue, tend to heal faster than those through cartilage, which is poorly vascularized. Areas of the body that are subject to movement also have slower healing times. For example, the tongue may take 1 to 2 months to heal, the nasal septum 2 to 3 months, and the tragus of the ear 3 to 4 months. High ear piercings through the cartilage also can take 3 to 4 months to heal. Navel piercings have the longest healing time (up to 12 months) because of friction and moisture from clothing and often are associated with the most complications.

As with tattooing, not all states have regulations and safety standards in place for body piercing and, if they do exist, local governing bodies do not consistently enforce them. Universal precautions should be strictly practiced, and adolescents need to be familiar with these guidelines as well as know how to find a reputable piercer prior to obtaining body art.

Because no formal training programs exist for piercers, many learn by video or apprenticeship. In general, practitioners in studios have completed an apprenticeship and have more training than those in cosmetic shops, malls, or ear-piercing kiosks. They also are more experienced in piercing sites other than the ears and may be a member of the Association of Professional Piercers (APP). The APP is a nonprofit organization dedicated to the education, health, and safety of body piercing for the public. It has developed self-regulatory policies for the industry, standards for membership in their organization, and annual conferences on health and safety issues. Membership includes at least 1 year of piercing experience, documented training in blood-borne pathogens and cardiopulmonary resuscitation, and certification in first aid. Members also must show photographic proof of a medical-grade autoclave in the piercing studio and send in spore test results from the autoclave. To help document this, a detailed video of the studio is required along with copies of all aftercare education given to clients. Once this process is completed, the member receives a certificate to mount in the studio.

Current legislation regarding minors and piercing is regulated by individual states, and in some states, such as California, there is an exclusion of ear piercing performed with "piercing guns" from the definition of body piercing. With regard to minors, the APP requires that the parent or legal guardian as well as the minor show proof of identification prior to signing the consent form for body piercing. In addition, nipple or genital piercings are not performed on anyone younger than 18 years.

Evaluation

History

All teenagers should be interviewed alone, after their parent or legal guardian has had an opportunity to discuss their concerns with the health care provider (see Chapter 5). A visible tattoo or body piercing allows the health care provider to inquire about the circumstances surrounding the body art at the beginning of the interview in contrast to body art noted in an inconspicuous area of the body during the physical examination. Whether parental consent was obtained prior to the procedure should be addressed directly because this issue could be a basis for familial conflict both currently and in the future. The type of facility where the tattoo or piercing was obtained should be reviewed, along with whether universal precautions were followed. A general review of systems should be performed to exclude systemic conditions such as viral hepatitis as well as any other complications related to obtaining the tattoo or piercing. Specific questions about the area of the body that has been pierced also should be reviewed (Questions Box). For example, the teenager with tongue piercing should be asked if he or she has problems with mastication, swallowing, loss of taste or movement, or permanent numbness.

It has been reported that amateur or self-administered tattoos are associated with increased psychosocial problems including substance abuse at a younger age, hard drug use, lower academic achievement (ie, grades), and a greater number of tattoos overall.

Other studies have shown, however, that not all adolescents and young adults with tattoos or body piercing engage in high-risk behavior (Box 121-1). Successful academic achievement and close family support have been reported in both tattooed and non-tattooed college students. Despite the fact that they are permanent, more than 50% of academically successful high school students with consistently good grades have reported an interest in tattoos.

Whether body art is seen as an expression of individuality, rebellious behavior, or succumbing to peer pressure, the presence of a tattoo or body piercing on an adolescent probably warrants an in-depth psychosocial assessment for both risk-taking behavior and possible exposure to a viral infection such as hepatitis C.

Questions

Tattoo and Body Piercing

- When was the tattoo or body piercing obtained?
- Did the teenager obtain the parent or legal guardian's consent prior to obtaining the tattoo or piercing?
- Is the adolescent satisfied with the tattoo or piercing?
- Was the tattoo or body piercing placed by a professional?
- Where was the studio located? Was it licensed? Was it clean "like a medical facility"?
- Did the tattooist or piercer wash their hands before gloving? Use new disposable gloves? Open all equipment in front of the teen?
- For tattoos, did the tattooist remove a sterile needle and tube set from a new envelope? Did he or she pour new ink in a new disposable container?
- For body piercing, did the piercer use individually wrapped sterile needles? Did he or she use a method not involving a piercing gun?
- Did the teen receive aftercare education, including written material?

Physical Examination

The routine physical examination in most adolescents with a tattoo or body piercing is completely normal unless there has been a past complication with the tattoo or piercing or there is a current problem. Poor aftercare and hygiene can prolong healing time in body piercings. In addition, smoking can delay the healing time associated with oral piercings. If the teen has recently had a tongue piercing performed, a larger barbell will be seen through the tongue. Larger barbells initially are placed with tongue piercing to accommodate the swelling associated with the procedure. Later the barbell is replaced with a shorter rod.

Both infectious and noninfectious complications from tattoos and body piercings can be seen and are listed in Box 121-2. While local infection occurs in only approximately 5% of tattoos, infectious complications have been reported in as many as 30% of body piercings. Signs of infection include erythema, warmth, swelling, and pain at the site, in addition to drainage in some cases. Rarely, a fluctuant, fluid-filled mass is seen if an abscess has developed.

Because some of the noninfectious complications can be related to the type of metal found in the jewelry, knowledge of this specific information is useful with body piercing. Only jewelry made from surgical stainless steel, titanium, solid 14k or 18k gold, or solid platinum should be used to avoid allergic dermatitis. Certain metals such as nickel, cobalt, and chromium have been associated with the development of contact dermatitis in sensitive individuals. Permanent makeup also has been reported to cause severe allergic contact dermatitis that can take from months to years to completely heal. The reported reactions included tenderness, itching, and "bumps" at the site of the permanent makeup application. Hypersensitivities to dyes or pigments from a professional tattoo also can appear as an

> ### Box 121-1. The Association Between Body Modification and High-Risk Behavior in Teens
>
> Numerous studies have been conducted to explore the association between high-risk behavior and body modification in adolescents. To date, while there are no definitive answers, research has shown
> - Adolescents with tattoos and/or body piercings were more likely to have engaged in risk-taking behaviors and at greater degrees of involvement than those without either. Risk-taking behaviors included disordered eating behavior, gateway drug use (cigarettes, alcohol, and marijuana), hard drug use (cocaine, crystal methamphetamine, and ecstasy), sexual activity, and suicide. Additionally, violence was associated with males having tattoos and with females having body piercings. Gateway drug use was associated with younger age of both tattooing and body piercing. (Carroll ST, Riffenburgh RH, Roberts TA, Myhre EB. Tattoos and body piercings as indicators of adolescent risk-taking behaviors. *Pediatrics*. 2002;109:1021–1028.)
> - Adolescents with body modification had 3.1 times greater odds of problem substance use compared with those without body modification. (Brooks TL, Woods ER, Knight JR, Shrier LA. Body modification and substance use in adolescents: is there a link? *J Adolesc Health*. 2003;32:44–49.)
> - Tattooing was significantly associated with older age, living in a single-parent household, and lower socioeconomic status. There also was greater involvement in sexual intercourse; higher levels of substance abuse in themselves as well as their peers, increased violent behaviors, and school problems. (Roberts TA, Ryan SA. Tattooing and high-risk behavior in adolescents. *Pediatrics*. 2002;110:1058–1063.)
> - A correlation between body piercing in teens and increased rate of sexual intercourse, smoking, marijuana use, school truancy, running away, suicidal ideation/attempts, and peer substance use. (Armstrong ML, Roberts AE, Owen DC, Koch JR. Contemporary college students and body piercing. *J Adolesc Health*. 2004;35:58–61.)

erythematous outline of the original work. This also can occur with temporary tattoos from henna, which is approved as a hair dye and not for use on the skin. Its use has been associated with severe contact dermatitis, especially if an additive containing phenylenediamine is mixed with the henna to give the normal red-brown paste an additional black and blue color.

Keloids and hypertrophic scars can appear as a flesh-colored mass at the area of the tattoo or piercing and differ in their timing and resolution. A hypertrophic scar generally appears within 6 weeks of the tattooing or piercing, is confined to the margins of the wound, and has a tendency to regress spontaneously. In contrast, a keloid may present as long as 1 year after the initial wound, often grows beyond the border of the wound, and persists. Keloids are seen primarily in African American and Asian patients and can cause an itching or burning sensation that may prompt referral for removal.

Box 121-2. Complications of Tattoos and Body Piercing: Infectious and Noninfectious

Tattooing Complications

Infectious

Bacterial etiologies
- Local skin infections
  — Superficial pyodermas
  — *Staphylococcus aureus*
- Systemic infections
  — Syphilis
  — *Mycobacterium tuberculosis*
  — *Mycobacterium leprae*
  — Chancroid
  — Tetanus
  — Endocarditis

Viral etiologies
- Human papillomavirus
- Hepatitis B and C
- Human immunodeficiency virus (HIV)

Noninfectious
- Hypersensitivity to dyes or pigments
- Allergic granulomas
- Malignant melanoma and basal cell carcinoma at tattoo site
- Keloid formation
- Swelling and burning during magnetic resonance imaging

Body Piercing Complications

Infectious

Bacterial etiologies
- *S aureus*
- *Pseudomonas aeruginosa*
- Group A beta-hemolytic streptococcus
  — Cellulitis
  — Septic arthritis
  — Acute glomerulonephritis
  — Erysipelas
  — Endocarditis
- *M tuberculosis*
- *Clostridium tetani*

Viral etiologies
- Hepatitis B and C
- HIV

Noninfectious

Body jewelry, in general
- Artifact on radiographs

High ear piercing
- Pinna deformity

Tongue piercing
- Airway obstruction
- Chipped/cracked teeth
- Interference with mastication/swallowing
- Permanent numbness
- Articulation disorders
- Loss of taste/movement
- Oral mucosa inflammation

Lip piercing
- Injury to salivary ducts
- Aspiration of jewelry

Navel piercing
- Allergic dermatitis

Nipple piercing
- Trauma/avulsion of nipple

Genital piercing
- Tissue inflammation in sexual partner
- Scarring
- Interruption of urinary flow (in males)

Laboratory

In general, laboratory studies are not necessary if the adolescent is not engaged in high-risk behavior and is certain that universal precautions were followed when the tattoo or piercing was placed. In most cases, however, the teen may be uncertain and not remember the details. If this is the case, a serum test for viral hepatitis B and C should be obtained because it has been reported that hepatitis C virus is found in approximately 30% of people with tattoos compared with 3.5% of people without them. Additionally, an antibody test for human immunodeficiency virus (HIV) should be sent as it continues to be a major public health concern with regard to the industry. However, there have been no definitive documented cases of HIV transmission from tattooing or body piercing in the literature to date.

A serum test for syphilis also should be sent because unlike HIV, transmission of this and other sexually transmitted infections has been reported from tattooing or piercing.

If there is evidence of abscess formation such as what may be seen with perichondritis, a specimen of the purulent fluid should be obtained and sent for culture and antimicrobial sensitivities.

Management

Although not ordinarily requested by most adolescents, tattoo removal or modification is available for the patient that no longer wants their tattoo or is unhappy with its current appearance. Even with the newer techniques, however, tattoo removal is difficult, and only about 70% of tattoos can be completely cleared because of impurities in tattoo pigments, different ink densities and depths, and the presence of certain metals in the dyes. More importantly, the cost for tattoo removal is not negligible; while the cost for tattoo placement might be $50 to $100, it can cost as much as $1,000 for its removal. Techniques for removal include laser treatments, dermabrasion, salabrasion (using a salt solution), scarification, and surgical removal using tissue expanders. Camouflaging also can be performed: a new pattern is made using skin-toned pigments or the tattoo is modified and made into another one. For instance, the name of a person can be incorporated into a new tattoo of an animal. Certain nonprofit organizations also offer tattoo removal to ex-gang members as a part of their employment and educational services.

Although it seems counterintuitive, removal of jewelry is not recommended if a piercing appears infected. The concern is that, without a wick or surgical drain, any potential space left at the site when the jewelry is removed could result in the development of an abscess. Instead, the adolescent should be instructed to leave the jewelry in place to allow drainage of the wound, use warm compresses, and clean the area with an antimicrobial soap and water. The use of topical antibiotic ointments is controversial because they can be occlusive and contribute to delayed healing.

Oral antibiotic coverage against skin staphylococcus and streptococcal species should be administered if the tattoo or piercing appears superficially infected and other measures have not been effective. More aggressive treatment is required if the piercing site involves the cartilage such as with high-ear piercings. Auricular infections can occur even after the use of strict antiseptic techniques and may appear a few weeks after the initial piercing. The cartilaginous helical area of the ear is particularly prone to infection because it is poorly vascularized and takes a long time to heal. Additional antimicrobial coverage against *Pseudomonas aeruginosa* is essential in these cases, along with diligent follow-up to monitor the initial response to oral antibiotic therapy. Currently, oral fluoroquinolones offer good antipseudomonal as well as anti-staphylococcal coverage and penetrate cartilage well. Inpatient hospitalization for intravenous antimicrobial therapy and subsequent drainage of the site may be required for moderate or unresponsive infections. Early recognition of perichondritis and its appropriate treatment are essential to prevent the development of a persistent infection as well as to minimize a permanent auricular deformity. In addition, timely consultation with a plastic surgeon or otolaryngologist early in the course of the suspected infection is recommended for early incision and drainage of a perichondrial abscess, appropriate wound care, and possible reconstruction of any disfigurement.

Role of the Primary Care Provider

For the adolescent who has not yet obtained a tattoo or piercing, or who already has one and is contemplating the placement of another, education is essential. The practitioner should inquire where the adolescent plans to have the procedure performed and educate them regarding what key questions to ask and how to find a reputable studio. Additional information such as the APT and APP Web sites should be shared with the teenager, and written materials that contain the safety guidelines should be given to the adolescent at the visit. Teenagers are often reluctant to ask their health care providers for information about obtaining tattoos and piercings and almost never contact them if they believe they may have a complication associated with tattooing or piercing. Instead, they tend to ask their peers or contact the establishment where the tattoo or piercing was initially placed. Primary care providers should be a nonjudgmental resource during health maintenance visits to ensure the adolescent's continued health and safety. Additionally, the appearance of an uncommon medical condition such as unexplained hepatitis, endocarditis, or toxic shock in the adolescent patient warrants careful consideration of a possible complication related to tattooing or body piercing.

Prognosis

Most teens experience no adverse effects from body modification. Complications, while uncommon, are usually amenable to medical management. Risk-taking behavior that may occur in conjunction with body modification may carry long-term sequelae.

CASE RESOLUTION

Because the presence of one tattoo puts this adolescent at risk for obtaining another, the primary care provider should review safety guidelines for obtaining a tattoo and body piercing with the adolescent and offer the teenager educational material and/or Web site references to reinforce the discussion. The immunization status of the teenager also should be checked, with particular attention to tetanus and hepatitis A and B. Additionally, while alone with the teenager, the provider should review their concern regarding the adolescent's current high-risk behavior and its possible consequences.

Selected References

Armstrong ML, Murphy KP. Tattooing: another adolescent risk behavior warranting health education. *Appl Nurs Res.* 1997;10:181–189

Armstrong ML, Caliendo C, Roberts AE. Genital piercings: what is known and what people with genital piercings tell us. *Urol Nurs.* 2006;26:173–179

Armstrong ML, Roberts AE, Owen DC, Koch JR. Contemporary college students and body piercing. *J Adolesc Health.* 2004;35:58–61

Association of Professional Piercers. www.safepiercing.org

Association of Professional Tattooists. www.safe-tattoos.com

Beers MS, Meires J, Loriz L. Body piercing: coming to a patient near you. *Nurs Pract.* 2007;32:55–60

Braverman PK. Body art: piercing, tattooing, and scarification. *Adolesc Med.* 2006;17:505–519

Brooks TL, Woods ER, Knight JR, Shrier LA. Body modification and substance use in adolescents: is there a link? *J Adolesc Health.* 2003;32:44–49

Carroll ST, Riffenburgh RH, Roberts TA, Myhre EB. Tattoos and body piercings as indicators of adolescent risk-taking behaviors. *Pediatrics.* 2002;109:1021–1028

Greif J, Hewitt W, Armstrong ML. Tattooing and body piercing. *Clin Nurs Res.* 1999;8:368–385

Jervis PN, Clifton NJ, Woolford TJ. Ear deformity in children following high ear-piercing: current practice, consent issues and legislation. *J Laryngol Otol.* 2001;115:519–521

Larzo MR, Poe SG. Adverse consequences of tattoos and body piercings. *Pediatr Ann.* 2006;35:187–192

Laumann AE, Derick AJ. Tattoos and body piercing in the United States: a national data set. *J Am Acad Dermatol.* 2006;55:413–421

Meltzer DI. Complications of body piercing. *Am Fam Physician.* 2005;72:2029–2034

More DR, Seidel JS, Bryan PA. Ear-piercing techniques as a cause of auricular chondritis. *Pediatr Emerg Care.* 1999;15:189–192

Nicoletti A. Teens, tattoos and body piercing. *J Pediatr Adolesc Gynecol.* 2004;17:215–216

Roberts TA, Ryan SA. Tattooing and high-risk behavior in adolescents. *Pediatrics.* 2002;110:1058–1063

Stewart GM, Thorp A, Brown L. Perichondritis—a complication of high ear piercing. *Pediatr Emerg Care.* 2006;22:804–806

Straetemans M, Katz LM, Belson M. Adverse reactions after permanent make-up procedures. *N Engl J Med.* 2007;356:2753

Childhood Obesity

Charlotte W. Lewis, MD, MPH

CASE STUDY

An 11-year-old girl is brought to your office by her mother to discuss their concerns about the child's weight, which is 59 kg (130 lb). Her height is 140 cm (55 in), giving her a body mass index (BMI) of 30 kg/m² (>95th percentile for age). The rest of the physical examination, including vital signs, is normal. The mother, who also is overweight, says she doesn't want her daughter to "end up like me." The patient says she would like to lose weight because she is tired of the other children at school making fun of her for being fat. The history reveals that this patient is an only child who lives with her single mother in low-income housing in a large urban city. The mother works the day shift as a nurse's aide at a nearby nursing home. Because the mother is often tired, meals are simple and often consist of prepackaged foods such as Danish pastry for breakfast and frozen dinners for supper. At school, the girl buys her lunch, which usually consists of whole milk, a bag of chips, and a cookie. After school, the girl goes home, where she watches television and snacks on chips and soda until her mother arrives home from work. The mother does not allow her daughter to play outside because the neighborhood is unsafe.

Questions

1. How is obesity defined and measured?
2. How does genetic susceptibility influence a person's risk for obesity?
3. What is the relationship between childhood and adult obesity?
4. What are the complications of obesity?
5. How can obesity be treated?

Childhood obesity is of significant concern because overweight children are more likely to be overweight as adults and at increased risk for a number of chronic conditions. In addition, the psychosocial toll that being obese exacts on affected adults and children cannot be overemphasized. Obese children are often shunned by their peers at school and have difficulty making friends, while obese adolescents complete less schooling, go on to have lower household incomes, and are more likely to live in poverty than their non-obese counterparts. The primary care provider is in an ideal position to counsel families whose children are at risk for obesity and to assist children who are obese.

Defining obesity presents certain challenges. Ideally, a measure of obesity would correlate with adiposity and predict morbidity and mortality. Unfortunately, an inexpensive and widely available method that meets these criteria is not yet available. Body mass index (BMI: weight in kilograms/[height in meters]²) is the best and most widely used surrogate measure for obesity. Standards for adults have established a BMI of 25 or greater as overweight based on the increased risk of morbidity and mortality above this level. Adults with BMIs of 30 or greater are classified as obese. There are fewer data about the interpretation of BMI in children. However, BMI is the preferred method for assessing degree of obesity in children, although other criteria are also used (DX Box). Experts classify children at 85% to 95% of BMI-for-age as **at risk for overweight** and child at greater than 95% of BMI-for-age as **overweight** (the term *overweight* is used because BMI is technically not a direct measure of adiposity, however,

in this chapter and elsewhere the terms *overweight* and *obesity* are used interchangeably). As children grow older and mature, they change in proportion, bone mass, and lean-to-fat tissue composition, and their BMI changes as well. After about 1 year of age, BMI-for-age values begin to decline and continue to do so during the preschool years until the BMI reaches a minimum around 4 to 6 years of age, before rising throughout the remainder of childhood, into adolescence and adulthood. This phenomenon of increasing BMI after the nadir in the preschool years is referred to as **adiposity rebound.**

Dx Obesity

- Body mass index ≥95th percentile for age (>85 percentile = at risk)
- Weight-for-height ≥95 percentile
- >120% of ideal body weight for height and age

Epidemiology

The prevalence of obesity is on the rise in developed countries. In the previous 20 years, the percentage of overweight children and adolescents in the United States tripled, reaching 17.1% in 2003 to 2004. Hispanics, African Americans, and Native Americans are disproportionately affected. Prevention and treatment of obesity is important to avoid health risks that affect the individual and are costly to society as a whole. In the United States, the overall spending associated with overweight and obesity was $93 billion in 2002 dollars, half of which was publicly financed through Medicare or Medicaid.

Clinical Presentation

Obese children usually present to the physician in 1 of 2 ways. The parents or the child may come in concerned that the child is overweight. The physician must then consider the growth parameters and BMI-for-age to make an appropriate determination of the child's overweight status. Alternatively, the family may have little concern that their child is overweight, and in fact some parents believe that a "pudgy" child is a healthy child. However, measurement of the child's height and weight and determination of the BMI-for-age during the examination indicate that the child is indeed overweight or gaining weight more rapidly than expected and will soon be overweight.

Pathophysiology

Our understanding of the pathophysiology of obesity continues to evolve. Certain neurohormones affect appetite, satiety, and the balance between fat storage and energy production. Nevertheless, in the end, obesity results when energy intake exceeds expenditure. The storage of excess calories was an advantage to our ancestors who faced intermittent food shortage; however, in our current setting where food is generally widely and consistently available and opportunities for physical activity are reduced, this predisposition to store excess calories has contributed to increasing rates of obesity.

It is known from twin and other studies that susceptibility to obesity is influenced substantially by **genetics.** Yet the magnitude of recent increases in obesity rates suggests the importance of **behavioral** and **environmental** factors as well. National surveys indicate that Americans are consuming more calories now than they were 35 years ago. This trend is likely related to increasingly widespread and ready availability of calorically dense foods. Surveys also tell us that Americans of all ages are less physically active than in the past. The reasons for this are myriad and include changes in transportation patterns, household work demands, and shifts in the workforce from manufacturing to more sedentary service-oriented jobs. Children have decreased opportunities for activity owing to safety concerns; parental work habits; the availability of television, computers, and other electronic toys; and reduced availability of physical education in school and after-school recreation programs.

Differential Diagnosis

Most children who present to physicians as overweight have primary obesity (resulting from excessive caloric intake and/or decreased activity). Only a small proportion of overweight children will have an organic cause, although parents may initially inquire about an organic etiology to their child's obesity. A thorough history, physical examination, and evaluation of growth parameters will help differentiate primary from organic obesity in most cases. While children with primary obesity tend to have normal or increased height-for-

age, children with an organic etiology, such as hypothyroidism, are shorter than normal or have a delayed rate of linear growth. Certain genetic syndromes, such as Prader-Willi syndrome, pseudo-hypoparathyroidism, and Laurence-Moon-Biedl syndrome, are associated with obesity. However, children with these syndromes have other findings, such as developmental delay, dysmorphic features, and short stature, which are usually readily identifiable during the physical examination.

Evaluation

History

The history should include the age of the child, parental weights, and lifestyle information (Questions Box). Knowledge of a child's birth weight and gestational age may also be helpful. Full-term babies weighing more than 9 lbs are at increased risk of obesity. Paradoxically, prematurity is also a risk factor for subsequent obesity. Breastfeeding has been shown to have a dose-dependent protective effect against future obesity. A diet history, for example, using the 24-hour recall method (Box 122-1) is helpful to

---

Questions

Obesity

- Is there a family history of obesity, hypertension, diabetes, or hyperlipidemia?
- Where does the child live? With whom does the child live?
- Are there kitchen facilities in the home (eg, refrigerator, microwave, hot plate, stove, and oven)?
- How often does the child/family go to fast food or other restaurants?
- Who does the shopping and food preparation? Are there financial problems, time limitations?
- What are the child's usual daily activities?
  — How does the child get to/from school?
  — What does the child do at recess, lunch, physical education class?
  — What does the child do after school?
  — What activities does the child do on the weekend?
  — What activities are participated in as a family?
- How much time does the child spend watching television? Playing with video games or on the computer?
- Who gives the parents advice on how to feed the child?
- What does the parent/child think about the child's weight? What do other family members think about the child's weight?
- Does the child get teased or ostracized because of weight?
- Has the child tried to lose weight before? How?
- Some additional questions for older children/adolescents include
  — Has the child/teen participated in fad dieting? Fasting? Laxative use? Diuretic use?
  — Has the child/teen used drugs to lose weight (illicit, over the counter, or prescription)?
  — Has the child/teen used nutritional supplements for weight loss?
  — Has the child/teen ever binged? Purged?
  — Does the child/teen use tobacco? Alcohol?

understand the dietary factors contributing to the child's overweight status as well as to identify areas for potential change. In addition, a history of signs or symptoms of complications of obesity should be elicited. For example, a teen may complain of hip pain suggestive of a slipped capital femoral epiphyses (SCFE). There may be a history of snoring, apneic pauses followed by gasping for breath during sleep, and daytime sleepiness indicating sleep disordered breathing and necessitating further evaluation for obstructive sleep apnea (OSA). A history of irregular menstrual periods is useful in the evaluation for polycystic ovary syndrome (PCOS).

Physical Examination

The accurate measurement of height and weight using appropriate equipment and plotting growth parameters on a growth chart are essential components of well-child care. In addition to allowing assessment of the child's weight, height, and rate of growth relative to other children, the revised 2000 growth curves (developed by the US National Center for Health Statistics and available at www.cdc.gov/growthcharts/) enable the physician and other health providers to evaluate BMI-for-age (for children ≥2 years) relative to other children of the same gender. Children should also be examined for any dysmorphic features suggestive of an underlying syndromic diagnosis.

The clinician should assess for potential complications of obesity when examining the overweight child. While many complications of obesity do not manifest until adulthood, overweight children are at risk for a number of conditions, including hypertension, hyperlipidemia, type 2 diabetes, nonalcoholic fatty liver disease, OSA, and orthopedic problems such as Blount disease and SCFE. One-third to one-half of overweight children will have evidence of **metabolic syndrome,** a cluster of traits that include hyperinsulinemia, obesity, hypertension, and hyperlipidemia. The higher the BMI-for-age, the greater the risk that the child or teen will have metabolic syndrome. Blood pressure should be accurately measured with an appropriate-sized cuff and compared with age-based standards. The physician should be alert for additional physical findings. The skin should be examined for acanthosis nigricans, the velvety pigmented lesion commonly found on the neck or axilla, which is associated with insulin resistance in overweight children, and for hirsutism, which in an obese adolescent girl may indicate the presence of PCOS. The musculoskeletal examination should focus on assessment for Blount disease, SCFE, or other degenerative joint diseases.

Laboratory Tests

Except for the rare case where an organic etiology of obesity is suspected, laboratory studies are of limited utility in the initial evaluation of the obese child. If a genetic condition is suspected, an evaluation by a geneticist may lead to a high-resolution karyotype and other genetic tests as directed by the suspected syndrome. Thyroid function studies or cortisol levels may be considered if an underlying endocrinologic disorder is suspected. More often, laboratory studies may be needed to evaluate for potential complications of obesity. It is recommended that adolescents with a BMI that exceeds the 85th percentile have fasting glucose and insulin levels and a fasting lipid panel assessed. Some experts also recommend checking liver enzymes. If the fasting glucose is abnormal, a glucose tolerance test is indicated. Clinicians may want to consider these tests in younger children with more severe overweight (eg, >99th percentile BMI-for-age), or for children with a family history of type 2 diabetes or hyperlipidemia. Children with a history of sleep-disordered breathing should be considered for a sleep study.

Imaging Studies

Radiologic studies are indicated when orthopedic complications of obesity such as Blount disease or SCFE are suspected. An echocardiogram for evaluation of ventricular hypertrophy is a consideration in children with long-standing hypertension (left ventricle may be affected) or OSA (right ventricle may be affected).

Management

The treatment of obesity is one of the most challenging areas in medicine today. Intervention is complicated because it is more than an individual's dietary intake, physical activity level, and genetic endowment that influence the development of obesity. Family beliefs and behaviors as well as community attitudes, practices, priorities, and resources also play a critical and often underappreciated role. These many factors must be considered as we plan obesity prevention and treatment programs. Recommending that a patient "go on a diet," particularly if the patient is a child or teen, is unlikely to be successful if the effect of the family and community on eating and physical activity is not also addressed. A focus on dieting or restricting an individual's dietary intake, in isolation of other factors, as a means of promoting weight loss has proven to be a dismal failure. More than 90% of patients who lose weight through dieting will ultimately regain it. Surgical and medical treatments for obesity, although increasingly marketed even for teens, are fraught with risks for complications and side effects.

The care of the *child* who is obese is further complicated beyond even consideration of the child's family and community. As a growing being, a child's growth potential and development may be compromised if obesity treatment is not managed carefully. Not all children who are obese will go on to be obese adults, providing an additional reason for a cautious approach. The pediatrician's first task is to determine a child's future risk for obesity. This is largely determined by the child's age and history of parental obesity; however, race/ethnicity may also play a role. Obese children younger than 3 years without obese parents are at low risk for future obesity. These children should be monitored but, for the most part, do not require intervention. Between the ages of 3 and 5 years, parental obesity substantially increases the risk of a child becoming an obese adult. The chance of adult obesity in an obese preschooler with at least one obese parent is 62%. In older children, the child's own obesity is an increasingly important predictor of adult obesity, regardless of whether the parents are obese. The probability that an overweight child older than 6 years will be obese as an adult is 50%, regardless of parental obesity status. Children determined to be at high risk for future obesity require close attention and active intervention by the clinician.

The practitioner's goal in caring for the obese child may not be weight loss but rather normal linear growth while slowing weight gain or maintaining weight. The only safe means of obesity treatment for children is behavior and lifestyle modification, the aims of which are to promote healthful eating, increased physical activity, and development of a healthy body image and self-esteem. Consideration of these goals is particularly important given the increasing number of children and teens who are overly focused on their weight or who participate in unhealthy weight loss practices including laxative abuse, induced vomiting, and fasting (see Chapter 120).

Behavior and lifestyle modification for obesity must be tailored for the individual child, family, and community. Before any intervention will be successful, the child and family must be ready to make a change. **Motivational interviewing** techniques can be helpful in determining and promoting a family's readiness to make changes, which are meant to be adopted as a permanent part of the child's and family's lifestyle. Because it is difficult to modify ingrained habits and behaviors related to food and activity, patients and their families require ongoing support and attention from their clinicians as they attempt to incorporate recommended changes into their lives. Negotiating acceptable lifestyle changes is an important first step for the clinician. Changes need to be realistic and acceptable to the patient and their family. Recommendations are unlikely to be implemented if they are inconsistent with a patient's and family's values, culture, and resources. For example, a child's participation in an after-school sports program may not be a realistic option if a family cannot afford the fees or transportation to and from the program is not available.

Understanding that good nutrition is important does not necessarily translate into healthy eating. For example, a person may know to limit fat and sodium but not know which foods are high in these ingredients or how to prepare foods to limit their content. It can be helpful to families to plan their daily menus and activity schedule in advance. Asking families to adhere as closely as possible to specific dietary and exercise plans until these changes become part of a family's routine can promote longer-term success. Most families need additional education on appropriate serving sizes, healthful food preparation, interpreting food labels, and making healthy food choices. A dietitian can be very helpful in the planning, education, and follow-up needed for families to be successful in these efforts.

Suggestions for clinicians to help their families toward a healthier lifestyle are listed in Box 122-2. Some items on this list involve changes in a single aspect of the diet, such as reducing the intake of juice. Restricting other sugar-sweetened beverages is also important. A growing body of evidence demonstrates an association between the consumption of sugar-sweetened beverages and overweight; limiting these beverages has successfully promoted weight loss in overweight teens. Other suggestions in Box 122-2 are more complex and involve providing a plan for healthy eating and physical activity. Guides to a healthier lifestyle are readily available. Examples include the US Department of Agriculture (USDA) Food and Nutrition Service "MyPyramid" (www.mypyramid.gov) and "MyPyramid for Kids," which expand on the original Pyramid Food Plan to encourage an individualized approach to healthy eating and promote increased physical activity. *Dietary Guidelines for Americans* is published jointly every 5 years by the Department of Health and Human Services and the USDA. The guidelines provide advice for people 2 years and older about how good dietary habits can promote health and reduce risk for major chronic diseases (www.healthierus.gov/dietaryguidelines/). These sites provide educational material appropriate for families and training materials for health professionals. Family and patient support groups and organized programs for overweight children may also be helpful. Data on effectiveness of specific programs aimed at overweight children are limited, and no program has yet been shown superior. Thus it behooves the clinician to know the details, costs, and track record of available local programs for appropriate referral of overweight children and their families.

Box 122-2. 10 Ways to Help Families Toward a Healthier Lifestyle

1. Learn as much as you can about the child's and family's usual diet and activity pattern so that you can negotiate changes that will be acceptable.
2. Provide families with a guide for healthy eating. Educate families on interpretation of nutrition information on food labels.
3. Educate families on foods that are high in fat and calories. Have them try alternative methods of food preparation (eg, baking or broiling rather than frying).
4. Encourage intake of "unprocessed" foods such as fresh fruits and vegetables and whole-grain products. Limit processed and prepackaged foods and snacks, and keep these out of the house as much as possible.
5. Help families come up with low-fat, nutritious snacks they can keep on hand.
6. After 1 year of age, switch from a bottle to a cup.
7. For children older than 2 years, change to low-fat or fat-free milk. Limit milk to 16 to 24 oz per day after the first year of life.
8. Limit juice to less than 6 oz per day. Limit soda to special occasions.
9. Limit television to less than 1 hour per day. Limit other sedentary activities such as playing video and computer games.
10. Incorporate physical activity into the child's and family's daily routine. Find a sport that the child enjoys and can master.

Prevention

Prevention of obesity is our best option for reversing the growing epidemic of obesity and obesity-related comorbidity. Prevention of obesity should be a priority for all clinicians who care for children and should focus on 3 broad areas: (1) anticipatory guidance starting at a young age on the importance of healthful eating and regular physical activity; (2) reinforcement with families of the importance of a healthy attitude toward food, eating, and body image; and (3) advocacy for public health measures to increase opportunities for healthful eating and regular physical activity within our communities.

Prognosis

Sadly, average American life expectancy is currently projected to decrease, owing to the increasing incidence of diseases associated with obesity such as diabetes. Taken together, poor diet and sedentary lifestyles are estimated to contribute to 300,000 excess deaths per year, rivaling smoking as a preventable cause of premature death. Obese children who remain obese into adulthood are at greatly increased risk for complications including hypertension, cardiovascular disease, gallbladder disease, diabetes, some types of cancer, degenerative arthritis, and obstructive sleep apnea.

CASE RESOLUTION

The opening vignette describes an overweight girl. She is at substantial risk for remaining obese into adulthood based on her present weight and her mother's history of obesity. Working with a dietitian, the mother and her daughter learn about the components of a healthy diet. They plan meals and snacks that are healthy and easily prepared in advance. The girl begins to make her own lunch each night before school. Rather than whole milk, the mother buys nonfat milk and no longer keeps juice, cookies, chips, or soda around the house. A social worker helps find an after-school program at the nearby YMCA. The patient starts attending and, with some special attention from the coach, finds she enjoys basketball and would like to try out for the junior high school team next year. The mother wants to exercise more, and so the girl and her mother go for nightly walks around the track at the local high school.

Over the next 6 months, you follow the girl and her mother closely. The most recent growth parameters show that the girl has maintained her weight at 59 kg but has grown 5 cm to 145 cm, giving her a body mass index of 28. The mother has lost 5 lb during this period, and both are excited about continuing their new lifestyle.

Selected References

American Academy of Pediatrics Committee on Nutrition. Policy statement: prevention of pediatric overweight and obesity. *Pediatrics*. 2003;112:424–430

American Academy of Pediatrics Council on Sports Medicine and Fitness and Council on School Health. Policy statement: active healthy living: prevention of childhood obesity through increased physical activity. *Pediatrics*. 2006;117:1834–1842

Daniels SR, Arnett DK, Eckel RH, et al. Overweight in children and adolescents: pathophysiology, consequence, prevention and treatment. *Circulation*. 2005;111:1999–2012

Dietz WH, Lee J, Wechsler H, Malepati S, Sherry B. Health plans' role in preventing overweight in children and adolescents. *Health Aff (Millwood)*. 2007;26:430–440

Freedman DS, Mei Z, Srinivasan SR, Berenson GS, Dietz WH. Cardiovascular risk factors and excess adiposity among overweight children and adolescents: the Bogalusa Heart Study. *J Pediatr*. 2007;150:12–17.e2

Institute of Medicine, Committee on Prevention of Obesity in Children and Youth. *Preventing Childhood Obesity: Health in the Balance*. Washington, DC: National Academy of Sciences; 2004

Divorce

Carol D. Berkowitz, MD

CASE STUDY

A 7-year-old girl who has been your patient for 5 years is brought in by her mother with abdominal pain that occurs on a daily basis and is not associated with any other symptoms. The pain is periumbilical. In obtaining the history, you learn that the father has moved out of the home and the parents are planning a divorce. The mother believes that her daughter's symptoms may relate to the impending divorce, and she wants to know what else to expect.

Questions

1. What are the problems faced by children whose parents are undergoing divorce?
2. What are the age-related reactions of children in families undergoing divorce?
3. What is the role of pediatricians in counseling families undergoing divorce?
4. What anticipatory guidance can be offered about custody and remarriage?
5. How can pediatricians help stepfamilies adjust?

Divorce represents the **"death"** of a marriage, and in some ways may be more devastating for children than the death of a parent. When a parent dies, that parent becomes idealized in the mind of children, but when parents divorce, the noncustodial parent is often devalued. In fact, each parent is frequently devalued by the other. For children, parents are no longer the idealized figures that they once were. The challenge for pediatricians is to maintain a neutral position. This may be particularly difficult because much of the contact has been with one parent rather than the other, usually the mother.

Pediatricians play a specific role in managing children going through a parental divorce because other resources are few. **Extended families** are no longer available to provide help. Religious institutions have often failed to assume a counseling role in this area; some religions view divorce unfavorably. Most families do not seek out mental health services unless the problems are overwhelming. Therefore, it is important for pediatricians to become involved in anticipatory guidance of families undergoing divorce. This guidance focuses on preparing children and families for times ahead. In addition, practitioners serve as child advocates. The parents themselves are so consumed by their emotional turmoil that they are often not available or are not even aware of the stress and trauma their children are experiencing. Physicians should be aware of the effect of the divorce on children and their subsequent psychological development. In addition, pediatricians can help as new families form, assisting the transition of caretakers into the role of stepparents.

Epidemiology

Divorce currently affects nearly 50% of marriages. **Ethnic differences** exist; 38% of European American compared with 75% of African American children's parents divorce prior to the children's 18th birthday. The US Office of National Statistics reported 895,189 divorces for 2004, a figure that probably is lower than the actual number of cases because not all states report their data. Divorce usually occurs in the first 14 years of marriage (mean: 7.8 years). Approximately 1 million children per year are affected by divorce. Nearly one-third of all children live in households in which parents are divorced or remarried. Children between the ages of 3 and 8 years are the major age group affected. Children involved with parental divorce take 2½ to 3 years to regain their equilibrium and master a sense of control. Divorce usually results in a decline of **economic resources** to mothers and children. In the first year after divorce, income is reduced to 58% of the pre-divorce level. Even after 5 years, income for mothers and children is only 94% of the pre-divorce amount; for intact couples, income has risen to 130% during that period. Decreased income is often associated with multiple moves to more affordable housing along with change in schools and loss of friends. More affordable neighborhoods may not provide the same resources and environment to which the children were previously accustomed.

Types of custody include **single-parent custody, joint custody, joint legal custody,** and **joint physical custody,** where parents have physical access to the child with equal frequency. **Birds-nest custody** is joint custody where children remain in the home and parents take turns moving in and out. Many states now allow for joint custody. Joint custody is associated with higher levels of involvement by the biological father, increased child support payments, and greater paternal satisfaction. Issues of **remarriage** and **stepsiblings** are also important. Eighty percent of divorced men and 75% of divorced women remarry, and 40% of these remarriages end in divorce. As a result of the high rate of remarriage, 1 in 3 children in the United States has a stepparent. Eighty-six percent of stepfamilies include the biological mother and a stepfather. Children in stepfamilies often have to readjust to differing roles in differing households and differing relationships between their biological parents, stepparents, biological siblings, and stepsiblings.

Psychophysiology

The experience that children have following parental divorce is influenced by many factors, including the individual child's **temperament** and **personality.** An easygoing child with strong self-esteem and a positive outlook fairs better than the child with a difficult temperament and less positive personality traits. The reaction to divorce also depends, to a large extent, on the age of the child (Table 123-1). In general, children do not have the cognitive ability to understand the meaning of divorce until they are 9 or 10 years of age.

Table 123-1. Children's Reaction to Divorce	
Age	*Symptoms*
2½–4 y	• Regressive behavior
3½–5 y	• Aggressive behavior
5–6 y	• Whiny, immature behavior
6 y–adolescence	• Disequilibrium • Depression • Somatic complaints • Poor school performance

Children up to the age of 2 years experience **sleeping** and **feeding disturbances,** as well as spitting up and clinginess. Between the ages of 2½ and 4 years, children usually manifest **regressive behavior.** They become needy and dependent, and their behavior is characterized by irritability, whining, crying, fearfulness, increased separation anxiety, and sleep problems. Both aggression and regression, particularly in the area of toilet training, may develop. One-third of children in this age group continue to exhibit regressive behavior 1 year after divorce.

Preschool-aged children between the ages of 3½ and 5 years often show more aggressive patterns of behavior with hitting, biting, and temper tantrums. Regressive behavior may also be seen. Young children feel particularly responsible for their parents' divorce (ie, the parents are divorcing the child). At this point in development, children experience what Piaget has referred to as an egocentric way of thinking. Self-blame, decreased self-esteem, and a high level of fantasy, particularly about parental reunion, are apparent. Approximately 1 year after divorce, 65% of these children still show decreased levels of functioning.

Children who are 5 to 6 years of age are often **depressed** and may exhibit immature behavior. Girls in this age group seem to handle a divorce more poorly than boys. Two-thirds of girls are less well-adjusted 1 year after the divorce, as opposed to only about one-fourth of boys. These children seem moody and daydream. They may also be whiny and have temper tantrums.

School-aged children between the age of 6 years and adolescence seem to experience profound disequilibrium, with feelings of shame, anger, and loneliness. This anger may be manifested by antisocial behavior. Older children also talk about an overwhelming feeling of sadness and grief. Their somatic complaints include headache, abdominal pain, and an increase in symptoms of preexisting medical conditions such as asthma. Sometimes the somatic complaints of children, particularly those in the school-aged group, are attributed by one parent to the poor living conditions at the other parent's household.

It is important for physicians to anticipate that 50% of children involved in parental divorce show a deterioration in their school performance. Therefore, the school should be notified about the divorce and changes in family structure. Decreased school performance is attributed to decreased ability to concentrate, sadness, and depression.

Parental divorce is particularly difficult for adolescents, who describe it as "extraordinarily painful." The experience is worse for younger adolescents. During the first stages of divorce, they experience a personal sense of abandonment and a loss of parental love. Older adolescents are concerned about their future potential as marital partners. They also feel anxious about financial security, especially money for college. **De-idealization** of both parents is precipitous. Adolescent girls do better than boys early on, but this reverses with time. This pattern is referred to as a **sleeper effect** or **delayed effect,** with girls subsequently feeling rejected and unattractive as they reinterpret their parents' divorce with their additional maturation. Divorce during adolescence sometimes leads to **precocious sexual activity** or risk- or thrill-seeking behavior. Adolescents from divorced families are more likely to experience teenage parenthood. Adolescent girls from divorced families are less likely to succeed academically than girls from families where there has not been a divorce. In addition, the adolescent may turn to alcohol or drug use to help cope with the stress of parental divorce. Boys may engage in illegal activities such as burglary.

Differential Diagnosis

Children who present with complaints including headache, abdominal pain, enuresis, and poor school performance should always be assessed for environmental factors that may be contributing to their symptomatology. When evaluating a child with suspected **somatic complaints,** it is appropriate to consider organic etiologies.

Many parents who are undergoing a divorce do not appreciate the impact the divorce is having on their children. They are often caught up in their own personal feelings and are not aware of their children's symptomatology. In addition, divorcing parents actually experience a deterioration in their physical and mental well-being, and divorced mothers have an increased rate of illness.

Evaluation

The focus of the evaluation should be on the interviewing process. Determination of the full extent of the impact of the home factors on children's symptomatology may take several visits. It is not appropriate to pursue extensive laboratory tests without first adequately determining what changes are occurring within the household.

History

The medical evaluation of children experiencing a parental divorce should include a review of the medical history and a discussion with the child of factors of change (Questions Box). This may help open up a discussion that reveals that the parents are in the process of divorce or that the father has moved out of the household.

Questions

Divorce

- Is there anything different about the child's house now?
- Who lives in the house?
- How are things going between the parents?
- Has the child shown any regressive or aggressive behaviors?
- Has the child been eating and sleeping normally?
- How is the child doing in school?

Physical Examination

Any symptom or specific complaint, such as headache or abdominal pain, should also be addressed (see Chapters 100 and 104). Depression and the risk for suicide should also be evaluated (see Chapter 126). A complete physical examination is usually warranted because children who are experiencing stress may also develop stress-related medical problems.

Laboratory Tests

Some simple baseline laboratory studies may be warranted, particularly in children who have complaints such as abdominal pain or enuresis. These tests may include a complete blood count or urinalysis.

Management

Management of children whose family is undergoing divorce is complex. In addition to treating any somatic complaints that may be related to the divorce, physicians play a key role in anticipatory guidance. Children need to understand that they didn't cause the divorce and that they will not be able to "cure" it. Physician involvement before parents actually separate helps. Initially, physicians should advise parents about how to talk to children and what to expect in terms of their reaction. It is important for parents to tell children that they are separating from one another and not from the children. As stated previously, parents undergoing a divorce are in so much turmoil that they themselves may not see their children's problems. In addition, their parenting skills may suffer, and routine

procedures such as meals and bedtime may become disrupted, sporadic, and irregular.

Box 123-1 summarizes advice to parents. **When, how, who,** and **what** to tell should be discussed. Generally, children should be told of impending divorce by both parents with support from the extended family. Unfortunately, studies report that 80% of preschoolers were told by one parent.

Box 123-1. Talking to Children About Divorce

Who
- Who tells? Both parents
- Who is told? Children, physicians, teachers, neighbors

When
- Before either parent leaves
- Age-dependent
- Older children: weeks ahead
- Younger children: days ahead

How
- Calmly, with emotional control

Where
- Privately, in the home

What
- Stress that children are not to blame; that the divorce is between parents, not between parents and children; it is the parents who cannot get along.
- Explain expected living arrangements.

When to tell depends on children's ages. Younger children should be told a few days before the actual separation. Older children should be told at least several weeks before. Practitioners should advise parents about **how** to tell. Displays of emotion are permissible. Parents should be encouraged to show their emotions, but not to the extent that they appear overwhelmed or uncontrollable.

Who to tell includes not only the children but also the neighbors and the school, so that the feeling of shame or secrecy is less. **What** to tell involves freeing the children of any blame for the divorce and answering their questions.

It is important for physicians not to become involved in custody disputes, but if they are asked to give an opinion, they should try to evaluate the parenting skills of both parents. In the past, custody was given to the mother in 90% of cases, but this is now decreasing. Questions that physicians should ask themselves when advising about custody include What are the emotional ties between parents and children? Do children indicate a preference for one parent? Children may be overwhelmed by feelings of loyalty and be torn if asked to choose one parent over the other, which makes this a difficult problem. What is the capacity of each parent to provide emotional and physical support for children? It is important to consider a need for continuity, and it is vital to keep conditions as close as possible to the pre-divorce situation. Children should not have to move. Living arrangements need to be reassessed on a periodic basis.

Physicians should be aware of the factors that support joint custody. Joint custody tends to maintain a parent-child attachment, and children experience less of a sense of loss. They have more cognitive and social stimulation. Joint custody relieves the burden of single parenthood, and parents who have joint custody are less likely to use children as bargaining tools. Parents themselves are freer to enter into different relationships and are less emotionally dependent on their children. Although physicians should not become involved in monetary issues, concerns related to payment and cost of medical care are appropriate to discuss. Practitioners should consider involving noncustodial parents in children's health care. Such parents could be notified if medical problems occur.

Pediatricians may also be helpful in counseling noncustodial parents about interacting with children. Unfortunately contact with noncustodial parents may decrease rapidly following a divorce. While 25% of children have weekly visits with their noncustodial father, 20% of children see their father only several times a year or not at all. In general, visitation should reflect previous relationships as closely as possible. Noncustodial parents should be advised not to become camp counselors who focus on fun and games but to be influential figures who help the children meet the challenges of normal living such as completing homework and doing chores and tasks. It is also important for noncustodial parents to be consistent. If a meeting is planned, the parents must show up. Although the parents are no longer married, they can still be co-parents rather than rivals. Noncustodial parents should be encouraged to participate in school and sports activities.

Custodial parents may attribute children's somatic complaints to poor care while under visitation with noncustodial parents. Allegations related to abuse, most often sexual abuse, may also arise. These allegations should be taken seriously. An appropriate medical and psychological evaluation is necessary (see Chapter 116). The most difficult situations involve allegations of sexual abuse of preverbal children, where conclusions may be contingent on the physical findings, which are usually inconclusive.

Issues related to parental dating and remarriage should be addressed at an early stage. Parents should be advised that pediatricians may be a resource in helping families readjust. Remarriage is often a difficult time for children because they experience feelings of rejection secondary to displacement by stepparents. Grandparents may also be a source of support.

The pediatrician can also serve as a resource for stepparents. Although stepparents do not have legal rights to consent for medical care of their stepchildren, they should become familiar with the children's medical history. Stepparents grow into their parenting role, and it takes 2 to 7 years for families to become blended. The pediatrician can help families adjust by recommending books or giving referrals to organizations such as Stepfamily Association of America (www.sfhelp.org) or National Stepfamily Resource Center (www.stepfamilies.info).

Prognosis

The prognosis for children undergoing a parental divorce depends, in part, on the degree of dysfunction that existed in the family before separation and the ability of the children to communicate their concerns. Supportive intervention by family, friends, and physicians is key to facilitating the necessary adjustment. Being a child of divorced and remarried parents has been likened to having dual citizenship. The experience is rewarding if the countries are not at war with one another.

CASE RESOLUTION

The case history shows that functional somatic complaints are not uncommon, especially in school-aged children of divorced parents. The mother and her daughter should be advised about how stressful divorce is for children. A careful medical examination may reassure both the mother and child about the child's physical well-being. Issues related to custody, financial responsibility, and the need for consistency should all be addressed. In addition, the pediatrician should refer the family to outside agencies if necessary.

Selected References

Behrman RE. Children and divorce: overview and analysis. *Future Child.* 1994;4:4–14

Bryner CL. Children of divorce. *J Am Board Fam Pract.* 2001;14:178–183

Cohen GJ, American Academy of Pediatrics Committee on Psychosocial Aspects of Child and Family Health. Helping children and families deal with divorce and separation. *Pediatrics.* 2002;110:1019–1023

Dell ML. Divorce—are you ready to help? *Contemp Pediatr.* 1995;12:57–68

Emery RE, Coiro MJ. Divorce: consequences for children. *Pediatr Rev.* 1995; 16:306–310

Hetherington EM. Divorce and the adjustment of children. *Pediatr Rev.* 2005; 26:163–169

Storksen I, Roysamb E, Moum T, Tambs K. Adolescents with a childhood experience of parental divorce: a longitudinal study of mental health and adjustment. *J Adolesc.* 2005;28:725–739

Books for Parents

Clapp G. *Divorce and New Beginnings: A Complete Guide to Recovery, Solo Parenting, Co-Parenting, and Stepfamilies.* Hoboken, NJ: John Wiley & Sons; 2000

Garon RJ. *Talking to Your Children about Separation and Divorce: A Handbook for Parents.* Columbia, MD: National Family Resiliency Center, Inc.; 1999

School-Related Violence

Elizabeth A. Edgerton, MD, MPH

CASE STUDY

A mother brings her 9-year-old son, Alex, in complaining of recurrent abdominal pain. His pain has become so severe that Alex misses school frequently. He denies any vomiting or diarrhea. His weight has been stable over the last 6 months. Alex's mother reports that lately he seems more withdrawn and passive. He used to be engaged in his schoolwork but now with his frequent absences has lost interest in school. His mother says he is often anxious or nervous about new situations.

Questions

1. How does school-related violence affect children's health and well-being?
2. What is the relationship between bullying and adult criminal behavior?
3. What is cyberbullying?
4. What are strategies to address school-related violence?
5. What can pediatricians do to help address violence in the school, home, and communities?

Violence is defined as an act of aggression that can be **physical, sexual,** or **psychological** and is usually deliberate and intended to cause harm. Its form, level of severity, and frequency are impacted by biological, individual, clinical, intrapersonal, situational, and sociocultural factors. Categorization of violence is also dependent on the relationship of the perpetrator and victim, as well as their ages. Domestic or **intimate partner violence** occurs among individuals in an established relationship, **child abuse** predominately occurs between an adult and a minor, and **bullying** is usually between peers. From a developmental perspective, bullying may be the earliest form of violence promulgated by children and can progress to intimate partner violence, **criminal delinquency, suicide,** or **homicide** in adolescence and adulthood. While violence may be considered a social issue, it impacts the physical and mental health of all of those involved. The primary care physician has unique opportunities to prevent violence and identify those potentially at risk.

Prevalence

Suicide and homicide represent the most lethal forms of violence. Suicide and homicide are responsible for approximately one-fourth of deaths among persons aged 10 to 24 years in the United States. Approximately 3 million youths are at risk for suicide, with 37% of at-risk individuals attempting to kill themselves (see Chapter 126). Suicide is the third leading cause of death among 15- to 24-year-olds, and over the last 20 years has increased 100% among 10- to 14-year-olds. It is estimated that approximately 12 youths die each day in the United States from suicide. Homicide is also increasing among children and adolescents. According to the Centers for Disease Control and Prevention, homicide is the fifth leading cause of death for youths 10 to 14 years of age and the second leading cause of death for 15- to 19-year-olds in the United States.

In 2004 emergency department data documented that more than 750,000 youth aged 10 to 24 were treated for injuries sustained due to violence. Nationwide surveys of high school students note that 33% report being in a physical fight one or more times in the 12 preceding months. An additional 17% reported carrying a weapon such as a gun, knife, or club on one or more of the 30 days preceding the survey. Furthermore, 6% of students reported not going to school on one or more days in the 30 days preceding the survey because they felt unsafe at school or on their way to and from school.

Those that admitted to being bullies in middle school had at least one criminal conviction by age 24 years, and 35% to 40% had 3 or more convictions by 24 years of age compared with 10% among control boys who were neither bullies nor victims as children. The aggressive antisocial behavior of bullying seems to contribute to future serious criminal behavior. Many of the recent killing sprees in the United States were committed by individuals who as children felt they were victimized. A review of 37 mass school shootings found more than two-thirds of perpetrators felt they had been persecuted, bullied, threatened, or attacked; often, they were acting out of revenge.

In a national survey of 6th- to 10th-grade students, approximately 30% reported moderate or frequent involvement in bullying; this could include being the bully, the victim, or both (known as the *bully-victim*). Those who reported being a bully or victim were more likely to carry weapons to school, as well as to be involved in frequent fights. Bullying itself is most common in the early school years. Initially, boys are more likely than girls to be involved in bullying. This gender gap decreases in middle and high school, as does the prevalence of bullying. Boys tend to participate in physical and verbal bullying, while girls use more subtle and indirect forms of bullying such as alienation or ostracizing.

Risk factors associated with violence are complex and involve the individual, family, peers, and community (Box 124-1). Demonstrated risk factors associated with violent behavior include exposure to violence as a witness or victim, childhood aggression and **antisocial behavior, substance abuse, depressed mood,** and **hyperactivity.** Protective factors include academic achievement and parent-family connectedness. Families that provide positive and consistent discipline and supervision can prevent involvement in violence.

Box 124-1. Risk Factors Associated With Violence

Individual Risk Factors[a]
- History of violent victimization or involvement
- Attention deficit, hyperactivity, or learning disorders
- History of early aggressive behavior
- Involvement with drugs, alcohol, or tobacco
- Low IQ
- Poor behavioral control
- Deficits in social, cognitive, or information-processing abilities
- High emotional distress
- History of treatment for emotional problems
- Antisocial beliefs and attitudes
- Exposure to violence and conflict in the family

Family Risk Factors
- Authoritarian childrearing attitudes
- Harsh, lax, or inconsistent disciplinary practices
- Low parental involvement
- Low emotional attachment to parents or caregivers
- Low parental education and income
- Parental substance abuse or criminality
- Poor family functioning
- Poor monitoring and supervision of children

Peer/School Risk Factors
- Association with delinquent peers
- Involvement in gangs
- Social rejection by peers
- Lack of involvement in conventional activities
- Poor academic performance
- Low commitment to school and school failure

Community Risk Factors
- Diminished economic opportunities
- High concentrations of poor residents
- High level of transience
- High level of family disruption
- Low levels of community participation
- Socially disorganized neighborhoods

---

[a]Adapted from the Centers for Disease Control and Prevention. Youth Violence Fact Sheet. www.cdc.gov/ncipc/factsheets/yvfacts.htm.

Bullying

Recently more attention and formal research regarding bullying is occurring in the United States. Tragic mass killing events, especially those at schools, coupled with reports of the perpetrators being victims or bullies during childhood, has raised the awareness of the seriousness of bullying as an early form of violence. Bullying has been extensively studied in Europe. Research, especially by Dr Olweus from Norway, demonstrates the serious consequences of this early form of aggression. Unfortunately, many parents, teachers, and health professionals still see bullying as a normal behavior of children.

Bullying is a type of aggression in which the intent of the behavior is to cause harm or disturb an individual. An imbalance of power exists with the more powerful attacking the less powerful. Opposed to what might be called "normal childhood conflicts," bullying occurs repeatedly over time. Bullying does not occur in isolation, but rather in an environment that supports the behavior. Participants include the bully, the victim, and the bystander. The bully is often an aggressive individual that uses violence to dominate others; he or she has little empathy for their victim. In contrast to common perception, bullies do not have poor self-esteem, but rather have a strong desire to control others. The victim may be more passive and anxious. This individual is often less secure than their peers and may be lonely, playing alone at school. When they are attacked by a bully, they usually withdraw rather than retaliate. A minority of youth may be classified as a bully-victim or a provocative victim. These individuals are both anxious and aggressive; while they are primarily victims of bullying, they may provoke the bully.

Bullying predominately occurs in a school environment, during recess, at lunch, or on the way to or from school. Children often do not report bullying to adults for both fear of and retaliation by the bully and the concern of disbelief by the adult. Studies demonstrate that adults underestimate the prevalence of bullying events compared with student reports. Clinicians need to consider this when asking the parent or child about bullying.

Consequences of Bullying

Bullying impacts the physical and mental health of all of those involved. Fear and anxiety about the school environment is most common. This can progress to avoidance of school, low self-esteem, and depression. Children with chronic illness are more vulnerable because they may suffer worsened body image with frequent teasing. In adulthood, higher rates of depression and poor self-esteem are seen among individuals with a history of being bullied. Strong associations in adolescence and early adulthood have been made between bullying and suicide and murder. The child who was victimized may react later in life with self-destructive acts or lethal retaliation.

A prospective cohort study of children 9 to 11 years of age in the Netherlands found that victims of bullying had significantly higher chances of developing new psychosomatic and psychosocial problems compared with children who were not bullied. A larger proportion of victims had underlying depression and anxiety prior to being bullied but still suffered significant psychosomatic and psychological problems after being bullied. Common complaints included depression, anxiety, abdominal pain, sleeping problems, headache, feeling tense, bed-wetting, feeling tired, and poor appetite. These complaints were present significantly more among children who had been victims of bullying.

Bystanders are also impacted because bullying distracts from the learning environment. Furthermore, they develop strategies to avoid being bullied that can include avoiding the restroom and staying home. One study reported that 1 in 5 secondary school children avoid restrooms out of fear at school. Another study stated that 7% of eighth graders stay home at least 1 day a month out of fear of other students.

Longitudinal studies report that bullies and bully-victims go on to more criminal activity than their counterparts. One study of Finnish boys reported 9% being bullies in childhood. These same individuals accounted for 37% of criminal activity in the study when the individuals reached adulthood. Bullies were more likely to commit occasional infractions while bully-victims were more likely to commit repeated offenses. Among bullies that participated in criminal activity, they were more likely to have underlying psychiatric symptoms. Other studies suggest that bullies have higher rates of conduct disorder.

In recent years there have been increasing reports of cyberbullying, where modern technology is used to pester, annoy, harass, and intimidate others, or to spread derogatory comments through chat rooms or other Internet sites. This represents yet another new problem related to computers (see Chapter 8).

Role of the Primary Care Physician

Childhood bullying is a complex abusive behavior with demonstrated serious consequences. Physicians are poised to identify at-risk individuals, screen for psychiatric comorbidities associated with bullying, counsel families, and advocate for school-based interventions. Because bullies or victims will not identify themselves as such, physicians need a systematic approach to screen for this early form of violence. Integrating screening during anticipatory guidance may be optimal for toddlers and school-aged children, while assessing risk factors at well- and acute-care visits may be needed for adolescents.

Multiple instruments have been used in a research setting for identifying bullying or associated internalizing or externalizing symptoms, but they have not been widely implemented in the primary care setting. Screening younger patients requires conversations with the child and family members. For adolescents, the use of the psychosocial interview **HEADDSSS** (home environment, employment and education, activities, diet, drugs, sexual activity/sexuality, suicide and depression, safety) may be useful in screening for high-risk behaviors and risk factors for violence (see Chapter 5).

When questioning a family about bullying, keep in mind that children will often not tell their parents that bullying occurred. When parents are told about bullying they may consider the situation as being normal behavior for young people and dismiss the event. Multiple forms of bullying exist. These include physical fights, verbal or cyber (text messaging or e-mail) harassment, and social isolation. Boys are more commonly involved in physical and verbal bullying while girls are more often involved in manipulative forms of bullying. As children become adolescents, intimate partner violence, suicide, and homicide are more likely consequences of bullying.

Prevention efforts need to focus on the individual, family, and community. In early childhood, parents can model for children appropriate social interaction, how to resolve conflict, and how to manage frustration and anger. School-wide bullying prevention programs are effective and should be advocated. The key components of these programs include involvement of the whole school and a long-term commitment to changing the social and behavioral norms. For older children and adolescents, identifying psychiatric symptoms and providing the appropriate intervention may prevent more serious violent behavior. At the individual level, physicians and parents can counsel children who are bullies or victims regarding appropriate behaviors (Box 124-2).

Box 124-2. Physician's Role

- Be vigilant for signs and symptoms of bullying and other psychosocial trauma and distress in children and adolescents.
- Increase awareness of the social and mental health consequences of bullying and other aggressive behaviors.
- Screen for psychiatric comorbidities in at-risk youth, and provide appropriate referrals for treatment for affected youth.
- Counsel affected youth and their families on effective intervention programs and coping strategies.
- Advocate for family, school, and community programs and services for victims and perpetrators for bullying and other forms of violence and aggression.

In a randomized controlled study, Borowsky and colleagues demonstrated the effectiveness of identifying at-risk youth aged 7 to 15 years of age in a primary care setting and of providing a **family-level intervention** to reduce violent behavior and injuries among youth. Families that received the telephone-based intervention focusing on positive parenting reported decreased parent-reported bullying, physical fighting, fight-related injuries requiring medical care, and child-reported victimization by bullying.

The Maternal and Child Health Bureau in partnership with other federal agencies developed a resource kit on bullying, which is available online at www.stopbullyingnow.hrsa.gov. Online vignettes are directed at children in their preteen years and are geared toward helping the youth identify what role they might have in bullying and what appropriate behavior might allow them to better handle the situation. Printed resources are available for parents and teachers. For adolescents, the Centers for Disease Control and Prevention launched **"Choose Respect,"** a Web-based program on relationships available online at www.chooserespect.org. It provides tools for adolescents to identify healthy peer relationships and appropriate responses if they are concerned about intimate partner violence.

Physicians are a vital component of youth violence prevention (Box 124-3). Prevention begins early in the child's development by providing positive reinforcement of appropriate pro-social behavior. Bullying is an early form of aggression. In and of itself bullying may seem harmless, but longitudinal studies as well as analysis of mass school shootings demonstrate the large impact aggression early in life can have on the future well-being of children, adolescents, and adults. Successful interventions require cooperation by parents, teachers, students, and health professionals.

Box 124-3. Individual-Level Prevention Strategies

Advice for Victims of Bullying

- Resist reacting to the bully; hold your frustration and anger.
- Walk away from the situation; ignore the bullying.
- Avoid retaliation or bullying back.
- Tell an adult.
- Talk about the bullying event with your family.
- Use a buddy system at school and traveling to and from school.
- Develop friendships by joining social organizations.

Management of Bullies

- Reinforce that bullying is a serious problem.
- Set limits and provide consequences for acts of aggression.
- Emphasize tolerance for people's differences; everyone deserves respect.
- Determine whether friends are also involved in bullying; seek a group intervention.
- Provide positive reinforcement for appropriate behavior.
- Work closely with schoolteachers and staff regarding behavior modification.
- Emphasize that it's the "behavior" that is not acceptable.

CASE RESOLUTION

Victims of bullying often present with psychosomatic symptoms such as headache or abdominal pain. Once organic etiologies have been ruled out, further questioning should focus on psychosocial stresses. Alex's abdominal pain is worse in the morning before going to school. When asked specifically about bullying, Alex states that a few of his classmates tease him and rough him up each day on his way to school. In the last few weeks they are text messaging him about how they are going to haze him the next day. Alex has not told anyone about the experience because he thought he would be viewed as a coward. Alex shares that he would rather avoid going to school than face potential bullying.

The physician needs to assure Alex that it is not his fault that he is a victim of bullying. Prevention should include interventions at the individual, family, and school level. Alex should walk away from the conflict when possible and not feel uncomfortable about reporting the event to school staff. He may want to find a friend to walk to school with. His family needs to understand that bullying is not just a normal kid behavior. He should be encouraged to talk about bullying events and jointly identify solutions. The school should be notified about the event and encouraged to promote a non-bullying school environment.

Selected References

Anderson M, Kaufman J, Simon TR, et al. School-associated violent deaths in the United States: 1994–1999. *JAMA.* 2001;286:2695–2702

Borowsky IW, Mozayeny S, Stuenkel K, Ireland M. Effects of a primary care-based intervention on violent behavior and injury in children. *Pediatrics.* 2004;114:e392–e399

Copelan R. Assessing the potential for violent behavior in children and adolescents. *Pediatr Rev.* 2006;27:e36–e41

Fekkes M, Pijpers FIM, Fredriks AM, Vogels T, Verloove-Vanhorick SP. Do bullied children get ill, or do ill children get bullied? A prospective cohort study on the relationship between bullying and health-related symptoms. *Pediatrics.* 2006;117:1568–1574

Lyznicki J, McCaferee MA, Robinowitz CB. Childhood bullying: implications for physicians. *Am Fam Physician.* 2004;70:1723–1728

Nansel T, Overpeck, M, Haynie DL, Ruan WJ, Scheidt PC. Relationships between bullying and violence among US youth. *Arch Pediatr Adolesc Med.* 2003;157:348–353

Olweus D. *Bullying at School: What We Know and What We Can Do.* Cambridge, MA: Blackwell; 1993

Resnick MD, Ireland M, Borowsky I. Youth violence perpetration: what protects? What predicts? Findings from the National Longitudinal Study of Adolescent Health. *J Adolesc Health.* 2004;35:424.e1–e10

Sourander A, Jensen P, Rönning JA, et al. Childhood bullies and victims and their risk of criminality in late adolescence: the Finnish From a Boy to a Man Study. *Arch Pediatr Adolesc Med.* 2007;161:546–552

Disaster Preparedness

Elizabeth A. Edgerton, MD, MPH

CASE STUDY

A family comes in for their children's well-child visit with their 9-month-old daughter who has complex congenital heart disease and their 7-year-old son. The mother is concerned after a recent tornado in the next town resulted in prolonged power outages and what the family might do in this situation. Their daughter needs daily breathing treatments and often requires oxygen at nighttime. She is on multiple medications and a special formula. All of her specialty doctors are at the children's hospital, which is more than an hour from their house. She is also concerned because her husband has a seizure disorder that requires medication. She asks whether the family should stay together in a disaster or separate to get her daughter to the children's hospital.

Questions

1. How should families prepare for disasters, particularly natural ones known to occur in their area?
2. What should be included in disaster preparedness kits? How should medications for all family members be included?
3. When should families consider getting a generator?
4. How can families notify the utility company that they need to be flagged for priority return of service during a power outage?
5. What is the role of the local hospital and emergency medical services provider when families have children with special health care and critical medical needs?
6. What should the pediatrician recommend to families about children's immunization records and important medical history?
7. How do you assess for the impact of traumatic events on children and their families?

Disaster preparedness is not a new concept in our society. We have always had natural disasters such as earthquakes and hurricanes. The potential of war or pandemic infections has been present for decades. In the past these threats were managed by the state and federal programs. With increasing population density, global warming, international trade, and terrorist threats, our view of disaster preparedness is broadening to include natural disaster; chemical, biological, and radioactive exposure; and emerging pandemic infections. Recent major disasters, including man-made events such as terrorist attacks in New York City and natural events such as hurricane Katrina, demonstrate the vulnerability of a community and the need for extensive local preparation for potential disasters. In both of these disasters, the community response in the first hours to days was vital to the well-being of others. While the state and federal systems are a vital component of disaster preparedness, communities may play a greater role than in the past.

Children are more vulnerable than adults during a disaster. Studies from refugee camps have found that children younger than 5 years had a higher mortality rate than the crude mortality rate of adults during the emergency situation. Children are reliant on others for food, shelter and, importantly, for psychological support. Their immune systems are often less mature; this puts them at greater risk of infection. Their unique nutritional needs put them at risk for malnutrition. Developmentally, they are at risk for acute and long-term psychological trauma from a disaster. The impact of being separated from their families can be devastating. Furthermore, children are at increased risk for exposure from chemical, biological, and radiation disasters due to their unique physiology. Infants and children have higher minute ventilation, resulting in increased inhalation of aerosolized agents. Their smaller height increases their exposure to high-vapor density agents, which are in higher concentrations closer to the ground. Infants' and children's skin is more permeable due to less keratinization; they also have a larger surface area to body mass ratio. As a result, exposed children receive a higher dose of transdermally absorbed toxins than adults exposed under identical circumstances.

A public health emergency occurs when the event exceeds the ability of community resources to provide routine care. This can be a result of any type of disaster. Preparedness experts suggest looking at public health emergencies from what is called an **all-hazards approach.** This approach focuses on the key elements that are needed to ensure that routine care can still be provided during a disaster. Specific case scenarios that occur rarely, such as chemical or radiation exposure, will require access to specialized resources that may be impractical to stockpile or are limited in availability. From a practical view, it is more effective to have the essential resources that are needed across all types of disasters. The primary care pediatrician plays a vital role in disaster preparedness on the local, regional, and national level, not only as a medical service provider but also as an advocate to the special needs of children.

Pediatrician's Role With Families

Pediatricians serve as a resource to families in preparation for disasters. Disaster preparedness can be incorporated into the primary care pediatrician's anticipatory guidance with families. Pediatricians may need to assess a family's level of readiness for a disaster and then tailor their anticipatory guidance accordingly. It is important for families to realize that everyone is susceptible to some type of disaster whether natural, chemical, biological, or radiation. Pediatricians need to ensure families understand the importance of preparation as well as the special needs of children during a disaster. Families should prepare an emergency kit that provides up to 3 days of basic essentials, including food, water, and clothing. Families need to include formula and diapers for infants and any daily medications for all family members. Copies of immunization and general medical information can be useful as well as pictures of family members in case the family unit is separated. Parents need to be prepared to handle non-emergent problems because medical care may be limited to the seriously ill and injured. If a family needs acute medical care, children may have to be treated in adult facilities; alternatively, for the family unit to remain together, adults within the family may need to be treated in pediatric facilities. The more information families can provide about any medical conditions requiring attention, the easier it will be to receive appropriate care in a disaster.

Families of children with special needs are especially vulnerable following a disaster because access to routine medical care may not be available. Common supplies such as a feeding tube may be in short supply or unavailable during a disaster. Families should not only have a sufficient supply of medication, but a surplus of medical equipment and nutritional supplements if necessary. Families with a child on a ventilator or who is oxygen dependent should notify the local utilities to flag their address for priority status during power outages. These families would also benefit by notifying their local emergency medical services (EMS) and local hospital of their child's medical needs. The American Academy of Pediatrics (AAP) has **emergency information forms** that can be completed with the pediatrician and should be part of the emergency preparedness kit. Families can also contact the National Organization on Disability and Emergency Preparedness (www.nod.org) or Family Voices (www.familyvoices.org) for more detailed information regarding preparing for a disaster with a special needs child. Some communities have developed systems where posters are disseminated that are to be placed in the window specifying if any occupant may require special services from EMS should a disaster or terrorist attack occur.

After a disaster, children and adolescents may have chronic problems depending on the type of disaster. Such problems need to be addressed case by case. What is universal among all types of disasters is that there is a psychological impact on children. Multiple studies of various types of disasters demonstrate the increase in mental health symptoms among children and adolescents exposed to a disaster. This is true even if a family is not directly impacted by the disaster but is exposed to the event within the community, on the television, or via the Internet. Children may present with somatic complaints such as headaches and stomachaches, or may not want to participate in their normal activities. Long-term effects include depression, anxiety, aggression, and substance abuse. Age-appropriate discussions should be encouraged along with validation of the child's concerns while ensuring their individual safety. Post-traumatic stress disorder should be considered in patients with persistent symptoms that are not responding to family support. Families and health care providers can obtain further information through the AAP (www.aap.org) and the Substance Abuse and Mental Health Services Administration (www.samhsa.gov).

Pediatrician's Role in the Community

Pediatricians can participate in both the disaster preparedness planning as well as community surveillance to identify potential disasters. Many state and regional disaster preparedness plans are tailored for an adult population and may not consider the special needs of children. From an operational standpoint, it is more effective to have one plan that can take into consideration the needs of multiple vulnerable populations rather than have separate disaster preparedness plans for each population. Pediatricians can serve as consultants about local preparation, providing guidance about children's medical, nutritional, and psychological needs. For example, more staffing is required when caring for younger children, especially infants. Infants require formula and a sterile water supply, and young children require frequent meals. Ideally, children need to be with their caregiver, but if this is not possible then a child advocate needs to be with the child at all times. Children may not respond well to new environments and disaster protocols. The simple process of decontamination can be devastating to a young child without a parent. A child may have concerns about being sprayed with water or refuse to disrobe in front of strangers. This may impact the success of decontamination for children and adolescents. While adults may have similar issues, it is presumed they will comply with protocols; however, such compliance is less predictable in a pediatric population. Other issues may need to be addressed, such as providing for increased staffing in adult facilities caring for children, as well as the need for those facilities to stockpile pediatric supplies. Facilities also need to plan for children arriving without a caregiver and the need to establish an identification system allowing children to be reunited with their families. This was a significant problem for children displaced during hurricane Katrina. Refugee camps often use digital cameras to photograph children on arrival as a way to reunite families. Recommendations include photographing children in their original clothing.

Triage systems need to take into account physiological differences of children as well as their psychological response to strangers. They may not be able to communicate their complaint, and because their vital signs are normally different from those of adults, medical personnel accustomed to working with adults may misinterpret their findings, resulting in children being over-triaged (judged to be sicker than they are). Stockpiling of medications for biological, chemical, or radiation disasters needs to take into consideration dosing differences in children compared with adults. Suspensions of medications will need to be available in addition to pill forms. Furthermore, many of the recommended antidotes and treatments are not approved for use in the pediatric population. Policies regarding the risks and benefits of their use in disasters should be established.

Pediatricians can also assist schools in developing disaster preparedness plans should a disaster occur during the school day.

Pediatrician's Role in Disaster Surveillance and Management

Pediatricians function as key public health workers. Their knowledge and diligence aids in local and regional surveillance for potential chemical, biological, and radiation disasters. Families are more likely to seek care from their pediatrician than an emergency department for early symptoms during and after a disaster. Although it is beyond the scope of this chapter to provide details about signs and symptoms following every type of disaster, the following section highlights important concepts in identifying and treating patients with exposures to chemical and biological agents and radiation.

Chemical exposures usually result in immediate symptoms and require special protection for emergency personnel as well as decontamination for the victims. Nerve agents, the most toxic of chemical agents, inhibit the enzyme acetylcholinesterase, resulting in accumulation of acetylcholine and excessive cholinergic stimulation in smooth muscles, exocrine glands, skeletal muscle, and preganglionic fibers. Symptoms include increased salivation, lacrimation, urination, gastric distress, and emesis, referred to as the **SLUDGE toxidrome.** Vesicant exposure leads to irreversible damage to mucous membranes, skin, and the respiratory system that occurs within minutes of exposure, often without any antecedent symptoms. Agents include mustard and lewisite. Cyanide is another common chemical agent, known for its "bitter almond" taste. Agents other than nerve agents usually do not result in severe mortality but rather incapacitate the victim.

Biological agents include bacteria, viruses, and preformed toxins. These agents are easy to disperse and, thus, can affect large populations. Unlike chemical exposures, the onset of symptoms is delayed by hours to days, and symptoms are more difficult to distinguish from common ailments. Secondary transmission of the infection is also of concern. Management of biological disaster requires detailed surveillance and containment of exposed populations.

Although there are far too many biological agents to discuss in any detail in a brief chapter, a few of particular relevance for disaster planning are mentioned here. **Anthrax,** from *Bacillus anthracis,* is a Gram-positive sporulating rod, which presents with severe influenza-like symptoms with a high case fatality rate. Fever and dyspnea associated with a widened mediastinum are common and may progress to shock. Ciprofloxacin and doxycycline are recommended for prophylaxis and treatment among adults, but ciprofloxacin is not approved by the US Food and Drug Administration (FDA) for children younger than 18 years and doxycycline is contraindicated in children younger than 8 years. Clinicians need to consider consulting with experts to assist in assessing the risks and benefits associated with using these medications. Among the viruses, variola, more commonly known as **small pox,** is of concern. After its global eradication in 1980, children were no longer immunized, leaving all children and most adults susceptible to the virus. Similar to varicella, it presents with vesicles with umbilicated centers but is associated with a higher mortality rate of 3% to 30% among non-immunized individuals. Exposure to **botulinum toxin,** one of the most potent toxins, results in cranial nerve disturbances, descending paralysis, and respiratory distress. **Ricin,** derived from the castor bean, is another potent toxin. Inhalation results in fever, cough, and pulmonary edema, often resulting in death within days. Ingestion presents with severe vomiting and diarrhea, resulting in hypovolemic shock. There is no antidote or treatment for these biological toxins. For a complete list of biological agents, presenting symptoms, and potential treatment and/or prophylaxis, clinicians should consult the Centers for Disease Control and Prevention (www.cdc.gov).

Radiation exposure may occur as a result of damage to a facility that contains nuclear material, detonation of a nuclear weapon, or dispersal of nuclear material by a radioactive dispersal device. Ionizing radiation, high-frequency energy, presents the greatest health risk. It causes chromosomal breaks in cells that can persist for years. There are 5 types of ionizing radiation that have specific characteristics, behaviors, and toxicities: alpha particles, beta particles, gamma rays, x-rays, and neutrons. Alpha particles have limited ability to penetrate, but when inhaled or ingested can cause damage to epithelial tissues. Beta particles usually are used in a medical setting or are a by-product of nuclear reactors, have greater penetration, and can cause skin damage as well as internal damage. Gamma rays and x-rays are part of the electromagnetic spectrum. Gamma rays are high-energy and cause significant damage. This type of radiation would be seen after a nuclear detonation or from radioactive materials. Much less common are neutrons, which can produce 10-fold more damage than gamma rays. Furthermore, exposure is classified as external, internal, whole body, and partial body. The effects of radiation can be directly on target tissue, or indirectly due to free radicals created by the radiation. Tissue sensitivity is based on the cell's rate of division and level of differentiation. The most sensitive to least is as follows: lymphoid>gastrointestinal>reproductive>dermal>bone marrow>nervous system. The severity of exposure is also dependent on the dose of radiation, type of radiation, and age of victim.

Radiation exposure is quantified by the amount of energy absorbed (the *rad,* for radiation absorbed dose) and the relative biological effectiveness of doses (RBE) based on the type of ionizing radiation. The *rem* is the product of the rad and RBE. Under the International System of Units, the rad and rem are being replaced by the gray (1 Gy = 100 rad) and sievert (1 Sv = 100 rem). Radiation exposure from common radiographic procedures can range from 0.00005 to 0.0001 Sv (5–10 mrem) for a chest x-rays and 0.05 Sv (5,000 mrem) for a computed tomography scan.

The symptoms associated with radiation exposure depend on the total exposure. Nausea and vomiting can present with exposures of 0.75 to 1.0 Gy, and lymphoid and bone marrow suppression with exposures of 3.0 to 6.0 Gy. The mean lethal dose, the radiation dose for which half of the population is expected to die within 60 days, is 4.0 Gy. Long-term effects of radiation include increased incidence of cancer and psychological distress. Evacuation is the ideal intervention to decrease exposure, but may not be feasible in highly populated areas. Seeking shelter can greatly decrease the level of exposure, with large cement structures providing the best protection. The use of potassium iodide is effective in exposures to radioactive iodine, which is associated with nuclear power facilities. It can be dispensed in a pill form, and home suspensions can be made for pediatric patients. Dosage is based on level of radiation exposure and the age of the patient. Clinicians should consult the FDA (www.fda.gov) or the Nuclear Regulatory Commission to determine the appropriate dosage of potassium iodide depending on the level of radiation exposure. For individuals seeking medical care, containment and decontamination are essential. Removal of clothing and washing the skin with warm water is very effective. Supportive medical care is essential in managing patients with radiation exposure. Radiation results in significant immune suppression, neutropenia, and lymphopenia, which last for weeks. Clinicians should be aggressive in managing infections and consider treatments to increase bone marrow regeneration.

In addition to caring for patients, the pediatrician needs to take into consideration the well-being of his or her family as well as that of the office staff. During a disaster, office staff may not be able to come to work. For those able to report to work, extra supplies of food and water need to be available in case they are not able to return to their homes. An office disaster plan should be implemented with emergency contacts and preparation for the staff's basic needs. Basic medical supplies should be available to care for patients during a disaster. Depending on the type and severity of the disaster, access to the office facility may be prohibited. Plans for backup of patient medical records should be implemented as well as alternative sites in which medical services can be delivered.

Clinicians need to review their medical liability policies regarding providing care in a disaster situation. Most policies only provide coverage of care that is provided in the office setting. Good Samaritan laws vary in each state regarding what level of protection is provided to the health care worker. The AAP recommends that during a disaster situation, pediatricians who volunteer do so under the auspices of an official disaster agency or recognized relief organization to ensure the greatest protection from liability.

Conclusion

Pediatricians have a vital role in pre-disaster, disaster, and post-disaster management. The essential components of disaster management are to provide for all basic human requirements, reduce an individual's vulnerability to disasters and, once a disaster has occurred, reduce the exposure risk. Pediatricians can educate and

assist families in preparing for disasters. In addition, they can guide communities in their disaster preparedness planning to address and plan to accommodate the particular vulnerabilities of children. As with other health care providers, pediatricians also can contribute to the essential medical and public health workforce during a disaster. Pediatricians can access the most current guidelines and recommendations through multiple professional and governmental resources. It is imperative for the practitioner to have easy access to phone numbers and Web sites specific to pediatric disaster preparedness and response for the relevant local, state, and federal agencies.

CASE RESOLUTION

The family is relieved to discuss the importance of preparing for a disaster. They now have an idea of what is involved in disaster preparation (emergency kit with food, water, and medication) and feel less vulnerable. They will complete an emergency medical information form for the kit and call their local utility company to identify their house as a priority during a power failure. The mother shares with the pediatrician that her son has been sleeping less since the tornado and does not want to go to school because he is afraid of being away from the family. The pediatrician encourages the family to discuss his fears while ensuring his safety. Having the son participate in making the emergency kit and creating a family plan may help. A follow-up visit is scheduled to reassess his symptoms and decide if a further intervention is needed.

Selected References

Agency for Healthcare Research and Quality. *Pediatric Terrorism and Disaster Preparedness: A Resource for Pediatricians.* www.ahrq.gov/research/pedprep/pedresource.pdf. Accessed May 21, 2007

American Academy of Pediatrics Committee on Environmental Health. Radiation disasters and children. *Pediatrics.* 2003;111:1455–1466

American Academy of Pediatrics Committee on Pediatric Emergency Medicine, Committee on Medical Liability. Pediatrician's liability during a disaster. *Pediatrics.* 2000;106:1492–1493

Auf der Heide E. The importance of evidence-based disaster planning. *Ann Emerg Med.* 2006;47:34–49

Family Voices. Emergencies and Disasters: Keeping Children and Youth with Special Health Care Needs Safe. www.familyvoices.org/info/emergencies.php. Accessed May 21, 2007

Hagan JF, American Academy of Pediatrics Committee on Psychosocial Aspects of Child and Family Health and Task Force on Terrorism. Psychosocial implications of disaster or terrorism on children: a guide for the pediatrician. *Pediatrics.* 2005;116:787–795

Melter FA, Voelz GL. Major radiation exposure—what to expect and how to respond. *N Engl J Med.* 2002;346:1554–1561

Adolescent Depression and Suicide

Monica Sifuentes, MD

CASE STUDY

A 15-year-old girl is brought to your office by her mother with the chief complaint of easy fatigability. The mother is concerned because her daughter is always tired, although several other physicians have told her that the girl is healthy. The adolescent, who states no complaints or concerns, appears very shy. She is currently in the 10th grade, likes school, receives average grades, and speaks both English and Spanish. The mother, a single parent, moved to the United States from El Salvador approximately 2 years ago with her 2 daughters. They are currently living with relatives in a 2-bedroom apartment. The mother is employed as a housekeeper, and the patient and her sister help their mother clean homes on weekends. During the week they make dinner for the rest of the family as a means of contributing to the rent. When you speak to the girl alone, she acknowledges she has a few friends at school and adamantly denies any drug, alcohol, or tobacco use. She has never been sexually active and reports no history of sexual or physical abuse. The girl's physical examination is entirely normal, although her affect appears somewhat flat.

Questions

1. What is the significance of nonspecific symptoms, such as fatigue, during adolescence?
2. What factors contribute to depression in adolescents?
3. What are the classic signs and symptoms of depression in adolescents?
4. What are some important historical points to cover when interviewing adolescents with suspected depression?
5. How is the risk of suicide assessed in adolescent patients?
6. How should suicidal behavior (ie, suicide attempts) be managed in adolescents?

Depression has been identified as one of the multiple risk factors that predispose adolescents to suicide. However, not all teenagers who try to take their own life are depressed and, conversely, not all depressed adolescents attempt suicide. This distinction is important to keep in mind when evaluating adolescents for either depression or suicidal behavior. Early identification of risk factors in the susceptible adolescent along with early intervention for those with depressive symptoms will hopefully benefit the teenager at risk for suicide and allow the primary care pediatrician to provide the first line of intervention for their adolescent patient experiencing emotional distress.

Epidemiology

Depression

The exact prevalence of depression in adolescents is difficult to determine because depression is both an illness and a symptom. Depressive symptoms have been reported in as many as 50% of girls and 40% of boys in the 14- to 15-year age group. The overall prevalence of depression as an illness is approximately 5%; mild depression is reported in 13% to 28% of teens, moderate depression in 7%,

and severe depression in 1.3%. Depression occurs more commonly in adolescents than in prepubertal children and is more frequent in females than males after puberty.

Several risk factors contribute to the development of depressive disorders in adolescents (Box 126-1). Certain psychiatric conditions also are associated with depression, including anxiety disorders, eating disorders, substance abuse, conduct disorders, and borderline personality disorders.

Suicide and Suicidal Behavior

Suicide is the third-leading cause of death in the United States in individuals 10 to 24 years of age; only motor vehicle crashes and homicides result in more deaths in young people. In 1960 the annual suicide rate in this age group was 5.2 per 100,000, and by 1990 it had more than doubled to 13.2 per 100,000. In particular, the 1990 suicide rate for 15- to 19-year-old adolescents was 11.1 per 100,000, triple that of 1960. It has been stated that for every suicide that is completed successfully, 50 to 100 suicides are attempted.

According to the 2006 Youth Risk Survey of the Centers for Disease Control and Prevention, 16.9% of all students in grades 9 to

12 nationwide had seriously considered attempting suicide during the previous 12 months. Approximately 13% of these students had made specific suicide plans, more than 50% of students with suicide plans reported attempting to take their lives, and 2.3% of the individuals who attempted suicide required medical attention. Overall, female students were much more likely than male students to have considered attempting suicide (22% vs 12%). Rates also differ by race and ethnicity, with African American teenagers having lower suicide rates than white youth, and African American females having the lowest suicide rate of all adolescents. American Indian/Alaska Native males have the highest suicide rate among this age group.

Several risk factors associated with adolescent suicide have been identified (Box 126-2). Although adolescent females are more likely to attempt suicide than males, males are more likely to succeed (ratio of 4:1 boys to girls). This fact may result from the lethality of the methods, such as firearms or hanging, that males usually choose. While females are more likely to ingest pills, the role of firearms is increasing. The availability of firearms and alcohol, which varies from state to state, greatly contributes to the occurrence of suicide. Up to 45% of individuals who have committed suicide show some evidence of intoxication at the time of death. Although most suicide attempts are impulsive, studies have shown that adolescents often have communicated their suicidal intent or ideation to someone before the attempt. Fifty percent of adolescents who attempt suicide have sought medical care within the preceding month and 25% within the preceding week. In contrast, only one-third have received previous mental health care.

Clinical Presentation

Depressed or suicidal adolescents may visit physicians for a variety of clinical reasons, but rarely do they seek professional assistance for feeling "depressed." They may present with seemingly non-emergent complaints and a flat affect or with multiple somatic concerns and an anxious appearance. Additionally, the teen may have frequent visits to the primary care practitioner's office for acute conditions that on first glance seem unrelated but later indicate possible substance abuse or a mood disorder. Some adolescents are accompanied by a

family member or friend, which initially may make the teen reticent to discuss psychosocial issues with the provider. Occasionally the teenager is referred by school officials for educational problems such as truancy, delinquency, or school failure.

Pathophysiology

Like other complex psychiatric conditions, the etiology of depression seems to be multifactorial, with a strong genetic and psychosocial/environmental basis. The **genetic basis** of depression is supported by statistics that indicate that 25% of children who take their own lives have a family member or close relative that has committed suicide. Similarly, a family history of major depression is a significant risk factor for the development of depression in children. Studies suggest the incomplete penetrance of a dominant gene as a possible etiology for this finding. Regardless of the exact mechanism, genetic influences establish the adolescent's vulnerability for depression. Specific **environmental events** or familial stresses can occur in an adolescent's life that may precipitate a depressive episode, such as the loss of a loved one or parental divorce. Other events such as physical or sexual abuse also can trigger depression in a susceptible teen. Although the "final common pathway" to depression can be quite variable, affected youth respond in one of several ways: irritability, diminished interest or pleasure in activities or relationships, changes in cognitive functioning, or impairments in multiple areas of daily living. Major depressive disorder (MDD) is diagnosed when the symptoms last for at least 2 weeks and there is a change in usual function. Changes can be manifested by poor academic performance, school attendance issues (including truancy and disruptive behaviors), and difficulties with peer and familial relationships (see Box 126-1).

Differential Diagnosis

The differential diagnosis of depression includes any condition that may affect the patient's nutritional status and lead to malnourishment (Dx Box). Examples include cancer, tuberculosis, and eating disorders such as anorexia nervosa. In addition, endocrine disorders such as hypothyroidism, hyperthyroidism, and Addison disease can mimic depression. Central nervous system (CNS) pathology, although rare, includes tumors, infections, postconcussive syndromes, and cerebrovascular accidents. Concomitant systemic illnesses such as systemic lupus erythematosus, diabetes mellitus, and acquired immunodeficiency syndrome can have CNS manifestations that may be mistaken for an isolated episode of depression. Illicit substance abuse and alcoholism also should be investigated as a possible source for the depressive symptoms because many teenagers may self-medicate to cope with an underlying comorbid disorder. Comorbid conditions such as early-onset bipolar disorder can present initially with depressive symptoms. In fact, 20% to 40% of children that have MDD eventually develop bipolar disorder. Other psychiatric diagnoses to consider include adjustment disorders, uncomplicated bereavement, separation anxiety, and dysthymia, which is more chronic and less severe than major depression. Lastly, side effects of both prescribed and over-the-counter medications may produce clinical symptoms consistent with depression and therefore should be excluded in the differential diagnosis.

Dx Adolescent Depression

- Depressed or irritable mood
- Decreased interest in most daily activities, including school
- Significant weight changes
- Sleep problems
- Psychomotor agitation or retardation
- Low energy or fatigue
- Feelings of worthlessness or guilt
- Diminished ability to concentrate or think
- Preoccupation with death or suicide

Evaluation

History

The assessment of an adolescent for depressive symptoms is an important part of any routine encounter, but the diagnosis of depression may be difficult to make after just one interview. At the initial visit, a complete psychosocial or **HEADDSSS** assessment (home, employment and education, activities, diet, drugs, sexual activity/sexuality, suicide and depression, safety) should be performed on all adolescents (see Chapter 5). The parent or guardian should be included during the first part of the interview to review their observations and concerns regarding their adolescent's behavior and mood. The teenager then should be interviewed alone, and a thorough history of recent feelings, behaviors, and attitudes should be obtained (Questions Box: Adolescent Depression). Mood changes should be noted; a labile affect can be a symptom of ongoing depression. Physicians should keep in mind that patients who are malnourished for any reason can have a depressed or seemingly flat affect. A full psychiatric assessment also should be completed to obtain information about a possible comorbid condition. This includes features of psychosis, anxiety disorders, disruptive behaviors, and mania. Information about a family history of psychiatric illness or substance abuse, including alcoholism, also should be reviewed with both the teenager as well as the parent/guardian.

Questions: Adolescent Depression

- Does the adolescent occasionally feel sad or "blue" and not understand why?
- Does the adolescent have unexplained crying spells?
- Does the adolescent feel "mad," "bored," or "grouchy"?
- Does the adolescent seem inappropriately jovial?
- Have there been any recent losses in the adolescent's life that may explain his or her feelings?
- Is the adolescent having trouble with concentration or memory?
- Does the adolescent have trouble falling asleep at night or have early morning awakening?
- Has the adolescent lost weight recently or shown any disinterest in food?
- Does the adolescent have feelings of hopelessness and have any desire to hurt himself or herself? Has the adolescent made any previous suicide attempts?
- Do the parents or siblings have a history of drug or alcohol use?
- Is there a family history of affective disorders? What has been their response to treatment?
- Is there a history of family violence?

To identify youth at risk for suicide, practitioners must inquire about specific areas of adolescents' lives including a history of sexual/physical abuse, violence, or neglect and current interpersonal conflicts. Feelings of hopelessness, agitation, and impulsivity should be identified, along with frequent thoughts of suicide. It has been reported that having frequent thoughts of suicide is the best predictor of suicide attempts. Adolescents who are suspected of being at risk for suicide must be questioned directly about suicidal ideation, specifically whether they have a plan in mind and access to firearms, medications, or other means of suicide. Previous suicide attempts also need to be reviewed with the teenager because 35% to 45% of adolescents that complete suicide have a positive history of a previous attempt. Nonlethal suicide gestures or other methods of self-inflicted harm should never be taken lightly or minimized. As is recommended in other arenas, initial questions should be non-specific and become more specific as the interview proceeds, especially if answers to the previous questions are positive (Questions Box: Adolescent Suicide).

Questions

Adolescent Suicide

- Is the adolescent on any prescribed medications (eg, phenobarbital)?
- Is the adolescent experiencing any psychiatric difficulties, social maladjustments, or family or environmental challenges (eg, recent parental divorce, school expulsion)?
- Does the adolescent have a history of symptoms of depression, conduct problems, or psychosis?
- How is the adolescent progressing in school?
- Does the adolescent have a history of substance abuse?
- Does the adolescent have any legal problems?
- Does the adolescent suffer any social isolation or have interpersonal conflicts with family or friends?
- Has the adolescent suffered any personal losses recently?
- Has there recently been a suicide in the school or community?
- Are there any family problems such as abuse or neglect?
- Has the adolescent ever thought that life was not worth living?
- Does the adolescent ever feel hopeless?
- Has the adolescent ever thought of hurting himself or herself?
- Does the adolescent have a previous history of suicide attempts?
- Does the adolescent presently have a plan for suicide?
- Does the adolescent have access to firearms, medications, or other means of suicide?

Promises to maintain confidentiality with depressed adolescents who are considered at risk for suicide are discouraged because parental involvement is strongly advised. Precipitating and motivating factors for any previous suicide attempts should be determined prior to the development of a treatment plan. More importantly, the lethality of previous attempts must be evaluated.

Physical Examination

A thorough physical examination and a review of systems should be completed to rule out a chronic medical condition or an organic etiology for nonspecific complaints. If patients have a history of sexual abuse, assault, or sexual activity, a genital examination should be performed to evaluate for sexually transmitted infections. In most cases, the physical examination may be of little yield in the adolescent with a true affective disorder. However, a careful detailed neurologic examination, including a mental status examination, is essential to perform and document as normal.

Laboratory Tests

No routine laboratory studies are recommended, although some authors advocate screening tests to rule out organic etiologies for depression and to serve as baseline parameters if pharmacotherapy

is indicated. A complete blood count with differential, glucose, electrolytes, blood urea nitrogen, creatinine, liver function tests (LFTs), and thyroid function tests may be considered. Psychometric testing may help rule out a concomitant learning disability or attention-deficit/hyperactivity disorder (ADHD). Although tricyclic antidepressants (TCAs) are no longer considered first-line therapy in the adolescent who is depressed, a baseline electrocardiogram (ECG) should be performed to rule out conduction defects if a TCA is prescribed for the adolescent with a comorbid disorder of ADHD. The ECG should be repeated as the TCA dose is increased. In addition, LFTs should be obtained and followed while on this particular therapy. Screening for substance abuse should be considered if significant use is suspected.

Imaging Studies

Radiographic imaging, such as computed tomography of the head or magnetic resonance imaging of the brain, generally is not indicated in the evaluation of depression if organic etiologies have been excluded.

Management

Depression

If depressive symptoms are associated with an adjustment disorder and if family, peers, or school factors are impacted, **supportive counseling** is indicated. The duration and depth of counseling depends, in part, on how comfortable the primary care practitioner feels performing this task and how receptive the youth and his or her family are to this intervention. Identification of the specific problem, exploration of the teen's response to the problem, and development of a reasonable solution with the adolescent and the parents may be helpful to improve adherence to psychotherapy. **Psychological referral** should be initiated if patients require more prolonged treatment, the degree of depression seems to worsen, suicidality becomes an issue and additional mental health consultation is needed, or a comorbid condition is suspected.

If family difficulties or dysfunction is the major issue, family members and the physician or counselor should meet to assess the magnitude of the problem and the motivation required to address it. Physicians should use this opportunity to educate both adolescents and families about the signs and symptoms of depression and the undeniable impact that depression has on school functioning, family and peer relationships, and social interactions. The need for individual cognitive-behavioral therapy as well as family therapy should be discussed as well as the effectiveness of psychiatric medication in the appropriate setting. Attention to parental mental health and to understanding the strategies necessary to manage the adolescent's irritability and isolation also are extremely important.

Immediate **psychiatric consultation and referral** are indicated if adolescents have severe depressive features that interfere with daily functioning or if they are suicidal, homicidal, or psychotic. Ensuring the adolescent's safety is the priority. A mental health referral is also appropriate if supportive counseling by the primary care physician has been ineffective or when the depression is recurrent or chronic. In some cases, the primary care provider may believe that the adolescent requires pharmacologic therapy but has little experience in prescribing psychotropic medications.

Psychiatric intervention generally includes **pharmacotherapy** (eg, selective serotonin reuptake inhibitors [SSRIs]) in conjunction with psychotherapy because most cases of depression include psychological, social, and environmental components. Although much attention has been given to safety concerns regarding the use of antidepressant medications among children and adolescents, SSRIs are considered first-line medications for the treatment of depression in teenagers (see Chapter 114). Two of them, fluoxetine (Prozac) and paroxetine (Paxil), have been well studied in double-blind, randomized, placebo-controlled trials to reduce depressive symptoms in this age group and are generally well tolerated with minimal or no side effects. The side effects tend to be dose related, and most subside with time (1–2 weeks) or with a decrease in dosage. Common adverse effects include headache, abdominal pain, diarrhea, sleep changes, and jitteriness or agitation. Serious behavioral symptoms, such as aggression, hostility, and impulsivity, must be reviewed with a psychiatrist.

The "black box" warning to antidepressant medications was added by the US Food and Drug Administration in 2004 stating that children and adolescents treated with these drugs are more likely to become suicidal. This caution should be put in context with the risks of untreated depression and discussed openly with the parent or guardian and the adolescent. Prior to starting the medication, informed consent must be obtained from the parent or guardian as well as assent from the teenager. Patients should be observed closely for worsening of symptoms, suicidality, or unusual changes in behavior. Families should be educated regarding the importance of close follow-up and immediate, open communication with the provider if these symptoms should occur. Initially, the adolescent should be seen weekly during the first 4 weeks of therapy, with a gradual increase in the interval between visits. An adequate trial of SSRIs is reported to be at least 4 to 6 weeks. Frequent medication adjustments are not advised, and tapering of paroxetine prior to discontinuation is recommended because withdrawal effects include agitation and increased depression.

Tricyclic antidepressants should be avoided in the treatment of depression in adolescents because studies have failed to show their effectiveness more than placebo, and they are associated with potentially life-threatening side effects, especially if intentionally ingested in a greater than recommended dose.

Suicide and Suicidal Behavior

Adolescents who are considered at risk for suicide must be asked directly at every visit if they are, in fact, suicidal and if they have a plan (Questions Box: Adolescent Suicide). Response to this inquiry determines whether adolescents will be treated on an inpatient or outpatient basis. In most cases, the adolescent with no previous suicide attempts, ambivalence regarding suicidal thoughts, no real intent to die, and a good family support system may be managed as an **outpatient.** In patients who deny current suicidal ideation, a written or verbal "no suicide" contract can be made between the physician or psychologist and the adolescent, although research does not support the conclusion that such contracts actively prevent suicide. The patient is asked to agree to contact the clinician, parent, or another responsible adult if he or she feels a suicidal urge or experiences suicidal intent. The precipitants for possible suicidality must be reviewed, and alternative methods for coping should be rehearsed with the teenager. In addition, all potential means of suicide, particularly firearms and toxic medications, must be removed from the home or place of residence. It is not enough to "secure" firearms; they must be removed. Referral to a therapist is recommended as soon as possible. Preferably, this should be arranged while adolescents are in the office, and they should be given a definite time and date for the appointment. Ideally, the therapist should meet with the family before the first appointment with the adolescent alone. Detoxification from drugs or alcohol, if necessary, also should be addressed.

Because all suicidal threats, gestures, or ideations by adolescents must be taken seriously, emergent psychiatric referral is required for most of these individuals. Adolescents judged to be at serious risk for suicide should be managed as **inpatients** and admitted to a pediatric or adolescent unit for 24 to 48 hours of observation. The purpose of this brief hospitalization is 3-fold: (1) to stabilize patients medically, if necessary; (2) to observe and evaluate patient-family dynamics; and (3) to impress on patients and families that the attempt has been recognized and taken seriously. Intervention requires the involvement of mental health professionals in addition to social services. Transfer to an inpatient psychiatric treatment center is indicated for those adolescents who are judged by mental health consultants to have serious suicidal intentions or an underlying psychiatric illness.

Prognosis

The risk of recurrence of major depression in adolescents who have recovered is substantial. One study reports that 5% of patients relapse within 6 months of recovery, 12% within 1 year, and an estimated 33% within 4 years. Higher rates of recurrence have been reported, however, with approximately 70% of teens with MDD experiencing another depressive episode within 5 years. In addition, youth who have a depressive disorder have a 4-fold risk of the same disorder as an adult. Prepubertal-onset depression is associated with an approximately 30% risk of developing future bipolar disorder or mania.

The risk of repeated suicidal behavior seems to be greatest within the first 3 months following the initial attempt. Reported reattempt rates are 6% to 15% in the first 1 to 3 years following the initial attempt.

CASE RESOLUTION

In the case history presented at the beginning of this chapter, the girl's symptoms may be indicative of depression because she has a flat affect and seems to be somewhat isolated (insufficient time for friends and just recently moved to the United States). She seems to be at low risk for suicide, however. The physician should nonetheless inquire about symptoms of depression and ask her directly about suicidality, and then make arrangements to follow the girl's condition closely. If depression is confirmed at future visits or if she becomes suicidal, both she and her family should be referred to a mental health professional for immediate consultation and intervention.

Selected References

Adler RS, Jellinek MS. After teen suicide: issues for pediatricians who are asked to consult to schools. *Pediatrics.* 1990;86:982–987

American Academy of Child and Adolescent Psychiatry. Practice parameter for the assessment and treatment of children and adolescents with suicidal behavior. *J Am Acad Child Adolesc Psychiatry.* 2001;40;24S–51S

Bolfek A, Janowski JJ, Waslick B, Summergrad P. Adolescent psychopharmacology: drugs for mood disorders. *Adolesc Med Clin.* 2006;17:789–808

Borowsky IW, Ireland M, Resnick MD. Adolescent suicide attempts: risks and protectors. 2001;107:485–493

Brookman RR, Sood AA. Disorders of mood and anxiety in adolescents. *Adolesc Med Clin.* 2006;17:79–95

Campbell AT. Consent, competence, and confidentiality related to psychiatric conditions in adolescent medicine practice. *Adolesc Med Clin.* 2006;17:25–47

Copelan R. Assessing the potential for violent behavior in children and adolescents. *Pediatr Rev.* 2006;27:e36–e41

Eaton DK, Kann L, Kinchen S, et al. Youth risk behavior surveillance—United States, 2005. *MMWR Surveill Summ.* 2006;55:1–108

Grossman DC, Mueller BA, Riedy C, et al. Gun storage practices and risk of youth suicide and unintentional firearm injuries. *JAMA.* 2005;293:707–714

Hatcher-Kay C, King CA. Depression and suicide. *Pediatr Rev.* 2003;24:363–370

Jellinek MS, Snyder JB. Depression and suicide in children and adolescents. *Pediatr Rev.* 1998;19:255–264

Lewisohn PM, Clarke GN, Seeley JR, Rohde P. Major depression in community adolescents: age at onset, episode duration, and time to recurrence. *J Am Acad Child Adolesc Psychiatry.* 1994;33:809–818

Shain BN, American Academy of Pediatrics Committee on Adolescence. Suicide and suicide attempts in adolescents. *Pediatrics.* 2007;120:669–676

Slap GB, Vorters DF, Khalid N, Marqulies SR, Forke CM. Adolescent suicide attempters: do physicians recognize them? *J Adolesc Health.* 1992;13:286–292

Woods ER, Lin YG, Middleman A, Beckford P, Chase L, DuRant RH. The associations of suicide attempts in adolescents. *Pediatrics.* 1997;99:791–796

Chronic Diseases of Childhood and Adolescence

127. Cancer in Children 779

128. Chronic Kidney Disease/Chronic Renal Failure 787

129. Diabetes Mellitus 795

130. Juvenile Idiopathic Arthritis/Collagen Vascular Disease 801

131. Nephrotic Syndrome 809

132. Seizures and Epilepsy 817

Cancer in Children

Wendy Y. Tcheng, MD

CASE STUDY

A 10-year-old boy has a history of intermittent fevers of 102.2°F (39.0°C) for 1 month. For 2 days, he has experienced increasing shortness of breath with rapid respirations. His face is dusky and plethoric, and the veins in his neck are prominent. The remainder of the examination is normal.

The blood count is normal, but the erythrocyte sedimentation rate is 110. A chest x-ray reveals a large mediastinal mass.

Questions
1. What signs and symptoms are associated with malignant conditions in children?
2. What oncological emergencies require immediate attention?
3. What factors correlate with the development of cancer in children?

Epidemiology

Approximately 1 in 350 individuals in the United States will develop a cancer before the age of 20 years. Cancer is the leading cause of death by disease in children younger than 15 years in the United States, with more than 2,700 children dying of cancer per year. Approximately 9,500 new cases of pediatric cancer are expected to occur within this age group annually. Acute leukemia is the most common childhood cancer diagnosis, followed by brain tumors, lymphomas, neuroblastoma, nephroblastoma, and other less common pediatric solid tumors (Figure 127-1).

Environmental factors, genetic predisposition, and developmental processes all play a role in influencing the cancer risk of a child. Case-control epidemiology studies looking for the causes of pediatric cancer have evaluated foods, prenatal exposures of parents and affected offspring, electromagnetic fields, radon, and various other environmental factors with no conclusive evidence of causality to date. Although many environmental factors are known to induce carcinogenesis, such as ionizing and ultraviolet radiation, stilbestrol, and androgen, these agents do not seem to play a significant role in childhood cancer. Infectious agents such as Epstein-Barr virus, papillomavirus type 5, and hepatitis B are associated with the development of certain types of cancer, but they seem to play a minimal role in the initiation events that trigger childhood malignancy. Inheritance of mutations in tumor suppressor genes such as the retinoblastoma gene or the p53 gene predispose affected children in families with these mutations to particular malignancies at a greater frequency and an earlier age than in unaffected individuals.

Although the macroscopic causes of pediatric cancer are not well elucidated, significant research progress has been made in determining some of the cellular and subcellular events that either actively trigger or fail to prevent malignancy. Most malignant cells have a genetic makeup that differs from the constitutional karyotype of the host. Thus while most cancers are not heritable, they seem to result from a genetic error or abnormality that occurs in the process of normal growth and development. An initiation event seems to alter or knock out one allele of a gene pair, and a second event results in loss of heterozygosity for that genetic locus. A good example is the p53 tumor suppressor gene—p53 is a recessive gene whose protein product acts to induce cell cycle arrest or apoptosis in response to DNA damage. Either an inherited abnormality of p53 or a serendipitous accident to p53 can cause heterozygosity for that gene. If a second event knocks out complete function of p53, a DNA-damaged cell can escape the signal to arrest its growth or to undergo apoptosis. The result can be a malignant transformation that allows the abnormal cell to grow unchecked.

Clinical Presentation (Table 127-1)

The signs and symptoms of childhood cancer are varied, often nonspecific at the start, and can mimic many common pediatric conditions. Children with **leukemia** commonly complain of generalized bone pain and can present with symptoms related to anemia, thrombocytopenia, or neutropenia. Mucosal bleeding, particularly from the gums, can be seen in children with acute myeloblastic leukemia (AML). Disseminated intravascular coagulation is characteristic of AML, especially acute promyelocytic leukemia. Children with leukemia often have hepatosplenomegaly and lymphadenopathy on examination. Superior vena cava (SVC) syndrome may occur in a child with an anterior mediastinal mass, seen most frequently in acute lymphoblastic leukemia (ALL). Children with SVC syndrome typically present with respiratory distress, plethora, and cyanosis due to compression of the mediastinal mass on the trachea and blockage of venous return and lymphatic drainage. Symptoms of SVC syndrome

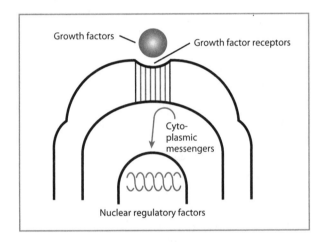

Figure 127-1. A. Leading causes of death in children between the ages of 1 and 14 years. (Adapted from US Vital Statistics.) **B.** Distribution of cancers in children younger than 15 years of age. (Reproduced with permission from Pizzo PC, Pollack DA. *Principles and Practice of Pediatric Oncology*. Philadelphia, PA: J. B. Lippincott; 1993:4; adapted from Surveillance, Epidemiology and End Results Program.) Abbreviations: HIV, human immunodeficiency virus; CNS, central nervous system.

can rapidly progress over a period of hours to pleural or pericardial effusion and respiratory arrest. Involvement of the central nervous system by leukemia can result in signs of increased intracranial pressure (ICP) (ie, headache, vomiting, hypertension, seizures, cranial neuropathies). With hyperleukocytosis, tumor lysis syndrome can occur, either spontaneously or with the initiation of chemotherapy. Tumor lysis syndrome occurs as a result of breakdown of tumor cells and release of metabolic by-products. It is characterized by a metabolic triad of hyperuricemia, hyperkalemia, and hyperphosphatemia, which places a child at risk for renal dysfunction or failure secondary to precipitation of urate or calcium phosphate crystals.

Children with **brain tumors** can present with diverse signs and symptoms, depending on the anatomical location of the tumor (infratentorial, supratentorial, or brain stem), age of the child (eg, infants with open sutures), and presence and degree of increased ICP. Infratentorial tumors, which are more common in children, typically present with gaze palsies, cerebellar signs (especially truncal ataxia), dysmetria, or vomiting. Supratentorial tumors can cause seizures, upper motor neuron signs (ie, hemiparesis, asymmetrical hyperreflexia, clonus), sensory changes, behavioral changes, decreased school performance, and disorders of the midbrain (Parinaud syndrome—paralysis of upward gaze). Signs and symptoms of ICP are often in the forefront of complaints, with both infratentorial and supratentorial tumors. Headaches, morning or persistent vomiting, lethargy, sun-downing (eyes deviating downwards like a sun setting on the horizon), loss of developmental milestones in infants, and change in school performance in older children all warrant close evaluation.

Children with spinal cord involvement from a primary spinal tumor or paraspinal tumor may present with persistent back pain, intense radicular pain, local bony tenderness of the affected vertebrae, weakness, abnormal reflexes, abnormal dermatomal sensory examination, and subtle symptoms of bowel or bladder

Figure 127-2. Pathway of stimulated cell proliferation. Cellular proliferation can be modified by extracellular signals, such as growth factors, that interact with receptors on the surface membrane. These receptors can be transmembrane proteins that transduce the regulatory signal through the membrane, which initiates an intracellular cascade of molecular messages that culminates in the alteration of nuclear proteins. This regulates the expression of genes important for cellular proliferation and tumorigenesis. (Reproduced with permission from Pizzo PC, Pollack DA. *Principles and Practice of Pediatric Oncology*. Philadelphia, PA: J. B. Lippincott; 1993:64.)

dysfunction. Suspicion of a spinal neurologic deficit constitutes a true oncological emergency for which timely, appropriate consultation must be sought.

Lymphomas in children can be divided pathologically into either Hodgkin or non-Hodgkin lymphoma. Children with **Hodgkin disease** classically have a protracted history (often at least 2–3 months) of enlarging lymphadenopathy, sometimes in association with constitutional symptoms (ie, "B" symptoms) that include fever, night sweats, and weight loss greater than 10% of body weight. **Non-**

Table 127-1. Signs and Symptoms of Childhood Cancer		
Disease	*Symptoms*	*Signs*
Leukemia	Fatigue Bone pain Fever, infection Petechiae, purpura, bleeding Disseminated intravascular coagulation Superior vena cava (SVC) syndrome Headache Seizures Oliguria/anuria	Anemia Neutropenia Thrombocytopenia Lymphadenopathy Hepatosplenomegaly Mediastinal mass Petechiae, purpura Papilledema Cranial neuropathies Renal failure

Brain tumors	Supratentorial tumors
	    Seizures
	    Visual dysfunction
	    Unilateral motor dysfunction
	
	Infratentorial tumors
	    Deficits of balance
	    Difficulty breathing
	
	Increased intracranial pressure
	    Headache
	    Vomiting
	    Diplopia
	    Motor weakness
	    Loss of developmental milestones
		Upper motor neuron signs
		Marcus Gunn pupils
		Parinaud syndrome
		Diabetes insipidus
		
		Appendicular dysmetria
		Sixth nerve palsy
		Cranial neuropathies
		Horner syndrome
		
		Papilledema
		Systemic hypertension
		Sixth nerve palsy
		"Setting sun" sign
		Large head size

Lymphoma		

Non-Hodgkin	Supradiaphragmatic (lymphoblastic)
	    Respiratory difficulty, cough
	    SVC syndrome
	    Enlarged/enlarging lymph nodes
	
	Infradiaphragmatic (small, non-cleaved)
	    Abdominal obstruction
	    Intussusception
	    Abdominal distension
		Mediastinal mass +/− effusions
		Lymphadenopathy
		
		Abdominal mass
		Hepatosplenomegaly
		
		Obstructive jaundice

Hodgkin	Constitutional symptoms (fever, weight loss, pruritus)	Lymphadenopathy +/− matted nodes
Neuroblastoma	Abdominal mass Skin nodules Proptosis, "raccoon eyes" Nystagmus Diarrhea Spinal cord compression symptoms	Hypertension Hepatosplenomegaly Horner syndrome
Rhabdomyosarcoma	Related to primary site	

Table 127-1. Signs and Symptoms of Childhood Cancer, continued		
Lymphoma, continued		

Wilms tumor	Rapid development of abdominal swelling
	Painless hematuria
		Abdominal mass
		Hypertension
		Associated congenital anomalies
		    Aniridia
		    Hemihypertrophy
		    Urogenital anomalies

Ewing sarcoma	Painful swelling of bone Constitutional symptoms (fever, fatigue)	
Osteosarcoma	Painful swelling of bone	

Hodgkin lymphoma often can be subdivided into 2 categories: lymphoblastic and non-lymphoblastic. Children with **lymphoblastic lymphoma** often present with supradiaphragmatic disease and may have cervical or supraclavicular lymphadenopathy, sometimes in association with a mediastinal mass or SVC syndrome. Central nervous system disease in such children is associated with signs of increased ICP. Patients with small, non-cleaved, **non-lymphoblastic lymphoma** of the Burkitt or non-Burkitt type often present with intra-abdominal disease, intussusception, abdominal obstruction, hepatosplenomegaly, and obstructive jaundice. Children with Burkitt lymphoma may also present with isolated jaw tumors. In addition, patients with lymphoma can manifest any of a number of paraneoplastic syndromes. These include idiopathic thrombocytopenic purpura, autoimmune hemolytic anemia, nephrotic syndrome, and peripheral neuropathies, which may be mediated by abnormal and lymphoma-driven humoral or cell-mediated processes. Children with lymphomas are also at risk for tumor lysis syndrome as described for leukemia. In general, patients may either have entirely normal blood counts or a mild anemia, but occasionally their bone marrow may be infiltrated, giving a clinical picture consistent with leukemia with anemia, thrombocytopenia, or neutropenia.

Neuroblastoma, the most common extracranial soft tissue tumor, is of sympathetic ganglionic cell origin and as such can present as intra-adrenal or extra-adrenal (paraspinal) abdominal masses; posterior (paraspinal) mediastinal masses; cervical masses; or in some cases with disseminated disease of the liver, spleen, skin, bone, and bone marrow. Because these tumors produce excess catecholamine analogs, children may have hypertension, diarrhea, nystagmus, opsomyoclonus (random dysconjugate eye movements), and cerebellar ataxia. Proptosis and hemorrhage due to metastases behind the orbit can result in periorbital ecchymoses. A mediastinal tumor may be associated with unilateral Horner syndrome due to compression of cranial nerve VII. Children with widespread disease, especially those older than 2 years, may have infiltration of the bone marrow leading to pancytopenia and severe bony pain.

Rhabdomyosarcoma, another soft tissue sarcoma of childhood, presents primarily with signs and symptoms related to whether the tumor has developed in the head and neck, chest, abdomen/pelvis, or extremities. One classic presentation, sarcoma botryoides, occurs when the tumor is located in the vagina or uterus and the patient presents with vaginal bleeding and a grape-like mass at the introitus. **Nephroblastoma** or **Wilms tumor,** which arises in the kidney, usually appears as an abdominal mass that sometimes rapidly enlarges as the result of hemorrhage. Painless hematuria may be present, even in the absence of an abdominal mass. Children may have hypertension and associated congenital anomalies including aniridia, hemihypertrophy, and various urogenital conditions.

The **bone sarcomas** that occur in children include Ewing sarcoma, osteosarcoma, and other rarer sarcomas. All bone tumors appear as growing, painful swellings of bone; patients with Ewing sarcoma may also have associated constitutional symptoms such as low-grade fever, fatigue, and weight loss.

Pathophysiology

The pathophysiology of carcinogenesis has its origins in genetic mutation. The entire process of cancer development is incompletely understood but begins with a series of sequential genetic mutations that affect the complex processes that control cell growth, differentiation, and death. Growth factors are often responsible for exogenous stimulation of proliferation, and growth factor receptors transduce this signal into the cell via cytoplasmic second messengers such as protein kinase C and activated *ras* proteins, which in turn transmit the signal to nuclear regulatory factors. These factors ultimately regulate transcription of new RNA and protein, resulting in the desired cellular response of either stimulation or inhibition of growth. Dysregulation of growth via mutations in genes controlling all of these steps has been identified in tumors. Similar aberrations in genes regulating differentiation and cell death have also been described.

Cancer's threat to a living organism lies in its uncontrolled growth (Figure 127-2). By growing unchecked and invading, compressing, and metastasizing to vital organs, malignant cells threaten normal life functions and cause symptoms specific to the affected area of the body.

Differential Diagnosis

The differential diagnoses for some of the common childhood complaints that may suggest an underlying malignancy will be discussed. **Lymphadenopathy** is a common pediatric complaint and is most frequently due to infections (see Chapter 73). Acute bacterial adenitis, usually involving the head and neck region, is typically associated with local signs of inflammation such as erythema, warmth, and tenderness. Cervical adenopathy due to viral illness is typically bilateral, and the lymph nodes are usually mobile, soft, and non-tender. Generalized lymphadenopathy or regional lymphadenopathy characterized by firm, matted, rubbery lymph nodes should raise the suspicion for an underlying malignancy. Lymphadenopathy that is persistent or progressive, despite empiric antibiotic therapy or resolution of infectious symptoms, also merits further evaluation for malignancy. Leukemia often presents with generalized lymphadenopathy, usually in association with hepatosplenomegaly and abnormal laboratory findings. Lymphoma typically presents with regional lymphadenopathy, often in the cervical or mediastinal region, in conjunction with other signs of systemic illness. Metastatic disease (neuroblastoma, rhabdomyosarcoma) may also present with regional lymphadenopathy. Nonmalignant causes of neck masses that can be mistaken for cervical lymphadenopathy include structural anomalies such as branchial cleft cysts or cystic hygromas (see Chapter 67).

Bone and joint pain are common complaints in children with acute leukemia, because of bone marrow involvement, and may be generalized. This presentation can be confused with various rheumatologic conditions. Localized bone pain is a common presentation for children with primary bone cancers (osteosarcoma, Ewing sarcoma) and is often attributed by the child or parents to some trauma. It is not unusual for the diagnosis to be delayed several months. Differential diagnosis includes infection (osteomyelitis), trauma, musculoskeletal conditions, and benign bone lesions.

Headache is a common complaint facing the general pediatrician, and few of these headaches are caused by intracranial brain tumors. When evaluating a child with headaches, signs to raise the index of suspicion for a brain tumor include persistent vomiting, recurrent morning headaches or headaches that awaken the child, worsening headaches, associated neurologic abnormalities, and visual changes (papilledema on examination). In infants, increasing head size, sundowning, and loss of acquired developmental milestones are red flags. The differential diagnosis for headaches in children is broad and includes infections (meningitis, sinusitis), migraines, hydrocephalus, hemorrhage, and seizures.

An **abdominal mass** in an infant or child is always concerning and merits an evaluation. The most common malignant causes for an abdominal mass in this age range include neuroblastoma, nephroblastoma (Wilms tumor), hepatoblastoma, non-Hodgkin lymphoma (ie, Burkitt lymphoma), sarcomas, and germ cell tumors. Massive hepatosplenomegaly due to leukemic or lymphomatous infiltration can also be palpated as an abdominal mass. Nonmalignant etiologies of an abdominal mass may include hepatomegaly or splenomegaly, renal cysts, hemangiomas, or constipation.

Pancytopenia or **single cytopenias** are always worrisome for a malignancy involving the bone marrow. Acute leukemia is the most common malignancy involving the bone marrow and often presents with leukopenia, anemia, thrombocytopenia, or in combination. Any malignancy that can metastasize to the bone marrow

(neuroblastoma, lymphoma, Ewing sarcoma, rhabdomyosarcoma) can also produce pancytopenia or depression of one of the cell lines due to replacement of the bone marrow. Pancytopenia can occur as a primary bone marrow failure syndrome, such as Fanconi anemia, or as an acquired aplastic anemia due to infections (post-hepatitis), drugs (chloramphenicol, anticonvulsants), radiation, or idiopathic causes. Transient mild depression of the cell lines (most often leukopenia or anemia) due to infectious causes is very common during childhood.

Evaluation

History

The history should focus on the duration and evolution of symptoms as well as the presence or absence of constitutional symptoms (eg, anorexia, fever, night sweats, weight loss). The impact of the symptoms on daily activities (eg, school attendance, sports) should be determined and will clue the physician to the scope of the illness. Recent or persistent infections, medications, or unusual environmental exposures (eg, ionizing radiation) should also be ascertained (Questions Box). Relevant medical history should be considered. A previous cancer diagnosis would raise the index of suspicion for relapse or a secondary malignancy. Certain immunodeficiencies and genetic syndromes are associated with an increased risk for malignancy (eg, trisomy 21 syndrome and leukemia) and should also be considered. A family history of childhood cancers or genetic syndromes is also important.

> ## Questions
>
> ### Cancer
>
> - How long has the child had the symptoms?
> - Does the child have a family history of cancer?
> - Does the child have a history of constitutional symptoms (eg, fever, weight loss)?
> - Does the child have a history of recent onset of pallor, fever, bleeding, pain, swelling, hematuria, or malaise?
> - Has the child been attending school or participating in routine activities?
> - Has the child been exposed to any environmental toxins?

Physical Examination

A thorough physical examination is essential, with particular attention to symptomatic areas (see Table 127-1). In general, the lymph nodes should be carefully assessed for enlargement or malignant characteristics (firm, fixed, rubbery nodes) and the abdomen for organomegaly or masses. The skin should be evaluated for the presence of pallor, petechiae, or purpura that would suggest anemia or thrombocytopenia. A thorough search for signs of infection or persistent infection should be performed and, if present, may reflect bone marrow disease with neutropenia. Neurologic symptoms, including headache, vomiting, or focal complaints, warrant a full neurologic examination. Increased ICP may manifest as papilledema, sixth nerve palsy, or systemic hypertension. In infants, increased ICP can manifest with a large head size, full fontanelles, or sun-downing. A complaint of back pain also merits a full neurologic examination with close attention to any signs of spinal cord compression, suggesting a possible spinal or paraspinal mass.

Laboratory Tests (Table 127-2)

In a child with nonspecific or constitutional symptoms concerning for malignancy, it is reasonable to begin with a screening complete blood count, peripheral blood smear, and comprehensive chemistry panel (electrolytes, renal and liver function). If a malignancy is suspected, a lactate dehydrogenase can be useful as a nonspecific

marker for increased cell turnover. If leukemia or lymphoma is suspected, evaluation for tumor lysis syndrome (by checking uric acid, potassium, phosphate, and calcium) should be performed. In addition, certain tumors secrete or synthesize characteristic markers and metabolites that are pathognomonic for their diagnosis. For example, elevated levels of the sympathetic neurotransmitter metabolites vanillylmandelic acid and homovanillic acid are found in the urine of individuals with neuroblastoma or pheochromocytoma. The substances α-fetoprotein, β-human chorionic gonadotropin, and carcinoembryonic antigen are sometimes secreted in the blood, urine, or cerebrospinal fluid of patients with malignant teratomas. Detection of these proteins in body fluids can also be an indicator of response

Table 127-2. Diagnostic Tests and Imaging Studies Used in the Evaluation of Childhood Cancer

Disease	Diagnostic Tests	Imaging Studies
Leukemia	Bone marrow aspirate and biopsy Cytogenetic analysis of bone marrow CBC with platelet count, differential PT, PTT, fibrinogen Serum electrolytes, Ca, PO$_4$ BUN, creatinine, uric acid, LDH CSF cell count, cytology	Chest x-ray (look for mediastinal mass)
Brain tumors	None usually indicated except in case of suspected teratoma: serum and CSF α-fetoprotein, β-human chorionic gonadotropin, carcinoembryonic antigen	MRI of brain with gadolinium MRI of spine for selected tumors
Lymphoma	Bone marrow aspirate and biopsy CSF cell count and cytology Serum LDH, electrolytes, Ca, PO$_4$ ESR, ferritin	Gallium scan, PET scan CT chest, abdomen, pelvis
Neuroblastoma	Serum ferritin CBC with platelet count Serum electrolytes, liver and renal panel Serum LDH Bone marrow aspirate and biopsy	CT or MRI of primary tumor site CT of chest, abdomen, pelvis, (+/– head) with contrast Bone scan MIBG scan
Rhabdomyosarcoma	CBC with platelet count Liver and renal panel Bone marrow aspirate and biopsy CSF cell count and cytology (head and neck primary tumors only)	CT or MRI of primary tumor site CT of chest, abdomen, pelvis Bone scan
Nephroblastoma (Wilms tumor)	Urinalysis	CT of primary tumor site Ultrasound of inferior vena cava CT of chest Bone scan
Ewing sarcoma	ESR CBC with platelet count Bone marrow aspirate and biopsy Serum LDH	CT or MRI of primary tumor site CT of chest Bone scan
Osteosarcoma		MRI of primary tumor site CT of chest Bone scan

Abbreviations: CBC, complete blood count; PT, prothrombin time; PTT, partial thromboplastin time; Ca, calcium; PO$_4$, phosphate; BUN, blood urea nitrogen; LDH, lactate dehydrogenase; CSF, cerebrospinal fluid; MRI, magnetic resonance imaging; ESR, erythrocyte sedimentation rate; PET, positron emission tomography; CT, computed tomography; MIBG, metaiodobenzylguanidine.

to therapy or relapse. Other laboratory values, such as ferritin or erythrocyte sedimentation rate, have prognostic value with certain tumors (see Table 127-2).

Imaging Studies

Radiographic studies are a necessity in the initial evaluation and staging of childhood cancers. Once the diagnosis of malignancy has been confirmed, appropriate imaging studies to assess the local and metastatic spread of the disease should be performed before the initiation of therapy. The type of studies performed depends on the specific malignancy and its associated pattern of metastatic spread. Common studies performed include x-rays, computed tomography (CT), magnetic resonance imaging, and gallium or positron emission tomography (PET) scans. For leukemias and lymphomas, an initial chest x-ray is necessary to evaluate for a mediastinal mass (most commonly seen in T-cell leukemia/lymphoma). Additional imaging is typically not necessary for leukemia; however, lymphomas warrant further diagnostic imaging for staging (CT, gallium, or PET scans). Required imaging for evaluation of specific childhood cancers is provided in Table 127-2.

Pathology

The initial diagnosis of a malignancy or its relapse, regardless of clinical likelihood, must be documented pathologically before treatment is initiated. The only exception to this rule is radiologic evidence of a brain stem tumor, which for all intents and purposes is consistent with the diagnosis of brain stem glioma. Even when a child is in respiratory distress (ie, with SVC syndrome secondary to a mediastinal mass), coordinated efforts must be made by the pediatrician, oncologist, intensivist, pathologist, and surgeon to obtain pathology specimens before the initiation of therapy. In less emergent situations, children with suspected malignancies should, when at all possible, be referred to an experienced pediatric surgeon associated with a children's cancer center for evaluation of biopsy versus surgery. Collection of fresh tissue at biopsy for specialized genetic tests and tumor banking can contribute significantly to a complete pathologic diagnosis.

Management

Because the management of specific childhood cancers is beyond the scope of this chapter, the discussion will focus on the general principles of pediatric oncological management. The primary therapeutic modalities for the treatment of childhood cancer include **chemotherapy, surgery, radiation therapy,** and **stem cell transplantation.** However, the evolving field of **cancer-targeted therapies** promises to change the way pediatric oncologists treat childhood cancer in the future. Conventional, cytotoxic anticancer therapy is likened to a "shotgun" approach in which both cancer cells and normal cells are subject to toxicity. The effects of therapy on normal tissues and organs can manifest acutely (limiting dose) or in the long term (affecting quality of life). As more and more children are surviving childhood cancer, the late effects of therapy are increasingly

evident, further emphasizing the need for cancer-targeted therapy and a reduction of treatment-related toxicities.

Any child with a suspected malignancy should be referred to a pediatric cancer center if possible. Optimal outcome depends on several factors: correct pathologic diagnosis; careful medical management, including administration of chemotherapy and monitoring of side effects; precision customization of radiation fields if radiation therapy is necessary; optimal surgical resection, if indicated; and therapeutic ability and experience with administration of treatment to small children. Centers that specialize in the treatment of pediatric cancer are experienced in the diagnosis and treatment of rare malignancies and are thus best equipped to treat affected children. In addition, the standard of care for children with cancer is treatment according to research study protocols from national collaborative research groups (Children's Oncology Group), available at most specialized pediatric cancer centers. Posttreatment analysis of children treated on protocols at specialized pediatric cancer centers have 4-year disease-free survival rates that are significantly better than those of children treated outside this setting. Similarly, treatment of adolescents and young adults on protocols at specialized pediatric cancer centers yields better outcomes than those treated by oncologists who typically treat adults.

In the interest of cost-containment and convenience as well as children's well-being, it is often more feasible for children to be closer to home between chemotherapy cycles. Primary care physicians should be familiar with the management of various infectious complications to which children undergoing cancer therapy are subject. Fever in children with neutropenia (absolute neutrophil count <500/cm^3) requires a different therapeutic approach than fever in otherwise normal children. Until proven otherwise, children with fever and neutropenia (usually induced by chemotherapy, sometimes in combination with radiation therapy) must be assumed to have a serious bacterial infection. They should be treated accordingly, with hospitalization, intravenous (IV) antibiotics, thorough examination for site of infection, and careful hemodynamic monitoring. Initial treatment consists of antibiotic coverage for *Staphylococcus aureus,* gram-negative enteric organisms, and *Pseudomonas aeruginosa* (eg, ceftazidime with or without gentamicin, vancomycin). Additional coverage for anaerobic infection (eg, mucositis), viral infection (eg, herpes stomatitis, varicella), and other pathogens (eg, fungi) depends on the child's treatment history and clinical findings.

The placement of indwelling central venous catheters is standard in cancer therapy in pediatrics, making frequent venous access for both diagnostic and therapeutic purposes more easily tolerated by children. External catheters (Broviac, Hickman) or internal subcutaneous catheters (Port-a-Caths) are selected depending on the underlying diagnosis and intensity of therapy. All indwelling catheters are at risk for infection, either from contamination of blood (line infections) or infections around the catheter site itself (tunnel infection). Most central line infections can be treated with IV antibiotic therapy; however, certain pathogens (fungi) are difficult to clear and require line removal. Central venous catheters may also be complicated with thromboses requiring local thrombolytic therapy.

Prognosis

The prognosis for children with all forms of cancer has dramatically improved over the past 4 decades. Nearly 80% of children diagnosed with cancer can expect to be long-term survivors. Figure 127-3 shows the improvement in cure rates for ALL, the most common childhood cancer. This success is largely due to the efforts of national collaborative group science and treatment protocols. However, with increased survivorship, new concerns have arisen with respect to the long-term effects of treatment, the risks of secondary malignancies, and complex social and psychological issues. In a large study of childhood cancer survivors, adults treated for a childhood cancer in the 1970s and 1980s were 3 times more likely than their siblings to have developed a chronic health condition. Continued multidisciplinary surveillance of childhood cancer survivors through adulthood will help to optimize a favorable outcome. As research efforts focus on cancer-targeted therapies that minimize treatment-related toxicities (acute and long term), the complex issues that face many childhood cancer survivors will hopefully be mitigated.

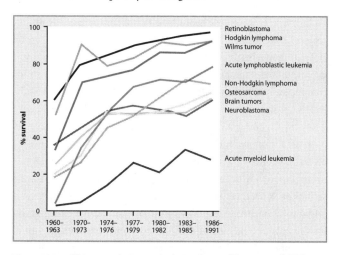

Figure 127-3. Five-year relative survival rates for specific cancers of children (0–14 years), 1973–2001. Data are from the Surveillance, Epidemiology, and End Results (SEER) program regions (9 areas). (From Pizzo PA, Poplack DG. *Principles and Practice of Pediatric Oncology.* Philadelphia, PA: Lippincott Williams & Wilkins; 2001:5, Figure 1.5 A and B.)

Selected References

Golden CB, Feusner JH. Malignant abdominal masses in children: quick guide to evaluation and diagnosis. *Pediatr Clin North Am.* 2002;49:1369–1392

Meck MM, Leary M, Sills RH. Late effects in survivors of childhood cancer. *Pediatr Rev.* 2007;27:257–263

Poplack DG. Acute lymphoblastic leukemia. In: Pizzo PA, Poplack DG, eds. *Principles and Practice of Pediatric Oncology.* 5th ed. Philadelphia, PA: Lippincott Williams & Wilkins; 2006

Pui CH, Schrappe M, Ribeiro RC, Niemeyer CM. Childhood and adolescent lymphoid and myeloid leukemia. *Hematology Am Soc Hematol Educ Program.* 2004:118–145

Ullrich NJ, Pomeroy SL. Pediatric brain tumors. *Neurol Clin.* 2003;21:897–913

Chronic Kidney Disease/ Chronic Renal Failure

Walter Jimenez, MD, and Isidro B. Salusky, MD

CASE STUDY

During a consultation for diarrhea and dehydration the pediatrician notes that a 7-year-old boy has concomitant growth retardation. His parents report decrease in appetite as well as in physical activity level over the last few months associated with bed-wetting, despite having been previously potty trained. His medical history is significant for multiple episodes of fever due to supposed ear infections during his first years of life and one episode of urinary tract infection without further studies. After hydration the physical examination reveals a pale and short patient (height 101 cm, <5th percentile) with blood pressure above 99th percentile for age, gender,

and height. Routine laboratories reveal anemia, a serum creatinine of 1.4, and 3+ proteinuria.

Questions

1. What are the relevant questions to ask about medical and family history in children who present with **chronic kidney disease (CKD)?**
2. How would you estimate the renal function?
3. What additional diagnostic tests should be performed to determine the etiology of the renal failure?
4. What are the approaches to the management of children with CKD?

Renal failure can affect synthesis and regulation of **erythropoietin; renin; 1,25-dihydroxycholecalciferol; acid-base; electrolytes; water;** and excretion or "clearance" of **wasting products.** Currently **glomerular filtration rate (GFR)** is the best method to detect, evaluate, and manage chronic kidney disease (CKD). The GFR varies according to gender, age, and body size and reflects the amount of plasma cleared by the kidney (Box 128-1). Early recognition of children with CKD is important in order to prevent the complications associated with the progressive decline in renal function. The signs and symptoms of CKD in children are nonspecific; thus it is vital that the primary medical caretaker, usually the pediatrician or family practitioner, recognize the earliest signs and symptoms and institute proper medical care. Prompt referral to a pediatric nephrologist must be made, and follow-up consultations by both physicians should be performed regularly to optimize the management of these children.

Depending on the GFR, the physician can classify kidney function in 5 stages as defined by the National Kidney Foundation (Table 128-1). Stages 1 and 2 are defined with GFR of more than 90 mL/min/1.73 m^2, and 60 to 89 mL/min/1.73 m^2 respectively. The staging of CKD provides guidelines for the management of these patients because there are specific primary and comorbid conditions associated with the primary cause of renal failure as well as those that are associated with progression of CKD. Indeed, the reduction of some of those associated factors may reduce the risk factors for cardiovascular disease (CVD). Particular importance should be placed on managing **proteinuria, acidosis, anemia, hypertension,** and **metabolic bone disease** among others. Once GFR declines to 15 to 29 mL/min/1.73 m^2 (stage 4), patients and families should be prepared for **renal replacement therapy** and **renal transplantation. End-stage renal disease (ESRD** or stage 5) is defined as GFR less than 15 mL/

Box 128-1. Creatinine Clearance
Measured from a 24-hour urine collection
$$Cl = \frac{\text{Urine creatinine [mmol/L]} \times \text{Volume of urine [mL]}}{\text{Time of urine sampling [min]} \times \text{Plasma creatinine [mmol/L]}}$$
Cl (normalized for 1.73 m^2) = Cl × 1.73/body surface area
Estimated by a spot urine (Schwartz formula)
Cl = k × Height [cm]/Plasma creatinine [mg/dL]
K = 0.7 adolescent boy, 0.55 child or adolescent girl, 0.45 infant

Table 128-1. Classification of Chronic Kidney Disease	
Stage	Glomerular Filtration Rate (mL/min/1.73 m^2)
1	≥90
2	60–89
3	30–59
4	15–29
5	≤15

min/1.73 m² or the need of **dialysis/transplant.** The staging of CKD is based on estimation of GFR but also additional factors are considered in the overall management of the patient, and the characteristics of the growth curve are very important in the assessment of the consequences of renal failure in childhood. All children with CKD should be referred early to pediatric nephrologists in order to carefully facilitate the future steps in the care of the patient and family. In adult patients with CKD, the late referral was found to be associated with increased rates of morbidity and mortality.

Epidemiology

The incidence of CKD in children is unknown. Current estimates are based on the number of children accepted for dialysis and renal transplantation; however, some children do not require dialysis or transplantation until adulthood. In 2006 the North American Pediatric Renal Transplant Cooperative Study (NAPRTCS) reported 6,405 patients with an estimated GFR 75 mL/min/1.73m² or less. The causes of CKD can be broadly categorized into 2 main groups: congenital and acquired. Congenital conditions such as **obstructive uropathy, aplasia/hypoplasia/dysplasia, reflux nephropathy, polycystic kidney disease,** and **prune belly syndrome** accounted for the majority (55%). Among the acquired conditions, **focal and segmental glomerulosclerosis** are the most prevalent diagnoses, accounting for 8.7%, with African Americans having a worse prognosis. Overall males are more affected.

Clinical Presentation

Children with CKD often present with no, or nonspecific, symptoms, and the abnormality is detected during routine health examinations or screening. For a small percentage of these patients, CKD is inadvertently discovered when they present with another illness such as diarrhea and dehydration. Patients may be referred to the physician because of **growth retardation, hypertension,** or **anemia** (Dx Box). Frequently, a history of recurrent episodes of fever without a source, or partially treated urinary tract infections (UTIs) secondary to undiagnosed vesicoureteral reflux, is uncovered. Children may complain of vague generalized symptoms, including malaise, anorexia, and vomiting, which may be associated with advanced renal failure.

Dx **Chronic Kidney Disease**

- Growth retardation/growth failure
- Anemia
- Bone disease
- Metabolic acidosis

Growth Failure

Failure to thrive is the hallmark of CKD in children, and the degree of growth retardation varies according to the age of presentation. Indeed, because maximal growth occurs during the early years in life, children with congenital renal problems are most affected. In the NAPRTCS study, height deficits were greatest for children younger than 5 years, with nearly 50% below the third percentile for age and gender. In addition, children with more severe degrees of affected renal function tended to have greater height deficits. Sexual development is often delayed in affected patients.

Anemia

The anemia of CKD is normochromic and normocytic. Insufficient erythropoietin production occurs when the GFR is less than 30 mL/min/1.73 m². Anemia is frequently accompanied by decreased serum iron levels, increased total iron binding capacity, and low reticulocyte counts. Dialysis patients are predisposed to develop bleeding tendencies because of platelet dysfunction.

Metabolic and Water/Electrolyte Abnormalities

Children with congenital abnormalities such as obstructive uropathy and/or renal dysplasia may develop polyuria due to inability to concentrate urine, and salt wasting may become a prominent feature as well as polydipsia. Thus a history of **bed-wetting** may be a clue in the diagnosis of CKD. However, children with advanced CKD may have impaired sodium excretion leading to water retention and, consequently, fluid overload and hypertension. **Hyperkalemia** is not an unusual component of CKD, and it becomes evident when the GFR falls below 10 mL/min/1.73 m². **Hypokalemia** is a less common problem and may be secondary to excessive diuretic use or strict dietary restriction.

Metabolic acidosis is mainly caused by the overall decrease in ammonia excretion by a reduced number of nephrons. Decreased excretion of titratable acid and bicarbonate wasting in cases of proximal renal tubular acidosis may play a role as well. Oral base therapy should be used to maintain a bicarbonate level in plasma above 20 mEq/L in order to facilitate skeletal growth.

Glucose intolerance may occur in some children with CKD despite elevated insulin levels. The linear correlation between a decline in renal function and insulin resistance even at early stages of CKD has been shown in adults. More than 50% of children develop **hyperlipidemia** by the time they reach ESRD. The characteristic plasma lipid abnormality is a moderate **hypertriglyceridemia.** There is also a high prevalence of **hypercholesterolemia** and low levels of high-density lipids and albumin. These derangements have a role in the developing of CVD.

Renal Osteodystrophy

The development of bone disease begins early in the course of CKD and if untreated progresses to bone pain; bone deformities; and extraskeletal calcifications in vessels, skin, and visceral organs. Clinical manifestations include growth retardation and skeletal deformities including **genu valgum, ulnar deviation of the hands, pes varus,** and **slipped capital femoral epiphyses.**

Hypertension

The incidence of **hypertension** in children varies from 38% to 78%. Prolonged hypertension may accelerate deterioration of renal function. An acute rise in blood pressure usually results in seizures in children. Other manifestations include headache, congestive heart failure, nerve palsies and, not uncommonly, cerebral hemorrhage. Hypertension is frequently seen in children with CKD secondary to polycystic kidney disease or chronic glomerulonephritis.

Cardiac Dysfunction

Congestive heart failure may be a prominent clinical finding associated with fluid overload, uncontrollable hypertension, severe anemia, or presence of uremic cardiomyopathy. Left ventricular hypertrophy diagnosed by echocardiographic assessment is present in 3 of 4 adults with CKD, with anemia and hypertension being the principal predisposing factors. Such findings are seen even in the pediatric population, with a prevalence of 10% to 20% in CKD stages 3 and 4.

Neurologic Dysfunction

Children with CKD may have **impaired neurodevelopment** related to the age of presentation. Memory deficits, lack of concentration, depression, and weakness may occur. Children younger than 5 years are most affected because significant brain growth and maturation occur during the early years of life. Children who are severely uremic may suffer from global developmental retardation and seizures. Unless neurodevelopmental delays are recognized promptly and early intervention is instituted, problems are most often progressive.

Pathophysiology

Regardless of the type of initial injury to the kidney, hyperfiltration and tubulointerstitial damage are the final common pathways of glomerular destruction. Hyperfiltration occurs as a response by the residual glomeruli to compensate the loss of nephrons. The reduced filtration results in increased production of **renin** and **angiotensin-converting enzyme (ACE)**. The resulting vasoconstriction of the efferent arteriole increases the hydrostatic pressure on the capillary wall, leading to a compensatory higher filtration rate but also to protein transit across the wall. Proteinuria recruits inflammatory cells and upregulates proinflammatory and pro-fibrotic genes. Protein overload in the tubular cells stimulates their differentiation into myofibroblasts, thus favoring fibrosis. The inflammatory cascade activates at the same time as the complement cascade, leading to additional kidney damage. The interstitial fibrosis impairs oxygenation of the tubular cells; the chronic hypoxia then further activates the renin-angiotensin system. The activation of fibroblasts by hypoxia is another stimulus to the differentiation of the tubular cells. Reducing intraglomerular pressure, proteinuria, and the consequent tubulointerstitial fibrosis is the rationale for prescribing ACE inhibitors or angiotensin receptor blockers (ARBs) in order to slow the rate of progression of CKD.

Multiple factors are involved in the pathogenesis of growth retardation in children with CKD, and the most predominant are deficient calorie and protein intake, decreased erythropoietin production, metabolic acidosis, decreased serum level of **insulin-like growth factor I,** peripheral resistance to growth hormone due to decreased levels of growth hormone–binding proteins and growth hormone receptors, and metabolic bone disease associated with progression of CKD. A particularity of renal osteodystrophy in children is the alteration of the growth plate cartilage architecture, another possible detrimental element in the growth failure.

The development of **renal osteodystrophy** is also multifactorial. The reduced renal mass results in a decreasing synthesis of 1,25-**dihydroxycholecalciferol;** the stimulus to absorb calcium from the gut decreases concomitantly. The resulting hypocalcemia and the lack of feedback by vitamin D stimulate the production of parathyroid hormone (PTH), facilitating the rapid mobilization of calcium and phosphorus from the skeleton, thus normalizing the serum calcium. However, there is skeletal resistance to PTH when CKD advances. The cycle is aggravated by an early alteration in the regulation of PTH gene transcription and a reduction in the calcium sensing receptor in the parathyroid glands. **Hyperparathyroidism** and resulting high bone turnover produces fibrosis in bone, which is also called **osteitis fibrosa.** Hyperphosphatemia develops when the few remaining nephrons lose the ability to excrete the daily load of phosphorus from diet; it is a late phenomenon, mainly in stages 4 and 5. The external administration of vitamin D and its derivatives can suppress such bone remodeling, but if not adequately monitored can result in low turnover bone disease (adynamic bone). Serum PTH and alkaline phosphatase levels are generally lower when compared with patients with secondary hyperparathyroidism. In the past, aluminum-containing phosphate binders were the main factors involved in the pathogenesis of osteomalacia and adynamic bone, but currently the use of large doses of calcium-based binders and active vitamin D sterols are implicated. The presence of abnormal calcium-phosphate metabolism, hyperparathyroidism in association with other traditional risk factors as hypertension, hyperlipidemia, hyperhomocysteinemia, anemia, and oxidative stress are also associated with CVD, the leading cause of death in ESRD. In young adults with childhood-onset CKD, the prevalence of coronary artery calcification can be as high as 92% when evaluated by sequential computed tomography (CT) scan with electrocardiogram (ECG) gating.

Differential Diagnosis

A variety of kidney problems, whether congenital, hereditary, acquired, or metabolic, may result in CKD. It is necessary to differentiate between acute and chronic renal failure at initial presentation because the therapeutic strategies may differ. In infants and children, congenital and anatomical malformations account for the largest percentage of patients who progress to chronic renal failure. These malformations include hypoplastic/dysplastic kidneys, obstructive uropathy, and reflux nephropathy. Patients with CKD present with retarded linear growth and signs of clinical and radiographic evidence of renal osteodystrophy. In advanced disease the renal ultrasound frequently reveals small, shrunken kidneys. The hereditary diseases most commonly encountered are hereditary nephritis (Alport syndrome), branchio-oto-renal syndrome (BOR), and juvenile nephronophthisis. Acquired diseases such as chronic glomerulonephritis, membranoproliferative glomerulonephritis, and focal and segmental glomerulosclerosis affect a large percentage of older children who progress to CKD. Anemia, hypertension, and fluid and electrolyte abnormalities are often associated with either chronic or acute renal failure.

Although specific cures are not available for most of these renal conditions, it is essential to perform a complete diagnostic workup to determine the etiology of the renal problem. Such information may identify the presence of an inherited problem that may require genetic counseling and, in some cases, anticipation of problems associated with renal transplantation. Some renal diseases may recur immediately after renal transplantation (eg, focal segmental glomerulosclerosis); parents and children must be informed early about this possibility in preparation for future strategies for renal transplantation.

Evaluation

Complete evaluation of children presenting with renal failure must be performed in order to differentiate whether the condition is acute or chronic because management strategies may differ in these conditions.

History

A thorough history must be obtained, including a complete and detailed family history that may provide some clues to the diagnosis of the patient's condition (Questions Box).

Physical Examination

A complete physical examination is required. Height and weight must be measured accurately, and the result must be plotted in the same growth curve as in healthy children. The weight can be overestimated if fluid retention is present. Blood pressure, using the appropriate cuff size, must be taken by the primary physician. Blood pressure must be compared with 50th percentile for age, gender, and height (www.nhlbi.nih.gov). The presence of tachycardia, heart murmurs, or adventitious heart sounds that may indicate uncompensate anemia or cardiac or pericardial involvement must be noted. Gross eye examination should be performed, including fundal examination, to assess for evidence of chronic hypertension. In addition, macular abnormalities and hearing problems may provide clues to a heritable disease (eg, Alport syndrome). Any ear abnormalities (eg, preauricular pits or ear tags) accompanied by hearing deficits are usually associated with some form of renal disease (eg, BOR). Undescended testes may be evident in some children with urogenital problems.

Laboratory Tests

For the initial laboratory workup, complete blood count, electrolytes, blood urea nitrogen, creatinine, calcium, phosphorus, and urinalysis must be obtained (Figure 128-1). Glomerulonephritides usually

---

Questions

Chronic Renal Failure

- Does the child have
  — Abnormalities on prenatal ultrasound such as hydronephrosis or polyhydramnios/oligohydramnios?
  — A history of prolonged illness, pallor, weakness, vomiting, or loss of appetite, and the age of presentation?
  — Any history of headaches or visual or hearing problems?
  — Any history of hematuria, proteinuria (foamy or bubbling urine), urinary tract infections, or episodes of fever with unknown source?
  — Impaired growth or development compared with siblings and other children?
  — Any problems with micturition, such as dribbling or weak stream?
  — Polyuria or polydipsia?
  — Daytime or nighttime enuresis?
- Does any family member have
  — Any kidney diseases (including hematuria, proteinuria, kidney cysts, urinary tract infections) or have they undergone any urology surgery?
  — Need of dialysis or kidney transplantation?
  — History of ear/hearing or eye abnormalities?

---

present with numerous red blood cells, white blood cells, proteinuria, and a variety of casts in the urine. In cases of proteinuria, quantified excretion should be estimated by a protein-creatinine ratio in a spot urine sample. A ratio greater than 0.2 is abnormal and is well correlated with urinary protein excretion greater than 4 mg/m^2/h in a 24-hour urine collection. In nephrotic syndrome, the proteinuria is usually greater than 40 mg/m^2/h. Immunologic studies including C_3, C_4, antinuclear antibody, and anti–double-stranded DNA should be obtained if the renal disease suggests the presence of an immune complex–mediated nephritis (eg, systemic lupus erythematosus, post-infectious glomerulonephritis, or membranoproliferative glomerulonephritis).

Imaging Studies

Ultrasound is by far one of the best radiographic tools in the assessment of patients with CKD. Renal ultrasound yields important information (eg, kidney size, echogenicity, presence of hydronephrosis or stones) that may help establish the diagnosis of the renal disease. The presence of small kidneys usually indicates chronic disease that may date back to fetal development. Increased echogenicity with normal kidney size indicates the presence of medical renal disease in more than 90% of cases.

A **voiding cystourethrogram** (VCUG) is indicated in patients with recurrent UTIs in order to diagnose vesicoureteral reflux and evaluate the anatomy of the upper urinary tract. The use of the spiral CT scan in the evaluation of patients with renal failure has increased

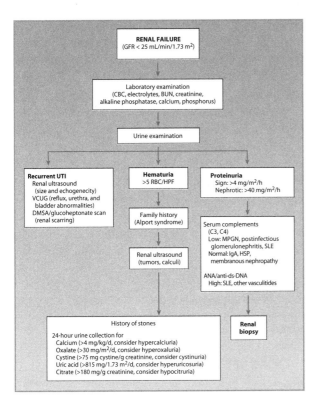

RENAL FAILURE
(GFR < 25 mL/min/1.73 m²)

↓

Laboratory examination
(CBC, electrolytes, BUN, creatinine,
alkaline phosphatase, calcium, phosphorus)

↓

Urine examination

Recurrent UTI
Renal ultrasound
(size and echogenecity)
VCUG (reflux, urethra, and
bladder abnormalities)
DMSA/glucoheptonate scan
(renal scarring)

Hematuria
>5 RBC/HPF

Family history
(Alport syndrome)

Renal ultrasound
(tumors, calculi)

Proteinuria
Sign: >4 mg/m²/h
Nephrotic: >40 mg/m²/h

Serum complements
(C3, C4)
Low: MPGN, postinfectious
glomerulonephritis, SLE
Normal: IgA, HSP,
membranous nephropathy

ANA/anti-ds-DNA
High: SLE, other vasculitides

History of stones
24-hour urine collection for
Calcium (>4 mg/kg/d, consider hypercalciuria)
Oxalate (>30 mg/m²/d, consider hyperoxaluria)
Cystine (>75 mg cystine/g creatinine, consider cystinuria)
Uric acid (>815 mg/1.73 m²/d, consider hyperuricosuria)
Citrate (>180 mg/g creatinine, consider hypocitruria)

Renal biopsy

Figure 128-1. Initial diagnostic workup of a pediatric patient with chronic renal failure. Abbreviations: GFR, glomerular filtration rate; CBC, complete blood count; BUN, blood urea nitrogen; UTI, urinary tract infection; VCUG, voiding cystourethrogram; DMSA, dimercaptosuccinic acid; RBC, red blood cell; HPF, high-power field; MPGN, membranoproliferative glomerulonephritis; SLE, systemic lupus erythematosus; IgA, immunoglobulin A; HSP, Henoch-Schönlein purpura; ANA, antinuclear antibodies; ds, double-stranded.

over the last few years. This procedure requires relatively less time than the standard CT scan and can be used to evaluate the kidney parenchyma, and the upper and lower urinary tract.

Nuclear imaging of the kidneys has provided vital information in the workup of children with CKD. In general, nuclear studies are not routinely done unless specifically indicated. Measurement of the GFR may be helpful, although it does not have a significant impact on the long-term management of children with chronic renal failure. Glomerular filtration rate measurements can be performed using technetium (Tc)-99m-DTP, which yields an estimate of the GFR within 5% of the true value. In some centers, the newer Tc-99m-MAG3 is being used to evaluate the renal plasma flow, whereas Tc-99m-DMSA is currently done to assess renal parenchymal involvement in both acute pyelonephritis and recurrent UTIs. This nuclear imaging study provides an excellent image of the renal parenchyma, and is frequently used in the detection of renal scars in patients with recurrent UTIs. Significant renal parenchymal scars portend the development of hypertension later in life.

Management

The management of children with CKD has markedly improved over the last 2 decades. Newer modes of treatment and early intervention have made great improvements in the lifestyles and psychological well-being of affected children. These patients must be managed by a multidisciplinary team involving the primary care physician and nephrologists, nurses, social services, nutritionists, and psychologists. Such management includes treatment of the primary disease and comorbid conditions, optimizing growth, slowing the progression and preserving residual renal function, preventing CVD, and preparing for renal replacement therapy and renal transplantation as CKD progresses. Available measures to retard the progression toward ESRD and cardiovascular mortality include strict control of hypertension; prevention of obesity; control of proteinuria with ACE inhibitors or ARB administration; maintaining normal levels of serum calcium/phosphorus/PTH; and prompt control of infections, anemia, and hyperlipidemia.

Dietary management remains an important and challenging part in the overall management of children with CKD. Frequently, these children are anorectic and require supplementation with fat, carbohydrates, and protein. Some patients, especially younger children, may require enteral feeding by nasogastric or gastrostomy tube in order to meet their daily nutritional requirements. Children with CKD should receive the recommended daily allowance for protein and calories according to age and gender; adjustments need to be made depending on weight gain. Protein restriction is not advised; studies have shown that restriction of protein intake does not retard the progression of renal failure in these patients. In patients with hypertension, appropriate salt intake must be given. Infants and children with congenitally obstructed and dysplastic kidneys often have polyuria, salt wasting, and acidosis. Sodium chloride or sodium bicarbonate must be administered to these children, and their required daily fluid intake may be higher to maintain normal intravascular volume.

Recombinant human growth hormone therapy has improved the management of growth retardation in children with CKD. It is indicated when despite correction of anemia, PTH, metabolic acidosis, and adequate caloric intake, the height is less than 2 SDs below that expected for age and gender. The response to treatment is better if initiated before dialysis. Response during the first year correlates with final height. Growth hormone administration is continued until the patient reaches the 50th percentile for mid-parental height or renal transplant is achieved. The use of recombinant human erythropoietin in the anemia associated with CKD has become a standard of treatment. The correction of anemia results in improved appetite, increased physical activity and, more importantly, avoidance of the risks associated with blood transfusion. Prior to the availability of erythropoietin, most patients received frequent blood transfusions, increasing their risks of infection, transfusion reaction, and development of antibodies. The goal is to keep the hemoglobin between

11 to 12 g/dL. Iron stores are assessed by transferrin saturation and ferritin levels and should be maintained between 20% to 50% and 200 to 800 ng/mL respectively.

Most children with CKD do not become hyperkalemic unless their renal function falls below 10 mL/min/1.73 m². Initially dietary intervention may be sufficient, but this is difficult in infants and small children whose diet is limited to formula and only a few solid foods. Pharmacologic interventions (eg, diuretics, polystyrene sulfone) are used to manage hyperkalemia in these children. In situations where there is an acute rise in serum potassium level, emergent measures must be implemented (Box 128-2). Intravenous and inhaled β₂-agonists (eg, albuterol) acutely decrease serum potassium level by facilitating intracellular potassium uptake. If hyperkalemia is unresponsive to conservative medical measures, dialysis must be performed immediately.

Box 128-2. Treatment of Hyperkalemia

- Calcium gluconate, 0.5 mL/kg of 10% solution, or calcium chloride, 0.2 mL/kg of 10% solution (intravenous [IV])
- Sodium bicarbonate, 2 mEq/kg/dose (IV)
- Glucose-insulin solution, 0.5 g/kg glucose with 0.25 U of insulin per gram of glucose (IV, monitor serum glucose closely)
- Diuretics (loop diuretics; do not use potassium-sparing diuretics): furosemide, 1 mg/kg/dose (IV)
- Polystyrene sulfonate (Kayexalate), 1 g/kg/dose orally (if awake) or rectally (do not use in patients with any gastrointestinal problems or anomalies)
- Dialysis (if hyperkalemia persists despite the above measures)

The use of a **diuretic** may be indicated in cases of fluid overload and hyperkalemia (potassium-sparing diuretics such as spironolactone should not be used). Diuretic therapy should not be used in patients with disturbed concentrating and diluting mechanisms because some of these children may have polyuria and develop dehydration on diuretic therapy.

For chronic management, antihypertensive medications should be started in children if blood pressure levels are above age-matched controls and after failure of conservative therapy, such as dietary changes. Drugs currently used to treat hypertension in children with CKD include ACE inhibitors, diuretics, adrenergic blockers, peripheral vasodilators, and calcium channel blockers. As mentioned previously, treatment with ACE inhibitors has been shown to be beneficial in reducing the degree of proteinuria and, thus, decreasing the associated hyperfiltration and tubulointerstitial fibrosis associated with hyperfiltration. Caution must be exercised when ACE inhibitors are used in patients with a solitary kidney and in those with renal artery stenosis because these medications can acutely decrease kidney function and precipitate hyperkalemia in patients with renal failure. Sexually active adolescent females must be informed about the adverse effects of ACE inhibitors in pregnancy, including renal agenesis in the fetus. Calcium channel blockers, especially nifedipine, have been used in cases of severe

hypertension because of their rapid onset of action. However, great caution must be exercised because blood pressure may acutely decline in these patients. For patients with poor adherence to daily oral medications, clonidine is currently available in the form of transdermal patches. However, patients should be warned of rebound hypertension and central nervous system side effects if the patch is removed abruptly. Patients with long-standing hypertension must have regular ECGs to evaluate left ventricular hypertrophy, and serial ophthalmologic examinations to follow eye-ground changes. If hypertension is secondary to fluid overload and salt retention, aggressive fluid removal with diuretic therapy should be added. Pericarditis, however, is usually a manifestation of severe uremia and may require pericardiocentesis. In some instances, the lack of response to medical management may be used as an additional criterion for the initiation of dialysis therapy (Box 128-3).

Box 128-3. Indications for Initiation of Dialysis

Severe fluid overload
- Congestive heart failure
- Uncontrollable hypertension

Uremic neuropathy
- Paresthesia

Electrolyte abnormalities unresponsive to medical management
- Intractable metabolic acidosis
- Hyperkalemia

Pericarditis

Severe renal osteodystrophy
- Extra-skeletal calcification
- Severe skeletal deformities

Progressive malnutrition and severe growth retardation, especially in the first year of life

Severe anemia or bleeding diathesis

There is increasing concern regarding the management of **lipid disturbances** due to their role in the progression of CKD. At present, no recommendations have been made about the use of lipid-lowering agents in children with hypercholesterolemia and hypertriglyceridemia because of reported liver and muscle toxicity associated with some of these medications. Further studies are warranted to test the efficacy and safety of these medications in the pediatric population.

For the management of renal osteodystrophy, dietary phosphorus restriction (ie, <800 mg/dL) is reinforced in children with CKD but generally is not well followed because of unpalatability of food. As such, calcium-containing phosphate-binding medications have become integral in the management of these patients. Aluminum-containing phosphate-binding agents are infrequently used today because of the risk of aluminum toxicity. Precautions must be taken in children who are concomitantly treated with citrate-containing medications (eg, sodium citrate) because citrate enhances the absorption of aluminum and, thus, enhances the risk for aluminum intoxication. Recent developments in the understanding of the interaction between vitamin D, PTH, and the calcium sensing receptor have led to novel treatment modalities for patients with CKD. Vitamin D, in the form of calcitriol, alfacalcidol, and doxercalciferol, has been used in the treatment of children with CKD. Earlier studies with vitamin D therapy demonstrated increases in linear growth in children with CKD; however, recent studies have not shown the same findings. In addition, concerns about a more rapid deterioration of renal function have also been addressed in these patients. To avoid these complications, certain biochemical markers including calcium, phosphorus, alkaline phosphatase, and PTH levels (intact assay) must be followed closely in any child being treated with any vitamin D preparation and calcium-containing salts. The use of large doses of calcium-based binders has been found to be associated with increased risk for vascular calcifications. Thus calcium- and metal-free phosphate binders, such as sevelamer HCL, have been shown to be effective phosphate binders in children treated with dialysis. Such compounds have not been used in pediatric patients with CKD prior to dialysis.

Children with CKD and their siblings and household contacts should receive all of the standard vaccines including varicella, influenza, and *Streptococcus pneumoniae*. Patients on immunosuppressive treatment due to glomerulonephritis or after transplant should not receive live virus vaccines. Every attempt to administer live virus vaccines such as measles, mumps, and rubella and varicella should be done before transplantation. Because children with CKD have a decreased ability to mount an immunologic response, repeated vaccination in order to induce protective serum antibody titers may be needed in dialyzed patients.

Review of all medications should be performed at every visit in order to adjust the dosages according to kidney function, detect possible adverse effects on the progression of the disease, and identify any drug interaction. Monitoring therapeutic dosage may be desirable when using antibiotics, anticonvulsants, digoxin, theophylline, and anticoagulants. In patients with reduced GFR, maintenance doses can be adjusted by increasing the interval between doses, reducing the individual dose, or both. Special care should be taken when using antibiotics such as aminoglycosides and vancomycin, as well as nonsteroidal anti-inflammatory drugs, because of possible detrimental effects on residual kidney function.

Prognosis

The prognosis of children with CKD has changed in the last 2 decades. Options for dialysis (hemodialysis or peritoneal dialysis) and kidney transplantation (deceased or living-related donor) must be discussed prior to occurrence of ESRD. Technical advances in dialysis allow the pediatric nephrologists to offer dialysis options to children of any age and have made long-term survival possible while children await renal transplantation.

Kidney transplantation is the ultimate treatment for children with CKD. Improvements in immunosuppressive medications and availability of other therapeutic strategies have considerably increased patient and graft survival after kidney transplantation. Full rehabilitation should be achieved after these children have undergone successful renal transplantation.

CASE RESOLUTION

The patient at the beginning of this chapter presents with a glomerular filtration rate of 40 mL/min/1.73 m² estimated by the Schwartz formula. The initial evaluation reveals hematocrit 28% (normal 36–48), a low serum bicarbonate (17 mEq/L, normal 22–26), hypocalcemia (8 mg/dL, normal 8.6–10), hyperphosphatemia (7 mg/dL, normal 2.7–4.5), and elevated parathyroid hormone (PTH) 700 pg/mL (normal 10–65). Diagnostic workup shows bilateral ureteral reflux on the voiding cystourethrogram. Small size and increased echogenicity of both kidneys are found on ultrasonography. Management of the primary disease is started with antibiotic prophylaxis to prevent further urinary tract infections, and the patient is referred to pediatric urology. Measures to slow the progression to end-stage renal disease are initiated involving dietary intervention and treatment of comorbid conditions, including bicarbonate for metabolic acidosis, iron and recombinant human erythropoietin for anemia, and calcium carbonate as a phosphate binder/calcium supplement. The hypertension associated with proteinuria is best treated with an angiotensin-converting enzyme inhibitor. Growth hormone will be considered once the acidosis, PTH, and anemia are corrected. Immunizations are up to date. An appointment with the pediatric nephrology team is scheduled.

Selected References

Boydstun II. Chronic kidney disease in adolescents. *Adolesc Med Clin.* 2005;16:185–199

Chan JC, McEnery PT, Chinchilli VM, et al. A prospective, double-blind study of growth failure in children with chronic renal insufficiency and the effectiveness of treatment with calcitriol versus dihydrotachysterol. The Growth Failure in Children with Renal Disease Investigators. *J Pediatr.* 1994;124:520–528

Daschner M. Drug dosage in children with reduced renal function. *Pediatr Nephrol.* 2005;20:1675–1686

Fine RN, Kohaut E, Brown D, Kuntze J, Attie KM. Long-term treatment of growth retarded children with chronic renal insufficiency, with recombinant human growth hormone. *Kidney Int.* 1996;49:781–785

Haffner D, Wuhl E, Schaefer F, Nissel R, Tonshoff B, Mehls O. Factors predictive of the short- and long-term efficacy of growth hormone treatment in prepubertal children with chronic renal failure. The German Study Group for Growth Hormone Treatment in Chronic Renal Failure. *J Am Soc Nephrol.* 1998;9:1899–1907

Hogg RJ, Furth S, Lemley KV, et al. National Kidney Foundation's Kidney Disease Outcomes Quality Initiative clinical practice guidelines for chronic kidney disease in children and adolescents: evaluation, classification, and stratification. *Pediatrics.* 2003;111:1416–1421

Ismail N. Use of erythropoietin, active vitamin D3 metabolites, and alkali agents in predialysis patients. *Am J Kidney Dis.* 1997;17:270–284

Kuizon BD, Salusky IB. Growth retardation in children with chronic renal failure. *J Bone Miner Res.* 1999;14:1680–1690

Neuhaus TJ. Immunization in children with chronic renal failure: a practical approach. *Pediatr Nephrol.* 2004;19:1334–1339

Sanchez CP, Goodman WG, Salusky IB. Prevention of renal osteodystrophy in predialysis patients. *Am J Med Sci.* 1999;317:398–404

Sedman A, Friedman A, Boineau F, Strife CF, Fine R. Nutritional management of the child with mild to moderate chronic renal failure. *J Pediatr.* 1996;129:S13–S18

Diabetes Mellitus

Jennifer K. Yee, MD, and Catherine S. Mao, MD

CASE STUDY

A 7-year-old girl presents with a 3-week history of nocturnal polyuria. Her mother reports that her daughter seems to have lost weight in the past 2 months although she has had a good appetite. Laboratory tests reveal that the girl's serum sodium level is 130 mEq/L; potassium, 3.2 mEq/L; glucose, 324 mg/dL; and 1+ ketones. Urinalysis reveals specific gravity of 1.025 and moderate glucose and ketones. Her height and weight are slightly below normal for her age, and the remainder of her physical examination is unremarkable.

Questions

1. What is the pathophysiology of type 1 and type 2 diabetes?
2. What are diagnostic criteria for differentiating type 1 and type 2 diabetes?
3. What are the objectives of therapeutic interventions in children with diabetes?
4. What diagnostic evaluations are used in the ongoing management of diabetes?
5. What are the acute and chronic complications associated with diabetes?
6. What is the role of "tight glycemic control" in children and adolescents?

Diabetes mellitus is the second most common chronic illness after asthma among children in developed countries. Diabetes mellitus is a metabolic imbalance that results from insulin deficiency, impairment of insulin action, or both. Advancement in the knowledge about the pathophysiology supports the assessment that diabetes is a heterogeneous disease involving immunologic, environmental, and genetic factors. This has led to a categorization of diabetes based on its pathophysiology rather than the therapeutic intervention. Diabetes associated with absolute insulin deficiency and impaired beta cell function is called **type 1** (previously juvenile onset or insulin-dependent), and diabetes associated with insulin resistance as well as impaired beta cell function is called **type 2** (previously adult-onset or non–insulin-dependent).

Epidemiology

In the past more than 97% of children with diabetes presented with type 1 diabetes mellitus (DM1), with an overall incidence of 18 in 100,000 cases per year. Recently, 2 population-based studies showed a dramatic increase in the number of older children and adolescents presenting with type 2 diabetes mellitus (DM2). One study reviewed newly diagnosed cases of diabetes over a 12-year period and found that DM2 made up 4% of such cases before 1992, and 16% in 1994 in one midwestern metropolitan area. Among adolescents, the relative incidence of DM2 increased from 3% to 10% before 1992 to 33% in 1994. By 1999 the proportion of diabetes in children and adolescents attributed to DM2 ranged from 8% to 45% depending on the geographic location. In addition, the populations affected by DM1 and DM2 seem to differ. Type 1 diabetes mellitus is seen equally among girls and boys, with the highest incidence among white youth. Type 2 diabetes mellitus is more prevalent among girls and has the highest incidence among African American, Mexican American, and Native American populations. The peak age of presentation for DM1 is between 5 and 15 years of age. Less is known about DM2 in children, but previous studies show a mean age of 13.8 years at presentation.

Clinical Presentation

Children can vary in their clinical presentation from being asymptomatic to having fulminate metabolic imbalance (Dx Box). Type 1 diabetes mellitus commonly presents with a classic triad of polydipsia, polyuria, and polyphagia. The most consistent presenting complaint is increased urinary frequency, manifested as nighttime polyuria or secondary enuresis. Alterations in appetite and thirst are most commonly recognized when disease onset occurs in the preschool years (probably because parents are most able to monitor eating and drinking behaviors during the first few years of life).

Dx Diabetes Mellitus

- Symptoms (polydipsia, polyuria, and polyphagia) together with a random plasma glucose higher than 200 mg/dL
- Fasting blood glucose higher than 126 mg/dL (confirmed on a subsequent day)
- Oral glucose tolerance test with 2-hour peak plasma glucose higher than 200 mg/dL

Weight loss can be variable but is more common in DM1 than DM2. Diabetic ketoacidosis (DKA) occurs at the time of initial presentation up to 45% in DM1 and 14% in DM2, and presents with vomiting, polyuria, dehydration, and Kussmaul respirations. Children and adolescents with DM2 also report having the classic triad of symptoms, but are often identified through screening urinalysis. Type 2 diabetes mellitus is highly associated with obesity (body mass index ≥85th percentile [see Chapter 122]), acanthosis nigricans, and having a first-degree relative with DM2.

Pathophysiology

Type 1 diabetes mellitus affects patients with an absolute insulin deficiency due to autoimmune destruction of the beta cells of the pancreas. The disease process is thought to be triggered by an environmental factor such as a virus or toxin in genetically susceptible individuals. The exposure occurs in early childhood, but disease progression can be variable. More than 90% of affected individuals carry either human leukocyte antigen (HLA) DR3 or DR4. Discordance of disease among twins supports the theory that DM1 involves an environmental exposure in genetically susceptible individuals. Twin studies show evidence of a preclinical autoimmune process, which also has predictive value in identifying susceptible individuals at risk for developing DM1. Immune changes include an increase in activated T-cells expressing HLA-DR, islet cell antibodies (ICA), insulin autoantibodies, and glutamic acid decarboxylase antibodies (Table 129-1).

Table 129-1. Predictive Tests for Individuals Susceptible to Type 1 Diabetes[a]	
Immunologic Marker(s)	*Risk of Developing Type 1 Diabetes (Within 5–8 y)*
Islet cell antibodies (ICA)	25%–70%
Insulin autoantibodies (IAA)	Variable (may not be specific to islet cell tissue)
Reduced first-phase insulin release	100%
ICA and IAA	90%
Human leukocyte antigen with index case	25%–30%

[a]Individuals with first-degree relative with type 1 diabetes.

Disordered immune function, in which some antigenic components of pancreatic islet cells are not recognized as self, seems to be the pathogenic mechanism for the development of DM1. It is generally believed that at least 90% of beta cell mass must be destroyed before problems with glycemic regulation are manifest. Endogenous insulin deficiency, occurring as a natural consequence of islet cell destruction, results in the inappropriate use of carbohydrate. Cellular uptake of glucose by liver, muscle, and adipose tissue is blocked. Synthesis of glycogen, protein, and fat is reduced, and a catabolic state marked by lipolysis, proteolysis, and ketone body formation

ensues. Increased serum glucose and ketones present an overwhelming osmotic load to the kidneys, resulting in urinary losses of volume and cations (Na^+, K^+, NH_4).

The autoimmune phenomena described previously are not evident in DM2 as demonstrated by the absence of ICAs. This disease, which is characterized by resistance to insulin, may assume different presentations in childhood. The more traditional form of DM2 presents in older children and adolescents and is highly associated with obesity and having a first-degree relative with DM2.

Differential Diagnosis

The diagnosis is usually straightforward given the symptomatology, except in children who present at a very young age. Although the onset of diabetes is rare before 1 year of age, the disease does occur but with nonspecific symptoms (eg, irritability, vomiting, tachypnea, and poor weight gain). Chemotherapeutic agents (eg, L-asparaginase) and a variety of medications (eg, corticosteroids, diuretics, oral contraceptives, diphenylhydantoin, epinephrine) may induce glucose intolerance. Glycosuria without evidence of ketosis or elevated blood glucose occurs in certain renal conditions (eg, Fanconi syndrome, carbohydrate malabsorption syndromes, heavy metal intoxication). Transient hyperglycemia, with or without glycosuria, may occur in response to physiological stress (eg, burns, trauma, hyperosmolar dehydration). In most of these cases, glucose regulation returns to normal within several days.

Evaluation

Evaluation should focus both on the diagnosis of diabetes (hyperglycemia) and the category because DM1 or DM2 can have different treatment modalities and disease courses.

History

The history should focus both on classic symptomatology and whether there is a family history of diabetes. Up to 80% of youth with DM2 will report a positive family history of diabetes, compared with 20% of youth with DM1. In addition, exogenous causes of diabetes should be ruled out. Obtaining a history of viral infections or chemical exposures during early childhood may be useful (Questions Box).

Questions

Insulin-Dependent Diabetes Mellitus

- Is the child having increased urination (eg, nighttime urination, unusual bed-wetting)?
- Is the child drinking or eating more than usual?
- Has the child experienced any weight loss?
- Has the child been taking or had access to any kind of medications (eg, corticosteroids, L-asparaginase, diuretics ["water pills"], birth control pills)?
- Are there any family members with diabetes (first- or second-degree relatives)?

Physical Examination

Growth parameters should be measured and plotted on standard growth curves. Obesity is present in 96% of DM2 youth, compared with 24% of DM1 youth. Even when obese, patients with diabetes may lose weight at the time of presentation. Youth with uncomplicated DM1 may have an unrevealing physical examination, while those with DM2 may have physical findings associated with obesity. One study demonstrated that 60% of adolescents with DM2 had acanthosis nigricans and 32% had hypertension at presentation. An intercurrent infection may trigger the symptomatology and should always be sought in cases of ketoacidosis. Children who present with ketoacidosis may have evidence of vomiting, dehydration, Kussmaul respirations and, in severe cases, altered mental status.

Laboratory Tests

Initial laboratory tests should include evaluation of the serum and urine for glucose and ketones. For patients presenting in DKA, evaluation should also include a full chemistry panel to assess for metabolic acidosis, hypokalemia, and serum osmolality. Once the diagnosis of diabetes is suspected, further testing can assist in categorizing the type of diabetes. Tests include insulin levels and C-peptide (a marker of insulin levels) levels. Both insulin and C-peptide levels are usually higher in patients with DM2 because they have insulin resistance rather than an absolute insulin deficiency. Insulin reserve can be measured by determining the basal and stimulated levels of C-peptide (>0.6 ng/mL basal level, >1.5 ng/mL 90 minutes after nutritional supplement such as Sustacal). In categorizing diabetes, it is important to note that some with DM1 can have insulin reserves up to 2 years after diagnosis.

Oral glucose tolerance tests may be necessary to confirm the diagnosis of diabetes in cases in which the onset of symptoms is not obvious. Two-hour postprandial values in excess of 200 mg/dL or fasting glucose of 126 mg/dL or higher are evidence of diabetes. The introduction of the intravenous glucose tolerance test with measurement of first-phase insulin release has allowed early diagnosis of individuals at risk for the disease prior to development of symptoms.

To assess children who are at risk for DM2, screening may be done every 2 years starting at age 10 years or at the onset of puberty (whichever comes first) and may be done using fasting plasma glucose (as recommended by the American Diabetes Association) and/or by oral glucose tolerance test (as recommended by the World Health Organization). The children who should be screened are those who meet criteria for obesity and have 2 or more of the following risk factors: family history of DM2 in first- or second-degree relatives, at-risk race/ethnicity (African American, Asian/Pacific Islander, Native American, Hispanic), or associated signs and symptoms of insulin resistance (acanthosis nigricans, dyslipidemia, hypertension, polycystic ovarian syndrome).

Management

Early diagnosis together with a comprehensive program of education and aggressive management are essential to prevent acute and long-term complications. Long-term objectives of therapeutic intervention in children with diabetes are (1) to facilitate normal physical growth and psychological and sexual maturation, (2) to promote normoglycemia through regulation of glucose metabolism, (3) to prevent acute complications (ie, hypoglycemia, ketoacidosis), (4) to prevent or delay long-term sequelae, and (5) to accommodate physiological changes that alter therapeutic needs (eg, exercise, adolescence, intercurrent illness).

Effective management requires a multidisciplinary team of professionals skilled in handling the myriad issues that arise for families and children with diabetes. Most clinics specializing in the care of children with diabetes include a nurse educator, dietitian, social worker, psychologist or counselor, and a pediatric endocrinologist. In settings where such special care centers are available, the primary care physician serves as a key adjunct, underscoring the importance of ongoing patient-family involvement in disease management and ensuring optimal growth, development, and nutrition. In the absence of special care centers, the primary care physician assumes responsibility for all aspects of management, including the treatment of acute complications, monitoring compliance and control, and surveillance for long-term complications.

Effective therapeutic intervention is based on individual needs for energy, insulin, and exercise. A number of factors, including physical growth, insulin requirement, glycemic control, and activity level, influence those needs and must be assessed on a regular basis. For DM1, insulin therapy is the mainstay of management, whereas DM2 therapeutic options include weight control through diet and exercise (see Chapter 122), oral hypoglycemic agents, and insulin. Oral hypoglycemic agents can lower blood glucose by increasing insulin secretion, increasing insulin action, decreasing hepatic glucose output, or decreasing nutrient absorption. These agents include sulfonylureas and other insulin secretogogues, metformin, thiazolidinediones, and acarbose. While DM2 may initially be managed with exogenous insulin, metformin is the oral agent prescribed most often for DM2 in children and adolescents. A newer class of medication acts by an incretin effect and increases glucose-dependent insulin secretion. These medications include exenatide (administered by injection) and a drug that inhibits dipeptidyl-peptidase-4, thereby prolonging the effect of endogenous insulin release after a meal. Similar to most drugs for the treatment of DM2, these newer drugs do not have a pediatric indication.

Insulin

The purpose of insulin therapy is to enable children to approach normoglycemia in response to adequate amounts of food, insulin, and exercise. The amount of daily insulin required is dependent on the child's age, weight, and development. On average for DM1, children younger than 5 years require 0.6 to 0.8 U/kg, children between 5 to 11 years of age require 0.75 to 0.9 U/kg, and 12- to 18-year-olds require 0.8 to 1.5 U/kg in a 24-hour period. Within 3 to 4 months of diagnosis, most individuals experience a partial remission, or "honeymoon" phase, during which time their insulin requirements decline dramatically. Conversely, illness, anxiety, and adolescence (ie, pubertal changes) may cause the insulin requirement to increase. Even under conditions of increased need, reported daily insulin dosages in excess of 2 U/kg of body weight should stimulate investigations into patient compliance.

A number of insulin regimens currently in use take advantage of the variable onset of action of the different insulin preparations (Table 129-2). The new insulin analogs are monomers of insulin rather than insulin aggregates. They provide a rapid onset and a shorter duration of action. This allows for easier adjustment of insulin dose depending on the child's appetite because the injection can be given immediately before the meal. Children with newly diagnosed diabetes should use semisynthetic or recombinant human insulin preparations to minimize the possibility of allergic reactions. Any change in insulin preparation should be undertaken cautiously and only under medical supervision because brands vary in strength, purity, and glycemic response.

Morning hyperglycemia may result from 1 of 2 phenomena, which must be distinguished because the appropriate therapeutic responses are opposite. The **dawn phenomenon** probably involves a nocturnal surge of growth hormone, resulting in hyperglycemia that is present during the night (2–4 am) and is sustained until morning. The treatment involves increasing the evening dose of intermediate-acting insulin. In the **Somogyi phenomenon,** morning glucose is high as a physiological response to nighttime hypoglycemia. Treatment of this condition requires decreasing the evening intermediate-acting insulin or increasing the carbohydrate content of a bedtime snack.

Adolescents require special consideration. The sexual maturation

Table 129-2. Commonly Used Insulin Preparations[a]

Type	Onset of Action	Duration of Effect
Short-acting		
Insulin analog: lispro, aspart	15–20 min	2–4 h
Regular	30 min	5–12 h
Intermediate-acting (zinc or protamine)		
Neutral protamine Hagedorn	1.5–2.5 h	18–24 h
Long-acting		
Glargine	70 min	22–24 h
Detemir	1.5–2.5 h	20–24 h

[a]Twice-daily injections: Two-thirds of the total daily dose before breakfast made up of intermediate- and short-acting insulin in 2:1 ratio. One-third before dinner made up of intermediate- and short-acting insulin in 1:1 ratio.

Basal bolus: Intermediate-/long-acting insulin at bedtime with regular insulin or short-acting insulin analog before each meal.

process occurs in the setting of relative insulin resistance, other hormonal alterations, and a burden of developmental tasks, which make glycemic control problematic at best. Daily insulin requirements may increase to 1.5 to 2 U/kg during adolescence, but return to prepubertal levels at the end of the teenage years. Particular efforts must be made to ensure physical and psychological growth in the context of these special tasks. Dietary manipulation and consideration of alternative (usually more intensive) insulin and monitoring regimens is critical for successful glycemic control during this challenging period.

External infusion pumps are not widely used in young children because of the danger of mechanical malfunction (leading to hypoglycemia or hyperglycemia). Their use may be considered, however, in children with unstable diabetes or severe, chronic, intercurrent illness.

Glucose Monitoring

Self-monitoring of glycemic response through the in-home assessment of blood glucose levels is critical to effective therapy. The introduction of reflectance meters (glucometers) has obviated the need for inaccurate, visually read strips of glucose-sensitive paper. Patients who are taking insulin should measure glucose 3 to 7 times daily. Most endocrinologists advocate testing before each meal and at bedtime during the first year after diagnosis. Testing may also be done at 2 am to test for hypoglycemia or hyperglycemia. Depending on the age of the child, an acceptable range for glycemic control is 80 to 150 mg/dL. Additional short-acting insulin may be given to correct for high blood glucose. Patients also need to monitor their urine for ketones whenever their blood glucose readings exceed 240 mg/dL.

Glycosylated hemoglobin (HbA_{1C}) measurements reflect glucose control over the preceding 2 to 3 months. The normal value is 4% to 6% of total hemoglobin. Glycosylated hemoglobin values less than 7% are excellent, between 7% to 8% are good, between 8% to 10% are average, and more than 10% are poor. The Diabetes Control and Complications Trial studied the effect of different levels of glycemic control on the complications of diabetes. Although the study only included pediatric patients 13 years or older, the study did show that patients with "tight glycemic control" had lower HbA_{1C} levels and fewer long-term complications than patients not tightly controlled. Adolescents with tight glycemic control had a greater risk of hypoglycemic events than the control group, a fact that must be taken into consideration in determining the ideal glycemic control for a child. In general, tight glycemic control is not recommended for children younger than 5 years; for older children, glycemic control should be individually tailored. Whenever children's routines undergo dramatic change, stepped-up home monitoring and medical consultation are advisable. Caution should be used in interpreting HbA_{1C} values in infants and others in whom fetal hemoglobin or other hemoglobin variants are present because these hemoglobin variants may falsely elevate or lower the value of HbA_{1C}. Although compliance with intensive regimens is an indisputable challenge (particularly as responsibility for management shifts from parent to child), increasing evidence underscores the importance of tight glycemic control.

Nutrition

The timing, amount, and types of foods eaten for meals and snacks should be relatively consistent from one day to the next to match the relative constancy of the exogenous insulin. Daily caloric requirements should be distributed in the following way: carbohydrate, 50% to 55% (<10% in the form of sucrose); protein, 20% to 25%; and fat, 25% to 30% (6%–8% polyunsaturated, <10% saturated). The distribution of these calories should be approximately 25% for breakfast, 25% for lunch, 30% for dinner, and 20% for snacks. Snacks are an important part of the nutrition regimen for children with diabetes. Most nutritionists recommend 3 snacks for young children (between meals and at bedtime) and 2 for older children. Some investigators promote the ingestion of cornstarch at bedtime as a means of stabilizing the serum glucose. Dietary discipline is a tremendous challenge for many children. Introducing one change at a time may make such dietary manipulations more acceptable over the long run. In addition, establishing healthy eating habits requires availability of healthy choices in the child's environment. Cooperation from the school and home enhances the likelihood of a child developing healthy eating practices.

Carbohydrate counting is an important part of matching insulin requirements to nutritional intake. For patients on multiple daily insulin injection schedules, there is flexibility in tailoring each dose of insulin based on the carbohydrate content of each meal or snack. For patients on twice-daily insulin injection regimens, consistent carbohydrate content of the meals and snacks is important in maintaining blood glucose levels. Learning carbohydrate counting takes time for the patient and families, and they need ongoing nutrition support to become familiar and comfortable with how different foods affect their blood glucose levels.

Exercise

Exercise contributes to glucose control by facilitating the use of glucose without the assistance of insulin. If not carefully undertaken on a regular basis, exercise can precipitate acute hypoglycemia. Physical activity enhances the body's sensitivity to insulin and can even decrease the daily insulin requirement. Thoughtful planning of exercise involves compensatory changes in food intake and insulin doses. For example, extra energy intake at bedtime may offset the nighttime hypoglycemia that accompanies late afternoon exercise. Seasonal physical activities may necessitate an adjustment in the insulin regimen at certain times of the year.

Education

The role of education is pivotal to the successful management of diabetes in childhood and throughout life. During childhood, educational efforts must be focused on the entire family unit. Affected children must be involved as early as possible and in ways that are developmentally appropriate. The process should involve the early introduction of basic survival information, such as insulin

therapy and management of complications. This can be followed by more detailed information, including strategies to reduce long-term sequelae.

Prognosis

Diabetic ketoacidosis is the major cause of morbidity and mortality in children and adolescents, followed by **hypoglycemia.** Clinical signs of hypoglycemia in older children include shakiness, blurred vision, and dysarthria. Concerns about the neurodevelopmental impact of hypoglycemia in young children have led to the recommendation of more liberal glycemic control in early onset disease. Diabetic ketoacidosis, precipitated by an intercurrent infection or poor compliance, is a metabolic derangement that always requires urgent medical attention and often necessitates hospitalization. Replacement of fluids, attention to electrolyte abnormalities, and insulin therapy are the mainstays of treatment in the face of this complication.

Long-term complications include **proliferative retinopathy, nephropathy, peripheral and autonomic neurologic impairment,** and **early onset of cardiovascular disease.** Ophthalmologic evaluation, overnight urine protein measurement, and a detailed neurologic examination should occur once or twice each year depending on the duration of disease. Intensive therapeutic intervention results in significant reduction in retinopathy, nephropathy, and cardiac and peripheral vascular disease. Preliminary evidence warrants consideration of such therapy with the expectation of benefit in long-term outcomes.

CASE RESOLUTION

The girl in the opening case history is admitted to the hospital to help determine appropriate insulin dosing. She and her family require ongoing education. Careful management is necessary to optimize normal growth and development as well as delay or prevent long-term sequelae.

Selected References

Fagot-Campagna A, Saaddine JB, Engelgau MM. Is testing children for type 2 diabetes a lost battle? *Diabetes Care.* 2000;23:1442–1443

Fellar LA, Schrader K, Nansel TR. Healthy eating practices: perceptions, facilitators, and barriers among youth with diabetes. *Diabetes Educ.* 2007;33:671–679

Hannon TS, Gunfor N, Arslanian S. Type 2 diabetes in children and adolescents: a review for the primary care provider. *Pediatr Ann.* 2006;35:880–887

Kaufman FR. Type 2 diabetes in children and youth. *Endocrinol Metab Clin North Am.* 2005;34:659–676

Leslie RDG, Elliott RB. Early environmental events as a cause of IDDM: evidence and implications. *Diabetes.* 1994;43:843–850

Libman I, Arslanian S. Prevention and treatment of type 2 diabetes in youth. *Horm Res.* 2007;67:22–34

Pinhas-Hamiel O, Zeitler P. Acute and chronic complications of type 2 diabetes mellitus in children and adolescents. *Lancet.* 2007;369:1823–1831

Pinhas-Hamiel O, Zeitler P. The global spread of type 2 diabetes mellitus in children and adolescents. *J Pediatr.* 2005;146:693–700

Report of the Expert Committee on the Diagnosis and Classification of Diabetes Mellitus. *Diabetes Care.* 1997;20:1183–1197

Scott CR, Smith JM, Cradock MM, Pihoker C. Characteristics of youth-onset noninsulin-dependent diabetes mellitus and insulin-dependent diabetes mellitus at diagnosis. *Pediatrics.* 1997;100:84–91

Silverstein J, Klingensmith G, Copeland K, et al. Care of children and adolescents with type 1 diabetes: a statement of the American Diabetes Association. *Diabetes Care.* 2005;28:186–212

Tamborlane WV, Ahern J. Implications and results of the diabetes control and complications trial. *Pediatr Clin North Am.* 1997;44:285–300

Tamborlane WV, Bonfig W, Boland E. Recent advances in treatment of youth with type 1 diabetes: better care through technology. *Diabet Med.* 2001;18:864–870

Juvenile Idiopathic Arthritis/ Collagen Vascular Disease

Elizabeth A. Edgerton, MD, MPH

CASE STUDY

A 4-year-old girl is evaluated for pain in the legs and arms for 4 months' duration. Symptoms began with pain and swelling in the left elbow. Initially she was diagnosed with a bad sprain and was treated with a course of nonsteroidal anti-inflammatory drugs. The ankle improved, but it still caused occasional discomfort. About 2 months ago, the child was evaluated for painful knees and was diagnosed with growing pains. She has had no history of trauma, fevers, or rashes, but her activity level has decreased since the symptoms began. The mother has noted swelling in all 3 of the joints at one time or another but reports no redness. On physical examination the vital signs are normal. Both knees are swollen but not erythematous. Her range of motion in the knees and elbow is decreased.

Questions

1. What findings are indicative of juvenile idiopathic arthritis?
2. How can the clinical history and laboratory evaluation assist in determining the subtype of juvenile idiopathic arthritis?
3. What are the long-term outcomes for patients with juvenile idiopathic arthritis?
4. What similar clinical findings are present in other collagen vascular diseases?
5. What types of agents are used in the treatment of juvenile idiopathic arthritis?

Collagen is a protein that represents 30% of the body's protein and is glue-like, shaping the structure of tendons, bones, and connective tissues. Malfunctioning of the immune system can affect these structures and result in what is termed *collagen vascular disease*. Diseases categorized as collagen vascular diseases include juvenile idiopathic arthritis (JIA), systemic lupus erythematosus (SLE), dermatomyositis (DM), and scleroderma (SD). While primarily known as collagen vascular diseases, they are also considered a subset of connective tissue disorders with a prominent immune component referred to as diffuse connective tissue diseases. They are also included in the category of secondary vasculitides.

An abnormal autoimmune reaction is common to all of these disorders, and it is not until specific vascular damage within an organ system occurs that more characteristic symptoms allow for diagnosis. Furthermore, the prevalence of these disorders is difficult to determine since their symptoms may overlap and no diagnostic gold standard exists. Each disease, though, has characteristic clinical presentations and serologic findings that guide in diagnosis. Treatment usually requires the use of anti-inflammatory and immunosuppressive therapy. Morbidity and mortality are dependent on the level and duration of inflammation, the target organs affected, and secondary complications that may arise from treatment.

Epidemiology

In JIA the predominant symptom is chronic arthritis that presents in children younger than 16 years. Juvenile idiopathic arthritis is the most common pediatric rheumatologic disease and one of the more common chronic diseases of childhood. The estimated worldwide incidence is 0.8 to 22 per 100,000 and the prevalence is 7 to 400 per 100,000 children. It is most prevalent among non-Hispanic whites. The International League of Associations for Rheumatology (ILAR) system is used for classification of the disease. Based on presenting symptoms, serology, age, gender, race, and/or ethnicity, the disease is divided into the following subtypes: oligoarthritis, polyarthritis, systemic, enthesitis-related, and psoriatic arthritis in decreasing frequency. Clinically, symptoms may change over time leading to a reclassification of a patient's subtype of JIA.

The incidence of SLE varies greatly by gender and ethnicity, with females and Hispanics, African Americans, Native Americans, and individuals from Southeast and South Asia most commonly affected. For individuals with onset before the age of 19 years, the incidence is approximately 6 to 18.9 per 100,000 among white females, 20 to 30 per 100,000 among African Americans females, and 16 to 36.7 per 100,000 among Puerto Rican females. The male-female ratio varies from 1:4 to 1:7 depending on the ethnicity of the cohort. Five- and

10-year survival rates have improved to as high as 100% and 86% respectively among pediatric patients. Survival is impacted by organ involvement, with those with renal and central nervous system (CNS) involvement fairing worse.

The incidence of juvenile DM is 2.5 to 4.1 per million among children younger than 17 years. It is predominantly seen in white, non-Hispanic individuals (65%). Median age of presentation is 7 years of age, with girls affected more often. The clinical presentation and course of juvenile DM is less severe than of adult-onset DM.

Overall, the annual incidence of systemic SD is 0.45 to 1.9 per 100,000 with a prevalence of 15 to 24 per 100,000. Scleroderma is very rare in childhood, with fewer than 10% of all patients younger than 20 years. While the adult-onset disease has a strong female predominance, gender and age specifics have not been identified in the juvenile form. Localized SD is 10-fold more common than systemic SD based on data from rheumatology referrals. Few epidemiological studies exist, but the overall prevalence of localized SD is estimated to be 1 in 100,000.

Clinical Presentation

Collagen vascular diseases may present with a variety of symptoms including joint pain or swelling, skin rashes, kidney disease, or neuropsychiatric problems depending on the specific disorder.

Differential Diagnosis

The differential diagnosis of collagen vascular diseases includes JIA, SLE, DM, and SD.

Juvenile Idiopathic Arthritis

The diagnosis of JIA is based on the clinical symptoms during the first 6 months following presentation (Dx Box).

Dx **Juvenile Idiopathic Arthritis**

- Systemic: arthritis with daily fevers, rash, and general malaise
- Oligoarthritis: arthritis affecting 1 to 4 joints in the first 6 months
- Polyarthritis: arthritis affecting more than 5 joints in the first 6 months
- Enthesitis-related: arthritis and/or enthesitis and presence of human leukocyte antigen-B27
- Psoriatic: arthritis and psoriasis or arthritis and dactylitis, nail abnormalities, and family history of psoriasis

The ILAR system of classification defines the following subtypes: systemic, oligoarthritis (persistent and extended) polyarthritis rheumatoid factor positive and negative, enthesitis-related arthritis, psoriatic arthritis, and other. Each subtype has varying clinical symptoms and long-term complications.

The **systemic form** is present in 10% to 20% of patients with JIA and is associated with the greatest morbidity and mortality. This subtype lacks gender, age, or HLA association seen among other subtypes. It is characterized by fever, rash, lymphadenopathy, hepatosplenomegaly, and serositis. The arthritis may present with or separate from these other symptoms. Classically the fever peaks twice a day and is associated with an evanescent rash that consists of discrete salmon-colored macules seen predominantly on the trunk and proximal extremities. The arthritis is polyarticular, affecting both large and small joints, and is present within the first 6 months of symptoms.

Up to 37% of patients develop chronic disease with destructive arthritis while the others may experience disease remission. Predictors of poor prognosis are age younger than 6 years at diagnosis, disease duration of more than 5 years, and persistence of systemic symptoms requiring treatment. Overall mortality is 0.3% in North America. A rare but life-threatening complication is macrophage activation syndrome. Patients present with hepatosplenomegaly, lymphadenopathy, and purpura and may progress to multiorgan failure. Sedimentation rate is low in macrophage activation syndrome in contrast to elevated during a disease exacerbation. Treatment involves steroids and immunosuppressive therapy. Triggers to macrophage activation syndrome include viral infections and addition or change in medications such as nonsteroidal anti-inflammatory drugs, sulfasalazine, and etanercept.

Oligoarticular JIA is the most common form. Arthritis is present in fewer than 5 joints during the first 6 months of disease. Often the large joints of the lower extremities are affected, and children may present with single joint involvement. Oligoarticular JIA is divided into persistent and extended forms, the latter associated with more severe disease course. Extended oligoarticular JIA can only be diagnosed after the first 6 months of symptoms in which patients suffer involvement of greater than 5 joints. Individuals, especially girls, who are antinuclear antibody (ANA)–positive have an increased risk of uveitis (asymptomatic). The American Academy of Pediatrics suggests frequent screening examinations because the uveitis can result in significant ophthalmologic morbidity. Among individuals with persistent oligoarticular JIA, 75% report remission of disease while only 12% of those with extended subtype report remission, with the remaining continuing to suffer symptoms into adulthood.

Polyarticular JIA presents with involvement of 5 or more joints during the first 6 months of disease. Rheumatoid factor (RF) negative disease is the more common subtype and tends to present in early childhood while RF positive disease presents later. Rheumatoid factor positive patients are often adolescent girls with symmetrical small joint disease and characteristic subcutaneous nodules. The arthritis is erosive and results in boutonniere deformities (proximal interphalangeal joint flexion and distal interphalangeal joint hyperextension) and swan-neck deformities (proximal interphalangeal joint hyperextension and distal interphalangeal joint flexion). Uveitis is present in approximately 10% of patients.

Enthesitis-related arthritis is characterized by inflammation where tendons insert at the bone. It usually affects the axial and peripheral skeleton. This subtype includes patients with ankylosing spondylitis and reactive arthritis associated with inflammatory bowel disease. Ankylosing spondylitis generally affects boys 8 years or older. This subtype is RF and ANA negative. Extra-articular symptoms include anterior uveitis, which is acute and painful in contrast to uveitis seen in oligoarticular and polyarticular arthritis, which is more insidious in onset.

Psoriatic JIA occurs in patients with chronic arthritis and psoriasis or those who meet 2 of the following criteria: dactylitis, nail pitting or onycholysis, and family history of psoriasis. Peak onset is in middle childhood. The arthritis, which is asymmetrical, may present before the psoriatic rash, making the diagnosis difficult. Up to 17% of patients will have asymptomatic uveitis and require routine slit-lamp examinations for diagnosis.

Systemic Lupus Erythematosus

Diagnosis of SLE is based on both clinical and laboratory findings and exclusion of other autoimmune diseases. Most patients have at least 4 of 11 of the American College of Rheumatology Classification Criteria for SLE. Criteria can be present over any period together or in isolation. Median age of presentation among pediatric patients is approximately 12 years of age. Patients usually present with constitutional symptoms such as fever, fatigue, weight loss, and systemic inflammation as demonstrated by lymphadenopathy and hepatosplenomegaly. The most common organs affected are skin and musculoskeletal and renal systems and their level of involvement directs treatment decisions.

A predominant feature of SLE is the rash. **Mucocutaneous involvement** includes classical malar rash or butterfly rash that spares the nasolabial folds, photosensitivity, and discoid rash. Approximately 10% to 30% of patients will have painless oral and nasal ulcers. Most patients also have some level of **musculoskeletal involvement** that includes arthritis, arthralgia, or tenosynovitis. The arthritis is usually a symmetrical polyarthritis affecting both small and large joints. In contrast to JIA, this arthritis is usually non-erosive as demonstrated radiographically, but clinically appears more painful. Musculoskeletal pain can be secondary to treatment resulting in what is called pain amplification syndrome attributed to glucocorticoid therapy.

Neuropsychiatric manifestations affect 20% to 70% of patients with SLE. This variation is due to the difficulty of diagnosing the often vague and varied symptoms. Headache is the most common symptom and can be isolated or be part of a constellation of other neurologic symptoms. Headaches that are refractory to treatment may be secondary to active CNS vasculitis, increased intracranial pressure, or cerebral vein thrombosis. Elevated levels of lupus anticoagulant (LAC) are usually present with cerebral vein thrombosis and are an indication for emergent imaging. Psychosis manifested by visual and tactile hallucinations may be present in 30% to 50% of patients. Psychotic symptoms will usually present with other neurologic symptoms. Imaging studies of the CNS provide little assistance in diagnosis. When psychosis is in isolation, secondary effects of glucocorticoids need to be considered. More difficult to delineate is cognitive impairment, which may present as a broad range of symptoms ranging from confusion and difficulty concentrating to coma. Other less common neurologic symptoms include seizures, movement

disorders including chorea, and cranial nerve abnormalities.

Lupus nephritis is present in 29% to 80% of patients, with most presenting during the first year of diagnosis. In contrast, less than 10% of patients suffer from renal vasculitis. Prognosis for patients is based on the histologic classification of nephritis as established by the World Health Organization using renal biopsy (class I–V). Unfortunately, clinical markers (proteinuria, hematuria, creatinine level) may not correspond to histologic classifications, but when renal function is impaired patients have class III or IV disease. Hypertension is common along with lupus nephritis and, when present with peripheral edema, carries a worse prognosis. Overall survival for patients with renal involvement has improved. The 5-year survival for class IV is 88% to 93% and 10-year survival of 85%.

Hematologic manifestations including anemia, thrombocytopenia, and leukopenia may be present in 50% to 75% of patients. Patients have a normochromic normocytic anemia typical of anemia of chronic disease. Of patients who are Coombs positive, only 10% suffer significant hemolysis. Thrombocytopenia is present in 15% of patients. Patients with chronic autoimmune idiopathic thrombocytopenic purpura (AITP) with antinuclear antibodies have a greater risk of developing SLE, as do patients with Evan syndrome (AITP and Coombs positive anemia). Leukopenia is thought to represent a general marker of disease activity.

Cardiac manifestations of SLE most often affect the pericardium. Patients suffering from pericarditis complain of chest pain exacerbated by positional changes. Up to 50% of patients have Libman-Sacks endocarditis, which results in sterile verrucous vegetations, putting them at risk for subacute bacterial endocarditis. The major cardiac mortality associated with SLE is premature arthrosclerosis; this is attributed to the chronic inflammation.

Pleuropulmonary disease is seen in 25% to 75% of patients with SLE. Again the variation in prevalence is due to the lack of specificity of symptoms. Pleuritic chest pain secondary to effusion can be a presenting symptom. Abnormal pulmonary function tests are common among asymptomatic patients. Patients can suffer acute respiratory failure secondary to SLE or opportunistic infection. **Gastrointestinal (GI) symptoms** are difficult to distinguish from the disease process versus adverse side effects of treatment. Abdominal pain can be secondary to peritoneal inflammation (serositis), vasculitis, pancreatitis, malabsorption, pseudo-obstruction, paralytic ileus, or direct bowel involvement (enteritis). **Endocrine abnormalities** can also be the result of the disease process or adverse effects of treatment. Hypothyroidism is associated with the presence of antithyroid antibodies while diabetes is secondary to steroid use. Delayed puberty and menstrual abnormalities are a consequence of chronic disease. Female patients managed with cyclophosphamide can suffer secondary ovarian failure.

Serologic presence of **ANA** is universal among patients with SLE. These include anti-DNA (60%–70%), anti-RNA–binding proteins (70%–90%), anti-U1RNP and anti-SM antibodies (40%–50%). Anti-Ro and La antibodies (30%) are seen less frequently. Anticardiolipin (50%) and LAC (20%) are the most common antiphospholipid antibodies. The greatest risk of thrombosis is associated with LAC rather than with the other antiphospholipid antibodies.

Inflammatory Myopathies

Inflammatory myopathies are rare conditions in pediatrics but are discussed here because their symptoms overlap with other collagen vascular diseases. **Juvenile DM** is the most common myopathy presenting with rash and muscle weakness. It is a vasculopathy resulting from intimal proliferation of small blood vessels. Skin and muscle are the primary systems affected, but the vasculopathy can target any organ. **Juvenile polymyositis** is an idiopathic myositis without the dermatologic manifestations.

Patients present with proximal muscle weakness of the shoulders, hips, neck flexors, and abdominal musculature. Muscle tenderness and inflammation are less common. Patients can have both positive Gower (using one's hands to go from a supine to a standing position) and Trendelenburg (see Chapter 88) signs. Muscle weakness may also present with swallowing difficulties. When arthritis is present it is mild, transient, and non-erosive. As with other autoimmune diseases, fever, malaise, anorexia, and weight loss can be associated with disease activity.

Further diagnostic evaluation is essential in confirming the diagnosis of juvenile DM. Muscle biopsy may show necrosis, atrophy, or inflammatory exudates. Electromyogram may or may not be abnormal. Evaluation of muscle enzymes often shows an elevated creatinine phosphokinase, aldolase, and/or lactate dehydrogenase.

The clinical course is varied, and multiple organ systems can be affected. Patients develop dystrophic calcinosis on the extremities. Although a characteristic finding of DM, it is usually not present at the time of diagnosis. Lipodystrophy, a progressive and symmetrical loss of subcutaneous fat, affects approximately 14% to 25% of patients. Patients may suffer esophageal dysmotility and malabsorption. Vasculopathy of the GI tract may result in pain, bleeding, or perforation. One-third of patients may have respiratory weakness during their disease course, primarily following an asymptomatic restrictive pattern. Up to 78% of patients have decreased ventilatory capacity. Although rare, patients are at increased risk of aspiration secondary to pharyngeal muscle weakness and to pneumonia secondary to immunosuppressive therapy.

Rash is critical for the diagnosis of DM and can occur prior to or after the presentation of muscle weakness. The heliotrope eyelid rash and Gottron papules are pathognomonic for DM. Eyelid or facial edema may be present with the rash, which may also have a malar component that includes nasolabial folds, in contrast to systemic lupus. Gottron papules or collodion patches are flat-topped, violaceous or red papules that can be scaly. They are seen predominantly on the extremities (extensor aspect of knuckles, elbows, knees, and medial malleoli). Nail bed changes demonstrating vasculopathy are also present. Neurologic symptoms are rare, but may present as generalized tonic-clonic seizures. Unlike adult-onset DM, malignancy is uncommon in juvenile dermatomyositis.

Scleroderma

Juvenile SD is characterized by the presence of hard skin before age 16. Localized SD involves only the skin and related tissues while systemic SD is a multisystem autoimmune disorder.

In **systemic SD,** skin, musculoskeletal system, GI tract, lungs, and heart are the organs most commonly affected. While the skin and musculoskeletal systems are the most common among pediatric cases, disease complications of the cardiopulmonary system are associated with the greatest mortality.

The diagnosis of systemic SD is based on the presence of major criteria that include sclerosis and/or induration, sclerodactyly, or Raynaud phenomenon in addition to minor criteria of the targeted organ systems. Diagnosis is often delayed due to the slow onset of disease and the initial subtlety of symptoms. Characteristic presentation starts with Raynaud phenomenon with associated tightening, thinning, and atrophy of the skin overlying the hands and face. Cutaneous changes start with edema, followed by induration and finally sclerosis. The skin becomes tightened by contractures and atrophy, giving the appearance of being hard, waxy, and tight. There may be either hypopigmentation or hyperpigmentation, and deposits of calcium may appear in the subcutaneous skin.

Musculoskeletal symptoms are the next most common symptom among patients and usually occur near the onset of disease. Arthralgias are usually mild and transient. Patients may suffer joint contractures over the proximal interphalangeal joints and elbows. Muscle inflammation occurs in approximately 38% of pediatric cases.

Up to 40% of patients will eventually have upper GI involvement. Dysphasia is caused by esophageal dysmotility or gastroesophageal reflux. Half of patients suffer small bowel involvement. Functional tests demonstrate GI abnormalities even among asymptomatic patients. Similarly, patients may have pulmonary involvement as demonstrated by abnormal function but initially appear asymptomatic. As the disease progresses, patients develop dry, hacking cough with dyspnea on exertion. A rare but severe complication is interstitial pulmonary fibrosis. Cardiac involvement is less common but is the primary cause of morbidity. Cardiac fibrosis leads to conduction defects, arrhythmias, and impaired ventricular function. Aggressive immunosuppressive therapy is required when the cardiomyopathy is severe.

As with many of the collagen vascular diseases, patients will have ANA (80%). Approximately 20% to 30% of patients have Scl-70 (antitopoisomerase I), in contrast to adult onset in which only 7% of patients have this antibody. Approximately 25% of pediatric patients will have blood indices consistent with the normocytic normochromic anemia of chronic disease.

Localized Scleroderma

Similar to systemic SD, **localized SD** is secondary to abnormalities of fibroblast regulation, collagen production, and autoimmune regulation. Localized SD predominantly affects the skin and only occasionally involves other organs. Localized SD is divided into

5 subtypes: plaque morphea, generalized morphea, bullous morphea, linear SD, and deep morphea. **Morphea** are areas of indurated, waxy skin with an ivory center and violaceous halo and are most commonly found on the trunk. When they become confluent they are classified as generalized morphea. **Linear SD** is the most common form of localized SD among children and adolescents. One or more linear streaks are present on the extremities. These cutaneous changes can extend into the subcutaneous tissue and muscle leading to significant deformities. Linear lesions on the face or head are referred to as *coup de saber* SD. Deep morphea involves subcutaneous morphea, eosinophilic fasciitis, and morphea profunda, in which the entire skin is thickened and feels bound down. This form is the least common and considered the most disabling.

The presence of extra-cutaneous involvement in cases of localized SD raises the controversial issue of whether localized SD can transition to systemic SD. Approximately 25% of patients with juvenile localized SD have extra-cutaneous involvement, most commonly articular. Diagnosis is based on clinical presentation and skin biopsy. Antinuclear antibodies and antihistone antibodies may be present. Approximately 13% of patients will have anticardiolipin antibodies, but unlike SLE their presence is not associated with thrombosis. Cosmetic appearance is often the focus of disease management. Systemic treatment is reserved primarily for subtypes with significant disability such as linear SD and deep morphea.

Pathophysiology

Autoimmune diseases result from an alteration in the selection, regulation, or death of T-cells or B-cells, which results in an abnormal response to a particular antigen. Genetic factors increase an individual's vulnerability but are not sufficient for disease expression. It is the interplay of environmental triggers and genetic susceptibility that leads to clinical manifestations. In JIA, the T-cell arm of the cell-dependent inflammation is best understood. It supports many of the clinical and biochemical factors into the subtypes of JIA. T-cells are dependent on the major histocompatibility complex (MHC) to recognize an antigen. HLA types that have been classically associated with certain subtypes of JIA play a role in the presentation of a specific antigen. Studies of synovial fluid in JIA patients demonstrate specific families, or cohorts, of T-cells depending on the subtype of JIA. Furthermore, each subtype of JIA has a specific T-cell response with key inflammatory mediators and secondary effects. Current theory suggests that JIA is linked to an antigen-specific response in the synovial fluid. Systemic lupus erythematosus is characterized by abnormal autoantibody production against nucleic acids, especially double-stranded DNA. The T-cell and B-cell receptor-signaling pathways may be abnormal, as well as have an abnormal clearance of self-antigens, resulting in autoactivation of lymphocytes. In SD, autoantibodies target topoisomerase, centromeric proteins, and RNA polymerases, resulting in dysregulated fibroblast activation. Over-expression of MHC I is a major component of inflammatory myopathies. Local injury of vessels and muscles results from complement-mediated immune response and soluble adhesion molecules.

The molecular understanding of JIA has increased greatly, providing insight to the disease process and leading to a new classification system for the disease. Juvenile idiopathic arthritis is the result of an inflammatory process in the synovial fluid of a joint. The inflammatory process consists of an innate inflammatory phase and a cell-dependent phase. Initially there is an egress of cells and proteins from the bloodstream. The inflammation progresses with migration of neutrophils and monocytes to the location of tissue injury. Cell-dependent inflammation involves both T cells and B cells. T cells are dependent on MHC to recognize an antigen. Furthermore, each subtype of JIA has a specific T-cell response with key inflammatory mediators and secondary effects. While B-cells are known to play a role in the pathogenesis of JIA based on their presence in synovial fluid, their specific mechanisms of action are only hypothesized.

Evaluation

History

The history should clearly delineate the duration and the extent of the symptoms (Questions Box). Has there been joint involvement and, if so, which joints? Do the joints ache and are there also visible changes such as swelling and erythema? Are the symptoms more pronounced at specific times of the day, such as in the morning on arising? Has the patient experienced weakness? If so, which muscle groups are most affected? Has the patient had a rash? What is the nature and location of the rash? What other symptoms are present, such as headache, fever, fatigue, and weight loss?

> **Questions**
> **Juvenile Idiopathic Arthritis/Collagen Vascular Disease**
> - Has the child ever had any swelling, warmth, or redness of joints?
> - Does the child have difficulty walking or running? If so, does it occur at any particular time of the day?
> - Has the family noticed any type of skin rash or skin changes?
> - Has the child had any eye complaints?
> - Has the child had any recent illnesses such as gastroenteritis?
> - Has the child traveled recently or been bitten by a tick?

Physical Examination

Patients should undergo a complete physical examination that includes a full assessment of the skin, all joints, flexibility of the spine, the strength of the muscles, and a neuropsychiatric assessment. Lymphadenopathy should be noted as well as the presence of organomegaly. Patients suspected of having JIA should also undergo a slit lamp examination of the eyes.

Laboratory Tests

In general laboratory testing includes a complete blood count, erythrocyte sedimentation rate, urinalysis, and other studies as determined by the differential diagnosis. Patients suspected of having SLE should have an anti-DNA, anti-RNA–binding protein, anti-U1RNP and anti-SM antibodies determined. Electrocardiograms and echocardiograms are appropriate in patients with SLE suspected of having cardiac involvement. Patients with inflammatory myopathies should have creatine phosphokinase, aldolase, and lactate dehydrogenase levels. Electromyogram and muscle biopsy may also be undertaken.

Imaging Studies

Imaging studies such as computed tomography scans and magnetic resonance imaging are rarely abnormal in patients with SLE and neuropsychiatric symptoms.

Management

The management of collagen vascular diseases varies with the specific condition.

Juvenile Idiopathic Arthritis

The objective of treatment for JIA is to control pain and inflammation while preserving function and normal growth, development, and well-being. Physical and occupational therapy are essential to maintain function. Medications used for the treatment of JIA include nonsteroidal anti-inflammatory drugs (NSAIDs), disease-modifying antirheumatic drugs (DMARDs), and tumor necrosis factor inhibiting agents. Corticosteroids are reserved for patients with serious systemic manifestations and are not considered ideal for long-term use in JIA secondary to the side effects. Most patients respond to the various NSAIDS, although the time to respond may vary greatly. Only nonspecific cyclooxygenase inhibitors are approved for pediatric use. Individuals with persistent joint disease require DMARDs, with methotrexate being the most common. Clinical improvement may not be seen for 1 to 6 months, but eventually 70% of patients will respond. Gastrointestinal disturbances are the most commonly seen side effects, with hepatotoxicity being rare. Sulfasalazine is another DMARD that is especially effective in patients with enthesitis-related JIA. Etanercept is a biological agent that is a tumor necrosis factor receptor antagonist reserved for patients not responding to methotrexate.

Systemic Lupus Erythematosus

A multidisciplinary team is essential to care for patients with SLE. Specific therapies are tailored to the symptoms, severity, and level of response. Initial treatment of musculoskeletal symptoms, primarily arthritis, is with NSAIDs combined with an antimalarial drug such as hydroxychloroquine. Resistant symptoms may require steroids or methotrexate. Treatment of neuropsychiatric manifestations is based on symptoms and severity. These include steroids, immunosuppressive medications (azathioprine or cyclophosphamide), antiepileptics, and antidepressants. The treatment of renal manifestations is based on the histologic classification of renal involvement. Medications include steroids and immunosuppressive agents and may also include angiotensin-converting enzyme inhibitors to

decrease proteinuria. In practice, patients at risk for thrombosis may be treated with low-dose aspirin, although not all studies support the efficacy.

Complications of treatment with glucocorticoid steroids include avascular necrosis of the femoral head, affecting approximately 10% of patients. Furthermore, patients are at increased risk for osteoporosis due to low calcium and vitamin D intake and diminished physical activity. A severe complication of SLE is antiphospholipid antibody syndrome with severe microangiopathic thrombolytic changes, resulting in thrombosis to multiple organs. It is primarily associated with elevated antibody levels of lupus anticoagulant. It can occur anywhere in the body and can be difficult to recognize. Although antiphospholipid antibodies can be present in patients with JIA, DM antiphospholipid antibody syndrome is rare.

Dermatomyositis

Methotrexate is the primary medication for treatment of DM. Corticosteroids are often used when initiating treatment due to the slow onset of clinical improvement with methotrexate. Methylprednisolone pulses, immunoglobulin intravenous and cyclophosphamide are reserved for nonresponsive cases or severe exacerbations.

Systemic Scleroderma

As with other collagen vascular disease, the treatment of systemic SD focuses on optimal function and control of inflammation. Many of the medications used in SD lack rigorous evaluations regarding efficacy. Immunosuppressive agents that are often used include methotrexate, mycophenolate, and cyclophosphamide in severe cases. Glucosteroids are primarily effective for the inflammatory phase of muscle involvement or edematous phase of cutaneous disease. Vasodilator agents, especially calcium channel blockers, are used for symptomatic relief of Raynaud phenomenon. Few studies exist on the long-term survival of patients with juvenile systemic sclerosis. Clinically, as the skin tightens and contractures progress, the disease becomes extremely disabling. Cardiac, renal, and pulmonary disease progressions are most often responsible for premature death. The extent of sclerosis may be a prognostic factor.

Prognosis

Making the diagnosis of a collagen vascular disease requires a thorough history and physical examination, as well as a broad differential diagnosis. While there is no gold standard for diagnosing these diseases, each type has characteristic symptoms and laboratory findings as well as specific ages for presentation. Consultation with rheumatologists, neurologists, nephrologists, and infectious disease specialists may be required to assist in the final diagnosis.

Likewise, the care of a child with a collagen vascular disease also requires a multidisciplinary approach involving a primary care physician, rheumatologist, and subspecialists with expertise in affected target organs. The role for the primary care physician is to ensure optimal function of the patient as well as prevention of long-term disease and treatment sequelae. Because many of the agents used to manage collagen vascular disease have significant side effects, it is vital for the primary care physician to be well versed with a patient's medication regimen. Patients with collagen vascular disease often suffer from growth failure either from the disease process or its treatment. Ensuring appropriate diet and physical activity is vital. Supplementation with calcium and vitamin D is beneficial to prevent osteoporosis. Periodic ophthalmologic screening is essential for patients with uveitis. In the long term, patients with collagen vascular disease are at a higher risk for cardiovascular disease (CVD) secondary to chronic inflammation. They may require annual cardiovascular risk assessments that include lipid profiles. While pediatric patients often don't have other CVD risk factors, it is important to ensure healthy behaviors. Individuals that have suffered thrombolytic events or are at high risk for thrombosis may benefit from low-dose aspirin prophylaxis. As with any patient with a chronic disease, maintaining a feasible quality of life is essential. Disease management for patients suffering from collagen vascular disease is a balance of optimal function, minimal complications, and improved quality of life.

CASE RESOLUTION

The young girl in the case scenario has a presentation consistent with oligoarthritic juvenile idiopathic arthritis based on the number of involved joints (3 joints) and her age (between 1 and 5 years). She has a number of laboratory studies including a complete blood count, erythrocyte sedimentation rate, rheumatoid factor, and antinuclear antibodies (ANA). Her ANA is positive. She is referred to a pediatric ophthalmologist for an eye examination to determine if she has uveitis. She is also referred to a pediatric rheumatologist for assistance in managing her disease and a physical therapist to address her limitation of motion.

Selected References

Allen E, Farewell VT, Isenberg DA, Gordon C. A statistical analysis of the interrelationships between disease activity in different systems in systemic lupus erythematosus. *Rheumatology (Oxford)*. 2006;45:308–313

Benseler SM, Silverman ED. Systemic lupus erythematosus. *Pediatr Clin North Am*. 2005;52:443–467

Berkun Y, Padeh S, Barash J, et al. Antiphospholipid syndrome and recurrent thrombosis in children. *Arthritis Rheum*. 2006;55:850–855

Cassidy J, Kivlin J, Lindsley C, Nocton J; American Academy of Pediatrics Section on Rheumatology and Section on Ophthalmology. Ophthalmologic examinations in children with juvenile rheumatoid arthritis. *Pediatrics*. 2006;117:1843–1845

Compeyrot-Lacassagne S, Feldman BM. Inflammatory myopathies in children. *Pediatr Clin North Am*. 2005;52:493–520

LeBovidge JS, Lavigne JV, Donenberg GR, Miller ML. Psychological adjustment of children and adolescents with chronic arthritis: a meta-analytic review. *J Pediatr Psychol*. 2003;28:29–39

Martini G, Foeldvari I, Russo R, et al. Systematic scleroderma syndromes in children: clinical and immunological characteristics of 181 patients. *Arthritis Rheum*. 2003;48:S512

Niehues T, Horneff G, Michels H, Hock MS, Schuchmann L; Working Groups Pediatric Rheumatology Germany (AGKJR); Pediatric Rheumatology Austria. Evidence-based use of methotrexate in children with rheumatic diseases: a consensus statement of the Working Groups Pediatric Rheumatology Germany (AGKJR) and Pediatric Rheumatology Austria. *Rheumatol Int*. 2005;25:169–178

Oen K, Malleson PN, Cabral DA, et al. Early predictors of longterm outcome in patients with juvenile rheumatoid arthritis: subset-specific correlations. *J Rheumatol*. 2003;30:585–593

Ravelli A, Martini A. Antiphospholipid syndrome. *Pediatr Clin North Am*. 2005;52:469–491

Ruperto N, Buratti S, Duarte-Salazar C, et al. Health-related quality of life in juvenile-onset systemic lupus erythematosus and its relationship to disease activity and damage. *Arthritis Rheum*. 2004;51:458–464

Stark LJ, Davis AM, Janicke DM, et al. A randomized clinical trial of dietary calcium to improve bone accretion in children with juvenile rheumatoid arthritis. *J Pediatr*. 2006;148:501–507

Sullivan KE. Inflammation in juvenile idiopathic arthritis. *Pediatr Clin North Am*. 2005;52:335–357

Tseng CE, Buyon JP, Kim M, et al. The effect of moderate-dose corticosteroids in preventing severe flares in patients with serologically active, but clinically stable, systemic lupus erythematosus: findings of a prospective, randomized, double-blind, placebo-controlled trial. *Arthritis Rheum*. 2006;54:3623–3632

Weiss JE, Howite NT. Juvenile idiopathic arthritis. *Pediatr Clin North Am*. 2005;52:413–442

Zulian F. Scleroderma in children. *Pediatr Clin North Am*. 2005;52:521–545

Nephrotic Syndrome

Elaine S. Kamil, MD

CASE STUDY

A 2-year-old boy is brought to the office because of abdominal distention. He has just recovered from a runny nose that lasted a week, with no fever or change in activity. His mother complains that his eyelids were very swollen that morning, and she says that his thighs look "fat." She has noticed that he has fewer wet diapers. He has always been a healthy child, and his immunizations are up to date. The family has a history of asthma and allergic rhinitis. Physical examination shows an active 2-year-old boy. Head and neck examination is clear, except for a few shotty anterior cervical lymph nodes and some minimal periorbital edema. Chest examination reveals some decreased breath sounds at the bases. The abdomen is moderately distended; bowel sounds are active and a fluid wave is detectable. There is 2+ pitting edema of the lower legs, extending up to the knees. The urine has a specific gravity of 1.030; pH 6; 4+ protein; and trace, nonhemolyzed blood. Microscopic examination shows 4 to 6 red blood cells per high-power field and 10 to 20 hyaline and fine granular casts per low-power field.

Questions

1. What is the differential diagnosis of edema and ascites in previously healthy young children?
2. What criteria are used to determine if nephrotic children require hospitalization or can be managed as outpatients?
3. What laboratory evaluation and therapy are instituted initially?
4. What are the important issues to address in parent education?
5. What is the prognosis of young children with nephrotic syndrome?

Although nephrotic syndrome is not a common childhood disease, every pediatrician can expect to care for 1 to 3 nephrotic children at some time. Nephrotic syndrome may have serious or even fatal complications, and the disease tends to follow a chronic, relapsing course. Thus it is important for the pediatrician to become familiar with the signs and symptoms of the disease and with the most current treatment modalities aimed at keeping affected children healthy and active.

Nephrotic syndrome occurs when an individual excretes a sufficient quantity of plasma proteins, primarily albumin, in the urine to cause hypoalbuminemia. Substantial urinary protein losses, hypercholesterolemia, and hypoalbuminemia characterize nephrotic syndrome. The condition is usually accompanied by obvious edema, but occasionally edema is not clinically detectable (Dx Box).

In children, proteinuria of more than 40 mg/m^2/h (>50 mg/kg in 24 hours) is considered nephrotic range proteinuria. (In adult-sized patients, proteinuria of more than 3.5 g in 24 hours is associated with

nephrotic syndrome.) Collection of a 24-hour urine sample is cumbersome in children, and the urinary total protein/creatinine ratio (U TP/CR) done on a random urine sample, preferably a first morning urine, is a useful alternative. Whereas a ratio greater than 3.5 is considered nephrotic range proteinuria in adults with normal renal function, a ratio greater than 1.0 is considered diagnostic in children (see Chapter 82). Twenty-four–hour urine protein losses (g/m^2/d) in children can be estimated by multiplying the U TP/CR by 0.63.

Epidemiology

Minimal change disease (MCD) is the most common form of nephrotic syndrome in childhood. The annual prevalence of new cases of nephrotic syndrome is 2 in 100,000 to 3 in 100,000 children in the population younger than 16 years. The cumulative prevalence of this chronic disease is 16 in 100,000. Ninety percent of childhood cases are not associated with any systemic disease, and two-thirds of cases of childhood nephrotic syndrome present before age 5 years. The ratio of boys to girls with nephrotic syndrome is 2:1. By late adolescence, both sexes are equally affected.

Clinical Presentation

The typical child presenting with nephrotic syndrome is a preschool-aged boy who is brought to the physician because he appears swollen to the parents. Some children are active and relatively asymptomatic despite the edema, whereas others may be very uncomfortable, with

---

Dx Nephrotic Syndrome

- Heavy proteinuria (>40 mg/m^2/h or 50 mg/kg/24 h in children)
- Hypoalbuminemia
- Hypercholesterolemia
- Edema

markedly swollen eyelids, abdominal discomfort, scrotal or labial edema, and even respiratory compromise. Usually children have a history of preceding infection, most typically an upper respiratory infection (URI). Occasionally children develop diarrhea secondary to edema of the bowel wall.

Occasionally children with nephrosis are critically ill due to peritonitis, bacteremia, or (rarely) a major thrombotic episode. Because their immune state is compromised, rapid evaluation and treatment of children with these complications of nephrotic syndrome are essential for survival. The primary peritonitis associated with nephrotic syndrome may be confused with an acute abdomen, such as may be seen with appendicitis. Some children who are experiencing a severe relapse have hypotensive symptoms secondary to intravascular volume depletion.

Pathophysiology

The exact cause of MCD and focal segmental glomerulosclerosis (FSGS) is not known. Although this is controversial, many nephrologists believe that FSGS may result from severe, treatment-resistant MCD. The best current theory postulates that some stimulus (usually infectious) causes a clone of lymphocytes or monocytes to proliferate and produce one or more cytokines that are toxic to the glomerular epithelial cells (podocytes), cells that maintain the glomerular basement membranes. The cytokine induces a reduction in the net negative charge across the glomerular basement membrane. The constituents of this membrane and of the chemicals coating the glomerular epithelial and endothelial cells normally bear a net negative charge. The presence of these negatively charged chemicals creates a charge-selective barrier to filtration. This barrier plays a significant role in the ultrafiltration of macromolecules present in the plasma, enhancing the filtration of molecules bearing a positive electrical charge and retarding the filtration of molecules bearing a negative electrical charge. During episodes of relapse, patients with MCD show a breakdown in the normal charge-selective barrier to filtration, often resulting in massive proteinuria. Kidney biopsies from patients with nephrotic syndrome demonstrate a net reduction in anionic sites during periods of relapse. In addition, some children have mutations in podocyte proteins such as nephrin and podocin that lead to nephrotic syndrome.

Evidence indicating that the proteinuria in the MCD or FSGS patient may be due to some soluble factor is 3-fold. (1) Some patients who develop end-stage renal disease from idiopathic nephrotic syndrome (particularly FSGS) have experienced a relapse of the nephrotic syndrome with massive proteinuria immediately after transplantation of a normal kidney. (2) Infusion of peripheral blood mononuclear cell products from nephrotic children induces albuminuria in rats. (3) Removal of serum proteins by adsorption to a protein A Sepharose column has led to remission of proteinuria in some patients who have experienced a recurrence of nephrotic syndrome after transplantation. The remission of the proteinuria after treatment with immunosuppressive medication provides further evidence that the nephrotic syndrome is mediated in some way by the immune system.

Normal adults are able to synthesize 12 g of albumin per day in the liver, and adults with nephrotic syndrome may synthesize 14 g of albumin per day. Therefore, the **hypoproteinemia** characteristic of nephrotic syndrome cannot be explained completely by measured amounts of urinary protein losses (about 3.5 g/d). The difference between the hepatic synthetic capacity for albumin and the measured urinary losses can be explained by protein catabolism in the kidney. Renal tubular epithelial cells reabsorb filtered plasma proteins and catabolize them to amino acids, which then reenter the amino acid pool of the body. Thus the magnitude of losses of plasma proteins at the glomerular level is far greater than the amount measured in a 24-hour urine sample.

The **hypoalbuminemia** seen in nephrotic syndrome is a result of the massive proteinuria, and the **hypercholesterolemia** occurs as a consequence of the hypoalbuminemia. The hyperlipidemia is partially the result of a generalized increase in hepatic protein synthesis that also involves the overproduction of lipoproteins. In addition, less lipid is transported into the adipose tissue, because the activity of lipoprotein lipase is reduced in adipose tissue during active nephrotic syndrome. Hyperlipidemia is most pronounced in children with MCD. Serum albumin and serum cholesterol are generally inversely correlated.

Differential Diagnosis

Nephrotic syndrome is considered either primary or secondary. Primary nephrotic syndrome is not associated with a systemic disease. Secondary nephrotic syndrome is a feature of a systemic disease such as anaphylactoid purpura or systemic lupus erythematosus (SLE). Most children with nephrotic syndrome have the primary form of the disease.

Children with primary nephrotic syndrome are also classified according to their response to steroid therapy. Affected individuals may be categorized as steroid-sensitive, steroid-dependent, or steroid-resistant. Typically, children who are steroid-sensitive and remain so have MCD although, strictly speaking, a renal biopsy must be performed before the diagnosis of MCD is made. Sensitivity to or dependence on corticosteroids is a critical factor in determining a child's prognosis.

Nephrotic syndrome is also classified by the appearance of the glomeruli on renal biopsy. A summary of the histologic lesions

Table 131-1. Distribution of Histologic Type by Age of Onset in Children With Nephrotic Syndrome					
Age (y)	MCD[a]	FSGS	MN	MPGN	Other GN
1–4	95%	3%	2%	—	—
4–8	75%	15%	1%	7%	2%
8–16	52%	15%	2%	25%	6%

Abbreviations: MCD, minimal change disease; FSGS, focal segmental glomerulosclerosis; MN, membranous nephropathy; MPGN, membranoproliferative glomerulonephritis; other GN, other forms of glomerulonephritis.

[a]MCD remains the dominant histologic type through mid-adolescence but becomes relatively less important in later childhood and adolescence.

causing nephrotic syndrome appears in Table 131-1. About 95% of young children with nephrotic syndrome have MCD. In these children, light microscopy shows normal-appearing glomeruli. Immunofluorescent microscopy is generally negative but may show some mesangial immunoglobulin (Ig) M deposits, and electron microscopy simply shows foot process effacement of the podocytes. In individuals with FSGS, light microscopy may show enlarged glomeruli and glomeruli with segments of sclerosis. Immunofluorescence may reveal some IgM and complement in the sclerotic segments, and electron microscopy shows areas of foot process effacement of podocytes. Biopsies performed later in the disease course show some totally sclerotic glomeruli, areas of interstitial fibrosis, and atrophy. Several recent series have noted an apparent increase in the incidence of FSGS among nephrotic children.

Other primary renal diseases that can cause nephrotic syndrome in children include membranous nephropathy, membranoproliferative glomerulonephritis, IgA nephropathy and other forms of chronic glomerulonephritis, congenital nephrotic syndrome, and diffuse mesangial proliferative glomerulonephritis. Chronic hepatitis B infection may cause membranous nephropathy or membranoproliferative glomerulonephritis. Rarely, post-streptococcal acute glomerulonephritis and other forms of postinfectious acute glomerulonephritis may also cause nephrotic syndrome. With the exception of congenital nephrotic syndrome, all of these diseases show (1) the presence of immune deposits in the glomerular mesangial regions or along the glomerular basement membrane and (2) some element of cellular proliferation, which may be severe. In these disease states, the presence of nephrotic syndrome is indicative of marked injury to the glomerular capillary wall. Infants with congenital nephrotic syndrome, Finnish type, have a mutation of the gene encoding the nephrin molecule, a podocyte protein with a large extracellular domain that is an integral part of the glomerular slit diaphragm. These infants have massive proteinuria beginning in utero and have severe nephrotic syndrome presenting in the first month of life.

Because of the varying distribution of edema fluid at presentation, nephrotic syndrome may be confused with sinusitis or an allergic reaction (periorbital edema), obesity (ascites), or an abdominal mass (ascites). Other causes of generalized edema, such as congestive heart failure or liver disease, can be easily excluded.

Evaluation

History

The clinical evaluation should include a careful history (Questions Box).

Physical Examination

A complete physical examination is necessary. Blood pressure should be monitored because hypertension or hypotension may occur. The extent of the peripheral and central edema, including swelling of the eyelids, should be assessed. The physician should obtain a reliable, overall impression of the child's level of comfort and activity. The examination should also include a careful search for

infection, particularly life-threatening infections such as pneumonia or peritonitis. Examination of the head and neck should focus on signs of recent infection such as otitis media. The presence of dullness to percussion at the bases of the thorax is consistent with large pleural effusions. Ascites may be minimal or massive. With severe ascites, scrotal or labial edema may occur. If the child has a history of abdominal pain, a careful check for signs of peritoneal irritation should be made. The skin should be inspected for infection and rashes.

Laboratory Tests

The laboratory evaluation of children with nephrotic syndrome begins with a urinalysis. The dipstick shows 3+ or 4+ protein, although a dilute urine may be only 2+. Microscopic hematuria may be present in up to 25% of children with MCD. The presence of associated glycosuria in a nephrotic child who is not on steroid therapy raises a concern for FSGS. Careful microscopic examination is necessary. Casts are seen frequently because urinary proteins precipitate in the tubules. The casts are hyaline, fine, and coarse granular. White blood cell (WBC) casts are sometimes seen because some children with nephrotic syndrome may also have increased amounts of leukocytes in their urine. Large amounts of red blood cells (RBCs) and RBC casts are not seen in uncomplicated MCD and, if present, indicate another cause for the nephrotic syndrome. If RBC casts are seen together with substantial hematuria, an antistreptolysin-O titer should be added to the preliminary evaluation. A random U TP/CR should be done to determine whether children have nephrotic range proteinuria.

If the urine shows only proteinuria, with perhaps some microscopic hematuria, blood tests should include a complete blood count (CBC), serum creatinine and blood urea nitrogen (BUN), electrolytes, serum calcium, serum albumin, cholesterol, complement component 3 (C3), and antinuclear antibody (ANA). The CBC may show a high hematocrit from hemoconcentration because many children experience volume contraction as a complication of hypoproteinemia. Children may also have very high platelet counts (sometimes >1 million/μL). The BUN and creatinine help assess renal function.

A hyperchloremic metabolic acidosis is sometimes seen. The serum albumin and cholesterol are required to differentiate nephrotic syndrome from other edematous states. A low level of C3 is associated with other renal diseases such as membranoproliferative glomerulonephritis, acute postinfectious glomerulonephritis, and SLE. The ANA is useful in screening for SLE and other collagen vascular diseases. Hepatitis B serology is helpful in children who come from a population at risk for hepatitis B infection, such as recent immigrants from Southeast Asia or children of intravenous (IV) drug abusers. Although not part of the routine laboratory evaluation, measurement of quantitative Ig often shows low IgG levels and elevated IgM levels. The febrile child should also have blood and urine cultures, and if there are signs of peritoneal irritation, a culture of peritoneal fluid.

Imaging Studies

Chest x-rays help assess the severity of pleural effusions in children with marked ascites and respiratory compromise.

Management

Hospitalization

The decision to admit a child with nephrotic syndrome to the hospital is determined by the child's functional status. All children with severe edema compromising ambulation or respiration should be admitted. Other indications for admission include unstable vital signs, fever, marked oliguria, and severe hemoconcentration (hematocrit >48%–50%).

Most children with nephrotic syndrome are hospitalized for control of edema or treatment of a complication such as infection. The management of children in relapse is aimed at minimizing edema and preventing complications until the disease can be controlled with immunosuppressive therapy. Intake, output, and weight need to be closely monitored. Blood pressure should be followed, although hypertension is not common. If children have a fever (temperature: >100.7°F [38.2°C]), blood and urine cultures should be obtained and antibiotics started pending culture results. If signs of peritoneal inflammation are evident, paracentesis should also be performed to obtain samples of the ascites fluid for Gram stain, cell count, and culture. Broad-spectrum antibiotics should be given to cover respiratory pathogens, especially pneumococcus, and enteric pathogens. All children who are newly diagnosed with nephrotic syndrome should have a purified protein derivative test because immunosuppression associated with steroid therapy may facilitate reactivation of tuberculosis infection.

Intravenous albumin (25%) should be used selectively because albumin infusions are very expensive, and the infused albumin is excreted very rapidly in the urine. Infusions are indicated in children with marked ascites, scrotal or labial edema, or significant pleural effusions. They are also helpful in maintaining blood pressure and renal perfusion in septic children with nephrotic syndrome. The usual dose is 1 g/kg, up to 25 g, infused over 2 to 4 hours, with close monitoring of blood pressure. Furosemide (1 mg/kg intravenously) is usually administered post-infusion. The albumin infusions may be repeated every 12 to 24 hours as necessary. If children with oliguria fail to increase their urine output after the first or second albumin infusion, they need to be evaluated immediately for the presence of acute renal failure (see Chapter 55). The albumin-induced mobilization of edema fluid in nephrotic children with acute tubular necrosis can precipitate pulmonary edema.

Supportive Therapy

Diet

Because sodium plays a key role in edema formation, children with nephrotic syndrome should be placed on a no-added-salt diet that limits dietary sodium to 2 or 3 g/d. Technically, sodium restriction is indicated only during times of relapse, but a constant no-added-salt diet helps entire families maintain a consistent regimen. In general, fluid restriction is not necessary except in unusual circumstances (eg, a steroid-resistant patient with persistent edema). Although earlier teachings recommended the use of high-protein diets, newer research has shown that these diets may actually increase urinary protein losses.

Activity

In the past, children with nephrotic syndrome were treated with bed rest because the supine position somewhat reduces urinary protein losses. No evidence shows that bed rest has a significant impact on children's clinical state, however. Therefore, most pediatric nephrologists recommend that children be allowed full activity. Boys with marked scrotal edema may be more comfortable resting in bed while diuresis is being initiated. Children with nephrotic syndrome should not be isolated from other children and should be allowed to attend school.

Diuretics

Diuretics are often helpful in children in relapse, particularly in children with steroid-resistant disease. Serum potassium levels, as well as clinical signs of intravascular volume, should be monitored. If children have moderate intravascular volume contraction, the injudicious use of diuretics could precipitate hypotension and increase the risk of thrombosis and acute tubular necrosis. The most commonly used diuretic is furosemide (1–2 mg/kg per dose given orally or intravenously). Spironolactone is sometimes added to the diuretic regimen for its potassium-sparing effect.

Long-term Management

The goal of long-term management is induction and maintenance of remission from active nephrotic syndrome. At the same time, the side effects of medications should be minimized. Spontaneous remission may eventually occur in children with MCD, but the 70% historical mortality rate makes waiting for a spontaneous remission unacceptable. Remissions are induced and maintained with the use of immunosuppressive medications. Figure 131-1 summarizes an

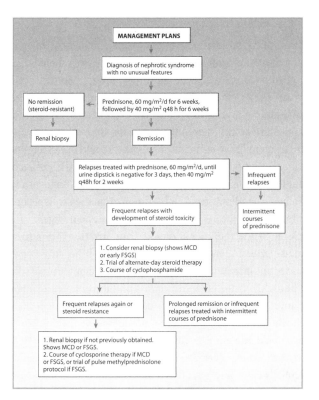

Figure 131–1. Management of nephrotic syndrome in children. Abbreviations: q, every; MCD, minimal change disease; FSGS, focal segmental glomerulosclerosis.

approach to the overall management of nephrotic syndrome with these agents. A list of commonly used medications and dosages appears in Table 131-2.

Corticosteroids and Alkylating Agents

More than 90% of children with primary nephrotic syndrome respond to corticosteroid therapy. Steroids are, therefore, both diagnostic and therapeutic because failure to respond to steroids can be a marker for disease other than MCD. Even so, some children with MCD are steroid-resistant at some time in their disease. Steroids can be started in children who are newly diagnosed with nephrotic syndrome if they have no signs of systemic disease, no more than microscopic hematuria, a normal C3 (or results pending), and normal renal function. Acute infection should be managed with specific antimicrobial therapy to avoid infection-related steroid resistance.

Prednisone is usually started at 60 mg/m²/d. It can either be given once a day, in the morning, or divided into 2 or 3 daily doses. If first episodes of nephrotic syndrome are treated with a prolonged course of corticosteroids (60 mg/m²/d for 6 weeks followed by 40 mg/m²/48 h for an additional 6 weeks), the children are subsequently less likely to follow a frequently relapsing course. Newly diagnosed children younger than 4 years are less likely to experience frequent relapses if their every-other-day steroids are tapered off over a 6-month period. Proteinuria resolves within 2 weeks in many children with MCD and by 4 weeks in more than 90%. Serum albumin normalizes soon after proteinuria clears, but hypercholesterolemia may take many weeks to return to normal.

The pediatrician can easily manage steroid-sensitive children, but children with more difficult nephrotic syndrome should be managed in conjunction with the pediatric nephrologist. Children with relapses are treated with daily prednisone (60 mg/m²) until the urine is protein-free for 3 days. This regimen is followed by 2 weeks of 40 mg/m² every other morning. An increased incidence of side effects (eg, cushingoid appearance, hypertension, obesity, glucose intolerance, cataracts, osteopenia, decreased growth rate) occurs when children require frequent courses of prednisone therapy. In frequently relapsing children, a chronic course of alternate-day steroid therapy may eliminate relapses and reduce steroid toxicity. Usually prednisone 60 mg/m² is given every other morning initially. The dose is then gradually tapered over several months to the lowest dose that keeps the child in remission.

If alternate-day steroid therapy fails to maintain remission, cyclophosphamide or chlorambucil is administered. Either of these alkylating agents may induce long-lasting remission in children with steroid-dependent or frequently relapsing nephrotic syndrome. Either agent is started while children are on steroid therapy, and the steroids are gradually tapered during the course of treatment with the alkylating agent. In the past a diagnostic renal biopsy was routine prior to starting an alkylating agent. Many pediatric nephrologists now consider such therapy in steroid-sensitive or steroid-dependent children without a biopsy, however, provided that renal function is normal. Initially a daily dose of cyclophosphamide (2 mg/kg) was recommended for 8 weeks. However, a 12-week course is more likely to induce prolonged remission and still be safe.

Potential toxicities of cyclophosphamide include bone marrow suppression with increased risk of infection; alopecia; hemorrhagic cystitis; gonadal toxicity; and possibly a small but indeterminately increased risk of developing a malignancy at some time. Complete blood counts should be monitored weekly, and parents should be cautioned about the increased risk of overwhelming varicella infections in children who have not yet had a varicella infection

Table 131-2. Treatment Options in Childhood Nephrotic Syndrome		
Medication	**Dose**	***Length of Therapy***
Prednisone	60 mg/m²/d	Varies
Cyclophosphamide	2–3 mg/kg/d (cumulative dose <200 mg/kg)	12 weeks
Chlorambucil	0.15–0.2 mg/kg/d (cumulative dose ≤8.2 mg/kg)	8 weeks
Cyclosporine	3 mg/kg every 12 h, monitor levels	Varies
Levamisole[a]	2.5 mg/kg every other day	Varies
Mycophenolate mofetil	20 mg/kg every 12 h	Varies
Tacrolimus	0.1mg/kg every 12 h, monitor levels	Varies

[a]Levamisole is no longer recommended for childhood nephrotic syndrome in the United States.

or vaccination. The dose should be withheld if the WBC count falls below 4,000/μL and restarted when the WBC returns to or exceeds 4000/μL. Alopecia and hemorrhagic cystitis are rare when the recommended dose is used. A 12-week course of cyclophosphamide (2 mg/kg/d) does not seem to increase the risk of infertility, but longer courses are associated with oligospermia, aspermia, and ovarian dysfunction. Postpubertal individuals may be at greater risk for gonadal toxicity than prepubertal children.

When steroid-sensitive or steroid-dependent children have failed to achieve prolonged remission after cyclophosphamide therapy, a diagnostic renal biopsy should be performed. Renal biopsy is indicated early in the course of illness for steroid-resistant children. If FSGS is identified on biopsy, treatment may involve a prolonged course of IV methylprednisolone therapy, cyclosporine, or tacrolimus. Therapeutic options for children with MCD who continue to be steroid-dependent after a course of cyclophosphamide include treatment with mycophenolate mofetil, cyclosporine, tacrolimus, or levamisole. Although cyclosporine is more likely to induce prolonged remission, it only maintains remission while being administered. Children trade steroid dependence for cyclosporine dependence. Nevertheless, for children with steroid toxicity, a 6- to 12-month course of cyclosporine allows resolution of the adverse effects of steroids and is generally well tolerated when administered by an experienced physician. Side effects such as hirsutism and gingival hyperplasia are frequent at the onset of therapy. These effects regress as the dose is decreased or the drug is discontinued, however. Hypertension is not uncommon. The most common metabolic abnormality seen with cyclosporine use is hypomagnesemia. Long-term therapy may lead to significant nephrotoxicity and, rarely, patients experience liver toxicity. Tacrolimus, like cyclosporine, is a calcineurin inhibitor. It has a similar toxicity profile to cyclosporine, but it does not cause gingival hyperplasia or hirsutism.

Because of potential toxicity, cyclosporine and tacrolimus should only be prescribed by a physician familiar with the drug. Dosing requirements may change with remission and relapse, and the family and physician should be aware of several drug interactions. Any medication interfering with the cytochrome P-450 enzyme system in the liver, such as erythromycin, greatly increases cyclosporine levels and should be used only under extraordinary circumstances. Diarrhea may increase tacrolimus blood levels to a toxic range. Children who require prolonged treatment with cyclosporine or tacrolimus should have follow-up kidney biopsies performed after a year or two of therapy to assess for any nephrotoxicity.

Nephrotic children who fail to achieve a good remission with immunosuppressive therapy are given supportive therapy with angiotensin-converting enzyme inhibitors or angiotensin blockers, which reduce proteinuria and have also been shown to reduce the progression of glomerulosclerosis. These medications are also first-line therapy for nephrotic children who develop hypertension. Other supportive measures for children with persistent edema include sodium restriction and the chronic use of diuretics.

Immunization Issues

Because of the unusual susceptibility to pneumococcal infections, children with nephrotic syndrome older than 2 years should receive the pneumococcal vaccine, even if they have previously received Prevnar. The vaccine is best administered while the children are in remission, but it produces protective titers even in children who are on alternate-day steroid therapy at the time of immunization. Patients on multiple immunosuppressives should have their pneumococcal antibody titers measured, and a second dose of vaccine should be administered if they fail to seroconvert. Influenza vaccine should be administered each autumn to children with nephrotic syndrome using the age-appropriate schedule and dosage.

Some of the routine childhood immunizations (diphtheria-tetanus-pertussis, *Haemophilus influenzae* type b, hepatitis B, poliovirus vaccine inactivated) should be administered by the usual schedule but while children are in remission (see Chapter 23). Some controversy exists concerning the use of live virus vaccines in children who require long-term immunosuppressive therapy. No vaccines should be administered if children are currently being treated with an alkylating agent. The measles-mumps-rubella vaccine could potentially cause a relapse. Based on the limited data on the use of varicella vaccine in nephrotic children, it is probably safe to administer varicella vaccine while the children are in remission and not on immunosuppressive medications.

Parent Education

Because nephrotic syndrome follows a chronic, relapsing course, parent education is essential for effective long-term management. Parents need to be instructed about using urinary dipsticks (Albustix) to monitor protein excretion. Generally urine dipsticks should be used daily during periods of active relapse and when medication is being tapered. Otherwise, the dipstick should be checked whenever children have infections, including URIs, whenever they look "puffy," and weekly when asymptomatic.

Weight should also be monitored, especially during relapse. Children should be weighed each morning when they awaken. Urine output should be measured in more difficult cases. As parents become more familiar with the nephrotic syndrome, they may become partners with the physician about medication changes. Parents should also contact the physician about "danger signs" such as fever (temperature: >100.7°F [38.2°C]), significant abdominal pain, or exposure to varicella. If children do not have protective antibodies against varicella and if they are taking any immunosuppressive medication (including prednisone), the varicella-zoster Ig should be administered within 72 hours of exposure to varicella. If varicella infection develops, IV acyclovir should be instituted.

Prognosis

In the pre-antibiotic era, nephrotic syndrome was frequently fatal, usually because of overwhelming infection. After the introduction of antibiotics, the mortality rate fell. The use of corticosteroids has led to a further reduction in mortality. Currently the mortality rate is about 5%, almost exclusively due to infections from encapsulated organisms or from thrombosis. The greatest risk of death in children with nephrotic syndrome (approaching 50% over 20 years in some series) is among the children with resistance to corticosteroid therapy.

The long-term outlook for most children with nephrotic syndrome is favorable, particularly for steroid-sensitive patients. Relapses often disappear by the completion of puberty. Occasionally individuals continue to have relapses into adulthood. Approximately 20% of children with steroid-sensitive MCD still experience relapses 15 years after the onset of their disease. Disease recurrence is highly unlikely if 8 years pass without a relapse. Less than 10% of initially steroid-sensitive children with nephrotic syndrome develop end-stage renal disease. This occurs almost exclusively in children with FSGS. Focal segmental glomerulosclerosis may recur after kidney transplants, particularly in young children with aggressive FSGS.

CASE RESOLUTION

In the opening scenario, the child most likely has minimal change disease. He appears stable enough to be managed as an outpatient and should be placed on a salt-restricted diet and prednisone. The overall prognosis depends on a close interaction among the parents, pediatrician, and consulting pediatric nephrologist.

Selected References

Arbeitsgemeinschaft für Paëdiatrische Nephrologie. Short versus standard prednisone therapy for initial treatment of idiopathic nephrotic syndrome in children. *Lancet.* 1988;1:380–383

Bayazit AK, Noyan A, Cengiz N, Anarat A. Mycophenolate mofetil in the children with multidrug-resistant nephrotic syndrome. *Clin Nephrol.* 2004;61:25–29

Bernard DB. Extrarenal complications of the nephrotic syndrome. *Kidney Int.* 1988;33:1184–1202

Eddy AA, Schnaper HW. The nephrotic syndrome: from the simple to the complex. *Semin Nephrol.* 1998;18:304–316

Filler G. Treatment of nephrotic syndrome in children and controlled trials. *Nephrol Dial Transplant.* 2003;18(suppl 6):vi75–vi78

Guan N, Ding J, Zhang J, et al. Expression of nephrin, podocin, α-actinin, and WT-1 in children with nephrotic syndrome. *Pediatr Nephrol.* 2003;18:1121–1127

Gulati S, Sharma AP, Sharma RK. Changing trends in histopathology in childhood nephrotic syndrome. *Am J Kidney Dis.* 1999;34:646–650

Hodson EM, Knight JF, Willis NS, Craig JC. Corticosteroid therapy for nephrotic syndrome in children. *Cochrane Database Syst Rev.* 2005;1:CD001533

Lewis MA, Baildom EM, Davis N, Houston IB, Postlethwaite RJ. Nephrotic syndrome: from toddlers to twenties. *Lancet.* 1989;1:255–259

Loeffler K, Gowrishankar M, Yiu V. Tacrolimus therapy in pediatric patients with treatment-resistant nephrotic syndrome. *Pediatr Nephrol.* 2004;19:281–287

Mendoza SA, Reznik VM, Griswold WR, Krensky AM, Yorgin PD, Tune BM. Treatment of steroid-resistant focal segmental glomerulosclerosis with pulse methylprednisolone and alkylating agents. *Pediatr Nephrol.* 1990;4:303–307

Minimal change nephrotic syndrome in children: deaths during the first 5 to 15 years' observation. Report of the International Study of Kidney Disease in Children. *Pediatrics.* 1984;73:497–501

Niaudet P, Gagnadoux MF, Broyer M. Treatment of childhood steroid-resistant idiopathic nephrotic syndrome. *Adv Nephrol.* 1998;28:43–61

Quien RM, Kaiser BA, Deforest A, et al. Response to the varicella vaccine in children with nephrotic syndrome. *J Pediatr.* 1997;131:688–690

Vester U, Kranz B, Zimmerman S. Cyclophosphamide in steroid-sensitive nephrotic syndrome: outcome and outlook. *Pediatr Nephrol.* 2003;18:661–664

Seizures and Epilepsy

Kenneth R. Huff, MD

CASE STUDY

A 6-year-old boy is evaluated for unusual episodic behaviors. The previous week his mother was awakened by the boy's brother and found her son lying in bed unresponsive and drooling, with his head and eyes averted to the right, his right arm slightly raised, and his body stiff. His face was jerking intermittently. When the paramedics arrived, the boy's posturing and movements had stopped. After the event he could speak but was somewhat incoherent. He was taken to the local emergency department, where his examination and mental status were normal. Screening blood and urine tests were normal, and he was discharged, with instructions to see his pediatrician for further recommendations.

His father remembers 2 or 3 other episodes of a somewhat different nature in the past month. These occurred as the boy was being put to bed. They involved some body stiffening and facial grimacing, with the mouth slightly open and the tongue twisted and deviated to one side. The child could not speak but appeared to be trying to talk. The

episodes lasted 20 to 30 seconds. Afterward the boy was his usual self and could tell his father what had been said to him.

The child has had no intercurrent illnesses or abnormal behavior apart from these "spells," and he has lost no abilities. A paternal cousin and grandfather had seizures during childhood but "grew out of them." The examination is completely normal.

Questions

1. How likely is it that episodic behavior such as that noted in the opening case represents a seizure?
2. What historical data about an event support the diagnosis of a seizure disorder?
3. How does the electroencephalogram help in classifying the type of seizure disorder?
4. What rationale should be used to formulate short-term and long-term treatment plans?

Seizures are a common medical problem in children. Diagnosing an episode that does not contain generalized convulsing movements as a seizure is sometimes problematic, however. Seizures are defined as episodic, stereotypical behavior syndromes of abrupt onset with loss of voluntary control by the patient, resulting in loss of responsiveness and rarely provoked by external stimuli. Frequently the occurrence of this behavior correlates with interictal brain electrical discharges on electroencephalogram (EEG), and the behavioral ictus (seizures) should match temporally with a period of electrical hypersynchrony if it occurs during the EEG recording.

A detailed history of the nature of the episodic behavior from an eyewitness is paramount, both in making the diagnosis of a seizure disorder and in elucidating the type of seizure problem. The EEG is most often an adjunct to diagnosis. It is abnormal in many individuals who do not have clinical seizures and it may be normal interictally in many patients with clinical seizures because of its sampling limitations. Special techniques can sometimes help alleviate these limitations.

The type of seizure problem is important information in devising the management plan. Seizures can simply be classified as primary generalized seizures or partial seizures. However, some partial seizures can secondarily generalize, thereby clinically mimicking primary generalized seizures. Distinguishing these entities illustrates the importance of eyewitness information. Many treatment

options are available, but the therapeutic plan must be individualized to the child's seizure type to optimize seizure control and minimize side effects. With appropriate treatment, most children with seizure disorders are not handicapped scholastically or socially and can enjoy normal lives.

Epidemiology

About 0.5% to 1.0% of all children experience at least one afebrile seizure. Recurrent seizures can occur as a component of a static encephalopathy after brain malformation or dysgenesis, encephalitis or meningitis, metabolic disorder, hypoxic-ischemic injury, or severe head trauma. Such secondary or symptomatic seizures make up approximately one-third of childhood epilepsies. The remaining two-thirds of epileptic seizures occur presumably as part of a genetic epileptic syndrome. As genetic knowledge increases, eventually it may no longer be true that most often seizures occur in children without any known cause or association.

Clinical Presentation

Children present with a history of an episode of abrupt onset characterized by a loss of ability to respond to external stimuli (Dx Box). They may experience various sensory phenomena before losing

Dx Seizures

- Abrupt loss of responsiveness
- Rhythmic clonic movements
- Sustained changes in posture or tone
- Simple automatic movements
- Staring without change in tone
- Simultaneous change in cerebral electrical activity (repetitive discharges)

consciousness and may be sleepy following convulsive movements. During the seizure, observers may note only an akinetic or staring spell or dramatic, rhythmic spasms of the face, extremities, or torso, depending on the type of seizure. Major motor seizures are frequently also associated with autonomic system changes, including changes in skin vascular supply causing color change, sweating, saliva production, and loss of sphincter control. Most seizure episodes are not provoked or attenuated by environmental factors (except for the provocative factors of fever, intercurrent illness, and sleep deprivation). Between episodes, children's general physical and neurologic examination may be entirely normal.

Pathophysiology

A seizure represents a sudden, synchronous depolarizing change in the electrical activity of a network of neurons that becomes widely propagated over the cortex, affecting awareness, responsiveness to external stimuli, and motor control. The propagation may be enhanced by defects in cell ion channels. Partial seizure disorders may result from a focal cortical lesion, such as a glial scar or dysplasia caused by a remote insult (eg, an infarct), or dysgenesis or cortical dysplasia that disrupts the electrical circuitry; displays retained prenatal cells and immature synaptic properties; and allows for periodic, abnormal transmission of impulses.

Exactly what initiates the synchronous depolarization of the neurons and the propagation is not well understood. Several physiological mechanisms, including neuronal circuitry, membrane ion channel abnormalities, neurotransmitter production metabolism or uptake, and perhaps glial support mechanisms are probably involved. An understanding of the mechanism involved in familial epilepsy syndromes awaits the definition of the various gene products and their functions. An example is cryptogenic West syndrome (infantile spasms), an "interneuronopathy," which has been associated with several genes including LIS1, DCX, and ARX (sometimes resulting in lissencephaly), which are important in GABAergic interneuron development. Another example is the neuronal voltage-gated sodium channel alpha subunit type 1 gene, which is mutated in the mild phenotype of generalized epilepsy with febrile convulsions plus and also mutated in the much worse phenotype of severe myoclonic epilepsy of infancy.

Seizure Types

Seizures can be simply classified as either **primary generalized seizures,** which include grand mal, generalized tonic-clonic convulsions, and petit mal (absence) seizures (so named because of the child's complete loss of awareness at the outset of the episode), or **partial seizures,** which include focal motor, psychomotor, and other partial disorders (Box 132-1). The examples presented here should not be considered an exhaustive list of seizure syndromes but some of the more important types encountered in practice.

Box 132-1. Classification of Epileptic Seizures

Partial seizures (seizures beginning locally)
- Elementary symptoms: focal seizures
- Complex symptoms: psychomotor seizures
- Partial seizures evolving secondarily to generalized seizures

Generalized seizures (bilaterally symmetrical; onset not local)
- Absence seizures (petit mal): typical and atypical
- Tonic-clonic seizures
- Tonic seizures
- Myoclonic seizures (minor motor)
- Atonic seizures (drop attacks)
- Infantile spasms

Unclassified seizures (includes neonatal "subtle" seizures)

Most seizures in older children result from a partial seizure disorder. **Psychomotor seizures** are partial seizures that have a wide range of ictal behaviors, including focal clonic jerking, aversive or asymmetrical hypertonic posturing, and more complex stereotypic fumbling or fingering behaviors. The seizures are usually preceded by a sensory aura or emotional manifestations and may be followed by postictal drowsiness. In some instances, children have partial sensory awareness during seizures. In other cases, however, they are completely unconscious. The initial partial motor manifestations may not be observed before they rapidly generalize. Partial seizures are more often associated with focal brain pathologic processes, including traumatic lesions, infarcts, malformations, infections (eg, viral infections or cerebral cysticercosis), and hippocampal sclerosis (seen on magnetic resonance imaging [MRI]).

Benign epilepsy syndromes occur in children with normal developmental history, respond well to therapy, and remit without sequelae. **Rolandic seizures** are a relatively common partial seizure syndrome that sometimes is familial and has a good prognosis for not lasting into adulthood. These episodes commonly occur when children are drowsy or awakening. Sensory auras precede the motor manifestations, which involve the tongue, mouth, or face and which can sometimes generalize to the rest of the body. The clinical syndrome is accompanied by a characteristic focal EEG discharge over the central temporal region of the scalp. Other benign syndromes include **benign familial infantile seizures, benign infantile seizures with mild gastroenteritis,** and **Panayiotopoulos syndrome,**

which is characterized by paroxysmal autonomic dysfunctions such as vomiting and other gastrointestinal (GI) motility problems, pallor, mydriasis, and cardiorespiratory and thermoregulatory abnormalities (lasting up to 30 minutes) ending often in generalized convulsing and largely occurring in sleep.

An **absence seizure** may sometimes be difficult to distinguish from a partial seizure (Table 132-1). The absence spell is a brief (2–15 seconds) loss of consciousness without loss of tone. Staring into space and minor movements such as lip smacking or semipurposeful-appearing movements of the hands are often the only observed behaviors. There is no postictal period. Because absence seizures occur multiple times a day and children are often unaware of them, parents may dismiss the subtle behavior change and inattention as daydreaming; however, these seizures may adversely affect learning. Hyperventilation, a useful diagnostic test that can be performed in the office, may provoke absence seizures. The EEG is confirmatory and distinguishes classic petit mal seizures with 3-per-second spike-wave discharges from variant syndromes. The classic petit mal is more often familial with dominant gene transmission, age-specific manifestation between 4 and 16 years, and sensitivity to ethosuximide; the atypical variant has a poorer prognosis for early resolution and is more resistant to anticonvulsant therapy.

Table 132-1. Partial Complex Versus Absence Seizures

	Partial Complex	*Absence*
Aura	Frequent	None
Loss of consciousness	Sometimes partial	Complete
Motor movements	Sometimes complex	Blinking or none
Postictal state	Frequent	None
Duration	>30 seconds	<15 seconds
Frequency	Few per month to few per day	Many per hour or day
Hyperventilation provoked	No	Yes
Electroencephalogram	Variably localized discharge or normal	3/s spike-wave generalized
Prognosis past adolescence	Frequently persists	Rarely occurs

A number of age-related seizure syndromes exist, perhaps related to maturational events in brain circuitry. Although the appearance of these syndromes is stereotypical, in most cases the prognosis depends on the etiologic diagnosis.

Neonatal seizures may be tonic, focal clonic, or multifocal clonic. The seizure problem is less often primary, and a vigorous search for an etiology of the seizure is more often successful than with older children. Problems commonly leading to neonatal seizures include hemorrhage (germinal matrix in the premature infant or subarachnoid from birth trauma in older neonates); hypoxic-ischemic damage from asphyxia; infections producing postnatal sepsis/meningitis or prenatal encephalitis; birth trauma; drug withdrawal in the infant of a substance-abusing mother; metabolic problems including hypoglycemia, hypocalcemia, or hypomagnesemia in the infant of a diabetic mother; amino or organic acidopathies occurring a few days after feedings have begun; and congenital brain malformations.

Infantile spasms are an age-related seizure syndrome with typical movements of flexion contraction of the trunk with the head bowed or sudden raising of the arms sometimes accompanied by a cry. These behaviors occur stereotypically several times in succession in a series. This syndrome occurs in infants between 3 months and 2 years of age. Another perhaps related but rarer syndrome of serial spasms, **Ohtahara syndrome,** occurs at a younger neonatal age and is associated with structural brain abnormalities and characterized by a different EEG pattern, but carries a similar ominous prognosis for impaired intellectual development. A third syndrome in older children that is also associated with a different but characteristic EEG pattern, **Lennox-Gastaut syndrome,** has the same poor prognosis for seizure control and cognitive development but produces several different behavioral seizure types, including tonic, absence, and drop attacks. Different types of brain lesions in these age groups (including focal lesions) can result in the same generalized seizure syndromes. Examples include tuberous sclerosis; neonatal ischemia, hemorrhage, or meningitis; and major central nervous system (CNS) malformations. These disorders most often present in the context of a moderate to severe learning disability.

Differential Diagnosis

Seizures are distinguished from non-epileptic paroxysmal disorders on the basis of history. The circumstances of place and time as well as details about the nature of the behavior are important pieces of data. **Syncope** is often preceded by symptoms of lightheadedness, nausea, tinnitus, and eventually a gradual darkening of vision sometimes without total loss of auditory perception. The syncopal episode is also frequently situational, unlike a seizure. It occurs when children are in hot, stuffy environments; when they have been standing in one place for a long time; or when they see or experience a painful event such as an injection or phlebotomy. Boys may experience micturition syncope standing in the bathroom shortly after arising in early morning.

Breath-holding spells are characterized by apnea and loss of responsiveness accompanied by either cyanosis or pallid skin. Breath-holding spells are also situational. Infants or children are often upset or crying just before such spells. They may be frightened by a seemingly minor injury or angry after a toy is taken away or they are disciplined. Children may then throw themselves backward and stiffen, and they may even have a few clonic jerks (see Chapter 38).

Selective attention is frequently mistaken for minor motor or absence seizures. This behavior often occurs when children are involved in passive activities (eg, watching television, playing a video game, or daydreaming) and do not respond to verbal stimuli such as hearing their own name called. Generally, the attention lapses do not occur during talking or eating; seizures will occur, however, even during these activities.

Epileptic seizures must also be differentiated from **pseudoseizures,** which actually occur most often in patients who have true seizures. Such episodes may resemble true seizures quite well, the psychodynamics of secondary gain or other motivation for the behavior may not be apparent, the "need" for attention may have some legitimacy, and the standard EEG often is not helpful. Pseudoseizures should be suspected in children who have witnessed seizures in relatives or close friends, who have seizures that recur in the same situations, whose seizure frequency is not decreased with therapeutic levels of anticonvulsants, and whose seizures appear "suggestible." Diagnosis can often be supported in complicated cases by simultaneous video EEG monitoring, which will show a lack of correlation of electrical abnormalities with the behavior in question. Postictal serum prolactin level also may be normal, and psychological assessment may detect underlying emotional problems related to prior trauma (eg, sexual abuse or other major psychological trauma). The prognosis of pseudoseizures in children generally is better than in adults and relates to the more acute psychosocial genesis of the problem in most children.

Paroxysmal events in sleep may also be a challenge for accurate diagnosis because the motor behaviors of non–rapid eye movement sleep or other **parasomnias** may mimic nocturnal frontal lobe epileptic seizures. Video EEG polysomnography will also help distinguish these as the former will not be associated with ictal discharges. Infantile gastroesophageal reflux (Sandifer syndrome) may look like brief epileptic tonic spasms, but should have a consistent temporal relationship to feeding. Benign paroxysmal vertigo occurs in the infant or toddler and presages migraine later in childhood but does not cause loss of responsiveness.

Evaluation (Box 132-2)

History

The history should determine the exact events surrounding the seizure episode. A detailed history of the nature of the behavior from an eyewitness is extremely important (Questions Box). The physician must

---

Box 132-2. Initial Evaluation of Seizure Patients

- Eyewitness account of the episode
- Description of children's own experiences before, during, and after the episode if they are articulate enough
- History from caregiver concerning remote injuries to the nervous system, progressive neurologic symptoms, or intercurrent illness
- Careful neurologic examination looking for signs of cerebral hemisphere lateralization
- Brain imaging study when a partial seizure is observed, a crescendo history of neurologic symptoms is obtained, focal neurologic signs are found on interictal examination, or the postictal encephalopathy persists too long
- Waking and sleep electroencephalogram with hyperventilation

---

Questions

Seizures

- Where was the child and what was he or she doing when the episode began?
- Did the child experience a loss of responsiveness?
- Did the child show any warning behavior or aura (eg, a cry, a facial expression of fear, irritability)?
- Did any part of the child's body become stiff? Was any shaking or jerking apparent?
- What did the child's eyes do and was saliva produced at the mouth?
- Did the child's skin change color?
- Did the child experience a loss of sphincter control?
- How long did the episode last?
- Has the child been well recently?
- Did the child have a complicated birth, head trauma, meningitis, or other previous brain damage?
- Have episodes of a similar nature occurred previously? If so, when did they begin and how frequently do they occur?
- Has the child's development and school experience progressed normally?
- Does the child have any relatives who have had seizures?

---

determine whether children experienced any loss of their normal level of responsiveness. Most often this change in mental status is abrupt, although a warning behavior or aura that lasts for a few seconds may precede complete loss of responsiveness. The warning behavior or aura may be a cry, an expression of fear or anxiety, or nonspecific irritability. If children are articulate, they may be able to describe a discrete sensory phenomenon or relate a less distinct or even indescribable sensation.

A change in muscle tone and activity is frequently associated with the abrupt change in mental status unless the spell is an absence seizure. Most often, the tone is increased with general extensor posturing, more focal hypertonicity, or more complex torsion or "aversive" upper-body posturing. The patient may fall if not supported. Rhythmic jerking or clonic movements (focal or general), including the trunk, limbs, face, and eyes, may occur concomitantly. Respirations may involve rhythmic grunting or nearly imperceptible movements. Swallowing may not occur, so that saliva pools or forms bubbles at the lips. Autonomic changes including skin color change (circumoral cyanosis), increased pulse, and loss of sphincter control frequently occur with major motor spells. The ictal period generally lasts 30 seconds to 2 minutes, although observers frequently overestimate this time. Postictal periods of sleepiness or lethargy may occur. Their length is often correlated with the length or intensity of the seizure.

Children and those around them are often unaware of the occurrence of absence seizures. Often an observant teacher brings the child's problem to a physician's attention. During a spell, a child has no change in tone or clonic movements and may have only subtle facial or hand movements. The episode lasts only a few seconds, and there are no preictal or postictal behaviors.

Historical information can also help determine potential etiologies of the seizure problem. A known distant brain insult or a hereditary disposition may be related to the cause. A progressive encephalopathy history indicates a need for a degenerative disease investigation.

Physical Examination

Children should be examined carefully for focal neurologic signs, particularly cerebral hemisphere-related asymmetries. The examination should include a developmental assessment and mental status examination. The physician should look for signs of potential genetic problems, such as dysmorphic features or organ malformations, which often correlate with cerebral dysgenesis; abnormal skin pigmentation or vessels, suggesting a neurocutaneous disorder; and organomegaly or bony abnormalities, indicating the possibility of a storage disorder. Children who are old enough to cooperate should be asked to hyperventilate to provoke an absence spell if the history is suggestive of this type of seizure.

Laboratory Tests

An EEG should be requested to help with the diagnosis of the type of seizure disorder. In children with partial seizure disorders, the interictal discharge is helpful in localizing the initial site of abnormal electrical activity. A sleep record is often essential for observing abnormalities. If a normal waking EEG is obtained and seizures continue to recur, it is sometimes useful to increase the likelihood of sleep during the record by prior sleep deprivation. Special techniques (eg, prolonged monitoring with telemetry or special anatomical electrode placements) can sometimes help overcome the standard EEG limitations of sample time and inaccessible areas of cerebral cortex. It should be noted, however, that even the standard EEG is rarely normal in petit mal disorders.

Historical information can frequently guide the need for metabolic tests. A blood sugar determination should be done acutely, but electrolytes are rarely abnormal in older children who have been well prior to the seizure. Neonates and infants with recurrent unexplained seizures should have metabolic screening including organic acid and amino acid levels and a diagnostic/therapeutic trial of pyridoxine. Tissue biopsy histologic analysis and specific assays may be indicated when physical signs suggest possible storage or metabolic etiologies.

Imaging Studies

Magnetic resonance imaging scans are particularly helpful if a progression in neurologic symptoms or signs has occurred, if there is a history of prior neurologic insult, if an asymmetry of strength or tone is noted on examination, or if signs of dysgenesis are present in other parts of the body. Even in the absence of these factors, partial or focal seizures have a higher yield of abnormal imaging results than do febrile seizures or petit mal disorders, which have a low yield. Acutely, intravenous contrast should generally be given because loss of focal blood-brain barrier with an inflammatory or neoplastic lesion can help with diagnosing the cause of the seizure.

Children with recurrent or resistant seizures should have an MRI scan, particularly when surgical treatment is under consideration. Coronal MRI scans can detect mesial temporal sclerosis, a lesion in the hippocampus seen in chronic temporal lobe epilepsy, and 20% of these will have had febrile seizures. Helpful additional modalities in studying surgical candidates include ictal positron emission tomography (PET) using fluorodeoxyglucose, interictal PET using α-methyl-L-tryptophan, single photon emission computerized tomography, functional MRI, and magnetoencephalography. These studies help define the nature of damaged or epileptic cortex and differentiate it from normal cortex.

Management

When there has been an episode of loss of consciousness or tone with potential recurrence, families need to be cautioned about the risks of submersion, falls from high places, and accidents with operating machinery including motor vehicles. However, anticonvulsants are the mainstay of management of seizure disorders (Table 132-2). At the same time the clinician must realize seizures and antiepileptic drugs affect brain development and could have long-term consequences, such as altered cognition and epilepsy susceptibility. (This observation may be especially true in the case of neonatal seizures where the seizures themselves may contribute to adverse outcomes; the standard treatment of phenobarbital has been shown in some models to be inhibitory of learning.) Anticonvulsants are prescribed if the risk of recurrence of seizures, particularly prolonged seizures, is significant based on seizure classification and individual factors. A known structural lesion or the clinical situation and EEG may suggest a higher recurrence risk. The choice of anticonvulsant depends on age, gender, neurologic diagnosis, seizure type and epilepsy syndrome, other conditions or medications, and social factors. The doses and combination of anticonvulsants prescribed for children depend on a balance of seizure resistance, risk of recurrence, and potential toxicity of medication. The initial goal is control with a single medication and as little toxicity as possible.

Oxcarbazepine and carbamazepine are often recommended for partial seizures. Toxicity is generally mild or nonexistent; adverse effects include GI upset, dizziness, and headache. Carbamazepine has been known to aggravate idiopathic generalized and myoclonic epilepsies, however. Phenytoin is also effective for partial types of seizures, and it can be given intravenously for status epilepticus. Phenobarbital is effective in neonatal seizures but may have deleterious effects on behavior and learning in older children. Ethosuximide is used for the relatively rare classical petit mal seizures. Valproic acid is used for more common atypical petit mal and other seizure disorders resistant to other anticonvulsants. It should not be used in a woman who might conceive because of an increased risk of fetal neural tube defects, however. Felbamate is also effective in many difficult to treat epilepsy syndromes, although a related incidence of severe bone marrow suppression and liver toxicity has limited its use. Other anticonvulsants including gabapentin, lamotrigine, vigabatrin, topiramate, zonisamide, and levetiracetam have proven

Table 132-2. Drugs Useful for Treating Seizures

Seizure Type	Dose	Toxic Symptoms/Side Effects
Partial Seizures		
Carbamazepine	Approx 15 mg/kg/d	Gastrointestinal distress, headache
Phenytoin	4–8 mg/kg/d	Ataxia, nystagmus, bone changes
Primidone	12–25 mg/kg/d	Drowsiness, ataxia
Oxcarbazepine	30 mg/kg/d	Drowsiness
Lamotrigine	4–7 mg/kg/d	Dizziness, sedation, rash (Stevens-Johnson syndrome)
Gabapentin	4–8 mg/kg/d	Somnolence, ataxia
Vigabatrin	15–50 mg/kg/d	Drowsiness, visual field defects
Topiramate	6–10 mg/kg/d	Weight loss, sedation, speech disturbance
Zonisamide	4–6 mg/kg/d	Sedation
Levetiracetam	20–30 mg/kg/d	Behavior or personality change
Neonatal Seizures		
Phenobarbital	5–6 mg/kg/d	Lethargy, irritability, osteopenia
Generalized Seizures		
Valproic acid	20–60 mg/kg/d	Tremors, hair loss, thrombocytopenia, weight gain
Felbamate	45 mg/kg/d	Insomnia, anorexia, bone marrow aplasia
Topiramate	6–10 mg/kg/d	Weight loss, sedation, speech disturbance
Clorazepate	0.1–0.4 mg/kg/d	Drowsiness
Clonazepam	0.15 mg/kg/d	Drowsiness, ataxia
Absence Seizures		
Ethosuximide	30 mg/kg/d	Nausea, hiccups
Valproic acid	20–60 mg/kg/d	Tremors, hair loss, thrombocytopenia, weight gain
Infantile Spasms		
Adrenocorticotropic hormone	40 U/m^2	Increased appetite, irritability, acne
Valproic acid	20–60 mg/kg/d	Tremors, hair loss, thrombocytopenia, weight gain
Vigabatrin	15–50 mg/kg/d	Drowsiness, visual field defects

effective. Gabapentin and levetiracetam are useful as adjunctive agents because of their lack of interaction with other anticonvulsants. Lamotrigine is useful in both partial and primary generalized seizure disorders. Vigabatrin is useful in infantile spasms when caused by tuberous sclerosis. Topiramate is effective in partial seizures, generalized seizures, and Lennox-Gastaut syndrome. Zonisamide and levetiracetam are effective in both partial and generalized seizure disorders.

Periodic monitoring of efficacy and side effects is essential in children who take medication daily on a long-term basis. A log of seizure frequency helps assess medication efficacy. Gastrointestinal and neurologic symptoms (sedation and ataxia) are the most common side effects. The perception of symptoms being related to the medication as well as the actual presence of side effects or toxicity both contribute to the complex issue of compliance. Serum drug levels are useful in monitoring compliance, dosage, and the likelihood that symptoms are the result of drug side effects. Organ toxicity (bone marrow, liver, and pancreas) must be considered and monitored with many

medications. Hypersensitivity reactions and Stevens-Johnson syndrome usually, but do not always, occur within 2 months of beginning the medication. Drug interactions can be important and can include the liver cytochrome P450-inducing potential of barbiturates and the potential of other medications, such as erythromycin, to inhibit other liver detoxification systems, such as that involved with carbamazepine metabolism, which produce acutely high levels and clinical toxicity. Recent onset of educational problems in a child with epilepsy deserves aggressive evaluation, both for determining a common etiology to the underlying seizure condition and for assessing medication toxicity or long-term effects.

Non-medication therapeutic options are also available for refractory cases. The ketogenic diet has success in about 50% of cases but requires considerable knowledge and commitment. The vagal nerve stimulator delivers a regular electrical stimulus afferently to the CNS and also allows for an abortive intervention by the caretaker with an external magnet. It is also effective in about 50% of cases, and when this occurs less medication may be used, allowing a better overall quality of life. Intracranial surgery for epilepsy in childhood must sometimes be considered. Children with seizure-associated syndromes including Sturge-Weber syndrome, Rasmussen encephalitis, catastrophic seizure disorders of early childhood such as infantile spasms related to a localized zone of epileptogenic cerebral tissue, and hamartomatous cortex–producing seizures have benefitted most, but patients with refractory partial seizure disorders, including temporal lobe epilepsy, may also be candidates. Extensive pre-surgical imaging and physiological monitoring are necessary for resective surgery candidates.

Prognosis

In general, approximately two-thirds of children who have experienced a tendency for seizure recurrence have a good prognosis for prevention of further recurrence and little or no problem with side effects of medication. They can lead normal lives without handicap. The etiologic diagnosis is the most important prognostic factor. The type of epilepsy, EEG findings, child's age, difficulty of initial seizure control, and time since the last seizure are also important. Some seizure types have intrinsically poor prognoses. For example, infantile spasms are prognostically ominous because even in the absence of a metabolic diagnosis, children frequently suffer temporary brain growth and developmental arrest unless the seizures are controlled with medication. About 10% to 25% of children, most often those with generalized symptomatic epilepsies, frequent seizures, high anticonvulsant use, and early onset of epilepsy, show some intellectual decline. Partial complex disorders and the atypical variant of petit mal disorders sometimes have a poorer prognosis for early resolution and may be more resistant to treatment with anticonvulsants. However, some of the seizure syndromes with a familial tendency such as rolandic seizures and typical petit mal seizures have a relatively good prognosis for both control by medication and ultimate complete resolution.

The individualized decision to discontinue medication is often complex. The prognosis for recurrence of seizures, the parents' and children's reactions to seizures and to the prospect of their recurrence, and social factors such as school participation may all contribute to the decision. Children and parents must be aware that none of the prognostic factors, whether considered individually or in combination, are absolute predictors of seizure recurrence or non-recurrence in a given child.

CASE RESOLUTION

The boy described in the case history at the beginning of the chapter had a generalized seizure when he was taken to the emergency department. The previous episodes recalled by the father had characteristics of partial seizures. The tonic-clonic seizure was probably a secondary generalized rather than a primary generalized seizure. The possibility of rolandic seizures is suggested by the circumstances of the prior episodes, drowsiness, "facial" or "oral" symptomatology, and the family history. This diagnosis was confirmed by electroencephalogram. Oxcarbazepine was prescribed. The boy experienced no side effects or seizure recurrences and was successfully able to discontinue the medication 3 years later.

Selected References

Camfield P, Camfield C. Pediatric epilepsy: an overview. In: Swaiman K, Ashwal S, Ferriero D, eds. *Pediatric Neurology: Principals and Practice.* 4th ed. Philadelphia, PA: Elsevier; 2006

Clancy R. The newborn drug development initiative workshop: summary proceedings from the neurology group on neonatal seizures. *Clin Ther.* 2006;28:1342–1352

Faught E. Epilepsy case studies. *Neurol Clin.* 2006;24:291–307

Glauser T, Ben-Menachem E, Bourgeois B, et al. ILAE treatment guidelines: evidence-based analysis of antiepileptic drug efficacy and effectiveness as initial monotherapy for epileptic seizures and syndromes. *Epilepsia.* 2006;47:1094–1120

Haslam RHA. Nonfebrile seizures. *Pediatr Rev.* 1997;18:39–49

Kato M. A new paradigm for West syndrome based on molecular and cell biology. *Epilepsy Res.* 2006;70(suppl 1):S87–S95

Koh S, Menkes J, Sankar R, Wu J. Paroxysmal disorders. In: Menkes J, Sarnat H, Maria B, eds. *Child Neurology.* 7th ed. Philadelphia, PA: Lippincott, Williams & Wilkins; 2006

Marsh ED, Brooks-Kayal AR, Proter BE. Seizures and antiepileptic drugs: does exposure alter normal brain development? *Epilepsia.* 2006;47:1999–2010

Pellock J, Dodson WE, Bourgeois B. *Pediatric Epilepsy Diagnosis and Therapy.* 2nd ed. New York, NY: Demos; 2001

Index

Page numbers followed by "t" indicate a table. Page numbers followed by "f" indicate a figure. Page numbers followed by "b" indicate a box.

A

Abdominal pain, 607–612
  adolescents, 610
  children, 609–610
  clinical presentation, 608
  differential diagnosis, 608–610
  epidemiology, 607
  evaluation, 610–611
  infants, 608–609
  management, 611
  pathophysiology, 607–608
  prognosis, 611
Abdominal trauma, 277–280
Abilify, 704t
Abnormal follicular keratinization, 652
ABR, 344
Absence seizure, 819, 819t
Abuse. *See* Failure to thrive (FTT); Physical abuse; Sexual abuse
Accommodative esotropia, 363
Accutane, 655
Acetabuloplasty, 534
Acetaminophen, 640t
Achalasia, 577
ACHES, 163, 163b
Acne, 651–655
  classification, 652t
  clinical presentation, 651–652
  epidemiology, 651
  evaluation, 652–653
  management, 653–655
  pathophysiology, 652
  prognosis, 655
Acquired coagulation inhibitors, 423
Acquired paralytic strabismus, 361
Acquired strabismus, 363
Acrodermatitis enteropathica, 665
Activated charcoal, 312t, 313
Active immunization, 118
Acute conjunctivitis, 369
Acute diarrhea, 595
Acute headaches, 639
Acute intermittent porphyria, 609
Acute kidney injury (AKI), 303–307. *See also* ARF/AKI
Acute necrotizing ulcerative gingivitis, 333
Acute OM (AOM), 335, 335b
Acute poststreptococcal glomerulonephritis, 481
Acute pyelonephritis, 491
Acute renal failure, 303–307. *See also* ARF/AKI
Acute tubular necrosis (ATN), 304
Acyclovir, 671, 715t

Addiction, 729
ADHD, 695–700. *See also* Attention-deficit/hyperactivity disorder (ADHD)
Adiposity rebound, 753
Adolescent depression and suicide, 771–776
Adolescents
  abdominal pain, 610
  body modification, 745–751
  depression, 771–776
  Down syndrome, 147–148
  eating disorders, 737–743
  health maintenance, 121–128
  immunization, 117, 123
  Internet usage, 33–34
  nutritional needs, 66–67
  substance abuse, 729–735
  suicide, 771–776
  talking with, 19–22
  vaginitis, 501t
  vegetarianism, 67
  vomiting, 578
Adrenocorticotropic hormone, 822t
Alcohol, 732t
All-hazards approach, 767
Allergic conjunctivitis, 369
Allergic contact dermatitis, 664, 669
Allergic disease, 387–392
  clinical presentation, 387
  differential diagnosis, 388
  epidemiology, 387
  evaluation, 389–390
  management, 390–391
  pathophysiology, 387–388
  prevention, 391
  prognosis, 391
Allergic rhinitis, 387, 389
Alopecia areata, 657, 660
α-thalassemias, 413
Alport syndrome, 482
ALTE, 253
Amastia, 522, 522f
Ambiguous genitalia, 467–471
  classification/causes, 469t
  clinical presentation, 467–468
  differential diagnosis, 468
  epidemiology, 467
  evaluation, 469
  gender assignment, 470
  management, 470
  pathophysiology, 468
  prognosis, 471
  treatment, 470–471

Amenorrhea, 516
Aminoaciduria, 486
Amitriptyline, 640t
Amphetamine, 699, 732t
Amrinone, 269
Anabolic steroids, 732t
Anagen effluvium, 660
Anaphylactoid purpura, 481
Anaphylaxis, 388, 389
Anemia, 411–418
  differential diagnosis, 412–416
  epidemiology, 411, 412b
  evaluation, 416–417
  macrocytic, 415
  management, 417
  microcytic, 413, 415
  normocytic, 415–416
  pathophysiology, 412
  prognosis, 417
Angioedema, 388, 389
Angular cheilitis, 332
Anion gap, 311
Ankyloglossia, 331
Ankylosing spondylitis, 802
Anodontia, 83
Anogenital anatomy, 714f
Anogenital examination, 714f
Anorexia nervosa, 737–743
Antalgic gait, 561
Anterior open bite, 83
Anterior uveitis, 370
Anthralin, 671
Anthrax, 769
Anti-reflux procedures, 585
Antidotes, 313, 314t
Antipyretics, 683
Anxiety, 207–211
AOM, 335, 335b
Aphthous ulcers, 331
Aplasia cutis congenita, 659
Apophysitis, 556
Apparent life-threatening event (ALTE), 253
Appendicitis, 610
Applied behavior analysis, 692b
ARF/AKI, 303–307
  clinical presentation, 303–304
  diagnostic indices, 305t
  differential diagnosis, 305
  epidemiology, 303
  etiology, 304b
  evaluation, 305–306
  intrinsic disorders, 304–305
  management, 306–307

ARF/AKI, *continued*
postrenal disorders, 304
prerenal disorders, 304
prognosis, 307
Arginine vasopressin (AVP), 295
Ariprazole, 704t
ARPANET, 31
Arterial blood gases, 439, 445
ASDs, 687–693. *See also* Autism spectrum disorders (ASDs)
Aspart, 798t
Asperger syndrome, 687
Asthma, 393–401. *See also* Wheezing and asthma
Asymmetrical tonic neck reflex, 88b
Athelia, 522
ATN, 304
Atopic dermatitis, 659, 665, 668, 668f
Attention-deficit/hyperactivity disorder (ADHD), 695–700
clinical presentation, 695
differential diagnosis, 697, 697b
DSM-IV, 695b
educational interventions, 699
epidemiology, 695
evaluation, 697–698
management, 698–700
pathophysiology, 696–697
stimulant medications, 699b
Atypical antipsychotics, 704–705
Autism spectrum disorders (ASDs), 687–693
alternative treatments, 692
associated medical conditions, 689b
clinical presentation, 688
disorders that co-occur with autism, 689b
disorders that mimic autism, 689b
DSM-IV, 687b
epidemiology, 688
evaluation, 689–691
excuses for unusual behavior, 690b
interventions, 691
management, 691
pathophysiology, 688–689
pharmacotherapy, 692
prognosis, 692
red flags, 688b
techniques used for treatment, 692b
Automated auditory brain stem response (ABR), 344
Autoregulation, 282
Avita, 653
AVP, 295
Azithromycin, 715t

B

Baby trichs, 213
Back pain, 567–572. *See also* Musculoskeletal disorders of neck and back
Bacteremia, 229. *See also* Fever and bacteremia
Bacterial conjunctivitis, 369
Bacterial vaginosis, 501t, 715t
Bacteriuria, 491
BAER, 344
Bag-valve mask, 244
Balanitis, 58

Barbiturates, 732t
Barlow (dislocation) test, 533f
Battered child syndrome, 707
Bedwetting, 219–222
Behavior. *See* Discipline
Behavioral analysis, 692b
Behavioral observation audiometry, 344
Benign migratory glossitis, 331
Benzathine penicillin, 715t
Benzodiazepines, 732t
Benzoyl peroxide, 653
Bernard-Soulier syndrome, 422
β-thalassemias, 413
β-thalassemias intermedia, 413
β-thalassemias major, 413
BHS, 203–205
Bilateral heart failure, 444
Bilious vomiting, 576
Bilirubin pathway, 614f
Bilirubin-reducing lights, 618
Biological agents, 769
Biomedical informatics, 27
Birth defect associations, 319
Biting, 214
Black box warning, 37
Blackhead, 652
Bleeding disorders, 419–426
clinical presentation, 419
differential diagnosis, 421–423
epidemiology, 419
evaluation, 424–425
inherited *vs* acquired, 420t
management, 425–426
pathophysiology, 420–421
prognosis, 426
Blepharitis, 368
Blount disease, 545
Body modification (tattooing/body piercing), 745–751
body piercing, 746–747
clinical presentation, 746
complications, 749b
epidemiology, 745–746
evaluation, 747–750
high-risk behavior, 748b
management, 750
prognosis, 750
role of primary care provider, 750
tattoos, 746
Body piercing, 745–751. *See also* Body modification (tattooing/body piercing)
Bohn nodules, 332
Bone sarcomas, 782
Botulinum toxin, 769
Botulinum toxin type A, 646
Bowlegs and knock-knees, 543–546
Brachycephaly, 325, 325f, 326f
Brain stem auditory evoked response (BAER), 344
Brain tumors, 780, 781t, 784t
Branding, 745
BRAT diet, 599
Breast development, 162f

Breast disorders, 521–528. *See also* Disorders of the breast
Breast milk jaundice, 614
Breastfeeding, 71–73
benefits, 71–72
contraindications, 72
epidemiology, 71
lactation, 71
management, 72
problems, 72–73
resources for mother, 73
twins, 53
Breastfeeding jaundice, 614
Breath-holding spells (BHS), 203–205
Buck teeth, 83
Bulimia nervosa, 737–743
Bullous impetigo, 679–680
Bullying, 763–766
Byler syndrome, 617

C

CAH, 577
Calcipotriene, 671
Caloric intake, 720
Caloric method, 293, 294t
Cancer, 779–786
clinical presentation, 779–782
diagnostic tests, 784t
differential diagnosis, 782–783
epidemiology, 779
evaluation, 783–785
imaging studies, 784t
management, 785
pathophysiology, 782
prognosis, 786
signs/symptoms, 781–782t
Candida albicans, 501t
Candidiasis, 664
Canker sores, 331
Capsulorrhaphy, 534
Caput succedaneum, 658
Car seats, 170t
Carbamazepine, 822t
Cardiac syncope, 259
Cardiogenic shock, 266, 266t
Cardiovascular system, 431–463
chest pain, 449–454
congestive heart failure, 443–448
cyanosis in the newborn, 437–441
heart murmurs, 433–436
hypertension, 455–463
Cat-scratch disease, 379
Cathartics, 312t, 313
CDR, 28
CDSS, 28
Cefixime, 715t
Ceftriaxone, 715t
Celiac disease, 598
Central precocious puberty, 523
Cephalhematoma, 658
Cerebral contusion, 282
Cerebral palsy, 92, 156, 562

Cervical lymphadenopathy, 427
Cervicitis, 507
Chalazion, 369
Chapter authors. *See* Contributors
Charcoal hemoperfusion, 313
Chemical exposures, 769
Chemical urethritis, 184
Chest pain, 449–454
    cardiac causes, 451b
    clinical presentation, 449
    differential diagnosis, 450b, 451
    epidemiology, 449
    evaluation, 451–453
    management, 453
    pathophysiology, 450–451
    prognosis, 454
Chest x-ray, 440, 445
Chickenpox, 679
Child abuse. *See* Failure to thrive (FTT); Physical
    abuse; Sexual abuse
Child advocacy, 7–9
Childhood obesity, 753–757
    clinical presentation, 754
    diet history, 755b
    differential diagnosis, 754
    epidemiology, 753
    evaluation, 754–755
    healthier lifestyle, 755b
    management, 755–756
    pathophysiology, 754
    prevention, 757
    prognosis, 757
Children with special health care needs, 155–159
    clinical presentation, 156
    differential diagnosis, 156
    epidemiology, 155–156
    evaluation, 156–157
    management, 157–159
    pathophysiology, 156
    prognosis, 159
Chlamydia, 503–504, 715t
Chlamydia trachomatis, 501t
Chlamydial conjunctivitis, 369
Chlorambucil, 813t
Chronic daily headaches, 639
Chronic diarrhea, 595
Chronic diseases, 777–823
    cancer, 779–786
    collagen vascular disease, 801–807
    diabetes mellitus, 795–800
    epilepsy, 817–823
    kidney disease, 787–793
    nephrotic syndrome, 809–815
    renal failure, 787–793
    seizures, 817–823
Chronic kidney disease/chronic renal failure,
    787–793
    clinical presentation, 788–789
    diagnostic workup, 791
    differential diagnosis, 789–790
    epidemiology, 788
    evaluation, 790–791

    initiation of dialysis, 792b
    management, 791–793
    pathophysiology, 789
    prognosis, 793
    treatment of hyperkalemia, 792b
Chronic OME, 336
Chronic progressive headaches, 639
Chronic pyelonephritis, 491
Chronic recurrent headaches, 639
Chronic suppurative OM, 336
Cimetidine, 585t
Circumcision, 57–61
    benefits, 58–59
    clinical presentation, 57
    complications, 59b, 60
    contraindications, 59–60
    differential diagnosis, 58
    epidemiology, 57
    evaluation, 58
    management, 59–60
    parent counseling, 59
    pathophysiology, 57
    procedure, 60
    prognosis, 58
    risks/complications, 59
CKD, 787–793. *See also* Chronic kidney disease/
    chronic renal failure
Cleft lip, 324f
Cleft palate, 323
Clinical data repository (CDR), 28
Clinical decision support system (CDSS), 28
Clomipramine, 646
Clonazepam, 822t
Clorazepate, 822t
Closed comedo, 652
Clotrimazole, 500, 671
Clubfoot, 540
Cluster headaches, 639
Cocaine, 724, 732t
Cochlear implant, 345
Colic, 189–193
Collagen, 801
Collagen vascular disease, 801–807
    clinical presentation, 802
    dermatomyositis (DM), 804, 806
    epidemiology, 801–802
    evaluation, 805–806
    inflammatory myopathies, 804
    juvenile idiopathic arthritis (JIA), 802–803, 806
    management, 806
    pathophysiology, 805
    prognosis, 806–807
    scleroderma, 804–805, 806
    systemic lupus erythematosus (SLE), 803, 806
Collagen-vascular disorders, 422
Colon, 602
Comedones, 652
Community pediatrics, 8
Compensated shock, 265, 272
Complete blood count, 445
Computerized provider order entry, 28
Concussion, 282

Conditioned play audiometry, 344
Conductive hearing loss, 342
Confidentiality, 28
Congenital adrenal hyperplasia (CAH), 577
Congenital clubfoot, 540
Congenital deafness, 341
Congenital epulis, 331
Congenital glaucoma, 375–376
Congenital metatarsus varus, 540
Congenital paralytic strabismus, 361
Congenital strabismus, 362
Congenital syphilis, 665
Congenital thrombocytopenias, 423
Congestive heart failure, 443–448
    clinical presentation, 443
    differential diagnosis, 444
    epidemiology, 443
    evaluation, 444–445
    management, 446–447
    pathophysiology, 444
    prognosis, 447
Conjugate vaccines, 118
Conjugated hyperbilirubinemia, 615–616
Conjunctivitis, 369, 389
Constipation, 601–606
    clinical presentation, 601–602
    differential diagnosis, 603–604
    epidemiology, 601
    evaluation, 604
    management, 605
    pathophysiology, 602–603
    physical examination, 604–605
    prognosis, 605
    referral to gastroenterologist, 605
Contraceptive methods, 165–166
Conventional audiometric testing, 344
Coombs test, 417
Corneal light reflex test, 364
Corticosteroids, 250, 269
Cough, 403–408
Cough reflex, 404f
CPK, 634
CRAFFT questions, 733b
Craniofacial anomalies, 323–329
    clinical presentation, 324
    differential diagnosis, 326
    epidemiology, 323
    evaluation, 327–328
    management, 328
    pathophysiology, 324–325
    prognosis, 329
Craniosynostosis, 324
Crigler-Najjar syndrome type I, 615
Crigler-Najjar syndrome type II, 617
Crohn disease, 597
Crossbite, 83
Croup. *See* Stridor and croup
Croup score, 249t
Crusted scabies, 669
Crying, 189–193
Crystal methamphetamine, 732t
Cushing triad, 283

Cyanosis in the newborn, 437–441
Cyberbullying, 32
Cyclic vomiting, 578
Cyclophosphamide, 813t
Cyclosporine, 813t
Cyproheptadine, 640t
Cystic fibrosis, 598
Cystic hygromas, 381
Cystitis, 491
Cysts, 652

D

Dacryocystitis, 373, 374
Dacryostenosis, 374
Data, 27
Database, 27
Dawn phenomenon, 798
DDH, 531–535, 562
Decontamination, 312–313
Defecation, 602
Deformations, 318
Delayed effect, 760
Dennie sign, 389
Dental disorders. *See* Oral health and dental
        disorders
Dental lamina cysts, 332
Dentinogenesis imperfecta, 84
Depo-Provera, 165
Depression, 771–776
Deprivational amblyopia, 362
Dermatologic disorders, 649–684
        acne, 651–655
        diaper dermatitis, 663–666
        hair/scalp disorders, 657–662
        morbilliform rashes, 673–678
        papulosquamous eruptions, 667–672
        vesicular exanthema, 679–684
Dermatomyositis (DM), 804, 806
Desmopressin, 222
Detemir, 798t
Developmental delays, 89, 92
Developmental dysplasia of the HIP (DDH),
        531–535, 562
Developmental evaluation, 93
Developmental field defect, 319
Developmental screening, 93
Developmental surveillance, 93
Dexamethasone, 291, 640t
Dextromethorphan, 730
Diabetes mellitus, 609, 795–800
        clinical presentation, 795–796
        differential diagnosis, 796
        education, 799
        epidemiology, 795
        evaluation, 796–797
        exercise, 799
        glucose monitoring, 798
        insulin, 797–798
        management, 797–799
        nutrition, 799
        pathophysiology, 796
        predictive tests, 796t
        prognosis, 799

Diabetic ketoacidosis, 799
Diamond-Blackfan anemia, 416
Diaper dermatitis, 663–666
Diarrhea, 595–599
        clinical presentation, 595
        definitions, 595
        differential diagnosis, 596–598
        epidemiology, 595
        evaluation, 598–599
        management, 599
        pathophysiology, 596
        prognosis, 599
Diffuse axonal injury, 282
Digoxin, 446
Dihydroergotamine, 640t
Dihydroxycholecalciferol, 789
Diphenylhydantoin, 640t
Direct laryngoscopy, 250
Disaster preparedness, 767–770
Discipline, 193–197
        defined, 193
        differential diagnosis, 194
        evaluation, 194–195
        ignoring, 196
        physician-parent interactions, 193
        problem behaviors, 194
        prognosis, 196
        psychophysiology, 194
        redirection, 195
        removal of privileges, 196
        scolding, 195–196
        spanking, 195
        time-out, 196
Discoid lupus erythematosus, 660
Discolored teeth, 83
Diskitis, 563
Disorders of hair and scalp, 657–662
        clinical presentation, 658
        differential diagnosis, 658–660
        epidemiology, 657
        evaluation, 660–661
        management, 661–662
        pathophysiology, 658
        prognosis, 662
        scalp disorders with hair loss, 659–660
        scalp disorders with no hair loss, 658–659
Disorders of the breast, 521–528
        causes of breast masses, 525b
        causes of galactorrhea, 524b
        causes of gynecomastia, 525b
        clinical presentation, 523
        differential diagnosis, 524–525
        epidemiology, 521–523
        evaluation, 525–527
        management, 527
        normal breast development, 523
        pathophysiology, 523–524
        prognosis, 527
Disruptions, 318
Dissociative shock, 266t, 267
Distributive shock, 266, 266t
Divorce, 759–762

DM, 804, 806
Dobutamine, 268
Dopamine, 268
Down syndrome, 143–148. *See also* Trisomy
Doxycycline, 654, 715t
Drug allergies, 36
Drug dosing, 37, 38t
Drug-induced gingival hyperplasia, 332
DUB, 514–515, 519, 519t
Duchenne muscular dystrophy, 631
Dynamic hallucis abductus, 540
Dysautonomia, 578
Dysfunctional uterine bleeding (DUB), 514–515,
        519, 519t
Dyshidrotic eczema, 680
Dyskinetic cerebral palsy, 92
Dysmenorrhea, 514, 518
Dysmorphic child, 317–321
        clinical presentation, 318
        differential diagnosis, 318–319
        epidemiology, 317–318
        evaluation, 319–320
        management, 320
        pathophysiology, 318
        prognosis, 320
Dysplasias, 318

E

Early childhood caries (ECC), 83
Eating disorders, 737–743
EBV, 676
ECC, 83
ECG, 435, 440
Echocardiography, 440
Ecstasy, 732t
Ectodermal dysplasia, 660
Edematous children, 485
Egg-allergic child, 117
EHR, 28
EI, 674, 675
Electrocardiogram (ECG), 435, 440
Electrolyte disturbances. *See* Fluid and electrolyte
        disturbances
Electromyography (EMG), 632, 634t
Electronic health record (EHR), 28
Electronic medical record (EMR), 28
Encopresis, 223–226
End-stage renal disease (ESRD), 787
Endoscopy with biopsy, 583
Enterovirus infections, 675
Enteroviruses, 674
Enthesitis-related arthritis, 802
Enuresis, 219–222
Environmental deprivation, 717
Environmental FTT, 718
Epididymitis, 505–507
Epidural hematomas, 282
Epiglottitis, 349
Epilepsy, 817–823. *See also* Seizures and epilepsy
Epinephrine, 268
Epiphora, 373–376
Epistaxis, 355–359. *See also* Nosebleed
Epstein pearls, 332

Ergotamine, 640t
Eruption hematoma, 82
Erythema infectiosum (EI), 674, 675
Erythromycin, 585t, 671, 715t
Erythromycin gel, 654
Esotropia, 362
ESRD, 787
Ethosuximide, 822t
Everted foot, 539
Evoked otoacoustic emissions, 344
Ewing sarcoma, 782, 782t, 784t
Exanthem subitum, 674
Excessive training, 373–376
Exchange transfusion, 618
Exogenous pigments, 479t
Expiratory stridor, 247
Expressive milestones, 96t
External tibial torsion, 541
Extrahepatic biliary atresia, 616
Eye infections, 367–372. *See also* Infections of the eye
Eyelid infections, 368–369

F

Face tent, 244, 244f
Factor XI deficiency, 422
Factor XIII deficiency, 422
Failure to thrive (FTT), 717–721
    caloric intake, 720
    clinical presentation, 718
    defined, 717
    differential diagnosis, 718
    epidemiology, 718
    evaluation, 719–720
    management, 720–721
    parenting issues, 721
    pathophysiology, 718
    prognosis, 721
Fainting, 259–263. *See also* Syncope
Family orientation, 3
Famotidine, 585t
FAS, 724
FASD, 724
Fears, 207–211
Febrile seizures, 237–240
    clinical presentation, 237–238
    differential diagnosis, 238
    epidemiology, 237
    evaluation, 239
    management, 239–240
    pathophysiology, 238
    prognosis, 240
    simple *vs* complex seizures, 238t
Feeding. *See* Nutritional needs
Felbamate, 822t
Female breast development, 162f
Female pubic hair development, 162f
Femoral shortening, 534
Fetal alcohol spectrum disorders (FASD), 724
Fetal alcohol syndrome (FAS), 724
Fever and bacteremia, 229–235
    clinical presentation, 230
    differential diagnosis, 231
    epidemiology, 229–230

evaluation, 231–233
    infectious causes, 231b
    low-risk criteria—young infants, 234b
    management, 233–234
    pathophysiology, 230
    prognosis, 234
    risk factors, 231b
Fever of unknown origin (FUO), 231
Fibroma, 332
Fifth disease, 674
First contact, 3
FISH analysis, 320
Fissured tongue, 331
Floor time, 692b
Fluconazole, 662
Fluid and electrolyte disturbances, 293–302
    epidemiology, 293–295
    evaluation, 296–298
    fluid needs in illness, 294–295
    maintenance requirements, 293–294
    management, 298–301
    oral rehydration, 300–301
    parenteral fluid therapy, 299
    pathophysiology, 295–296
    potassium replacement, 300
    prognosis, 301
Fluorosis, 83
Fluoxetine, 640t, 646
Fluphenazine, 646
Focal segmental glomerulosclerosis (FSGS), 810
Food allergy, 388, 390
Foot progression angle during gait, 538
Formula, 64t
Formula concentration, 720
46XX DSD, 467
46XX testicular DSD, 469t
46XY complete gonadal dysgenesis, 467
46XY DSD, 467
Foster care, 137–141
FSGS, 810
FTT, 717–721. *See also* Failure to thrive (FTT)
Functional fecal retention with encopresis, 223
FUO, 231
Furosemide, 446

G

Gabapentin, 822t
Galactorrhea, 524
Gastric lavage, 312, 312t
Gastroesophageal reflux (GER), 581–586
    anti-reflux procedures, 585
    clinical presentation, 581–582
    differential diagnosis, 582
    epidemiology, 581
    evaluation, 583–584
    GERD, contrasted, 581
    lifestyle changes, 584
    management, 584–585
    medications, 584–585, 585t
    non-reflux causes of vomiting, 582b
    pathophysiology, 582
    prognosis, 585

Gastroesophageal reflux disease (GERD), 581
Gastrointestinal bleeding, 587–593
    causes, 590t
    children, 591–592
    clinical manifestations, 589t
    clinical presentation, 587–588
    differential diagnosis, 589–592
    epidemiology, 587
    evaluation, 588
    infants, 590–591
    management, 592–593
    neonates, 589–590
    pathophysiology, 588
    procedural management, 593b
    prognosis, 593
    resuscitation, 592–593
Gastrointestinal disorders, 573–627
    abdominal pain, 607–612
    constipation, 601–606
    diarrhea, 595–599
    gastroesophageal reflux, 581–586
    gastrointestinal bleeding, 587–593
    infectious hepatitis, 621–627
    jaundice, 613–619
    vomiting, 575–579
Generalized lymphadenopathy, 427
Genital ulcers, 508–509
Genital warts, 509–510
Genitourinary disorders, 465–528
    ambiguous genitalia, 467–471
    disorders of the breast, 521–528
    hematuria, 477–483
    inguinal lumps and bumps, 473–476
    menstrual disorders, 513–520
    proteinuria, 485–489
    sexually transmitted infections, 503–511
    urinary tract infections, 491–495
    vaginitis, 497–501
Genu valgum, 544
Genu varum, 544
Geodon, 704t
GER, 581–586. *See also* Gastroesophageal reflux (GER)
GERD, 581
GFR, 787
GI bleeding, 587–593. *See also* Gastrointestinal bleeding
Gianotti-Crosti syndrome, 674, 676
Gifted children, 105–108
Giggle incontinence, 184
Gilbert disease, 617
Gingivitis, 331–334
Glanzmann thrombasthenia, 422
Glargine, 798t
Glasgow Coma Scale, 275b, 283t, 284t
Glaucoma, 375–376
Glomerular diseases, 481–482
Glomerular filtration rate (GFR), 787
Glomerulonephritis, 481
Glucose-6-phosphate dehydrogenase deficiency, 415
Glucose intolerance, 788
Glucose monitoring, 798

Gonadectomy, 470
Gonorrhea, 504
Granuloma gluteale infantum, 664
Grasp reflex, 88b
Gross hematuria, 477
Growing pains, 547–553. *See also* Orthopedic injuries and growing pains
Guanfacine, 646
Gynecomastia, 522, 522f, 525b

H
H2RA, 584
Habit covariance, 216
Haddon matrix, 169–170, 170t
Haggerty, Robert, 7, 8
Hair-grooming syncope, 259
Hair/scalp disorders, 657–662
Haloperidol, 646
Hand-foot-and-mouth disease (HFMD), 675, 679
HBIG, 625
Head lice, 659
Head trauma, 281–286
    clinical presentation, 281
    CT scan, 284b
    epidemiology, 281
    evaluation, 283–285
    Glasgow Coma Scale, 283t, 284t
    management, 285–286
    pathophysiology, 281–282
    prevention, 286
    prognosis, 286
    types of head injuries, 282
Headache, 637–641
    acute, 638
    chronic progressive, 638
    chronic recurrent, 638
    clinical presentation, 637
    differential diagnosis, 638
    drugs, 640t
    epidemiology, 637
    evaluation, 639
    management, 639–640
    pathophysiology, 638
    prognosis, 641
HEADDSSS, 20, 21, 516
Health informatics, 27
Hearing aids, 345
Hearing impairment, 341–346
    causes of childhood deafness, 343b
    clinical presentation, 342
    differential diagnosis, 343
    epidemiology, 341
    evaluation, 343–345
    management, 345–346
    newborn hearing screening, 343
    pathophysiology, 342–343
    prognosis, 346
    types of hearing loss, 342
Heart murmurs, 433–436
Heel-bisector, 538
Height suppression, 702
Hematologic and vascular disorders, 609

Hematuria, 477–483
    causes, 478t
    clinical presentation, 478
    differential diagnosis, 479
    epidemiology, 477
    etiology, 477t
    evaluation, 479–481
    glomerular diseases, 481–482
    management, 482
    pathophysiology, 478–479
    pigmenturia, distinguished, 479t
    prognosis, 482
    urinary calcium-creatinine ratios, 479t
Hemodialysis, 313
Hemoglobin H disease, 413
Hemoglobinuria, 479t
Hemolytic anemias, 415
Hemolytic uremic syndrome (HUS), 482, 591
Hemophilia, 422
Hemophilia C, 422
Henoch-Schönlein purpura, 591
Hepatitis, 621–627
Hepatitis A, 622, 625
Hepatitis B, 622–623, 625–626
Hepatitis B immunoglobulin (HBIG), 625
Hepatitis C, 623, 626
Hepatitis D, 623, 626
Hepatitis E, 623
Hereditary spherocytosis, 415–416
Heroin, 732t
Herpangina, 332
Herpes genitalis, 715t
Herpes simplex virus (HSV), 679
Herpes simplex virus type 2 (HSV-2), 504
Herpes zoster, 680
Herpetic infections of the eye, 370
Heterotropia, 362
HFMD, 675, 679
High pulmonary blood flow (HPBF) group, 438
Higher-order multiples. *See* Twins and higher-order multiples
Hip dysplasia, 531–535
Hip rotation, 538
HIS, 28
Hodgkin disease, 780, 781t, 784t
Hordeolum, 368
Hormone replacement therapy, 470
Hospital information system (HIS), 28
HPBF group, 438
HPV, 504
HSV, 679
HSV-2, 504
Human-computer interaction, 28
Human papillomavirus (HPV), 504
HUS, 482, 591
Hydrops fetalis, 413
Hyperbilirubinemia, 614–616
Hypercalciuria, 479
Hypercholesterolemia, 788, 810
Hyperkalemia, 788, 792b
Hyperlipidemia, 788
Hypernatremic dehydration, 295

Hyperoxia challenge, 439
Hyperparathyroidism, 789
Hypertension, 455–463
    blood pressure levels, 457–458t, 459–460t
    causes, 461b
    clinical presentations, 456
    definitions, 456t
    differential diagnosis, 456
    epidemiology, 455–456
    etiology, 456
    evaluation, 456–462
    laboratory evaluation, 462b
    management, 462
    normal blood pressure, 455
    pathophysiology, 456
    prevention, 463
    prognosis, 462–463
Hypertonic dehydration, 296f
Hypertriglyceridemia, 788
Hypoalbuminemia, 810
Hypodontia, 82
Hypoglycemia, 799
Hypokalemia, 788
Hyponatremic dehydration, 296
Hypoproteinemia, 810
Hypotonia, 631–636
    approach to the diagnosis, 633t
    clinical presentation, 631
    differential diagnosis, 632–633
    epidemiology, 631
    evaluation, 633–635
    laboratory tests, 634–635, 634t
    management, 635–636
    pathophysiology, 632
    prognosis, 636
Hypotonic dehydration, 296f
Hypovolemic shock, 266, 266t

I
IAA, 796t
Ibuprofen, 640t
ICA, 796t
Idiosyncratic reaction, 703
IgA nephropathy, 481
Ignoring, 196
IIS, 29
Imipramine, 222
Immune-mediated anemias, 416
Immunization, 115–120
    active, 118
    adolescents, 117, 123
    adverse events, 119
    egg-allergic child, 117
    immunocompromised child, 116
    international persons, 117
    Internet sources of information, 119t
    passive, 117–118
    precautions/contraindications, 119
    pregnancy, 116
    special-risk populations, 116
    vaccination schedule, 115–116
    vaccine received in other countries, 118

Immunization information system (IIS), 29
Immunocompromised child, 116
Impetigo, 664
Implanon, 165
In-toeing, 537–542
Inactivated vaccines, 118
Increased intracranial pressure, 287–292
    clinical presentation, 288
    differential diagnosis, 289
    epidemiology, 287–288
    evaluation, 290
    management, 290–291, 292b
    pathophysiology, 288–289
    prognosis, 292
Infant formula, 64t
Infantile exotropia, 362
Infantile glaucoma, 375–376
Infantile strabismus, 362
Infants of substance-abusing mothers, 723–726
Infections of the eye, 367–372
    clinical presentation, 367
    differential diagnosis, 367–370
    epidemiology, 367
    evaluation, 370–371
    management, 371–372
    pathophysiology, 367
    prognosis, 372
Infectious hepatitis, 621–627
Inflammatory bowel disease, 597
Inflammatory diarrhea, 596
Inflammatory myopathies, 804
Informatics, 27–30
Information, 27
Information system, 27
Ingestions, 309–314
    anticipatory guidance and prevention, 314
    antidotes, 313, 314t
    clinical presentation, 309
    decontamination, 312–313
    differential diagnosis, 309–310
    epidemiology, 309
    evaluation, 310–312
    laboratory tests, 311, 311b
    management, 312–314
    pathophysiology, 309
    potentially fatal substances, 314b
    prognosis, 314
    supportive care, 313
    toxidromes, 311t
Inguinal lumps and bumps, 473–476
Inhalants, 732t
Inherited coagulation deficiencies, 423
Injury prevention, 169–173
    advocacy, 172
    car seats, 170t
    counseling, 171–172
    epidemiology, 169
    Haddon matrix, 169–170, 170t
    passive/active interventions, 170–171
    recent recommendations, 172
    TIPP, 171, 171t

Innocent vibratory murmur, 434
Inspiratory stridor, 247
Insulin, 797–798
Insulin autoantibodies (IAA), 796t
Interface, 28
Intermittent exotropia, 363
Internal femoral torsion, 541
Internal tibial torsion, 540
International adoptees, 129–135
    clinical presentation, 130–131
    epidemiology, 129–130
    evaluation, 132–133
    health care issues, 131–132
    Internet as source of information, 130t
    management, 133–134
    pediatrician's role, 134–135
    prognosis, 134
Internet usage, 31–34
Interoperability, 28
Interstitial nephritis, 479
Intra-esophageal pH monitoring, 583
Intracranial hemorrhage, 639
Intraosseous cannulation technique, 279
Intravenous immunoglobulin, 635
Intussusception, 591, 609
Inverted foot, 539
Iron deficiency, 413, 417
Irreversible shock, 272
Irritable bowel syndrome, 597
Irritant contact dermatitis, 664
Irritant dermatitis, 669
Islet cell antibodies (ICA), 796t
Isometheptene mucate, 640t
Isonatremic/isotonic dehydration, 296f
Isotonic/isonatremic dehydration, 296f
Isotretinoin, 655
Itraconazole, 662
Ivermectin, 671

J
Jacobi, Abraham, 7
Jaundice, 613–619
    clinical presentation, 613
    differential diagnosis, 614–617
    epidemiology, 613
    evaluation, 617–618
    hyperbilirubinemia, 614–616
    management, 618
    neonates, 614–616
    pathophysiology, 614
    prognosis, 618
Jervell and Lange-Nielsen syndrome, 261
JIA, 564, 802–803, 806
Juvenile DM, 804
Juvenile idiopathic arthritis (JIA), 564, 802–803, 806
Juvenile polymyositis, 804
Juvenile polyps, 591

K
Kawasaki disease, 674, 675–676, 677
Kerion, 660
Kidney failure, 787–793. See also Chronic kidney
        disease/chronic renal failure
Kindergarten readiness skills, 110b
Kinky hair syndrome, 660
Knock-knees, 543–546
Knowledge, 27
Koebner phenomenon, 669
Koplik spots, 675f

L
Labial adhesions, 712
Labial fusion, 184
Laboratory information system, 28
Laboratory tests, 4
Lamotrigine, 822t
Langerhans cell histiocytosis, 665
Language development, 95–99
Lansoprazole, 585t
Lateral tibial torsion, 541t
LCPD, 564
Left-sided failure, 444
Leg length discrepancy, 562
Legg-Calvé-Perthes disease (LCPD), 564
Leukemia, 779, 781t, 784t
Leukoplakia, 331
Levamisole, 813t
Levetiracetam, 822t
Lice, 659
Lichen planus, 660, 669
Lichen sclerosus et atrophicus, 712
Lichen striatus, 669
Limp, 561–566
    clinical presentation, 561
    defined, 561
    differential diagnosis, 561–564
    epidemiology, 561
    evaluation, 564–565
    management, 565
    pathophysiology, 561
    prognosis, 566
Lindane, 671
Linear SD, 805
Lipid disturbances, 792
Lispro, 798t
Literacy, 101–104
Live-attenuated vaccines, 118
Liver biopsy, 618
Localized lymphadenopathy, 427
Localized scleroderma, 804–805
Long bone, 549f
Long bone fracture patterns, 549t
Long QT syndrome, 261, 261t
Longitudinal care, 3
Loose anagen syndrome, 660
Low pulmonary blood flow (LPBF) group, 438
LPBF group, 438
LSD, 732t
Lupus nephritis, 803
Lymph node drainage patterns, 428t

Lymphadenitis, 379
Lymphadenopathy, 378, 427–430, 782
Lymphoblastic lymphoma, 782
Lymphoma, 780

M
Macrocytic anemias, 415
Male genital/pubic hair development, 163f
Malformations, 318
Malocclusion, 83
Malware, 33
Mannitol, 291
Marijuana, 730, 732t
Mastitis, 73
Maternal substance abuse during pregnancy,
   723–726
MCD, 809
Mean corpuscular hemoglobin (MCH), 417
Measles, 673, 674
Mebendazole, 500
Meckel diverticulum, 591, 610
Medial femoral torsion, 541t
Medial tibial torsion, 541t
Medical informatics, 27
Membranous nephropathy, 481
Menkes syndrome, 660
Menstrual disorders, 513–520
   amenorrhea, 516
   clinical presentation, 514
   differential diagnosis, 516, 516b
   dysfunctional uterine bleeding (DUB), 514–515,
      519, 519t
   dysmenorrhea, 514, 518
   epidemiology, 513
   evaluation, 516–518
   gynecologic history, 517b
   management, 518–519
   normal menstrual cycle, 514, 515f
   pathophysiology, 514–516
   premenstrual syndrome, 515–516, 519
   prognosis, 519
   vaginal discharge, 516
Mesangial proliferative glomerulonephritis, 481
Mescaline, 732t
Mesenteric adenitis, 609
Mesial temporal sclerosis (MTS), 240
Metabolic acidosis, 788
Metabolic syndrome, 705, 755
Metalloporphyrin, 618
Metatarsus adductus, 540
Metatarsus primus varus, 540
Methadone, 732t
Methamphetamine, 724
Methotrexate, 806
Methylphenidate, 699
Metoclopramide, 585t
Metronidazole, 715t
MI, 17, 17t, 756
Miconazole, 500, 671
Microcephaly, 325
Microcytic anemias, 413, 415
Microhematuria, 477–482
Microscopic hematuria, 477

Microtia, 324
Middle-child syndrome, 179
Migraine, 637–641. *See also* Headache
Milrinone, 269
Mineralocorticoids, 291
Minimal change disease (MCD), 809
Minocycline, 654
Mixed dentition, 82
Mixed FTT, 717
Mixed gonadal dysgenesis, 467
Mongolian spots, 708
Monilethrix, 660
Monitoring software, 33
Monotropy, 54
Morbidity. *See* New morbidity
Morbilliform rashes, 673–678
   clinical presentation, 674
   differential diagnosis, 674–676
   epidemiology, 673–674
   evaluation, 676–677
   management, 677–678
   pathophysiology, 674
   prognosis, 678
Morgan line, 389
Morning-after pill, 165–166
Moro reflex, 88b
Morphea, 805
Motility disorders, 596
Motivational interviewing (MI), 17, 17t, 756
MPGN, 481
MTS, 240
Mucocele, 332
MUDPILES, 311
Multichannel intraluminal impedance, 584
Multifactorial or mixed FTT, 717
Multiple-dose charcoal, 313
Munchausen syndrome by proxy, 707
Muscle biopsy, 634t, 635
Muscle enzymes, 634t
Musculoskeletal disorders of neck and back, 567–572
   causes of back pain, 570b
   causes of scoliosis, 569b
   causes of torticollis, 569b
   clinical presentation, 568
   differential diagnosis, 569
   epidemiology, 567–568
   evaluation, 570–571
   management, 571–572
   pathophysiology, 568–569
   prognosis, 572
Mushrooms, 732t
Mycophenolate mofetil, 813t
Myoglobinuria, 479t

N
Nail biting, 214
NAIT, 423
Naproxen, 640t
Nasal sponge, 358
Nasal tampon, 358
Nasolacrimal duct obstruction, 373–375
Natal teeth, 83
Nausea, 576

Neck deformity, 567–572. *See also* Musculoskeletal
   disorders of neck and back
Neck masses, 377–385
   clinical presentation, 377
   congenital lesions, 381
   differential diagnosis, 378–381
   epidemiology, 377
   evaluation, 381–382
   lymphadenopathy/lymphadenitis, 378–379
   management, 382–384
   pathophysiology, 378
   prognosis, 384
   trauma, 380
   tumors, 379
Necrotizing enterocolitis, 597
Neisseria gonorrhoeae, 501t, 715t
Neonatal alloimmune thrombocytopenia
   (NAIT), 423
Neonatal breast hypertrophy, 523
Neonatal conjunctivitis, 369
Neonatal cyanosis, 437–441
Neonatal examination/screening, 41–50
   common physical findings, 44
   core screening disorders, 48t
   differential diagnosis, 48–49
   discharge planning/counseling, 44
   imaging studies, 44
   laboratory tests, 43–44
   management, 44
   neonatal nursery visit, 41–42
   neurologic examination, 43
   newborn screening, 47–50
   pediatric prenatal visit, 41
   perinatal history, 42
   physical examination, 42–43
   specimen collection/handling, 49
Neonatal teeth, 83
Neoplastic disease, 564
Nephroblastoma, 782, 782t, 784t
Nephrotic syndrome, 809–815
   clinical presentation, 809–810
   differential diagnosis, 810–811
   epidemiology, 809
   evaluation, 811–812
   histologic type, 810t
   immunization issues, 814
   management, 812–814
   medication, 813t
   parent education, 814
   pathophysiology, 810
   prognosis, 814–815
Nerve conduction velocity, 635
Neurally mediated syncope, 259
Neuroblastoma, 781t, 782, 784t
Neurocardiogenic syncope, 259
Neurogenic bladders, 184
Neurogenic shock, 266
Neuroleptic malignant syndrome, 705
Neurologic disorders, 629–647
   headache, 637–641
   hypotonia, 631–636
   tics, 643–647

Nevus sebaceous, 659
New morbidity, 685–776
 abuse, 707–716
 ADHD, 695–700
 autism, 687–694
 body piercing, 745–751
 bullying, 763–766
 depression, 771–776
 disaster preparedness, 767–770
 divorce, 759–762
 eating disorders, 737–744
 FTT, 717–722
 maternal substance abuse, 723–728
 obesity, 753–758
 psychopharmacology, 701–706
 school violence, 763–766
 sexual abuse, 711–716
 substance abuse, 729–736
 suicide, 771–776
 tattooing, 745–751
Nicotine, 732t
Night terrors, 78, 78t
Nightmares, 78, 78t
Nitroprusside, 269
Nodules, 652
Non-epiphyseal plate fractures, 549f
Non-hemorrhage meningeal irritation, 639
Non-Hodgkin lymphoma, 780, 781t, 782, 784t
Non-lymphoblastic lymphoma, 782
Non-paralytic strabismus, 361
Non-rapid eye movement (NREM) sleep, 76
Non-rebreathing mask, 244, 244f
Non-retentive encopresis, 223
Noncardiac syncope, 259
Nonimmune hemolytic anemias, 416
Nonorganic FTT, 717
Norepinephrine, 268
Normal development, 88–92
Normal menstrual cycle, 514, 515f
Normocephaly, 325f
Normocytic anemias, 415–416
Nose picking, 214
Nosebleed, 355–359
 clinical presentation, 355
 differential diagnosis, 356–357
 epidemiology, 355
 evaluation, 357
 management, 357–358
 pathophysiology, 356
 prognosis, 359
NREM sleep, 76
Nursemaid's elbow, 547–553
Nutritional needs, 63–69
 adolescents, 66–67
 evaluation, 67–68
 formula, 64t
 infants, 64–66
 liquid foods, 64–65
 problems, 68
 requirements of normal children, 63–64
 solid foods, 65–66
Nystatin, 671

O
Obesity, 753–757. See also Childhood obesity
Obsessive-compulsive disorder (OCD), 703
Obstructive shock, 266t, 267
Obstructive sleep apnea syndrome (OSAS), 78–79
Occlusion therapy, 365
Occult bacteremia, 229
OCD, 703
Olanzapine, 704t
Older children. See Adolescents
Oligoarticular JIA, 802
OM, 335–339. See also Otitis media (OM)
Omeprazole, 585t
Open comedo, 652
Opium, 732t
Oral acyclovir, 683
Oral antistaphylococcal therapy, 683
Oral candidiasis, 331
Oral griseofulvin, 661
Oral health and dental disorders, 81–86
 clinical presentation, 81–83
 differential diagnosis, 84
 epidemiology, 81
 evaluation, 84
 management, 85
 pathophysiology, 81–86, 83–84
 prevention, 85
 prognosis, 85
 risk factors, 81
 tooth brushing, 85
Oral lesions, 331–334
Oral rehydration, 300–301
Oral rehydration therapy (ORT), 298, 301t
Orbital cellulitis, 370
Organic FTT, 717
ORT, 298, 301t
Orthopedic disorders, 529–572
 bowlegs and knock-knees, 543–546
 developmental hip dysplasia, 531–535
 in-toeing and out-toeing, 537–542
 limp, 561–566
 neck/back disorders, 567–572
 orthopedic injuries and growing pains, 547–553
 sports-related acute injuries, 555–559
Orthopedic injuries and growing pains, 547–553
 clinical presentation, 547–548
 differential diagnosis, 550
 epidemiology, 547
 evaluation, 550–552
 management, 552
 pathophysiology, 548–549
 prognosis, 552–553
Orthostatic proteinuria, 486
Ortolani and Barlow maneuvers, 532, 533f
OSAS, 78–79
Osgood-Schlatter disease (OSD), 564
Osler-Weber-Rendu syndrome, 356
Osmolar gap, 311
Osmotic diarrhea, 596
Osteitis fibrosa, 789
Osteomyelitis, 563

Osteosarcoma, 782, 782t, 784t
Otitis media (OM), 335–339
 antibiotics, 338b
 categories, 335–336
 clinical presentation, 336
 differential diagnosis, 337
 epidemiology, 336
 evaluation, 337
 management, 338–339
 pathophysiology, 336
 prevention, 338
 prognosis, 339
Otitis media with effusion, 335
Out-toeing, 537–542, 541
Overjet, 83
Overuse syndromes, 556
Ovotesticular DSD, 467
Oxcarbazepine, 822t
Oxybutynin, 222
Oxycephaly, 325f

P
P acnes, 652
p53, 779
Pacifiers, 216
PACS, 29
Pancreatitis, 609
Pancytopenia, 783
Papular-purpuric gloves and socks syndrome (PPGSS), 675, 676
Papules, 652
Papulosquamous eruptions, 667–672
Parachute reactions, 88b
Paralytic strabismus, 361
Paraphimosis, 58
Parasitic infestations, 609
Parenteral fluid therapy, 299
Parenteral infections, 609
Partial rebreathing mask, 244
Partial seizures, 818, 819t
Passive immunization, 117–118
Pavlik harness, 534
Pelvic inflammatory disease, 507–508, 510b
Peptic ulcers, 609
Perianal streptococcal disease, 664
Periodic leg movements, 79
Periorbital cellulitis, 370
Permethrin, 671
Persistent diarrhea, 595
Personal health record (PHR), 28
PFA-100 screen, 424
PHAILS, 313
Pharmacy information system, 28–29
Phencyclidine, 732t
Phenobarbital, 822t
Phenytoin, 822t
PHI, 28
Phimosis, 60
Phobias, 207–211
Phoria, 362
PHR, 28
Physical abuse, 707–710

Physiological jaundice, 613, 614

Physiological out-toeing, 541

Piaget's stages of cognitive development, 11t

Pica, 214

Picture archiving and communication system (PACS), 29

Picture exchange communication system, 692b

Pierre Robin syndrome, 323

Pimozide, 646

Pincer grasp, 89f

Pinworms, 500

Pityriasis alba, 668

Pityriasis rosea, 669

Pivotal response training, 692b

Placing reflex, 88b

Plagiocephaly, 325, 326f

Plan B, 166

Plaque-type psoriasis, 669

Plasmapheresis, 635

Platelet release defects, 422

Pleuropulmonary disease, 803

Pocket mask, 244, 244f

Poisoning. *See* Ingestions

Polyarticular JIA, 802

Polymastia, 521–522, 522f

Polythelia, 521, 521f, 522

Poor mixing group, 438

Porphyrins, 479t

Portal hypertension, 591

Posttraumatic headaches, 639

Postural reactions, 88

Potassium replacement, 300

Potentially fatal substances, 314b

PPE, 555

PPGSS, 675, 676

PPI, 584

PPPS murmur, 434

Practice management system, 28

Pre-hypertension, 456t

Prednisone, 662, 813, 813t

Premature thelarche, 522, 523–524

Premenstrual syndrome, 515–516, 519

Preparticipation physical evaluation (PPE), 555

Preseptal cellulitis, 370

Preterm infants, 149–154
  developmental assessment, 152
  developmental surveillance, 152b
  epidemiology, 149
  evaluation, 149–151
  immunization, 152–153
  laboratory tests, 151
  management, 151–153
  nutrition, 151–152
  physical examination, 150–151
  prognosis, 154
  vision/hearing, 153

Primary amenorrhea, 516

Primary care, 1–38
  child advocacy, 7–9
  informatics, 27–30
  Internet usage, 31–34
  principles of therapeutics, 35–38
  talking with adolescents, 19–22
  talking with children, 11–14
  talking with parents, 15–18
  telephone management, 23–25

Primary dentition, 82f

Primary dysmenorrhea, 514

Primary enuresis, 219

Primary herpetic gingivostomatitis, 332

Primary peritonitis, 609

Primary snoring, 79

Primary varicella-zoster virus (VZV), 679

Primidone, 822t

Primitive reflexes, 88, 88b

Principles of therapeutics, 35–38

Privacy, 28

Prolactin, 705

Propranolol, 640t

Prostaglandin E_1, 269

Protected health information (PHI), 28

Protective equilibrium response, 88b

Proteinuria, 485–489

Pseudoesotropia, 362, 363f

Psoriasis, 665

Psoriatic JIA, 803

Psychopharmacology, 701–705
  atypical antipsychotics, 704–705
  psychostimulants, 702
  serotonergic dopamine antagonists (SDAs), 704–705
  SNRIs, 702–703
  SSRIs, 703–704

Psychostimulants, 702

Pubic hair development, 162f, 163f

Pulmonary flow murmur, 434

Pulse oximetry, 439

Pustules, 652

Pyloric stenosis, 577

Pyogenic granuloma, 332

Pyrantel pamoate, 500

Pyruvate kinase deficiency, 415

Q

Quetiapine, 704t

R

Racemic epinephrine, 250

Radiation exposure, 769

Radioallergosorbent testing (RAST), 390

Radiology information system, 29

Rapid antigen detection test (RADT), 350

Rapid eye movement (REM) sleep, 76

Rashes. *See* Morbilliform rashes; Papulosquamous eruptions; Vesicular exanthema

RAST, 390

Receptive milestones, 96t

Recombinant human growth hormone, 791

Recurrent OM, 335

Recurrent UTI, 491

Redirection, 195

Reflexes, 88, 88b

Reflux disease, 581–586. *See also* Gastroesophageal reflux (GER)

Refractive amblyopia, 362

Regional lymphadenopathy, 427

Regurgitation, 575

REM sleep, 76

Removal of privileges, 196

Renal failure, 787–793. *See also* Chronic kidney disease/chronic renal failure

Renal osteodystrophy, 788, 789

Reproductive health, 161–167
  contraceptive methods, 165–166
  evaluation, 162–164
  female breast development, 162f
  female pubic hair development, 162f
  male genital/pubic hair development, 163f
  management, 164–166
  normal development, 161
  pelvic examinations, 164b

Respiratory distress, 241–245

Respiratory failure, 241

Restless leg syndrome, 79

Retching, 576

Retentive encopresis, 223

Retentive posture, 602f

Retin-A, 653

Retinoic acid, 653

Retrocochlear hearing loss, 342

Retropharyngeal abscess, 349

Rett syndrome, 687

Reye syndrome, 578

Rhabdomyosarcoma, 781t, 782, 784t

Rhythmic habits, 213–214

RICE, 558

Ricin, 769

Rickets, 545

Right-sided failure, 444

Righting reactions, 88b

Riley-Day syndrome, 578

Risperdol, 704t

Risperidone, 646, 704t, 705

Rizatriptan, 640t

Rocky Mountain spotted fever (RMSF), 674, 676

Rooting reflex, 88b

Roseola infantum, 674, 675

Rubella, 673, 675

Rule of 6 and 0.6, 269

Rumination, 575

S

Salter-Harris classification of epiphyseal plate fractures, 550f

Scabies, 659, 668f, 669, 680

Scalp disorders, 657–662. *See also* Disorders of hair and scalp

Scaphocephaly, 325, 325f, 326f

Scarification, 745

Scarlet fever, 674, 676

SCFE, 564
School readiness, 109–114
   causes of school failure, 111b
   clinical presentation, 110
   epidemiology, 109–110
   evaluation, 111–112
   kindergarten readiness skills, 110b
   management, 112–113
   pathophysiology, 110–111
   prognosis, 113
   signs of school difficulties, 110b
School-related violence, 763–766
Scintigraphy, 583
Scleroderma, 804–805, 806
Scolding, 195–196
Scoliosis, 567–572. *See also* Musculoskeletal
   disorders of neck and back
Screening bacteriuria, 491
SDAs, 704–705
Searching toe, 540
Seborrheic dermatitis, 658, 659, 661, 668f, 669
Seborrheic diaper dermatitis, 664
Secondary amenorrhea, 516
Secondary care, 4
Secondary dysmenorrhea, 514
Secondary enuresis, 219
Secondary syphilis, 660
Secretory diarrhea, 596
Security, 28
Seizures. *See* Febrile seizures
Seizures and epilepsy, 817–823
   clinical presentation, 817–818
   differential diagnosis, 819–820
   drugs, 822t
   epidemiology, 817
   evaluation, 820–821
   management, 821–823
   pathophysiology, 818–819
   prognosis, 823
   seizure types, 818–819
Selective norepinephrine reuptake inhibitors
   (SNRIs), 702–703
Selective serotonin reuptake inhibitors (SSRIs),
   703–704
Self-esteem, 175–178
Sensorineural hearing loss, 342
Septic arthritis, 563
Septic shock, 267
Seroquel, 704t
Serotonergic dopamine antagonists (SDAs), 704–705
Serpentine metatarsus adductus, 540
Sertraline, 646
Serum creatine phosphokinase (CPK), 634
Severe autoimmune hemolytic anemia, 417
Sexual abuse, 711–716
Sexually transmitted infections (STIs), 503–511
   cervicitis, 507
   clinical presentation, 504
   differential diagnosis, 505, 506b
   epidemiology, 503–504
   epididymitis, 505–507
   evaluation, 505

genital ulcers, 508–509
genital warts, 509–510
management, 510
pathophysiology, 505
pelvic inflammatory disease, 507–508, 510b
prognosis, 510
urethritis, 505–507
Sheppard-Towner Act, 7
Shock, 265–270, 272
Shunt study, 439
Sibling rivalry, 179–181
Sickle cell disease, 415, 564
SIDS. *See* Sudden infant death syndrome (SIDS)
Single cytopenias, 783
Sitting, 89f
Skewfoot, 540
Skin bridges, 60
SLE, 803, 806
Sleep, 75–80
   differential diagnosis, 77
   epidemiology, 75
   evaluation, 79
   good hygiene, 80b
   management, 79–80
   pathophysiology, 76–77
   prognosis, 80
Sleep cycle, 76
Sleep states, 76
Sleep tics, 214
Sleep-wake patterns, 76–77
Sleeper effect, 760
Sleeptalking, 78
Sleepwalking, 78
Slipped capital femoral epiphysis (SCFE), 564
SLUDGE toxidrome, 769
SMA, 631
Small pox, 769
Smith, Job Lewis, 7
SNRIs, 702–703
Social stories, 692b
Soiling, 223–226
Somogyi phenomenon, 798
Sore throat, 347–354
   antibiotics, 352t
   clinical presentation, 347–348
   differential diagnosis, 348–349
   epidemiology, 347
   evaluation, 349–350
   management, 350–353
   pathophysiology, 348
   prognosis, 353
Spanking, 195
Spasmodic croup, 248
Spastic cerebral palsy, 92
Speech-language auditory milestones, 344b
Spinal muscular atrophy (SMA), 631
Spironolactone, 446
Splenic sequestration, 417
Sports participation health record, 125–126f
Sports-related acute injuries, 555–559
   differential diagnosis, 556, 557b
   epidemiology, 555

evaluation, 557–558
management, 558
pathophysiology, 556
preparticipation physical evaluation (PPE), 555
prevention, 558–559
prognosis, 559
rehabilitation, 558b
Sprain, 556
SSRIs, 703–704
Stage 1 hypertension, 456t
Stage 2 hypertension, 456t
Standard, 28
Starling curve of cardiac output, 266f
Steatorrhea, 596
Step-down therapy, 584
Step-up therapy, 584
Stepping reflex, 88b
Still's murmur, 434
STIs, 503–511. *See also* Sexually transmitted
   infections (STIs)
Storage pool disorders, 422
Strabismic amblyopia, 362
Strabismus, 361–365
   clinical presentation, 361
   differential diagnosis, 362–363
   epidemiology, 361
   evaluation, 363–364
   management, 365
   pathophysiology, 361–362
   prognosis, 365
   vision testing, 364
Straddle injuries, 712
Strain, 556
Strawberry tongue, 676f
Stress fracture, 556
Stress incontinence, 184
Stridor and croup, 247–251
   causes of stridor, 248b
   croup score, 249t
   differential diagnosis, 248t
   epidemiology, 247
   evaluation, 248–249
   management, 250
   pathophysiology, 247–248
   prognosis, 250
Subdural hematomas, 282
Subspecialist care, 4
Substance abuse, 729–735
   clinical presentation, 730
   CRAFFT questions, 733b
   defined, 729
   differential diagnosis, 731
   epidemiology, 729–730
   evaluation, 731–734
   management, 734
   pathophysiology, 730
   prevention programs, 734
   prognosis, 734–735
   questionnaire, 731b
   questions to ask, 733b
   risk factors, 730
   substance and their toxicity, 732t

Substance use, 729
Sucking reflex, 88b
SUDC, 253
Sudden infant death syndrome (SIDS), 253–257
    child abuse, 255b
    clinical presentation, 254
    differential diagnosis, 255
    epidemiology, 253–254
    evaluation, 255–256
    management, 256
    pathophysiology, 254–255
    prognosis, 256–257
    risk factors, 254b
Sudden unexplained death in childhood (SUDC), 253
Suicidal ideation, 20
Suicide, 771–776
Sumatriptan, 640t
Supernumerary teeth, 83
Syncope, 259–263
    causes, 259b
    differential diagnosis, 261
    epidemiology, 259–260
    evaluation, 261–262
    management, 262
    pathophysiology, 260–261
    prognosis, 263
Syphilis, 504, 715t
Syrup of ipecac, 312, 312t
Systemic lupus erythematosus (SLE), 803, 806
Systemic SD, 804, 806

T

Tacrolimus, 813t
Talking with adolescents, 19–22
Talking with children, 11–14
Talking with parents, 15–18
Tar, 671
TAR syndrome, 423
Tattooing, 745–751. *See also* Body modification
    (tattooing/body piercing)
Tc-99m-DMSA, 791
Tc-99m-MAG3, 791
Tearing, 373–376
Teeth. *See* Oral health and dental disorders
Teeth grinding, 214
Teething, 82
Telemedicine, 29
Telephone advice, 25
Telephone history taking, 24
Telephone management, 23–25
Telogen effluvium, 660
Temper tantrums, 199–201
Tendinitis, 556
Tensilon test, 634t
Tension headaches, 639
Terbinafine, 662
Tetracycline, 654
Thalassemias, 413
The Injury Prevention Program (TIPP), 171, 171t
Thigh-foot axis, 538
Throat culture, 350
Thrombocytopenia—absent radius (TAR) syndrome,
    423

Thumb sucking, 213–217
Thyroglossal duct cysts, 381
Tics, 643–647
Time-limiting software, 33
Time-out, 196
Tinea amiantacea, 659
Tinea capitis, 657, 659, 661, 680
Tinea pedis, 680
TIPP, 171, 171t
Tobacco-associated keratosis, 331
Toddler's fracture, 561
Toe-to-heel gait, 561
Toilet training, 183–187
Tooth anatomy, 82f
Tooth brushing, 85
Topiramate, 640t, 822t
TORCHS, 615
Torticollis, 381, 567–572. *See also* Musculoskeletal
    disorders of neck and back
Torus palatinus, 331
Tourette syndrome, 643–647
Toxidromes, 311t
Traction alopecia, 660
Trained night crier, 77
Trained night feeder, 77
Transient erythroblastopenia of childhood, 416
Transient neonatal strabismus, 362
Transient synovitis, 562
Transmalleolar axis, 538
Trauma, 271–286
    abdominal, 277–280
    airway assessment and treatment, 273b
    breathing assessment and treatment, 274b
    circulation assessment and treatment, 274b
    clinical presentation, 272
    epidemiology, 271–272
    evaluation and management, 273–275
    Glasgow Coma Scale, 275b, 283t, 284t
    head, 281–286. *See also* Head trauma
    pathophysiology, 272–273
    prognosis, 275
Trendelenburg gait, 561
Tretinoin, 653
Trichobezoar, 660
Trichomonas, 715t
Trichomonas vaginalis, 501t
Trichotillomania, 213, 657, 660
Trigonocephaly, 325, 325f, 326f
Trisomy, 143–148
    adolescents, 147–148
    clinical presentation, 144
    counseling the family, 144b
    epidemiology, 143–144
    evaluation, 144
    growth charts, 146f
    health supervision, 145t
    infancy/early childhood, 145–147
    newborn period, 144–145
    pathophysiology, 144
    physical examination, 147b

Twins and higher-order multiples, 51–55
    breastfeeding, 53
    congenital malformations, 52
    epidemiology, 51
    history, 53
    laboratory tests, 53
    management, 53–55
    pathophysiology, 51–52
    perinatal complications, 52
    physical examination, 53
    postnatal complications, 53
    prognosis, 55
2-minute orthopedic examination, 124, 127t
Tympanometry curves, 98f

U

UGI, 583
Ultrasound, 790
Uncompensated shock, 265, 272
Unconjugated hyperbilirubinemia, 614–615
Underbite, 83
Upper gastrointestinal series (UGI), 583
Upper GI bleeding, 587–593. *See also* Gastrointestinal
    bleeding
Urethral prolapse, 712
Urethritis, 491, 505–507
Urgency incontinence, 184
Urinary alkalinization, 313
Urinary calcium-creatinine ratios, 479t
Urinary protein, 485–489
Urinary tract infections (UTIs), 491–495
    clinical presentation, 492
    differential diagnosis, 493
    epidemiology, 491–492
    evaluation, 493–494
    management, 494
    pathophysiology, 492–493
    prognosis, 494–495
Urticaria, 388, 389
UTIs. *See* Urinary tract infections (UTIs)

V

Vaccination. *See* Immunization
VACTERRL association, 319
Vaginal discharge, 516
Vaginitis, 497–501
Valgus angulation, 539
Valproic acid, 640t, 822t
Van der Woude syndrome, 323
Varus angulation, 539
Vasovagal syncope, 259
VCUG, 790
Vegetarianism, 67
Venous hum, 434
Venturi mask, 244
Verapamil, 640t
Vesicoureteral reflux, 492, 493f
Vesicular exanthema, 679–684
    approach to evaluation, 682f
    causes, 681b
    clinical presentation, 680
    differential diagnosis, 680–681

epidemiology, 679–680
evaluation, 681–682
management, 682–683
pathophysiology, 680
prognosis, 684
Vigabatrin, 822t
Vincent angina, 333
Violence, 763–766
Viral conjunctivitis, 369
Vitamin K deficiency, 423
Voiding cystourethrogram (VCUG), 790
Vomiting, 575–579
adolescents, 578
children, 577–578
clinical presentation, 575
defined, 575
differential diagnosis, 576–578
epidemiology, 575
evaluation, 578–579
infants, 577
management, 579
non-reflux causes, 582b
pathophysiology, 576
prognosis, 579
Von Willebrand disease, 422
VUR, 492
VZV, 679

W
Waddell triad, 272f
Wheezing and asthma, 393–401
asthma management plan, 400f
asthma severity, 397t
causes of wheezing, 394b
clinical presentation, 394
differential diagnosis, 395
epidemiology, 393–394
evaluation, 395–398
management, 398–400
pathophysiology, 394–395
pharmacologic therapy, 398b, 399–400
prognosis, 400
therapeutic goals, 399b
Whitehead, 652
Whole-bowel irrigation, 312t, 313
Wilms tumor, 782, 782t, 784t
Winter vomiting syndrome, 596
Wolff-Parkinson-White (WPW) syndrome, 261

Y
Yuzpe method, 166

Z
Zinc deficiency, 665
Ziprasidone, 704t
Zonisamide, 822t
Zyprexa, 704t